Volume I

The Cell

Contents at a Glance

Volume I

Volume II

Volume I

The Cell

S Kemper

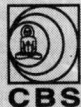

CBS Publishers & Distributors Pvt Ltd

New Delhi • Bengaluru • Chennai • Kochi • Kolkata • Mumbai

Bhopal • Bhubaneswar • Hyderabad • Jharkhand • Nagpur • Patna • Pune • Uttarakhand • Dhaka (Bangladesh)

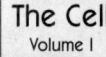

The Cell
Volume I

ISBN: 978-93-89261-68-4

First Edition: 2020

Published by Satish Kumar Jain and produced by Varun Jain for

CBS Publishers & Distributors Pvt Ltd

4819/XI Prahlad Street, 24 Ansari Road, Daryaganj, New Delhi 110 002, India.

Ph: 23289259, 23266861, 23266867   Fax: 011-23243014   Website: www.cbspd.com
e-mail: delhi@cbspd.com; cbspubs@airtelmail.in

Corporate Office: 204 FIE, Industrial Area, Patparganj, Delhi 110 092

Ph: 4934 4934   Fax: 4934 4935   e-mail: publishing@cbspd.com; publicity@cbspd.com

Branches

- **Bengaluru:** Seema House, 2975, 17th Cross, K.R. Road,
  Banasankari 2nd Stage, Bengaluru 560 070, Karnataka
  Ph: +91-80-26771678/79   Fax: +91-80-26771680   e-mail: bangalore@cbspd.com
- **Chennai:** 7, Subbaraya Street, Shenoy Nagar, Chennai 600 030, Tamil Nadu
  Ph: +91-44-26680620, 26681266   Fax: +91-44-42032115   e-mail: chennai@cbspd.com
- **Kochi:** 42/1325, 1326, Power House Road, Opposite KSEB Power House,
  Ernakulam 682 018, Kochi, Kerala
  Ph: +91-484-4059061-65   Fax: +91-484-4059065   e-mail: kochi@cbspd.com
- **Kolkata:** 6/B, Ground Floor, Rameswar Shaw Road, Kolkata-700 014, West Bengal
  Ph: +91-33-22891126, 22891127, 22891128   e-mail: kolkata@cbspd.com
- **Mumbai:** 83-C, Dr E Moses Road, Worli, Mumbai-400018, Maharashtra
  Ph: +91-22-24902340/41   Fax: +91-22-24902342   e-mail: mumbai@cbspd.com

Representatives

• Bhopal	0-8319310552	• Bhubaneswar	0-9911037372	• Hyderabad	0-9885175004
• Jharkhand	0-9811541605	• Nagpur	0-9421945513	• Patna	0-9334159340
• Pune	0-9623451994	• Uttarakhand	0-9716462459	• Dhaka (Bangladesh)	01912-003485

Printed at: Mudrak, Noida, UP, India

Preface

Cells are the basic unit of life. In the modern world, they are the smallest known world that performs all of life's functions. All living organisms are either single cells, or are multicellular organisms composed of many cells working together. Cells are the smallest known unit that can accomplish all of these functions. Defining characteristics that allow a cell to perform these functions include: A cell membrane that keeps the chemical reactions of life together, at least one chromosome, composed of genetic material that contain the cell's *blueprints* and *software*, cytoplasm—the fluid inside the cell, in which the chemical processes of life occur. Thus, cells are the basic building blocks of living things. The human body is composed of trillions of cells, all with their own specialised function. Cells are the basic structures of all living organisms. Cells provide structure for the body, take in nutrients from food and carry out important functions. Cells group together to form tissues, which in turn group together to form organs, such as the heart and brain. Our cells contain a number of functional structures called organelles. These organelles carry out tasks such as making proteins, processing chemicals and generating energy for the cell. The nucleus is based at the centre of the cell and is the 'control room' for the cell. The genome is found within the nucleus.

This reference textbook *The Cell* is divided in two volumes. First volume contains five sections and 1 to 25 chapters.

Section I discusses *general considerations and biological aspects*. Chapter 1 is devoted to structure and function of the cell. Cells form the basis of all living things. They are the smallest single unit of life, from the simplest bacteria to blue whales and giant redwood trees. Chapter 2 deals with tools and techniques in cell biology. Chapter 3 concentrates on HeLa cells. These are possibly the best known of all cancer cell lines. HeLa cells have played an important role in many important medical discoveries, including the development of the Polio vaccine. Chapter 4 focuses on viruses and human cancer. Viruses are very small organisms; most can't even be seen with an ordinary microscope. They are made up of a small number of genes in the form of DNA or RNA surrounded by a protein coating.

Section II discusses *molecule and membrane*. Chapter 5 is devoted to molecules and biomolecules of cells. Chapter 6 deals with enzymes as biocatalysts. Enzymes are protein catalysts that increase the velocity of a chemical reaction and are not consumed during the reaction they catalyse. All enzymes contain a protein backbone. Chapter 7 focuses on cell membrane. The cell membrane, also known as the plasma membrane, is a double layer of lipids and proteins that surrounds a cell and separates the cytoplasm (the contents of the cell) from its surrounding environment.

Section III discusses *bioenergetics and metabolism*. Chapter 8 concentrates on bioenergetics. Bioenergetics is the subject of a field of biochemistry that concerns energy flow through living systems. This is an active area of biological research that includes the study of thousands of different cellular processes such as cellular respiration and the many other metabolic processes that can lead to production and utilisation of energy in forms such as adenosine triphosphate (ATP) molecules. Chapter 9 explains cell metabolism. Metabolic processes are concerned with all those biological or chemical reactions which can be carried out by the cell. Chapter 10 is devoted to electron transport and oxidative phosphorylation. The electron transport chain is a collection of membrane-embedded proteins and organic molecules. In prokaryotes, the electron transport chain components are found in the plasma membrane. Chapter 11 deals with photosynthesis. Photosynthesis is the process used by plants, algae and certain bacteria to harness energy from sunlight and turn it into chemical energy. Chapter 12 focuses on chemiosmotic theory. Chemiosmosis is the process of a molecule moving from high to low concentration, based on its charge and concentration inside a cell. Chapter 13 concentrates on antimetabolites and chemotherapy. An antimetabolite is a chemical that inhibits the use of a metabolite, which is another chemical that is part of normal metabolism.

Section IV discusses *fundamentals of molecular biology.* Chapter 14 is devoted to heredity, genes and DNA. Heredity, the sum of all biological processes by which particular characteristics are transmitted from parents to their offspring. The gene is the basic physical and functional unit of heredity. It consists of a specific sequence of nucleotides at a given position on a given chromosome that codes for a specific protein (or, in some cases, an RNA molecule). DNA stands for deoxyribose nucleic acid. This chemical substance is present in the nucleus of all cells in all living organisms. Chapter 15 deals with expression of genetic information. Gene expression is the process by which information from a gene is used in the synthesis of a functional gene product. These products are often proteins, but in non-protein coding genes such as rRNA genes or tRNA genes, the product is a functional RNA. Chapter 16 concentrates on recombinant DNA. Recombinant DNA, which is often shortened to rDNA, is an artificially made DNA strand that is formed by the combination of two or more gene sequences. Chapter 17 focuses on detection of nucleic acid and proteins. Chapter 18 explains gene function in eukaryotes. Gene is a part of DNA that specifies a protein/RNA. All the proteins/RNA are not required by the cell all the time. Some proteins are required at some time and yet other proteins are required at another time. Chapter 19 is devoted to DNA provirus hypothesis. A provirus is a virus genome that is integrated into the DNA of a host cell. In the case of bacterial viruses (bacteriophages), proviruses are often referred to as prophages. Chapter 20 deals with RNA interference. RNA interference (RNAi) is a post-transcriptional, highly conserved process in eukaryotes that leads to specific gene silencing through degradation of the target mRNA. This mechanism is mediated by double-stranded RNA (dsRNA) that is homologous in sequence to the silenced gene.

Section V discusses *genomes, proteomics and system biology.* Chapter 21 explains genomes and transcriptomes. Genomics focuses on the dynamic aspects such as gene transcription, translation and protein – protein interactions, as opposed to the static aspects of the genomic information such as DNA sequence or structures. The transcriptome is the set of all RNA molecules in one cell or a population of cells. It is sometimes used to refer to all RNAs, or just mRNA, depending on the particular experiment. Chapter 22 focuses on proteomics. Proteomics is the large-scale study of proteins, particularly their structures and functions. Proteins are vital parts of living organisms, as they are the main components of the physiological metabolic pathways of cells. The proteome is the entire set of proteins, produced or modified by an organism or system. Chapter 23 concentrates on system biology. Systems biology is the study of the interactions and behaviour of the components of biological entities, including molecules, cells, organs, and organisms. Chapter 24 is devoted to human genomes. Human genome, all of the approximately three billion base pairs of deoxyribonucleic acid (DNA) that make up the entire set of chromosomes of the human organism. Chapter 25 deals with synthetic biology. Synthetic biology is a new interdisciplinary area that involves the application of engineering principles to biology. It aims at the redesign and fabrication of biological components and systems that do not already exist in the natural world.

Diagrams, figures, tables and index supplement the text. All topics have been covered in a cogent and lucid style to help the reader grasp the information quickly and easily.

It may not be wrong to hold that the present reference textbook *The Cell* is a complete treatise on this subject. It is an essential reading for BTech (environmental biotechnology/microbiology/food microbiology/biomedical and biochemical engineering) and students pursuing BSc/MSc course in biotechnology and microbiology. Besides students, this book will prove useful to industrialists and consultants in their respective fields.

This reference textbook also caters to the requirement of the syllabus prescribed by various universities for undergraduate and postgraduate courses in the above subjects. It has been prepared with meticulous care, aiming at making the book error-free. Constructive suggestions are always welcome from the readers of this book.

S Kemper

Contents

Section II
MOLECULE AND MEMBRANE

Section III
BIOENERGETICS AND METABOLISM

Section IV
FUNDAMENTALS OF MOLECULAR BIOLOGY

19. DNA Provirus Hypothesis 391–400

20. RNA Interference 401–419

Section V
GENOMES, PROTEOMICS AND SYSTEM BIOLOGY

21. Genomes and Transcriptomes 423–446

22. Proteomics 447–454

23. System Biology 455–465

SECTION I

General Considerations and Biological Aspects

Chapter 1

Structure and Function of The Cell

INTRODUCTION

Cells form the basis of all living things. They are the smallest single unit of life, from the simplest bacteria to blue whales and giant redwood trees. Differences in the structure of cells and the way that they carry out their internal mechanisms form the basis of the first major divisions of life, into the three kingdoms of *Archaea* (ancient bacteria), *Eubacteria* (modern bacteria) and *Eukaryota* (everything else, including us). An understanding of cells is therefore vital in any understanding of life itself.

Both living and non-living things are composed of molecules made from chemical elements such as carbon, hydrogen, oxygen, and nitrogen. The organisation of these molecules into cells is one feature that distinguishes living things from all other matter. The cell is the smallest unit of matter that can carry on all the processes of life.

1. Every living thing from the tiniest bacterium to the largest whale - is made of one or more cells.

2. Before 17 BC, no one knew that cells existed, since they are too small to be seen with the naked eye. The invention of the microscope enabled Robert Hooke, and Anton van Leuwenhoek to see and draw the first 'cells', a word coined by Hooke to describe the cells in a thin slice of cork, which reminded him of the rooms where monks lived.

3. The idea that all living things are made of cells was put forward in about 1840 and in 1855 came Cell theory, i.e. 'cells only come from other cells' – contradicting the earlier theory of spontaneous generation'.

Cell theory consists of three principles:

1. All living things are composed of one or more cells.

2. Cells are the basic units of structure and function in an organism.

3. Cells come only from the replication of existing cells.

The modern version of the cell theory includes the ideas that:

1. Energy flow occurs within cells.

2. Heredity information (DNA) is passed on from cell to cell.

3. All cells have the same basic chemical composition.

3

Cell diversity: Cell type diversity refers to the range of different cell types that comprise a tissue or organism. Cell type diversity arises during the development of the nervous system as a result of the acts of cell intrinsic and extrinsic factors controlling cell fate determination.

CELL SIZE

1. A few types of cells are large enough to be seen by the unaided eye. The human egg (ovum) is the largest cell in the body, and can (just) be seen without the aid of a microscope.
2. Most cells are small for two main reasons:
   (a) The cell's nucleus can only control a certain volume of active cytoplasm.
   (b) Cells are limited in size by their surface area to volume ratio. A group of small cells has a relatively larger surface area than a single large cell of the same volume. This is important because the nutrients, oxygen, and other materials a cell requires must enter through it surface. As a cell grows larger at some point its surface area becomes too small to allow these materials to enter the cell quickly enough to meet the cell's need.

INTERNAL ORGANISATION OF CELL

1. Cells contain a variety of internal structures called organelles.
2. An organelle is a cell component that performs a specific function in that cell.
3. Just as the organs of a multicellular organism carry out the organism's life functions, the organelles of a cell maintain the life of the cell.
4. There are many different cells, however, there are certain features common to all cells.
5. The entire cell is surrounded by a thin cell membrane. All membranes have the same thickness and basic structure.
6. Organelles often have their own membranes too once again, these membranes have a similar structure.
7. The nucleus, mitochondria and chloroplasts all have double membranes, more correctly called envelopes.
8. Because membranes are fluid mosaics, the molecules making them up – phospholipids and proteins move independently. The proteins appear to 'float' in the phospholipids bilayer and thus membranes can thus be used to transport molecules within the cell, e.g. endoplasmic reticulum.
9. Proteins in the membrane can be used to transport substances across the membrane, e.g. by facilitated diffusion or by active transport.
10. The proteins on the outside of cell membranes identify us as unique.

PROKARYOTES

Prokaryotes are single-celled organisms that lack a membrane-enclosed nucleus. Most prokaryotes have similar anatomies: A rigid cell wall surrounding a cell membrane that encloses the cytoplasm. The cell's single chromosome is condensed to form a nucleoid. *Escherichia coli*, the biochemically most well-characterised organism, is a typical prokaryote. Prokaryotes have quite varied nutritional requirements. The chemolithotrophs metabolise inorganic substances. Photolithotrophs, such as cyanobacteria, carry out photosynthesis. Heterotrophs, which live by oxidising organic substances, are classified as aerobes if they use oxygen in this process and as anaerobes if some other oxidising agent serves as their terminal electron acceptor. Traditional prokaryotic classification schemes are rather arbitrary because of poor correlation between bacterial form and metabolism. Sequence comparisons of nucleic acids and proteins, however, have established that all life-forms can be classified into three domains of evolutionary descent: the *Archaea* (archaebacteria) (Fig. 1.1), the Bacteria (eubacteria) and the *Eukarya* (eukaryotes) (Fig. 1.2).

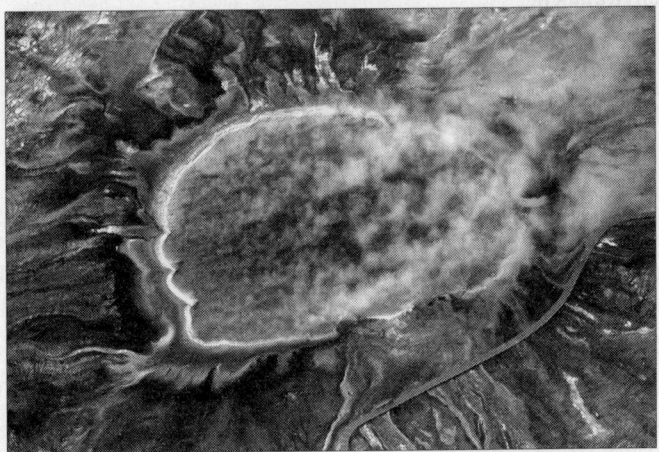

Fig. 1.1: *Archaea.*

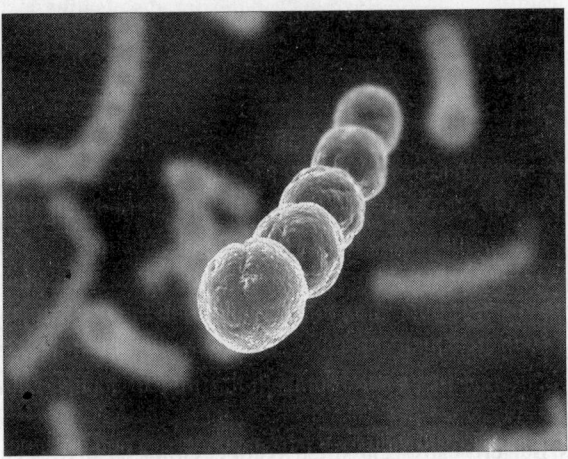

Fig. 1.2: *Eukarya.*

Cell structure

Like all cells, a prokaryotic cell is bounded by a plasma membrane that completely encloses the cytosol and separates the cell from the external environment. The plasma membrane, which is about 8 nm thick, consists of a lipid bilayer containing proteins. Although prokaryotes lack the membranous sub-cellular organelles characteristic of eukaryotes, their plasma membrane may be infolded to form mesosomes. The mesosomes may be the sites of deoxyribonucleic acid (DNA) replication and other specialised enzymatic reactions. In photosynthetic bacteria, the mesosomes contain the proteins and pigments that trap light and generate adenosine triphosphate (ATP). The aqueous cytosol contains the macromolecules [enzymes, messenger ribonucleic acid (mRNA), transfer (tRNA) and ribosomes], organic compounds and ions needed for cellular metabolism. Also within the cytosol is the prokaryotic 'chromosome' consisting of a single circular molecule of DNA which is condensed to form a body known as the nucleoid (Fig. 1.3). Many bacterial cells have one or more tail-like appendages known as flagella which are used to move the cell through its environment.

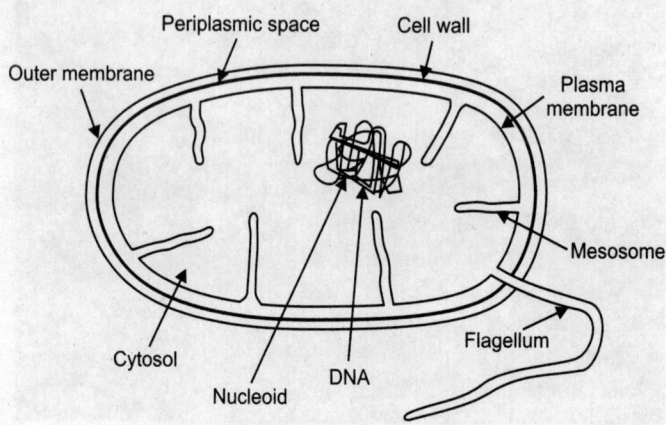

Fig. 1.3: Prokaryote cell structure.

Bacterial cell wall

To protect the cell from mechanical injury and osmotic pressure, most prokaryotes are surrounded by a rigid 3–25 nm thick cell wall (Fig. 1.3). The cell wall is composed of peptidoglycan, a complex of oligosaccharides and proteins. The oligosaccharide component consists of linear chains of alternating *N*-acetylglucosamine (GlcNAc) and *N*-acetylmuramic acid (NAM) linked β(1–4). Attached via an amide bond to the lactic acid group on NAM is a D-amino acid—containing tetrapeptide. Adjacent parallel peptidoglycan chains are covalently cross-linked through the tetrapeptide side-chains by other short peptides. The extensive cross-linking in the peptidoglycan cell wall gives it its strength and rigidity. The presence of D-amino acids in the peptidoglycan renders the cell wall resistant to the action of proteases which act on the more commonly occurring L-amino acids, but provides a unique target for the action of certain antibiotics such as penicillin. Penicillin acts by inhibiting the enzyme that forms the covalent cross-links in the peptidoglycan, thereby weakening the cell wall. The β(1–4) glycosidic linkage between NAM and GlcNAc is susceptible to hydrolysis by the enzyme lysozyme which is present in tears, mucus and other body secretions. Bacteria can be classified as either Gram-positive or Gram-negative depending on whether or not they take up the Gram stain. Gram-positive bacteria (e.g. *Bacillus polymyxa*) have a thick (25 nm) cell wall surrounding their plasma membrane, whereas Gram-negative bacteria (e.g. *Escherichia coli*) have a thinner (3 nm) cell wall and a second outer membrane (Fig. 1.4). In contrast with the plasma membrane, this outer membrane is very permeable to the passage of relatively large molecules (molecular weight >1000 Da) due to porin proteins which form pores in the lipid bilayer. Between the outer membrane and the cell wall is the periplasm, a space occupied by proteins secreted from the cell.

EUKARYOTES

Eukaryotic cells, which are far more complex than those of prokaryotes, are characterised by having numerous membrane-enclosed organelles. The most conspicuous of these is the nucleus, which contains

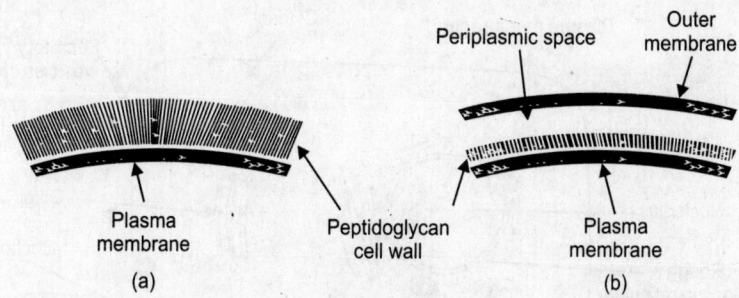

Fig. 1.4: Cell wall structure of: (a) Gram-positive and (b) Gram-negative bacteria.

the cell's chromosomes and the nucleolus, where ribosomes are assembled. The endoplasmic reticulum is the site of synthesis of lipids and of proteins that are destined for secretion. Further processing of these products occurs in the Golgi apparatus. The mitochondria, wherein oxidative metabolism occurs, are thought to have evolved from a symbiotic relationship between an aerobic bacterium and a primitive eukaryote. The chloroplast, the site of photosynthesis in plants, similarly evolved from a cyanobacterium. Other eukaryotic organelles include the lysosome, which functions as an intracellular digestive chamber and the peroxisome, which contains a variety of oxidative enzymes including some that generate H_2O_2. The eukaryotic cytoplasm is pervaded by a cytoskeleton whose components include microtubules, which consist of tubulin; microfilaments which are composed of actin; and intermediate filaments, which are made of different proteins in different types of cells. Eukaryotes have enormous morphological diversity on the cellular as well as on the organismal level. They have been classified into four kingdoms: Protista, Plantae, Fungi and Animalia. The pattern of embryonic development in multicellular organisms partially mirrors their evolutionary history (Fig. 1.5).

Prokaryotes vs Eukaryotes

Organisms whose cells normally contain a nucleus are called Eukaryotes, those (generally smaller) organisms whose cells lack a nucleus and have no membrane-bound organelles are known as Prokaryotes.

PARTS OF THE EUKARYOTIC CELL

The structures that make up a Eukaryotic cell are determined by the specific functions carried out by the cell. Thus, there is no typical Eukaryotic cell. Nevertheless, Eukaryotic cells generally have three main components: A cell membrane, a nucleus, and a variety of other organelles.

Cell Membrane

Cell membranes protect and organise cells. All cells have an outer plasma membrane that regulates not only what enters the cell, but also how much of any given substance comes in. Unlike prokaryotes, eukaryotic cells also possess internal membranes that encase their organelles and control the exchange of essential cell components. Both types of membranes have a specialised structure that facilitates their gatekeeping function.

1. A cell cannot survive if it is totally isolated from its environment. The cell membrane is a complex barrier separating every cell from its external environment.
2. This 'Selectively Permeable' membrane regulates what passes into and out of the cell.
3. The cell membrane is a fluid mosaic of proteins floating in a phospholipid bilayer.

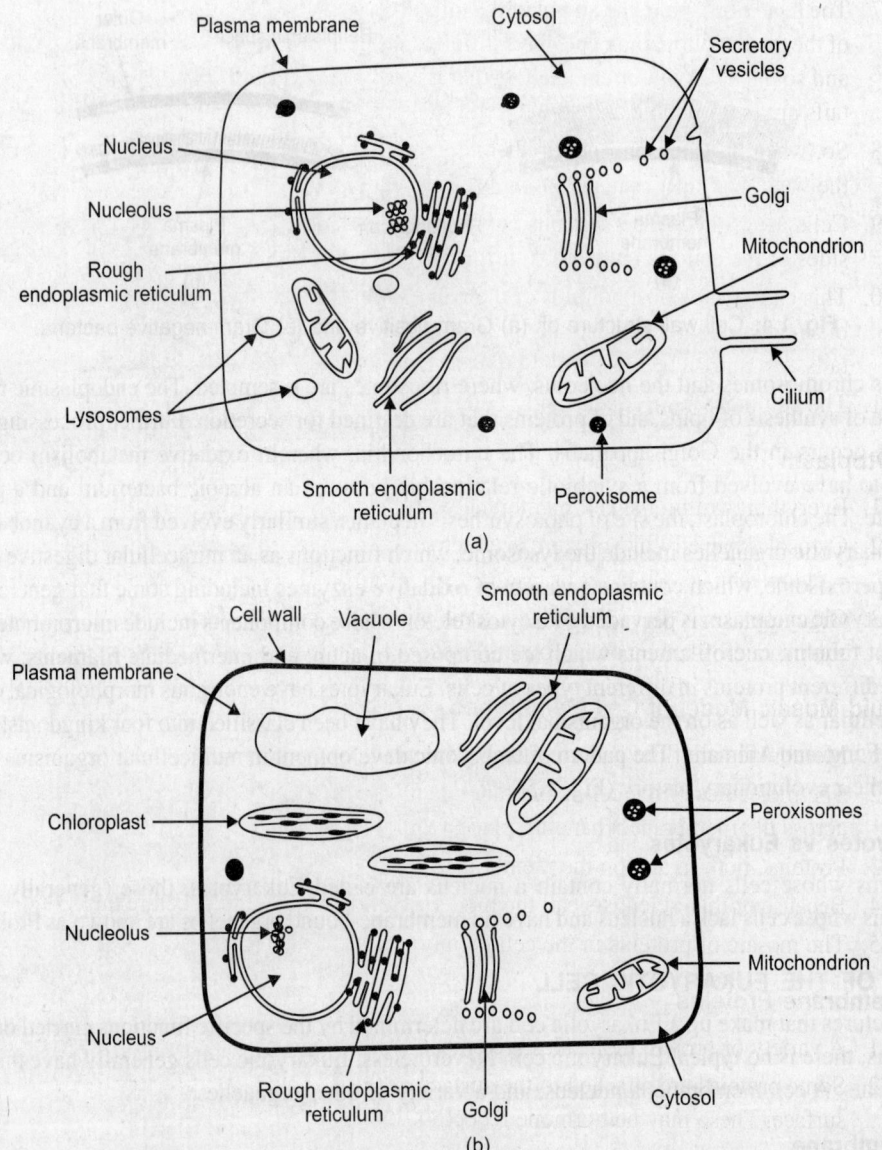

Fig. 1.5: Eukaryote cell structure: (a) structure of a typical animal cell and (b) structure of a typical plant cell.

4. The cell membrane functions like a gate, controlling which molecules can enter and leave the cell.

5. The cell membrane controls which substances pass into and out of the cell. Carrier proteins in or on the membrane are specific, only allowing a small group of very similar molecules through. For instance, α- glucose is able to enter, but β-glucose is not. Many molecules cannot cross at all. For this reason, the cell membrane is said to be selectively permeable.

6. The rest of the cell membrane is mostly composed of phospholipid molecules. They have only two fatty acid 'tails' as one has been replaced by a phosphate group (making the 'head').

7. The head is charged and so polar, the tails are not charged and so are non-polar. Thus the two ends of the phospholipid molecule have different properties in water. The phosphate head is hydrophyllic and so the head will orient itself so that it is as close as possible to water molecules. The fatty acid tails are hydrophobic and so will tend to orient themselves away from water.

8. So, when in water, phospholipids line up on the surface with their phosphate heads sticking into the water and fatty atails pointing up from the surface.

9. Cells are bathed in an aqueous environment and since the inside of a cell is also aqueous, both sides of the cell membrane are surrounded by water molecules.

10. This causes the phospholipids of the cell membrane to from two layers, known as a phospholipid bilayer. In this, the heads face the watery fluids inside and outside the cell, whilst the fatty acid tails are sandwiched inside the bilayer.

11. The cell membrane is constantly being formed and broken down in living cells.

Cytoplasm

1. Everything within the cell membrane which is not the nucleus is known as the cytoplasm.

2. Cytosol is the jelly-like mixture in which the other organelles are suspended, so cytosol + organelles = cytoplasm.

3. Organelles carry out specific functions within the cell. In Eukaryotic cells, most organelles are surrounded by a membrane, but in Prokaryotic cells there are no membrane-bound organelles.

Fluid Mosaic Model of Cell Membranes

1. Membranes are fluid and are rather viscous – like vegetable oil.

2. The molecules of the cell membrane are always in motion, so the phospholipids are able to drift across the membrane, changing places with their neighbour.

3. Proteins, both in and on the membrane, form a mosaic, floating in amongst the phospholipids.

4. Because of this, scientists call the modern view of membrane structure the 'Fluid Mosaic Model'.

5. The mosaic of proteins in the cell membrane is constantly changing.

Membrane Proteins

1. A variety of protein molecules are embedded in the basic phospholipid bilayer.

2. Some proteins are attached to the surface of the cell membrane on both the internal and external surface. These may be hormone receptors, enzymes or cell recognition proteins (or antigens)

3. Other proteins are embedded in the phospholipid bilayer itself. These are often associated with transporting molecules from one side of the membrane to the other and are referred to as carrier proteins.

4. Some of these form channels or pores through which certain substances can pass (facilitated diffusion), whilst others bind to a substance on one side of the membrane and carry it to the other side of the membrane (active transport).

5. Proteins exposed to the cell's external environment often have carbohydrates attached to them which act as antigens (e.g. blood groups A and B – group AB has both, group O has neither).

6. Some viruses may also bind here too.

Nucleus

1. The nucleus is normally the largest organelle within a Eukaryotic cell. But it is NOT the 'brain' of the cell.

2. Prokaryotes have no nucleus, having a nuclear body instead. This has no membrane and a loop of DNA - cccDNA - and no chromatin proteins).

3. The nucleus contains the cell's chromosomes (human, 46, fruit fly 6, fern 1260) which are normally uncoiled to form a chromatinic network, which contain both linear DNA and proteins, known as histones. These proteins coil up (dehydrate) at the start of nuclear division, when the chromosomes first become visible.

4. Whilst most cells have a single nucleus some cells (macrophages, phloem companion cells) have more than one and fungi have many nuclei in their cytoplasm – they are coenocytic (= common cytoplasm throughout).

5. The nucleus is surrounded by a double membrane called the nuclear envelope, which has many nuclear pores through which mRNA, and proteins can pass. These dimples make it look like a golf ball.

6. Most nuclei contain at least one nucleolus (plural, nucleoli). The nucleoli are where ribosomes are synthesised. Ribosomes translate mRNA into proteins.

7. When a nucleus prepares to divide, the nucleolus disappears.

PARTS OF PROKARYOTIC CELLS

Higher eukaryote has multiple organs to perform specific functions such as liver, kidney and heart. Organs have specific tissues and each tissue is composed of cells. 'Cell is the structural and functional unit of life' and it contains all necessary infrastructures to perform all functions. Based on cellular structure, cells are classified as prokaryotic and eukaryotic cells. In most of the cases, prokaryotes are single cells where as eukaryotes are either single cells or part of multi-cellular tissues system.

Structure of Prokaryotic Cells

A prokaryotic cell is much simpler and smaller than eukarotic cells. It lacks membrane bound organelles including nucleus. The description of different structural feature of prokaryotic cells is as follows:

Outer flagella

A. *flagellum* attached to the bacterial capsule is a central feature of most of the prokaryotic cell especially motile bacteria. It provides motion or locomotion to the bacteria and be responsible for chemotaxis of bacteria. Movement of bacteria towards a chemical gradient (such as glucose) is known as chemotaxsis. Flagellum is a part of cell wall and its motion is regulated by motor protein present inside the cell. Flagellar motion is an energy consuming process and governed by ATPase present at the bottom of the shaft. It is made up of protein flagellin and reduction or suppression of flagellar protein reduces bacterial infectivity (pathogenicity) and ability to grow.

Bacterial surface layers

Bacteria posses 3 anatomical barriers to protect the cells from external damage. Bacterial capsule is the outer most layer and made up of high molecular weight polysaccharides. It is impermeable to the water or other aqueous solvent and it is responsible for antigenicity of bacterial cells. Cell wall in bacteria and its response to gram staining is the basis of classification of bacterial species. Cell wall composition in Gram –ve and Gram +ve bacteria is different. Bacterial cell wall has different constituents and be responsible for their reactivity towards gram stain.

Peptidoglycan layer: Peptidoglycan layer is thick in gram +ve bacteria and thin in gram –ve bacteria. Peptidoglycan is a polymer of NAG (*N*-acetyl-glucosamine) and NAM (*N*-acetyl-muramic glucosamine) linked by a β-(1,4) linkage. Sugar polymer are attached to peptide chain composed of amino acids, L-alanine, D-glutamic acid, L-lysine and D-alanine. Peptide chain present in one layer cross linked to the next layer to form a mesh work and be responsible for physical strength of cell wall. Peptidoglycan synthesis is targeted by antibiotics such as pencillin where as lysozyme (present in human saliva or tears) degrades the peptidoglycan layer by cleaving glycosidic bond connecting NAG-NAM to form polymer.

Lipoteichoic acids: Lipoteichoic acid (LTA) are only found in gram +ve bacteria cell wall and it is an important antigenic determinant.

Lipopolysaccharides: Lipopolysaccharides (LPS) are found only in gram –ve bacterial cell wall and it is an important antigenic determinant.

Cytosol and other organelles

Prokaryotic cells do not contains any membrane bound organelle. The organelles are present in cytosol such as ribosome (70S), genetic material where as electron transport chain complexes are embedded within the plasma membrane.

Chromosome and extra chromosomal DNA

Prokaryote cell contains genetic material in the form of circular DNA, known as 'bacterial chromosome'. It contains genetic elements for replication, transcription and translation. Bacterial chromosome follows a rolling circle mode of DNA replication. The genes present on chromosome does not contains non coding region (introns) and it is co-translated to protein. Besides main circle DNA, bacteria also contains extra circular DNA known as 'plasmid'. Presence of plasmid containing resistance gene confers resistance towards known antibiotics. Exchange of extra-chromosomal DNA between different bacterial strains is one of the mechanisms responsible for spread of antibiotic resistance across the bacterial population.

Bacterial plasmid: Plasmid are widely been used for cloning of foreign DNA into the bacteria as host strain. Before getting into the details of discussing bacterial plasmid we will discuss the basic properties of plasmids.

Different forms of plasmids: Bacterial plasmid is a double stranded circular DNA exists in 3 different forms (Fig. 1.6). If the both strands of circular double strands are intact then it is called as covalently closed circles (CCC) where as if one of the strand has nick, then it acquire the conformation of open circle DNA (OC, DNA). During the isolation of plasmid DNA from bacteria, covalently closed circular DNA losses few number of turns and as a result it acquire supercoiled configuration. The interchange between these different forms are possible under the *in vitro* or *in vivo* conditions, such as DNA gyrase produces additional turn into the circular DNA to adopt supercoiled conformation.

Features of different plasmids: There are minimum molecular components to assemble bacterial plasmid to perform the function of vector are as follows:

- Origin of replication: Like any other replicating DNA, plasmid DNA needs its own independent origin of replication to provide replication start site to make more copies. It decides the range of

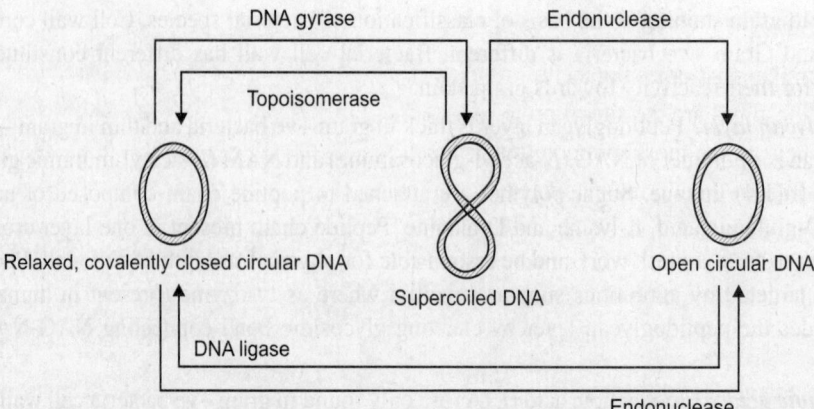

Fig. 1.6: Different forms of plasmids.

bacterial host strain can be use with the particular plasmid vector. The plasmids containing ori region from Col E1 can be able to grow in limited bacterial species such as *E. coli*, etc. In contrast, plasmid containing ori from RP4 or RSF1010 can be able to grow in gram (–) bacteria and gram (+) bacteria.

- Selection marker: Selection marker in the form of either antibiotic resistance gene or enzymatic gene is essential to give phenotypic changes in host after entry of the plasmid.

- Promoter: Plasmid replication in host is performed by the host provided proteins such as DNA gyrase, helicase, polymerase and DNA ligase. But proteins required for conferring antibiotic resistance or enzyme use for selecting transformed host cells is present on plasmid and a promoter adjacent is required to express genes present on plasmid DNA. In addition, promoter is also needed to express gene present on foreign DNA.

Mitochondria

1. Mitochondria are found scattered throughout the cytosol, and are relatively large organelles (second only to the nucleus and chloroplasts).

2. Mitochondria are the sites of aerobic respiration, in which energy from organic compounds is transferred to ATP. For this reason they are sometimes referred to as the 'powerhouse' of the cell.

3. ATP is the molecule that most cells use as their main energy 'currency'.

4. Mitochondria are more numerous in cells that have a high energy requirement - our muscle cells contain a large number of mitochondria, as do liver, heart and sperm cells.

5. Mitochondria are surrounded by two membranes, indicating that they were once free-living organisms that have become mutualistic and then a part of almost every eukaryotic cell (not RBC's and xylem vessels).

   (a) The smooth outer membrane serves as a boundary between the mitochondria and the cytosol.

   (b) The inner membrane has many long folds, known as cristae, which greatly increase the surface area of the inner membrane, providing more space for ATP synthesis to occur.

6. Mitochondria have their own DNA, and new mitochondria arise only when existing ones grow and divide. They are thus semi-autonomous organelles.

Ribosomes

1. Unlike most other organelles, ribosomes are not surrounded by a membrane.
2. Ribosomes are the site of protein synthesis in a cell.
3. They are the most common organelles in almost all cells.
4. Some are free in the cytoplasm (Prokaryotes), others line the membranes of rough ER.
5. They exist in two sizes: 70s are found in all Prokaryotes, chloroplasts and mitochondria, suggesting that they have evolved from ancestral Prokaryotic organisms. They are free-floating. 80s found in all eukaryotic cells – attached to the rough ER (they are rather larger).
6. Groups of 80s ribosomes, working together, are known as a polysome.

Endoplasmic Reticulum (ER)

1. The ER is a system of membranous tubules and sacs.
2. The primary function of the ER is to act as an internal transport system, allowing molecules to move from one part of the cell to another.
3. The quantity of ER inside a cell fluctuates, depending on the cell's activity. Cells with a lot include secretory cells and liver cells.
4. The rough ER is studded with 80s ribosomes and is the site of protein synthesis. It is an extension of the outer membrane of the nuclear envelope, so allowing mRNA to be transported swiftly to the 80s ribosomes, where they are translated in protein synthesis.
5. The smooth ER is where polypeptides are converted into functional proteins and where proteins are prepared for secretion. It is also the site of lipid and steroid synthesis, and is associated with the Golgi apparatus. Smooth ER has no 80s ribosomes and is also involved in the regulation of calcium levels in muscle cells, and the breakdown of toxins by liver cells.
6. Both types of ER transport materials throughout the cell.

Golgi Apparatus

1. The Golgi apparatus is the processing, packaging and secreting organelle of the cell, so it is much more common in glandular cells.
2. The Golgi apparatus is a system of membranes, made of flattened sac-like structures called cisternae.
3. It works closely with the smooth ER, to modify proteins for export by the cell.

Lysosomes

1. Lysosomes are small spherical organelles that enclose hydrolytic enzymes within a single membrane.
2. Lysosomes are the site of protein digestion – thus allowing enzymes to be recycled when they are no longer required. They are also the site of food digestion in the cell, and of bacterial digestion in phagocytes.
3. Lysosomes are formed from pieces of the Golgi apparatus that break off.
4. Lysosomes are common in the cells of Animals, Protoctista and even Fungi, but rare in plants.

Centriole

1. This consists of two bundles of microtubules at right-angles to each other.

2. Each bundle contains 9 tubes in a very characteristic arrangement
3. At the start of mitosis and meiosis, the centriole divides, and one half moves to each end of the cell, forming the spindle.
4. The spindle fibres are later shortened to pull the chromosomes apart.

Cytoskeleton

1. Just as your body depends on your skeleton to maintain its shape and size, so a cell needs structures to maintain its shape and size.
2. In animal cells, which have no cell wall, an internal framework called the cytoskeleton maintains the shape of the cell, and helps the cell to move.
3. The cytoskeleton consists of two structures:
   (a) Microfilaments (contractile). They are made of actin, and are common in motile cells.
   (b) Microtubules (rigid, hollow tubes – made of tubulin).
4. Microtubules have three functions:
   (a) To maintain the shape of the cell.
   (b) To serve as tracks for organelles to move along within the cell.
   (c) They form the centriole.

Cilia and Flagellae

1. Cilia and Flagellae are structures that project from the cell, where they assist in movement.
2. Cilia (*sing. cilium*) are short, and numerous and hair-like.
3. Flagellae (sing. flagellum) are much longer, fewer, and are whip-like.
4. The cilia and flagellae of all Eukaryotes are always in a '9 + 2' arrangement that is characteristic.
5. Protoctista commonly use cilia and flagellae to move through water.
6. Sperm use flagellae (many, all fused together) to swim to the egg.
7. Cilia line our trachea and bronchi, moving dust particles and bacteria away from the lungs.

PLANT CELL STRUCTURES

1. Most of the organelles and other parts of the cell are common to all Eukaryotic cells. Cells from different organisms have an even greater difference in structure.
2. Plant cells have three additional structures not found in animal cells:
   (a) Cellulose cell walls.
   (b) Chloroplasts (and other plastids).
   (c) A central vacuole.

Cellulose Cell Wall

1. One of the most important features of all plants is presence of a cellulose cell wall.
2. Fungi such as Mushrooms and Yeast also have cell walls, but these are made of chitin.
3. The cell wall is freely permeable (porous), and so has no direct effect on the movement of molecules into or out of the cell.

4. The rigidity of their cell walls helps both to support and protect the plant.

5. Plant cell walls are of two types: (i) primary (cellulose) cell wall: While a plant cell is being formed, a middle lamella made of pectin, is formed and the cellulose cell wall develops between the middle lamella and the cell membrane. As the cell expands in length, more cellulose is added, enlarging the cell wall. When the cell reaches full size, a secondary cell wall may form and (ii) secondary (lignified) cell wall: The secondary cell wall is formed only in woody tissue (mainly xylem). The secondary cell wall is stronger and waterproof and once a secondary cell wall forms, a cell can grow no more – it is dead.

Vacuoles

1. The most prominent structure in plant cells is the large vacuole.

2. The vacuole is a large membrane-bound sac that fills up much of most plant cells.

3. The vacuole serves as a storage area, and may contain stored organic molecules as well as inorganic ions.

4. The vacuole is also used to store waste. Since plants have no kidney, they convert waste to an insoluble form and then store it in their vacuole - until autumn.

5. The vacuoles of some plants contain poisons (e.g. tannins) that discourage animals from eating their tissues.

6. Whilst the cells of other organisms may also contain vacuoles, they are much smaller and are usually involved in food digestion.

Chloroplasts (and other Plastids)

1. A characteristic feature of plant cells is the presence of plastids that make or store food.

2. The most common of these (some leaf cells only!) are chloroplasts – the site of photosynthesis.

3. Each chloroplast encloses a system of flattened, membranous sacs called thylakoids, which contain chlorophyll.

4. The thylakoids are arranged in stacks called grana.

5. The space between the grana is filled with cytoplasm-like stroma.

6. Chloroplasts contain ccc DNA and 70S ribosomes and are semi-autonomous organelles.

7. Other plastids store reddish-orange pigments that colour. Table 1.1 shows function of various type of components of cells.

MULTICELLULAR ORGANISATION

In a unicellular organism, one cell carries out all of the functions of life. In contrast, most cells in a multicellular organism are specialised to perform one or a few functions – more efficiently. Because of cell specialisation, the cells of multicellular organisms depend on other cells in the organism for their survival.

TISSUE, ORGANS AND ORGAN SYSTEMS

1. In most multicellular organisms, we find the following organisation:

    (a) Cellular level: The smallest unit of life capable of carrying out all the functions of living things.

    (b) Tissue level: A group of cells that performs a specific function in an organism.

Table 1.1: Function of various type of components of cells.

Organelle	Location	Description	Function
Cell wall	Plant, not animal	Outer layer rigid, strong, stiff made of cellulose	Support (grow tall) protection allows H_2O, O_2, CO_2 to pass into and out of cell
Cell membrane	Both plant/animal	Plant - inside cell wall animal - outer layer; cholesterol selectively permeable movement	support protection controls of materials in/out of cell barrier between cell and its environment maintains homeostasis controls cell activities
Nucleus	Both plant/animal	Large, oval	Controls movement of materials in/out of
Nuclear membrane	Both plant/animal	Surrounds nucleus selectively permeable	nucleus
Cytoplasm	Both plant/animal	Clear, thick, jellylike material and organelles found inside cell membrane	Supports/protects cell organelles
Endoplasmic reticulum (ER)	Both plant/animal	Network of tubes or membranes	Carries materials through cell produces proteins
Ribosome	Both plant/animal	Small bodies free or attached to ER	Breaks down sugar molecules into energy
Mitochondrion	Both plant/animal	Bean-shaped with inner membranes	store food, water, waste (plants need to
Vacuole	Plant - few/large Animal - small	fluid-filled sacs	store large amounts of food)
Lysosome	Plant - uncommon animal - common	Small, round, with a membrane	Breaks down larger food molecules into smaller molecules digests old cell parts
Chloroplast	Plant, not animal	Green, oval usually containing chlorophyll (green pigment)	Uses energy from sun to make food for the plant (photosynthesis)

(c) Organ level: Several different types of tissue that function together for a specific purpose.

(d) Organ system level: Several organs working together to perform a function. The different organ systems in a multicellular organism interact to carry out the processes of life.

2. Plants also have tissue and organs, although they are arranged somewhat differently from those of animals, e.g. vascular tissue.

3. The four plant organs are: (i) roots, (ii) stems, (iii) leaves and (iv) flowers.

Colonial Organisations

1. A colonial organisation is a collection of genetically identical cells that live together in a closely connected group.

2. Many of the cells of the colony carry out specific functions that benefit the whole colony.

3. Colonial organisms (e.g. sponges, coral) appear to straddle the border between a collection of unicellular organisms and a true multicellular organism. They lack tissues and organs, but do exhibit the principle of cell specialisation.

MODEL ORGANISM

A model organism is a non-human species that is extensively studied to understand particular biological phenomena, with the expectation that discoveries made in the model organism will provide insight into the workings of other organisms. Model organisms are *in vivo* models and are widely used to research human disease when human experimentation would be unfeasible or unethical. This strategy is made possible by the common descent of all living organisms, and the conservation of metabolic and developmental pathways and genetic material over the course of evolution.

Studying model organisms can be informative, but care must be taken when extrapolating from one organism to another. In researching human disease, model organisms allow for better understanding the disease process without the added risk of harming an actual human. The species chosen will usually meet a determined taxonomic equivalency to humans, so as to react to disease or its treatment in a way that resembles human physiology as needed. Although biological activity in a model organism does not ensure an effect in humans, many drugs, treatments and cures for human diseases are developed in part with the guidance of animal models. There are three main types of disease models: homologous, isomorphic and predictive. Homologous animals have the same causes, symptoms and treatment options as would humans who have the same disease. Isomorphic animals share the same symptoms and treatments. Predictive models are similar to a particular human disease in only a couple of aspects, but are useful in isolating and making predictions about mechanisms of a set of disease features.

The use of animals in research dates back to ancient Greece, with Aristotle (384–322 BCE) and Erasistratus (304–258 BCE) among the first to perform experiments on living animals. Discoveries in the 18th and 19th centuries included Antoine Lavoisier's use of a guinea pig in a calorimeter to prove that respiration was a form of combustion, and Louis Pasteur's demonstration of the germ theory of disease in the 1880s using anthrax in sheep.

Research using animal models has been central to many of the achievements of modern medicine. It has contributed most of the basic knowledge in fields such as human physiology and biochemistry, and has played significant roles in fields such as neuroscience and infectious disease. For example, the results have included the near-eradication of polio and the development of organ transplantation, and have benefited both humans and animals. From 1910 to 1927, Thomas Hunt Morgan's work with the fruit fly *Drosophila melanogaster* identified chromosomes as the vector of inheritance for genes. *Drosophila* became one of the first, and for some time the most widely used, model organisms, and Eric Kandel wrote that Morgan's discoveries 'helped transform biology into an experimental science.' *D. melanogaster* remains one of the most widely used eukaryotic model organisms. During the same time period, studies on mouse genetics in the laboratory of William Ernest Castle in collaboration with Abbie Lathrop led to generation of the DBA (dilute, brown and non-agouti) inbred mouse strain and the systematic generation of other inbred strains. The mouse has since been used extensively as a model organism and is associated with many important biological discoveries of the 20th and 21st centuries.

In the late 19th century, Emil von Behring isolated the diphtheria toxin and demonstrated its effects in guinea pigs. He went on to develop an antitoxin against diphtheria in animals and then in humans, which resulted in the modern methods of immunisation and largely ended diphtheria as a threatening disease. The diphtheria antitoxin is famously commemorated in the Iditarod race, which is modelled after the delivery of antitoxin in the 1925 serum run to Nome. The success of animal studies in producing the diphtheria antitoxin has also been attributed as a cause for the decline of the early 20th-century opposition to animal research in the United States.

Subsequent research in model organisms led to further medical advances, such as Frederick Banting's research in dogs, which determined that the isolates of pancreatic secretion could be used to treat dogs with diabetes. This led to the 1922 discovery of insulin and its use in treating diabetes, which had previously meant death. John Cade's research in guinea pigs discovered the anticonvulsant properties of lithium salts, which revolutionised the treatment of bipolar disorder, replacing the previous treatments of lobotomy or electroconvulsive therapy. Modern general anaesthetics, such as halothane and related compounds, were also developed through studies on model organisms, and are necessary for modern, complex surgical operations. In the 1940s, Jonas Salk used rhesus monkey studies to isolate the most virulent forms of the polio virus, which led to his creation of a polio vaccine. The vaccine, which was made publicly available in 1955, reduced the incidence of polio 15-fold in the United States over the following five years. Albert Sabin improved the vaccine by passing the polio virus through animal hosts, including monkeys; the Sabin vaccine was produced for mass consumption in 1963, and had virtually eradicated polio in the United States by 1965. It has been estimated that developing and producing the vaccines required the use of 100,000 rhesus monkeys, with 65 doses of vaccine produced from each monkey. Sabin wrote in 1992, 'Without the use of animals and human beings, it would have been impossible to acquire the important knowledge needed to prevent much suffering and premature death not only among humans, but also among animals.'

Other 20th-century medical advances and treatments that relied on research performed in animals include organ transplant techniques, the heart-lung machine, antibiotics, and the whooping cough vaccine. Treatments for animal diseases have also been developed, including for rabies, anthrax, glanders, feline immunodeficiency virus (FIV), tuberculosis, Texas cattle fever, classical swine fever (hog cholera), heartworm, and other parasitic infections. Animal experimentation continues to be required for biomedical research, and is used with the aim of solving medical problems such as Alzheimer's disease, AIDS, multiple sclerosis, spinal cord injury, many headaches, and other conditions in which there is no useful *in vitro* model system available.

Models are those organisms with a wealth of biological data that make them attractive to study as examples for other species and/or natural phenomena that are more difficult to study directly. Continual research on these organisms focus on a wide variety of experimental techniques and goals from many different levels of biology—from ecology, behaviour and biomechanics, down to the tiny functional scale of individual tissues, organelles and proteins. Inquiries about the DNA of organisms are classed as genetic models (with short generation times, such as the fruitfly and nematode worm), experimental models, and genomic parsimony models, investigating pivotal position in the evolutionary tree. Historically, model organisms include a handful of species with extensive genomic research data, such as the NIH model organisms.

Often, model organisms are chosen on the basis that they are amenable to experimental manipulation. This usually will include characteristics such as short life-cycle, techniques for genetic manipulation (inbred strains, stem cell lines, and methods of transformation) and non-specialist living requirements. Sometimes, the genome arrangement facilitates the sequencing of the model organism's genome, for example, by being very compact or having a low proportion of junk DNA (e.g. yeast, arabidopsis, or pufferfish). When researchers look for an organism to use in their studies, they look for several traits. Among these are size, generation time, accessibility, manipulation, genetics, conservation of mechanisms, and potential economic benefit. As comparative molecular biology has become more common, some researchers have sought model organisms from a wider assortment of lineages on the tree of life.

Phylogeny and Genetic Relatedness

The primary reason for the use of model organisms in research is the evolutionary principle that all organisms share some degree of relatedness and genetic similarity due to common ancestry. The study of taxonomic human relatives, then, can provide a great deal of information about mechanism and disease within the human body that can be useful in medicine. Various phylogenetic trees for vertebrates have been constructed using comparative proteomics, genetics, genomics as well as the geochemical and fossil record. These estimations tell us that humans and chimpanzees last shared a common ancestor about 6 million years ago (mya). As our closest relatives, chimpanzees have a lot of potential to tell us about mechanisms of disease (and what genes may be responsible for human intelligence). However, chimpanzees are rarely used in research and are protected from highly invasive procedures. The most common animal model is the rodent. Phylogenetic trees estimate that humans and rodents last shared a common ancestor ~80–100 mya. Despite this distant split, humans and rodents have far more similarities than they do differences. This is due to the relative stability of large portions of the genome; making the use of vertebrate animals particularly productive. Genomic data is used to make close comparisons between species and determine relatedness. As humans, we share about 99% of our genome with chimpanzees (98.7% with bonobos) and over 90% with the mouse. With so much of the genome conserved across species, it is relatively impressive that the differences between humans and mice can be accounted for in approximately six thousand genes (of ~30,000 total). Scientists have been able to take advantage of these similarities in generating experimental and predictive models of human disease.

Types of Many Model Organisms

There are many model organisms. One of the first model systems for molecular biology was the bacterium *Escherichia coli*, a common constituent of the human digestive system. Several of the bacterial viruses (bacteriophage) that infect *E. coli* also have been very useful for the study of gene structure and gene regulation (e.g. phages Lambda and T4). However, it is debated whether bacteriophages should be classified as organisms, because they lack metabolism and depend on functions of the host cells for propagation. In eukaryotes, several yeasts, particularly *Saccharomyces cerevisiae* (baker's or budding yeast), have been widely used in genetics and cell biology, largely because they are quick and easy to grow. The cell cycle in a simple yeast is very similar to the cell cycle in humans and is regulated by homologous proteins. The fruit fly *Drosophila melanogaster* is studied, again, because it is easy to grow for an animal, has various visible congenital traits and has a polytene (giant) chromosome in its salivary glands that can be examined under a light microscope. The roundworm *Caenorhabditis elegans* is studied because it has very defined development patterns involving fixed numbers of cells, and it can be rapidly assayed for abnormalities.

Disease Models

Animal models serving in research may have an existing, inbred or induced disease or injury that is similar to a human condition. These test conditions are often termed as animal models of disease. The use of animal models allows researchers to investigate disease states in ways which would be inaccessible in a human patient, performing procedures on the non-human animal that imply a level of harm that would not be considered ethical to inflict on a human.

The best models of disease are similar in etiology (mechanism of cause) and phenotype (signs and symptoms) to the human equivalent. However complex human diseases can often be better understood in a simplified system in which individual parts of the disease process are isolated and examined. For instance, behavioural analogues of anxiety or pain in laboratory animals can be used to screen and test new drugs for the treatment of these conditions in humans. A 2000 study found that animal models concorded (coincided on true positives and false negatives) with human toxicity in 71% of cases, with 63% for nonrodents alone and 43% for rodents alone. In 1987, Davidson and others suggested that selection of an animal model for research be based on nine considerations.

These include (i) appropriateness as an analog, (ii) transferability of information, (iii) genetic uniformity of organisms, where applicable, (iv) background knowledge of biological properties, (v) cost and availability, (vi) generalisability of the results, (vii) ease of and adaptability to experimental manipulation, (viii) ecological consequences, and (ix) ethical implications.

Animal models can be classified as homologous, isomorphic or predictive. Animal models can also be more broadly classified into four categories: (i) experimental, (ii) spontaneous, (iii) negative, (iv) orphan. Experimental models are most common. These refer to models of disease that resemble human conditions in phenotype or response to treatment but are induced artificially in the laboratory.

Spontaneous models

Spontaneous models refer to diseases that are analogous to human conditions that occur naturally in the animal being studied. These models are rare, but informative. Negative models essentially refer to control animals, which are useful for validating an experimental result. Orphan models refer to diseases for which there is no human analog and occur exclusively in the species studied. The increase in knowledge of the genomes of non-human primates and other mammals that are genetically close to humans is allowing the production of genetically engineered animal tissues, organs and even animal species which express human diseases, providing a more robust model of human diseases in an animal model.

Animal models observed in the sciences of psychology and sociology are often termed animal models of behaviour. It is difficult to build an animal model that perfectly reproduces the symptoms of depression in patients. Depression, as other mental disorders, consists of endophenotypes that can be reproduced independently and evaluated in animals. An ideal animal model offers an opportunity to understand molecular, genetic and epigenetic factors that may lead to depression. By using animal models, the underlying molecular alterations and the causal relationship between genetic or environmental alterations and depression can be examined, which would afford a better insight into pathology of depression. In addition, animal models of depression are indispensable for identifying novel therapies for depression.

Important Model Organisms

Model organisms are drawn from all three domains of life, as well as viruses. The most widely studied prokaryotic model organism is *Escherichia coli* (*E. coli*), which has been intensively investigated for over 60 years. It is a common, gram-negative gut bacterium which can be grown and cultured easily and inexpensively in a laboratory setting. It is the most widely used organism in molecular genetics, and is an important species in the fields of biotechnology and microbiology, where it has served as the host organism for the majority of work with recombinant DNA.

Simple model eukaryotes include baker's yeast (*Saccharomyces cerevisiae*) and fission yeast (*Schizosaccharomyces pombe*), both of which share many characters with higher cells, including those of humans. For instance, many cell division genes that are critical for the development of cancer have been discovered in yeast. *Chlamydomonas reinhardtii*, a unicellular green alga with well-studied genetics, is used to study photosynthesis and motility. *C. reinhardtii* has many known and mapped mutants and expressed sequence tags, and there are advanced methods for genetic transformation and selection of genes. *Dictyostelium discoideum* is used in molecular biology and genetics, and is studied as an example of cell communication, differentiation, and programmed cell death. Among invertebrates, the fruit fly *Drosophila melanogaster* is famous as the subject of genetics experiments by Thomas Hunt Morgan and others.

They are easily raised in the lab, with rapid generations, high fecundity, few chromosomes, and easily induced observable mutations. The nematode *Caenorhabditis elegans* is used for understanding the genetic control of development and physiology. It was first proposed as a model for neuronal development by Sydney Brenner in 1963, and has been extensively used in many different contexts since then. *C. elegans* was the first multicellular organism whose genome was completely sequenced, and as of 2012, the only organism to have its connectome completed.

Arabidopsis thaliana is currently the most popular model plant. Its small stature and short generation time facilitates rapid genetic studies, and many phenotypic and biochemical mutants have been mapped. *A. thaliana* was the first plant to have its genome sequenced.

Among vertebrates, guinea pigs (*Cavia porcellus*) were used by Robert Koch and other early bacteriologists as a host for bacterial infections, becoming a byword for 'laboratory animal,' but are less commonly used today. The classic model vertebrate is currently the mouse (*Mus musculus*). Many inbred strains exist, as well as lines selected for particular traits, often of medical interest, e.g. body size, obesity, muscularity, and voluntary wheel-running behaviour. The rat (*Rattus norvegicus*) is particularly useful as a toxicology model, and as a neurological model and source of primary cell cultures, owing to the larger size of organs and suborganellar structures relative to the mouse, while eggs and embryos from *Xenopus tropicalis* and *Xenopus laevis* (African clawed frog) are used in developmental biology, cell biology, toxicology, and neuroscience. Likewise, the zebrafish (*Danio rerio*) has a nearly transparent body during early development, which provides unique visual access to the animals internal anatomy during this time period. Zebrafish are used to study development, toxicology and toxicopathology, specific gene function and roles of signalling pathways.

Other important model organisms and some of their uses include: T4 phage (viral infection), *Tetrahymena thermophila* (intracellular processes), maize (transposons), *hydras* (regeneration and morphogenesis), cats (neurophysiology), chickens (development), dogs (respiratory and cardiovascular systems), *Nothobranchius furzeri* (aging), and non-human primates such as the rhesus macaque and chimpanzee (hepatitis, HIV, Parkinson's disease, cognition, and vaccines).

Selected model organisms

The organisms below have become model organisms because they facilitate the study of certain characters or because of their genetic accessibility. For example, *E. coli* was one of the first organisms for which genetic techniques such as transformation or genetic manipulation has been developed. The genomes of all model species have been sequenced, including their mitochondrial/chloroplast genomes. Model organism databases exist to provide researchers with a portal from which to download sequences (DNA, RNA, or protein) or to access functional information on specific genes, for example the sub-cellular localisation of the gene product or its physiological role.

Limitations of model organism

Many animal models serving as test subjects in biomedical research, such as rats and mice, may be selectively sedentary, obese and glucose intolerant. This may confound their use to model human metabolic processes and diseases as these can be affected by dietary energy intake and exercise.

Similarly, there are differences between the immune systems of model organisms and humans that lead to significantly altered responses to stimuli, although the underlying principles of genome function may be the same.

Unintended bias

Some studies suggests that inadequate published data in animal testing may result in irreproducible research, with missing details about how experiments are done omitted from published papers or differences in testing that may introduce bias. Examples of hidden bias include a 2014 study from McGill University in Montreal, Canada which suggests that mice handled by men rather than women showed higher stress levels. Another study in 2016 suggested that gut microbiomes in mice may have an impact upon scientific research.

Alternatives

Ethical concerns, as well as the cost, maintenance and relative inefficiency of animal research has encouraged development of alternative methods for the study of disease. Cell culture, or *in vitro* studies, provide an alternative that preserves the physiology of the living cell, but does not require the sacrifice of an animal for mechanistic studies. Human, inducible pluripotent stem cells can also elucidate new mechanisms for understanding cancer and cell regeneration. Imaging studies (such as MRI or PET scans) enable non-invasive study of human subjects. Recent advances in genetics and genomics can identify disease-associated genes, which can be targeted for therapies. Ultimately, however, there is no substitute for a living organism when studying complex interactions in disease pathology or treatments.

Ethics

Debate about the ethical use of animals in research dates at least as far back as 1822 when the British Parliament enacted the first law for animal protection preventing cruelty to cattle. This was followed by the Cruelty to Animals Act of 1835 and 1849, which criminalised ill-treating, over-driving, and torturing animals. In 1876, under pressure from the National Anti-Vivisection Society, the Cruelty to Animals Act was amended to include regulations governing the use of animals in research. This new act stipulated that (i) experiments must be proven absolutely necessary for instruction, or to save or prolong human life, (ii) animals must be properly anesthetised, and (iii) animals must be killed as soon as the experiment is over. Today, these three principles are central to the laws and guidelines governing the use of animals and research. In the US, the Animal Welfare Act of 1970 set standards for animal use and care in research. This law is enforced by APHIS's Animal Care programme.

In academic settings in which NIH funding is used for animal research, institutions are governed by the NIH Office of Laboratory Animal Welfare (OLAW). At each site, OLAW guidelines and standards are upheld by a local review board called the Institutional Animal Care and Use Committee (IACUC). All laboratory experiments involving living animals are reviewed and approved by this committee. In addition to proving the potential for benefit to human health, minimisation of pain and distress, and timely and humane euthanasia, experimenters must justify their protocols based on the principles of Replacement, Reduction and Refinement. Replacement refers to efforts to engage alternatives to animal use. This includes the use of computer models, non-living tissues and cells, and replacement of 'higher-order' animals (primates and mammals) with 'lower' order animals (e.g. cold-blooded animals, invertebrates, bacteria) wherever possible. Reduction refers to efforts to minimise number of animals used during the course of an experiment, as well as prevention of unnecessary replication of previous experiments. To satisfy this requirement, mathematical calculations of statistical power are employed to determine the minimum number of animals that can be used to get a statistically significant experimental result. Refinement refers to efforts to make experimental design as painless and efficient as possible in order to minimise the suffering of each animal subject.

Chapter 2

Tools and Techniques in Cell Biology

INTRODUCTION

The following chapter covers some of the commonly used cell biology techniques. Cell/tissue culture in the same way that bacteria and other simple organisms can be grown in the laboratory outside their normal environment, cells and tissues from more complicated organisms can be cultured as well. The techniques are slightly different, and the culture media are more complex to reflect the complex internal environment inside the host from which the cells are derived, however cell and tissue culture is a powerful tool which provides an almost limitless supply of test material for researchers to use without resorting to using whole organisms. In addition, the controlled conditions in cell and tissue culture allow researchers to carry out experiments with a lower number of variables which may affect the outcome of the test. Cell culture may use cells removed directly from an organism (primary culture), or it may use lines of cultured cancer cells. The benefit of the latter approach is that cancer cells continue to divide, while primary cultures cease dividing after a number of cycles.

PREPARATION OF CELLS FOR IMMUNOFLUORESCENCE

Using routine brightfield microscopy, a reasonable amount of detail in the cell can be determined. Large structures such as the nucleus (and its nucleoli) and vacuoles are easily distinguished inside the cell with even fairly rudimentary microscopes. Some other structures can also be demonstrated with the careful use of dyes and stains which give a colour based on chemical reactions with cellular components, and this forms the basis of cytochemistry (on individual cells) and histochemistry (on thin sections of tissue). However, even these methods are not nearly specific enough to properly demonstrate the wide variety of subcellular structures and materials. Immunofluorescence is a technique which uses the highly specific binding of antibodies to their target antigens as a way of demonstrating materials and structures inside cells. Before any immunofluorescence procedures can be carried out on the cells, they must be properly prepared. The cells have been grown on a coverslip placed on the bottom of a culture plate. When a new culture is needed, a suspension of cells is prepared with the cells floating around inside the cell culture medium. The number of cells per unit volume (generally per millilitre of medium) can be calculated using cell counters and a specific number of cells added to a dish containing culture medium by adding the correct volume of cell suspension (e.g. if the density of cells in the suspension is 100,000 cells/mL and you needed 100,000 cells to start a culture, you would add 1mL of suspension). The exact seeding density depends on the reproductive rate of the cells you are using and how dense you want the culture to be in the time you have.

When the cells are added to the culture dish, they sink to the bottom and attach through proteins embedded in the cell membrane. Cells that have attached to the bottom of the dish take on the appearance of a fried egg, with the nucleus as the yolk and the cytoplasm as the white. Cells only release from the bottom of the flask when they are in the process of dividing, becoming spherical as they carry out mitosis. The cells have been added to a 6-well culture plate. In each well, a number of coverslips were added to the wells prior to the addition of the cells. When the cells settled to the bottom of the well, some landed on the coverslip. This means that the cells can be easily removed from the well and treated while on the coverslip, and eventually the coverslip containing the cells can be mounted onto a microscope slide for observation. The coverslips have been previously treated with Poly-L-Lysine, a peptide which acts as a cellular 'glue' and assists in holding the cells (including mitotic cells which have rounded up) onto the coverslip.

At several times during the course of the immunofluorescence procedures, cells will need to be washed. This is usually done by replacing the liquid in the well they are contained in with phosphate buffered isotonic saline, a solution of sodium chloride at 9 g/L in a buffer which keeps the pH at a physiological level of around 7.2. Because the cells are stuck to the coverslip, the liquid can be gently removed and replaced with a solution which does not put the cells under osmotic stress.

Once cells die (which starts to occur once their nutrients and ideal growing conditions have been removed), they start to break down and lose their structure and integrity. A typical live cell taken through the processes needed for immunofluorescence would have started the breakdown process by the time the techniques have been completed. Therefore the cells must be preserved prior to undergoing antibody treatment. This process is called fixation, and is the same technique used to preserve biological specimens in museums. Fixation relies on 'freezing' the proteins in place using a chemical process rather than temperature. The tertiary structure of proteins is maintained by weak hydrogen bonds between the side chains of the amino acids that make up the proteins. These hydrogen bonds are easily broken by increases in temperature or changes in pH, resulting in a loss of protein structure called denaturation. Formalin is a buffered solution of the gas formaldehyde which forms permanent covalent cross-links between protein chains and locks them into their tertiary structure, regardless of minor changes in temperature or pH, and thus preserves the structure of the cell. In this investigation, you will use a type of formalin called *para*-formaldehyde to fix the cells, although other fixatives like ice cold methanol can also be used.

Once cells have been washed, fixed in *para*-formaldehyde and washed again, they must then be permeablised. The antibodies used for immunofluorescence are large protein molecules which cannot cross the cell membrane, so the cell membrane must be removed. It is very important that the cells must be fixed prior to permeablisation, otherwise the cell will burst.

To understand why it is important to fix the cells, it may help to imagine the cell as a dome tent filled with cooked spaghetti (with the nucleus as a beach ball inside it, perhaps). The shape of the cell is maintained by structural proteins such as Tubulin, represented in our analogy by the cooked spaghetti, while the whole shape of the cell is maintained by the cell membrane, represented by the fabric of the tent itself. If you were to cut away the tent fabric (removing the cell membrane through permeablisation), all of the spaghetti would fall out and spill onto the ground. Washing the cell would then have the effect of hosing the mess away.

Fixing the cells would be like drying the spaghetti out. It would shrink slightly and revert back to its state prior to cooking, however it would be in the same position it was in when the drying occurred. The tent fabric (cell membrane) could then be removed and you would be left with a mound of dried spaghetti in the same shape as the tent, but without the tent around it (Fig. 2.1). Chemical fixation does make some changes to the proteins in the cell, however enough of the original structure is often left to retain some of the proteins' functions, including the ability of the proteins to bind antibodies and the fluorescence characteristics of green fluorescent protein (both of which are vital for this investigation.

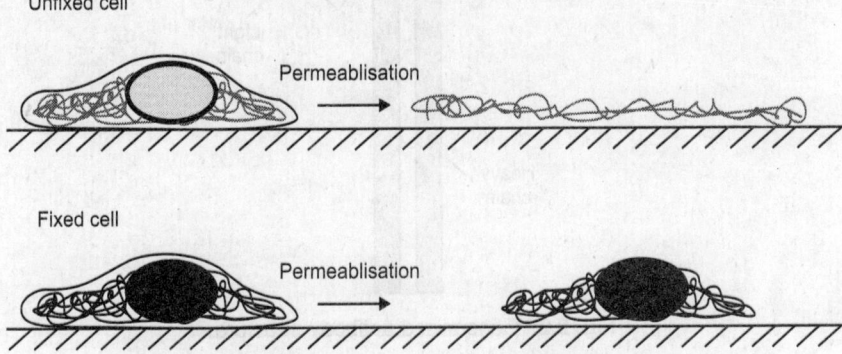

Fig. 2.1: Fate of unfixed and fixed cells following permeablisation.

The cells will be permeablised using a detergent (Triton X100). Detergents work by solublising lipids in water, and since the cell membrane is made up of lipid molecules, the Triton X100 in this method removes the lipids from the membrane, allowing large molecules such as antibodies to enter the cell and bind to proteins inside. At the same time as they are permeablised, the cells will be blocked. Blocking involves the addition of a solution of proteins (usually bovine serum albumin, or BSA). Cells may contain proteins which can bind onto antibodies and other proteins non-specifically, rather than the antibodies specifically binding onto their target proteins. The BSA 'soaks up' these non-specific binding sites, ensuring that the only way the antibodies can bind is via their specific targets. Once permeablised, blocked and washed once more, the cells are ready to be treated with antibodies.

Antibodies and Immunofluorescence

Antibodies are large, complex proteins made by specific immune cells in the body (the plasma cells, which are derived from populations of B lymphocytes). Antibodies are produced in response to the presence of an agent in the body which the immune system recognises as being not from the body. These agents are usually foreign materials, such as proteins on the surface of microbes, although in some cases the immune system may target the body's own proteins, causing autoimmune diseases such as Type I Diabetes and Rheumatoid Arthritis.

Antibodies are composed of four peptide chains (two light chains and two heavy chains) arranged like a capital letter 'Y' (Fig. 2.2). Most of an antibody's structure is constant between antibodies (with some variation between different classes), however at the ends of the 'arms' of the Y is a small, highly variable region made up of a region of the light and heavy chains. It is changes in the shape of this region which determines the difference between antibodies. The shape of this variable region is such that it fits around and binds very specifically to a region on the material it is raised against. The area which it binds to is called the epitope, while the material where the epitope is found is called the

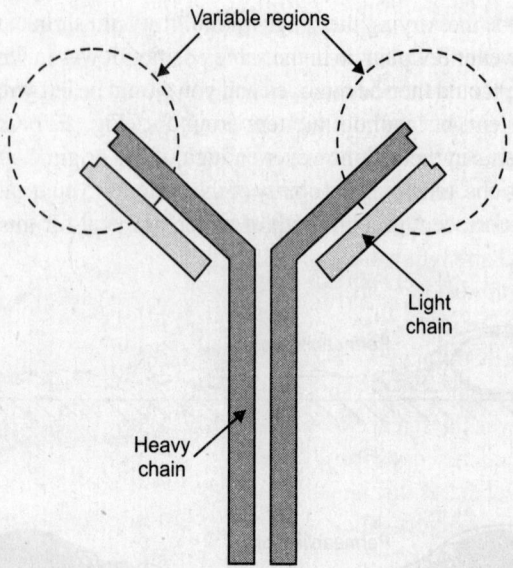

Fig. 2.2: Generalised antibody structure.

antigen. A different antibody is made in response to each epitope on each antigen, with the variable regions confirming exactly to each epitope. This means that antibodies are made which bind very specifically to particular epitopes on antigens. This specificity is so high that two antibodies can be generated which can tell the difference between two versions of the same protein, one which has a phosphate group attached and one which does not. This high level of specificity makes antibodies extremely useful in detecting particular proteins, and is used in techniques such as diagnosis of disease agents in the blood, western blotting, immunohistochemistry, and, of course, immunofluorescence.

Antibodies are made in animals, or in cell lines derived from those animals. To generate an antibody against a particular protein, samples of that protein are injected into a test animal. A better antibody response is generated if the target protein comes from a different species to the animal used to raise the antibody as the host animal would recognise the protein as being foreign. For example, if you are interested in using antibodies to detect a human protein, you would use a non-human animal such as a mouse, rabbit or goat to raise the antibody. Once the animal starts making the antibody, it can be recovered from the animal's blood and purified for use. In some cases the lines of plasma cells which are making the antibody can be isolated and fused with a cancer cell, making a hybridoma cell line which has the immortality of the cancer cells and the antibody-generating properties of the plasma cells. This means that the antibodies can be produced in culture without the need for using further animals.

The technique you will be using is indirect immunofluorescence. Direct immunofluorescence involves chemically combining a fluorescent dye directly to the primary antibody raised against the protein you are interested in. The antibody, with its fluorescent label binds, onto the target protein in the cell, essentially colouring the target protein with the label. Direct immunofluorescence is not often used now, as it would involve making a range of differently labelled antibodies for every protein studied in laboratories. In addition, the sensitivity of the technique is low, as there is only one label for each binding site.

With indirect immunofluorescence, the primary antibody is left unlabelled. It still binds to the target protein, however it must be itself demonstrated using a labelled secondary antibody. This secondary antibody is generated in the same way as the primary antibody, however its target is antibodies from the species in which the primary antibody has been raised. For example, if the primary antibody was raised in a mouse, the labelled secondary antibody would be raised in another species against mouse antibodies (e.g. goat anti-mouse). This allows laboratories to have a wide selection of primary antibodies directed against any protein they might be working on, and then a smaller selection of labelled secondary antibodies directed against the species the primary antibodies were raised in (e.g. anti-mouse, anti-rat, anti-goat, anti-chicken, etc.). In addition, because multiple labelled secondary antibodies can bind to a single primary antibody, the signal strength is higher, resulting in greater sensitivity.

If primary antibodies from different species are used, then multiple proteins can be targeted in the one cell. The only limits are the number of species available and the range of dyes used. For example, a mouse derived primary antibody against protein A could be used alongside a goat derived primary antibody against protein B, so long as the anti-mouse and anti-goat secondary antibodies had different coloured labels. Microscopy is the science of producing and observing images of objects that cannot be seen by the unaided eye. A microscope is an instrument that produces the image. The primary function of a microscope is to resolve, that is distinguish, two closely spaced objects as separate. The secondary function of a microscope is to magnify. Microscopy has developed into an exciting field with numerous applications in biology, geology, chemistry, physics, and technology.

ELECTRON MICROSCOPIC EXAMINATION OF MICRO-ORGANISMS

Depending upon the microscope used and the preparation technique, an entire intact organism, or thin slices through the interior of the sample can be examined by electron microscopy. The electron beam can pass through very thin sections of a sample (transmission electron microscopy) or bounced off of the surface of an intact sample (scanning electron microscopy). Samples must be prepared prior to insertion into the microscope because the microscope operates in a vacuum. Biological material is comprised mainly of water and so would not be preserved, making meaningful interpretation of the resulting images impossible. For transmission electron microscopy, where very thin samples are required, the sample must also be embedded in a resin that can be sliced. For scanning electron microscopy, a sample is coated with a metal (typically, gold) from which the incoming electrons will bounce. The deflected electrons are detected and converted to a visual image. This simple-sounding procedure requires much experience to execute properly.

Samples for transmission electron microscopy are processed differently. The sample can be treated, or fixed, with one or more chemicals to maintain the structure of the specimen. Chemicals such as glutaraldehyde or formaldehyde act to cross-link the various constituents. Osmium tetroxide and uranyl acetate can be added to increase the contrast under the electron beam. Depending on the embedding resin to be used, the water might then need to be removed from the chemically fixed specimen. In this case, the water is gradually replaced with ethanol or acetone and then the dehydrating fluid is gradually replaced with the resin, which has a consistency much like that of honey. The resin is then hardened, producing a block containing the sample. Other resins, such as Lowicryl, mix easily with water. In this case, the hydrated sample is exposed to gradually increasing concentrations of the resins, to replace the water with resin. The resin is then hardened.

Sections a few millionths of a meter in thickness are often examined by electron microscopy. The sections are sliced off from a prepared specimen in a device called a microtome, where the sample is passed by the sharp edge of a glass or diamond knife and the slice is floated off onto the surface of a volume of water positioned behind the knife-edge. The slice is gathered onto a special supporting grid.

Often the section is exposed to solutions of uranyl acetate and lead citrate to further increase contrast. Then, the grid can be inserted into the microscope for examination.

Samples can also be rapidly frozen instead of being chemically fixed. This cryopreservation is so rapid that the internal water does not form structurally disruptive crystals. Frozen thin sections are then obtained using a special knife in a procedure called cryosectioning. These are inserted into the microscope using a special holder that maintains the very cold temperature.

Thin sections (both chemically fixed and frozen) and whole samples can also be exposed to antibodies in order to reveal the location of the target antigen within the thin section. This technique is known as immunoelectron microscopy. Care is required during the fixation and other preparation steps to ensure that the antigenic sites are not changed so that antibody is still capable of binding to the antigen.

Frozen samples can also be cracked open by allowing the sample to strike the sharp edge of a frozen block. The crack, along the path of least chemical resistance, can reveal internal details of the specimen. This technique is called freeze-fracture. Frozen water can be removed from the fracture (freeze-etching) to allow the structural details of the specimen to appear more prominent. Samples such as viruses are often examined in the transmission electron microscope using a technique called negative staining. Here, sample is collected on the surface of a thin plastic support film. Then, a solution of stain is flowed over the surface. When the excess stain is carefully removed, stain will pool in the surface irregularities. Once in the microscope, electrons will not pass through the puddles of stain, producing a darker appearing region in the processed image of the specimen. Negative staining is also useful to reveal surface details of bacteria and appendages such as pili, flagella and spinae. A specialised form of the staining technique can also be used to visualise genetic material. Electron microscopes exist that allow specimens to be examined in their natural, water-containing state. Examination of living specimens has also been achieved. The so-called high-vacuum environmental microscope is finding an increasing application in the examination of microbiological samples such as biofilms.

MICROSCOPY AND CULTURE

To determine the cause of an infection, it may be necessary to grow body fluids and tissue samples in a laboratory. This is done in order to identify and assess bacteria and fungal infections. When using microscopy, it is possible to find and identify micro-organisms and analyse samples to diagnose diseases in tissue samples.

1. The micro-organisms that cause sickness (pathogens) are separated into several different groups, according to their type. The most important are viruses, bacteria and chlamydia (virus-like bacterium). Other groups include eggs and larvae from different parasites and protozoa (which are one-celled parasites such as an amoeba).

2. The standard way to identify bacteria is through using a culture (bacteria grown in the laboratory). In this process a non-contaminated group, which can be identified, is purified and assessed as a comparison.

3. Fungi can also be grown and purified in the same way as bacteria, but this procedure is not often used.

4. It is more difficult to analyse viruses and chlamydia, which require more advanced laboratory examinations. Some viruses and other micro-organisms are so difficult to culture that it is necessary to examine the person's blood (serum) for antibodies against the micro-organism.

5. Worms, larvae, eggs and protozoans are clearly visible under a microscope and can easily be identified by a trained microbiologist without further examination.

Bacterial Culture

All the body's exterior surfaces (hair and skin) and interior areas such as the mucous membranes in the nose and throat, intestines, stomach and sexual organs, contain many bacteria. These bacteria are harmless under normal circumstances. Many of them are even part of a healthy functioning body and keep away harmful bacteria. If a doctor thinks that a patient is infected by a bacterium, they will usually take a sample from the place they think is infected. If, for instance, it is in the intestine, a sample may be taken from the stools. If it is in the bladder or the kidneys, a urine sample will be taken, and so on. This sample—along with the patient's details—will then be sent to be cultured at a microbiology laboratory.

There are many different ways to grow a culture in the laboratory. Samples can be taken from blood or saliva, for example. It is also possible to take samples from the mouth, skin, outer ear canal, throat, wounds and other areas of the body.

How is a Culture Produced?

When the sample arrives at the laboratory, it is spread out on a special gel, e.g. agar, in a plastic bowl (culture dish), which is then covered with a lid. Extracts of live substances such as meat, bread or chocolate may be added to the gel in order to give it more nourishment. If the sample is thought to hold a particular bacterium, the gel can be mixed with specific substances that encourage the growth of this particular bacterium and suppress the growth of others.

The test is then placed in a heating cupboard at approximately 100°F (about 35°C) the temperature at which disease-causing bacteria thrive best. Often, several different bacteria will grow, but the one that causes the disease (the pathogen) will be dominant compared to the non-pathogen.

How is Microscopy of Bacteria Performed?

The bacteria are taken and spread on a small glass plate (microscope slide), which can be placed under a microscope, and then dried. After that, it is possible to stain the bacteria. Often a special kind of stain called the Gram-stain is used, which will determine whether the bacteria are Gram-positive or Gram-negative—see below. It should be noted that the following list does not include all Gram-positive and Gram-negative bacteria, and only the most frequent diseases are described.

Gram-positive bacteria

1. *Staphylococci*: These may cause pneumonia, toxic shock syndrome, wound infections and pimples.
2. *Streptococci*: These may cause blood poisoning, sore throat, and infection of the inside of the heart.
3. *Anthrax*, *Bacilli* and *Clostridium*: These may cause tetanus and gangrene.

Gram-negative bacteria

1. *Salmonella*, *Shigellosis* and *Campylobacter*: These may infect the stomach-intestine canal.
2. *Legionella*: This may cause legionnaires' disease.
3. *Meningococcus*: This may cause cerebrospinal meningitis.
4. *Gonorrhoea* bacteria: This may cause gonorrhoea.

Apart from those mentioned above, many Gram-negative bacteria cause urinary tract infections and blood poisoning in chronically ill people. There are several other ways of identifying bacteria. All bacteria from the intestines, both the natural ones and those that cause diseases, are Gram-negative and look practically the same under a microscope.

They can, however, be identified because they are capable of making different kinds of sugar ferment, and so can be distinguished from one another.

How is Fungal and Protozoan Microscopy Performed?

1. Micro-organisms that are only a little bit bigger than bacteria can be identified by using microscopy. Thrush (oral candidiasis) can be identified using a sample from the mouth or the sexual organs.
2. Protozoa that may cause amoebic dysentery (infection in the intestines), malaria or trichomonas (a sexually transmitted disease that causes a vaginal infection) can be isolated from stools, blood sample and discharge.
3. Parasites such as roundworm and hookworm can often be identified through eggs or worms in the stools.
4. Micro-organisms that are smaller than bacteria, such as chlamydia, rickettsiay and viruses can be identified through blood samples that are then analysed for antibodies against the micro-organism.

How is a Cell and Tissue (Histology) Test Performed?

Use of the microscope is very important in the study of tissue structure and cells with unusual appearances. It is, for example, possible to diagnose cancer, as cancer cells very often have an unusual shape and form irregular patterns. When the pathologist receives a biopsy (tissue sample) it is separated into small pieces that are dipped into formalin or a similar fixing chemical.

The fixed tissue is then placed in paraffin before being cut into extremely thin slices, which can be placed under a microscope. The paraffin is then removed, and the tissue is stained to make the microscopic details easier to see. Then it is ready for microscopy. If certain types of cells are expected to be present, the sample can be stained in colours that are particularly helpful in detecting them.

Unfortunately, it can sometimes take up to a week before the result of a tissue test is ready. Sometimes it takes even longer if the sample needs further staining. In an emergency, the result can be ready within half an hour, as the tissue can be frozen before it is cut into slices. This may be necessary if the patient urgently needs an operation for which the results of the test are crucial.

SAMPLING OF AIRBORNE MICRO-ORGANISMS

Sampling of airborne micro-organisms aims at their removal from air on to the surface for further microscopic examination or culturing to observe post-growth development. It is conducted for various purposes and may be qualitative or quantitative. Qualitative sampling refers of the percentage contribution of different types of micro-organisms in air spora and one can determine the specific nature of micro-organisms within some related group in qualitative analysis. Qualitative sampling refers to different type of micro-organisms in air spora and one can actually determine their concentration in sampled air by quantitative analysis. The sampling methods vary greatly depending upon individual interest.

EXAMINATION OF UNSTAINED BACTERIA

Bacteria can be best examined and studied under the microscope. It may be desirable to examine unstained bacteria to determine their biologic grouping, motility, and reaction and chemicals or specific sera. These properties may be determined in a hanging drop preparation or in a wet mount. A few species of bacteria that cannot be stained by the methods to be discussed are often examined by darkfield illumination.

Hanging Drop Preparation

To examine bacteria using the microscope in a hanging drop method, one must use an inoculating loop for transferring the material to be examined to, a cover glass to fit over and a hanging drop slide. The inoculating loop is made by a piece of fine wire about three inches in length. One end is fastened in a handle and the other end is fashioned into a loop about one inch in diameter. Platinum, Nichrome V or tungsten alloy are used for making inoculating loops because repeatedly heating these metals in a flame to sterilise them does not at the same time destroy them, and the wire loop cools quickly after being heated. A hanging drop slide on the other hand is a thick glass slide with a circular concavity or depression as its center. A cover glass or cover slip is a piece of very thin glass about 7/8 inch square.

To make the preparation, the first thing to do is to spread a small amount of petroleum jelly around the concavity of the slide. If the specimen to be examined is a culture growing on a solid medium or material such as thick pus, take up a loopful of specimen with the wire loop and mix thoroughly with a drop of sterile isotonic saline solution placed in the center of the cover glass. If bacteria growing in a liquid medium are to be examined, transfer a drop of the fluid to the cover glass by means of the wire loop. Place the hanging drop slide over the cover glass in such a way that the center of the depression lies over the drop. The petroleum jelly seals the cover glass to the slide, holds it in place, and prevents evaporation. Invert the slide now so that the drop to be examined hangs from the bottom of the cover glass but does not touch the surface of the concavity at any point.

The preparation is ready for examination under a microscope. Examine with the 4 mm high dry lens, and reduce the amount of light passing through it by partly closing the diaphragm of the substage condenser of the microscope. Examine all parts of the drop, but the best areas for microscopic study are usually near the edges where cells in a single layer are more evenly dispersed in the fluid medium. When hanging drop preparations are observed, brownian motion and flowing of organisms in currents in the microscope should not be mistaken for true motility. Care must be taken when one is viewing a hanging drop with the microscope's oil-immersion objective that the contamination from the specimen is not spread and that the microscope objective is not soiled either from the specimen or from the ring of petroleum jelly. Another thing to remember is that the inoculating loop must be sterilised immediately before and after each transfer of material containing bacteria for examination under a microscope. Since hanging drop preparations contain living bacteria, discard the slide and cover glass into a suitable container of disinfectant after the microscope examination is finished.

Wet Mount

Another method in used in the examination of unstained bacteria with the use of the microscope is the wet mount method. It is similar to the hanging drop preparation except that an ordinary microslide is used instead of the thick hanging drop slide with its central depression, and the fluid specimen spreads to fill the narrow space between cover glass and microslide. Many of the applications are the same.

Darkfield Illumination

To examine certain delicate bacteria that are invisible in the living state in the light microscope, dark-field illumination is the best method to use. Dark field illumination is ideal in the study of delicate bacteria that cannot be stained by standard methods or bacteria that are so distorted by staining as to lose their identifying characteristics. Its greatest usefulness is in the demonstration of Treponema pallidum in chancres and other syphilitic lesions, but it is of value in the examination of many other organisms as well. The suitably prepared specimen to be examined under the microscope is placed on a microslide and covered with a cover slip. Sealing the cover glass to the slide with a ring of melted paraffin prevents the cover glass from slipping and accidental infection of the fingers.

Dark-field illumination depends on the use of a substage condenser so constructed that the light rays do not pass directly through the object being examined, as is the case with an ordinary condenser, but strike it from the sides at almost a right angle to the objective of the microscope. The microscopic field becomes a dark background against which bacteria or other particles appear as bright silvery objects. A similar effect is seen when a beam of light enters a darkened room and renders visible particles of dust that cannot be seen in a better lighted room.

BRIGHT FIELD AND DARK FIELD MICROSCOPY

Bright Field Microscopy

Bright field microscopy is the simplest of all the optical microscopy illumination techniques. Sample illumination is transmitted (i.e. illuminated from below and observed from above) white light and contrast in the sample is caused by absorbance of some of the transmitted light in dense areas of the sample. Bright field microscopy is the simplest of a range of techniques used for illumination of samples in light microscopes and its simplicity makes it a popular technique. The typical appearance of a bright field microscopy image is a dark sample on a bright background, hence the name.

Light path

The light path of a bright field microscope is extremely simple, no additional components are required beyond the normal light microscope setup.

The light path therefore consists of:
1. Transillumination light source, commonly a halogen lamp in the microscope stand.
2. Condenser lens which focusses light from the light source onto the sample.
3. Objective lens which collects light from the sample and magnifies the image.
4. Oculars and/or a camera to view the sample image.

Bright field microscopy may use critical or Köhler illumination to illuminate the sample. Bright field microscopy typically has low contrast with most biological samples as few absorb light to a great extent. Stains are often required to increase contrast which prevents use on live cells in many situations. Bright field illumination is useful for samples which have an intrinsic colour, for example chloroplasts in plant cells.

Dark Field Microscopy

Dark field microscopy (dark ground microscopy) describes microscopy methods, in both light and electron microscopy, which exclude the unscattered beam from the image. As a result, the field around the specimen (i.e. where there is no specimen to scatter the beam) is generally dark.

Light microscopy applications

In optical microscopy, darkfield describes an illumination technique used to enhance the contrast in unstained samples. It works by illuminating the sample with light that will not be collected by the objective lens, and thus will not form part of the image. This produces the classic appearance of a dark, almost black, background with bright objects on it.

Advantages and disadvantages: Dark field microscopy is a very simple yet effective technique and well suited for uses involving live and unstained biological samples, such as a smear from a tissue culture or individual water-borne single-celled organisms. Considering the simplicity of the setup, the quality of images obtained from this technique is impressive.

The main limitation of dark field microscopy is the low light levels seen in the final image. This means the sample must be very strongly illuminated, which can cause damage to the sample. Dark field microscopy techniques are almost entirely free of artifacts, due to the nature of the process. However the interpretation of dark field images must be done with great care as common dark features of bright field microscopy images may be invisible, and vice versa.

While the dark field image may first appear to be a negative of the bright field image, different effects are visible in each. In bright field microscopy, features are visible where either a shadow is cast on the surface by the incident light, or a part of the surface is less reflective, possibly by the presence of pits or scratches. Raised features that are too smooth to cast shadows will not appear in bright field images, but the light that reflects off the sides of the feature will be visible in the dark field images.

FLUORESCENCE MICROSCOPE

A fluorescence microscope is an optical microscope used to study properties of organic or inorganic substances using the phenomena of fluorescence and phosphorescence instead of, or in addition to, reflection and absorption. The term 'fluorescence microscope' is colloquially synonymous with epifluorescence microscope but also refers to microscope designs such as the confocal microscope which also use fluorescence to generate the image.

All fluorescence microscopy methods share the same principle. A sample is illuminated with light of a one wavelength which causes fluorescence in the sample. The light emitted by fluorescence, which is at a different, longer, wavelength than the illumination, is then detected through a microscope objective. Two filters are normally used in this technique, an illumination (or exitation) filter which ensures the illumination is near monochromatic and at the correct wavelength, and a second emission (or detection) filter which ensures none of the exitation light source reaches the detector. Fluorescence microscopy takes is a fundamentally different to generating a light microscope image compared to transmitted or reflected white light techniques such as phase contrast and differential interference. These two contrasting optical microscopy methods give very different but complementary data.

The specimen is illuminated with light of a specific wavelength (or wavelengths) which is absorbed by the fluorophores, causing them to emit light of longer wavelengths (i.e. of a different colour than the absorbed light). The illumination light is separated from the much weaker emitted fluorescence through the use of a spectral emission filter. Typical components of a fluorescence microscope are a light source (xenon arc lamp or mercury-vapour lamp), the excitation filter, the dichroic mirror (or dichromatic beamsplitter), and the emission filter. The filters and the dichroic are chosen to match the spectral excitation and emission characteristics of the fluorophore used to label the specimen. In this manner, the distribution of a single fluorophore (colour) is imaged at a time. Multi-colour images of several types of fluorophores must be composed by combining several single-colour images.

Most fluorescence microscopes in use are epifluorescence microscopes (i.e. excitation and observation of the fluorescence are from above (*epi–*) the specimen). These microscopes have become an important part in the field of biology, opening the doors for more advanced microscope designs, such as the confocal microscope and the total internal reflection fluorescence microscope (TIRF).

Epifluorescence Microscopy

The majority of fluorescence microscopy, especially in the life sciences, is epifluorescence microscopy. The excitatory light is passed from above (or, for inverted microscopes, from below), through the objective lens and then onto the specimen instead of passing it first through the specimen. The fluorescence in the specimen gives rise to emitted light which is focused to the detector by the same objective that is used for the excitation. Since most of the excitatory light is transmitted through the specimen, only reflected excitatory light reaches the objective together with the emitted light and this method therefore gives an improved signal to noise ratio. An additional filter between the objective and the detector can filter out the remaining excitation light from fluorescent light (Fig. 2.3).

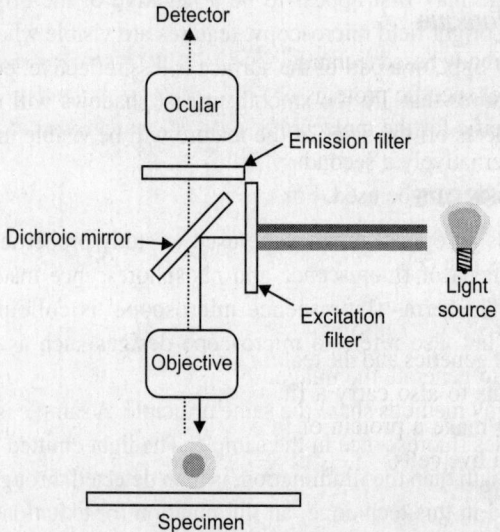

Fig. 2.3: Schematic of a fluorescence microscope.

Light Sources

Fluorescence microscopy requires intense, near-monochromatic, illumination which some widespread light sources, like halogen lamps cannot provide. There are two main types of light source used, xenon arc lamp or mercury-vapour lamps with an excitation filter and lasers. Lasers are most widely used for more complex fluorescence microscopy techniques like confocal microscopy and total internal reflection fluorescence microscopy while xenon and mercury lamps with an exitation filter are commonly used for widefield epifluorescence microscopes.

Sample Preparation

In order for a sample to be suitable for fluorescence microscopy it must be fluorescent. There are several methods of creating a fluorescent sample, the main techniques are labelling with fluorescent stains or, in the case of biological samples, expression of a fluorescent protein. Alternatively the intrinsic fluorescence of a sample (i.e. auto-fluorescence) can be used. In the life sciences fluorescence microscopy is a powerful tool which allows the specific and sensitive staining of a specimen in order to detect the distribution of proteins or other molecules of interest. As a result there is a diverse range of techniques for fluorescent staining of biological samples.

Biolocal fluorescent stains

Many fluorescent stains have been designed for a range of biological molecules. Some of these are small molecules which are intrinsically fluorescent and bind a biological molecule of interest. Major examples of these are nucleic acid stains like DAPI and Hoescht which bind the minor groove of DNA, thus labelling the nuclei of cells. Others are drugs or toxins which bind specific cellular structures and have been derivitised with a fluorescent reporter. A major example of this class of fluorescent stain is fluorescently labelled-phalloidin which is used to stain actin fibres in mammalian cells. There are many fluorescent reported molecules, called fluorophores such as fluorescein and DyLight 488, which can be chemically linked to a different molecule which binds the target of interest within the sample.

Immunofluorescence technique

Immuofluorescence is an antibody based technique which uses the highly specific binding of an antibody to its antigen in order to label specific proteins or other molecules within the cell. A sample is treated with a primary antibody specific for the molecule of interest. A fluorophore can be directly conjugated to the primary antibody. Alternatively a secondary antibody, conjugated to a fluorophore, which binds specifically to the first antibody cam be used. For example a primary antibody raised in a mouse which recognises tubulin combined with a secondary anti-mouse antibody derivatised with a fluorophore could be used to label microtubules in a cell.

Fluorescent proteins

The modern understanding of genetics and the techniques available for modifying DNA allows scientists to genetically modify proteins to also carry a fluorescent protein reporter. In biological samples this allows a scientist to directly make a protein of interest fluorescent. The protein location can then be directly tracked, including in live cells.

Limitations

Fluorophores lose their ability to fluoresce as they are illuminated in a process called photobleaching. Photobleaching occurs as the fluorescent molecules accumulate chemical damage from the electrons excited during fluorescence. Photobleaching can severely limit the time over which a sample can be observerd by fluorescent microscopy. Several techniques exist to reduce photobleaching such as the use of more robust fluorophores, by minimising illumination or by using photoprotective a scavenger chemicals. Fluorescence microscopy with fluorescent reporter proteins has enabled analysis of live cells by fluorescence microscopy, however cells are susceptible to phototoxicity, particularly with short wavelength light. Furthermore fluorescent molecules have a tendency to generate reactive chemical species when under illumination which enhances the phototoxic effect.

Unlike transmitted and reflected light microscopy techniques fluorescence microscopy only allows observation of the specific structures which have been fluorescently labelled. For example observing a tissue sample prepared with a fluorescent DNA stain by fluorescent microscopy only reveals the organisation of the DNA within the cells and reveals nothing else about the cell morphologies.

DIRECT FLUORESCENT ANTIBODY

Direct fluorescent antibody (DFA or dFA) (also known as 'direct immunofluorescence') is a laboratory test that uses antibodies tagged with fluorescent dye that can be used to detect the presence of micro-organisms. This method offers straightforward detection of antigens using fluorescently labelled antigen-specific antibodies. Because detection of the antigen in a substrate of patient sample (cellular smear, fluid or patient-inoculated culture medium) is the goal, DFA is seldom quantitative. This is the main test used to detect rabies in animals and requires the examination of brain tissue.

IMMUNOFLUORESCENCE

Immunofluorescence is a technique used for light microscopy with a fluorescence microscope and is used primarily on biological samples. This technique uses the specificity of antibodies to their antigen to target fluorescent dyes to specific biomolecule targets within a cell, and therefore allows visualisation of the distribution of the target molecule through the sample. Immunofluorescence is a widely used example of immunostaining and is a specific example of immunohistochemistry that makes use of fluorophores to visualise the location of the antibodies. Immunofluorescence can be used on tissue sections, cultured cell lines or individual cells, and may be used to analyse the distribution of proteins, glycans, and small biological and non-biological molecules. Immunofluoresence can be used in combination with other, non-antibody methods of fluorescent staining, for example, use of 4′,6-diamidino-2-phenylindole (DAPI) to label DNA. Several microscope designs can be used for analysis of immuno-fluorescence samples, the simplest is the epifluorescence microscope, and the confocal microscope is also widely used. Various super-resolution microscope designs that are capable of much higher resolution can also be used.

TRANSMISSION ELECTRON MICROSCOPE

The transmission electron microscope (TEM) operates on the same basic principles as the light microscope but uses electrons instead of light. What you can see with a light microscope is limited by the wavelength of light. TEMs use electrons as 'light source' and their much lower wavelength makes it possible to get a resolution a thousand times better than with a light microscope.

You can see objects to the order of a few angstrom (10^{-10} m). For example, you can study small details in the cell or different materials down to near atomic levels. The possibility for high magnifications has made the TEM a valuable tool in both medical, biological and materials research.

Magnetic Lenses Guide the Electrons

A 'light source' at the top of the microscope emits the electrons that travel through vacuum in the column of the microscope. Instead of glass lenses focusing the light in the light microscope, the TEM uses electromagnetic lenses to focus the electrons into a very thin beam. The electron beam then travels through the specimen you want to study. Depending on the density of the material present, some of the electrons are scattered and disappear from the beam. At the bottom of the microscope the unscattered electrons hit a fluorescent screen, which gives rise to a 'shadow image' of the specimen with its different parts displayed in varied darkness according to their density. The image can be studied directly by the operator or photographed with a camera. TEMs are capable of imaging at a significantly higher resolution than light microscopes, owing to the small de Broglie wavelength of electrons. This enables the instruments user to examine fine detail—even as small as a single column of atoms, which is tens of thousands times smaller than the smallest resolvable object in a light microscope. TEM forms a major analysis method in a range of scientific fields, in both physical and biological sciences. TEMs find application in cancer research, virology, materials science as well as pollution and semiconductor research.

At smaller magnifications TEM image contrast is due to absorption of electrons in the material, due to the thickness and composition of the material. At higher magnifications complex wave interactions modulate the intensity of the image, requiring expert analysis of observed images. Alternate modes of use allow for the TEM to observe modulations in chemical identity, crystal orientation, electronic structure and sample induced electron phase shift as well as the regular absorption based imaging.

SCANNING ELECTRON MICROSCOPY

The scanning electron microscope (SEM) uses a focused beam of high-energy electrons to generate a variety of signals at the surface of solid specimens. The signals that derive from electron-sample interactions reveal information about the sample including external morphology (texture), chemical composition, and crystalline structure and orientation of materials making up the sample. In most applications, data are collected over a selected area of the surface of the sample, and a 2-dimensional image is generated that displays spatial variations in these properties.

Areas ranging from approximately 1 cm to 5 microns in width can be imaged in a scanning mode using conventional SEM techniques (magnification ranging from 20X to approximately 30,000X, spatial resolution of 50 to 100 nm). The SEM is also capable of performing analyses of selected point locations on the sample, this approach is especially useful in qualitatively or semi-quantitatively determining chemical compositions (using EDS), crystalline structure, and crystal orientations (using EBSD). The design and function of the SEM is very similar to the EPMA and considerable overlap in capabilities exists between the two instruments.

Fundamental Principles of Scanning Electron Microscopy

Accelerated electrons in an SEM carry significant amounts of kinetic energy, and this energy is dissipated as a variety of signals produced by electron-sample interactions when the incident electrons are decelerated in the solid sample. These signals include secondary electrons (that produce SEM images), backscattered electrons (BSE), diffracted backscattered electrons (EBSD that are used to determine crystal structures and orientations of minerals), photons (characteristic X-rays that are used for elemental analysis and continuum X-rays), visible light (cathodoluminescence—CL), and heat. Secondary electrons and backscattered electrons are commonly used for imaging samples: secondary electrons are most valuable for showing morphology and topography on samples and backscattered electrons are most valuable for illustrating contrasts in composition in multiphase samples (i.e. for rapid phase discrimination).

X-ray generation is produced by inelastic collisions of the incident electrons with electrons in discrete ortitals (shells) of atoms in the sample. As the excited electrons return to lower energy states, they yield X-rays that are of a fixed wavelength (that is related to the difference in energy levels of electrons in different shells for a given element). Thus, characteristic X-rays are produced for each element in a mineral that is 'excited' by the electron beam. SEM analysis is considered to be 'non-destructive', that is, X-rays generated by electron interactions do not lead to volume loss of the sample, so it is possible to analyse the same materials repeatedly.

Scanning Electron Microscopy Instrumentation—How Does It Work?

Essential components of all SEMs include the following:

1. Electron source (Gun).
2. Electron lenses.
3. Sample stage.
4. Detectors for all signals of interest.

5. Display/Data output devices.
6. Infrastructure requirements:
    (a) Power supply.
    (b) Vacuum system.
    (c) Cooling system.
    (d) Vibration-free floor.
    (e) Room free of ambient magnetic and electric fields.

Schematic drawing of the electron and X-ray optics of a combined SEM–EPMA are shown in Fig. 2.4. SEMs always have at least one detector (usually a secondary electron detector), and most have additional detectors. The specific capabilities of a particular instrument are critically dependent on which detectors it accommodates.

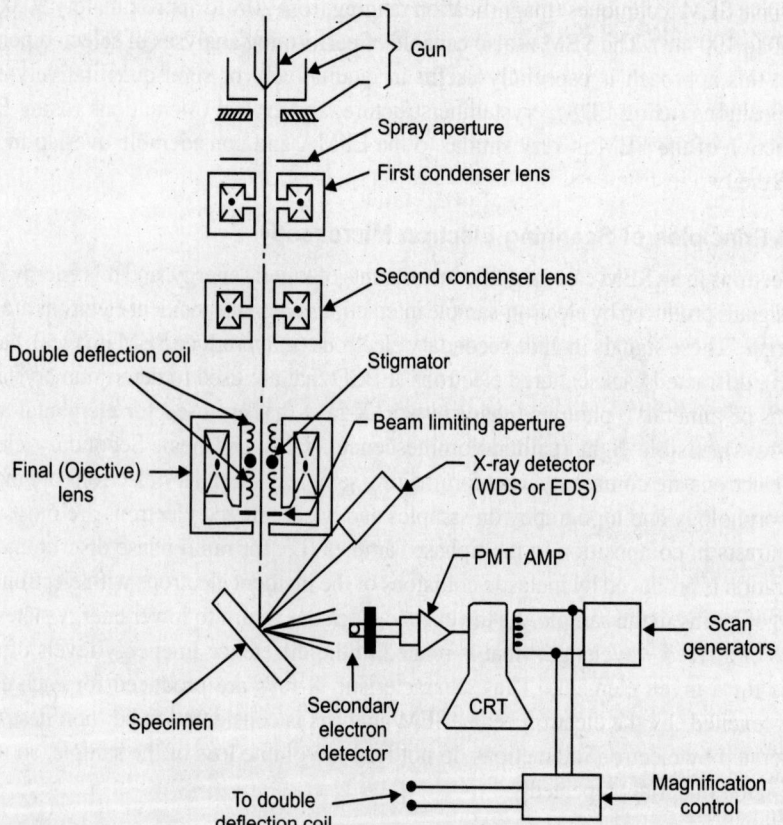

Fig. 2.4: Schematic drawing of the electron and X-ray optics of a combined SEM–EPMA.

Strengths and Limitations of Scanning Electron Microscopy (SEM)

Strengths

There is arguably no other instrument with the breadth of applications in the study of solid materials that compares with the SEM. The SEM is critical in all fields that require characterisation of solid materials. While this contribution is most concerned with geological applications, it is important to note that these applications are a very small subset of the scientific and industrial applications that exist for this instrumentation. Most SEM's are comparatively easy to operate, with user-friendly 'intuitive' interfaces. Many applications require minimal sample preparation. For many applications, data acquisition is rapid (less than 5 minutes/image for SEI, BSE, spot EDS analyses). Modern SEMs generate data in digital formats, which are highly portable.

Limitations

Samples must be solid and they must fit into the microscope chamber. Maximum size in horizontal dimensions is usually on the order of 10 cm, vertical dimensions are generally much more limited and rarely exceed 40 mm. For most instruments samples must be stable in a vacuum on the order of 10^{-5}–10^{-6} torr. Samples likely to outgas at low pressures (rocks saturated with hydrocarbons, 'wet' samples such as coal, organic materials or swelling clays, and samples likely to decrepitate at low pressure) are unsuitable for examination in conventional SEM's. However, 'low vacuum' and 'environmental' SEMs also exist, and many of these types of samples can be successfully examined in these specialised instruments. EDS detectors on SEM's cannot detect very light elements (H, He, and Li), and many instruments cannot detect elements with atomic numbers less than 11 (Na). Most SEMs use a solid state X-ray detector (EDS), and while these detectors are very fast and easy to utilise, they have relatively poor energy resolution and sensitivity to elements present in low abundances when compared to wavelength dispersive X-ray detectors (WDS) on most electron probe microanalysers (EPMA). An electrically conductive coating must be applied to electrically insulating samples for study in conventional SEM's, unless the instrument is capable of operation in a low vacuum mode.

PREPARATION FOR LIGHT-MICROSCOPE EXAMINATION

Two general techniques are used to prepare specimens for light-microscope examination. One is to suspend organisms in a liquid (the wet-mount or the hanging-drop techniques), and the other is to dry, fix, and stain films or smears of the specimen.

Wet Mount and Hanging Drop

The hanging drop and wet mount techniques allow for observation of living organisms. The wet mount tend to dry out quickly under the heat of the microscope light, it is simpler to perform than the wet mount, but it is useful for short-term observation only. The hanging drop is a more complex technique, but it allows for longer-term observation and more reliable observation of motility. These techniques are usually performed without the addition of any stains, therefore, the organisms can be difficult to see. Reduce the illumination on your microscope as much as you can while still allowing yourself enough light to observe the organism. If you use these techniques to observe motility, be sure you can tell the difference between motility and brownian motion. Vibration of the cell is caused by the cell colliding with water molecules. True motility allows the cell to move in different directions and across larger areas.

Examination of micro-organisms in wet preparation is desirable in the following instances:

1. The morphology of spiral bacteria is greatly distorted when these bacteria are dried and stained, they should be examined in living condition. For example, in the examination of serous exudates suspected of containing the spirochete that causes syphilis, the wet preparations are examined by dark-field microscopy. This provides a sharp contrast between the organisms and the dark background. The normal arrangement of cells can also be better determined in a wet preparation.

2. The observation of bacteria to determine whether or not they are motile obviously requires that they be suspended in a liquid medium, free to move about.

3. To observe cytological changes occurring during cell division and to determine the rate at which the division occurs, the organisms must be examined in the living state (i.e. wet mount). Spore formation and germination must also be observed in living cells.

4. Some cell inclusion bodies, e.g. vacuoles and lipid material, can be observed readily by this method.

When wet preparations are examined by bright-field microscopy, it is extremely important to control the light source. The reason is that the lack of a stain makes the cells less distinctly visible, adjustment of the intensity of the light source can enhance their visibility. Partially closing the substage condenser diaphragm helps to increase contrast, however, some resolving power is lost. Dark-field and phase-contrast microscopy offer the distinct advantage of providing both high contrast and high resolving power for examination of unstained preparations.

Staining

Staining is an auxiliary technique used in microscopy to enhance contrast in the microscopic image. Stains and dyes are frequently used in biology and medicine to highlight structures in biological tissues for viewing, often with the aid of different microscopes. Stains may be used to define and examine bulk tissues (highlighting, for example, muscle fibres or connective tissue), cell populations (classifying different blood cells, for instance), or organelles within individual cells.

In biochemistry it involves adding a class-specific (DNA, proteins, lipids, carbohydrates) dye to a substrate to qualify or quantify the presence of a specific compound. Staining and fluorescent tagging can serve similar purposes. Biological staining is also used to mark cells in flow cytometry, and to flag proteins or nucleic acids in gel electrophoresis. Staining is not limited to biological materials, it can also be used to study the morphology of other materials for example the lamellar structures of semi-crystalline polymers or the domain structures of block copolymers.

In vivo vs in vitro staining

In vivo staining is the process of dyeing living tissues—in vivo means 'in life' (compare with in vitro staining). By causing certain cells or structures to take on contrasting colour(s), their form (morphology) or position within a cell or tissue can be readily seen and studied. The usual purpose is to reveal cytological details that might otherwise not be apparent, however, staining can also reveal where certain chemicals or specific chemical reactions are taking place within cells or tissues.

In vitro staining involves colouring cells or structures that are no longer living. Certain stains are often combined to reveal more details and features than a single stain alone. Combined with specific protocols for fixation and sample preparation, scientists and physicians can use these standard techniques as consistent, repeatable diagnostic tools. A counterstain is stain that makes cells or structures more visible, when not completely visible with the principal stain.

For example, crystal violet stains only Gram-positive bacteria in Gram-staining. A safranin counterstain is applied which stains all cells, allowing the identification of Gram-negative bacteria as well. Often these stains are called vital stains. They are introduced to the organism while the cells are still living. However, these stains are eventually toxic to the organism, some more so than others. To achieve desired effects, the stains are used in very dilute solutions ranging from 1:5000 to 1:5,00,000. Note that many stains may be used in both living and fixed cells.

In vitro methods

Preparation: The preparatory steps involved depend on the type of analysis planned, some or all of the following procedures may be required.

1. Fixation: Which may itself consist of several steps—aims to preserve the shape of the cells or tissue involved as much as possible. Sometimes heat fixation is used to kill, adhere, and alter the specimen so it will accept stains. Most chemical fixatives (chemicals causing fixation) generate chemical bonds between proteins and other substances within the sample, increasing their rigidity. Common fixatives include formaldehyde, ethanol, methanol, and/or picric acid. Pieces of tissue may be embedded in paraffin wax to increase their mechanical strength and stability and to make them easier to cut into thin slices.

2. Permeabilisation: Permeabilisation involves treatment of cells with (usually) a mild surfactant. This treatment will dissolve the cell membranes, and allow larger dye molecules access to the cell's interior.

3. Mounting: Mounting usually involves attaching the samples to a glass microscope slide for observation and analysis. In some cases, cells may be grown directly on a slide. For samples of loose cells (as with a blood smear or a pap smear) the sample can be directly applied to a slide. For larger pieces of tissue, thin sections (slices) are made using a microtome, these slices can then be mounted and inspected.

Staining proper: At its simplest, the actual staining process may involve immersing the sample (before or after fixation and mounting) in dye solution, followed by rinsing and observation. Many dyes, however, require the use of a mordant: a chemical compound which reacts with the stain to form an insoluble, coloured precipitate. When excess dye solution is washed away, the mordanted stain remains. Most of the dyes commonly used in microscopy are available as certified stains. This means that samples of the manufacturer's batch have been tested by an independent body, the Biological Stain Commission and found to be meet or exceed certain standards of purity, dye content and performance in staining techniques. These standards are published in detail in the journal Biotechnic and Histochemistry. Many dyes are inconsistent in composition from one supplier to another. The use of certified stains eliminates a source of unexpected results.

Negative staining: A simple staining method for bacteria which is usually successful even when the 'positive staining' methods detailed below fail, is to employ a negative stain. This can be achieved simply by smearing the sample on to the slide, followed by an application of nigrosin (a black synthetic dye) or Indian ink (an aqueous suspension of carbon particles). After drying, the micro-organisms may be viewed in bright field microscopy as lighter inclusions well-contrasted against the dark environment surrounding them. Note: negative staining is a mild technique which may not destroy the micro-organisms therefore it is unsuitable for studying pathogens.

Specific techniques

Gram-staining: Gram-staining is used to determine Gram-status to classify bacteria broadly. It is based on the composition of their cell wall. Gram-staining uses crystal violet to stain cell walls, iodine as a mordant, and a fuchsin or safranin counterstain to mark all bacteria. Gram-status is important in medicine, the presence or absence of a cell wall will change the bacterium's susceptibility to some antibiotics.

Gram-positive bacteria stain dark blue or violet. Their cell wall is typically rich with peptidoglycan and lacks the secondary membrane and lipopolysaccharide layer found in Gram-negative bacteria.

On most Gram-stained preparations, Gram-negative organisms will appear red or pink because they are counterstained. Due to presence of higher lipid content, after alcohol-treatment, the porosity of the cell wall increases, hence the CVI complex (crystal violet-iodine) can pass through. Thus, the primary stain is not retained. Also, in contrast to most Gram-positive bacteria, Gram-negative bacteria have only a few layers of peptidoglycan and a secondary cell membrane made primarily of lipopolysaccharide.

Ziehl-Neelsen stain: Ziehl-Neelsen staining is used to stain species of Myco-bacterium tuberculosis that do not stain with the standard laboratory staining procedures like Gram-staining. The stains used are the red coloured Carbol fuchsin that stains the bacteria and a counter stain like Methylene blue or Malachite green.

Haematoxylin and eosin (H&E) staining: Microscopic view of a histologic specimen of human lung tissue stained with hematoxylin and eosin. Haematoxylin and eosin staining protocol is used frequently in histology to examine thin sections of tissue. Haematoxylin stains cell nuclei blue, while eosin stains cytoplasm, connective tissue and other extracellular substances pink or red. Eosin is strongly absorbed by red blood cells, colouring them bright red. In a skilfully made H & E preparation the red blood cells are almost orange, and collagen and cytoplasm (especially muscle) acquire different shades of pink. When the staining is done by a machine, the subtle differences in eosinophilia are often lost.

Papanicolaou staining: Papanicolaou staining or Pap staining, is a frequently used method for examining cell samples from various bodily secretions. It is frequently used to stain Pap smear specimens. It uses a combination of haematoxylin, Orange G, eosin Y, Light Green SF yellowish, and sometimes Bismarck Brown Y.

PAS staining: Periodic acid-Schiff staining is used to mark carbohydrates (glycogen, glycoprotein, proteoglycans). It is used to distinguish different types of glycogen storage diseases.

Masson's trichrome: Masson's trichrome is (as the name implies) a three-colour staining protocol. The recipe has evolved from Masson's original technique for different specific applications, but all are well-suited to distinguish cells from surrounding connective tissue. Most recipes will produce red keratin and muscle fibres, blue or green staining of collagen and bone, light red or pink staining of cytoplasm, and black cell nuclei.

Romanowsky stains: The Romanowsky stains are all based on a combination of eosinate (chemically reduced eosin) and methylene blue (sometimes with its oxidation products azure A and azure B). Common variants include Wright's stain, Jenner's stain, Leishman stain and Giemsa stain. All are used to examine blood or bone marrow samples. They are preferred over H&E for inspection of blood cells because different types of leukocytes (white blood cells) can be readily distinguished. All are also suited to examination of blood to detect blood-borne parasites like malaria.

Silver staining: Silver staining is the use of silver to stain histologic sections. This kind of staining is important especially to show proteins (for example type III collagen) and DNA. It is used to show both substances inside and outside cells. Silver staining is also used in temperature gradient gel electrophoresis.

Differential staining

Differential staining is a general term that can refer to a number of specific processes. Generally, it is used to describe staining processes which use more than one chemical stain. Using multiple stains can better differentiate between different micro-organisms or structures/cellular components of a single organism. Differential staining also describes medical process used to detect abnormalities in the proportion of different white blood cells in the blood. The process or results are called a WBC differential. This test is useful because many diseases alter the proportion of certain white blood cells. By analysing these differences in combination with a clinical exam and other lab tests, medical professionals can diagnose disease. One commonly recognisable use of differential staining is the Gram-stain. Gram-staining uses two dyes: Crystal violet and Fuchsin (the counterstain) to differentiate between Gram-positive bacteria (large Peptidoglycan layer on outer surface of cell) and Gram-negative bacteria.

Common biological stains

Different stains react or concentrate in different parts of a cell or tissue, and these properties are used to advantage to reveal specific parts or areas. Some of the most common biological stains are listed below. Unless otherwise marked, all of these dyes may be used with fixed cells and tissues, vital dyes (suitable for use with living organisms) are noted.

Acridine orange: Acridine orange (AO) is a nucleic acid selective fluorescent cationic dye useful for cell cycle determination. It is cell-permeable, and interacts with DNA and RNA by intercalation or electrostatic attractions. When bound to DNA, it is very similar spectrally to fluorescein. Like fluorescein, it is also useful as a nonspecific stain for backlighting conventionally stained cells on the surface of a solid sample of tissue (fluorescence backlighted staining).

Bismarck brown: Bismarck brown (also Bismarck brown Y or Manchester brown) imparts a yellow colour to acid mucins. Bismarck brown may be used with live cells.

Carmine: Carmine is an intensely red dye which may be used to stain glycogen, while Carmine alum is a nuclear stain. Carmine stains require the use of a mordant, usually aluminium.

Coomassie blue: Coomassie blue (also brilliant blue) nonspecifically stains proteins a strong blue colour. It is often used in gel electrophoresis.

Crystal violet: Crystal violet, when combined with a suitable mordant, stains cell walls purple. Crystal violet is an important component in Gram-staining.

DAPI: DAPI is a fluorescent nuclear stain, excited by ultraviolet light and showing strong blue fluorescence when bound to DNA. DAPI binds with A=T rich repeats of chromosomes. DAPI is also not visible with regular transmission microscopy. It may be used in living or fixed cells. DAPI-stained cells are especially appropriate for cell counting.

Eosin: Eosin is most often used as a counterstain to haematoxylin, imparting a pink or red colour to cytoplasmic material, cell membranes, and some extracellular structures. It also imparts a strong red colour to red blood cells. Eosin may also be used as a counterstain in some variants of Gram-staining, and in many other protocols. There are actually two very closely related compounds commonly referred to as eosin. Most often used is eosin Y (also known as eosin Y ws or eosin yellowish), it has a very slightly yellowish cast. The other eosin compound is eosin B (eosin bluish or imperial red), it has a very faint bluish cast. The two dyes are interchangeable, and the use of one or the other is more a matter of preference and tradition.

Thin Layer Chromatography

In thin layer chromatography or TLC the stationary phase consists of a thin layer of adsorbent like silica gel, alumina or cellulose on a flat carrier like a glass plate, a thick aluminum foil, or a plastic sheet. The process is similar to paper chromatography with the advantage of faster runs, better separations, and the choice between different adsorbents.

Column Chromatography

Column chromatography utilises a vertical glass column filled with some form of solid support with the sample to be separated placed on top of this support. The rest of the column is filled with a solvent which moves the sample through the column under the influence of gravity. Like other forms of chromatography, differences in rates of movement through the solid medium are translated to different exit times from the bottom of the column for the various elements of the original sample.

Gas-liquid Chromatography

Gas-liquid chromatography is based on a partition equilibrium of analyte between a liquid stationary phase and a mobile gas. It is useful for a wide range of non-polar analytes, but poor for thermally labile molecules.

Ion Exchange Chromatography

Ion exchange chromatography is a column chromatography that uses a charged stationary phase. It is used to separate charged compounds.

CELL FRACTIONTION

The eukaryotic cell contains many organelles, each of which performs one or more specialised functions, they are suspended within the cytoplasm and bounded by the plasma membrane. Each organelle has specific characteristics like size, shape and density which make it different from other organelles within the same cell. Because of these different features, individual types of organelles can be isolated from cells and studied. The technique of cell fractionation is employed in order to break up tissues and cells and isolate various organelles. The process of breaking the cells is called homogenisation and the subsequent isolation of organelles is called fractionation. Isolation of organelles requires the use of physical chemistry techniques, and these techniques can range from the use of simple sieves, gravity sedimentation or differential precipitation, to ultracentrifugation of fluorescent labeled organelles in computer generated density gradients.

One technique for isolating organelles is to homogenise cells in a blender. Homogenisation ruptures the cells freeing many of the organelles. To preserve the viability of the organelles, cells are homogenised in a phosphate buffered sucrose solution. Under carefully controlled conditions, organelles can continue to perform their functions outside of the cell for some time. In order to study specific organelles, homogenisation is followed by some procedure that can isolate one type of organelle from the others. This technique is differential centrifugation, a process by which homogenised cells are centrifuged at increasingly higher speeds and for increasingly longer periods of time. Centrifugation tends to isolate the cellular components in order of and may form interactions with it. Any substance that will react with (and thus bond to) the paper cannot be measured using this technique. The paper is then dipped into a suitable solvent (such as ethanol or water) and placed in a sealed container. As the solvent rises through the paper it meets the sample mixture which starts to travel up the paper with the solvent. Different compounds in the sample mixture travel different distances according to how strongly they interact with the paper. Paper chromatography takes some time and the experiment is usually left to complete for some hours.

The final chromatogram can be compared with other known mixture chromatograms to identify sample mixes. Two-way paper chromatography involves using two solvents and rotating the paper 90° in between. This is useful for separating complex mixtures of similar compounds.

Chapter 3

HeLa Cells

INTRODUCTION

When researchers want to obtain sufficient quantities of organisms to use in their studies, they may grow them up in a vat of broth containing all of the nutrients they need to survive. This is called culturing the organisms, and for many simple, free-living organisms such as bacteria or fungi, the process is relatively straightforward. These organisms often require very little in the way of specialised nutrients and so long as the culture conditions are suitable, they will undergo almost constant division, increasing their populations at an exponential rate.

If cells from a multi-cellular organism like a human are to be used in research, the culture methods are not nearly so simple. Firstly, cells from multi-cellular organisms have differentiated to such an extent that they can no longer survive without the complex systems of nutrients and stimuli provided by the other cells in the body. As a result, growing human cells in culture requires the use of growth media containing a complex mixture of basic nutrients and specific growth factors provided by the inclusion of serum (the liquid component of clotted blood). In addition, body cells spend most of their time carrying out the functions which allow them to play their roles within the body. This means that they are not constantly dividing - in many cases they must be stimulated to enter mitosis, and in some cases do not divide at all. As a result, human cells in culture often proliferate very slowly.

One solution to this problem is the use of cancer cells. One of the hallmarks of cancer is the loss of regulation of the cell cycle, leading to cells constantly passing through division cycles. This results in hyperproliferation of the cells, which in the body leads to the growth of tissue masses known as tumours. Cancer cell hyperproliferation means that they can be grown in culture for many generations, with further cultures able to be sub-cultured from the original – they are effectively immortal. This has led to the production of cancer cell lines, each of which was derived from a tumour recovered from an individual with cancer.

Most types of cancer have numerous cell lines which researchers can use to study the cancer in question. Each of these cell lines have particular characteristics dependent on the cancer from which they were derived, allowing researchers to select the line which most closely matches the situation they are working on. Unfortunately, being cancer cells, the cells contain errors and abnormalities which mean that they do not often behave as normal cells do, making them inappropriate models for normal cells, or even for cancers of other parts of the body. In addition, the same errors which remove the cell cycle controls in cancer cells may also remove mechanisms which regulate damage to the DNA, allowing mutations to accumulate in the cells which make them even more distinct from the cells from which they were derived

HELA CELLS

HeLa cells (Fig. 3.1) are possibly the best known of all cancer cell lines. They were originally recovered from a cervical cancer removed from a patient named *H*enrietta *La*cks in 1951. The cancer resulted from an infection by a strain of human papillomavirus (HPV18), and so the genome of these cells also contains the genome for this strain of HPV. HeLa was the first cell line to be successfully and continuously cultured *in vitro* and have been used widely around the world since the physician who first subcultured them made them and the techniques used to grow them freely available to scientists around the world. HeLa cells have played an important role in many important medical discoveries, including the development of the Polio vaccine.

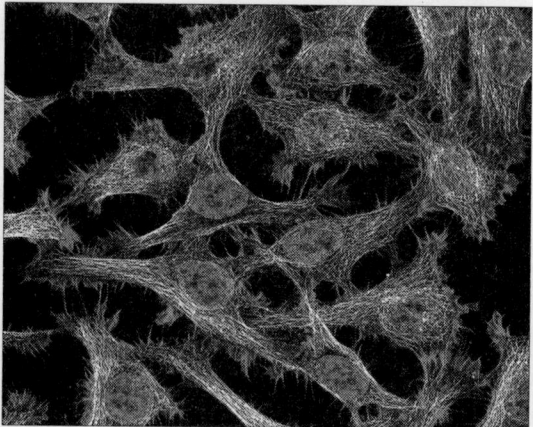

Fig. 3.1: HeLa cells.

Cell line: The cell line was derived from cervical cancer cells taken from Henrietta Lacks, who died from her cancer in 1951. The cells were propagated without Lacks' knowledge or permission by George Otto Gey. Initially, the cell line was said to be named after a 'Helen Lane' or 'Helen Larson', in order to preserve Lacks' anonymity. These cells are treated as cancer cells, as they are believed to have stemmed from Ms. Lacks' cervical cancer, but a debate still continues on the classification of the cells.

HeLa are considered 'immortal': they do not die of old age and can divide an unlimited number of times as long as basic cell survival conditions are met (i.e. being maintained and sustained in a suitable environment). There are many strains of HeLa cells as they continue to evolve by being grown in cell cultures, but all HeLa cells are derived from the same tumour cells removed from Lacks. It has been estimated that the total mass of HeLa cells today far exceeds that of the rest of Henrietta Lacks body.

Scientists would spend more time trying to keep the cells alive than performing actual research on them. Cells from Lacks's tumour behaved differently. As was custom for Gey's lab assistant, she labelled the culture 'HeLa', the first two letters of the patient's first and last name; this became the name of the cell line. These were the first human cells grown in a lab that were naturally 'immortal', meaning that they do not die after a set number of cell divisions (i.e. cellular senescence). These cells could be used for conducting a multitude of medical experiments—if the cells died, they could simply be discarded and the experiment attempted again on fresh cells from the culture. This represented an enormous boon to medical and biological research, as previously stocks of living cells were limited and took significant effort to culture.

The stable growth of HeLa enabled a researcher at the University of Minnesota hospital to successfully grow polio virus, enabling the development of a vaccine, and by 1952, Jonas Salk developed a vaccine for polio using these cells. To test Salk's new vaccine, the cells were put into mass production in the first-ever cell production factory.

In 1953, HeLa cells were the first human cells successfully cloned and demand for the HeLa cells quickly grew in the nascent biomedical industry. Since the cells first mass replications, they have been used by scientists in various types of investigations including disease research, gene mapping, effects of toxic substances on organisms, and radiation on humans. Additionally, HeLa cells have been used to test human sensitivity to tape, glue, cosmetics, and many other products.

Scientists have grown an estimated 50 million metric tons of HeLa cells, and there are almost 11,000 patents involving these cells. The HeLa cell lines are also notorious for invading other cell cultures in laboratory settings. Some have estimated that HeLa cells have contaminated 10–20% of all cell lines currently in use.

History HeLa Cells

The cells were propagated by George Otto Gey shortly before Lacks died of her cancer in 1951. This was the first human cell line to prove successful *in vitro*, which was a scientific achievement with profound future benefit to medical research. Gey freely donated these cells along with the tools and processes that his lab developed to any scientist requesting them simply for the benefit of science. Neither Lacks nor her family gave permission to harvest the cells but, at that time, permission was neither required nor customarily sought. The cells were later commercialised, although never patented in their original form. There was no requirement at that time (or at present) to inform patients or their relatives about such matters because discarded material or material obtained during surgery, diagnosis, or therapy was the property of the physician or the medical institution. This issue and Lacks situation were brought up in the Supreme Court of California case of Moore v. Regents of the University of California. The court ruled that a person's discarded tissue and cells are not his or her property and can be commercialised.

HeLa cells, like other cell lines, are termed 'immortal' in that they can divide an unlimited number of times in a laboratory cell culture plate as long as fundamental cell survival conditions are met (i.e. being maintained and sustained in a suitable environment). There are many strains of HeLa cells as they continue to mutate in cell cultures, but all HeLa cells are descended from the same tumour cells removed from Lacks. The total number of HeLa cells that have been propagated in cell culture far exceeds the total number of cells that were in Henrietta Lacks body.

Uses of HeLa Cells

- Develop virology—field of biology study of viruses
- Develop methods of freezing cells for storage
- Develop standardised methods for culturing cells

- Develop the first vaccine for polio.
- Develop methods for accurately determining the number of chromosomes in cells—beneficial for cancer research.
- Used to study effects of radiation.
- Used to study effects of deep sea pressure.
- Used to test safety of cosmetics and pharmaceuticals—replacing lab animals.
- Used in research on HIV (human immunodeficiency virus), the most common sexually transmitted disease—to help with developing treatments for AIDS (acquired immunodeficiency syndrome).
- Used in research on what causes ageing.
- Used in studying the effects of *salmonella* and *tuberculosis*.
- Used to determined that HPV (human papilloma virus Fig. 3.2) causes cancer.
- Used to help develop treatments for Parkinson's disease, influenza, leukemia, and hemophilia.

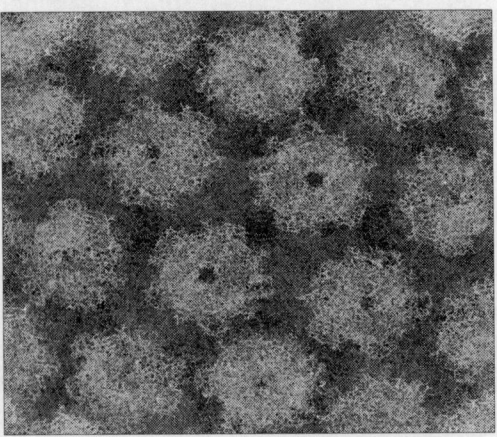

Fig. 3.2: Human papilloma virus.

Uses in research

HeLa cells were used by Jonas Salk to test the first polio vaccine in the 1950s. They were observed to be easily infected by poliomyelitis, causing infected cells to die. This made HeLa cells highly desirable for polio vaccine testing since results could be easily obtained. A large volume of HeLa cells were needed for the testing of Salk's polio vaccine, prompting the National Foundation for Infantile Paralysis (NFIP) to find a facility capable of mass-producing HeLa cells. In the spring of 1953, a cell culture factory was established at Tuskegee University to supply Salk and other labs with HeLa cells. Less than a year later, Salk's vaccine was ready for human trials.

HeLa cells were also the first human cells to be successfully cloned in 1953 by Theodore Puck and Philip I Marcus at the University of Colorado, Denver. Since that time, HeLa cells have 'continually been used for research into cancer, AIDS, the effects of radiation and toxic substances, gene mapping, and countless other scientific pursuits.' According to author Rebecca Skloot, by 2009, 'more than 60,000 scientific articles had been published about research done on HeLa, and that number was increasing steadily at a rate of more than 300 papers each month.'

HeLa cells have been used in testing how parvo virus infects cells of humans, dogs, and cats. These cells have also been used to study viruses such as the oropouche virus (OROV). OROV causes the disruption of cells in culture, where cells begin to degenerate shortly after they are infected, causing viral induction of apoptosis. HeLa cells have been used to study the expression of the papillomavirus E2 and apoptosis. HeLa cells have also been used to study canine distemper virus ability to induce apoptosis in cancer cell lines, which could play an important role in developing treatments for tumour cells resistant to radiation and chemotherapy.

HeLa cells have also been used in a number of cancer studies, including those involving sex steroid hormones such as estradiol, estrogen, and estrogen receptors, along with estrogen-like compounds such as quercetin and its cancer reducing properties. There have also been studies on HeLa cells, the effects of flavonoids and antioxidants with estradiol on cancer cell proliferation.

HeLa cells were used to investigate the phytochemical compounds and the fundamental mechanism of the anticancer activity of the ethanolic extract of mango peel (EEMP). EEMP was found to contain various phenolic compounds and to activate death of human cervical malignant HeLa cells through apoptosis, which suggests that EEMP may help to prevent cervical cancer as well as other types of cancers.

In 2011, HeLa cells were used in tests of novel heptamethine dyes IR-808 and other analogs which are currently being explored for their unique uses in medical diagnostics, the development of theranostics, the individualised treatment of cancer patients with the aid of PDT, co-administration with other drugs, and irradiation. HeLa cells have been used in research involving fullerenes to induce apoptosis as a part of photodynamic therapy, as well as in *in vitro* cancer research using cell lines. Further HeLa cells have also been used to define cancer markers in RNA, and have been used to establish an RNAi Based Identification System and Interference of Specific Cancer Cells. HeLa was shown in 2014 to be viable cell line for tumour xenografts in C57BL/6 nude mice, and was subsequently used to examine the *in vivo* effects of Fluoxetine and cisplatin on cervical cancer.

Analysis of HeLa Cells

Telomerase

The HeLa cell line was derived for use in cancer research. These cells proliferate abnormally rapidly, even compared to other cancer cells. Like many other cancer cells, HeLa cells have an active version of telomerase during cell division, which prevents the incremental shortening of telomeres that is implicated in ageing and eventual cell death. In this way, the cells circumvent the Hayflick limit, which is the limited number of cell divisions that most normal cells can undergo before becoming senescent.

Chromosome number

Horizontal gene transfer from human papillomavirus 18 (HPV18) to human cervical cells created the HeLa genome, which is different from Henrietta Lacks genome in various ways, including its number of chromosomes. HeLa cells are rapidly dividing cancer cells, and the number of chromosomes varied during cancer formation and cell culture. The current estimate (excluding very tiny fragments) is a 'hypertriploid chromosome number (3n+)' which means 76 to 80 total chromosomes (rather than the normal diploid number of 46) with 22–25 clonally abnormal chromosomes, known as HeLa signature chromosomes. The signature chromosomes can be derived from multiple original chromosomes, making challenging summary counts based on original numbering.

Researchers have also noted how stable these aberrant karyotypes can be: Human papillomaviruses (HPVs) are frequently integrated into the cellular DNA in cervical cancers. Researchers mapped by FISH five HPV18 integration sites: three on normal chromosomes 8 at 8q24 and two on derivative chromosomes, der(5)t(5;22;8)(q11;q11q13;q24) and der(22)t(8;22)(q24;q13), which have chromosome 8q24 material. An 8q24 copy number increase was detected by CGH. Dual-coulor FISH with a c-MYC probe mapping to 8q24 revealed colocalisation with HPV18 at all integration sites, indicating that dispersion and amplification of the c-MYC gene sequences occurred after and was most likely triggered by the viral insertion at a single integration site. Numerical and structural chromosomal aberrations identified by SKY, genomic imbalances detected by CGH, as well as FISH localisation of HPV18 integration at the c-MYC locus in HeLa cells are common and representative for advanced stage cervical cell carcinomas. The HeLa genome has been remarkably stable after years of continuous cultivation; therefore, the genetic alterations detected may have been present in the primary tumour and reflect events that are relevant to the development of cervical cancer.

Complete genome sequence

The complete genome of the HeLa cells was sequenced and published on 11 March 2013 without the Lacks family's knowledge. Concerns were raised by the family, so the authors voluntarily withheld access to the sequence data. Jay Shendure led a HeLa sequencing project at the University of Washington which produced a paper that had been accepted for publication in March 2013, but that was also put on hold while the Lacks family's privacy concerns were being addressed. On August 7, 2013, NIH director Francis Collins announced a policy of controlled access to the cell line genome based on an agreement reached after three meetings with the Lacks family. A data-access committee will review requests from researchers for access to the genome sequence under the criteria that the study is for medical research and the users will abide by terms in the HeLa Genome Data Use Agreement, which includes that all NIH-funded researchers will deposit the data into a single database for future sharing. The committee consists of six members including representatives from the medical, scientific, and bioethics fields, as well as two members of the Lacks family. In an interview, Collins praised the Lacks family's willingness to participate in this situation that was thrust upon them. He described the whole experience with them as 'powerful', saying that it brought together 'science, scientific history and ethical concerns' in a unique way.

Contamination

HeLa cells are sometimes difficult to control because of their adaptation to growth in tissue culture plates. Through improper maintenance, they have been known to contaminate other cell cultures in the same laboratory, interfering with biological research and forcing researchers to declare many results invalid. The degree of HeLa cell contamination among other cell types is unknown because few researchers test the identity or purity of already established cell lines. It has been demonstrated that a substantial fraction of in vitro cell lines are contaminated with HeLa cells; estimates range from 10% to 20%. Stanley Gartler and Walter Nelson-Rees were the first to publish on the contamination of various cell lines by HeLa.

Science writer Michael Gold wrote about the HeLa cell contamination problem in his book A Conspiracy of Cells. He describes Nelson-Rees's identification of this pervasive worldwide problem—affecting even the laboratories of the best physicians, scientists, and researchers, including Jonas Salk —and many possibly career-ending efforts to address it. According to Gold, the HeLa contamination problem almost led to a Cold War incident. The USSR and the USA had begun to cooperate in the war on cancer launched by President Richard Nixon, only to find that the exchanged cells were contaminated by HeLa. Gold contends that the HeLa problem was amplified by emotions, egos, and a reluctance to admit mistakes. Nelson-Rees explains:

It's all human an unwillingness to throw away hours and hours of what was thought to be good research worries about jeopardising another grant that's being applied for, the hurrying to come out with a paper first. And it isn't limited to biology and cancer research. Scientists in many endeavors all make mistakes, and they all have the same problems.

Rather than focus on how to resolve the problem of HeLa cell contamination, many scientists and science writers continue to document this problem as simply a contamination issue caused not by human error or shortcomings but by the hardiness, proliferating, or overpowering nature of HeLa. Recent data suggest that cross-contaminations are still a major ongoing problem with modern cell cultures. Taken directly from the International Cell Line Authentication Committee (ICLAC) webpage:

Regrettably, cross-contamination and misidentification are still common within the research community. Many cell lines were cross-contaminated during establishment; this means that all work using those cell lines has incorrectly used the contaminant – which may come from a different species or a different tissue. A cell line is considered to be misidentified if it no longer corresponds to the individual from whom it was first established. Many cases of misidentification are caused by cross-contamination, where another, faster growing, cell line is introduced into that culture.

New Species Proposal

HeLa was described by Leigh Van Valen as an example of the contemporary creation of a new species, dubbed Helacyton gartleri, due to their ability to replicate indefinitely, and their non-human number of chromosomes. The species was named after Stanley M. Gartler, whom van Valen credits with discovering 'the remarkable success of this species.' His argument for speciation depends on these points:

- The chromosomal incompatibility of HeLa cells with humans.
- The ecological niche of HeLa cells.
- Their ability to persist and expand well beyond the desires of human cultivators.
- HeLa can be defined as a species as it has its own clonal karyotype.

Van Valen proposed the new family Helacytidae and the genus Helacyton, as well as proposing a new species for HeLa cells in the same paper. However, this proposal has not been taken seriously by other prominent evolutionary biologists, nor by scientists in other disciplines. Van Valen's argument of HeLa being a new species does not fulfill the criteria for an independent unicellular asexually reproducing species because of the notorious instability of HeLa's karyotype and their lack of a strict ancestral-descendant lineage.

DIFFERENT BETWEEN NORMAL CELLS AND HELA CELLS

There are 3 major differences between normal cells and HeLa cells:

1. HeLa cells are cancerous. The difference between normal cells and HeLa cells is most visible when you look at the chromosomes (karyotype). HeLa cells, like many tumours, have error-filled genomes, with one or more copies of many chromosomes: a normal cell contains 46 chromosomes whereas HeLa cells contain 76 to 80 (ref) total chromosomes, some of which are heavily mutated (22–25), per cell. This is due to the Human Papillomavirus (HPV), the cause of nearly all cervical cancers. HPV inserts its own DNA into host cells and the additional DNA results in the production

of a p53-binding protein which inhibits it and prevents native p53 from repairing mutations and suppressing tumours, causing errors in the genome to accumulate as unchecked cellular divisions occur.

2. HeLa cells grow unusually fast, even considering their cancerous state. Indeed, HeLa cells grow easily and rapidly, doubling cellular count in only 24 hr, making them ideal for large scale testing. They grow so fast that they can contaminate and overtake other cell cultures. This is related to the fact that Henrietta Lacks had syphilis which results in an aggressive growth of cancer due to a weakened immune system. And in 2013, it was shown that the scrambled HPV genome inserted itself near the c-myc proto-oncogene in Henrietta's genome, causing its constitutive expression and the rapid replication of HeLa cells in her body.

3. HeLa cells are immortal, meaning they will divide again and again and again. This performance can be explained by the expression of an overactive telomerase that rebuilds telomeres after each division, preventing cellular ageing and cellular senescence, and allowing perpetual divisions of the cells.

The HeLa cell line was the first successful attempt at immortalizing human-derived cells *in vitro*. In the past, researchers spent more time trying to keep cells alive than performing actual experiments. Soon after his discovery, Dr. Gey was sharing this cell line with co-workers active in cancer research and other fields, all around the world. The HeLa cell line gave them the time and the possibility to conduct repeatable experiments on human cells, without testing directly on humans. And to this day, HeLa cells have saved countless lives, and many scientific landmarks (such as cloning, gene mapping, *in vitro* fertilisation, the polio vaccine) have used HeLa cells and owe everything to the life and death of Henrietta Lacks.

HeLa Cells as Immortal

Normally, human cell cultures die within a few days after a set number of cell divisions via a process called senescence. This presents a problem for researchers because experiments using normal cells cannot be repeated on identical cells (clones), nor can the same cells be used for extended study. Cell biologist George Otto Gey took one cell from Henrietta Lacks sample, allowed that cell to divide, and found the culture survived indefinitely if given nutrients and a suitable environment. The original cells continued to mutate. Now, there are many strains of HeLa, all derived from the same single cell.

Researchers believe the reason HeLa cells don't suffer programmed death is because they maintain a version of the enzyme telomerase that prevents gradual shortening of the telomeres of chromosomes. Telomere shortening is implicated in ageing and death.

Disadvantages of Using HeLa Cells

While the HeLa cell line has led to amasing scientific breakthroughs, the cells can also cause problems. The most significant issue with HeLa cells is how aggressively they can contaminate other cell cultures in a laboratory. Scientists don't routinely test the purity of their cell lines, so HeLa had contaminated many *in vitro* lines (estimated 10 to 20 per cent) before the problem was identified. Much of the research conducted on contaminated cell lines had to be thrown out. Some scientists refuse to allow HeLa in their labs in order to control the risk.

Another problem with HeLa is that it doesn't have a normal human karyotype (the number and appearance of chromosomes in a cell). Henrietta Lacks (and other humans) have 46 chromosomes (diploid or a set of 23 pairs), while the HeLa genome consists of 76 to 80 chromosome (hypertriploid, including 22 to 25 abnormal chromosomes). The extra chromosomes came from the infection by human papilloma virus that led to cancer. While HeLa cells resemble normal human cells in many ways, they are neither normal nor entirely human. Thus, there are limitations to their use.

INFORMED CONSENT FOR BIOSPECIMEN RESEARCH

Informed consent describes a process for enabling individuals to make voluntary decisions about participating in research with an understanding of the purpose, procedures, risks, benefits, and alternatives. Informed consent is premised on well-established ethical principles, including respect for persons, beneficence, and justice. Following from these principles, key aspects of informed consent include the provision of information about the research that a reasonable person would want to know, in a manner and language understandable to the person, and under conditions that are free from coercion or undue influence. Several approaches to informed consent for the research use of biospecimens have been suggested. Actual practice varies, as collections of biospecimens (or biobanks) are highly heterogeneous in terms of tissue type, procurement situation, and geographic, social, and historical context. Furthermore, regulations and guidelines concerning informed consent are not necessarily specific to biospecimen research, nor are they harmonised. As illustrated by current US regulations, the result has sometimes been ambiguity, inadvertent constraints on research access, and research proceeding without consent.

Current US Regulations

In the United States, federal regulations (known as the Common Rule) were developed in response to revelations of extreme research abuses of vulnerable populations; these regulations were designed primarily to protect human beings from physical risks involved in experimental research. They set forth provisions for informed consent and oversight by an institutional review board (IRB) that, with limited exceptions, must be met in federally funded research.

In terms of application to biospecimen research, the Common Rule defines a human subject as a living individual about whom an investigator obtains: (i) data through intervention or interaction with the individual or (ii) identifiable private information.

Thus, when an investigator interacts with a person to collect biospecimens specifically for research (e.g. for a particular study or to build a biobank), informed consent and IRB oversight are required. However, when an investigator uses only biospecimens that have already been collected for another purpose (e.g. for a clinical purpose, for an earlier study, or to build a biobank), no intervention or interaction with a person is involved. Furthermore, a fundamental strategy to protect confidentiality is to remove direct identifiers and replace them with a code, and take additional steps to ensure that researchers have no access to identifying information. For example, material transfer and data use agreements can prohibit access to the key that links the code to identifiers (the code cannot be derived from information about the person; thus, Henrietta Lacks's cells today would not be labelled HeLa), as well as any attempt to reidentify sample sources.

Under these conditions—when there is no intervention or interaction with the individuals who were the sources of the samples, and researchers cannot readily ascertain their identities—research can be determined not to involve human subjects, and thus informed consent is not required. There are other provisions that allow research using existing biospecimens to be classified as exempt from the regulations (e.g. if researchers do not record identifying information), in which case consent would not be required, as well as provisions for waiving the requirement to obtain consent (when research qualifies as nonexempt research involving human subjects but certain criteria are met). All of these situations require some level of IRB involvement, as investigators cannot make these determinations themselves. Rather, they must submit at least basic information to an IRB, at which point the IRB can assess the adequacy of confidentiality protections, and could choose to consider the scope of the original consent and whether reconsent is required.

Thus, if Henrietta Lacks were a patient in the United States today, biospecimens collected solely for her clinical care would not require her consent for use in research. Any part of such specimens remaining after all the analyses needed for her care were completed might be stored for generic teaching, quality assurance, and research purposes, as briefly disclosed in a general consent-to-treat form. Researchers seeking to study stored clinical specimens could do so without her consent if an IRB determines either that the proposed research does not involve human subjects (based primarily on their having no access to identifiers) or that it meets the criteria for exemption from the regulations or waiver of the requirement to obtain consent. An IRB-approved research protocol and informed consent (unless waived) would be required when researchers prospectively intend to use clinical specimens for a specific project, including plans for use of residual specimens as well as taking more tissue than is needed for clinical care (i.e. taking extra tissue for research purposes during a necessary clinical procedure). Collecting biospecimens from family members solely for research purposes would require an IRB-approved protocol and informed consent.

In summary, regulations originally intended to protect research participants from bodily harm have been interpreted and clarified through guidance and practice to apply to research on biospecimens, with identifiability as a pivotal factor. However, this rapidly evolving research arena has been accompanied by equally rapid confirmation that genomic data can never be truly anonymised. A steady stream of provocative studies has demonstrated that it is possible to discover the identities of individuals whose genomic data had otherwise been considered deidentified. These developments come at a time when public concern about biospecimen research and informed consent has already been stoked not only by the story of Henrietta Lacks, but also by lawsuits over the research use of newborn screening samples and biospecimens from indigenous populations.

Proposed US Regulations

In September 2015, the federal government published a notice of proposed rulemaking (NPRM) to overhaul the Common Rule. Citing the changing research landscape, including the volume and diversity of studies, analytic sophistication, and growing use and global sharing of massive electronic data sets, the stated goals of the NPRM are to increase human subjects' ability and opportunity to make informed decisions, reduce potential for harm and increase justice by increasing the uniformity of protections, and facilitate promising research. Among the most significant changes are those proposed for biospecimen research:

- The definition of a human subject would be modified to include living individuals about whom an investigator obtains, uses, studies or analyses biospecimens, regardless of identifiability.
- With few exceptions, consent would be required for research use of all biospecimens—regardless of whether they were originally collected for research, clinical, or other purposes and whether they are deidentified (notably, consent would not be required for secondary research use of nonidentified private information, such as medical records).
- Consent would not be needed for each specific study, but rather could be obtained through broad consent for future unspecified research.
- The government would develop a broad consent template covering the storage of biospecimens and data for secondary research, as well as the use of stored materials for specific studies.

- In addition to basic elements of consent, additional required elements would cover commercial use and profit from study of biospecimens, return of individual research results, optional recontact, and widespread sharing, among others.

- Secondary use of biospecimens to establish a biobank would be exempt, subject only to limited IRB review to ensure that initial broad consent has been obtained and specified privacy and security safeguards are in place.

- Research using materials that have been stored for secondary use would be exempt from the regulations and required only to have safeguards in place. Investigators could use a to-be-created decision tool to make the exempt determination themselves.

HELA CELL LINES – ROBUST CELLULAR MODELS FOR *IN VITRO* TESTING

With all these characteristics, HeLa cells became progressively popular cellular models for life scientists willing to study mechanism of action of diseases or therapeutically active drug molecules. They have also been used to decipher cell signalling events such as DNA damage repair.

Recently, HeLa cells have been used to develop cellular models in which a specific gene of interest is silenced by genome editing. Several methods are available for gene editing.

SilenciX HeLa cells are tebu-bio's knockdown (KD) cell lines based on a unique siRNA Delivery system that enables the generation of syngenic, ready-to-use and stable cellular *in vitro* models stably silenced for a gene of interet. This technology has already been validated in numerous scientific articles covering various biological domains and applications such as DNA Repair, Epigenetics, Ubiquitination and the cell cycle, Drug discovery, cell signalling and mechanism of action studies.

ETHICAL ASPECTS OF HELA CELLS

Human biospecimens have played a crucial role in scientific and medical advances. Although the ethical and policy issues associated with biospecimen research have long been the subject of scholarly debate, the story of Henrietta Lacks, her family, and the creation of HeLa cells captured the attention of a much broader audience. The story has been a catalyst for policy change, including major regulatory changes proposed in the United States surrounding informed consent. These proposals are premised in part on public opinion data, necessitating a closer look at what such data tell us. The development of biospecimen policy should be informed by many considerations—one of which is public input, robustly gathered, on acceptable approaches that optimise shared interests, including access for all to the benefits of research. There is a need for consent approaches that are guided by realistic aspirations and a balanced view of autonomy within an expanded ethical framework.

Human biospecimens have played a crucial role in scientific and medical advances, and their continued widespread availability for research will be vital to realising the goals of precision medicine. Discoveries from biospecimen research have led to new understandings of human biology and targeted approaches to detecting and treating health conditions, as well as reducing the risk of future disease. In oncology research, for example, biospecimen use has increased dramatically in recent decades, helping illuminate molecular mechanisms that drive cancer and generating knowledge that, in some instances, has profound implications for risk assessment, diagnostic categorisation, and novel therapeutic strategies. The collection, storage, and research use of biospecimens and data, however, raise deep questions about informed consent, oversight, large-scale data sharing, privacy and confidentiality, commercialisation, access to research results, and the ability to withdraw. The success of this enterprise critically depends on addressing such concerns in ways that are acceptable to patients and the public, and on building and maintaining support, trust, and transparency. Although the ethical and policy issues associated with biospecimen research have long been the subject of scholarly analysis and debate, the publication of Rebecca Skloot's bestselling book The Immortal Life of Henrietta Lacks captured the attention of a much broader audience. The book is a popular teaching tool and book club favourite, and the book and its author have been the subject of numerous reviews, news stories, features, commentaries, profiles, and interviews.

The story of Henrietta Lacks, her family, and the creation of HeLa cells has been a catalyst for policy change, including major regulatory changes proposed in the United States for informed consent for biospecimen research. This review reflects on the role of the HeLa controversy and public opinion data more generally in the development of biospecimen research policy, and the need for informed consent approaches that are guided by realistic aspirations and a balanced view of autonomy within an expanded ethical framework.

To sum up, HeLa cells are important because they revolutionised the biotechnology research world—they were a relatively cheaper alternative that would actually stay alive, unlike previous cell lines.

They have been used to develop many treatments and drugs, such as the vaccine to prevent polio, chemotherapy drugs, in vitro fertilisation, and more. The cancer cells were the basis behind the discovery of the telomerase enzyme and that there are 46 chromosomes in the human genome, not 48. But perhaps most notably, HeLa cells have impacted fields other than biology. They've brought light important ethical questions, such as: Do patients have the right to know that their tissue has been extracted during sugery? If doctors take the cells out of a patient's body and culture them, who owns the cells? If such cells were ever commercialised, who gets the profits? These are some of the questions being debated right now, as the family of Henrietta Lacks, from whom the HeLa cells were first isolated, is seeking financial claims to the cells.

Chapter 4

Viruses and Human Cancer

INTRODUCTION

Cancer, also called malignancy, is an abnormal growth of cells. There are more than 100 types of cancer, including breast cancer, skin cancer, lung cancer, colon cancer, prostate cancer, and lymphoma. Symptoms vary depending on the type. Cancer treatment may include chemotherapy, radiation, and/or surgery. Cells are the basic units that make up the human body. Cells grow and divide to make new cells as the body needs them. Usually, cells die when they get too old or damaged. Then, new cells take their place. Cancer begins when genetic changes interfere with this orderly process. Cells start to grow uncontrollably. These cells may form a mass called a tumour. A tumour can be cancerous or benign. A cancerous tumour is malignant, meaning it can grow and spread to other parts of the body. A benign tumour means the tumour can grow but will not spread.

How cancer spreads: As a cancerous tumour grows, the bloodstream or lymphatic system may carry cancer cells to other parts of the body. During this process, known as metastasis, the cancer cells grow and may develop into new tumours. One of the first places a cancer often spreads is to the lymph nodes. Lymph nodes are tiny, bean-shaped organs that help fight infection. They are located in clusters in different parts of the body, such as the neck, groin area, and under the arms.

Cancer may also spread through the bloodstream to distant parts of the body. These parts may include the bones, liver, lungs, or brain. Even if the cancer spreads, it is still named for the area where it began. For example, if breast cancer spreads to the lungs, it is called metastatic breast cancer, not lung cancer.

An estimated 15 per cent of all human cancers worldwide may be attributed to viruses, representing a significant portion of the global cancer burden. Both DNA and RNA viruses have been shown to be capable of causing cancer in humans. Epstein-Barr virus, human papilloma virus, hepatitis B virus, and human herpes virus-8 are the four DNA viruses that are capable of causing the development of human cancers. Human T lymphotrophic virus type 1 and hepatitis C viruses are the two RNA viruses that contribute to human cancers. Close study of viruses and human cancer has led to optimism for the development of new strategies for the prevention of the preceding infection that can lead to carcinogenesis. The presence of viral gene products in tumour cells that require them to maintain their unchecked proliferation also can provide important targets for directed therapies that specifically can distinguish tumour cells from normal cells. The inability of traditional cancer therapy, such as chemotherapy and radiation, to distinguish cancer cells from normal cells is a significant drawback and leads to toxicities for patients undergoing treatment. Targeted therapies directed against viral proteins or generate immune responses in order to either prevent infection or kill infected cells or cancer cells hold much promise for more effective and tolerable strategies.

VIRUSES THAT CAN LEAD TO CANCER

Viruses are very small organisms; most can't even be seen with an ordinary microscope. They are made up of a small number of genes in the form of DNA or RNA surrounded by a protein coating. A virus must enter a living cell and 'hijack' the cell's machinery in order to reproduce and make more viruses. Some viruses do this by inserting their own DNA (or RNA) into that of the host cell. When the DNA or RNA affects the host cell's genes, it can push the cell toward becoming cancer.

In general, each type of virus tends to infect only a certain type of cell in the body. (For example, the viruses that cause the common cold only infect the cells lining the nose and throat.) Several viruses are linked with cancer in humans. Our growing knowledge of the role of viruses as a cause of cancer has led to the development of vaccines to help prevent certain human cancers. But these vaccines can only protect against infections if they are given before the person is exposed to the cancer-promoting virus.

HUMAN TUMOUR VIRUSES

Although it is convenient to consider human tumour viruses as a discrete group of viruses, these six viruses, in fact, have very different genomes, life cycles, and represent a number of virus families. The path from viral infection to tumourgenesis is slow and inefficient; only a minority of infected individuals progress to cancer, usually years or even decades after primary infection. Virus infection also is generally not sufficient for cancer, and additional events and host factors, such as immunosuppression, somatic mutations, genetic predisposition, and exposure to carcinogens must also play a role.

HEPATITIS B AND C VIRUSES

Hepatitis C virus is an enveloped RNA virus of the flavivirus family. It is capable of causing both acute and chronic hepatitis in humans by infecting liver cells. It is estimated that approximately 3 per cent of the world's population are hepatitis C carriers. Chronic infection with hepatitis C virus results in cirrhosis, which in turn can lead to primary hepatocellular carcinoma. Between 1 and 2 per cent of infected patients with subsequent compensated cirrhosis will develop primary hepatocellular carcinoma per year. Transmission of the virus occurs through the blood, with shared needles in intravenous drug abuse, sexual activity, and parturition being the primary routes.

The hepatitis B virus of the family hepadnaviridae is, by contrast, a DNA virus, but the features of its resulting disease share many similarities with hepatitis C virus. Hepatitis B virus also is a blood-borne pathogen that can result in acute and chronic hepatitis. Chronic hepatitis, that is infections lasting more than three months, can lead to cirrhosis and liver failure. Chronic infection also can lead to the development of hepatocellular carcinoma. Hepatitis B infections is a significant global health problem with an estimated 2 billion people infected and 1.2 million deaths per year attributed to subsequent hepatitis, cirrhosis and hepatocellular carcinoma. Hepatocellular carcinoma is an aggressive tumour that can occur in the setting of liver disease resulting from infections with hepatitis B and/or hepatitis C virus, although the exact mechanism of oncogenesis by these viruses is unclear. Diagnosis is usually made late in the course of liver disease and median survival ranges from six to 20 months after that time. The traditional foundation of treatment is surgical, whether tumour resection or transplantation. However, nonsurgical options such as percutaneous ethanol injection, transarterial embolisation, radiofrequency ablation, chemotherapy, and radiotherapy are also utilised. The choice of therapies frequently depends on the extent of disease and the amount of liver function the patient has in reserve.

Research into novel therapies have focused on the use of virally targeted and immunological strategies with an eye on preventing infection. Unfortunately, hepatitis C virus has proved to be poorly suited to vaccines because its genome possesses a very high mutation rate, especially in the hyper variable region of the genome coding for the envelope proteins allowing it to escape immune recognition and elimination by the host. There are 11 distinct genotypes and several subtypes identified.

The introduction of vaccines against hepatitis B virus in the early 1980s marked a major milestone with what might be considered the first cancer prevention vaccine, although the primary goal of this vaccine was to prevent hepatitis. Since that time, more than 110 countries have adopted a universal policy of immunising all new borns, according to the World Health Organisation. Additionally, countries that have successfully implemented this programme significantly have decreased the carrier rate and infection in their populations. However, vaccine coverage is often low in many developing countries due to the cost, lack of heath care infrastructure for delivery of the vaccine, and the need for three needle injections over six months. Even in some developed nations, universal vaccination has not been implemented because of the belief that it is a limited public health problem and the expense is not justified.

New challenges for combating hepatitis B infection center around efforts to address the limitations of the current vaccine: the need for multiple injections, the presence of up to 10 per cent non-responders to the vaccine, the discovery of hepatitis B virus S gene escape mutants in infants that were infected despite an adequate response to the vaccine, and the cost for developing nations. The current multiple dosing schedule is being addressed with attempts to combine it with other required vaccines or decrease the number of doses. Oral vaccination also is being investigated as a way to obviate the need for trained personnel to administer injections. The World Health Organisation estimates that from $14 to $20 billion will be needed to immunise children from the poorest countries from 2016–2020, which has prompted efforts from public and private organisations to advocate for funding to fill the need.

Medical therapy for patients infected with hepatitis B has focused on the use of interferon to reduce viral replication, which decreases the incidence of life-threatening liver complications in patients who respond to the treatment. Interferon alpha treatment is effective in 20 to 30 per cent of cases in inducing loss of the hepatitis Be antigen. However, the impact of interferon therapy on subsequent hepatocellular carcinoma rates is less clear. Interferon therapy is also limited by cost and side effects.

The limitations of interferon therapy have been partly circumvented with the use of targeted antiviral agents. Lamivudine has been shown in a large multicenter randomised placebo-controlled trial to be effective in reducing both the incidence of hepatic decompensation and the risk of hepatocellular carcinoma. Other antiviral agents continue to join the armamentarium, lamivudine, adefovir, entecavir, and telbivudine have been shown to be effective in hepatitis B disease.

These agents are nucleotide analogues that exploit the need for the hepatitis B virus to use reverse transcriptase to replicate viral DNA. Since these agents specifically target the viral replication machinery and are given orally, they are better tolerated. However, it has been observed that long-term therapy with lamivudine can lead to the emergence of genotypic resistance mutations, but this does not negate the benefits of lamivudine therapy in reducing the rates of hepatocellular carcinoma. The success of these therapies has reached the point where patients with advanced cirrhosis secondary to hepatitis B can be treated and transplanted without the development of hepatitis B in the transplanted liver.

Medical treatment of infection with hepatitis C has not progressed at the same speed. Pegylated interferon with ribavirin, an antiviral agent that may act as a nucleoside analogue and inhibitor of RNA dependent RNA polymerase, has been shown to be successful in eradicating infection in half of patients. However, therapy is expensive and side effects are significant. Phase II trials of oral antivirals such as protease inhibitors and polymerase inhibitors are currently under way. Unlike hepatitis B, treatment of hepatocellular carcinoma due to hepatitis C infection with transplantation almost always results in recurrent infection of the transplanted liver.

The search for targeted therapies that can block hepatitis C viral replication by selectively inhibiting viral replication has for many years been hampered by the lack of experimental infection systems, in either cell culture or animal models to test candidate therapies. The recent development of viral replicons, subgenomic RNAs that are expressed and autonomously replicate within cells, has led to the use of hepatitis C viral replicons that can replicate in human hepatoma cells lines and the development of mouse models of the disease. These advances may herald more rapid progress in the development of virally targeted therapies such as hepatitis C virus specific protease and polymerase inhibitors.

EPSTEIN-BARR VIRUS (EBV) AND HUMAN HERPESVIRUS 8 (HHV-8)

EBV and HHV-8 (also known as Kaposi sarcoma herpesvirus) are both herpesviruses that possess large double-stranded DNA genomes. As with all herpesviruses, they encode enzymes involved in DNA replication and repair and nucleotide biosynthesis. They also both possess the ability to establish latency in B lymphocytes and reactivate into the lytic cycle. Both also are associated with naturally occurring tumours in humans.

EBV is a ubiquitous virus that is most commonly known for being the primary agent for infectious mononucleosis. Up to 95 per cent of all adults are estimated to be seropositive, and most EBV infections are subclinical. EBV also is associated with a number of malignancies: B and T cell lymphomas, Hodgkin's disease, post-transplant lymphoproliferative disease, leiomyosarcomas, and nasopharyngeal carcinomas. Of these cancers, Burkitt's lymphoma, post-transplant lymphoproliferative disease, and leiomyosarcomas show an increased frequency in patients with immunodeficiency, suggesting a role for immuno surveillance in the suppression of malignant transformation.

The primary site of infection is the oropharyngeal cavity, and EBV is capable of infecting both B cells and epithelial cells and switching between the two. The major surface glycoprotein, gp350/220, binds to the cd21 receptor on B cells. Transformation of B cells is a highly efficient process requiring a large portion of the EBV genome, which becomes circular for replication and latency. Virus will directly enter the latent gene expression state with suppression of the lytic cycle. Production of a number of latent gene products are required for immortalisation.

Immune therapy of EBV-associated tumours has been target of research since standard therapy generally has entailed the use of multi-agent chemotherapy, radiation therapy, and surgery. This work has centered around adoptive transfer of EBV-specific cytotoxic T-cells and shown success but must overcome obstacles such as potential graft vs. host disease and resistance due to mutation of selected EBV epitopes. Vaccines capable of preventing primary EBV infection or boosting immune responses against EBV-associated tumours are under investigation. Much of the development thus far has focused on gp350/220 subunit vaccines, since it is one of the most abundant proteins on the virus coat and also the protein against which the human EBV neutralising antibody response is directed. Another strategy involves the use of a recombinant vaccinia viral vector to express an EBV membrane antigen. A successful vaccine would have the greatest impact in regions of the world that have an especially high incidence of specific malignancies. Burkitt's lymphoma is the most common childhood malignancy in the central part of Africa where EBV and malaria are considered cofactors in its carcinogenesis and 95 per cent of children are infected by age 3, compared to the United States, where infection is usually delayed until adolescence. Nasopharyngeal carcinoma is relatively rare but has an exceptionally high incidence in southern China, approaching more than 20 times greater than that of most populations.

In 1994, HHV-8 DNAwas identified in biopsies from tumours of a patient with Kaposi sarcoma, a relatively rare malignancy prior to the AIDS epidemic. In addition to it likely being an essential cofactor for the development of Kaposi sarcoma, HHV-8 also is believed to have a role in Castleman's disease and primary effusion lymphoma. The viral genome is expressed in these tumours and encodes transforming proteins and anti-apoptotic factors. The virus is also able to enhance the proliferation of microvascular endothelial cells. As with EBV, the predominant infected cell is the B lymphocyte, although here the lytic cycle is embraced rather than repressed. This may play a crucial role in the pathogenesis of Kaposis sarcoma by elaboration of viral and host cytokines promoting cell proliferation, angiogenesis, and enhancement of viral spread.

Targeted antiviral agents such as ganciclovir directed against viral DNA replication have had a dramatic affect on decreasing the incidence of Kaposi sarcoma in AIDS patients through both therapy and prophylaxis. Ganciclovir is phosphorylated into a GTP analog, which acts as a competive inhibitor of viral DNApolymerase resulting in termination of viral DNA elongation. Furthermore, a G protein coupled receptor (vGPCR) has been identified as a viral oncogene in HHV-8 infected cells that can exploit cell signalling pathways to induce transformation and angiogenesis. vGPCR also has been proposed as a target for novel molecular therapies because of its key role in disease progression. But the therapy regimen most responsible for the decreasing incidence of Kaposi sarcomamay well be the success of highly active antiretroviral therapy (HAART) regimens targeting HIV, since it was the emergence of HIV that led to the increasing incidence of Kaposi sarcoma.

HUMAN PAPILLOMAVIRUS (HPV)

HPV are small non-enveloped DNA tumor viruses that commonly cause benign papillomas or warts in humans. Persistent infection with high-risk subtypes of human papillomavirus (HPV) is associated with the development of cervical cancer. HPV infects epithelial cells, and, after integration in host DNA, the production of oncoproteins, mainly E6 and E7, disrupts natural tumor suppressor pathways and is required for proliferation of cervical carcinoma cells. HPV also is believed to play a role in other human cancers, such as head and neck tumors, skin cancers in immuno suppressed patients, and other anogenital cancers.

Cervical cancer is the second leading cause of cancer mortality in women worldwide, causing 240,000 deaths annually. Of approximately 490,000 cases reported each year, more than 80 per cent occur in the developing world, where effective but costly Pap smear screening programmes are not in place. Early precancerous changes and early cancers detected by Pap smears are effectively treated and cured with surgical therapy or ablation. In the absence of effective screening, the disease is detected late. Traditional therapeutic options for cervical cancer that have advanced beyond definitive surgical treatment are chemotherapy and radiation therapy, which are associated with many toxicities and do not offer a lasting cure. The immune system plays an important role in the prevention of persistent HPV infection and progression of precancerous lesions. Human papillomavirus is a poor natural immunogen; as a double stranded DNA virus, there is no RNA intermediate, nor does infection cause cytolysis, allowing initiation of innate immune responses. HPV mainly encodes non-secreted nucleoproteins, which are poorly cross-presented and compared to other viruses its non-structural proteins are expressed at low levels. However, genital infection with HPV is usually transient. Additionally, inadequate T cell responses may lead to failure to clear HPV infected cells. AIDS patients, renal transplant patients receiving immunosuppressive therapy, and individuals with T cell deficiencies have increased rates of HPV persistence, anogenital lesions, and cervical cancer.

In 2006, an effective prophylactic vaccine against HPV 16 and 18 based on virus like particles (VLP) of recombinant L1, the major capsid protein, was approved for use by the FDA based on clinical trials that demonstrated nearly 100 per cent protection from persistent infection through the generation of high levels of neutralising antibodies. Since these types are the causative agent of approximately 70 per cent of cervical cancers, development of such an effective vaccine holds much promise for the prevention of cervical cancer. However, the vaccine currently costs $360 for a complete course of three injections given over six months, does not provide protection against other high risk HPV types, will presumably have limited benefit to women already infected, and has an unknown duration of protection. Because of these limitations, therapeutic vaccination is being explored to treat women already infected and accelerate the impact of prophylactic vaccination in decreasing cervical cancer incidence. Traditional therapy for early cervical cancer and precancerous lesions involves surgical excision or ablation.

Therapeutic vaccination seeks to generate a population of cytoxic T cells that will recognise and kill tumor cells. Since patients with T cell deficiencies are known to be more susceptible to HPV infection and disease progression, boosting T cell responses to HPV may be crucial to a therapeutic immune strategy. In the case of cervical cancer, E6 and E7 oncoproteins are expressed in all malignancies and are not found in uninfected normal cells. Therefore, they represent ideal targets for a therapeutic immune response. A number of strategies to generate immune responses against these antigens are under investigation. Viral and bacterial vectors have been used in mouse models to generate immune responses. Vaccinia virus delivery of HPV 16 and 18 modified E6 and E7 proteins has demonstrated safety and specific immune responses in early clinical trials. DNA vaccination strategies also are under active investigation, and several are in various stages of clinical trials. Vaccination with plasmid DNA encapsulated in biodegradable micorparticles has shown histological and immunological responses when used to treat patients with high grade cervical dysplasia.

HUMAN T LYMPHOTROPIC VIRUS TYPE I (HTLV-1)

HTLV-1 is a slow transforming, single stranded RNA retrovirus and is associated with adult T-cell leukemia. It possesses a diploid genome similar to other retroviruses: two long terminal repeats flanking gag, pol, and env genes as well as a number of accessory genes. HTLV-1 has a worldwide distribution, with an estimated 12 to 25 million people infected. However, disease is only observed in less than 5 per cent of infected individuals. It is transmitted through blood transfusions, sexual contact, and during parturition. HTLV-1 displays a special tropism for CD4 cells, which clonally proliferate in adult T cell leukemia, though how this is effected is not known.

HTLV-1 infection has a very long latency period of 20 to 30 years, but once tumor formation begins, progression is rapid. Standard chemotherapy often can bring about an initial response with a partial or complete remission; however, relapse is common, and median survival is eight months. The HTLV-1 *Tax* gene has been postulated to play an important role in tumourgenesis through the activation of viral transcription and the hijacking of cellular growth and cell division machinery, but the mechanisms leading to adult T cell leukemia are not well understood. It has been suspected that HTLV-1 infection may not be sufficient to transform, and recent evidence suggests that the decreased diversity, frequency, and function of HTLV-1 specific CD8 T cells in the host may play an important part in the development of adult T cell leukemia. Therefore, targeted therapies using peptide, recombinant protein, DNA, and viral vectors with the goal of generating neutralising antibody against HTLV-1 and multivalent cytotoxic T cell response against *Tax* are under investigation.

The viruses reviewed here illustrate the diverse biological pathways to malignancy and the challenges of treating the resulting diseases. Yet the presence of the viral gene products in cancer and precancerous cells present attractive targets that may be exploited in novel therapies that distinguish these cells from normal cells. Antivirals such as lamuvidine used in heptatitis B and ganciclovir for Kaposi sarcoma specifically target the viral replication machinery. Targeting cancer cells specifically would have advantages over traditional modalities such as chemotherapy and radiation, which can include significant toxicities. Cervical cancer, because it retains HPV viral oncoproteins E6 and E7 and requires their continued expression for proliferation, provides an ideal model for cytotoxic immune therapies against these known antigens.

Given the prevalence of these cancers in the developing world and the limitations of health care infrastructure, strategies for vaccine design to prevent primary infection and targeted therapies for the treatment of disease must be carefully considered in this context. Use of needles, refrigeration, multiple doses, and cost are all significant barriers to the delivery of an effective vaccine. Cost, need for trained personnel and sophisticated equipment and facilities may impede global use of the most advanced targeted therapies. These challenges suggest that exploration of prophylactic strategies and development of specific, targeted therapies are both necessary to decrease this portion of the global cancer burden.

SECTION II

Molecule and Membrane

Chapter 5

Molecules and Biomolecules of Cells

INTRODUCTION

Cells form the basis of all living things. They are the smallest single unit of life, from the simplest bacteria to blue whales and giant redwood trees. Differences in the structure of cells and the way that they carry out their internal mechanisms form the basis of the first major divisions of life, into the three kingdoms of *Archaea* ('ancient' bacteria), *Eubacteria* ('modern' bacteria) and *Eukaryota* (everything else, including us). An understanding of cells is therefore vital in any understanding of life itself.

Cell biology is the study of cells and how they function, from the subcellular processes which keep them functioning, to the way that cells interact with other cells. Whilst molecular biology concentrates largely on the molecules of life (largely the nucleic acids and proteins), cell biology concerns itself with how these molecules are used by the cell to survive, reproduce and carry out normal cell functions.

MOLECULES AND BIOMOLECULES OF CELLS

Water

Water is very often a direct participant in the chemical reactions of living cells. Water is not only a solvent for many biomolecules but also plays a huge role in many reactions with biomolecules within living organisms. A prime example is the conversion of ADP to ATP, which is an essential process for storing energy in living organisms. In this process, a condensation reaction occurs which is characterised by the elimination of water when the reactant ADP couples with a phosphate group, water is thus a product in this reaction. When energy is needed, a type of hydrolysis reaction occurs where water is required to hydrate ATP to release the energy. When water acts as a reactant, such as in a hydrolysis reaction, the electron-rich oxygen will serve as a nucleophile.

Living organisms have effectively adapted to their aqueous environment and have even evolved means of exploiting the unusual properties of water. The high specific heat of water is useful to large terrestrial animals, because body water acts as a heat buffer, allowing the temperature of the organism to remain relatively constant as the air temperature fluctuates. But most fundamental to all living organisms is that many important biological properties of cell macro-molecules, particularly the proteins and nucleic acids, derive from their interactions with water molecules of the surrounding medium. The high specific heat of water is useful to cells and organisms because it allows water to act as a 'heat buffer', keeping the temperature of an organism relatively constant as the temperature of surrounding flactuants.

Thus, water is the most abundant compound in living organisms. Its relatively high freezing point, boiling point, heat of vapourisation and surface tension are the result of strong intermolecular attractions in the form of hydrogen bonding between neighbouring water molecules. Most of the recent theoretical and practical advances in the field of biology have been made in the area of biochemistry. Both teaching and research have been concentrating on understanding the complex web of chemical reactions that occur in every living cell. Cell biologists especially have tried to understand the chemical interactions between the various cellular components. Great progress has been made in understanding the ways in which the cell manipulates its chemical environment to manufacture new compounds and break down existing ones.

Special Properties and Behaviour of Water

Water is the most common molecule, whereas carbohydrates and protein are the most prevalent organic substances. Water not only makes up 70 to 90% of the weight of most forms of life, it also represents the continuous phase of living organisms. Because it is familiar and ubiquitous, water is often regarded as a bland, inert liquid, a mere space filler in living organisms.

Actually, however, it is a highly reactive substance with unusual properties that distinguish it strikingly from most other common liquids. We now recognise that water and its ionisation products, hydronium and hydroxide ions, are important determinants of the characteristic structure and biological properties of proteins and nucleic acids, as well as membranes, ribosomes and many other cell components. Water is so familiar, we generally consider it to be a rather bland fluid of simple character. It is, however, a chemically reactive liquid with such extraordinary physical properties that, if chemists had discovered it in recent times, it would undoubtedly have been classified as an exotic substance.

The properties of water are of profound biological significance. The structures of the molecules on which life is based—proteins, nucleic acids, lipids and complex carbohydrates—result directly from their interactions with their aqueous environment. The combination of solvent properties responsible for the intramolecular and inter-molecular associations of these substances is peculiar to water, no other solvent even resembles water in this respect. Although the hypothesis that life could be based on organic polymers other than proteins and nucleic acids seems plausible, it is all but inconceivable that the complex structural organisation and chemistry of living systems could exist in other than an aqueous medium. Indeed, direct observations on the surface of Mars, the only other planet in the solar system with temperatures compatible with life, indicates that it is devoid both of water and of life. Biological structures and processes can only be understood in terms of the physical and chemical properties of water.

Properties of Water

Physical properties and hydrogen bonding of water

Water has a higher melting point, boiling point, heat of vapourisation, heat of fusion and surface tension than such comparable hydrides as H_2S or NH_3 or for that matter, than most common liquids. All these properties indicate that the forces of attraction between the molecules in liquid water and thus its internal cohesion, are relatively high. For example, Table 5.1 shows that the heat of vapourisation of water is considerably higher than that of any of the other common liquids listed. The heat of vapourisation is a direct measure of the amount of energy required to overcome the attractive forces between adjacent molecules in a liquid so that individual molecules can escape from each other and enter the gaseous state.

Table 5.1: Heat of vapourisation of some common liquids at their boiling point (1.0 atmosphere).

Liquid	ΔH_{vap}, cal g^{-1}
Water	540
Methanol	263
Ethanol	204
n-Propanol	164
Acetone	125
Benzene	94
Chloroform	59

The strong intermolecular forces in liquid water are caused by the specific distribution of electrons in the water molecule. Each of the two hydrogen atoms shares a pair of electrons with the oxygen atom, through overlap of the 1s orbitals of the hydrogen atoms with two hybridised sp^3 orbitals of the oxygen atom. From spectroscopic and X-ray analyses the precise H—O—H bond angle is 104.5° and the average hydrogen-oxygen interatomic distance is 0.0965 nm. This arrangement of electrons in the water molecule gives it electrical asymmetry. The highly electronegative oxygen atom tends to withdraw the single electrons from the hydrogen atoms, leaving the hydrogen nuclei bare. As a result, each of the two hydrogen atoms has a local partial positive charge (designated δ^+). The oxygen atom, in turn, has a local partial negative charge (designated δ^-) located in the zone of the unshared orbitals.

Thus, although the water molecule has no net charge, it is an electric dipole. When two water molecules approach each other closely, electrostatic attraction occurs between the partial negative charge on the oxygen atom of one water molecule and the partial positive charge on a hydrogen atom of an adjacent water molecule. This is accompanied by a redistribution of the electronic charges in both molecules which greatly enhances their interaction. A complex electrostatic union of this kind is called a hydrogen bond. Because of the nearly tetrahedral arrangement of the electrons about the oxygen atom, each water molecule is potentially capable of hydrogen-bonding with four neighbouring water molecules. It is this property that is responsible for the great internal cohesion of liquid water.

CARBOHYDRATES

A carbohydrate is an organic compound which has the empirical formula $C_m(H_2O)_n$, that is, consists only of carbon, hydrogen and oxygen, with it in a 1:2:1 atom ratio. Carbohydrates can be viewed as hydrates of carbon, hence their name. Structurally however, it is more accurate to view them as polyhydroxy aldehydes and ketones. The term is most common in biochemistry, where it is a synonym of saccharide. The carbohydrates (saccharides) are divided into four chemical groupings: monosaccharides, disaccharides, oligosaccharides, and polysaccharides. In general, the monosaccharides and disaccharides, which are smaller (lower molecular weight) carbohydrates, are commonly referred to as sugars. While the scientific nomenclature of carbohydrates is complex, the names of the monosaccharides and disaccharides very often end in the suffix -ose. For example, blood sugar is the monosaccharide glucose, table sugar is the disaccharide sucrose, and milk sugar is the disaccharide lactose.

Carbohydrates perform numerous roles in living things. Polysaccharides serve for the storage of energy (e.g. starch and glycogen) and as structural components (e.g. cellulose in plants and chitin in arthropods). The 5-carbon monosaccharide ribose is an important component of coenzymes (e.g. ATP, FAD, and NAD) and the backbone of the genetic molecule known as RNA. The related deoxyribose is a component of DNA. Saccharides and their derivatives include many other important biomolecules that play key roles in the immune system, fertilisation, preventing pathogenesis, blood clotting, and development. In food science and in many informal contexts, the term carbohydrate often means any food that is particularly rich in the complex carbohydrate starch (such as cereals, bread and pasta) or simple carbohydrates, such as sugar (found in candy, jams and desserts). Carbohydrates are a class of biological molecules that contain primarily carbon (C) atoms flanked by hydrogen (H) atoms and hydroxyl (OH) groups (H-C-OH).

Carbohydrates have two major biochemical roles. For one, they act as a source of energy that can be released in a form usable by bodily tissues. Secondly, they serve as carbon skeletons that can be rearranged to form other molecules necessary for biological structures and functions. While carbohydrates are essential for the human diet, excessive consumption of particular types of carbohydrates correlates with obesity, diabetes, heart disease, and even drowsiness.

The carbohydrates found in candy or processed sugar can be very stimulating to the senses, but it is essential to use discipline in one's diet to avoid the complications of too many of the wrong types of carbohydrates. Some carbohydrates are small with molecular weights of less than one hundred, whereas others are true macromolecules with molecular weights in the hundreds of thousands.

The four categories of carbohydrates are classified by their number of sugar units:

1. Monosaccharides (mono- 'one', saccharide- 'sugar') are the monomers (small molecules that may bond chemically to form a polymer) out of which larger carbohydrates are constructed. Monosaccharides such as glucose, ribose, and fructose are simple sugars.

2. Disaccharides (di- 'two'), such as sucrose and lactose, are two monosaccharides linked together by covalent bonds.

3. Oligosaccharides (oligo- 'several') are made up of from 3 to 20 monosaccharides.

4. Polysaccharides (poly- 'many') are large polymers composed of hundreds or thousands of monosaccharides. Starch, glycogen, and cellulose are polysaccharides.

The general chemical formula for carbohydrates, $C(H_2O)$, gives the relative proportions of carbon, hydrogen, and oxygen in a monosaccharide (the proportion of these atoms are 1:2:1). This formula is characteristic of sugars and gave rise to the term carbohydrate because compounds of this sort were originally thought to be 'hydrates of carbon'. This term persists even though a carbohydrate definitely is not a hydrated carbon atom. For monosaccharides, the general formula is $(CH_2O)_n$, with n equal to the number of carbon atoms. In disaccharides, oligosaccharides, and polysaccharides, the molar proportions deviate slightly from the general formula because two hydrogens and one oxygen are lost during each of the condensation reactions that forms them. These carbohydrates have the more general formula $C_n(H_2O)_m$.

Type of Carbohydrates

Monosaccharides

The repeating units of polysaccharides are simple sugars called monosaccharides. There are two categories of sugars: aldosugars, with a terminal carbonyl group (a carbon atom double-bonded to an oxygen atom), and ketosugars, with an internal carbonyl group typically on the second carbon atom. Within these two groups, sugars are named according to the number of carbon atoms they contain. Most sugars have between three and seven carbon atoms and are termed triose (three carbons), tetrose (four carbons), pentose (five carbons), hexose (six carbons), or heptose (seven carbons). Figure 5.1 shows glucose as a

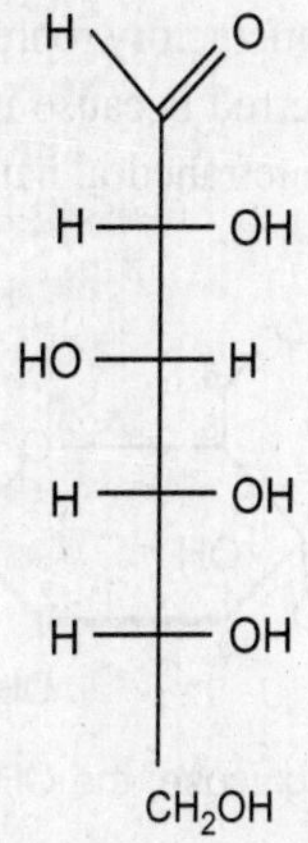

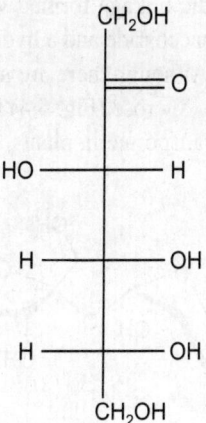

Fig. 5.1: Glucose as a straight-chain carbohydrate (Fischer projection). Glucose is an aldohexose because it has a terminal carbonyl group.

straight-chain carbohydrate (Fischer projection). Glucose is an aldohexose because it has a terminal carbonyl group. Glucose is an aldohexose, fructose is a ketohexose, and ribose is an aldopentose. Each carbon atom that supports a hydroxyl group (except for the first and last) is optically active, allowing a number of different carbohydrates with the same basic structure. For instance, galactose is an aldohexose but has different properties from glucose because the atoms are arranged differently. Figure 5.2 shows fructose as a straight-chain carbohydrate (Fischer projection). Fructose is a ketohexose because it has an internal carbonyl group.

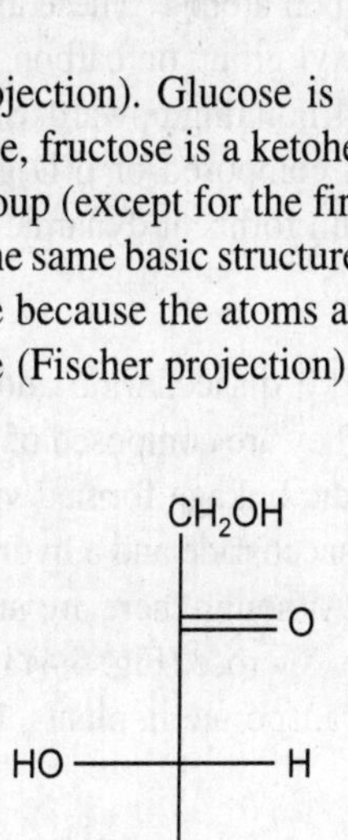

Fig. 5.2: Fructose as a straight-chain carbohydrate (Fischer projection). Fructose is a ketohexose because it has an internal carbonyl group.

The single most common monosaccharide is the aldohexose D-glucose, represented by the formula $C_6H_{12}O_6$. The carbons of glucose are numbered beginning with the more oxidised end of the molecule, the carbonyl group. In the cell, however, glucose exists in dynamic equilibrium between the linear and ring configurations. The ring form is the predominant structure because it is energetically more stable. This form results from the addition of the hydroxyl (OH) group on carbon atom 5 across the carbonyl group of carbon atom 1 (Fig. 5.3). A more satisfactory representation of glucose is shown in the Haworth projection. The Haworth projection is preferred because it indicates both the ring form and the spatial relationship between the carbon atoms. The tetrahedral nature of each carbon atom in the chain actually favours the ring formation of glucose.

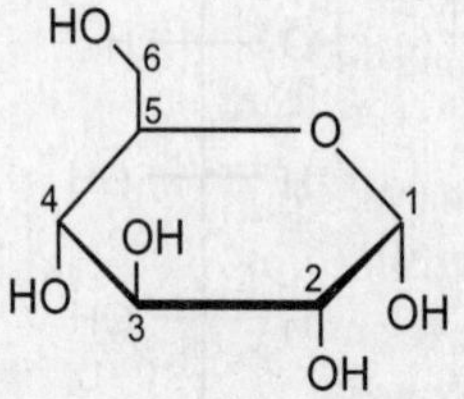

Fig. 5.3: Haworth projection of α-D-glucose, the OH group of carbon 1 points downwards.

The formation of the ring structure generates two alternative forms of glucose based on the spatial orientation of the hydroxyl group on carbon atom 1. These alternative forms of glucose are designated α and β and α-D-glucose has the hydroxyl group on carbon atom 1 pointing downward. β-D-glucose, has the hydroxyl group on carbon atom 1 pointing upward. Starch and glycogen are composed of α-D-glucose monomers whereas cellulose is composed of β-D-glucose monomers. Glucose interconverts between α-ring, β-ring, and straight-chain forms at dynamic equilibrium.

Disaccharides

Two joined monosaccharides are called a disaccharide and these are the simplest polysaccharides. Examples include sucrose and lactose. They are composed of two monosaccharide units bound together by a covalent bond known as a glycosidic linkage formed via a dehydration reaction, resulting in the loss of a hydrogen atom from one monosaccharide and a hydroxyl group from the other. The formula of unmodified disaccharides is $C_{12}H_{22}O_{11}$. Although there are numerous kinds of disaccharides, a handful of disaccharides are particularly notable. Sucrose (Fig. 5.4) is the most abundant disaccharide, and the main form in which carbohydrates are transported in plants. It is composed of one D-glucose molecule and one D-fructose molecule.

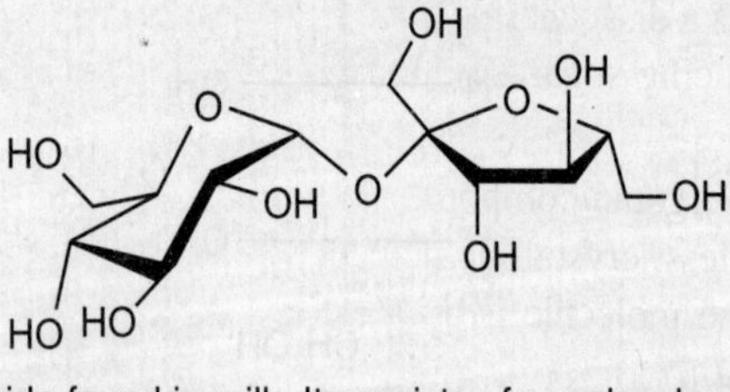

Fig. 5.4: Sucrose is a disaccharide found in milk. It consists of a molecule of D-galactose and a molecule of D-glucose bonded by α-1,4-glycosidic linkage.

The systematic name for sucrose, O-α-D-glucopyranosyl-(1→2)-D-fructofuranoside, indicates four things:

1. Its monosaccharides: Glucose and fructose.
2. How they are linked together: The oxygen on carbon number 1 (C1) of α-D-glucose is linked to the C_2 of D-fructose.

3. Their ring types: Glucose is a pyranose and fructose is a furanose.

4. The -oside suffix indicates that the anomeric carbon of both monosaccharides participates in the glycosidic bond.

Lactose, a disaccharide composed of one D-galactose molecule and one D-glucose molecule, occurs naturally in mammalian milk. The systematic name for lactose is O-β-D-galactopyranosyl-(1→4)-D-glucopyranose. Other notable disaccharides include maltose (two D-glucoses linked α-1,4) and cellulobiose (two D-glucoses linked β-1,4). Some of the important disaccharides are discussed below.

Cellobiose: Cellobiose is a disaccharide with the formula $[HOCH_2CHO(CHOH)_3]_2O$. The molecule is derived from the condensation of two glucose molecules linked in a β(1→4) bond. It can be hydrolysed by bacteria or cationic ion exchange resins to give glucose. Cellobiose has eight free alcohol (COH) groups and three ether linkages, which give rise to strong inter- and intramolecular hydrogen bonds.

It can be obtained by enzymatic or acidic hydrolysis of cellulose and cellulose rich materials such as cotton, jute or paper. Cellulose is a polymer of glucose units linked by β(1→4) bonds. Treatment of cellulose with acetic anhydride and sulphuric acid, gives cellobiose octoacetate, which cannot engage in hydrogen bonding and is soluble in nonpolar organic solvents.

Maltose: Maltose or malt sugar, is a disaccharide formed from two units of glucose joined with an α(1→4) bond. The isomer 'isomaltose' has two glucose molecules linked through an α(1→6) bond. Maltose is the second member of an important biochemical series of glucose chains. Maltose is the disaccharide produced when amylase breaks down starch. It is found in germinating seeds such as barley as they break down their starch stores to use for food. The addition of another glucose unit yields maltotriose, further additions will produce dextrins (also called maltodextrins) and eventually starch (glucose polymer). Maltose can be broken down into two glucose molecules by hydrolysis. In living organisms, the enzyme maltase can achieve this very rapidly. In the laboratory, heating with a strong acid for several minutes will produce the same result. Isomaltose is broken by isomaltase.

The production of maltose from germinating cereals, such as barley, is an important part of the brewing process. When barley is malted, it is brought into a condition in which the concentration of maltose-producing amylases has been maximised. Mashing is the process by which these amylases convert the cereal's starches into maltose. Metabolism of maltose by yeast during fermentation then leads to the production of ethanol and carbon dioxide.

Isomaltose: Isomaltose is a disaccharide similar to maltose, but with a α-(1-6)-linkage instead of the α-(1-4)-linkage. It is a reducing sugar. The linkage between the sugars is 1,6. Both of the sugars are glucose and pyranoses.

Sucrose: Sucrose is the organic compound commonly known as table sugar and sometimes called saccharose. A white, odourless, crystalline powder with a pleasing, sweet taste, it is best known for its role in human nutrition. The molecule is a disaccharide derived from glucose and fructose with the molecular formula $C_{12}H_{22}O_{11}$.

Trehalose: Trehalose, also known as mycose or tremalose, is a natural alpha-linked disaccharide formed by an α,α-1,1-glucoside bond between two α-glucose units. It can be synthesised by fungi, plants, and invertebrate animals. It is implicated in anhydrobiosis—the ability of plants and animals to withstand prolonged periods of desiccation. It has high water retention capabilities, and is used in food and cosmetics. The sugar is thought to form a gel phase as cells dehydrate, which prevents disruption of internal cell organelles, by effectively splinting them in position. Rehydration then allows normal cellular activity to be resumed without the major, lethal damage that would normally follow a dehydration/

rehydration cycle. Trehalose has the added advantage of being an antioxidant. Extracting trehalose used to be a difficult and costly process, but, recently, the Hayashibara company (Okayama, Japan) confirmed an inexpensive extraction technology from starch for mass production. Trehalose is currently being used for a broad spectrum of applications.

Trisaccharide: Trisaccharides are oligosaccharides composed of three mono-saccharides with two glycosidic bonds connecting them. Similar to the disaccharides, each glycosidic bond can be formed between any hydroxyl group on the component monosaccharides. Even if all three component sugars are the same (e.g. glucose), different bond combinations (regiochemistry) and stereochemistry (alpha- or beta-) result in trisaccharides that are diastereoisomers with different chemical and physical properties.

Homopolysaccharide: Homopolysaccharides are Polysaccharide (polymers) composed of a single type of sugar monomer. For example, cellulose is an unbranched homopolysaccharide made up of glucose monomers connected, via., beta-glycosidic linkages, glycogen is a branched form, where the glucose monomers are joined by alpha-glycosidic linkages.

Polysaccharide

Polysaccharides are polymeric carbohydrate structures, formed of repeating units (either mono- or di-saccharides) joined together by glycosidic bonds. These structures are often linear, but may contain various degrees of branching. Polysaccharides are often quite heterogeneous, containing slight modifications of the repeating unit. Depending on the structure, these macromolecules can have distinct properties from their monosaccharide building blocks. They may be amorphous or even insoluble in water.

When all the monosaccharides in a polysaccharide are the same type the polysaccharide is called a homopolysaccharide, but when more than one type of monosaccharide is present they are called heteropolysaccharides. Examples include storage polysaccharides such as starch and glycogen, and structural polysaccharides such as cellulose and chitin. Polysaccharides have a general formula of $C_x(H_2O)_y$ where, x is usually a large number between 200 and 2500. Considering that the repeating units in the polymer backbone are often six-carbon monosaccharides, the general formula can also be represented as $(C_6H_{10}O_5)_n$ where, $40 \leq n \leq 3000$. Some of important polysaccharide are discussed below.

Starches: Starches are glucose polymers in which glucopyranose units are bonded by alpha-linkages. It is made up of a mixture of Amylose (15–20 per cent) and Amylopectin (80–85 per cent). Amylose consists of a linear chain of several hundred glucose molecules and Amylopectin is a branched molecule made of several thousand glucose units (every chain 24–30 glucose unit). Starches are insoluble in water. They can be digested by hydrolysis, catalysed by enzymes called amylases, which can break the alpha-linkages (glycosidic bonds). Humans and other animals have amylases, so they can digest starches. Potato, rice, wheat, and maize are major sources of starch in the human diet. The formation of starches are the way that plants store glucose.

Glycogen: Glycogen is the molecule that functions as the secondary long-term energy storage in animal and fungi cells. It is made primarily by the liver and the muscles, but can also be made by glycogenesis within the brain and stomach.

Glycogen is the analogue of starch, a less branched glucose polymer in plants, and is commonly referred to as animal starch, having a similar structure to amylopectin. Glycogen is found in the form of granules in the cytosol in many cell types, and plays an important role in the glucose cycle. Glycogen forms an energy reserve that can be quickly mobilised to meet a sudden need for glucose, but one that is less compact than the energy reserves of triglycerides (lipids). In the liver hepatocytes, glycogen can compose up to 8 per cent of the fresh weight (100–120 g in an adult) soon after a meal. Only the glycogen stored in the liver can be made accessible to other organs. In the muscles, glycogen is found in a low concentration (1 to 2 per cent of the muscle mass). However, the amount of glycogen stored in the body, especially within the red blood cells, liver and muscles, mostly depends on physical training, basal metabolic rate and eating habits such as intermittent fasting. Small amounts of glycogen are found in the kidneys, and even smaller amounts in certain glial cells in the brain and white blood cells. The uterus also stores glycogen during pregnancy to nourish the embryo. As a meal containing carbohydrates is eaten and digested, blood glucose levels rise, and the pancreas secretes insulin. Glucose from the portal vein enters liver cells (hepatocytes). Insulin acts on the hepatocytes to stimulate the action of several enzymes, including glycogen synthase. Glucose molecules are added to the chains of glycogen as long as both insulin and glucose remain plentiful. In this postprandial or 'fed' state, the liver takes in more glucose from the blood than it releases. After a meal has been digested and glucose levels begin to fall, insulin secretion is reduced, and glycogen synthesis stops. When it is needed for energy, glycogen is broken down and converted again to glucose. Glycogen phosphorylase is the primary enzyme of glycogen breakdown. For the next 8–12 hr, glucose derived from liver glycogen will be the primary source of blood glucose to be used by the rest of the body for fuel.

Glucagon is another hormone produced by the pancreas, which in many respects serves as a counter-signal to insulin. When the blood sugar begins to fall below normal, glucagon is secreted in increasing amounts. It stimulates glycogen breakdown into glucose even when insulin levels are abnormally high.

Structural polysaccharides

Cellulose: The structural component of plants are formed primarily from cellulose. Wood is largely cellulose and lignin, while paper and cotton are nearly pure cellulose. Cellulose is a polymer made with repeated glucose units bonded together by beta-linkages. Humans and many other animals lack an enzyme to break the beta-linkages, so they do not digest cellulose. Certain animals can digest cellulose, because bacteria possessing the enzyme are present in their gut. The classic example is the termite.

Chitin: Chitin is one of many naturally occurring polymers. It is one of the most abundant natural materials in the world. Over time it is biodegradable in the natural environment. Its breakdown may be catalysed by enzymes called chitinases, secreted by micro-organisms such as bacteria and fungi, and produced by some plants. Some of these micro-organisms have receptors to simple sugars from the decomposition of chitin. If chitin is detected, they then produce enzymes to digest it by cleaving the glycosidic bonds in order to convert it to simple sugars and ammonia. Chemically, chitin is closely related to chitosan (a more water-soluble derivative of chitin). It is also closely related to cellulose in that it is a long unbranched chain of glucose derivatives. Both materials contribute structure and strength, protecting the organism.

Arabinoxylans: Arabinoxylans are the copolymers of two pentose sugars—arabinose and xylose.

Acidic polysaccharides: Acidic polysaccharides are polysaccharides that contain carboxyl groups, phosphate groups and/or sulphuric ester groups. Some other polysaccharides are also briefly discussed.

Amylose: Amylose is a linear polymer made up of D-glucose units. This polysaccharide is one of the two components of starch, making up approximately 20–30 per cent of the structure. The other component is amylopectin, which makes up 70–80 per cent of the structure. Because of its tightly packed structure, amylose is more resistant to digestion than other starch molecules and is, therefore, an important form of resistant starch which has been found to be an effective prebiotic. Amylose is made up of $\alpha(1{\to}4)$ bound glucose molecules. The carbon atoms on glucose are numbered, starting at the aldehyde (C=O) carbon, so in amylose, the 1-carbon on one glucose molecule is linked to the 4-carbon on the next glucose molecule [$\alpha(1\rightarrow4)$ bonds]. Unlike amylopectin, amylose is insoluble in water. It also reduces the crystallinity of amylopectin and how easily water can infiltrate the starch.

Amylopectin: Amylopectin is a soluble polysaccharide and highly branched polymer of glucose found in plants. It is one of the two components of starch, the other being amylose. Glucose units are linked in a linear way with $\alpha(1\rightarrow4)$ glycosidic bonds. Branching takes place with $\alpha(1\rightarrow6)$ bonds occurring every 24 to 30 glucose units. In contrast, amylose contains very few $\alpha(1\rightarrow6)$ bonds which causes it to be hydrolysed more slowly but have higher density.

Plants store starch within specialised organelles called amyloplasts. When energy is needed for cell work, the plant hydrolyses the starch releasing the glucose subunits. Humans and other animals that eat plant foods also use amylase, an enzyme that assists in breaking down amylopectin.

Amylopectin is highly branched, being formed of 2,000 to 2,00,000 glucose units. Its inner chains are formed of 20–24 glucose subunits.

Dextrin: Dextrins are a group of low-molecular-weight carbohydrates produced by the hydrolysis of starch or glycogen. Dextrins are mixtures of polymers of D-glucose units linked by α-(1,4) or α-(1,6) glycosidic bonds.

Dextrins can be produced from starch using enzymes like amylases, as during digestion in the human body and during malting and mashing or by applying dry heat under acidic conditions (pyrolysis or roasting). The latter process is used industrially, and also occurs on the surface of bread during the baking process, contributing to flavour, colour and crispness. Dextrins produced by heat are also known as pyrodextrins. During roasting under acid condition the starch hydrolyses and short chained starch parts partially rebranches with α-(1,6) bonds to the degraded starch molecule.

Dextrins are white, yellow or brown powders that are partially or fully water-soluble, yielding optically active solutions of low viscosity. Most can be detected with iodine solution, giving a red colouration, one distinguishes erythrodextrin (dextrin that colours red) and achrodextrin (giving no colour). White and yellow dextrins from starch roasted with little or no acid is called British gum. Yellow dextrins are used as water-soluble glues in remoistable envelope adhesives and paper tubes, in the mining industry as additives in froth flotation, in the foundry industry as green strength additives in sand casting, as printing thickener for batik resist dyeing and as binders in gouache paint.

Cellulose: Cellulose is an organic compound with the formula $(C_6H_{10}O_5)_n$, a polysaccharide consisting of a linear chain of several hundred to over nine thousand $\beta(1\rightarrow4)$ linked D-glucose units.

Cellulose is the structural component of the primary cell wall of green plants, many forms of algae and the oomycetes. Some species of bacteria secrete it to form biofilms. Cellulose is the most common organic compound on earth. About 33 per cent of all plant matter is cellulose (the cellulose content of cotton is 90 per cent and that of wood is 40–50 per cent). For industrial use, cellulose is mainly obtained from wood pulp and cotton. It is mainly used to produce paperboard and paper, to a smaller extent it is converted into a wide variety of derivative products such as cellophane and rayon. Converting cellulose from energy crops into biofuels such as cellulosic ethanol is under investigation as an alternative fuel source. Some animals, particularly ruminants and termites, can digest cellulose with the help of symbiotic micro-organisms that live in their guts. Humans can digest cellulose to some extent, however it is often referred to as 'dietary fibre' or 'roughage' (e.g. outer shell of maize) and acts as a hydrophilic bulking agent for feces.

Bacterial polysaccharides: Bacterial polysaccharides represent a diverse range of macromolecules that include peptidoglycan, lipopolysaccharides, capsules and exopolysaccharides, compounds whose functions range from structural cell-wall components (e.g. peptidoglycan), and important virulence factors (e.g. Poly-N-acetyl-glucosamine in *S. aureus*), to permitting the bacterium to survive in harsh environments (e.g. *Pseudomonas aeruginosa* in the human lung). Polysaccharide biosynthesis is a tightly regulated, energy-intensive process and understanding the subtle interplay between the regulation and energy conservation, polymer modification and synthesis, and the external ecological functions is a huge area of research. The potential benefits are enormous and should enable for example the development of novel antibacterial strategies (e.g. new antibiotics and vaccines) and the commercial exploitation to develop novel applications.

Bacterial capsular polysaccharides: Pathogenic bacteria commonly produce a thick, mucous-like, layer of polysaccharide. This capsule cloaks antigenic proteins on the bacterial surface that would otherwise provoke an immune response and thereby lead to the destruction of the bacteria. Capsular polysaccharides are water soluble, commonly acidic, and have molecular weights on the order of 100–1000 kDa. They are linear and consist of regularly repeating subunits of one to six monosaccharides. There is enormous structural diversity, nearly two hundred different polysaccharides are produced by *E. coli* alone. Mixtures of capsular polysaccharides, either conjugated or native are used as vaccines. Bacteria and many other microbes, including fungi and algae, often secrete polysaccharides as an evolutionary adaptation to help them adhere to surfaces and to prevent them from drying out. Humans have developed some of these polysaccharides into useful products, including xanthan gum, dextran, welan gum, gellan gum, diutan gum and pullulan.

Most of these polysaccharides exhibit interesting and very useful visco-elastic properties when dissolved in water at very low levels. This gives many foods and various liquid consumer products, like lotions, cleaners and paints, for example, a viscous appearance when stationary, but fluidity when the slightest shear is applied, such as when wiped, poured or brushed. This property is referred to as pseudoplasticity, or shear thinning. Aqueous solutions of the polysaccharide alone have a curious behaviour when stirred. After stopping, the swirl continues due to momentum, then stops, and then reverses direction briefly. This recoil demonstrates the elastic effect of the polysaccharide chains previously stretched in solution, returning to their relaxed state.

Cell-surface polysaccharides play diverse roles in bacterial ecology and physiology. They serve as a barrier between the cell wall and the environment, mediate host-pathogen interactions, and form structural components of biofilms. These polysaccharides are synthesised from nucleotide-activated precursors (called nucleotide sugars) and, in most cases, all the enzymes necessary for biosynthesis, assembly and transport of the completed polymer are encoded by genes organised in dedicated clusters within the genome of the organism. Lipopolysaccharide is one of the most important cell-surface polysaccharides, as it plays a key structural role in outer membrane integrity, as well as being an important mediator of host-pathogen interactions. The enzymes that make the *A-band* (homopolymeric) and *B-band* (heteropolymeric) *O*-antigens have been identified and the metabolic pathways defined. The exopolysaccharide alginate is a linear copolymer of β-1,4-linked D-mannuronic acid and L-guluronic acid residues, and is responsible for the mucoid phenotype of late-stage cystic fibrosis disease. The *pel* and *psl* loci are two recently discovered gene clusters that also encode exopolysaccharides found to be important for biofilm formation. Rhamnolipid is a biosurfactant whose production is tightly regulated at the transcriptional level, but the precise role that it plays in disease is not well understood at present. Protein glycosylation, particularly of pilin and flagellin, is a recent focus of research by several groups and it has been shown to be important for adhesion and invasion during bacterial infection.

Glycosaminoglycan: Glycosaminoglycans (GAGs) or mucopolysaccharides are long unbranched polysaccharides consisting of a repeating disaccharide unit. The repeating unit consists of a hexose (six-carbon sugar) or a hexuronic acid, linked to a hexosamine (six-carbon sugar containing nitrogen). Protein cores made in the rough endoplasmic reticulum are post-translationally modified by glycosyltransferases in the Golgi apparatus, where GAG disaccharides are added to protein cores to yield proteoglycans, the exception is the GAG hyaluronan, which is uniquely synthesised without a protein core and is 'spun out' by enzymes at the cell surface directly into the extracellular space. This family of carbohydrates is essential or important for life. GAGs form an important component of connective tissues. GAG chains may be covalently linked to a protein to form proteoglycans. Water sticks to GAGs, this is where the resistance to pressure comes from. The density of sugar molecules and the net negative charges attract cations, for example, Na^+, which, after the sodium binds, attracts water molecules.

Some examples, of glycosaminoglycan uses in nature include heparin as an anti-coagulant, hyaluronan as a component in the synovial fluid lubricant in body joints, and chondroitins, which can be found in connective tissues, cartilage, and tendons. Members of the glycosaminoglycan family vary in the type of hexosamine, hexose or hexuronic acid unit they contain (e.g. glucuronic acid, iduronic acid, galactose, galactosamine, glucosamine). They also vary in the geometry of the glycosidic linkage.

Oligosaccharide

An oligosaccharide is a saccharide polymer containing a small number (typically three to ten) of component sugars, also known as simple sugars (monosaccharides). The name is derived from the Greek word oligos, meaning 'a few', and from the Latin/Greek word sacchar which means 'sugar'. Oligosaccharides can have many functions, for example, they are commonly found on the plasma membrane of animal cells where they can play a role in cell-cell recognition. They are generally found either O- or N-linked to compatible amino acid side chains in proteins or to lipid moieties.

Fructo-oligosaccharides (FOS), which are found in many vegetables, consist of short chains of fructose molecules. (Inulin has a much higher degree of polymerisation than FOS and is a polysaccharide.) Galactooligosaccharides (GOS), which also occur naturally, consist of short chains of galactose molecules. These compounds can be only partially digested by humans. Oligosaccharides are often found as a component of glycoproteins or glycolipids and as such are often used as chemical markers, often for cell recognition. An example is ABO blood type specificity. A and B blood types have two different oligosaccharide glycolipids embedded in the cell membranes of the red blood cells, AB-type blood has both, while O blood type has neither.

Mannan-oligosaccharides (MOS) are widely used in animal feed to encourage gastrointestinal health and performance. They are normally obtained from the yeast cell walls of *Saccharomyces cerevisiae*. Some brand names are: CitriStim, Bio-Mos, SAF-Mannan, Y-MOS and Celmanax. When oligosaccharides are consumed, the undigested portion serves as food for the intestinal microflora. Depending on the type of oligosaccharide, different bacterial groups are stimulated or suppressed.

Clinical studies have shown that administering FOS, GOS or inulin can increase the number of these friendly bacteria in the colon while simultaneously reducing the population of harmful bacteria. Not all natural oligosaccharides occur as components of glycoproteins or glycolipids. Some, such as the raffinose series, occur as storage or transport carbohydrates in plants. Others, such as maltodextrins or cellodextrins, result from the microbial breakdown of larger polysaccharides such as starch or cellulose.

Glycoproteins

Glycoproteins are proteins that contain oligosaccharide chains covalently attached to polypeptide side-chains. The carbohydrate is attached to the protein in a cotranslational or post-translational modification.

This process is known as glycosylation. In proteins that have segments extending extracellularly, the extracellular segments are often glycosylated. Glycoproteins are often important integral membrane proteins, where they play a role in cell-cell interactions. Glycoproteins also occur in the cytosol, but their functions and the pathways producing these modifications in this compartment are less well-understood.

N-glycosylation and O-glycosylation: There are two types of glycoproteins:

1. In *N*-glycosylation, the addition of sugar chains can happen at the amide nitrogen on the side chain of the asparagine.

2. In *O*-glycosylation, the addition of sugar chains can happen on the hydroxyl oxygen on the side chain of hydroxylysine, hydroxyproline, serine, or threonine.

Examples: One example of glycoproteins found in the body is mucins, which are secreted in the mucus of the respiratory and digestive tracts. The sugars attached to mucins give them considerable water-holding capacity and also make them resistant to proteolysis by digestive enzymes.

Glycoproteins are important for white blood cell recognition, especially in mammals. Examples of glycoproteins in the immune system are:

1. Molecules such as antibodies (immunoglobulins), which interact directly with antigens.

2. Molecules of the major histocompatibility complex (or MHC), which are expressed on the surface of cells and interact with T cells as part of the adaptive immune response.

Other examples of glycoproteins include:

1. Glycoprotein IIb/IIIa, an integrin found on platelets that is required for normal platelet aggregation and adherence to the endothelium.

2. Components of the zona pellucida, which surrounds the oocyte, and is important for sperm-egg interaction.

3. Structural glycoproteins, which occur in connective tissue. These help bind together the fibres, cells, and ground substance of connective tissue. They may also help components of the tissue bind to inorganic substances, such as calcium in bone.

4. Glycoprotein-41 (gp41) and glycoprotein-120 (gp120) are HIV viral coat proteins.

Soluble glycoproteins often show a high viscosity, for example, in egg white and blood plasma.

Hormones: Hormones that are glycoproteins include:

1. Follicle-stimulating hormone.

2. Luteinising hormone.

3. Thyroid-stimulating hormone.

4. Human chorionic gonadotropin.

5. Alpha-fetoprotein.

6. Erythropoietin (EPO).

AMINO ACIDS AND PROTEINS

It is well known that cells utilise energy to overcome the general tendency toward disorder. No class of molecules in the cell is more important than the proteins in mediating the reactions and forming the structures that generate order in organisms. Proteins are the workhorses of the cell. The Swedish chemist Berzelius suggested the name 'protein', derived from the Greek noun *protios*, meaning 'holding the first place'. His suggestion was inspired by observations and deductions made by the Dutch chemist Gerardus

Mulder. Mulder had been able to extract very similar nitrogen-rich substances from both animal and plant sources and had guessed that these substances, whatever their other properties, must be important simply because their occurrence is so widespread and they are so abundant in tissues. Half and more of the dry weight of many cells is in fact protein.

Functions of Proteins

Most of the functions of proteins fall into the categories of binding, catalysis, conduction or transport, contraction, nutrition and/or structure. Often, a protein will have more than one of these functions and the categories are in any case not mutually exclusive. Consider some examples of binding. A protein that binds to a specific portion of a nucleic acid molecule may be able to control the expression of the genetic information encoded in nearby regions of that molecule. A cell surface protein receptor that binds insulin molecules may be able, in effect, to let the cell 'sense' the concentration of insulin in its environment, providing a link between the hormone and the hormone's action. Serum antifreeze proteins that are crucial to the survival of certain cold water fishes appear to act by binding to the surface of ice crystals.

The tremendous variety of chemical reactions within the cell must all be carried out within the narrow ranges of temperature, pH and so on, under which the cell is active. The cell does not have the option of using extremes of temperature or pH to facilitate a reaction. Instead, catalysts of specific reactions are used. Virtually all of the important catalysts of the cell are proteins: the enzymes. Enzymes, of course, bind the molecules on which they act, but they also transform them, breaking and making covalent and non-covalent bonds. Without enzymes, clearly there would be no metabolism. Some proteins facilitate the movement of compounds through cell membranes. The movement may be passive, a conduction of the substance through the membrane from a concentrated to a less concentrated solution. However, often the transport is active. In an energy-requiring process, a substance moves against a gradient of its concentration. Conduction and transport involve binding and contribute to such processes as nutrient uptake and nerve conduction.

Contraction is, of course, a property of muscles. Muscles are principally protein and it is the sliding motion of muscle proteins, one relative to the other, that is responsible for contraction of muscles. Some proteins contribute to motion and coordination directly through their contraction.

The storage proteins of seeds supply much of the necessary nitrogen and energy to support growth of the plant until it can be supported by photosynthesis. Prolamins, the most abundant class of cereal storage proteins, make up a significant fraction of the protein consumed by man and domestic animals. Collagen, a fibrous protein of skin and bone, is just one example of the many structural proteins. Thus, proteins influence almost every facet of the cell's activity.

Proteins as Polymers of Amino Acids

The abundance of proteins and their relatively high content of nitrogen, roughly 15 to 18 per cent by weight, brought them to the attention of pioneering biochemists. Nitrogen is an essential constituent of proteins because proteins are polymers of amino acids. Because the amino group is on the carbon atom adjacent to the carboxyl group, the amino acids having this general formula are known as α-amino acids. It is also apparent that if R in this structure is not equal to H, the α-carbon atom is asymmetric.

The α-amino acids are chiral or 'optically active' compounds. It is well-known that all the naturally occurring amino acids found in proteins have the same configuration. With respect to the reference compound for carbohydrates, D-glyceraldehyde, the amino acids that occur in proteins have the opposite or L-configuration. This relationship is shown in Structure 5.1 where, in the ball-and-stick model and the Fischer projection, the amino group of L-serine is on the left when the carboxyl group is written at the top of the formula. An early accomplishment in biochemistry was the conversion of L-serine into L-glyceraldehyde by a series of chemical reactions that did not modify the configuration of the α-carbon atom. In this way, the absolute configuration of L-serine was established. Other amino acids are compared, for absolute configuration about the α-carbon atom, to L-serine as the reference compound. (When reference is made to the absolute configuration of L-serine rather than to the actual optical rotation of the amino acid, the notation L_s is often used.) Note that the amino group is below the α-carbon atom in the structure of an L-amino acid when the carboxyl group is written to the right in the projection formula. As with the carbohydrates, it is important to stress that the use of L and D conventions refers only to the relative configuration of these compounds and does not provide any information regarding the direction in which these optically active compounds rotate polarised light. Note that the amino acids are represented in different ionic forms in Structures 5.1.

Ball-and-stick model

Fischer projection formula

L-Serine

D-Glyceraldehyde

Structure 5.1

The zwitterionic form of the amino acid, as represented in Structure 5.1, most closely represents the state of ionisation of the amino acids in solutions of neutral pH.

The fundamental structural unit of proteins is the α-amino acid is easily demonstrated by hydrolysing purified proteins by either chemical or enzymatic procedures. For example, a protein may be hydrolysed completely or nearly completely to its constituent amino acids in a period of 18 to 24 hr by the action of $6N$ HCl at 110°C in a sealed tube. Under these conditions, 17 of the 20 common protein amino acids are released in good yield. Isolating 17 distinct amino acids from a hydrolysate by crystallisation and other classical techniques of organic chemistry was a considerable accomplishment of pioneering biochemists. An amino acid analysis, which gives the relative amounts of the amino acids that survive the hydrolysis procedure, is an important step in the preliminary characterisation of a newly purified protein.

Early investigators realised, from certain physical properties of proteins, that they must be high molecular weight substances. High molecular weight substances already were well known in the chemistry laboratory. The tars that accumulate in some reactions and the colloidal substances formed by an electric arc between two metal electrodes under water are examples. Such high molecular weight substances are said to be 'polydisperse' because they are, in fact, mixtures of compounds of related chemical structure but highly variable size. Tars and colloidal substances, as well as haemoglobin and certain other oxygen-transporting proteins, all were examined by applying strong centrifugal fields to their solutions or suspensions. The relatively large size of the molecules in tars and proteins or the aggregates in colloidal substances caused them to move much more rapidly than low molecular solutes, such as salts, in the centrifugal field. However, purified proteins, such as haemoglobin, behaved very differently from tars and colloids. Only the proteins migrated in the centrifugal field in such a way as to give a sharp, discrete boundary. This was observed because proteins are high molecular weight compounds, meaning that they have a definite atomic composition. Each constituent of a tar or colloid will have its characteristic rate of sedimentation in the centrifugal field. However, since the constituents are of different sizes, no sharp, discrete boundary could be observed for these substances. The atomic composition of haemoglobin, stripped of its oxygen-bearing heme groups, is:

$$C_{2796}H_{4592}O_{832}N_{812}S_8$$

This atomic composition is typical of protein molecules, which usually are 30 to 33 per cent C, roughly 50 per cent H, 9 to 11 per cent O and 7 to 9 per cent N, with small amounts of S.

Primary Structure of Proteins

The covalent structure of a protein is essentially linear. Amino acids are connected together to form a chain, the connection being a peptide bond. The peptide bond is simply an amide bond between the carbonyl carbon of one amino acid and the amino nitrogen of another as shown below:

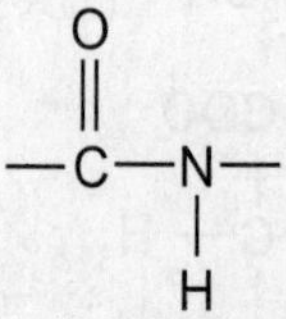

$$\begin{matrix} & O & & \\ & \parallel & & \\ -C & - & N & - \\ & & \mid & \\ & & H & \end{matrix}$$

Conceptually, the formation of the peptide bond may be considered to result from the removal of two protons and one oxygen atom (i.e. one molecule of water) from a pair of amino acids. In the reaction shown below, the oxygen atom may be considered to have been removed from the carboxylate group of amino acid 1 and two protons from the alkyl ammonium group of amino acid 2. The polypeptide character of a protein is shown in Fig. 5.5.

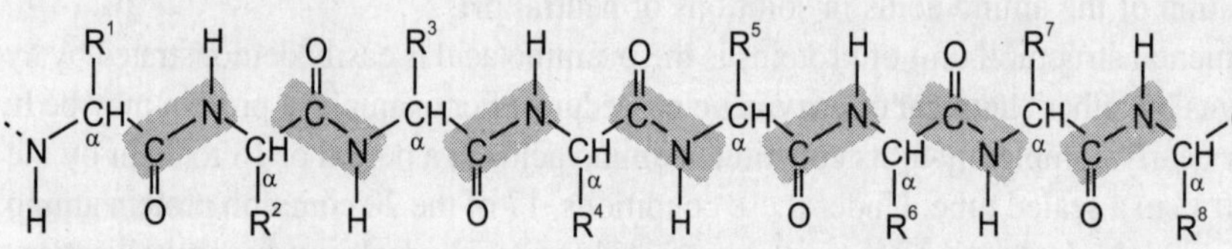

Fig. 5.5: A generalised structure of a polypeptide chain showing the linkage of adjacent amino acid residues through peptide bonds.

Obviously, there is no theoretical limit to the molecular weight attainable with such a chain structure and proteins vary in molecular weight from a few thousands to a few millions. When an amino acid has been incorporated into a polypeptide chain, it is referred to as an 'amino acid residue' rather than simply an amino acid. The reason for this is that water has been 'split out' in the process of forming the peptide bond, so that what remains does not correspond to the full structure of an amino acid. Twenty different amino acid residues account for the vast majority of protein structures. With the exception of the imino acid proline (whose structure follows), these all are α-amino acids, which means that they differ only in the R groups as given below:

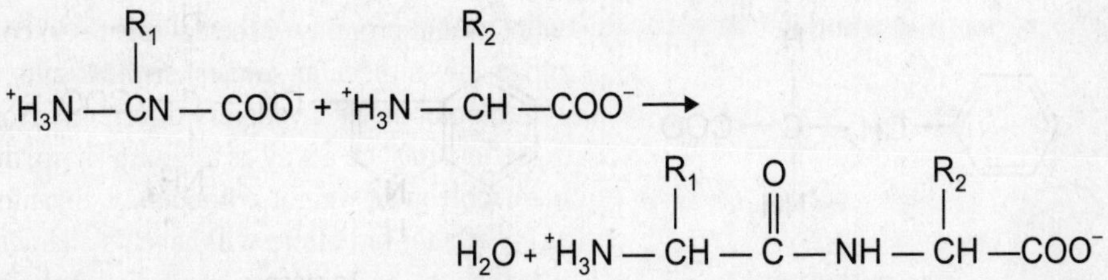

$$\overset{\displaystyle R_1}{\underset{\displaystyle |}{^+H_3N - CN - COO^-}} + \overset{\displaystyle R_2}{\underset{\displaystyle |}{^+H_3N - CH - COO^-}} \longrightarrow$$

$$H_2O + \overset{\displaystyle R_1}{\underset{\displaystyle |}{^+H_3N - CH}} - \overset{\displaystyle O}{\underset{\displaystyle ||}{C}} - NH - \overset{\displaystyle R_2}{\underset{\displaystyle |}{CH - COO^-}}$$

The average weight of a protein amino acid residue is approximately 110, which means that proteins have from a few tens to about ten thousand amino acid residues. The primary structure of a protein is simply the order of amino acid residues in the polypeptide chain. In the remainder of this section, we present the structures of the 20 common protein amino acids and of a few less common protein amino acids. These could be classified according to the chemical nature (aliphatic, aromatic, heterocyclic) of their R groups into appropriate sub-classes. More meaningful, however, is a classification-based on the polarity of the R group or residue because it emphasises the possible functional roles that the different amino acids can play in proteins and their possible contributions to the folding of the polypeptide chain. In this classification, the 20 amino acids commonly found in proteins may be described as:

1. Non-polar or hydrophobic.
2. Polar but uncharged.
3. Polar because of a negative charge at the physiological pH of 7.
4. Polar because of a positive charge at physiological pH.

Hydrophobic means 'water hating'. It is a term used to describe aliphatic and aromatic hydrocarbon compounds or portions of molecules or other chemical groups, that share the property of having only very limited solubility in water.

Amino Acids with Non-polar or Hydrophobic R Groups

This group contains amino acids with both aliphatic (alanine, valine, leucine, isoleucine, methionine) and aromatic (phenylalanine and tryptophan) residues that are understandably hydrophobic in character. One of the amino acids, proline, is unusual in that its nitrogen atom present is as a secondary rather than a primary amine. Thus, it is in fact an imino acid rather than an amino acid as shown below:

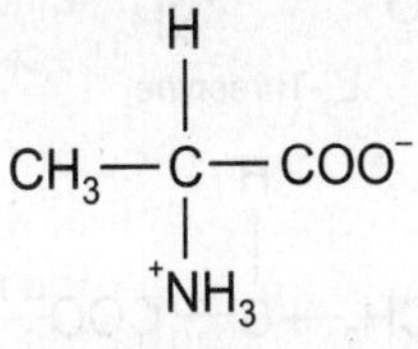

$$\overset{\displaystyle H}{\underset{\displaystyle ^+NH_3}{CH_3 - \overset{|}{\underset{|}{C}} - COO^-}} \qquad \overset{\displaystyle CH_3}{\underset{\displaystyle CH_3}{\diagdown}} \overset{\displaystyle H}{\underset{\displaystyle ^+NH_3}{CH - \overset{|}{\underset{|}{C}} - COO^-}} \qquad \overset{\displaystyle CH_3}{\underset{\displaystyle CH_3}{\diagdown}} \overset{\displaystyle H}{\underset{\displaystyle ^+NH_3}{CH - CH_2 - \overset{|}{\underset{|}{C}} - COO^-}}$$

$$L_s\text{-Alanine} \qquad\qquad L_s\text{-Valine} \qquad\qquad L_s\text{-Leucine}$$

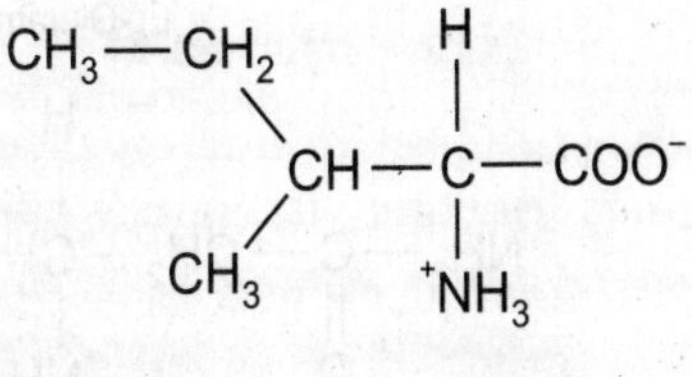

$$\overset{\displaystyle CH_3 - CH_2}{\underset{\displaystyle CH_3}{\diagdown\diagup}} \overset{\displaystyle H}{\underset{\displaystyle ^+NH_3}{CH - \overset{|}{\underset{|}{C}} - COO^-}} \qquad\qquad \begin{matrix} H_2C - CH_2 \\ | \quad\quad | \\ H_2C \quad CH - COO^- \\ \diagdown_{\underset{\displaystyle H_2}{N}}\diagup^{+} \end{matrix}$$

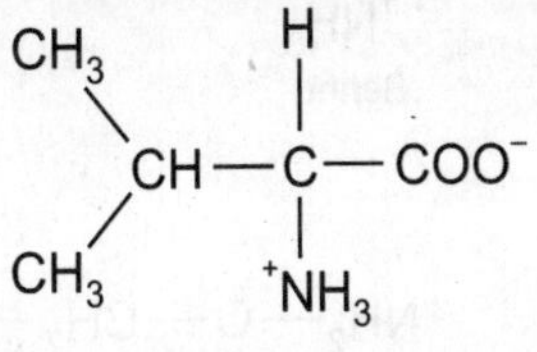

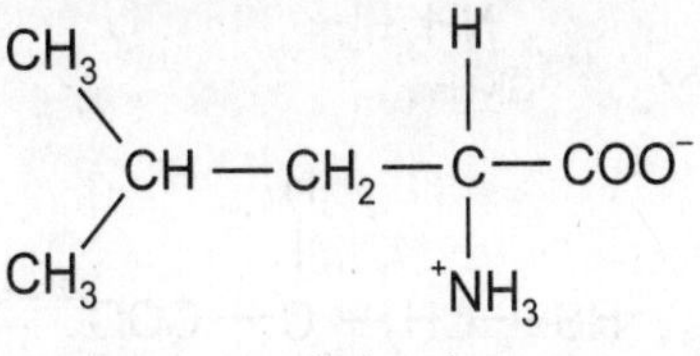

$$L_s\text{-Isoleucine} \qquad\qquad\qquad L_s\text{-Proline}$$

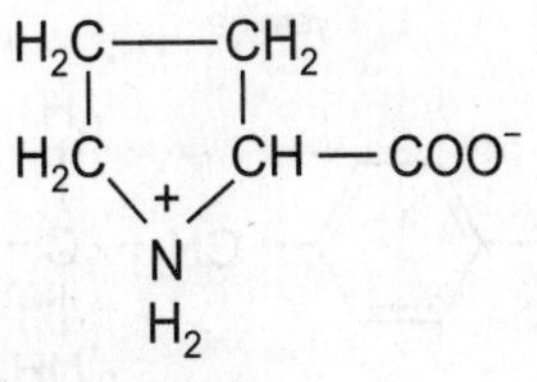

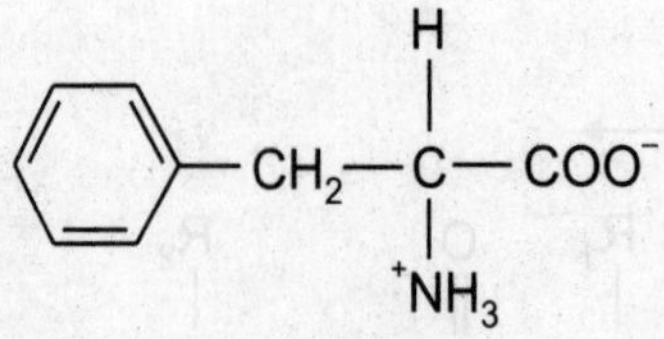

L_s-Phenylalanine

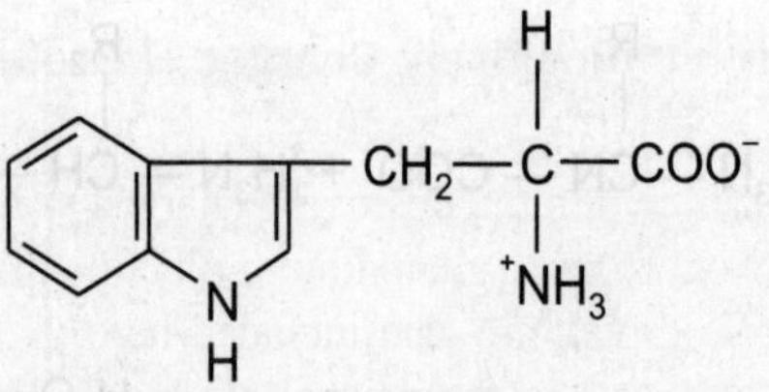

L_s-Tryptophan

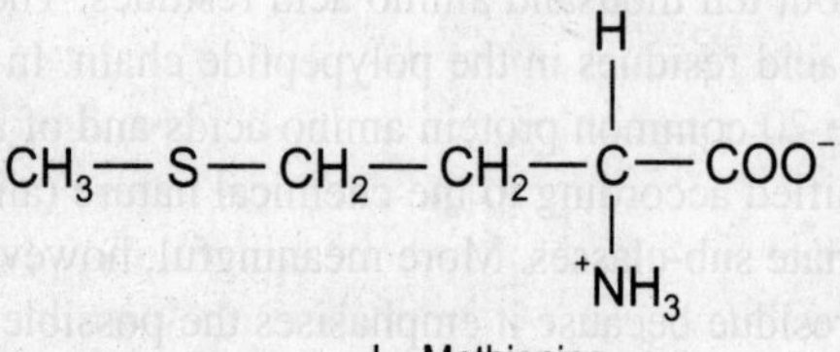

L_s-Methionine

$$CH_3 - S - CH_2 - CH_2 - \overset{\displaystyle H}{\underset{\displaystyle {}^+NH_3}{\overset{|}{\underset{|}{C}}}} - COO^-$$

Amino Acids with Polar, but Uncharged R Groups

Most of these amino acids contain polar R residues that can participate in hydrogen bond formation. A hydrogen bond is a highly ionic bond that results when two heteroatoms usually oxygen or nitrogen, but occasionally sulphur, share one proton. Several of the amino acids in this group possess a hydroxyl group (serine, threonine and tyrosine) or sulphydryl group (cysteine), while two (asparagine and glutamine) have amide groups.

Glycine, which lacks an R group, is included in this grouping because of its definite polar nature, a property it possesses because its carbonyl and amino nitrogen groups constitute such a large proportion of the mass of the glycine molecule. Both aliphatic and aromatic (tyrosine) compounds are included in this group as shown below:

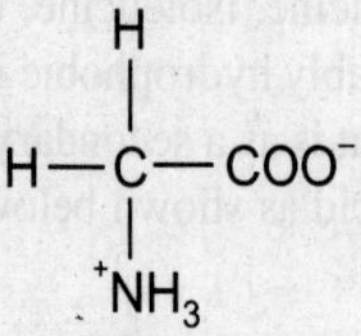

Glycine

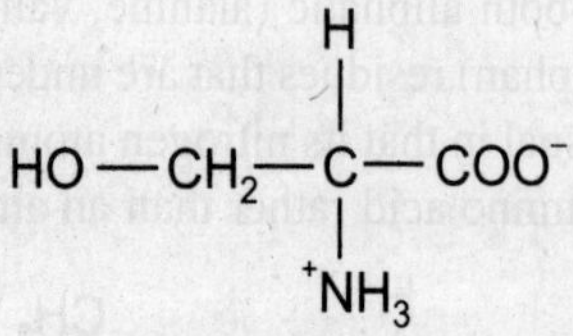

Serine

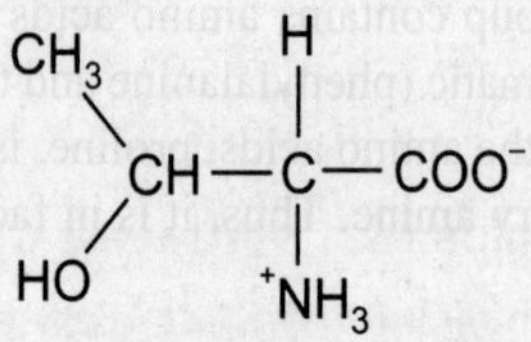

L_s-Threonine

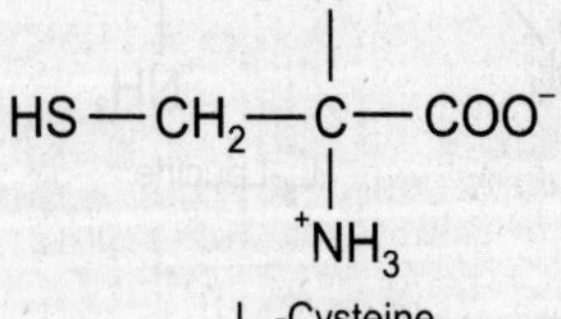

L_s-Cysteine

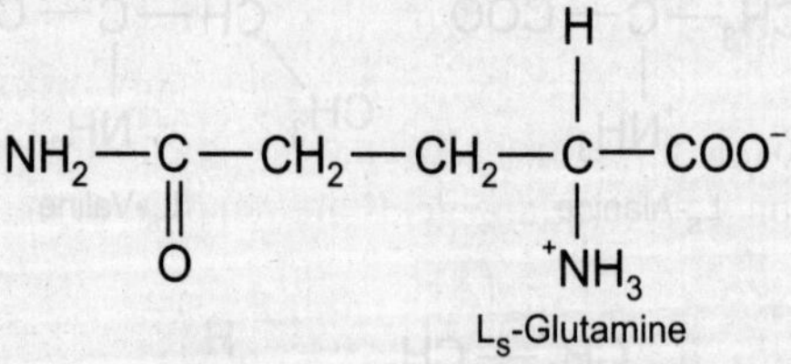

L_s-Glutamine

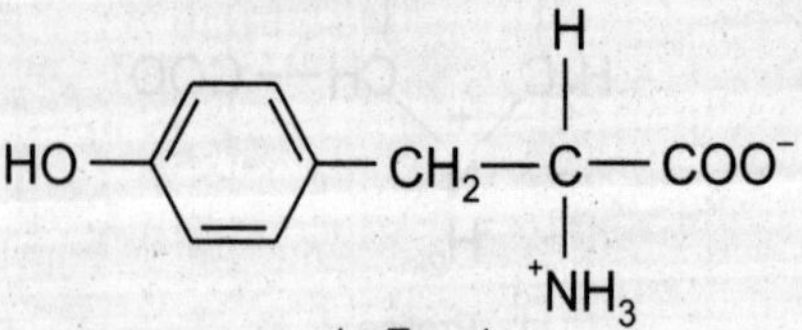

L_s-Tyrosine

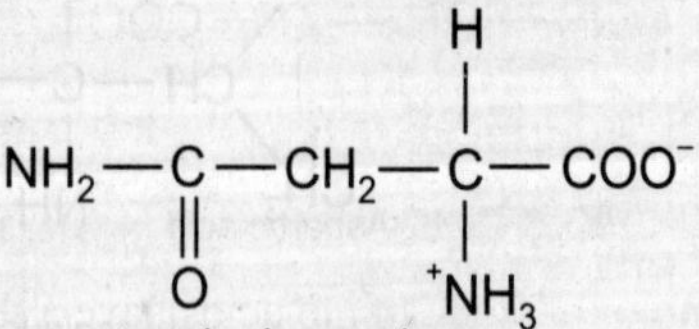

L_s-Asparagine

Amino Acids with Positively Charged R Groups

Three amino acids are included in this group. Lysine, with its second ε-amino group ($pK = 10.5$), will be more than 50 per cent in the positively charged state at any pH below the pK_a of that group. Arginine, containing a strongly basic guanidinium function ($pK_a = 12.5$) and histidine, with its weakly basic ($pK_a = 6.0$) imidazole group, are also included here. Note that histidine is the only amino acid that has a proton that dissociates in the neutral pH range. It is this characteristic that allows certain histidine residues to play an important role in the catalytic activities of some enzymes as shown below:

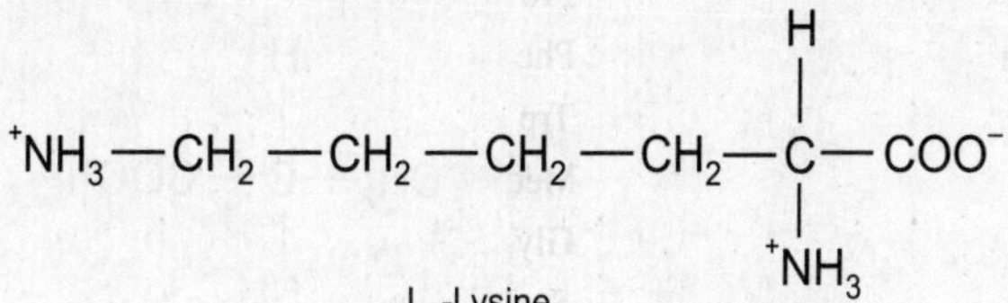

$$\overset{+}{N}H_3 - CH_2 - CH_2 - CH_2 - CH_2 - \overset{\overset{\displaystyle H}{|}}{\underset{\underset{\displaystyle \overset{+}{N}H_3}{|}}{C}} - COO^-$$

$$L_s\text{-Lysine}$$

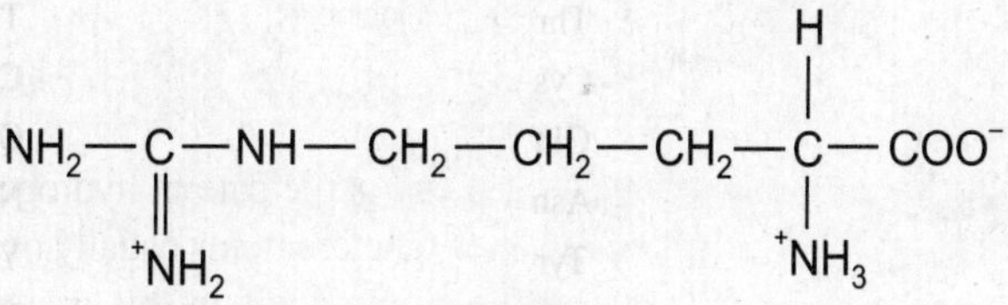

$$NH_2 - \overset{\overset{\displaystyle }{\|}}{\underset{\underset{\displaystyle \overset{+}{N}H_2}{}}{C}} - NH - CH_2 - CH_2 - CH_2 - \overset{\overset{\displaystyle H}{|}}{\underset{\underset{\displaystyle \overset{+}{N}H_3}{|}}{C}} - COO^-$$

$$L_s\text{-Arginine}$$

$$HC = C - CH_2 - \overset{\overset{\displaystyle H}{|}}{\underset{\underset{\displaystyle \overset{+}{N}H_3}{|}}{C}} - COO^-$$

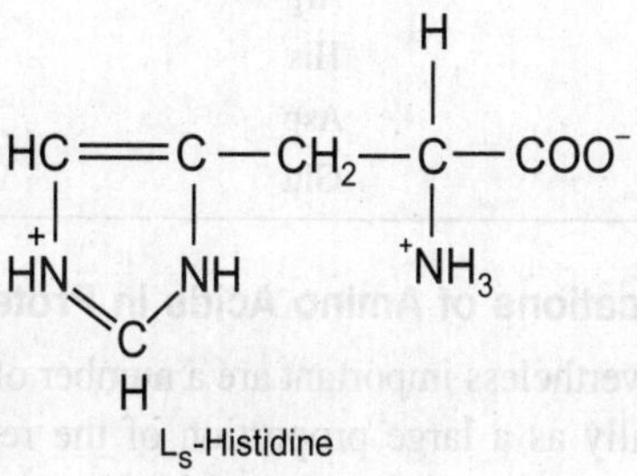

$$L_s\text{-Histidine}$$

Amino Acids with Negatively Charged R Groups

This group includes the two dicarboxylic amino acids, aspartic acid and glutamic acid. At neutral pH, their second carboxyl groups with pK_{a2}'s of 3.9 and 4.3, respectively, dissociate, giving a net charge of -1 to these compounds. These 20 amino acids constitute the bulk of the amino acids in the proteins of bacteria, plants and animals, illustrating the unity of living systems on our planet. The 20 side chains apparently provide a sufficient diversity of chemical reactivities and conformations of the polypeptide chain so that only these amino acids are required in most proteins as shown below:

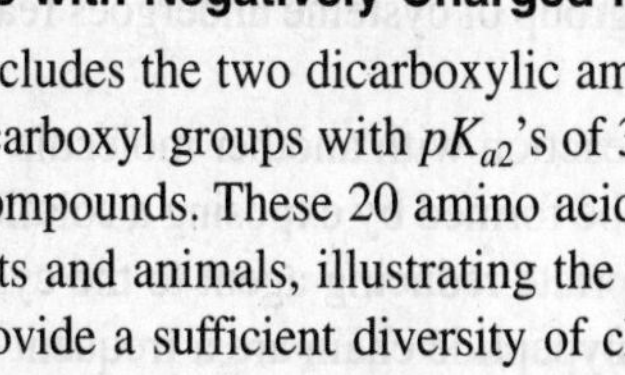

$$^-OOC - CH_2 - \overset{\overset{\displaystyle H}{|}}{\underset{\underset{\displaystyle \overset{+}{N}H_3}{|}}{C}} - COO^- \qquad ^-OOC - CH_2 - CH_2 - \overset{\overset{\displaystyle H}{|}}{\underset{\underset{\displaystyle \overset{+}{N}H_3}{|}}{C}} - COO^-$$

$$L_s\text{-Aspartic acid} \qquad\qquad L_s\text{-Glutamic acid}$$

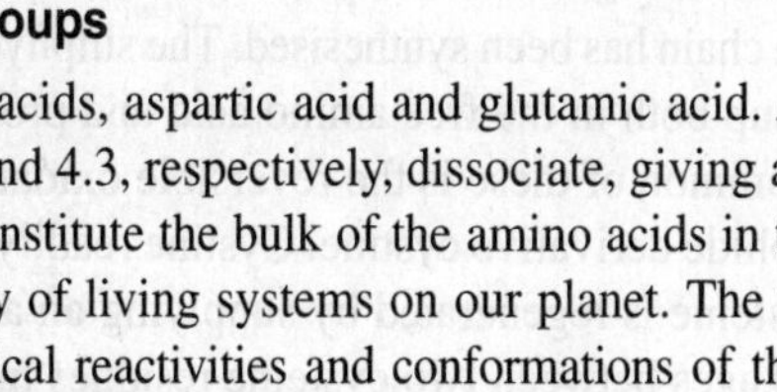

The 20 common protein amino acids have a standard set of three-letter and one-letter abbreviations for use in writing amino acid sequences in polypeptide chains (Table 5.2).

Table 5.2: Notations for 20 standard protein amino acids.

Amino acid	Three-letter symbol	One-letter symbol
Alanine	Ala	A
Valine	Val	V
Leucine	Leu	L
Isoleucine	Ile	I
Proline	Pro	P
Phenylalanine	Phe	F
Tryptophan	Trp	W
Methionine	Met	M
Glycine	Gly	G
Serine	Ser	S
Threonine	Thr	T
Cysteine	Cys	C
Glutamine	Gln	Q
Asparagine	Asn	N
Tyrosine	Tyr	Y
Lysine	Lys	K
Arginine	Arg	R
Histidine	His	H
Aspartate	Asp	D
Glutamate	Glu	E

Naturally Occurring Modifications of Amino Acids in Proteins

Less widely distributed but nevertheless important are a number of other amino acids that occur in only a few proteins, but occasionally as a large proportion of the residues in those few proteins. These additional amino acids are formed by modifications of the 20 common protein amino acids, usually after the polypeptide chain has been synthesised. The sulphydryl group of cysteine undergoes reactions typical of the –SH group both in the free amino acid and proteins.

The most common of these is the reversible oxidative reaction with another molecule of cysteine to form the disulphide derivative cystine. Cystine readily can be formed by exposing a solution of cysteine to oxygen. Cysteine is regenerated by supplying an appropriate reducing agent to the cystine solution. Disulphide linkages between two cysteine residues in a polypeptide chain are a frequent occurrence in protein structures, especially in proteins that are secreted into the extracellular environment where requirements of stability may be particularly stringent.

The ribonucleic acid degrading enzyme bovine pancreatic ribonuclease, for example, contains four disulphide bonds between four pairs of cysteine residues.

A second type of cysteine modification occurs in Cytochrome c, an electron transporting protein that contains an iron chelating heme group. Cytochrome c has a crucial role in biological reduction-oxidation reactions. Unlike many other heme proteins such as haemoglobin, cytochrome c covalently binds its heme group. Two cysteine residues are linked to the heme through thioether bonds. A second example of a protein amino acid that is modified in some proteins is proline, which is converted to hydroxyproline.

The structure to follow shows a disulphide bond connecting two portions of a polypeptide chain (or even two polypeptide chains):

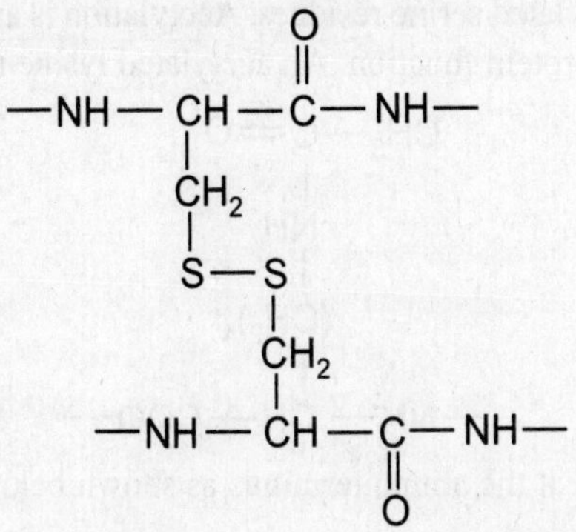

$$-NH-CH-\underset{\underset{O}{\|}}{C}-NH-$$
$$\qquad\ \ |$$
$$\qquad CH_2$$
$$\qquad\ \ |$$
$$\qquad S-S$$
$$\qquad\qquad |$$
$$\qquad\qquad CH_2$$
$$\qquad\qquad\ |$$
$$-NH-CH-\underset{\underset{O}{\|}}{C}-NH-$$

Hydroxyproline has a limited distribution in nature, but constitutes more than 12 per cent of the structure of collagen, an important structural protein of animals. Hydroxyproline also is an important constituent of the plant cell wall protein extensin and certain other plant proteins that appear to be involved in plant responses to pathogenic agents. The second amino acid shown here, hydroxylysine, also is a component of collagen.

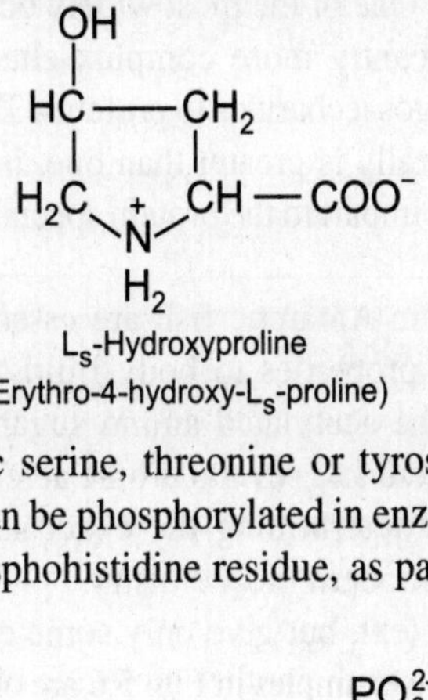

$$\begin{array}{c} OH \\ | \\ HC-CH_2 \\ H_2C\ \underset{\underset{H_2}{\overset{+}{N}}}{}\ CH-COO^- \end{array}$$

L$_s$-Hydroxyproline
(Erythro-4-hydroxy-L$_s$-proline)

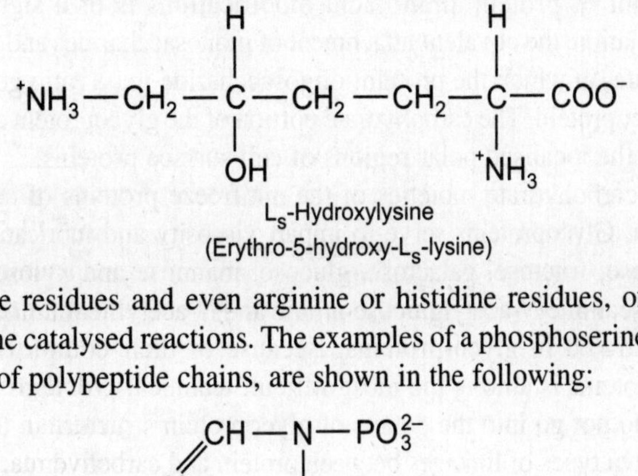

$$^+NH_3-CH_2-\underset{\underset{OH}{|}}{\overset{\overset{H}{|}}{C}}-CH_2-CH_2-\underset{\underset{^+NH_3}{|}}{\overset{\overset{H}{|}}{C}}-COO^-$$

L$_s$-Hydroxylysine
(Erythro-5-hydroxy-L$_s$-lysine)

Specific serine, threonine or tyrosine residues and even arginine or histidine residues, of certain proteins can be phosphorylated in enzyme catalysed reactions. The examples of a phosphoserine residue and a phosphohistidine residue, as part of polypeptide chains, are shown in the following:

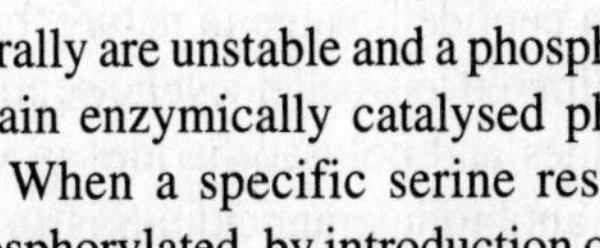

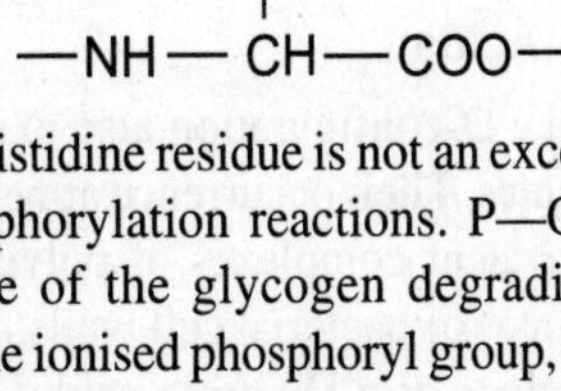

$$\begin{array}{c} PO_3^{2-} \\ | \\ O \\ | \\ CH_2 \\ | \\ -NH-CH-COO- \end{array}$$

$$\begin{array}{c} CH-N-PO_3^{2-} \\ N\diagup\qquad\qquad \\ CH=C \\ | \\ CH_2 \\ | \\ -NH-CH-COO- \end{array}$$

P—N bonds generally are unstable and a phosphohistidine residue is not an exception, it is an unstable intermediate in certain enzymically catalysed phosphorylation reactions. P—O bonds generally are much more stable. When a specific serine residue of the glycogen degrading enzyme glycogen phosphorylase is phosphorylated, by introduction of the ionised phosphoryl group, —OPO$_3^{2-}$, the enzyme is converted to a form that is much more active under physiological conditions. Many other examples are known of the regulation of the enzymic or other activity of proteins by phosphorylation, including proteins that bind to deoxyribonucleic acid and the glycolytic enzyme phosphoglucomutase. The milk protein casein contains many phosphorylated serine residues. Acetylation is another chemical modification that may result in the alteration of protein function. An acetylated lysine residue is presented here:

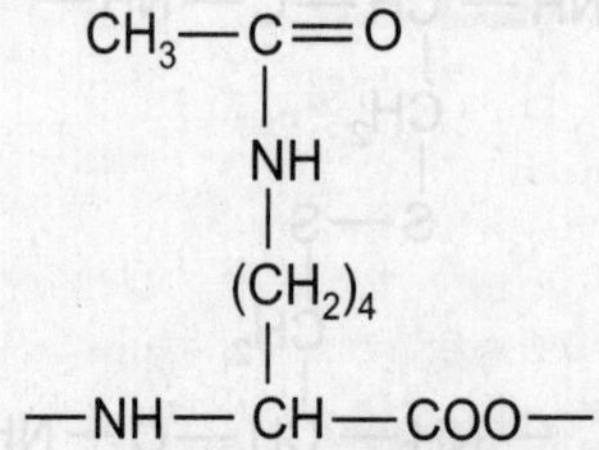

$$CH_3 - C = O$$
$$|$$
$$NH$$
$$|$$
$$(CH_2)_4$$
$$|$$
$$-NH-CH-COO-$$

Some proteins are acetylated at the amino terminus as shown below:

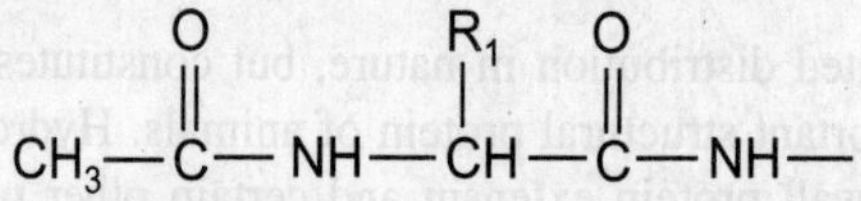

$$
\begin{array}{ccc}
O & R_1 & O \\
\| & | & \| \\
CH_3 - C - NH - CH - C - NH -
\end{array}
$$

Similarly, the polypeptide chain of some bacterial proteins begins with a formyl-methionine residue, which is a modification that occurs at the time of polypeptide synthesis rather than after. Methylation of amino groups also is an important modification of certain proteins. One of the most widely occurring and important of protein amino acid modifications is of a significantly more complex character. It is glycosylation, the covalent attachment of monosaccharides and oligosaccharides to proteins. The resulting conjugate, in which the protein: oligosaccharide mass ratio generally is greater than one, is referred to as a glycoprotein. The carbohydrate portion of the glycoprotein can impart to the protein special properties, such as the localised polar regions of cell surface proteins.

The carbohydrate moieties of the antifreeze proteins of certain Antarctic fish are essential to their function. Glycoproteins serve to impart viscosity and lubricating properties to body fluids and joints. Arabinose, fructose, galactose, glucose, mannose and xylose, the acetylated amino sugars N-acetyl-galactoseamine N-acetylglucose-amine and N-acetylneuraminic acid and several uronic acids have been demonstrated in glyco-proteins. Because of their complexity, determining the exact structures of glycoproteins is among the most difficult technical problems in modern biochemistry.

We do not go into the details of glycoprotein structure in this text, but give only some examples of the known types of linkages between protein and carbohydrate. The examples in Fig. 5.6 are of: (i) human red cell ABO blood group substances, (ii) immuno-globulins and (iii) the plant cell wall protein extensin. Note that in most instances, other monosaccharide residues will be bonded to the monosaccharide shown to create oligo-saccharide side chains and that only certain serine, threonine, asparagine and other such residues of a given glycoprotein actually will bear such an oligosaccharide side chain.

Non-protein Amino Acids

Amino acids having the D-configuration also exist in peptide linkage in nature, but not as components of large protein molecules. Their occurrence appears limited to smaller, cyclic peptides or as components of peptidoglycans (covalent complexes of polypeptides and polysaccharides in which the latter form the bulk of the conjugate) of bacterial cell walls. The antibiotic gramicidin-S is an example of a peptide that contains two residues of a D-amino acid, D-phenylalanine. Gramicidin-S also contains the non-protein amino acid L-ornithine, which is an important metabolic intermediate in the synthesis of amino

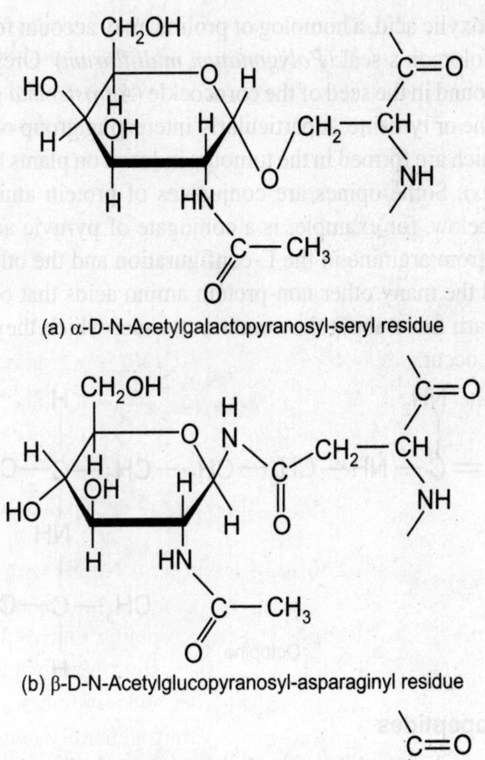

(a) α-D-N-Acetylgalactopyranosyl-seryl residue

(b) β-D-N-Acetylglucopyranosyl-asparaginyl residue

(c) β-L-Arabinofuranosyl-hydroxyprolyl residue

Fig. 5.6: Examples of carbohydrate-amino acid covalent linkages that have been found in glycoproteins: (a) an O-glycosidic bond between N-acetylgalactosamine and a serine residue, (b) an N-glycosidic bond between N-acetylglucosamine and an asparagine residue, and (c) an O-glycosidic bond between arabinose and a hydroxyproline residue.

acids and other compounds. D-Valine occurs in actinomycin-D, a potent inhibitor of RNA synthesis and D-alanine and D-glutamic acid are found in the peptidoglycan of the cell wall of gram-positive bacteria. An isomer of alanine, β-alanine, occurs free in nature and as a component of the vitamin pantothenic acid, co-enzyme A and acyl carrier protein. The quaternary amine creatine, a derivative of glycine, plays a fundamental role in the energy storage process in vertebrates, where it is phosphorylated and converted to creatine phosphate. In addition to these non-protein amino acids, for which metabolic roles have been described, several hundred other nonprotein amino acids have been detected as natural products. Higher plants are a particularly rich source of these amino acids. In contrast to the amino acids previously described, however, these compounds do not occur widely, but may be limited to a single species or only a few species within a genus. These non-protein amino acids are usually related to the protein amino acids as homologs or substituted derivatives.

Thus, L-azetidine-2-carboxylic acid, a homolog of proline, may account for 50 per cent of the nitrogen present in the rhizome of Solomon's seal (*Polygonatum multiflorum*). Orcylalanine (2,4-dihydroxy-6-methyl phenyl-L-alanine), found in the seed of the corncockle *(Agrostemma githago)*, may be considered as a substituted phenylalanine or tyrosine. A particularly interesting group of non-protein amino acids is found among the opines, which are formed in the tumours induced on plants by the crown gall bacterium, (*Agrobacterium tumefaciens*). Some opines are conjugates of protein amino acids and α-keto acids. Octopine structure shown below, for example, is a conjugate of pyruvic acid and arginine. It has two chiral centers: one derived from arginine in the L-configuration and the other from pyruvic acid in the D-configuration. These and the many other non-protein amino acids that occur in nature are presently being studied in order to learn more about the conditions under which they arise and their function in the organism in which they occur.

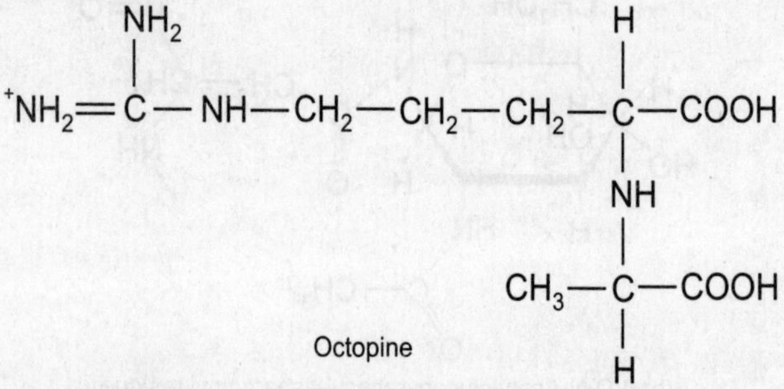

$$^+NH_2 = \overset{\overset{\displaystyle NH_2}{|}}{C} - NH - CH_2 - CH_2 - CH_2 - \underset{\underset{\displaystyle NH}{|}}{\overset{\overset{\displaystyle H}{|}}{C}} - COOH$$

$$CH_3 - \underset{\underset{\displaystyle H}{|}}{C} - COOH$$

Octopine

Biologically Active Oligopeptides

An oligopeptide, is simply a short polypeptide. It is composed of a small number of amino acids, sometimes arbitrarily stated as ten or fewer residues, joined by peptide bonds. Two amino acids joined by a peptide bond form a dipeptide, a peptide containing three amino acids is a tripeptide and so on. Sometimes the term peptide is substituted for 'oligopeptide'. We discuss a chemical property of peptides and then the structures of some biologically active peptides.

Like an α-amino acid, a peptide has an α-amino and an α-carboxyl group. It is of interest to note the changes in the pK_a values for these groups that occur when amino acid residues are incorporated into an oligopeptide. Thus, in small peptides, the α-carboxyl group generally has a pK_a value in the range 3 to 4, indicating that it is less acidic than the α-carboxyl group of a free amino acid (pK_a range of 1.7–2.4). In a peptide, the α-carboxyl group no longer has a protonated α-amino group in its immediate vicinity, making it more difficult to remove a proton from the carboxyl group. Thus, the α-carboxyl group becomes a weaker acid. Similarly, the α-amino group of a peptide becomes a weaker base, with a pK_a value in the range 7.5 to 8.5. This is outside the range of 9 to 11 observed for the α-amino groups of free amino acids. Peptides have roles as hormones, antibiotics, toxins and metabolic intermediates. An example of a metabolically important peptide is glutathione. Glutathione is a tripeptide that is ubiquitious in nature and in mammals is required to prevent oxidative damage to red blood cells. It has a structure that deviates from that of a standard peptide and that we use to illustrate the procedure for naming a simple peptide. The chemical name for glutathione is γ-glutamylcysteinyl glycine. The suffix -yl signifies the amino acid residue whose carboxyl group is linked in peptide linkage to the amino group of the next amino acid in the peptide. In the case of peptides containing glutamic (or aspartic) acid, the carboxyl group involved in the peptide linkage must be identified. In glutathione, it is the γ-carboxyl that is bound in the peptide linkage. This obviously is an unusual situation, for when glutamic acid (or aspartic acid) occurs in proteins, it is the α-carboxyl that is bound in peptide linkage. When no prefix is given, the α linkage is understood. A very important group of naturally occurring peptides is that of the peptide hormones, which are responsible for intercellular and interorgan communication. Tens of groups of peptide hormones are recognised. Vasopressin and oxytocin are nonapeptides that are formed in the pituitary gland and can assume a cyclical structure by forming disulphide linkages between the amino-terminal cysteine and a cysteine in the interior of the peptide.

Seven of the nine amino acids in the two peptides are identical. Nevertheless, the physiological effects are quite different. Oxytocin causes the contraction of smooth muscle, vasopressin causes a rise in blood pressure by constricting the peripheral blood vessels. The structures of these peptide hormones follow. One should identify the amino terminus and trace the course of the peptide chains of these hormones. Note that the carboxyl terminal residue of these peptides is the amide of glycine.

Carboxyl terminal amidation is almost unknown among proteins, but occurs frequently in naturally occurring peptides. Protection against proteinases of the carboxypeptidase type is a possible function. Insulin, produced by the pancreas, is a hormone consisting of two polypeptide chains containing a total of 51 amino acid residues. The synthesis of the peptide hormones discussed in this paragraph proceeds by proteolysis of polypeptide precursors. Several antibiotics are peptides of comparatively simple structure and are synthesised by mechanisms that are distinct from those of protein synthesis. Gramicidin and tyrocidin are examples of such compounds. Penicillin, another antibiotic, contains the valine and cysteine residues, but these are not linked by peptide bonds. Rather, a strained four-membered ring and a sulphur-containing ring are found. Synthetic peptides may also have biological activity. An especially simple example is the artificial sweetener Aspartame. Aspartame is L-aspartyl-L-phenylalanyl-methyl ester. It is approximately 200 times as sweet as sucrose and is considered to lack some of the unpleasant after-taste associated with other synthetic sweeteners.

Peptides now can be synthesised for research purposes. These find uses in studies on hormone activity, as substrates for enzymes and as 'immunogens', substances capable of eliciting antibodies when injected into animals. Sometimes, portions of the structure of a rare protein have been determined from analysis of its gene or microsequence analysis, but available quantities of the protein do not allow antibodies to be induced. A synthetic peptide that corresponds to the carboxyl terminal region of the protein or hydrophilic stretches of the polypeptide chain often will induce the desired antibodies. Usually, the synthetic peptide is conjugated to a protein such as serum albumin, to increase the efficiency of antibody production.

Forms that Proteins Take

Up to this point, we have discussed proteins primarily in terms of their covalent structure, the polypeptide chain. The essence of a protein's function and the diversity of functions that proteins have, resides in their ability to bring amino acid residues that are distantly arrayed along the peptide chain into contact in three-dimensional space. Proteins have not only a definite covalent structure, defined by the order of amino acids along the polypeptide chain, but also a definite three-dimensional structure. As we point out, the three-dimensional structure also is controlled primarily by the order of amino acid residues. The stability of these three-dimensional structures is the result of non-covalent bonding.

The positioning of reactive functional groups relative to one another in an environment of controlled polarity allows proteins to bind other molecules specifically, to become catalysts and to take on other functions. The general form of most proteins is globular, meaning that they are roughly spherical. The technique known as X-ray crystallography gives information about the three-dimensional structures of globular proteins and other macromolecules that can be crystallised or otherwise placed in orderly arrays. This complex and laborious method has revealed the three-dimensional structures of several tens of globular proteins with sufficient resolution to be able to locate all of the non-proton atoms. From X-ray crystallography results and other data, it appears that the interior of a globular protein is packed as tightly with amino acid residues as amino acids are packed in amino acid crystals. About 75 per cent of the available interior space is within the surfaces at which non-bonded atoms of the amino acid residues are expected to contact.

The remaining 25 per cent of the interior volume is sub-divided into spaces that, with few exceptions, are too small to accommodate a water molecule. The solvent in which the globular protein is dissolved appears to penetrate only a short distance from the protein surface in most instances. Since most of the side chains of amino acids are non-polar, the interior of the protein molecule is predominantly a polar. In fact, the polarity of an amino acid residue is a good predictor of its location in the three-dimensional structure of the molecule, with polar amino acids confined mainly to the exterior. When a polar amino acid side chain is located in the interior of a protein, the possibility of functional significance should be kept in mind. A surface location for hydrophobic amino acid side chains may indicate binding of lipids or other hydrophobic substances, possibly in a membrane or at the surface of another protein.

Ionic Charge of Protein Molecules

Since a protein may have both positively and negatively charged, ionised amino acid residues, the net charge on a protein may be negative or positive. Or the protein may have no net charge, depending on the pK_a values of the groups involved and the pH of the solution. The pH at which the protein has no net electric charge is termed the isoelectric point or pI. In solutions with pH values above the isoelectric point, the protein will have a net negative charge, at lesser pH values, it will be positively charged. More proteins have pI values below 7 than above 7, so that most proteins are negatively charged at neutral pH. A technique that takes advantage of the ionic charge of a protein molecule is electrophoresis.

One of the characteristics that the investigator would like to determine for a newly discovered protein is its mass. When the entire amino acid sequence becomes known, the exact molecular weight of the protein can be determined by summing the weights of the amino acid residues. However, generally this information will be available only late in the characterisation of the protein. It is surprising that the technique of polyacrylamide gel electrophoresis, which depends on the charge of the protein molecule, should also provide information about the size of a protein molecule. In fact, because it is such an easy and inexpensive technique, gel electrophoresis is commonly used for estimating protein molecular weights, especially in the preliminary stages of the characterisation of a protein.

The reader should be aware, however, that the molecular weights estimated by gel electrophoresis are just that, estimates. They are based on the comparison of the mobilities of the proteins under study and other proteins of known molecular weight. Amino acid sequence determination and certain physical methods such as sedimentation and diffusion, which will not be discussed here, give more reliable measures of the molecular weight.

LIPIDS

Lipids are of great importance to the body as the chief concentrated storage form of energy, besides their role in cellular structure and various other biochemical functions. As such, lipids are a heterogeneous group of compounds and therefore, it is rather difficult to define them precisely. Lipids may be regarded as organic substances relatively insoluble in water, soluble in organic solvents (alcohol, ether, etc.) actually or potentially related to fatty acids and utilised by the living cells. Unlike the polysaccharides, proteins and nucleic acids, lipids are not polymers. Further, lipids are mostly small molecules. They may be further fractionated by such techniques such as adsorption chromatography, thin layer chromatography and reverse phase chromatography. Fats, oils, certain vitamins and hormones and most non-protein membrane components are lipids. Lipids are water-insoluble organic biomolecules that can be extracted from cells and tissues by non-polar solvents, e.g. chloroform, ether or benzene.

There are several different families or classes of lipids but all derive their distinctive properties from the hydrocarbon nature of a major portion of their structure. Lipids have several important biological functions, serving: (i) as structural components of membranes, (ii) as storage and transport forms of metabolic fuel, (iii) as a protective coating on the surface of many organisms, and (iv) as cell-surface components concerned in cell recognition, species specificity and tissue immunity. Some substances classified among the lipids have intense biological activity, they include some of the vitamins and hormones. Although lipids are a distinct class of biomolecules, we shall see that they often occur combined, either covalently or through weak bonds, with members of other classes of biomolecules to yield hybrid molecules such as glycolipids, which contain both carbohydrate and lipid groups and lipoproteins, which contain both lipids and proteins. In such biomolecules the distinctive chemical and physical properties of their components are blended to fill specialised biological functions.

Classification of Lipids

Lipids have been classified in several different ways. The most satisfactory classification is based on their backbone structures (Table 5.3). The complex lipids, which characteristically contain fatty acids as components, include the acylglycerols, the phosphoglycerides, the sphingolipids and the waxes, which differ in the backbone structures to which the fatty acids are covalently joined. They are also called saponifiable lipids since they yield soaps (salts of fatty acids) on alkaline hydrolysis. The other great group of lipids consists of the simple lipids, which do not contain fatty acids and hence are non-saponifiable. Let us first consider the structure and properties of fatty acids, characteristic components of all the complex lipids.

Table 5.3: Classification of lipids.

Lipid type	Backbone
Complex (saponifiable)	
Acylglycerols	Glycerol
Phosphoglycerides	Glycerol 3-phosphate
Sphingolipids	Sphingosine
Waxes	Non-polar alcohols of high molecular weight
Simple (non-saponifiable)	
Terpenes	
Steroids	
Prostaglandins	

FATTY ACIDS

Although fatty acids occur in very large amounts as building-block components of the saponifiable lipids, only traces occur in free (unesterified) form in cells and tissues. Well over 100 different kinds of fatty acids have been isolated from various lipids of animals, plants and micro-organisms. All possess a long hydrocarbon chain and a terminal carboxyl group. The hydrocarbon chain may be saturated, as in palmitic acid or it may have one or more double bonds, as in oleic acid, a few fatty acids contain triple bonds. Fatty acids differ from each other primarily in chain length and in the number and position of their unsaturated bonds. They are often symbolised by a shorthand notation that designates the length of the carbon chain and the number, position and configuration of the double bonds. Thus palmitic acid (16 carbons, saturated) is symbolised 16:0 and oleic acid [18 carbons and one double bond (*cis*) at carbons 9 and 10] is symbolised $18:1^{D9}$. It is understood that the double bonds are *cis* unless indicated otherwise. The structures and symbols of some important saturated and unsaturated fatty acids and a few with unusual structures. Some generalisations can be made on the different fatty acids of higher plants and animals. The most abundant have an even number of carbon atoms with chains between 14 and 22 carbon atoms long, but those with 16 or 18 carbons predominate. The most common among the saturated fatty acids are palmitic acid (C_{16}) and stearic acid (C_{18}) and among the unsaturated fatty acids oleic acid (C_{18}). Unsaturated fatty acids predominate over the saturated ones, particularly in higher plants and in animals living at low temperatures. Unsaturated fatty acids have lower melting points than saturated fatty acids of the same chain length. In most monounsaturated (monoenoic) fatty acids of higher organisms there is a double bond between carbon atoms 9 and 10. In most polyunsaturated (polyenoic) fatty acids one double bond is between carbon atoms 9 and 10, the additional double bonds usually occur between the 9,10 double bond and the methyl-terminal end of the chain. In most types of polyunsaturated fatty acids the double bonds are separated by one methylene group, for example, —CH=CH—CH$_2$—CH= CH—, only in a few types of plant fatty acids are the double bonds in conjugation, that is, —CH=CH— CH=CH—. The double bonds of nearly all kinds of naturally occurring unsaturated fatty acids are in the *cis* geometrical configuration, only a very few are *trans*.

Metabolism of Lipids

In both plants and animals, lipids are stored in large amounts as neutral, highly insoluble triacylglycerol, they can be rapidly mobilised and degraded to meet the cell's demands for energy. In the complete combustion of a typical fatty acid, palmitic acid, there is a large negative free-energy change.

$$C_{16}H_{32}O_2 + 23O_2 \rightarrow 16CO_2 + 16H_2O \qquad \Delta G' = -2340 \text{ kcal/mole}$$

This negative change is due to the oxidation of the highly reduced hydrocarbon chain attached to the carboxyl group of the fatty acid. Of all the common foodstuffs, only the long-chain fatty acids possess this important chemical feature. Thus, lipids have quantitatively the best caloric value of all foods, that is, 9.3 kcal/g for lipids in contrast to 4.1 kcal/g for carbohydrates and proteins.

Lipids also function as important insulators of delicate internal organs. In addition, nerve tissue, plasma membrane and all membranes of sub-cellular particles such as mitochondria, endoplasmic reticulum and nuclei have complex lipids as essential components. Moreover, the vital electron transport system in mitochondria and the intricate structures found in chloroplasts, the site of photosynthesis, contain complex lipids in their basic architecture. Since, the chief storage form of available energy in the animal cell is the triacylglycerol molecule. When the caloric intake exceeds utilisation, excess food is invariably stored as fat, the body cannot store any other form of food in such large amounts. Carbohydrates are converted to glycogen, for example, but the capacity of the body to store this polysaccharide as a potential source of energy is strictly limited. In a normal liver, the average amount of glycogen is 5 to 6 per cent of the total weight and is skeletal muscle, the glycogen content averages only 0.4 to 0.6 per cent. Blood glucose is present at a level of 60 to 100 mg per 100 ml of whole blood. Only under pathological conditions are these values drastically altered.

Chapter 6

Enzymes as Biocatalysts

INTRODUCTION

Enzymes are protein catalysts that increase the velocity of a chemical reaction and are not consumed during the reaction they catalyse. All enzymes contain a protein backbone. In some enzymes this is the only component in the structure. However there are additional non-protein moieties usually present which may or may not participate in the catalytic activity of the enzyme. Covalently attached carbohydrate groups are commonly encountered structural features which often have no direct bearing on the catalytic activity, although they may well effect an enzyme's stability and solubility. Other factors often found are metal ions (cofactors) and low molecular weight organic molecules (coenzymes).

These may be loosely or tightly bound by noncovalent or covalent forces. They are often important constituents contributing to both the activity and stability of the enzymes. This requirement for cofactors and coenzymes must be recognised if the enzymes are to be used efficiently and is particularly relevant in continuous processes where there may be a tendency for them to become separated from an enzyme's protein moiety.

BIOLOGICAL CATALYSTS

This section discusses shared properties with chemical catalysts and differences between enzymes and chemical catalysts.

1. Shared properties with chemical catalysts:
   (a) Enzymes are neither consumed nor produced during the course of a reaction.
   (b) Enzymes do not cause reactions to take place, but they greatly enhance the rate of reactions that would proceed much slower in their absence. They alter the rate but not the equilibrium constants of reactions that they catalyse.

2. Differences between enzymes and chemical catalysts:
   (a) Enzymes are proteins.
   (b) Enzymes are highly specific and produce only the expected products from the given reactants, or substrates (i.e. there are no side reactions).

(c) Enzymes may show a high specificity toward one substrate or exhibit a broad specificity, using more than one substrate.

(d) Enzymes usually function within a moderate pH and temperature range.

Functions of Enzymes

Enzymes allow many chemical reactions to occur within the homeostasis constraints of a living system. Enzymes function as organic catalysts. A catalyst is a chemical involved in, but not changed by, a chemical reaction. Many enzymes function by lowering the activation energy of reactions. By bringing the reactants closer together, chemical bonds may be weakened and reactions will proceed faster than without the catalyst. The use of enzymes can lower the activation energy of a reaction. Enzymes can act rapidly, as in the case of carbonic anhydrase (enzymes typically end in the -ase suffix), which causes the chemicals to react 10^7 times faster than without the enzyme present. Carbonic anhydrase speeds up the transfer of carbon dioxide from cells to the blood. There are over 2000 known enzymes, each of which is involved with one specific chemical reaction. Enzymes are substrate specific. The enzyme peptidase (which breaks peptide bonds in proteins) will not work on starch (which is broken down by human-produced amylase in the mouth).

Enzymes are proteins. The functioning of the enzyme is determined by the shape of the protein. The arrangement of molecules on the enzyme produces an area known as the active site within which the specific substrates will 'fit'. It recognises, confines and orients the substrate in a particular direction.

Functions of Enzymes in Cells

Enzymes are proteins that do the everyday work within a cell. Their basic function is to speed up the process and efficiency of a reaction without themselves being consumed in the process. Enzymes are responsible for moving large parts of a cell's internal structure, such as pulling chromosomes apart when a cell divides. Enzymes make the energy molecules that are constantly needed for the cell to survive, and they break down molecules, recycle the old parts and make new molecules that allow the cell to grow.

Catalysts for change: Enzymes are catalysts, meaning they speed up the rate at which reactants interact to form products in a chemical reaction, while not being consumed in the reaction. They physically combine chemical reactants in a way that lowers the energy required for bonds to break and new bonds to form, making the formation of a product much faster. They lower what is called the activation energy of the reaction, or the amount of energy required for a hybrid of the reactants and products to form. The hybrid then becomes the product. Without enzymes, these chemical reactions would proceed at a rate that is hundreds to thousands of times slower.

Making energy: Living organisms store the energy required for daily life in the form of chemical energy. Adenosine triphosphate, or ATP, is the main form of chemical energy. ATP is a charged battery that can be discharged to release energy that powers the movement of enzymes. Enzymes are also required to make ATP, however. The main enzyme that produces ATP is called ATP Synthase, which is part of the electron transport chain in the mitochondria of cells. For every molecule of glucose that is broken down for energy, ATP Synthase makes about 32 to 34 ATP molecules.

Molecular motors: Enzymes are the protein machines that perform the day-to-day functions within cells. They deliver packages from one part of the cell to another. They pull chromosomes apart when the cell undergoes mitosis. They pull cilia, which are like the oars of a cell, to help cells move or to help cells move mucus up our airway into our throat. Common motor proteins are myosins, kinesins and dyneins.

These families of motor proteins catalyse the breakage of ATP into ADP (adenosine diphoshphate) to get the energy they need to do their grunt work.

Breaking and building: The cells that comprise organisms obtain energy by breaking down organic carbon compounds such as sugar, protein and fat. Breaking these molecules down into smaller parts is called catabolism, while building new molecules from these recycled smaller parts is called anabolism. Enzymes perform these functions at every step of the way. Energy sources such as glucose, a simple sugar, store a lot of energy. But the cell cannot access that energy to make ATP unless it is able to break the bonds within the glucose molecule.

CLASSIFICATION OF ENZYMES

Enzymes are divided into six major classes with several sub classes is shown in Table 6.1.

Table 6.1: Six major classes of enzymes and examples of their sub classes.

Classification	*Distinguishing feature*
1. Oxidoreductases	$A_{red} + B_{ox} \rightarrow A_{ox} + B_{red}$
Oxidases	Use oxygen as an electron acceptor but do not incorporate it into the substrate
Dehydrogenases	Use molecules other than oxygen (e.g. NAD^+) as an electron acceptor
Oxygenases	Directly incorporate oxygen into the substrate
Peroxidases	Use H_2O_2 as an electron acceptor
2. Transferases	$A–B + C \rightarrow A+B– C$
Methyltransferases	Transfer one-carbon units between substrates
Aminotransferases	Transfer NH_2 from amino acids to keto acids
Kinases	Transfer $PO_3\sim$ from ATP to a substrate
Phosphorylases	Transfer PO_{3-} from inorganic phosphate (P) to a substrate
3. Hydrolases	$A–B + H_2O \rightarrow A–H + B–OH$
Phosphatases	Remove $PO_3\sim$ from a substrate
Phosphodiesterases	Cleave phosphodiester bonds such as those in nucleic acids
Proteases	Cleave amide bonds such as those in proteins
4. Lyases	$A(XH)–B \rightarrow A–X+B–H$
Decarboxylases	Produce CO_2 via elimination reactions
Aldolases	Produce aldehydes via elimination reactions
Synthases	Link two molecules without involvement of ATP
5. Isomerases	Isomers have the same molecular formula but differ in their structural formula
Racemases	Interconvert L and D stereoisomers
Mutases	Transfer groups between atoms within a molecule
6. Ligases	$A+B+ATP \rightarrow A–B+ADP+Pi$
Carboxylases	Use CO_2 as a substrate
Synthetases	Link two molecules via an ATP-dependent reaction

EC 1 oxidoreductases: Catalyse the transfer of hydrogen or oxygen atoms or electrons from one substrate to another, also called oxidases, dehydrogenases, or reductases. Note that since these are 'redox' reactions, an electron donor/acceptor is also required to complete the reaction.

EC 2 transferases: Catalyse group transfer reactions, excluding oxido-reductases (which transfer hydrogen or oxygen and are EC 1). These are of the general form:

$$A–X + B \leftrightarrow BX + A$$

EC 3 hydrolases: Catalyse hydrolytic reactions. Includes lipases, esterases, nitrilases, peptidases/proteases. These are of the general form:

$$A–X + H_2O \leftrightarrow X–OH + HA$$

EC 4 lyases: Catalyse non-hydrolytic (covered in EC 3) removal of functional groups from substrates, often creating a double bond in the product, or the reverse reaction, i.e. addition of function groups across a double bond.

EC 5 isomerases: Catalyses isomerisation reactions, including racemisations and *cis-tran* isomerisations.

EC 6 ligases: Catalyses the synthesis of various (mostly C-X) bonds, coupled with the breakdown of energy-containing substrates, usually ATP.

NOMENCLATURE OF ENZYMES

Each enzyme is assigned two names. The first is its short, recommended name, convenient for everyday use. The second is the more complete systematic name, which is used when the enzyme must be identified without ambiguity.

Recommended Name

Most commonly used enzyme names have the suffix '*-ase*' attached to the substrate of the reaction, for example, glucosidase, urease, sucrase, or to a description of the action performed, for example, lactate dehydrogenase and adenylate cyclase.

[*Note:* Some enzymes retain their original trivial names, which give no hint of the associated enzymic reaction, for example, trypsin and pepsin.]

Systematic Name

The International Union of Biochemistry and Molecular Biology (IUBMB) developed a system of nomenclature in which enzymes are divided into six major classes, each with numerous subgroups. The suffix '*-ase*' is attached to a fairly complete description of the chemical reaction catalysed, for example D-*glyceraldehyde 3-phosphate: NAD oxidoreductase*. The IUBMB names are unambiguous and informative, but are sometimes too cumbersome to be of general use.

A skeletal outline of the IUB system is presented below:

1. Reactions and the enzymes that catalyse them form six classes, each having 4–13 subclasses.

2. The enzyme name has two parts. The first names the substrate or substrates. The second, ending in *-ase,* indicates the type of reaction catalysed.

3. Additional information, if needed to clarify the reaction, may follow in parentheses, e.g. the enzyme catalysing:

$$\text{L-malate} + NAD^+ = \text{Pyruvate} + CO_2 + NADH + H^+$$

is designated 1.1.1.37 L-malate: NAD^+ oxidoreductase (decarboxylating).

4. Each enzyme has a code number (EC) that characterises the reaction type as to class (first digit), subclass (second digit) and subsubclass (third digit). The fourth digit is for the specific enzyme.

Thus, EC 2.7.1.1 denotes class 2 (a transferase), subclass 7 (transfer of phosphate), sub-subclass 1 (an alcohol is the phosphate acceptor). The final digit denotes hexokinase, or ATP:D-hexose 6-phospho-transferase, an enzyme catalysing phosphate transfer from ATP to the hydroxyl group on carbon 6 of glucose.

Co-enzymes

Enzymes may be simple proteins, or complex enzymes. A complex enzyme contains a non-protein part, called as prosthetic group (co-enzymes). Co-enzymes are heat stable low molecular weight organic compound. The combined form of protein and the co-enzyme are called as holo-enzyme. The heat labile or unstable part of the holo-enzyme is called as apo-enzyme. The apo-enzyme gives necessary three dimensional structures required for the enzymatic chemical reaction. Co-enzymes are very essential for the biological activities of the enzyme. Co-enzymes combine loosely with apo-enzyme and are released easily by dialysis. Most of the co-enzymes are derivatives of vitamin B complex group of substance. One molecule of the co-enzyme with its enzyme is sufficient to convert a large group of substrate.

Co-enzymes are further divided into two groups. The first groups of co-enzymes are a part of reaction catalysed by oxidoreductase by donating or accepting hydrogen atoms or electrons.

The first group of co-enzymes are also called as co-substrates or secondary substrates. Because they are involved in counter-balance in change occurring in the substrate.

The second group of co-enzymes involves in reactions transferring groups other than hydrogen.

Difference between Catalysts and Enzymes

When compared to man made catalysts, enzymes have several unique properties.

1. They are extremely specific. Enzymes will catalyse reactions involving only one substrate or a very small group of structurally related substrates. Enzymes show:
   (a) Absolute specificity - working upon only a single substrate.
   (b) Group specificity - working upon a related group of molecules containing a specific functional group.
   (c) Linkage specificity - working on molecules that contain a specific type of chemical bond.
2. Enzymes are stereospecific. If a molecule exists as a pair of enantiomers, the enzyme will use only one of the pair as substrate and produce only one of the pair as the product. For example, the enzymes that are involved in amino acid metabolism and/or protein synthesis will only utilise the L-amino acids as substrates.
3. Reactions catalysed by enzymes produces only one product. Wasteful side reactions do not occur during enzyme catalysed reactions.
4. Enzymes are very much faster than man made catalysts. The best man made catalysts increase reaction rates about 10^7 fold, on average man made catalysts increase reaction rates 10^2 to 10^4 fold. Enzymes can enhance the rate from 10^{17} to 10^{20} fold when compared to the uncatalysed reaction.

ENZYMES AS BIOCATALYSTS

Improvement in the activity and usefulness of an existing enzyme or creation of a new enzyme activity by making suitable changes in its amino acid sequence is called enzyme engineering. When this approach is used to modify the properties of any protein, whether enzyme or nonenzyme, it is termed as protein engineering. Since enzymes are proteins, enzyme engineering is a part of the larger activity of protein engineering. Enzyme engineering utilises r-DNA technology to introduce the desired changes in amino acid sequences of enzymes. In addition, the level of production of an enzyme may be increased by introducing more copies of the gene into the concerned organism. The chief objective of enzyme engineering is to produce an enzyme that is more useful for industrial and other applications.

The various properties of an enzyme that may be modified to achieve this objective are as follows:

1. Improved kinetic properties.
2. Elimination of allosteric regulation.
3. Enhanced substrate and reaction specificity.
4. Increased thermostability.
5. Alteration in optimal pH.
6. Suitability for use in organic solvents.
7. Increased/decreased optimal temperature.

The structure and function of an enzyme molecule, for that matter of any protein molecule, are chiefly determined by its amino acid sequence, i.e. its primary structure. Therefore, any change in the properties of an enzyme is always reflected in its primary structure. Conversely, a change in the amino acid sequence should alter the properties of the enzyme. But, this is not always the case because the enzymatic properties, etc. are changed only when amino acid changes are introduced in certain critical regions of the protein. Therefore, it is of great importance to know the critical regions for the various functions of an enzyme and to be able to predict the effect of specific amino acid changes in these areas on the various functions. However, the present knowledge of the relationships between amino acid sequences, 3D structure of protein and properties of enzymes, obtained from a large database is only partially operative. It allows an explanation of the changes in structure and function on the basis of the changes in amino acid sequence, but it does not allow a dependable prediction of the influences of specific amino acid changes on the structure and function of the enzymes (Fig. 6.1). It may, however, be reasonable to anticipate that as more elaborate databases and improved softwares become available, it should become possible to predict with a far greater confidence the structural and functional changes in enzymes produced by the specified changes in their amino acid sequences. The effectiveness of enzyme engineering will be greatly enhanced then and this activity may have a tremendous influence on enzyme technology.

STEPS IN ENZYME ENGINEERING

The strategies for enzyme engineering and their theoretical considerations are quite involved. The steps involved in enzyme engineering (Fig. 6.2) are briefly described in as under.

1. The first step consists of isolation of the concerned enzyme and determination of its structure and properties. Both amino acid sequence and the 3D structure are usually obtained from X-ray diffraction, nuclear magnetic resonance (NMR), etc.

2. The data so obtained are analysed together with the database of known and putative structural effects of amino acid substitutions on enzyme structure and function. Molecular modelling is performed to determine a possible change in amino acid sequence for the desired improvement in the structure/function of an enzyme.

3. The next step consists of constructing a gene that will encode the amino acid sequence specified at the end of step 2. This is best achieved by isolation and cloning of the endogenous gene encoding the concerned enzyme and using this gene for site directed mutagenesis.

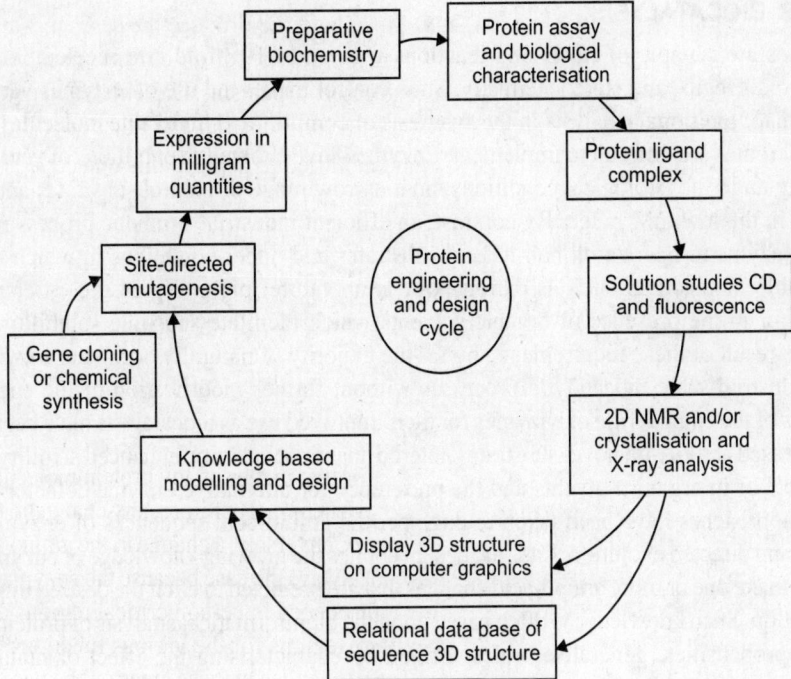

Fig. 6.1: Protein engineering and design cycle.

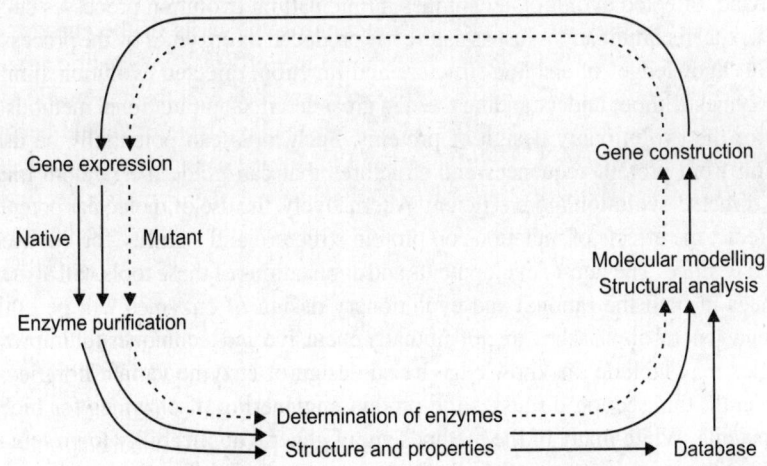

Fig. 6.2: Steps in enzyme engineering.

4. Once the appropriated gene is constructed, it is introduced and expressed in a suitable host, e.g. *E. coli*.

5. The recombinant or mutant enzyme so produced is isolated, purified and used for determination of its structure and properties. The information so obtained is added to the database. If the enzyme structure and function are not altered as desired, the next cycle of experimentation (step 2–5) is undertaken.

ENZYMES AS BIOCATALYSIS

Natural enzymes are capable of catalysing reactions with up to 10^{17}-fold rate accelerations and with exquisite control of regio- and stereochemistry. Such control makes the use of enzymes very attractive as an alternative to traditional catalysts in the synthesis of complex and highvalue molecules, especially where chemical routes are difficult to implement. Enzymes have evolved over billions of years to operate most effectively under physiological conditions, on a narrow range of natural substrates and usually at concentrations in the low mM range. By contrast, an efficient industrial synthetic process may require a biocatalytic enzyme to operate on non-natural substrates and under conditions in which the enzyme becomes unstable or inactive, such as extremes of temperature, pH and pressure, after repeated or prolonged use, or in the presence of organic solvents which facilitate substrate solubility or product extraction. As a result of these requirements, by far the majority of naturally occurring enzymes are not suitable for industrial-scale biocatalytic processes without further modification of the enzyme itself. Many examples of the engineering of enzymes for their improved use as biocatalysts have been published including: increased activity on novel substrates, altered enantioselectivity, enhanced stability at extreme temperatures, pH or in organic solvents and the preference for alternative enzyme cofactors.

Two broad approaches have been taken to engineer the amino-acid sequences of enzymes, namely rational design and directed evolution. Rational design applies the growing knowledge of enzyme structure and function to make one or more amino-acid changes that are predicted to elicit the desired improvements to enzyme function. Such knowledge is often based upon the bioinformatical analysis of protein sequences or amino-acid propensities, generalised rules derived by characterising the effect of mutations upon enzyme properties and by implementation of molecular potential functions that enable the effect of mutations upon structure to be predicted.

On the other hand, directed evolution techniques mimic natural evolution processes such as random mutagenesis and sexual recombination. Just as nature has produced its enzymes by the process of evolution without using any 'knowledge' of enzyme structure and function, directed evolution similarly permits us to engineer enzymes without understanding them in great detail. Computational methods also provide a valuable tool for the evolutionary design of proteins. Such tools can potentially be used to obtain useful information from protein sequences and structures that can guide the random mutagenesis of proteins making directed evolution more efficient. Alternatively, the use of molecular potential functions can be used to predict the effects of mutations on protein structure and stability for libraries of enzyme variants generated *in silico*. The latest developments and applications of these tools will also be discussed.

Recent advances in both the rational and evolutionary design of enzymes will be outlined below. However, these two general approaches are not mutually exclusive and techniques for improving directed evolution strategies may include the knowledge-based design of enzyme variant libraries, as will also be discussed. Overall, this section discusses the protein engineering of enzymes for biocatalysis and associated new patents. While many of the methods are of general applicability to protein engineering, only those of interest to modifying enzymes for biocatalysis are included. The final section brings together examples of the applications of protein engineering to various biocatalytic enzymes, particularly those appearing as published patents.

Rational Design Strategies

The degree of success of rational design studies depends largely on the enzyme property to be altered. For example, the expression level of a protein is readily improved by ensuring the use of the DNA codons for which the host cell has the greatest preference. Many successful studies have applied rational design to the improved conformational stability of enzymes, through the introduction of disulphide bonds, proline residues or the mutation of protein sequences towards the consensus for a given enzyme family. An alternative approach that uses combinatorial mutation towards the consensus sequence is discussed later as a directed evolution strategy. Since these successful applications, progressively more challenging goals have been achieved using rational design. An ability to improve the aqueous solubility of membrane-bound enzymes is of potential use in the application of these enzymes as biocatalysts and also for determining their three-dimensional structures which would critically enable further enzyme design work. An automated computational design strategy has recently been demonstrated to effectively solubilise two membrane-associated proteins, phospholamban and KcsA.

In the example of phospholamban (PLB), the researchers first predicted the sites for mutagenesis, in the absence of a PLB structure. They used the experimentally observed effects of mutations upon pentameric protein structure formation, to define a perturbation index as a sinusoidal function of residue position in helices. While one residue, F32, was mutated to a more chromogenic tyrosine residue to assist experimental characterisation, the remaining ten were subjected to an energy minimisation designed to optimise the net free energy, α-helical propensity and water solubility of the protein. Sequence diversity was introduced using a sequence entropy term in the potential function. In the PLB example, the new water-soluble variant was found to retain the pentameric form and degree of helical structure and also to be stabilised upon phosphorylation, in the same manner as the wild-type PLB. More recently, the formation of this water-soluble variant of PLB has subsequently enabled the crystal structure of its tetrameric form to be obtained, providing information about the PLB structure that was previously difficult to obtain. While the techniques described are limited to the solubilisation of helical membrane-associated proteins, there is a clear potential for the application of this approach to the solubilisation of membrane associated enzymes with highly α-helical content.

Some striking examples of the *de novo* design of protein structures have been achieved based on existing knowledge and using computational design algorithms. Computational design has been successfully used to introduce binding functionality into natural protein structures, such as the design of TNT, L-lactate, D-lactate and serotonin binding-sites into *Escherichia coli* periplasmic binding proteins (PBP) and also to redesign the DNA-sequence specificity of an endonuclease. Furthermore, computational design has been used to add binding functionality, such as calcineurin-binding, to protein scaffolds that were themselves obtained previously by rational design.

Enzyme functionality has also been introduced into protein scaffolds using computational design methods, demonstrating the potential application of such methods to biocatalysis. For example, the ability to hydrolyse paranitrophenyl acetate ester has been engineered into the catalytically inert thioredoxin protein scaffold. In a spectacular example, Hellinga and coworkers introduced triose phosphate isomerase (TIM) activity into the bacterial ribose-binding protein (RBP), a periplasmic receptor that has no known catalytic activity, using the computational design algorithm described above. The nascent enzyme functionality was then further improved by experimental directed evolution to achieve a rate enhancement of 3.4×10^5 over the uncatalysed reaction.

The *de novo* design of a protein structure that also has partial enzyme functionality has been demonstrated for a four-helix bundle with stoichiometric ferridoxase activity, obtained by introducing a diiron-binding site. However, the creation of an enzyme functionality that has an efficiency comparable with natural enzymes, remains elusive using rational design techniques alone, most likely due to the greater complexity of the problem and the reliance on static protein structure models and transition-state theory for predicting enzyme structure-function relationships. These models omit the potentially significant contributions of enzyme dynamics and quantum tunnelling towards catalysis. Recent efforts to study the function of enzymes using molecular dynamics simulations and experimental probes of structural dynamics are expected to lead to improved rational design methods for enzyme functionality. While the rational design of a highly efficient catalytic activity into an inert protein scaffold remains challenging, it is worth noting that the improvement of an existing enzyme activity using computational design methods has been recently demonstrated. In this example, the activity of chorismate mutase from *E. coli* was improved by 50% despite modelling an *ab initio* calculated transition-state structure bound into only a static active-site configuration of the enzyme.

Directed Evolution Strategies

While rational design methods seek to design beneficial mutations or protein sequences by applying empirically derived rules or theoretical models, directed evolution uses a combinatorial approach to create libraries of enzymes from which enhanced variants can be identified experimentally. The two most important aspects to consider when devising directed evolution programmes are: (i) the availability of suitable screening or selection-based methods for identifying 'hits' with improvements of the desired enzyme property and (ii) an appropriate mutagenesis strategy given the extent of change required in the target property and the existing availability of information relating to the target enzyme structure and function. These two aspects are discussed below along with recent related innovations that impact on the application of directed evolution to enzyme biocatalysis.

Screening and Selection Methods

For directed evolution to be successful and efficient, it is essential that good screening or selection tools are employed for accurately identifying enzymes with improvements in the desired properties. Furthermore, the screening or selection based method available for the target activity or enzyme property critically dictates the enzyme variant library size that can be practically tested and therefore, the most appropriate strategy for library design. In general, the ability to isolate variants from larger libraries will improve the chances of success in finding an enzyme with the desired enhanced properties. Screening methods analyse individual colonies cultured on agar plates, in microtitre plates, or in microfluidic chips and are typically used to screen in the range of 10^3–10^6 individual enzyme variants.

However, selection-based methods can use phage display, cell surface display, ribosomal display, or plasmid display, to isolate high-performing enzymes from libraries ranging up to 10^{14} variants. While selection-based methods enable much greater sequence diversity to be explored, they rely upon indirect selection for catalytic activity such as binding to transition-state analogues, whereas screening methods bring the advantage of direct evaluation of catalytic proficiency. Screening methods also permit enzyme variants to be assessed in accurately controlled and non-physiological environments which may otherwise prohibit the use of selection-based techniques.

The gap between library sizes that can be practicably analysed by screening and by selection-based techniques is gradually being diminished, for example by using fluorescence-activated cell-sorting (FACS) of cell surface displayed enzymes, capable of sorting up to 10^7 enzyme variants per hour. A recent high-throughput screening technique has been developed in which water-in-oil-in-water emulsion droplets are sorted by FACS as outlined in Fig. 6.3, to identify the best enzyme variants. This technique takes advantage of *in vitro* compartmentalisation, in which library encoding DNA and an *in vitro* transcription/translation reaction mixture create enzyme variants within an emulsion droplet. The droplets also contain a fluorogenic enzyme substrate, such that enzyme variants can then be assessed and sorted by FACS.

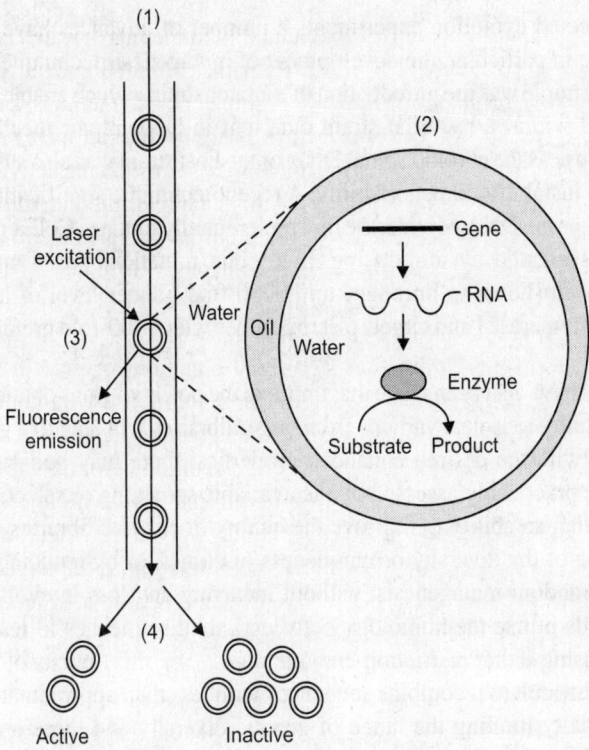

Fig. 6.3: Selection of active enzymes in double emulsion microdroplets by fluorescence-activated cell sorting (FACS): (1) water-in-oil-in-water emulsion droplets are passed through a fluorescence-activated cell sorter, (2) each of these double emulsion droplets contains a variant gene which is transcribed and translated to a mutant enzyme. Active enzymes convert fluorogenic substrate into fluorescent product. (3) laser excitation produces fluorescence for double emulsion droplets containing active enzyme and (4) droplets are sorted by FACS into those containing active and inactive enzyme variants.

The DNA that encodes the highest performing variants can then also be isolated from the same droplet and used for sequencing. In an alternative version of this technique, single bacterial cells expressing enzyme variants cytoplasmically or displayed on the cell surface, can be encapsulated in water-in-oil-in-water emulsions and screened by FACS.

Library Construction

The first methods of directed evolution employed mutagenesis that was targeted across entire genes by error-prone PCR or recombination of homologous genes by DNA shuffling. While these techniques provided the ground breaking benefits of being able to enhance the properties of enzymes without the need for any knowledge of the enzyme structure or its relationship to enzyme function, they still suffer from a number of deficiencies that present a barrier to their wider application. For example, the gains in enzyme activity or other desired properties obtained by these techniques, may not always sufficiently improve an industrial biocatalytic process such that an investment in them is seen as worthwhile. On the other hand, performing directed evolution experiments require a degree of experience sufficient to overcome the difficulties in creating large libraries with techniques that depends on inefficient DNA ligation reactions.

Since the early directed evolution experiments a number of advances have been made that help to overcome these issues, in particular, the development of mutagenesis techniques that avoid the need for DNA ligations. One example was the introduction of mutator strains which enable mutations to accumulate in plasmids harboured within a bacterial strain deficient in DNA repair mechanisms. However, such strains were of limited use as the chromo somal DNA of the host strain was also susceptible to mutagenesis, resulting in long-term instability in cell viability. A recent technique significantly reduces this problem by using a highly error-prone DNA polymerase that preferentially mutates ColE1 plasmids. The errorprone DNA polymerase was created by introducing three point mutations based upon homology with Taq polymerase I. It has been shown to introduce an 80000-fold greater level of mutagenesis on average, than wild-type DNA polymerase I and targets plasmid genes with a 400-fold preference over chromosomal gene mutagenesis.

Many developments have also been made that improve the potential gains obtained by directed evolution strategies. While the ability to isolate variants from larger libraries will lead to a greater chance of success in finding an enzyme with the desired enhanced properties, there may be limitations imposed by the library size that can be practically assessed by the available screening or selection-based methods. It is, therefore, recognised that an ability to improve the quality of enzyme libraries would be beneficial, for example, by promotion of the diversity or uniqueness of clones, or by reducing the number of enzyme residues subjected to random mutagenesis, without incurring any loss in evolutionary potential. Most DNA shuffling methods utilise the homology between parent sequences to reassemble fragments that have been generated using either restriction-enzyme digests, or short bursts of PCR.

Consequently it is difficult to recombine sequences with less than approximately 70% DNA sequence similarity, thus potentially limiting the range of genetic diversity and therefore, enzyme functionality that can be explored. Recent methods have enabled the non-homologous random recombination (NRR) of DNA sequences. While most NRR methods typically achieve only a single cross over, a few enable multiple cross overs to occur, including a technique in which DNA hairpins are added to a mixture of DNA fragments before reassembly by ligation with T4 DNA ligase. The use of T4 DNA ligase enables the recombination of DNA fragments independently of their homology, whereas the addition of the DNA hairpins, which can only ligate at one end, permits the range of DNA sequence lengths obtained to be carefully controlled.

In an alternative approach to NRR, a method that mimics exon shuffling has been described in an example which recombined two distantly related polymerase genes, to identify novel DNA polymerases. The approach, called structure-based combinatorial protein engineering (SCOPE), requires structural knowledge or sequence analysis of the parent enzymes to design PCR primers that enable recombination to occur at defined structural boundaries.

Amino-acid mutations introduced by traditional error-prone PCR tend to be biased towards those that can be obtained by single-base substitutions, typically accessing only 5.7 alternative residues on average. Greater sequence diversity can be obtained by applying saturation mutagenesis to one or more specific sites using degenerate oligonucleotides that encode for potentially all twenty amino-acids. In one approach, every single site in a protein can be systematically mutagenised independently to identify the optimal residues at each position. The best mutations can then be recombined with the aim of combining the enhancements endowed by each individual mutation.

Another recent method enables sequence saturation mutagenesis (SeSaM) to occur with less bias than error-prone PCR, at random positions within the targeted sequence, yet with only a single 1-3bp mutation appearing in each variant. The method creates random-length DNA gene fragments by PCR doped with α-phosphothioate nucleotides (dNTPaS) and selective cleavage of the sites of dNTPaS incorporation using iodine. The 3′ ends of each DNA fragment are then 'tailed' with typically 1–3 units of the universal base deoxyinosine (dITP), before elongation to the full length genes by PCR with a single-stranded template. A subsequent PCR to amplify the product allows promiscuous incorporation of standard bases at only the sites of dITP in the template DNA.

The incorporation of random saturation mutations at specific multiple sites provides the potential of identifying pairs of mutations that result in synergistic effects on enzyme properties. This type of library can be achieved using oligonucleotide PCR primers that encode for potentially all twenty amino-acids at each position, in a modification of the original Quikchange® protocol as supplied by Stratagene. The original protocol employs Pfu DNA polymerase to extend mutagenic primers annealed to a template plasmid. This then creates a non-methylated nicked plasmid progeny containing mutations defined by the oligonucleotide primers. Subsequent digestion with the methylated-DNA specific DpnI restriction enzyme then removes the methylated parental plasmid DNA that is obtained from cell lysates, leaving only the mutated plasmid DNA progeny. The improved method significantly enhances the ability to introduce mutations at multiple sites by including a blend of Pfu DNA polymerase with Taq polymerase, Pfu flap endonuclease (PfuFEN-1) and Taq DNA ligase in the Quikchange® PCR reaction. Adaptation of the Quikchange methods are also available for performing site-directed mutagenesis of genes in plasmids, with improved transformation directly into *Bacillus* strains and without the need for an intermediate transformation of *E. coli*.

Mutagenesis at specific sites of a plasmid DNA generally makes use of PCR for amplification of mutagenised DNA, as discussed in the examples above. However, the use of mismatch endonucleases, mixed with a proof-reading polymerase, dNTPs and a ligase, potentially obviates the PCR step by simply excising and repairing mismatched DNA in the heteroduplex formed between parental template plasmid and a mutagenic oligonucleotide. This new method presents an efficient alternative for site-directed mutagenesis and also for the recombination of point mutations from several gene variants.

The functionality represented by the standard twenty amino-acids may be limiting in terms of engineering novel enzyme functions. For example, the incorporation of nonnatural amino-acids into proteins may potentially permit enzyme chemistries that are not observed in nature. It is now possible, through ground breaking work, to incorporate nonnatural amino-acids into proteins at specific sites during their expression from bacterial cells. This was achieved by the directed evolution of a tyrosyl t-RNA synthetase to enable it to charge the t-RNA which is complementary to the little used amber codon TAG, with a non-natural amino-acid.

Identifying Target Sites for Mutagenesis

Alongside the development of techniques for creating different types of library as discussed above, the methods available for identifying key residues within an enzyme to target with mutagenesis have also advanced considerably. Decreasing the redundancy of enzyme libraries by targeting mutagenesis has the potential to allow more useful sequence space to be searched and makes more efficient use of the practical limits often imposed by the throughput of analytical tools. Two general approaches are taken. In the first, aligned sequence information from homologous enzymes can be used to identify residues that vary in nature, which may be linked to various enzyme properties. It has recently been observed that the consensus protein sequence for a particular enzyme has greater stability in many cases than the wild-type enzymes. A recent method for improving enzyme stability takes advantage of this observation by creating libraries of enzymes that contain variations only at sites that deviate from the consensus sequence. Interestingly, a similar method has also recently been used to invert the cofactor specificity of a lactate dehydrogenase enzyme from NAD^+ to $NADP^+$.

The second general approach for identifying key residues uses computational techniques, often though not necessarily, the same as those applied to rational design. In these examples, the conformational stabilities of enzyme variants generated *in silico*, are estimated. The degree of loss in conformational stability estimated by such a method has been shown to correlate well with mutagenic hot-spots that were determined experimentally and could therefore potentially be used for identifying amino acids in a protein that are tolerant to mutagenesis.

A similar concept has been used for pre-screening libraries *in silico* in a technique dubbed protein design automation (PDA), which eliminates sequences that are incompatible with the protein fold of the target enzyme. In this example, the 7×10^{23} potential variants created by *in silico* mutagenesis of nineteen active-site residues of β-lactamase, were reduced down to just 17,2800. The remaining variants were designed and screened experimentally in a single round of directed evolution to produce entirely novel enzyme variants with a 1280-fold increase in cefotaxime resistance.

Examples of Enzyme Engineering as Biocatalysis

Many enzymes have been modified by protein engineering methods and some recently patented examples are summarised below.

The targeted random mutagenesis of seven amino-acid residues of human butyrylcholinesterase expressed in mammalian cells, were recently used to evolve an increased activity towards cocaine hydrolysis. Such an enzyme has therapeutic potential for treating severe cases of cocaine toxicity. Seven residues that line the active-site gorge when aligned to the available structure of the homologous acetylcholinesterase, were chosen for mutagenesis. Previous biochemical data that identified sites important for cocaine hydrolysis were also used to guide the choice of the seven target sites. Several enzyme variants were found that had up to 100-fold greater activity towards cocaine hydrolysis than the wild-type butyrylcholinesterase.

Using a range of protein engineering techniques, including error-prone PCR, saturation mutagenesis and DNA shuffling, mutants of toluene 4-mono-oxygenase, toluene-oxylene mono-oxygenase and toluene-4-mono-oxygenase from various *Pseudomonads* have been obtained with improved activities towards benzene, toluene, nitrobenzene, nitrophenols, catechols, *o*-methoxy-phenol and *o*-cresol. Such biocatalytic reactions can be used in the synthesis of phenol, catechol, nitrophenols, nitrocatechols, 3-methoxy-catechol, 1,2,3-trihydroxybenzene, methoxyhydroquinone, methylhydroquinone, 4-methyl-resorcinol, methylhydroquinone and pyrogallol.

B12-dependent dehydratases with improved reaction kinetics have been obtained using error-prone PCR and oligonucleotide-directed mutagenesis to target the DhaB1 gene, encoding the α-subunit of glycerol dehydratase. Such enzymes are useful in the production of glycerol and 1,3-propanediol.

Nitrilases can be used in biocatalytic processes to convert nitriles to carboxylic acids. Recently, error-prone PCR has been used to generate mutants of an *Acidovorax facilis* (Fig. 6.4) nitrilase having improved activity towards 3-hydro-xynitriles. Isolated enzyme variants were capable of up to 1.9-fold improved activities when used to convert 3-hydroxynitrile to 3-hydroxycarboxylic acid, 3-hydroxyvalero-nitrile to 3-hydroxyvaleric acid, or 3-hydroxybutyronitrile to 3-hydroxybutyric acid.

In another example highlighting the general applicability of error-prone PCR, two carotenoid biosynthesis genes were simultaneously mutated randomly to improve the production of astaxanthin from beta-carotene. Targeting of the two enzymes, CrtO ketolase and CrtZ hydroxylase, simultaneously

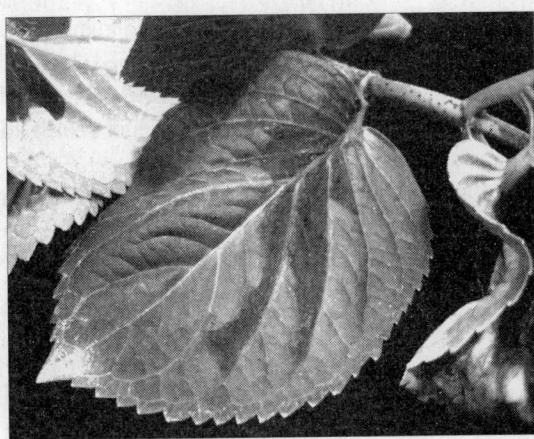

Fig. 6.4: *Acidovorax facilis.*

resulted in mutations within both genes and a net increase in the astaxanthin biosynthesis yield of up to 20% above that obtained with the wild-type enzyme pathway.

Error-prone PCR has also been used to improve the activity of 5'-xanthylic acid (XMP) aminase, which is potentially useful for the biocatalytic synthesis of 5'-guanylic acid (GMP) from XMP in microbial fermentations. Six improved mutants were found, with between two and six accumulated mutations and the best mutant having 3.8-fold greater activity resulting from three mutations. Xylanases are useful enzymes added to animal feed to aid the digestion of feed grains containing xylan. The growing need to sterilise the feed grain requires a xylanase enzyme that can retain activity after heat treatment, as well as being active at physiological digestive conditions (pH 3.5–5.0, 40°C). A recent patent has combined an engineered disulphide bond, previously introduced into a homologous xylanase enzyme and the Q162H mutation previously reported for xylanases.

Previously, the disulphide bond was shown to only marginally increase the xylanase thermostability, whereas the Q162H mutation had no effect on thermostability. However, the two mutations combined together result in a xylanase enzyme with a thermal denaturation midpoint increase of 14°C and which also retains 40% of the original activity after a 30 min treatment at 70°C and at least 30% activity at pH 3.5–6 and 40–60°C. A similar product, 5'-inosinic acid (IMP), is synthesised in an industrial process that uses mutant acid phosphatases from *E. blattae*, for which the phosphomonoesterase activity has been reduced to less than 40% of the wild-type enzyme due to the mutations G74D or I153T. Decreased esterase activity allows the mutant enzymes to synthesise IMP from inosine.

Another enzyme that can be used as a supplement to animal feeds is phytase. This enzyme is useful during digestion for releasing inorganic phosphate from phytate, which contains over 70% of the phosphate in plant material. A variant of the *E. coli* pH 2.5 acid phosphatase has been shown, rather unexpectedly, to exhibit increased phytase activity upon digestion of the enzyme with a mixture of trypsin and pepsin. Alpha-amylase is an enzyme that is commonly used for the degradation of starch during textile and paper desizing and also as a component of household detergents. Several examples of engineered alpha-amylases have been recently patented, including variants with improved activity and/or thermostability, solvent stability and resistance to multimerisation.

Polysaccharide lyases have potential uses in polysaccharide sequencing and degradation. A recent patent describes rationally designed variants of the polysaccharide lyase, chondroitinase B and also potential uses in the inhibition of anticoagulation, angiogenesis and maternal malarial infection. Active-site residues involved in catalysis and substrate binding were targeted by site-directed mutagenesis. While mutagenesis of the catalytic residues were damaging to enzyme activity, the mutation of a substrate binding arginine (R364) to alanine resulted in an altered product profile to that of wild-type enzyme after the digestion of dermatan sulphate.

In recent years, significant advances have been made in the understanding of protein structure and function that have also enabled rational design techniques to become more successful and further reaching than previously. In particular, the use of computational design algorithms with advanced features has made it possible to introduce nascent enzyme functionality into proteins and in at least one example, to improve the efficiency of an existing enzyme activity. Advances in rapid screening techniques, new methods for creating genetic diversity and computational tools for predicting hot-spots in protein sequences, have also pushed forward the boundaries that can be reached using directed evolution. The challenge now resides in refining computational methods for more accurate prediction of the effect of mutations on enzyme activity, potentially including the effects of protein dynamics. Meanwhile, improved understanding of natural enzyme evolution and better prediction of important residues within enzymes will enable directed evolution techniques to become much more powerful.

PECTIC ENZYMES

Pectic enzyme, also known as pectinase, is a protein that is used to break down pectin, a jelly like glue that holds plant cells together. In wines pectin can cause troublesome 'pectin haze' that is not easily cleared without the use of pectic enzymes. While this enzyme does occur naturally in grapes as well as yeast there is not enough of it to overcome the amount of pectin present in the must. Other sources of pectic enzyme include plants, bacteria and fungus. It turns out that fungus produces a special kind of pectic enzyme that is particularly adept at breaking down pectin even in the harsh environment created during fermentation. Most commercially sold pectic enzymes come from fungus.

Pectic enzymes may be purchased in a liquid form or as a powder at any home brewing supply store. Pectins are polysaccharides ubiquitous in the plant kingdom and constitute the major component of plant cell walls. The pectinases are a group of related enzymes capable of degrading pectin. Therefore, this group of enzymes have been used for decades in the food and wine making industry for the processing of fruit juices.

The pectinases are synthesised by plants and micro-organisms, the latter being used for industrial production. Micro-organisms are used to produce many enzymes of industrial interest in processes relatively inexpensive and environmentally friendly. Moreover, enzymatic catalysis is preferred over other chemical methods since it is more specific, less aggressive and generates less toxicity. Advances in biotechnology, especially in the fields of molecular biology and microbial genetics, have led to major advances in enzyme technology and have allowed, in many cases, the development of new producing strains and microbial enzymes. The production of pectinases may also benefit from these technologies.

This section reviews the characteristics of pectic substances, the types and mode of action of enzymes which degrade them and the main applications of commercial preparations of microbial pectinases in the food and wine making industry, followed by a review of new micro-organisms and pectolytic enzymes, evaluating new approaches to their production, marketing and use.

Pectic substances are polysaccharides of high molecular weight, with a negative charge, appearing mostly in the middle lamella and the primary cell wall of higher plants, found in the form of calcium pectate and magnesium pectate. They are formed by a central chain containing a variable amount although in high proportion of galacturonic acid residues linked through α-(1–4) glycosidic bonds partially esterified with methyl groups. The generic name of pectic substances is used for referring to four types of molecules: protopectin (pectic substance in intact tissue), pectinic acids (polygalacturonan containing >0–75% methylated galacturonate units), pectic acids (polygalacturonan that contains negligible amount of methoxyl groups) and pectins (pectinic acid with at least 75% methylated galacturonate units). Protopectines are insoluble in water, while the rest are wholly or partially soluble in water.

Pectic substances represent between 0.5–4% of fresh weight plant material. In addition to their role as cementing and lubricating agents in the cell walls of higher plants, they are responsible for the texture of fruits and vegetables during growth, maturation and their storage. Furthermore, pectic substances are involved in the interaction between plant hosts and their pathogens.

Pectins have numerous and important applications in the food and pharmaceutical industries. In the food sector, it is primarily used as a gelling agent, replacing sugars and/or fats in low-calorie food and as nutritional fibre. The pharmaceutical industry offers them as preparations to reduce cholesterol or to act as a lubricant in the intestines thus promoting normal peristaltic movement without causing irritation. In addition, these polysaccharides are used as drug delivery systems, which can also reduce the toxicity of these and make their activity longer lasting without altering their therapeutic effects.

Pectic Enzymes in Nature: Microbial Pectinases

The microbial world has shown to be very heterogeneous in its ability to synthesise different types of pectolytic enzymes with different mechanisms of action and biochemical properties. Pectic enzymes are produced by both prokaryotic micro-organisms, which primarily synthesise alkaline pectinases and by eukaryotic micro-organisms, mostly fungi that synthesise acid pectinases. There are many studies that have been conducted related to the characterisation of different microbial pectic enzymes concerning their mechanisms of action and biochemical properties. The optimal pHs that these enzymes may act range between 3.5–11, while the optimal temperatures vary between 40–75°C. Given the features of the substrate on which they act and the effect that is required of them, acidic and depolymerising pectinases are of great interest for the food industry although some applications such as the extraction of oils requires the alkaline ones.

Maceration products of plant tissues

The enzymatic maceration of plant tissues allows the transformation of these organised tissues in suspensions of intact cells that constitute the pulpy products that are used as a basis for preparing juices, nectars, baby food and some dairy products such as yoghurts. Enzyme preparations for this purpose contain cellulases, hemicellulases and pectic enzymes which should only act on the middle lamella of the plant tissue.

Biotechnological Aspects for Production of Microbial Pectic Enzymes

As discussed until now, there are numerous applications of microbial pectic enzymes in food and wine-making industry. Not surprisingly, the sales volume of these enzymes represents 25% of the enzymes that are commercialised in the food and alcoholic beverages industry. These many applications require one or more types of pectinases that must act in very different condition according to the process in which they are involved. For example, while in the extraction and clarification of fruit juice enzymes can be used at temperatures between 45–95°C, the wine industry employs temperatures below 15–10°C. Although most food applications pectinases have to act in a medium acid, in others, such as oil extraction, they should perform in a medium alkaline.

So far, commercial pectic enzymes are prepared only from cultures of filamentous fungi, mainly of the genus *Aspergillus*. Commercial products contain mainly a mix of polygalacturonase, pectin lyase and pectin methyl esterase. The use of different strains of *Aspergillus* and modification of substrates and culture conditions can lead to mixtures enriched in one type of enzyme.

However, these commercial pectic preparations are not always optimal for each process and its use is not without side effects and controversy. Thus, while pectin methyl esterase activity present in the samples may be necessary for the action of polygalacturonase in the case of pectin with a high degree of esterification, its action may lead to an undesirable increase of methanol in the products. Moreover, although the pectic enzymes are the most abundant in commercial mixtures, they can also contain other undesirable activities, such as in the case of making wine, polyphenoloxidases or cinnamyl esterases.

At present especially in recent years, the accumulated knowledge of new microbial pectolytic enzymes as well as methodological and technological advances can address the production and use of these enzymes with a different approach. The diversity of applications and conditions in which these enzymes must work also demand a large number of different enzymes capable of acting in such conditions. Even more interesting would be having more robust, broad-spectrum enzymes which allow for a more versatile use in different applications.

Considering the variety of enzymes, traditionally the majority of studies refer to the pectinases of *Erwinia* (Fig. 6.5) and *Bacillus* within the bacteria and various fungi especially *Aspergillus* although there has been a major advance in the description and characterisation of pectic enzymes produced by yeast in the last 15 years. In recent years there has been also a growing interest in studying pectic enzymes with very interesting properties from the point of view of their application. These include thermostable pectinases or pectinases with optimal activity at low temperatures.

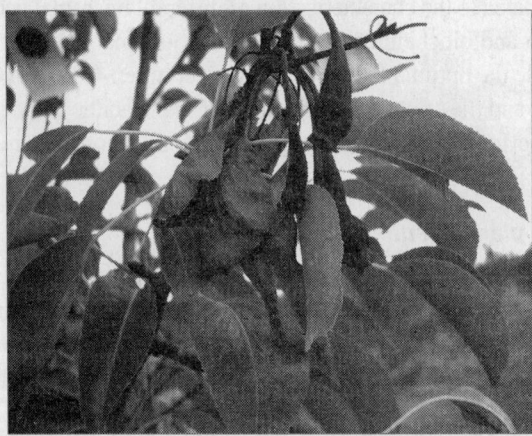

Fig. 6.5: Pectinases of *Erwinia*.

The possibility of producing different types of pectolytic enzymes separately and for later preparation of their mixtures in the proper proportions would allow to provide more suitable commercial preparations for each application and lacking undesirable activities. In this sense, micro-organisms such as some strains of yeast *Saccharomyces cerevisiae* and *Kluyveromyces marxianus* which produce only one type of enzyme or that constitutively synthesise it are of great interest. Similarly, obtaining constitutive mutants from producing strains allow the optimisation of production and contribute to making cost-effective production processes. Furthermore, these strains can be used to produce pectinases that accumulate together with other metabolites in the culture broth, which contributes favourable to the overall economy of the process. Heterologous expression of enzymes in prokaryotic or eukaryotic systems is a technique of great interest for the production of a single type of enzyme. Table 6.2 shows some of the many pectic enzymes, both from bacteria, yeast and fungi, which are rightly expressed in *Escherichia coli* and different species of yeast. Although *E. coli* is unable to carry out post-translational modifications of proteins, fungal pectolytic enzymes expressed in these bacteria are active.

Table 6.2: Microbial pectic enzymes expressed in different host strains.

Micro-organism gene origin	Type of enzyme	Host strain
Xanthomonas campestris	Pectate lyase Polygalacturonase	E. coli
Streptomyces coelicolour	Polygalacturonase	E. coli
Pseudoalteromonas haloplanktis ANT/505	Pectate lyase	E. coli
Thermotoga maritima	Exopolygalacturonase	E. coli
Burkholderia capacia	Endopolygalacturonase	E. coli
Phytophthora capsici	Pectate lyase	E. coli
Erwinia chrysantemy	Pectate lyase Polygalacturonase	S. cerevisiae
Aspergillus niger RH5344	Polygalacturonase	S. cerevisiae
Aspergillus aculeatus	Pectin methyl esterase	S. cerevisiae
S. cerevisiae IM1-8b	Endopolygalacturonase	S. cerevisiae
S. cerevisiae IM1-8b	Endopolygalacturonase	Schizosaccharomyces pombe
K. marxianus CECT1043	Endopolygalacturonase	P. pastoris
Bispora sp. MEY-1	Endopolygalacturonase	P. pastoris

However, one of the most interesting strategies seems to be the expression of pectinase genes in yeast, particularly in *Pichia pastoris*, in which very high levels of constitutive expression has been achieved. In some cases changes in glycosylation patterns conducted by yeast did not affect the activity and characteristics of recombinant pectinases, while other changes do occur with respect to the characteristics of the native protein, which even lead to enzymes with interesting properties for certain applications.

Thus, the enzymes that degrade the pectic substances play an essential role in the food and wine making industries because they are used to degrade the pectins that interfere with the extraction and clarification of fruit juices and oils as well as being important in the fermentation of coffee, cocoa and tea. Also, in the wine industry they play an important role by contributing to the release of the molecules responsible for aroma and colour, two of the major components that characterise a wine.

Traditionally, this industry uses different mixtures of pectolytic enzymes derived from fungi cultures, mainly of the genus *Aspergillus*, not always completely adequate for the processes they must carry out because of the type and concentration of different enzyme activities that they contain, not without undesirable effects due to other non-pectic enzymes that may be present in the mixtures.

The exploration of microbial biodiversity has allowed, especially in recent years, to identify and characterise new pectic-enzyme-producing micro-organisms with different biochemical characteristics, some potentially very interesting from the point of view of their application. Also, it has been technically possible, on the one hand, to select wild strains and constitutive mutants that produce a single enzyme, and, on the other hand, the heterologous expression in bacteria and yeast of numerous genes which encode pectic enzymes, obtaining producing strains of interest. All this opens the possibility of producing different pectic enzymes individually and preparing commercial mixtures of these, adapted to each process.

ENZYME APPLICATION IN MICROBIAL TECHNOLOGY

There are many enzymes employed in biotechnological operations. These include:

SI endonuclease: This enzyme is isolated from *Aspergilus cryzae* and it acts exclusively on ssDNA or RNA. It can break supercoiled DNA because it contains ss bubbles. It can also be used to distinguish supercoiled from both non-supercoiled, covalent circles and nicked circular DNA, both of which are resistant to the enzyme.

Restriction endonucleases: Restriction endonucleases are enzymes that cut DNA molecules at specific positions. It recognises 'foreign' (unmodified) DNA at a specific site and degrades it by internal cleavage. Most commonly used are the type II restriction enzymes, which cut within the recognition site. Some examples are EcoRI from *E. coli*, HindIII from *Haemophilus influenzae*, BamHI from *Bacillus amyloliquefaciens*, PstI from *Providencia stuartii*, SmaI from *Serratia marcescens*, Sau3A from *Staphylococcus aureus*, AluI from *Arthrobacter luteus*, TagI from *Thermus aquaticus* and HpaII from *Haemophilus parainfluenza*.

DNA polymerase I: It is primarily known as a 'repair' polymerase, which fills in single-stranded gaps. It is also involved in repair of the gaps formed on the lagging strand during replication. It also possesses both 5^I --- 3^I and 3^I --- 5^I exonuclease activity.

Klenow fragment of E. coli DNA polymerase 1: This enzyme is used for sequencing DNA using the Sanger Dideoxy System, filling the 3 recessed termini of restriction enzyme treated DNA and also used for labelling the termini of DNA fragments. The enzyme is also used for second strand cDNA synthesis in the cDNA procedures. 'Klenow fragment' is a proteolytic cleavage of DNA polymerase I. It leaves a fragment that is devoid of 5^I ---3^I exonuclease activity.

DNA polymerase III: This is the main 'replication' polymerase.

Helicase: It unwinds DNA, for example in conjugal plasmid transfer.

S1 nuclease: This enzyme degrades single-stranded DNA.

T4 DNA polymerase: This enzyme is used in the labelling of DNA fragments for use as hybridisation probes.

RNA polymerase: This enzyme synthesises RNA, using a DNA template.

Primase: This is a special RNA polymerase, which makes a short primer required for DNA synthesis.

Replicase: This is RNA-directed RNA polymerase used in replication of some RNA viruses.

Ribonuclease (RNase): This enzyme degrades RNA molecules.

Rnase H: This is a specific RNAse which cuts RNA---DNA hybrids. It is involved in replication of Col EI-like plasmid.

Exonuclease: This is an enzyme that removes nucleotides from the ends of DNA fragments. A 5^I----3^I exonuclease removes nucleotides from the 5^I end, while a 3^I ----5^I exonuclease removes nucleotides from the 3Iend. This enzyme recognises the terminal 5^I-phosphate of dsDNA for its exonuclease activity. Its primary use is the removal of protruding 5^I terminus from dsDNA which is needed for the terminal transferase tailing of DNA.

Exonuclease III: This enzyme is used for generating linear template DNA for the dideoxysequencing technique and generating staggered ends on dsDNA due to its 3^I---- 5^I exonuclease activity.

Ligases: It seals single-stranded gaps (nicks) in double-stranded DNA. It is also used for the formation of recombinant DNA molecules in gene cloning.

T4 DNA ligase: This enzyme catalysis the formation of a Phosphodiester bond between 3^I-OH and 5^I- phosphate ends in DNA using DNA molecules with cohesive ends as substrate.

Alkaline phosphatase: In gene cloning, this enzyme is used to remove phosphate groups from the 5^I end of DNA molecules and also used as a reporter gene for identification of secretion signals.

Polynucleotide kinase: It transfers a phosphate group from ATP to the 5^I OH end of DNA or RNA. T4 Polynucleotide kinase is an enzyme isolated from T4 infected *E. coli* and catalyses the transfer of-phosphate of ATP to a 5^I-OH end in DNA or RNA. It is also used for the labelling of 5^I termini of DNA for Maxam and Gilbert DNA sequencing and the phosphorylation of DNA lacking 5^I P termini.

Reverse transcriptase: This is RNA-directed DNA polymerase. It synthesises DNA (complementary DNA) using mRNA template. For example reverse transcriptase is an enzyme coded for by avian myeloblastosis virus which catalyses the synthesis of cDNA from an RNA template. It can also be used for the labelling of termini of DNA with extended 5I ends.

Topoisomerase: This is a class of enzymes that alters the conformation of DNA, for example by changing the degree of winding or super coiling.

Transposase: This enzyme catalysis the initial steps in transpositions.

Terminal transferase: This adds nucleotides to the 3^I end of DNA, without requiring a template strand.

Terminal deoxynucleotidyl transferase: This enzyme is isolated from calf thymus and catalyses the addition of dNTP to the 3^I -OH of DNA molecules. One of the primary uses of terminal transferase is the tailing of vectors and cDNA with complementary bases, thus permitting the cloning of the cDNA fragments. It can also be used for labelling of 3^I ends of DNA fragments.

IMMOBILISED ENZYMES AND IMMOBILISED CELLS

An immobilised enzyme is an enzyme attached to an inert, insoluble material—such as calcium alginate (produced by reacting a mixture of sodium alginate solution and enzyme solution with calcium chloride). This can provide increased resistance to changes in conditions such as pH or temperature. It also lets enzymes be held in place throughout the reaction, following which they are easily separated from the products and may be used again - a far more efficient process and so is widely used in industry for enzyme catalysed reactions. An alternative to enzyme immobilisation is whole cell immobilisation.

Immobilisation of Enzymes

Enzyme immobilisation may be defined as confining the enzyme molecules to a distinct phase from the one in which the substrates and the products are present; this may be achieved by fixing the enzyme molecules to or within some suitable material. It is critical that the substrates and the products move freely in and out of the phase to which the enzyme molecules are confined. Immobilisation of enzyme molecules does not necessarily render them immobile; in some methods of immobilisation, e.g. entrapment and membrane confinement, the enzyme molecules move freely within their phase, while in cases of adsorption and covalent bonding they are, in fact, immobile.

The materials used for immobilisation of enzymes, called carrier matrices, are usually inert polymers or inorganic materials. The ideal carrier matrix has the following properties: (i) low cost, (ii) inertness, (iii) physical strength, (iv) stability, (v) regenerability after the useful lifetime of the immobilised enzyme, (vi) enhancement of enzyme specificity, (vii) reduction in product inhibition, (viii) a shift in the pH optimum for enzyme action to the desired value for the process, and (ix) reduction in microbial contamination and non-specific adsorption. Clearly, most matrices possess only some of the above features. Therefore, carrier matrix for the immobilisation of an enzyme must be chosen with care keeping in view the properties and limitations of various matrices.

Methods of Immobilisation

The various methods used for immobilisation of enzymes may be grouped into the following four types: (i) adsorption, (ii) covalent bonding, (iii) entrapment, and (iv) membrane confinement. Methods of enzyme immobilisation is shown in Fig. 6.6.

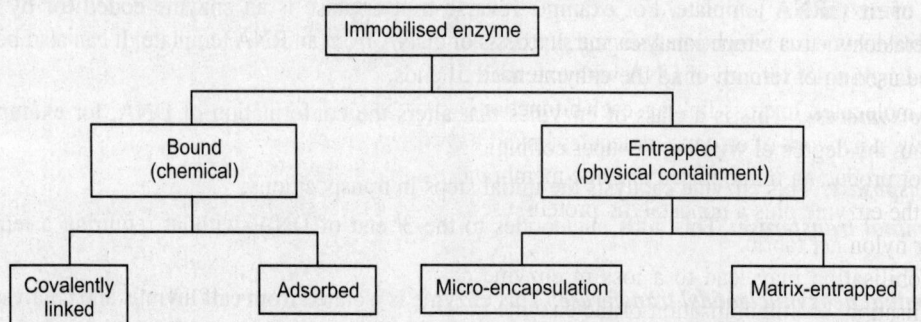

Fig. 6.6: Methods of enzyme immobilisation.

Adsorption

In case of adsorption, the enzyme molecules adhere to the surface of carrier matrix due to a combination of hydrophobic effects and the formation of several salt links per enzyme molecule. The binding of enzyme molecules to the carrier matrix is usually very strong, but it may be weakened during use by many factors, e.g. addition of substrate, pH or ionic strength. Therefore, the matrix should be carefully chosen keeping these factors in mind. Some of the commonly used matrices are, ion exchange matrices, porous carbon, clays, hydrous metal oxides, glasses, and polymeric aromatic resins. Ion exchange matrices are costly, but they can be readily regenerated (at the end of active life of the absorbed enzyme) by a simple operation, e.g. washing-off the adsorbed enzyme with a concentrated salt solution.

Adsorption of enzymes to the matrices is very easy and widely used. The enzyme is mixed with a suitable adsorbent under appropriate conditions of pH and ionic strength. After incubation for a sufficient period of time, the carrier is washed to remove unadsorbed enzyme molecules, and the immobilised enzyme is ready for use. This method usually produces a high loading (about 1 g enzyme/g matrix) of the enzyme.

Covalent binding

In this system the enzyme molecules are attached to the carrier matrix by formation of covalent bonds. As a result, the strength of binding is very strong, and there is no enzyme loss during use. The covalent bond formation occurs with the side chains of amino acids of the enzyme, their degree of reactivity being dependent on their charged status. The following relation is observed in reactivity:

$$-S^- > -SH > -O^- > -NH_2 > -COO^- > -OH \gg -NH_3^+$$

Lysine residues are the most useful in covalent binding of enzymes since they are usually exposed on the surface, are highly reactive and only very rarely occur at active sites of enzymes. Enzyme loading is quite low (ca. 0.02 g/g matrix); only in exceptional cases it may be as high as 0.3 g/g matrix.

The most commonly employed matrices are agarose, celluloses and polyacrylamides. Sepharose, an agarose, is available commercially as beads, is highly hydrophilic and is generally inert to microbial attack. On a research scale, it is activated by a treatment with cyanogen bromide which forms highly reactive intermediates with the –OH groups of sepharose; the enzyme molecules bind to these activated groups. However, cyanogen bromide is highly toxic so that it is not used commercially. Alternatively, sepharose is activated by treating it with chloroformates, carbodiimides, glutaraldehyde or other compounds. Treatment with trialkoxysilanes enables the use of such inert matrices as glass for covalent binding of enzymes.

Gluteraldehyde is a bifunctional reagent. It exists as an equilibrium mixture of monomer and oligomers It can be used to covalently bind the enzyme molecules or, alternatively, it can be used to cross-link enzyme molecules. In cross-linking, each bifunctional reagent molecule binds to two enzyme molecules; ultimately, a network of enzyme molecules linked together is produced. Glutaraldehyde is particularly useful for producing immobilised enzyme membranes for use in biosensors; this is achieved by cross-linking the enzyme plus a noncatalytic protein, used for dilution within a porous sheet; e.g. lens tissue paper or nylon net fabric.

Immobilisation may lead to a loss in enzyme activity due to the involvement of active site in immobilisation, or immobilisation of the enzyme in an orientation which either distorts the active site or renders it unavailable. This can be markedly reduced as follows. The enzyme is immobilised in the presence of saturating concentration of its substrate or a competitive inhibitor (such inhibitors bind to the active site). In such a situation, the active site is occupied and kept in the correct conformation while immobilisation, takes place; this minimises the involvement of active site as well as incorrect orientation of the enzyme molecules during immobilisation.

Entrapment

In this approach, enzyme molecules are held or entrapped within suitable gels or fibres and there mayor may not be covalent bond formation between the enzyme molecules and the matrix. A non-covalent entrapment may be viewed as putting the enzyme molecule in a molecular cage just as a caged bird/ animal. When covalent binding is also to be generated, the enzyme molecules are usually treated with a suitable reagent.

For example, acryloyl chloride is used to prepare lysine residues for binding by forming acryloyl amides; these are then copolymerised and cross-linked with acrylamide and bisacrylanide to form a gel containing the entrapped enzyme which may be used to form small beads or a film on a solid support. Enzymes may be entrapped within cellulose acetate fibres as follows. An emulsion of the enzyme and cellulose acetate is prepared in methylene chloride.

The emulsion is extruded as fibres into a solution of an aqueous precipitant. Entrapment in calcium alginate is the most widely used method for entrapment of microbial, animal and plant cells. Enzyme loading is very high (1 g/g gel or fibre). However, diffusion of the substrate to, the enzyme and of the product away from the enzyme creates difficulties.

Membrane confinement

Enzyme molecules, usually in an aqueous solution, may be confined within a semipermeable membrane which, ideally, allows a free movement in either direction to the substrates and products but does not permit the enzyme molecules to escape. A number of strategies are employed for this purpose which are briefly outlined below:

1. The reaction vessel may be partitioned into two chambers by a semipermeable membrane; one chamber contains the enzyme while the other has the substrate and the product.

2. Hollow-fibre membrane units contain the enzyme in their lumen or hollow space, and themselves are submerged in the substrate. This strategy provides an extremely large surface area per unit volume, e.g. > 20 m²/l, but is useful for only such substrates that are much smaller than the enzyme molecules. Hollow-fibres are costly, and can be used with a variety of enzymes including coenzyme regenerating systems.

3. Enzymes may be packed in microcapsules formed by a polymerisation reaction, e.g. by using 1, 6-diaminohexane. In addition, they may be enclosed within liposomes which are small spheres made up of concentric lipid membranes.

Each immobilisation strategy has some strong and some weak points which are summarised in Table 6.3.

Table 6.3: Comparison of the various features of the different immobilisation systems.

| Feature | Adsorption | Immobilisation system | | Membrane confinement |
		Covalent binding	Entrapment	
Matrices (examples)	Ion-exchange matrices, clays, glasses, etc.	Sepharose, cellulose, acrylamide, etc.	Acrylamide, cellulose acetate, etc.	Semipermeable membranes, e.g. hollow-fibres, lipsomes, etc.
Preparation	Simple	Difficult	Difficult	Simple
Immobilisation mechanism	Hydrophobic effects, salt links	Covalent bonds	Trapping in gel/fibre, even covalent bonds	Confinement in a semipermeable membrane
Binding force	Variable	Strong	Weak	Strong
Enzyme loading	High matrix)	Small (matrix)	–	–
Enzyme leakage during use	Yes	No	Yes	No
Applicability	Wide	Selective	Wide	Very wide
Problems during operation	High	Low	High	High
Matrix effects on enzyme	Yes	Yes	Yes	No
Diffusional barriers to substrate and product molecules	Absent	Absent	Large	Large
Protection from microbial attack	No	No	Yes	Yes
Cost	Low	High	Moderate	High

Effects of Immobilisation on Enzyme

Often kinetic behaviour of an immobilised enzyme may differ significantly from that of its free molecules. Different enzymes respond differently to the same immobilisation protocol. Therefore, a suitable immobilisation protocol has to be worked out for a given enzyme. The effects on enzyme kinetics (i.e. activity) may be due to the influence of matrix *per se* or due to conformational changes in the enzyme molecules induced by the procedure of immobilisation.

Immobilisation protocol may increase or decrease enzyme stability. When immobilisation produces a strain in the enzyme molecules, they become more prone to inactivation by higher temperatures, pH, etc. In contrast, binding of an enzyme molecule at several points without creating any strain in the enzyme molecule may lead to substantial stabilisation. This is primarily due to the physical prevention (due to multipoint binding) of large changes in the conformation of enzyme molecules which is essential for their inactivation. However, enzymes, whether free or immobilised, loose activity with time due to denaturation.

Advantage of Immobilisation

1. Enzymes are costly items, and can be used repeatedly only if they can be recovered from the reaction mixtures. Immobilisation permits their repeated use since such enzyme preparations can be easily separated from the reaction system.
2. The product is readily freed from the enzyme. This saves on the cost of downstream processing of the product.
3. Immobilised enzymes can be used in nonaqueous systems as well, which may be highly desirable in some cases.
4. Continuous production systems can be used, which is not possible with free enzymes.
5. Thermostability of some enzymes may be increased. For example, glucose isomerase denatures at 45°C in solution, but is stable for about 1 year even at 65°C when suitably immobilised.
6. Recovery of enzyme may also reduce effluent handling problems.
7. Enzymes can be used at much higher concentrations than free enzyme.

Disadvantage of Immobilisation

1. Immobilisation means additional cost. Therefore, it should be used only when there is a sound economic, safety or process advantages over soluble enzymes.
2. Immobilisation often adversely affects the stability and/or activity of the enzymes. In such cases suitable immobilisation protocols should be developed.
3. This approach can not be used when one of the substrates is insoluble.
4. Some immobilisation strategies present large problems in diffusion of the substrate to reach the enzyme.

METHODS FOR THE IMMOBILISATION OF CELLS

Three general methods are available for immobilising microbial cells.

1. Ionic binding to water-soluble ion-exchangers: Cells of *E. coli* and Azotobacter agile bound to Dowex-1 resin have been studied while mold spores have been bound to ion-exchange cellulose derivatives. In both cases successful demonstration of succinic acid oxidation and invertase activity

were demonstrated. This method is however not entirely satisfactory as enzymes may leak out following autolysis during continuous enzyme reaction.

2. Immobilisation in cross-linked chemicals: Microbial cells have been immobilised by cross-linking each other with bi-functional reagents such as glutaraldehyde. But non-cross-linking agents are equally effective.

3. Entrapment in a polymer matrix: This appears to be the most widely used method of immobilising cells. In this method the cells are entrapped in a polymer matrix where they are physically restrained. The following matrixes have been used: polyacrylamide, collagen, cellulose triacetate, agar, alginate and polystyrene.

Advantages of Immobilised Cells

Immobilised cells have the following advantages over conventional batch fermentation as well as over immobilised enzymes.

1. In batch fermentation, a significant proportion of the substrate is 'wasted' for the growth of the microbial population and for producing other substances other than enzymes required for the conversion at hand. Once the cells are immobilised however, they need to be offered nutrients for growth.

2. When cells are immobilised the reactions are more homogeneous and can be treated more like catalysts.

3. The lag period which occurs in a conventional batch fermentation is eliminated for the accumulation of products associated with non-growth phase of the cells.

4. It is more feasible to run immobilised cells continuously at high dilution rates without the risk of washout which would occur in a conventional continuous culture system.

5. Higher and faster yield is possible because of the greater density of cells, furthermore, toxic materials are continuously removed.

6. It is possible to recharge or resuscitate the cells by inducing growth and reproduction among resting cells.

7. A high capital cost is involved in installing, and operating a fermentor; in systems where comparison have been made, immobilised cells are cheaper than the conventional batch production.

8. The use of immobilised cells eliminates the need for enzyme extraction and purification. Furthermore, systems involving multi-enzyme reactions can occur more easily in intact cells harbouring these enzymes.

9. Immobilised cells are more suited to multiple step processes.

10. Cofactor regeneration is not a problem.

Immobilised cells are particularly appropriate under the following conditions:

- When the enzymes are intracellular: the use of immobilised cells would eliminate the need for breaking the cells for enzyme isolation.

- When extracted enzymes are unstable during or after immobilisation.

- When the micro-organism does not produce enzymes which can cause undesirable side reactions; or when such side-reaction producing enzymes can be readily inactivated.

- When the substrates and products are not high molecular weight substances.

Disadvantages of Immobilised Cells

Some of the disadvantages of the conventional system of cultivation of organisms spill over to the immobilised cell thus:

1. The cells may produce enzymes other than the one (s) sought.
2. Genetic changes, although with reduced likelihood in comparison with conventional fermentation, can also occur during immobilisation.
3. Immobilisation may result in the loss of a specific catalytic activity due to enzyme inactivation, resulting from the immobilisation process or to diffusional barriers hindering substrate access, or product removal from the organisms.
4. Cells located in the center of a cell flow may be deprived of nutrients or be inactivated by accumulating toxic wastes.
5. Contamination by other micro-organisms can occur.

PRACTICAL APPLICATION OF IMMOBILISED BIOLOGICAL CATALYST SYSTEMS

Immobilised enzymes and cells have been intensively studied in the hope that they can be used industrially. Only some of the expectations have been realised because of economic reasons. Soluble 'once only' enzymes marketed in the form of powder or liquids are available at low prices. Amylases and glucoamylases used in the starch industry are so low-priced comparatively that immobilised forms can hardly compete. The only immobilised enzyme currently used on a large scale is glucose isomerase used to produce about 2 million tons of high-fructose syrups around the world, but especially in the USA, Europe, and Japan. High fructose syrup competes successfully with sugar from beet or cane.

Several immobilised enzymes or whole cell processes are being applied in the Japanese pharmaceutical industry. These include L-amino acid from racemic acyl – D – L – amino acids, L-aspartic acid from ammonium fumarate, L-citrulline from L-arginine, and the production of 6-amino penicillanic acid (6-APA) for semi synthetic penicillin production. In the United States and Europe 6-APA is produced with immobilised enzymes. In Italy whole milk lactose hydrolysis is carried out by fibre entrapped lactase.

Many other applications are nearing the point in their development where they are ready for commercialisation: saccharification of starch by immobilised glucoamylase; cheese whey lactose hydrolysis by bound -galactosidase; beer chill-proofing, steroid transformations, protein-hydrolysis to improve digestibility. Industrial processes do not receive publicity rapidly and it is not unlikely that some of these may well have been commercialised already.

Immobilised cells have been used industrially in Japan for the transformations mentioned above except for L-amino acid isolation from racemic mixtures. The mostwidely employed use of immobilised cells however are glucose isomerisation and the hydrolysis of raffinose in beet sugar using mycelial pellets of the fungus *Mortierrella* sp. Raffinose (in beet molasses) is hydrolysed to sucrose and galactose by –galactosidase (mellibiase) produced by the fungus. The potentials of immobilised enzymes and cells are yet far from realised. When economic conditions permit them to become so, the whole process of fermentation as we know it today may be revolutionised and fermentors may become largely for the growth of cells for subsequent use in immobilised enzyme or cell production.

Immobilised Enzymes

Since the second half of the last century, numerous efforts have been devoted to the development of insoluble immobilised enzymes for a variety of applications. These applications can clearly benefit from use of the immobilised enzymes rather than the soluble counterparts, for instance as reusable heterogeneous biocatalysts, with the aim of reducing production costs by efficient recycling and control of the process as stable and reusable devices for analytical and medical applications as selective adsorbents for purification of proteins and enzymes as fundamental tools for solid-phase protein chemistry and as effective micro devices for controlled release of protein drugs. This is an enzyme that is physically confined while it carries out its catalytic function. This may occur naturally, as in the case of particulate enzymes, or it may be produced artificially by chemical or by physical methods.

In the chemical methods, the enzyme is linked covalently to a support. These methods include attachment of the enzyme to a water-insoluble support, incorporation of the enzyme into a growing polymer chain, or cross linking of the enzyme with a multifunctional low molecular weight reagent. In the physical methods, the enzyme is not linked covalently to a support. These methods include adsorption of the enzyme to a water-insoluble matrix, entrapment of the enzyme within either a water-insoluble gel or a microcapsule, or containment of the enzyme within special devices equipped with semi permeable membrane. Expensive enzymes can be recovered and used again. The enzyme can also be used in a variety of configurations of bioreactors that permit continuous operation.

Enzyme Immune System

Enzymes become part of the immune system (alpha-2-macroglobulin), working with it and facilitating its function. The modulation of growth factor binding properties of alpha-2-macroglobulin by enzyme therapy. Ingestion of proteinases was found to trigger the formation of intermediate forms of alpha-2-macro-globulin displaying high affinity of transforming growth factor- beta (TGF-β). Smith and others observed maximum binding of TGF-β 1–2 hr after bolus ingestion and steadily levelled off with time. They concluded that intestinal absorption of proteinase triggers the formation of TGF-β binding species of alpha 2 macroglobulin in blood mediated by this process of high concentrations of TGF-β might be reduced via enhanced clearance of alpha 2-macroglobulin TGF-β complexes. Thus, proteinase therapy may have beneficial effects in treatment of fibrosis and certain cancers accompanied by excessively high TGF-β concentrations. The oral therapy with proteolytic enzymes decreases excessive TGF-beta levels in human blood. In the study, they stated that therapy with oral proteolytic enzymes (OET) with combination drug products containing papain, bromelain, trypsin and chymotrypsin have been shown to be beneficial in clinical settings such as radio therapy induced fibrosis, bleomycin pneumotoxicity and immuno suppression in cancer, all of which are now-a-days knowned to be accompanied by excessive transforming growth factor-beta (TGF-β) production. Finally Smith and others concluded that their results support the concept that OET is beneficial in diseases characterised in part by TGF-β1 overproduction.

Enzymes as Markers for Disease

Some enzymes are found only in specific tissues or in a limited number of such tissues. For example, lactase dehydrogenase (LDH) has 2 different forms, called isozymes, in heart and skeletal muscle. Two forms differ slightly in amino acid composition and can be separated on the basis of charge as a result. Since LDH is a tetramer of four subunits, it too can exist in 5 different forms depending on the source of the subunits. An increase of any form of LDH in the blood indicates some kind of tissue damage. A heart attack can usually be diagnosed with certainty if there is an increase of LDH from heart. Also, there are different forms of Creatine Kinase (CK), an enzyme that occurs in the brain, heart and skeletal muscle. Appearance of the brain type can indicate a stroke or a brain tumour, whereas the heart type indicates a heart attack. After a heart attack, CK shows up more rapidly in the blood than LDH. Monitoring the presence of both enzymes extends the possibility of diagnosis, which is useful, since a very mild heart attack might be difficult to diagnose. An elevated level of the isozyme from heart in blood is a definite indication of damage to the heart tissue.

Another useful enzyme assayed is acetyl cholinesterase (AChE), which is important in controlling certain nerve impulses. Many pesticides affect this enzyme, so farm workers are often tested to be sure that they have not received inappropriate exposure to these important agricultural toxins. There are several enzymes that are typically used in the clinical laboratory to diagnose diseases. There are highly specific markers for enzymes active in the pancrease, red blood cells, liver, heart, brain, prostate gland and many of the endocrine glands. Since these enzymes are relatively easy to assay using automated techniques, they are part of the standard blood test veterinary and medical doctors are likely to need in the diagnosis and treatment/management of diseases.

Enzymes as Drug or Antibiotics

New antibiotics that are active against resistant bacteria have lived on earth for several billion years. During this time, they encountered in nature a wide range naturally occurring antibiotics or drugs. To survive, bacteria developed antibiotic resistance mechanism. Enzymes as drugs have two important features that distinguish them from all other types of drugs. First, enzymes often bind and act on their targets with great affinity and specificity. Second, enzymes are catalytic and convert multiple target molecules to the desired products. These two features make enzymes specific and potent drugs that can accomplish therapeutic biochemistry in the body that small molecules cannot. These characteristics have resulted in the development of many enzyme drugs for a wide range of disorders.

Enzymes in the Diagnosis of Pathology

The measurement of the serum levels of numerous enzymes has been shown to be of diagnostic significance. This is because the presence of these enzymes in the serum indicates that tissue or cellular damage has occurred resulting in the release of intracellular components into the blood. Hence, when a physician indicates that he/she is going to assay for liver enzymes, the purpose is to ascertain the potential for liver cell damage. Commonly assayed enzymes are the aminotransferases: alanine transaminase, ALT (sometimes still referred to as serum glutamate-pyruvate aminotransferase, SGPT) and aspartate amino-transferase, AST (also referred to as serum glutamate-oxaloacetate amino-transferase, SGOT), lactate dehydrogenase, LDH, creatine kinase, CK (also called creatine phosphokinase, CPK), gamma-glutamyl transpeptidase, GGT. Other enzymes are assayed under a variety of different clinical situations. Many enzymes are involved in the clinical diagnoses of various diseases in human and veterinary medicine. These enzymes facilitate or enhance rapid diagnoses of these diseases.

The classification of these enzymes is discussed below:

Alkaline phosphatase: Alkaline phosphatases were the earliest serum enzymes to be recognised to have clinical significance, when in the 1920s, it was discovered that they increase in bone and liver diseases . Since then, they have been the subject of more publications than any other enzyme. Alkaline phosphates are a group of isoforms which hydrolyse many types of phosphate esters, whose natural substrate or substrates are unknown. The term 'alkaline' refers to the optimal alkaline pH of this class of phosphatases *in vitro*. In both humans and animals, the major sources of ALPs are the liver, bone, kidney and placenta. In humans, it is involved in bone and hepatobiliary diseases. ALPs are also of diagnostic importance in animal diseases. Total serum ALP activity has diagnostic value in the hepatic and bone diseases in dogs and cats. It is of little value in hepatic diseases of horses and ruminants because of the broad range of reference values against which the patients' values must be compared. The range of serum ALP value in goats may be 10-fold with no evidence of hepatic damage. Values within the individual are fairly constant for sequential evaluation.

Creatine kinase: Creatine kinase isozymes are the most organspecific serum enzymes in clinical use. They catalyse the reversible phosphorylation of creatine by ATP to form creatine phosphate, the major storage form of high-energy phosphate required by muscle. Creatine kinases are found in many parts of the body like the heart, brain, skeletal muscle and smooth muscle but they have their highest specific activity in the skeletal muscle. In humans, creatine kinase is associated with myocardial infarction and muscle diseases. Increase in creatine kinase in cerebrospinal fluid has been associated with a number of disorders in dogs, cats, cattle and horses. The creatine kinase are such sensitive indicators of muscle damage that, generally, only large increases in serum activity are of clinical significance.

Alanine aminotransferase: It was formerly known as Glutamic Puruvate Transaminase, (GPT). It catalyses the reversible transamination of Lalanine and 2-oxoglutarate to pyruvate and glutamate in the cytoplasm of the cell. ALT can be found in the liver, skeletal muscle and heart. The greatest specific activity of ALT in primates, dogs, cats, rabbits and rats is in the liver. It is a well established, sensitive liver-specific indicator of damage. However, ALT in the tissues of pigs, horses, cattle, sheep or goats is too low to be of diagnostic value. It is used as an indicator of hepatopathy in toxicological studies which use small laboratory rodents as well as dogs.

Aspartate aminotransferase: It was formerly called Glutamic Oxaloacetic Transaminase, (GOT). It catalyses the transamination of L-aspartate and 2-oxoglutarate to oxaloacetate and glutamate. AST is found in skeletal muscle, heart, liver, kidney and erythrocytes and is associated with myocardial, hepatic parenchymal and muscle diseases in humans and animals. The presence of AST in so many tissues make their serum level a good marker of soft tissue but precludes its use as an organspecific enzyme. Red blood cells contain a large amount of AST which leaks into plasma before haemolysis is seen.

Sorbitol dehydrogenase (SDH): It is also called L-iditol dehydrogenase, (IDH). It catalyses the reversible oxidation of D-sorbitol to D-fructose with the cofactor NAD. The plasma activity is low in dog and horse plasma but appreciably greater in cattle, sheep and goat serum. Aside from the testes, it is found in appreciable amounts only in hepatocytes. As a result of this, an increase in plasma SDH is consistent with hepatocyte damage. SDH is liver specific in humans and all species of animals and hepatic injury appears to be the only source of increased SDH activity. Although SDH is liver specific in all species, the already established usage of ALT in dogs and cats has limited SDH as a diagnostic indicator of hepatocellular damage to horses, cattle, sheep and goats.

Lactate dehydrogenases (LDH): It catalyses the reversible oxidation of pyruvate to L(+) lactate with the cofactor NAD. The equilibrium favours lactate formation, but the preferred assay method is in the direction of pyruvate because pyruvate has an inhibitory effect on LDH. Lactate dehydrogenase has isoenzymes. LDH can be found in the heart, liver, erythrocyte, skeletal muscle, platelets and lymph nodes. In humans, it is involved in myocardial infarction, haemolysis and liver disease. LDH isoenzyme profiles were the first isoenzyme profiles used in clinical veterinary medicine in an attempt to detect specific organ damage. The introduction of more highly organspecific procedures has resulted in LDH no longer being in common use in veterinary medicine.

Cholinesterase (ChE): Serum cholinesterase activity is composed of two distinct cholinesterases. The major substrate is acetylcholine, the neurotransmitter found at the myoneural junction. Acetylcholinesterase

(AChE, EC 3.1.1.7) found at the myoneural junction is the true ChE and is essential in hydrolysing acetylcholine so that the junction can be re-established and prepared for additional signals. The myoneural junction AChE is also found in red blood cells (RBC), mouse, pig, brain and rat liver. Only a small amount of AChE is found in plasma. The ChE of plasma is a pseudocholine sterase, butyl-cholinesterase (ButChE, EC 3.1.1.8), which hydrolyses butyrylcholine four times faster than acetylcholine and is also located in white matter of the brain, liver, pancrease and intestinal mucosa. Decreases in ButChE have been reported in humans with acute infection, muscular dystrophy, chronic renal disease and pregnancy, as well as insecticide intoxification.

Lipase: Serum pancreatic lipases (EC 3.1.1.3, triacylglycerol lipase) catalyse the hydrolysis of triglycerides preferentially at the 1 and 3 positions, releasing two fatty acids and a 2-monoglyceride. Lipase can be found in the pancrease and hepatobiliary tract and is involved in pancreatitis and hepatobiliary disease.

Amylase: Amylases are calcium-dependent metalloenzymes that randomly catalyse the hydrolysis of complex carbohydrates, e.g. glycogen at the 1-4-linkages. The products of this action are maltose and limit dextrins. The enzyme is a Ca_2^+ metalloenzyme which requires one of a number of activator ions such as Cl-or Br-. Amylase can be found in the salivary glands, pancrease and ovaries and is used as a diagnostic aid for pancreatitis.

Glutamyltransferase: This is a carboxypeptidase which cleaves C-terminal glutamyl groups and transfers them to peptides and other suitable acceptors. It is speculated that GGT is associated with glutathione metabolism. The major sources are the liver and kidney and are involved in hepatobiliary disease and alcoholism. Cholestatic disorders of all species examined result in increased serum GGT activity.

Trypsin: Trypsins are serum proteases which hydrolyse the peptide bonds formed by lysine or arginine with other amino acids. The pancreas as the zymogen trypsinogen, which is converted to tyrosine by intestinal enterokinase or trypsin itself, secretes them.

Glutathione peroxidases: These are metalloenzymes containing four atoms of selenium per molecule of enzyme. They catalyse the oxidation of reduced glutathione by peroxide to form water and oxidised glutathione. Because of the high concentration of selenium in glutathione peroxidases, there is a good direct correlation between the amount of red blood cell GPx activity and the selenium concentration of other organs. Other enzymes with disease diagnosis applications are acid phosphatase (ACP), found in prostate and erythrocytes and are used in diagnosis of prostate carcinoma. Aldolase (ALD), found in skeletal muscle and heart and involved in muscle disease.

Glutamate dehydrogenase (GLDH), found in the liver is used to diagnose hepatic parenchymal disease. Hydroxybutyrate dehydrogenase (HBD), which is the heart form of lactate dehydrogenase is involved in myocardial infarction Just as enzyme assay is used to diagnose diseases in humans and animals, it may also be applied to the investigation of diseases in plants. For example, it has been found that an injury (either mechanical or pathogenic) results in a marked, localised increase in the activity of glucose-6-phosphate dehydrogenase, but not of glucose phosphate isomerase, indicating diversion of glucose break down from glycolysis to the pentose phosphate pathway.

Enzymes used in Immunoassay

Enzymes may also be used as an alternative to radio isotopes as markers in immunoassays have been used for the determination of a variety of proteins and hormones. The role of enzymes in immunoassay used to replace radio-isotopes as markers, since they are not hazardous to health and can be detected by techniques which are more generally available. Any enzyme with a sensitive and convenient assay procedure can be used for this purpose. Two common examples of enzyme immunoassay (EIA) procedures are enzyme-linked immunosorbent assay (ELISA) and enzyme-multiplied immunoassay test (EMIT). ELISA is a highly sensitive assay that can be used to detect either antigen or antibody. Applications of ELISA include diagnostics for non-infectious diseases involving hormones, drugs, serum components, oncofetal proteins, or autoimmune diseases, as well as diagnostics for infectious diseases caused by bacterial, viral, mycotic or parasitic organisms. The enzymes frequently used in ELISA are Horseradish peroxidase, alkaline phosphatase and β-galactosidase. In EMIT, the activity of malate dehydrogenase is assayed by standard enzyme methodology for the detection of thyroxine by enzyme-labelled immunoassay.

Enzymes as Therapeutic Agents

Enzymes have found a few applications as therapeutic agents. Some examples are transfusion of fresh blood or its active components in bleeding disorders, oral administration of digestive enzymes in digestive diseases (e.g. cystic fibrosis), administration of fibrinolytic enzymes (e.g. streptokinase) to recanalise blood vessels occluded by blood clots (thrombi) in thromboembolic disorders (e.g. pulmonary embolism, acute myocardial infarction), treatment of selected disorders of inborn errors of metabolism (e.g. *Gauchers disease*), and cancer therapy (e.g. L-asparaginase in acute lymphocytic leukemia). For enzymes to be therapeutically useful, they should be derived from human sources to prevent immunological problems. Although enzymes derived from human blood are readily obtainable, enzymes derived from tissues, which would be particularly useful in the treatment of inborn errors of metabolism, are difficult to obtain in adequate quantities. Transport of specific enzymes to target tissues is also a problem, but some recent advances and commercial applications (e.g. propagation of human tissue culture cell lines, isolation and cloning of specific genes) have the potential of overcoming these difficulties. Such techniques have been used in the production of peptide hormones such as somatostatin and insulin, interferon, and tissue plasminogen activator. In the treatment with enzymes or proteins, covalent attachment of an inert polymer polyethylene glycol (PEG) provides many therapeutic benefits.

These include slowing the clearance, diminished immunogeneity, prevention of degradation, and binding to antibody. PEG-enzyme therapy is used in the treatment of immunodeficiency disease caused by adenosine deaminase deficiency and PEG-interferon alfa complex (peginterferon alfa-2a) is used in treatment of chronic hepatitis C infection. Ultimately, however, when a gene is cloned, techniques will be developed to incorporate it into the genome of persons lacking the gene or having a mutated gene.

Chapter 7

Cell Membrane

INTRODUCTION

The cell membrane, also known as the plasma membrane, is a double layer of lipids and proteins that surrounds a cell and separates the cytoplasm (the contents of the cell) from its surrounding environment. It is selectively permeable, which means that it only lets certain molecules enter and exit. It can also control the amount of some substances that go into or out of the cell. All cells have a cell membrane. Despite differences in structure and function, all living cells in multicellular organisms have a surrounding cell membrane. As the outer layer of your skin separates your body from its environment, the cell membrane (also known as the plasma membrane) separates the inner contents of a cell from its exterior environment. This cell membrane provides a protective barrier around the cell and regulates which materials can pass in or out.

The cell membrane (also called the plasma membrane or plasmalemma) is one biological membrane separating the interior of a cell from the outside environment. The cell membrane surrounds all cells and it is semipermeable, controlling the movement of substances in and out of cells. It contains a wide variety of biological molecules, primarily proteins and lipids, which are involved in a variety of cellular processes such as cell adhesion, ion channel conductance and cell signalling. The plasma membrane also serves as the attachment point for the intracellular cytoskeleton and, if present, the extracellular cell wall.

FUNCTIONS OF CELL MEMBRANE

The cell membrane surrounds the protoplasm of a cell and, in animal cells, physically separates the intracellular components from the extracellular environment, thereby serving a function similar to that of skin. In fungi, some bacteria, and plants, an additional cell wall forms the outermost boundary, however, the cell wall plays mostly a mechanical support role rather than a role as a selective boundary. The cell membrane also plays a role in anchoring the cytoskeleton to provide shape to the cell, and in attaching to the extracellular matrix and other cells to help group cells together to form tissues. The barrier is differentially permeable and able to regulate what enters and exits the cell, thus facilitating the transport of materials needed for survival. The movement of substances across the membrane can be either passive, occurring without the input of cellular energy, or active, requiring the cell to expend energy in moving

127

it. The membrane also maintains the cell potential. Specific proteins embedded in the cell membrane can act as molecular signals that allow cells to communicate with each other. Protein receptors are found ubiquitously and function to receive signals from both the environment and other cells. These signals are transduced and passed in a different form into the cell. For example, a hormone binding to a receptor could open an ion channel in the receptor and allow calcium ions to flow into the cell. Other proteins on the surface of the cell membrane serve as 'markers' that identify a cell to other cells. The interaction of these markers with their respective receptors forms the basis of cell-cell interaction in the immune system.

Lipid Bilayer

The cell membrane consists primarily of a thin layer of amphipathic phospholipids which spontaneously arrange so that the hydrophobic 'tail' regions are shielded from the surrounding polar fluid, causing the more hydrophilic 'head' regions to associate with the cytosolic and extracellular faces of the resulting bilayer. This forms a continuous, spherical lipid bilayer (Fig. 7.1).

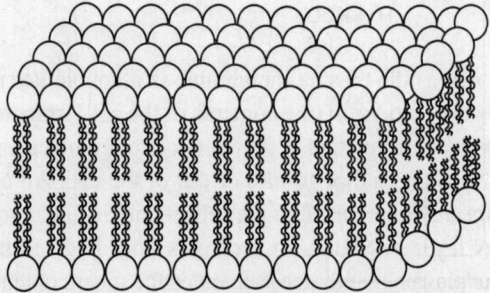

Fig. 7.1: Diagram of the arrangement of amphipathic lipid molecules to form a lipid bilayer. The polar head groups separate the grey hydrophobic tails from the aqueous cytosolic and extracellular environments.

The arrangement of hydrophilic heads and hydrophobic tails of the lipid bilayer prevent polar solutes (e.g. amino acids, nucleic acids, carbohydrates, proteins, and ions) from diffusing across the membrane, but generally allows for the passive diffusion of hydrophobic molecules. This affords the cell the ability to control the movement of these substances, via., transmembrane protein complexes such as pores and gates. Flippases and Scramblases concentrate phosphatidyl serine, which carries a negative charge, on the inner membrane. Along with *N*-acetyl Neuraminic acid (NANA), this creates an extra barrier to charged moieties moving through the membrane.

Membranes serve diverse functions in eukaryotic and prokaryotic cells. One important role is to regulate the movement of materials into and out of cells. The phospholipid bilayer structure (fluid mosaic model) with specific membrane proteins accounts for the selective permeability of the membrane and passive and active transport mechanisms. In addition, membranes in prokaryotes and in the mitochondria and chloroplasts of eukaryotes facilitate the synthesis of ATP through chemiosmosis.

Membrane polarity

The apical membrane of a polarised cell is the surface of the plasma membrane that faces the lumen. This is particularly evident in epithelial and endothelial cells, but also describes other polarised cells, such as neurons. The basolateral membrane of a polarised cell is the surface of the plasma membrane that forms its basal and lateral surfaces. It faces towards the interstitium, and away from the lumen.

'Basolateral membrane' is a compound phrase referring to the terms basal (base) membrane and lateral (side) membrane, which, especially in epithelial cells, are identical in composition and activity. Proteins (such as ion channels and pumps) are free to move from the basal to the lateral surface of the cell or vice versa in accordance with the fluid mosaic model. Tight junctions that join epithelial cells near their apical surface prevent the migration of proteins from the basolateral membrane to the apical membrane. The basal and lateral surfaces thus remain roughly equivalent to one another, yet distinct from the apical surface. Figure 7.2 shows alpha intercalated cell.

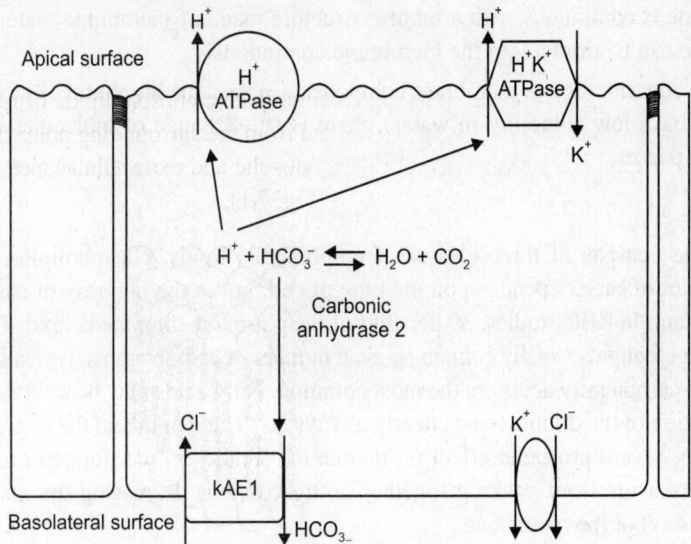

Fig. 7.2: Alpha intercalated cell.

Integral membrane proteins

The cell membrane contains many integral membrane proteins, which pepper the entire surface. These structures, which can be visualised by electron microscopy or fluorescence microscopy, can be found on the inside of the membrane, the outside or membrane spanning. These may include integrins, cadherins, desmosomes, clathrin-coated pits, caveolaes, and different structures involved in cell adhesion.

Membrane skeleton

The cytoskeleton is found underlying the cell membrane in the cytoplasm and provides a scaffolding for membrane proteins to anchor to, as well as forming organelles that extend from the cell. Indeed, cytoskeletal elements interact extensively and intimately with the cell membrane. Anchoring proteins restricts them to a particular cell surface, for example, the apical surface of epithelial cells that line the vertebrate gut and limits how far they may diffuse within the bilayer. The cytoskeleton is able to form appendage-like organelles, such as cilia, which are microtubule-based extensions covered by the cell membrane, and filopodia, which are actin-based extensions. These extensions are ensheathed in membrane and project from the surface of the cell in order to sense the external environment and/or make contact with the substrate or other cells. The apical surfaces of epithelial cells are dense with actin-based finger-like projections known as microvilli, which increase cell surface area and thereby increase the absorption rate of nutrients. Localised decoupling of the cytoskeleton and cell membrane results in formation of a bleb.

Composition of Cell Membrane

Cell membranes contain a variety of biological molecules, notably lipids and proteins. Material is incorporated into the membrane or deleted from it, by a variety of mechanisms:

1. Fusion of intracellular vesicles with the membrane (exocytosis) not only excretes the contents of the vesicle but also incorporates the vesicle membrane's components into the cell membrane. The membrane may form blebs around extracellular material that pinch off to become vesicles (endocytosis).
2. If a membrane is continuous with a tubular structure made of membrane material, then material from the tube can be drawn into the membrane continuously.
3. Although the concentration of membrane components in the aqueous phase is low (stable membrane components have low solubility in water), there is an exchange of molecules between the lipid and aqueous phases.

Lipids

The cell membrane consists of three classes of amphipathic lipids: phospholipids, glycolipids, and steroids. The amount of each depends upon the type of cell, but in the majority of cases phospholipids are the most abundant. In RBC studies, 30 per cent of the plasma membrane is lipid. The fatty chains in phospholipids and glycolipids usually contain an even number of carbon atoms, typically between 16 and 20. The 16- and 18-carbon fatty acids are the most common. Fatty acids may be saturated or unsaturated, with the configuration of the double bonds nearly always *cis*. The length and the degree of unsaturation of fatty acid chains have a profound effect on membrane fluidity as unsaturated lipids create a kink, preventing the fatty acids from packing together as tightly, thus decreasing the melting temperature (increasing the fluidity) of the membrane.

The ability of some organisms to regulate the fluidity of their cell membranes by altering lipid composition is called homeoviscous adaptation. The entire membrane is held together via noncovalent interaction of hydrophobic tails, however, the structure is quite fluid and not fixed rigidly in place. Under physiological conditions phospholipid molecules in the cell membrane are in the liquid crystalline state. It means the lipid molecules are free to diffuse and exhibit rapid lateral diffusion along the layer in which they are present. However, the exchange of phospholipid molecules between intracellular and extracellular leaflets of the bilayer is a very slow process. Lipid rafts and caveolae are examples of cholesterol-enriched microdomains in the cell membrane.

In animal cells cholesterol is normally found dispersed in varying degrees throughout cell membranes, in the irregular spaces between the hydrophobic tails of the membrane lipids, where it confers a stiffening and strengthening effect on the membrane.

Carbohydrates

Plasma membranes also contain carbohydrates, predominantly glycoproteins, but with some glycolipids (cerebrosides and gangliosides). For the most part, no glycosylation occurs on membranes within the cell, rather generally glycosylation occurs on the extracellular surface of the plasma membrane.

The glycocalyx is an important feature in all cells, especially epithelia with microvilli. Recent data suggest the glycocalyx participates in cell adhesion, lymphocyte homing, and many others. The penultimate sugar is galactose and the terminal sugar is sialic acid, as the sugar backbone is modified in the Golgi apparatus. Sialic acid carries a negative charge, providing an external barrier to charged particles.

Proteins

The cell membrane plays host to a large amount of protein that is responsible for its various activities. The amount of protein differs between species and according to function, however, the typical amount in a cell membrane is 50 per cent. These proteins are undoubtedly important to a cell: Approximately a third of the genes in yeast code specifically for them, and this number is even higher in multicellular organisms. The cell membrane, being exposed to the outside environment, is an important site of cell-cell communication. As such, a large variety of protein receptors and identification proteins, such as antigens, are present on the surface of the membrane. Functions of membrane proteins can also include cell-cell contact, surface recognition, cytoskeleton contact, signalling, enzymatic activity or transporting substances across the membrane. Most membrane proteins must be inserted in some way into the membrane. For this to occur, an *N*-terminus 'signal sequence' of amino acids directs proteins to the endoplasmic reticulum, which inserts the proteins into a lipid bilayer. Once inserted, the proteins are then transported to their final destination in vesicles, where the vesicle fuses with the target membrane.

Chemical Composition of Membrane

Membranes are lipid-protein assemblies in which the components are held together in a thin sheet by noncovalent bonds. As noted above, the core of the membrane consists of sheet of lipids arranged in a bimolecular layer. The lipid bilayer serves primarily as a structural backbone of the membrane and provides the barrier that prevent random movements of water-soluble materials into and out of the cell. The ratio of lipid to protein in a membrane varies, depending on the type of cellular membrane (plasma vs. endoplasmic reticulum vs. Golgi), the type of organism (bacterium vs. plant vs. animal), and the type of cell (cartilage vs. muscle vs. liver). For example, the inner mitochondrial membrane has a very high ratio of protein/ lipid in comparison to the red blood cell plasma membrane, which is high in comparison to the membranes of the myelin sheath that form a multilayered wrapping around a nerve cell. To a large degree these differences can be correlated with the basic functions of these membranes. The inner mitochondrial membrane contains the protein carriers of the electron-transport chain, and relative to other membranes, lipid is diminished. In contrast, the myelin sheath acts primarily as electrical insulation for the nerve cell it enclose, a function that is best carried out by a thick lipid layer of high electrical resistance with a minimal content of protein.

Membrane lipids

The three major classes of membrane lipids are phospholipids, glycolipids, and cholesterol.

Phospholipids: Phospholipids and glycolipids consist of two long, nonpolar (hydrophobic) hydrocarbon chains linked to a hydrophilic head group.

Glycolipids: The heads of glycolipids contain a sphingosine with one or several sugar units attached to it.

Fatty acids: The fatty acids (FAs) in phospho- and glycolipids usually contain an even number of carbon atoms, typically between 14 and 24.

Sphingosine: Sphingosine is an amino alcohol that contains a long, unsaturated hydrocarbon chain.

Cholesterol: Cholesterol occurs naturally in eukaryote cell membranes where it is biosynthesised from mevalonate via a squalene cyclisation of terpenoids. It is associated preferentially with sphingolipids in cholesterol-rich lipid rafts areas of the membranes in eukaryotic cells. Hopanoids serve a similar function in prokaryotes.

Functions of Mammalian Sphingolipids

Sphingolipids are commonly believed to protect the cell surface against harmful environmental factors by forming a mechanically stable and chemically resistant outer leaflet of the plasma membrane lipid bilayer. Certain complex glycosphingolipids were found to be involved in specific functions, such as cell recognition and signalling. The first feature depends mainly on the physical properties of the sphingolipids, whereas signalling involves specific interactions of the glycan structures of glycosphingolipids with similar lipids present on neighbouring cells or with proteins. Recently, relatively simple sphingolipid metabolites, such as ceramide and sphingosine-1-phosphate, have been shown to be important mediators in the signalling cascades involved in apoptosis, proliferation, and stress responses. Ceramide-based lipids self-aggregate in cell membranes and form separate phases less fluid than the bulk phospholipids. These sphingolipid-based microdomains, or 'lipid rafts' were originally proposed to sort membrane proteins along the cellular pathways of membrane transport. At present, most research focuses on the organising function during signal transduction.

Sphingolipids are synthesised in a pathway that begins in the ER and is completed in the Golgi apparatus, but these lipids are enriched in the plasma membrane and in endosomes, where they perform many of their functions. Transport occurs, via., vesicles and monomeric transport in the cytosol. Sphingolipids are virtually absent from mitochondria and the ER, but constitute a 20–35 molar fraction of plasma membrane lipids. There are several disorders of sphingolipid metabolism, known as sphingolipidoses. The most common is Gaucher's disease. Also of note is Fabry's disease, an X-linked recessive condition wherein a buildup of glycosphingolipids in lysosomes of various tissues is due to alpha-galactosidase deficiency. These patients tend to present with peripheral neuropathies and develop chronic renal conditions.

Yeast sphingolipids

Because of the incredible complexity of mammalian systems, yeast are sometimes used as a model organism for working out new pathways. These single-celled organisms are often more genetically tractable than mammalian cells, and strain libraries are available to supply strains harbouring almost any non-lethal open reading frame single deletion. The two most commonly used yeasts are *Saccharomyces cerevisiae* and *Schizosaccharomyces pombe*, although research is also done in the pathological yeast *Candida albicans* (Fig. 7.3).

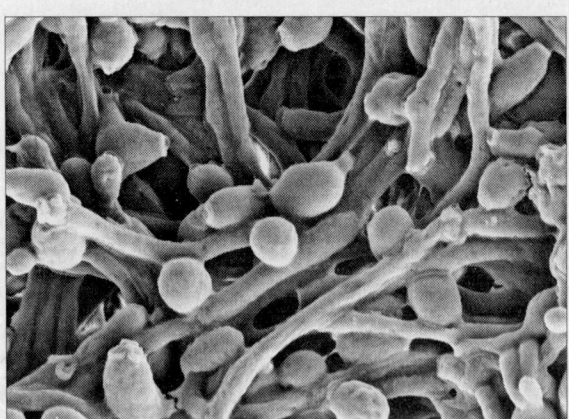

Fig. 7.3: *Candida albicans.*

Phases and phase transitions

At a given temperature a lipid bilayer can exist in either a liquid or a gel (solid) phase. All lipids have a characteristic temperature at which they transition (melt) from the gel to liquid phase. In both phases the lipid molecules are prevented from flip-flopping across the bilayer, but in liquid phase bilayers a given lipid will exchange locations with its neighbour millions of times a second. This random walk exchange allows lipid to diffuse and thus wander across the surface of the membrane. Unlike liquid phase bilayers, the lipids in a gel phase bilayer are locked in place (Fig. 7.4). The phase behaviour of lipid bilayers is largely determined by the strength of the attractive van der Waals interactions between adjacent lipid molecules. Longer tailed lipids have more area over which to interact, increasing the strength of this interaction and consequently decreasing the lipid mobility. Thus, at a given temperature, a short-tailed lipid will be more fluid than an otherwise identical long-tailed lipid.

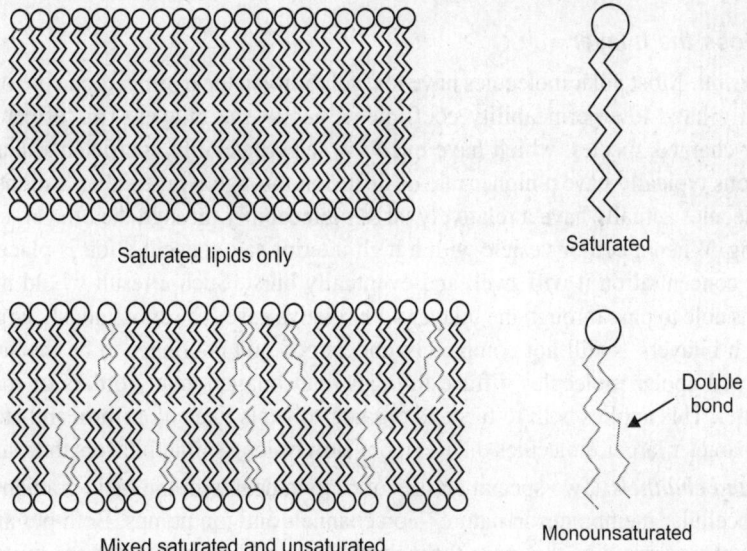

Fig. 7.4: Diagram showing the effect of unsaturated lipids on a bilayer. The lipids with an unsaturated tail disrupt the packing of those with only saturated tails. The resulting bilayer has more free space and is consequently more permeable to water and other small molecules.

Transition temperature can also be affected by the degree of unsaturation of the lipid tails. An unsaturated double bond can produce a kink in the alkane chain, disrupting the lipid packing. This disruption creates extra free space within the bilayer which allows additional flexibility in the adjacent chains. An example of this effect can be noted in everyday life as butter, which has a large percentage saturated fats, is solid at room temperature while vegetable oil, which is mostly unsaturated, is liquid. Most natural membranes are a complex mixture of different lipid molecules. If some of the components are liquid at a given temperature while others are in the gel phase, the two phases can coexist in spatially separated regions, rather like an iceberg floating in the ocean. This phase separation plays a critical role in biochemical phenomena because membrane components such as proteins can partition into one or the other phase and thus be locally concentrated or activated. One particularly important component of many mixed phase systems is cholesterol, which modulates bilayer permeability, mechanical strength and biochemical interactions.

Biological roles

Containment and separation: The primary role of the lipid bilayer in biology is to separate aqueous compartments from their surroundings. Without some form of barrier delineating 'self' from 'nonself' it is difficult to even define the concept of an organism or of life. This barrier takes the form of a lipid bilayer in all known life forms except for a few species of *archaea* which utilise a specially adapted lipid monolayer.

Signalling: Probably the most familiar form of cellular signalling is synaptic transmission, whereby a nerve impulse that has reached the end of one neuron is conveyed to an adjacent neuron via. the release of neurotransmitters. This transmission is made possible by the action of synaptic vesicles loaded with the neurotransmitters to be released. These vesicles fuse with the cell membrane at the presynaptic terminal and release its contents to the exterior of the cell. The contents then diffuse across the synapse to the post-synaptic terminal.

Transport across the bilayer

Passive diffusion: Most polar molecules have low solubility in the hydrocarbon core of a lipid bilayer and consequently have low permeability coefficients across the bilayer. This effect is particularly pronounced for charged species, which have even lower permeability coefficients than neutral polar molecules. Anions typically have a higher rate of diffusion through bilayers than cations. Compared to ions, water molecules actually have a relatively large permeability through the bilayer, as evidenced by osmotic swelling. When a cell or vesicle with a high interior salt concentration is placed in a solution with a low salt concentration it will swell and eventually burst. Such a result would not be observed unless water was able to pass through the bilayer with relative ease. The anomalously large permeability of water through bilayers is still not completely understood and continues to be the subject of active debate. Uncharged apolar molecules diffuse through lipid bilayers many orders of magnitude faster than ions or water. This applies both to fats and organic solvents like chloroform and ether. Regardless of their polar character larger molecules diffuse more slowly across lipid bilayers than small molecules.

Ion pumps and channels: Two special classes of protein deal with the ionic gradients found across cellular and subcellular membranes in nature—ion channels and ion pumps. Both pumps and channels are integral membrane proteins that pass through the bilayer, but their roles are quite different. Ion pumps are the proteins that build and maintain the chemical gradients by utilising an external energy source to move ions against the concentration gradient to an area of higher chemical potential.

Endocytosis and exocytosis: Some molecules or particles are too large or too hydrophilic to effectively pass through a lipid bilayer. Other molecules could pass through the bilayer but must be transported rapidly in such large numbers that channel-type transport is impractical. In both cases these types of cargo can be moved across the cell membrane through fusion or budding of vesicles. When a vesicle is produced inside the cell and fuses with the plasma membrane to release its contents into the extracellular space this process is known as exocytosis. In the reverse process a region of the cell membrane will dimple inwards and eventually pinch off, enclosing a portion of the extracellular fluid to transport it into the cell. Endocytosis and exocytosis rely on very different molecular machinery to function, but the two processes are intimately linked and could not work without each other.

Electroporation: Electroporation is the rapid increase in bilayer permeability induced by the application of a large artificial electric field across the membrane. Experimentally, electroporation is used to introduce hydrophilic molecules into cells. It is a particularly useful technique for large highly charged molecules such as DNA which would never passively diffuse across the hydrophobic bilayer core. Because of this, electroporation is one of the key methods of transfection as well as bacterial transformation. It has even been proposed that electroporation resulting from lightning strikes could be a mechanism of natural horizontal gene transfer.

Fusion: Fusion is the process by which two lipid bilayers merge, resulting in one connected structure. If this fusion proceeds completely through both leaflets of both bilayers, a water-filled bridge is formed and the solutions contained by the bilayers can mix. Alternatively, if only one leaflet from each bilayer is involved in the fusion process, the bilayers are said to be hemifused. Fusion is involved in many cellular processes, particularly in eukaryotes since the eukaryotic cell is extensively subdivided by lipid bilayer membranes. Exocytosis, fertilisation of an egg by sperm and transport of waste products to the lysosome are a few of the many eukaryotic processes that rely on some form of fusion. Even the entry of pathogens can be governed by fusion, as many bilayer-coated viruses have dedicated fusion proteins to gain entry into the host cell (Fig. 7.4). There are four fundamental steps in the fusion process. First, the involved membranes must aggregate, approaching each other to within several nanometers. Second, the two bilayers must come into very close contact (within a few angstroms). To achieve this close contact, the two surfaces must become at least partially dehydrated, as the bound surface water normally present causes bilayers to strongly repel. The presence of ions, particularly divalent cations like magnesium and calcium, strongly affects this step. One of the critical roles of calcium in the body is regulating membrane fusion. Third, a destabilisation must form at one point between the two bilayers, locally distorting their structures.

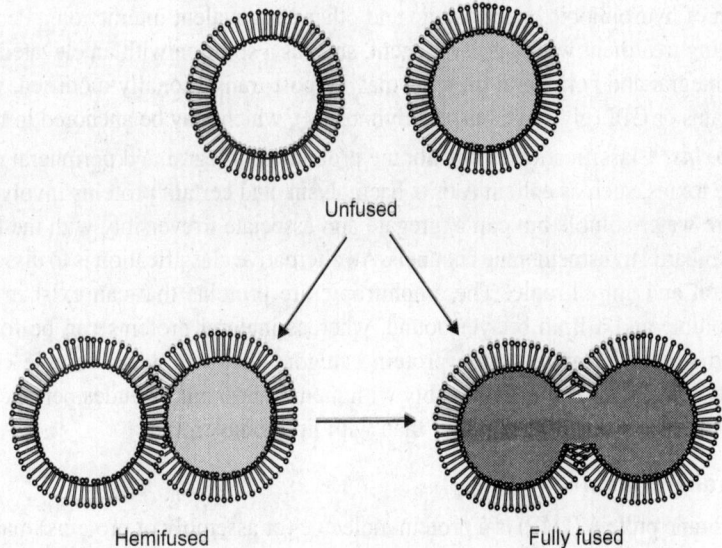

Unfused

Hemifused

Fully fused

Fig. 7.5: Illustration of lipid vesicles fusing showing two possible outcomes: hemifusion and full fusion. In hemifusion only the outer bilayer leaflets mix. In full fusion both leaflets as well as the internal contents mix.

STRUCTURE AND FUNCTIONS OF MEMBRANE PROTEINS

A membrane protein is a protein molecule that is attached to, or associated with the membrane of a cell or an organelle. More than half of all proteins interact with membranes.

Biological membranes consist of a phospholipid bilayer and a variety of proteins that accomplish vital biological functions. Structural proteins are attached to micro-filaments in the cytoskeleton which ensures stability of the cell. Cell recognition proteins allow cells to identify each other and interact. Such proteins are involved in immune response, for example. Membrane enzymes produce a variety of substances essential for cell function. Membrane receptor proteins serve as connection between the cell's internal and external environments. Finally, transport proteins play an important role in the maintenance of concentrations of ions. These transport proteins come in two forms: carrier proteins and channel proteins. Carrier proteins are involved in using the energy released from ATP being broken down to facilitate active transport and ion exchange. These processes ensure that useful substances are able to enter the cell and that toxic substances are pumped out of the cell. The main categories are— integral membrane proteins, peripheral membrane proteins and polypeptide toxins. Integral membrane proteins: Integral membrane proteins are permanently attached to the membrane. They can be defined as those proteins which require a detergent (such as SDS or Triton X-100) or some other apolar solvent to be displaced. They can be classified according to their relationship with the bilayer:

1. Transmembrane proteins span the entire membrane. The transmembrane regions of the proteins are either β-barrels or α-helical. The α-helical domains are present in all types of biological membranes including outer membranes. The β-barrels were found only in outer membranes of Gram-negative bacteria, lipid-rich cell walls of a few Gram-positive bacteria, and outer membranes of mitochondria and chloroplasts.

2. Integral monotopic proteins are permanently attached to the membrane from only one side.

Peripheral membrane proteins are temporarily attached either to the lipid bilayer or to integral proteins by a combination of hydrophobic, electrostatic and other noncovalent interactions. Peripheral proteins dissociate following treatment with a polar reagent, such as a solution with an elevated pH or high salt concentrations. Integral and peripheral proteins may be post-translationally modified, with added fatty acid or prenyl chains or GPI (glycosylphosphatidylinositol), which may be anchored in the lipid bilayer.

Polypeptide toxins: Classification of membrane proteins to integral and peripheral does not include some polypeptide toxins, such as colicin A or α-haemolysin, and certain proteins involved in apoptosis. These proteins are water-soluble but can aggregate and associate irreversibly with the lipid bilayer and form α-helical or β-barrel transmembrane channels. An alternative classification is to divide all membrane proteins to integral and amphitropic. The amphitropic are proteins that can exist in two alternative states: a water-soluble and a lipid bilayer-bound, whereas integral proteins can be found only in the membrane-bound state. The amphitropic protein category includes water-soluble channel-forming polypeptide toxins, which associate irreversibly with membranes, but excludes peripheral proteins that interact with other membrane proteins rather than with lipid bilayer.

Integral Membrane Protein

An integral membrane protein (IMP) is a protein molecule (or assembly of proteins) that is permanently attached to the biological membrane. Such proteins can be separated from the biological membranes only using detergents, nonpolar solvents or sometimes denaturing agents (Fig. 7.6). IMPs comprise a very significant fraction of the proteins encoded in an organism's genome. Three-dimensional structures of only ~160 different integral membrane proteins are currently determined at atomic resolution by X-ray crystallography or nuclear magnetic resonance spectroscopy due to the difficulties with extraction and crystallisation. In addition, structures of many water-soluble domains of IMPs are available in the Protein Data Bank. Their membrane-anchoring α-helices have been removed to facilitate the extraction and crystallisation.

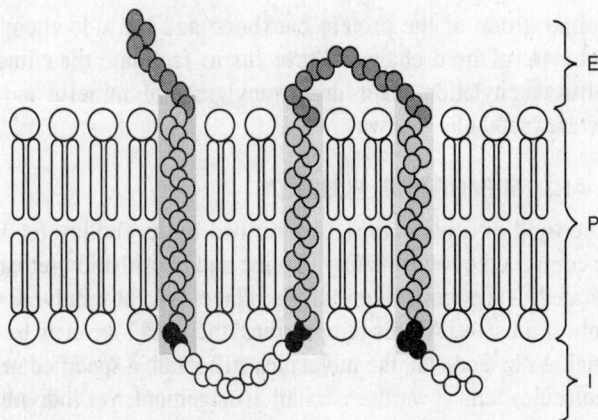

Fig. 7.6: Integral membrane protein. E = extracellular space, P = plasma membrane, I = intracellular space.

IMPs can be divided into two groups:

1. Transmembrane proteins.
2. Integral monotopic proteins.

The most common type of IMP is the transmembrane protein (TM), which spans the entire biological membrane. Single-pass membrane proteins cross the membrane only once, while multi-pass membrane proteins weave in and out, crossing several times. TM proteins can be categorised as Type I, which are positioned such that their amino-terminus is outside of the membrane or Type II, which have their carboxy-terminus outside of the membrane.

Peripheral Membrane Protein

Peripheral membrane proteins are proteins that adhere only temporarily to the biological membrane with which they are associated. These molecules attach to integral membrane proteins or penetrate the peripheral regions of the lipid bilayer. The regulatory protein subunits of many ion channels and transmembrane receptors, for example, may be defined as peripheral membrane proteins. In contrast to integral membrane proteins, peripheral membrane proteins tend to collect in the water-soluble component, or fraction, of all the proteins extracted during a protein purification procedure. Proteins with GPI anchors are an exception to this rule and can have purification properties similar to those of integral membrane proteins. Peripheral membrane proteins may interact with other proteins or directly with the lipid bilayer. In the latter case, they are then known as amphitropic proteins. Some proteins, such as G-proteins and certain protein kinases, interact with transmembrane proteins and the lipid bilayer simultaneously. Some polypeptide hormones, antimicrobial peptides, and neurotoxins accumulate at the membrane surface prior to locating and interacting with their cell surface receptor targets, which may themselves be peripheral membrane proteins.

Lipid-anchored Protein

In lipid-anchored proteins, a covalently attached fatty acid such as palmitate or myristate serves to anchor them to either face of the cell membrane. Examples include G-proteins and certain kinases. It is believed that the fatty acid chain inserts and assumes a place in the bilayer structure of the membrane alongside the similar fatty-acid tails of the surrounding lipid molecules. Potential points of attachment include the terminal amino group of the protein backbone and the side chain of cysteine residues. Prenylation is the attachment of lipid chains to proteins to facilitate their interaction with the cell membrane. Some important prenylation chains are geranylgeraniol, farnesol and dolichol, all products of the HMG-CoA reductase metabolic pathway.

MEMBRANE LIPIDS AND MEMBRANE FLUIDITY

The physical state of the lipid of a membrane is described by its fluidity (or viscosity). Consider a simple artificial bilayer composed of phosphatidylcholine and phosphatidyl-ethanolamine, whose fatty acids are largely unsaturated. If the temperature of the bilayer is kept relatively warm (e.g. 37°C), the lipid exists in a relatively fluid state. At this temperature, the lipid bilayer is best described as a two-dimensional liquid crystal. As in a crystal, the molecules still retain a specified orientation, in this case, the long axes of the molecules tend toward a parallel arrangement, yet individual phospholipids can rotate around their axis or move laterally within the plane of the bilayer. If the temperature is slowly lowered, a point is reached where the bilayer distinctly changes.

The lipid is converted from a liquid crystalline phase to a frozen crystalline gel in which the movement of the phospholipid fatty acid chains is greatly restricted. The temperature at which this change occurs is called the transition temperature. The transition temperature of a particular bilayer depends on the ability of the lipid molecules to be packed together, which depends in turn on the particular lipids of which it is constructed. The greater the degree of unsaturation of the fatty acids of the bilayer, the lower the temperature before the bilayer gels. Another factor that influences bilayer fluidity is fatty acid chain length. The shorter the fatty acyl chains of a phospholipid, the lower its melting temperature. The physical state of the membrane is also affected by cholesterol. The presence of cholesterol tends to abolish sharp transition temperatures and creates a condition of intermediate fluidity. In physiologic terms, cholesterol tends to increase the durability while decreasing the permeability of a membrane.

PLASMA MEMBRANE

The plasma membrane is a phospholipid bilayer membrane that separates the cell from its environment and regulates the transport of molecules and signals into and out of the cell. Embedded in the membrane are proteins that perform the functions of the plasma membrane. In addition to these universal functions, the plasma membrane has a more specific role in multicellular organisms. Glycoproteins on the membrane assist the cell in recognising other cells, in order to exchange metabolites and form tissues. Other proteins on the plasma membrane allow attachment to the cytoskeleton and extracellular matrix, a function that maintains cell shape and fixes the location of membrane proteins. Enzymes that catalyse reactions are also found on the plasma membrane. Receptor proteins on the membrane have a shape that matches with a chemical messenger, resulting in various cellular responses. The plasma membrane is not fixed or rigid structure, the molecules that compose the membrane are capable of laterally movement. This movement and the multiple components of the membrane are why it is referred to as a fluid mosaic. Smaller molecules such as carbon dioxide, water, and oxygen can pass through the plasma membrane freely by diffusion or osmosis. Larger molecules needed by the cell are assisted by proteins through active transport. The plasma membrane of a cell has multiple functions. These include transporting nutrients into the cell, allowing waste to leave, preventing materials from entering the cell, averting needed materials from leaving the cell, maintaining the pH of the cytosol, and preserving the osmotic pressure of the cytosol. Transport proteins which allow some materials to pass through but not others are used for these functions. These proteins use ATP hydrolysis to pump materials against their concentration gradients.

SECTION III

Bioenergetics and Metabolism

Chapter 8

Bioenergetics

INTRODUCTION

Living things require a continuous throughout of energy. For example, through photosynthesis, plants convert radiant energy from the sun, the primary energy source for life on earth, to the chemical energy of carbohydrates and other organic substances. The plants or the animals that eat them, then metabolise these substances to power such functions as the synthesis of biomolecules, the maintenance of concentration gradients and the movement of muscles. These processes ultimately transform the energy to heat, which is dissipated to the environment. A considerable portion of the cellular biochemical apparatus must therefore be devoted to the acquisition and utilisation of energy. For instance, although thermodynamics tells us that glucose and oxygen react with the release of copious amounts of energy, it does not indicate that this mixture is indefinitely stable at room temperature in the absence of the appropriate enzymes.

BIOENERGETICS AND THERMODYNAMICS

Bioenergetics is the subject of a field of biochemistry that concerns energy flow through living systems. This is an active area of biological research that includes the study of thousands of different cellular processes such as cellular respiration and the many other metabolic processes that can lead to production and utilisation of energy in forms such as Adenosine Triphosphate (ATP) molecules. Bioenergetics is the part of biochemistry concerned with the energy involved in making and breaking of chemical bonds in the molecules found in biological organisms.

Growth, development and metabolism are some of the central phenomena in the study of biological organisms. The role of energy is fundamental to such biological processes. The ability to harness energy from a variety of metabolic pathways is a property of all living organisms. Life is dependent on energy transformations, living organisms survive because of exchange of energy within and without.

In a living organism, chemical bonds are broken and made as part of the exchange and transformation of energy. Energy is available for work (such as mechanical work) or for other processes (such as chemical synthesis and anabolic processes in growth), when weak bonds are broken and stronger bonds are made. The production of stronger bonds allows release of usable energy.

Living organisms obtain energy from organic and inorganic materials. For example, lithotrophs can oxidise minerals such as nitrates or forms of sulphur, such as elemental sulphur, sulphites and hydrogen sulphide to produce ATP. In photosynthesis, autotrophs can produce ATP using light energy. Heterotrophs must consume organic compounds. These are mostly carbohydrates, fats and proteins. The amount of energy actually obtained by the organism is lower than the amount present in the food, there are losses in digestion, metabolism and thermo-genesis. Living things require a continuous throughput of energy. For example, through photosynthesis, plants convert radiant energy from the sun, the primary energy source for life on earth, to the chemical energy of carbohydrates and other organic substances.

The plants or the animals that eat them, then metabolise these substances to power such functions as the synthesis of biomolecules, the maintenance of concentration gradients and the movement of muscles. These processes ultimately transform the energy to heat, which is dissipated to the environment. A considerable portion of the cellular biochemical apparatus must therefore be devoted to the acquisition and utilisation of energy.

Thermodynamics is a marvellously elegant description of the relationships among the various forms of energy and how energy affects matter on the macroscopic as opposed to the molecular level, that is it deals with amounts of matter large enough for their average properties, such as temperature and pressure, to be well defined. Indeed the basic principles of thermodynamics were developed in the nineteenth century before the atomic theory of matter had been generally accepted. With a knowledge of thermo-dynamics we can determine whether a physical process is possible. Thermodynamics is therefore essential for under standing why macromolecules fold to their native conformations, how metabolic pathways are designed, why molecules cross biological membranes, how muscles generate mechanical force and so on. The list is endless. However, the thermodynamics does not indicate the rates at which possible processes actually occur. For instance, although thermodynamics tells us that glucose and oxygen react with the release of copious amounts of energy, it does not indicate that this mixture is indefinitely stable at room temperature in the absence of the appropriate enzymes.

The prediction of reaction rates requires, a mechanistic description of molecular processes. Yet thermodynamics is also an indispensable guide in formulating such mechanistic models because such models must conform to thermodynamic principles.

Thermodynamics, as it applies to biochemistry is most frequently concerned with describing the conditions under which processes occur spontaneously (by themselves). We shall consequently review the elements of thermodynamics that enable us to predict chemical and biochemical spontaneity: the first and second laws of thermodynamics, the concept of free energy and the nature of processes at equilibrium. Familiarity with these principles is indispensable for understanding many of the succeeding discussions in this chapter.

First Law of Thermodynamics: Energy is Conserved

In thermodynamics, a system is defined as that part of the universe that is of interest, such as a reaction vessel or an organism: the rest of the universe is known as the surroundings. A system is said to be open, closed or isolated according to whether or not it can exchange matter and energy with its surroundings, only energy or neither matter nor energy. Living organisms, which take up nutrients, release waste products and generate work and heat, are examples of open systems: if an organism were sealed inside an uninsulated box, it would, together with the box, constitute a closed system, whereas if the box were perfectly insulated, the system would be isolated.

Energy

The first law of thermodynamics is a mathematical statement of the law of conservation of energy: energy can be neither created nor destroyed:

$$\Delta U = U_{final} - U_{initial} = q - w \qquad \qquad ...(8.1)$$

Here U is energy, q represents the heat absorbed by the system from the surroundings and w is the work done by the system on the surroundings. Heat is a reflection of random molecular motion, whereas work, which is defined as force times the distance moved under its influence, is associated with organised motion. Force may assume many different forms, including the gravitational force exerted by one mass on another, the expansional force exerted by a gas, the tensional force exerted by a spring or muscle fiber, the electrical force of one charge on another or the dissipative forces of friction and viscosity. Processes in which the system releases heat, which by convention are assigned a *negative q*, are known as exothermic processes (Greek: *exo*, out of): those in which the system gains heat (*positive q*) are known as endothermic processes (Greek: *endon*, within). Under this convention, work done by the system against an external force is defined as a positive quantity. The SI unit of energy, the joule (J), is steadily replacing the calorie (cal) in modern scientific usage. The large caloric (Cal, with a capital C) is a unit favoured by nutritionists. The relationships among these quantities and other units, as well as the values of constants that will be useful throughout this chapter, are shown in Table 8.1.

Table 8.1: Thermodynamic units and constants.

Joule (J)

   1 J = 1 kg·m^2·S^{-2} 1 J = 1 C·V (coulomb volt)

   1 J = 1 N·M (Newton meter)

Calorie (cal)

   1 cal heats 1 gram of H_2O from 14.5 to 15.5°C

   1 cal = 4.184 J

Large calorie (Cal)

   1 Cal = 1 kcal   1 Cal = 4184 J

Avogadro's number (N)

   $N = 6.0221 \times 10^{23}$ molecules · mol^{-1}

Coulomb (C)

   $1\ C = 6.241 \times 10^{18}$ electron charges

Faraday (F)

   1 F = N electron charges

   1 F = 96485 C · mol^{-1} = 96,485 J·V^{-1}·mol^{-1}

Kelvin temperature scale (K)

   0 K = absoute zero   273.15 K = 0°C

Boltzmann constant (k_B)

   $k_B = 1.3807 \times 10^{-23}$ J·K^{-1}

Gas constant (R)

   R = Nk$_B$ R = 1.9872 cal·K^{-1}·mol^{-1}

   R = 8.3145 J·K^{-1}·mol^{-1} R = 0.08206 L·atm·K^{-1}·mol^{-1}

State functions are independent of the path a system follows: Experiments have invariably demonstrated that the energy of a system depends only on its current properties or state, not on how it reached that state. For example the state of a system composed of a particular gas sample is completely described by its pressure and temperature. The energy of this gas sample is a function only of these so called state functions (quantities that depend only on the state of the system) and is therefore a state function itself. Consequently, there is no net change in energy ($\Delta U = 0$) for any process in which the system returns to its initial state (a cyclic process).

Neither heat nor work is separately a state function because each is dependent on the path followed by a system in changing from one state to another. For example, in the process of changing from an initial to a final state, a gas may do work by expanding against an external force or do no work by following a path in which it encounters no external resistance.

If Equation 8.1 is to be obeyed, heat must also be path dependent. It is therefore meaningless to refer to the heat or work content of a system. To indicate this property, the heat or work produced during a change of state is never referred to as Δq or Δw but rather as just q or w.

Enthalpy

Any combination of only state functions must also be a state function. One such combination, which is known as enthalpy (Greek: enthalpein, to warm in), is defined

$$H = U + PV \qquad \qquad ...(8.2)$$

where, V is the volume of the system and P is its pressure. Enthalpy is a particularly convenient quantity with which to describe biological systems because under constant pressure, a condition typical of most biochemical processes, the enthalpy change between the initial and final states of a process, ΔH, is the easily measured heat that it generates or absorbs. To show this, let us divide work into two categories: pressure-volume (P–V) work, which is work performed by expansion against an external pressure ($P\Delta V$) and all other work (w'):

$$w = P\Delta V + w' \qquad \qquad ...(8.3)$$

Then, by combining Equations 8.1, 8.2 and 8.3, we see that:

$$\Delta H = \Delta U + P\Delta V = q_p - w + P\Delta V = q_p - w' \qquad \qquad ...(8.4)$$

where q_p is the heat transferred at constant pressure. Thus if $w' = 0$, as is often true of chemical reactions, $\Delta H = q_p$. Moreover the volume changes in most biochemical processes are negligible, so that the differences between their ΔU and ΔH values are usually insignificant.

We are now in a position to understand the utility of state functions. For instance, suppose we wished to determine the enthalpy change resulting from the complete oxidation of 1 g of glucose to CO_2 and H_2O by muscle tissue. To make such a measurement directly would present enormous experimental difficulties. For one thing, the enthalpy changes resulting from the numerous metabolic reactions not involving glucose oxidation that normally occur in living muscle tissue would greatly interfere with our enthalpy measurement. Since enthalpy is a state function, however, we can measure glucose's enthalpy of combustion in any apparatus of our choosing, say, a constant pressure calorimeter rather than a muscle and still obtain the same value. This, of course, is true whether or not we know the mechanism through which muscle converts glucose to CO_2 and H_2O, as long as we can establish that these substances actually are the final metabolic products. In general, the change of enthalpy in any hypothetical reaction pathway can be determined from the enthalpy change in any other reaction pathway between the same reactants and products. We stated earlier in the chapter that thermodynamics serves to indicate whether a particular process occurs spontaneously. Yet the first law of thermodynamics cannot, by itself, provide the basis for such an indication, as the following example demonstrates. If two objects at different temperatures are brought into contact, we know that heat spontaneously flows from the hotter object to the colder one, never *vice versa*. Yet either process is consistent with the first law of thermodynamics since the aggregate energy of the two objects is independent of their temperature distribution. Consequently, we must seek a criterion of spontaneity other than only conformity to the first law of thermodynamics.

Second Law of Thermodynamics: The Universal Trends Towards Maximum Disorder

When a swimmer falls into the water (a spontaneous process), the energy of the coherent motion of his body is converted to that of the chaotic thermal motion of the surrounding water molecules. The reverse process, the swimmer being ejected from still water by the sudden coherent motion of the surrounding water molecules, has never been witnessed even though such a phenomenon violates neither the first law of thermodynamics nor Newton's laws of motion.

This is because spontaneous processes are characterised by the conversion of order (in this case the coherent motion of the swimmer's body) to chaos (here the random thermal motion of the water molecules). The second law of thermodynamics, which expresses this phenomenon, therefore provides a criterion for determining whether a process is spontaneous. Note that thermodynamics says nothing about the rate of a process, that is the purview of chemical kinetics. Thus a spontaneous process might proceed at only an infinitesimal rate.

Spontaneity and disorder

The second law of thermodynamics states, in accordance with all experience, that spontaneous processes occur in direction that increase the overall disorder of the universe, that is, of the system and its surroundings. Disorder, in this context, is defined as the number of equivalent ways, W, of arranging the components of the universe. To illustrate this point, let us consider an isolated system consisting of two bulbs of equal volume containing a total of N identical molecules of ideal gas (Fig. 8.1). When the stopcock connecting the bulbs is open, there is an equal probability that a given molecule will occupy either bulb, so there are a total of 2^N equally probable ways that the N molecules may be distributed among the two bulbs. Since the gas molecules are indistinguishable from one another, there are only $(N + 1)$ different states of the system: those with $0,1,2 \ldots, (N - 1)$ or N molecules in the left bulb. Probability theory indicates that the number of (indistinguishable) ways, W_L, of placing L of the N molecules in the left bulb is:

$$W_L = \frac{N!}{L!(N-L)!}$$

The probability of such a state occurring is its fraction of the total number of possible states: $W_L/2^N$.

For any value of N, the state that is most probable, that is, the one with the highest value of W_L, is the one with half of the molecules in one bulb ($L = N/2$ for N even). As N becomes large, the probability that L is nearly equal to $N/2$ approaches unity: For instance, when $N = 10$, the probability that L is within 20% of $N/2$ (that is, 4, 5 or 6) is 0.66, whereas for $N = 50$, this probability (that L is in the range 20–30) is 0.88. For a chemically significant number of molecules, say $N = 10^{23}$, the probabilily that the number of molecules in the left bulb differs from those in the right by as insignificant a ratio as 1 molecule in every 10 billion is 10^{-434}, which, for all intents and purposes, is zero.

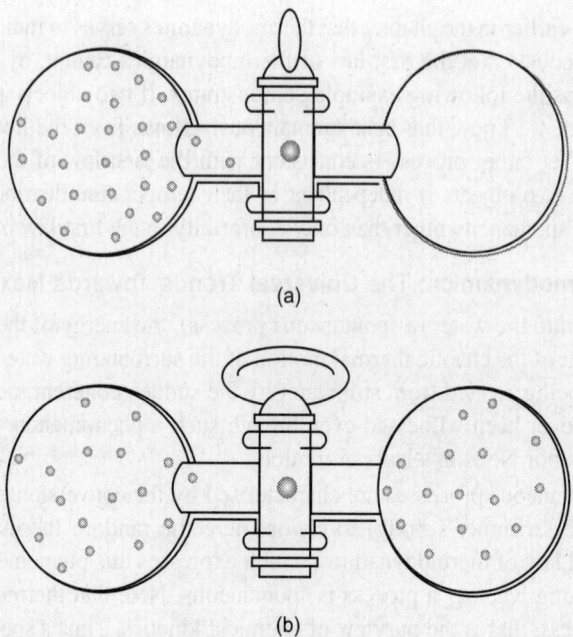

(a)

(b)

Fig. 8.1: Two bulbs of equal volumes connected by a stopcock. In (a) a gas occupies the left bulb, the right bulb is evacuated and the stopcock is closed. When the stopcock is opened and (b) the gas molecules diffuse back and forth between the bulbs and eventually become distributed, so that half of them occupy each bulb.

Therefore, the reason the number of molecules in each bulb of the system in Fig. 8.1b is always observed to be equal is not because of any law of motion, the energy of the system is the same for any arrangement of the molecules. It is because the aggregate probability of all other states is so utterly insignificant. By the same token, the reason that our swimmer is never thrown out of the water or even noticeably disturbed by the chance coherent motion of the surrounding water molecules is that the probability of such an event is nil. Consider a simple 'universe' consisting of a square array of 9 positions that collectively contain 4 identical 'molecules'. If the 4 molecules are arranged in a square, we shall call the arrangement a 'crystal', otherwise we shall call it a 'gas.' The total number of distinguishable arrangements of our 4 molecules in 9 positions is given by:

$$W = \frac{9 \cdot 8 \cdot 7 \cdot 6}{4 \cdot 3 \cdot 2 \cdot 1} = 126$$

Here, the numerator indicates that the first molecule may occupy any of the universe's 9 positions, the second molecule may occupy any of the 8 remaining unoccupied positions and so on, whereas the denominator corrects for the number of indistinguishable arrangements of the 4 identical molecules. Of the 126 arrangements this universe can have only 4 crystals (black squares). Thus, even in this simple universe, there is a more than 30-fold greater probability that it will contain a disordered gas, when arranged at random, than an ordered crystal.

Entropy

In chemical systems, W, the number of equivalent ways of arranging a system in a particular state, is usually inconveniently immense. For example, when the above twin-bulb system contains N gas molecules,

$W_{N/2} \approx 10^{N \ln 2}$ so that for $N = 10^{23}$, $W_{5 \times 10^{22}} \approx 10^{7 \times 10^{22}}$. In order to be able to deal with W more easily, we define, as did Ludwig Boltzmann in 1877, a quantity known as entropy (Greek: *en*, in + *trope*, turning):

$$S = k_B \ln W \qquad \qquad ...(8.5)$$

that increases with W but in a more manageable way.

Here k_B is the Boltzmann constant (Table 8.1). For our twin-bulb system, $S = k_B N \ln 2$, so the entropy of the system in its most probable state is proportional to the number of gas molecules it contains. Note that entropy is a state function because it depends only on the parameters that describe a state. The laws of random chance cause any system of reasonable size to spontaneously adopt its most probable arrangement, the one in which entropy is a maximum, simply because this state is so overwhelmingly probable. For example, assume that all N molecules of our twin-bulb system are initially placed in the left bulb (Fig. 8.1a, $W_N = 1$ and $S = 0$ since there is only one way of doing this). After the stopcock is opened, the molecules will randomly diffuse in and out of the right bulb until eventually they achieve their most probable (maximum entropy) state, that with half of the molecules in each bulb. The gas molecules will subsequently continue to diffuse back and forth between the bulbs, but there will be no further macroscopic (net) change in the system. The system is therefore said to have reached equilibrium. According to Equation 8.5, the foregoing spontaneous expansion process causes the system's entropy to increase. In general, for any constant energy process ($\Delta U = 0$), spontaneous process is characterised by $\Delta S > 0$. Since the energy of the universe is constant (energy can assume different forms but can be neither created nor destroyed), any spontaneous process must cause the entropy of the universe to increase:

$$\Delta S_{system} + \Delta S_{surroundings} = \Delta S_{universe} > 0 \qquad \qquad ...(8.6)$$

Equation 8.6 is the usual expression for the second law of thermodynamics. It is a statement of the general tendency of all spontaneous processes to disorder the universe, that is, the entropy of the universe tends toward a maximum.

The conclusions based on our twin-bulb apparatus may be applied to explain, for instance, why blood transports O_2 and CO_2 between the lungs and the tissues. Solutes in solution behave analogously to gases in that they tend to maintain a uniform concentration throughout their occupied volume because this is their most probable arrangement. In the lungs, where the concentration of O_2 is higher than that in the venous blood passing through them, more O_2 enters the blood than leaves it. On the other hand, in the tissues, where the O_2 concentration is lower than that in the arterial blood, there is net diffusion of O_2 from the blood to the tissues. The reverse situation holds for CO_2 transport since the CO_2 concentration is low in the lungs but high in the tissues. Keep in mind, however, that thermodynamics says nothing about the rates at which O_2 and CO_2 are transported to and from the tissues. The rates of these processes depend on the physicochemical properties of the blood, the lungs and the cardiovascular system.

Equation 8.6 does not imply that a particular system cannot increase its degree of order. As already explained a system can only be ordered at the expense of disordering its surroundings to an even greater extent by the application of energy to the system. For example, living organisms, which are organised from the molecular level upward and are therefore particularly well ordered, achieve this order at the expense of disordering the nutrients they consume. Thus, eating is as much a way of acquiring order as it is of gaining energy. A state of a system may constitute a distribution of more complicated quantities than those of gas molecules in a bulb or simple solute molecules in a solvent. For example, if our system consists of a protein molecule in aqueous solution, its various states differ, as we shall see, in the conformations of the protein's amino acid residues and in the distributions and orientations of its associated water molecules. The second law of thermodynamics applies here because a protein molecule in aqueous solution assumes its native conformation largely in response to the tendency of its surrounding water structure to be maximally disordered.

Measurement of entropy

In chemical and biological systems, it is impractical, if not impossible, to determine the entropy of a system by counting the number of ways, W, it can assume its most probable state. An equivalent and more practical definition of entropy was proposed in 1864 by Rudolf Clausius: For spontaneous processes

$$\Delta S \geq \int_{initial}^{final} \frac{dq}{T} \qquad \qquad ...(8.7)$$

where, T is the absolute temperature at which the change in heat occurs. The proof of the equivalence of our two definitions of entropy, which requires an elementary knowledge of statistical mechanics, can be found in many physical chemistry textbooks.

It is evident, however, that any system becomes progressively disordered (its entropy increases) as its temperature rises (e.g. Fig. 8.3). The equality in Equation 8.7 holds only for processes in which the system remains in equilibrium throughout the change, these are known as reversible processes. For the constant temperature conditions typical of biological processes, Equation 8.7 reduces to

$$\Delta S \geq \frac{q}{T} \qquad \qquad ...(8.8)$$

Thus the entropy change of a reversible process at constant temperature can be determined straightforwardly from measurements of the heat transferred and the temperature at which this occurs. However, since a process at equilibrium can only change at an infinitesimal rate (equilibrium processes are, by definition, unchanging), real processes can approach, but can never quite attain, reversibility. Consequently, the universe's entropy change in any real process is always greater than its ideal (reversible) value. This means that when a system departs from and then returns to its initial state via a real process, the entropy of the universe must increase even though the entropy of the system (a state function) does not change.

Free Energy: The indicator or Spontaneity

The disordering of the universe by spontaneous processes is an impractical criterion for spontaneity because it is rarely possible to monitor the entropy of the entire universe. Yet the spontaneity of a process cannot be predicted from a knowledge of the system's entropy change alone.

This is because exothermic processes ($\Delta H_{system} < 0$) may be spontaneous even though they are characterised by $\Delta S_{system} < 0$. For example, 2 mol of H_2 and 1 mol of O_2 when sparked, react in a decidedly exothermic reaction to form 2 mol of H_2O. Yet two water molecules, each of whose three atoms are constrained to stay together, are more ordered than are the three diatomic molecules from which they are formed. Similarly, under appropriate conditions, many denatured (unfolded) proteins will spontaneously fold to assume their highly ordered native (normally folded) conformations. What we really want, therefore, is a state function that predicts whether or not a given process is spontaneous. In this section, we consider such a function.

Gibbs free energy

The Gibbs free energy,

$$G = H - TS \qquad \qquad ...(8.9)$$

which was formulated by J. Willard Gibbs in 1878, is the required indicator of spontaneity for constant temperature and pressure processes. For systems that can only do pressure-volume work ($w' = 0$), combining Equations 8.4 and 8.9 while holding T and P constant yields

$$\Delta G = \Delta H - T\Delta S = q_p - T\Delta S \qquad \qquad ...(8.10)$$

But Equation 8.8 indicates that $T \Delta S \geq q$ for spontaneous processes at constant T. Consequently, $\Delta G \leq 0$ is the criterion of spontaneity we seek for the constant T and P conditions that are typical of biochemical processes. Spontaneous processes, that is, those with negative ΔG values, are said to be exergonic (Greek: *ergon*, work), they can be utilised to do work. Processes that are not spontaneous, those with positive ΔG values, are termed endergonic, they must be driven by the input of free energy. Processes at equilibrium, those in which the forward and backward reactions are exactly balanced are characterised by $\Delta G = 0$.

Note that the value of ΔG varies directly with temperature. This is why for instance the native structure of a protein, whose formation from its denatured form has both $\Delta H < 0$ and $\Delta S < 0$, predominates below the temperature at which $\Delta H = T\Delta S$ (the denaturation temperature), whereas the denatured protein predominates above this temperature. The variation of the spontaneity of a process with the signs of ΔH and ΔS is summarised in Table 8.2.

Table 8.2: Variation of reaction spontaneity (sign of ΔG) with the signs of ΔH and ΔS.

ΔH	ΔS	$\Delta G = \Delta H - T\Delta S$
−	+	The reaction is both enthalpically favoured (exothermic) and entropically favoured. It is spontaneous (exergonic) at all temperatures
−	−	The reaction is enthalpically favoured but entropically opposed. It is spontaneous only at temperatures $T = \Delta H/\Delta S$
+	+	The reaction is enthalpically opposed (endothermic) but entropically favoured. It is spontaneous only at temperatures above $T = \Delta H/\Delta S$
+	−	The reaction is both enthalpically and entropically opposed. It is unspontaneous (endergonic) at all temperatures

Free energy and work

When a system at constant temperature and pressure does non-P–V work, Equation 8.10 must be expanded to:

$$\Delta G = q_p - T\Delta S - w' \qquad \qquad ...(8.11)$$

or because $T\Delta S \geq q_p$ (Equation 8.8),

$$\Delta G \leq -w'$$

so that

$$\Delta G \geq -w' \qquad \qquad ...(8.12)$$

Since P–V work is unimportant in biological systems, ΔG for a biological process represents its maximum recoverable work. The ΔG of a process is therefore indicative of the maximum charge separation it can establish, the maximum concentration gradient it can generate, the maximum muscular activity it can produce and so on. In fact, for real processes, which can only approach reversibility, the inequality in Equation 8.12 holds, so that the work put into any system can never be fully recovered. This is inductive of the inherent dissipative character of nature. Indeed, as we have seen, it is precisely this dissipative character that provides the overall driving force for any change. It is important to reiterate that a large negative value of ΔG does not ensure a chemical reaction will proceed at a measurable rate. This depends on the detailed mechanism of the reaction, which is independent of ΔG. For instance, most biological molecules, including proteins, nucleic acids, carbohydrates and lipids, are thermodynamically unstable to hydrolysis but, nevertheless, spontaneously hydrolyse at biologically insignificant rates. Only with the introduction of the proper enzymes will the hydrolysis of these molecules proceed at a reasonable pace. Yet a catalyst, which by definition is unchanged by a reaction, cannot affect the ΔG of a reaction. Consequently, an enzyme can only accelerate the attainment of thermodynamic equilibrium, it cannot, for example, promote a reaction that has a positive ΔG.

Chemical Equilibria

The entropy (disorder) of a substance increases with its volume. For example, as we have seen for our twin-bulb apparatus (Fig. 8.1), a collection of gas molecules, in occupying all of the volume available to it, maximises its entropy. Similarly, dissolved molecules become uniformly distributed throughout their solution volume. Entropy is therefore a function of concentration. If entropy varies with concentration, so must free energy. Thus, as is shown in this section, the free energy change of a chemical reaction depends on the concentrations of both its reactants and its products. This phenomenon is of great biochemical significance because enzymatic reactions can proceed in either direction depending on the relative concentrations of their reactants and products. Indeed the directions of many enzymatically catalysed reactions depend on the availability of their substrates (reactants) and on the metabolic demand for their products (although most metabolic pathways operate unidirectionally).

Equilibrium constants

The relationship between the concentration and the free energy of a substance A, is approximately:

$$K_{eq} = \frac{[C]_{eq}^c \, [D]_{eq}^d}{[A]_{eq}^a \, [B]_{eq}^b} = e^{-\Delta G^\circ / RT} \qquad \qquad ...(8.13)$$

where $\overline{G}_A$ is known equivalently as the partial molar free energy or the chemical potential of A (the bar indicates the quantity per mole), $\overline{G}_A^o$ is the partial molar free energy of A in its standard state, R is the gas constant (Table 8.1) and $[A]$ is the molar concentration of A. Thus for the general reaction:

$$aA + bB \rightleftharpoons cC + dD$$

Since free energies are additive and the free energy change of a reaction is the sum of the free energies of the products less those of the reactants, the free energy change for this reaction is:

$$\Delta G = c\overline{G}_C + d\overline{G}_D - a\overline{G}_A - b\overline{G}_B \qquad \qquad ...(8.14)$$

Substituting this relationship into Equation (8.13) yields:

$$\Delta G = \Delta G^o + RT \, In\left(\frac{[C]^c [D]^d}{[A]^a [D]^b}\right) \qquad \qquad ...(8.15)$$

where, $\Delta G°$ is the free energy change of the reaction when all of its reactants and products are in their standard states. Thus the expression for the free energy change of a reaction consists of two parts: (i) a constant term whose value depends only on the reaction taking place and (ii) a variable term that depends on the concentrations of the reactants and the products, the stoichiometry of the reaction and the temperature. For a reaction at equilibrium, there is no net change because the free energy of the forward reaction exactly balances that of the backward reaction. Consequently $\Delta G = 0$, so that Equation 8.15 becomes:

$$\Delta G° = -RT \ln K_{eq} \qquad \qquad ...(8.16)$$

where K_{eq} is the familiar equilibrium constant of the reaction:

$$K_{eq} = \frac{[C]_{eq}^c \, [D]_{eq}^d}{[A]_{eq}^a \, [B]_{eq}^b} = e^{-\Delta G°/RT} \qquad \qquad ... (8.17)$$

and the subscript 'eq' in the concentration terms indicates their equilibrium values. (The equilibrium condition is usually clear from the context of the situation, so that equilibrium concentrations are often expressed without this subscript). The equilibrium constant of a reaction may therefore be calculated from standard free energy data and *vice versa*. Table 8.3 indicates the numerical relationship between $\Delta G°$ and K_{eq}.

Table 8.3: Variation of K_{eq} with $\Delta G°$ at 25°C.

K_{eq}	$\Delta G°(kJ \cdot mol^{-1})$
10^6	−34.3
10^4	−22.8
10^2	−11.4
10^1	−5.7
10^0	0.0
10^{-1}	5.7
10^{-2}	11.4
10^{-4}	22.8
10^{-6}	34.3

Note that a 10-fold variation of K_{eq} at 25°C corresponds to a 5.7 kJ·mol^{-1} change in $\Delta G°$, which is less than half of the free energy of even a weak hydrogen bond.

Equations 8.15 through 8.17 indicate that when the reactants in a process are in excess of their equilibrium concentrations, the net reaction will proceed in the forward direction until the excess reactants have been converted to products and equilibrium is attained. Conversely, when products are in excess, the net reaction proceeds in the reverse reaction so as to convert products to reactants until the equilibrium concentration ratio is likewise achieved.

Thus, as Le Chatelier's principle states, any deviation from equilibrium stimulates a process that tends to restore the system to equilibrium, all isolated system must therefore inevitably reach equilibrium. Living systems escape this thermodynamic *cul-de-sac* by being open systems. The manner in which the equilibrium constant varies with temperature is seen by substituting Equation 8.10 into Equation 8.16 and rearranging:

$$\ln K_{eq} = \frac{-\Delta H°}{(R)}\left(\frac{1}{T}\right) + \frac{\Delta S°}{R} \qquad \qquad ...(8.18)$$

where $H°$ and $S°$ represent enthalpy and entropy in the standard state. If $\Delta H°$ and $\Delta S°$ are independent of temperature, as they often are to a reasonable approximation, a plot of $\ln K_{eq}$ versus $1/T$, known as a van't Hoff plot, yields a straight line of slope $-\Delta H°/R$ and intercept $\Delta S°/R$. This relationship permits the values of $\Delta H°$ and $\Delta S°$ to be determined from measurements of K_{eq}, at two (or more) different temperatures.

Calorimetric data, which until recently have been quite difficult to measure for biochemical processes, are therefore not required to obtain the values of $\Delta H°$ and $\Delta S°$. Consequently, most biochemical thermodynamic data have been obtained through the application of Equation 8.18. However, the recent development of the scanning microcalorimeter has made the direct measurement of $\Delta H(q_p)$ for biochemical processes a practical alternative. Indeed, a discrepancy between the values of $\Delta H°$ for a reaction as determined calori-metrically and from a van't Hoff plot suggests that the reaction occurs via one or more intermediate states in addition to the initial and final states implicit in the formulation of Equation 8.18.

Standard free energy changes

Since only free energy differences, ΔG can be measured, not free energies themselves, it is necessary to refer these differences to some standard state in order to compare the free energies of different substances (likewise, we refer the elevations of geographic locations to sea level, which is arbitrarily assigned the height of zero). By convention, the free energy of all pure elements in their standard state of 25°C, 1 atm and in their most stable form (e.g. O_2 not O_3), is defined to be zero. The free energy of formation of any non-elemental substance, $\Delta G°_f$ is then defined as the change in free energy accompanying the formation of 1 mol of that substance, in its standard state, from its component elements in their standard states. The standard free energy change for any reaction can be calculated according to:

$$\Delta G° = \Sigma \Delta G°_f \text{ (products)} - \Sigma \Delta G°_f \text{(reactants)} \qquad ...(8.19)$$

Table 8.4 provides a list of standard free energies of formation, $\Delta G°_f$ for a selection of substances of biochemical significance.

Standard state conventions in biochemistry: The standard state convention commonly used in physical chemistry defines the standard state of a solute as that with unit activity at 25°C and 1 atm (activity is concentration corrected for non-ideal behaviour, for the dilute solutions typical of biochemical reactions in the laboratory, such corrections are small, so activities can be replaced by concentrations). However, because biochemical reactions usually occur in dilute aqueous solutions near neutral pH, a somewhat different standard state convention for biological systems has been adopted:

1. Water's standard state is defined as that of the pure liquid, so that the activity of pure water is taken to be unity despite the fact that its concentration is 55.5M. In essence, the [H_2O] term is incorporated into the value of the equilibrium constant. This procedure simplifies the free energy expressions for reactions in dilute aqueous solutions involving water as a reactant or product because the [H_2O] term can then be ignored.

2. The hydrogen ion activity is defined as unity at the physiologically relevant pH of 7 rather than at the physical chemical standard state of pH 0, where many biological substances are unstable.

3. The standard state of a substance that can undergo an acid-base reaction is defined in terms of the total concentration of its naturally occurring ion mixture at pH 7. In contrast, the physical chemistry convention refers to a pure species whether or not it actually exists at pH 0. The advantage of the biochemistry convention is that the total concentration of a substance with multiple ionisation states,

Table 8.4: Free energies of formation of some compounds of biochemical interest.

Compound	$-\Delta G°_f$ (kJ·mol^{-1})
Acetaldehyde	139.7
Acetate$^-$	369.2
Acetyl-CoA	374.1[a]
cis-Aconitate^{3-}	920.9
CO_2(g)	394.4
CO_2(aq)	386.2
HCO_3^-	587.1
Citrate^{3-}	1166.6
Dihydroxyacetone phosphate^{2-}	1293.2
Ethanol	181.5
Fructose	915.4
Fructose-6-phosphate^{2-}	1758.3
Fructose-1, 6-bisphosphate^{4-}	2600.8
Fumarate^{2-}	604.2
α-D-Glucose	917.2
Glucose-6-phosphate^{2-}	1760.2
Glyceraldehyde-3-phosphate^{2-}	1285.6
H^+	0.0
H_2(g)	0.0
H_2O(l)	237.2
Isocitrate^{3-}	1160.0
α-ketoglutarate^{2-}	798.0
Lactate$^-$	516.6
L-Malate^{2-}	845.1
OH^-	157.3
Oxaloacetate^{2-}	797.2
Phosphoenolpyruvte^{3-}	1269.5
2-Phosphoglycerate^{3-}	1285.6
3-Phosphoglycerate^{3-}	1515.7
Pyruvate$^-$	474.5
Succinate^{2-}	690.2
Succinyl-CoA	686.7[a]

[a] For formation from free elements + free CoA (co-enzyme A).

such as most biological molecules, is usually easier to measure than the concentration of one of its ionic species. Since the ionic composition of an acid or base varies with pH, however, the standard free energies calculated according to the biochemistry convention are valid only at pH 7.

Under the biochemistry convention, the standard free energy changes of substances are customarily symbolised by $\Delta G°'$ in order to distinguish them from physical chemistry standard free energy changes, $\Delta G°$ (note that the value of ΔG for any process, being experimentally measurable, is independent of the chosen standard state, i.e. $\Delta G = \Delta G'$). Likewise, the biochemical equilibrium constant, which is defined by using $\Delta G^{\circ\prime}$ in place of ΔG° in Equation 8.17, is represented by K'_{eq}.

The relationship between $\Delta G^{\circ\prime}$ and $\Delta^{\circ\prime}$ is often a simple one. There are three general situations:

1. If the reacting species include neither H_2O nor H^+, the expressions for $\Delta G^{\circ\prime}$ and ΔG° coincide.

2. For a reaction in dilute aqueous solution that yields nH_2O molecules:

$$A + B \rightleftharpoons C + D + nH_2O$$

Equations 8.16 and 8.17 indicate that:

$$\Delta G^{\circ\prime} = -RT \ \ln \ K_{eq} = -RT \ \ln\left(\frac{[C][D][H_2O]^n}{[A][B]}\right)$$

Under the biochemistry convention, which defines the activity of pure water as unity:

$$\Delta G^{\circ\prime} = -RT \ \ln \ K'_{eq} = -RT \ \ln\left(\frac{[C][D]}{[A][B]}\right)$$

Therefore,

$$\Delta G^{\circ\prime} = \Delta G^{\circ} + nRT \ \ln[H_2O] \qquad \qquad \ldots(8.20)$$

where, $[H_2O] = 55.5M$ (the concentration of water in aqueous solution), so that for a reaction at 25°C which yields 1 mol of H_2O, $\Delta G^{\circ\prime} = \Delta G^{\circ} + 9.96 \ kJ \cdot mol^{-1}$.

3. For a reaction involving hydrogen ions, such as:

$$A + B \rightleftharpoons C + HD$$
$$\Updownarrow$$
$$D^- + H^+$$

where,

$$K = \frac{[H^+][D^-]}{[HD]}$$

manipulations similar to those above lead to the relationship

$$\Delta G^{\circ\prime} = \Delta G^{\circ} - RT \ \ln(1 + K/[H^+]_0) + RT \ \ln[H^+]_0 \qquad \qquad \ldots(8.21)$$

where $[H^+]_0 = 10^{-7} \ M$, the only value of $[H^+]$ for which this equation is valid.

TYPES OF REACTIONS

An exergonic reaction is a spontaneous chemical reaction that releases energy. It is thermodynamically favoured, indexed by a negative value of ΔG (Gibbs free energy). Over the course of a reaction, energy needs to be put in, and this activation energy drives the reactants from a stable state to a highly energetically unstable transition state to a more stable state that is lower in energy. The reactants are usually complex molecules that are broken into simpler products. The entire reaction is usually catabolic. The release of energy (called Gibbs free energy) is negative (i.e. $-\Delta G$) because energy is released from the reactants to the products. An endergonic reaction is an anabolic chemical reaction that consumes energy. It is the opposite of an exergonic reaction. It has a positive ΔG because it takes more energy to break the bonds of the reactant than the energy of the products offer, i.e. the products have weaker bonds than the reactants. Thus, endergonic reactions are thermodynamically unfavourable. Additionally, endergonic reactions are usually anabolic. The free energy (ΔG) gained or lost in a reaction can be calculated as follows: $\Delta G = \Delta H - T\Delta S$ where ΔG = Gibbs free energy, ΔH = enthalpy, T = temperature (in kelvins), and ΔS = entropy.

EXAMPLES OF MAJOR BIOENERGETIC PROCESSES

Glycolysis is the process of breaking down glucose into pyruvate, producing two molecules of ATP (per 1 molecule of glucose) in the process. When a cell has a higher concentration of ATP than ADP (i.e. has a high energy charge), the cell can undergo glycolysis, releasing energy from available glucose to perform biological work. Pyruvate is one product of glycolysis, and can be shuttled into other metabolic pathways (gluconeogenesis, etc.) as needed by the cell. Additionally, glycolysis produces reducing equivalents in the form of NADH (nicotinamide adenine dinucleotide), which will ultimately be used to donate electrons to the electron transport chain.

Gluconeogenesis is the opposite of glycolysis, when the cell's energy charge is low (the concentration of ADP is higher than that of ATP), the cell must synthesise glucose from carbon- containing biomolecules such as proteins, amino acids, fats, pyruvate, etc. For example, proteins can be broken down into amino acids, and these simpler carbon skeletons are used to build/ synthesise glucose. The citric acid cycle is a process of cellular respiration in which acetyl coenzyme A, synthesised from pyruvate dehydrogenase, is first reacted with oxaloacetate to yield citrate. The remaining eight reactions produce other carbon-containing metabolites. These metabolites are successively oxidised, and the free energy of oxidation is conserved in the form of the reduced coenzymes $FADH_2$ and NADH. These reduced electron carriers can then be re-oxidised when they transfer electrons to the electron transport chain. Ketosis is a metabolic process whereby ketone bodies are used by the cell for energy (instead of using glucose). Cells often turn to ketosis as a source of energy when glucose levels are low, e.g. during starvation. Oxidative phosphorylation and the electron transport chain is the process where reducing equivalents such as NADPH, $FADH_2$ and NADH can be used to donate electrons to a series of redox reactions that take place in electron transport chain complexes. These redox reactions take place in enzyme complexes situated within the mitochondrial membrane. These redox reactions transfer electrons 'down' the electron transport chain, which is coupled to the proton motive force. This difference in proton concentration between the mitochondrial matrix and inner membrane space is used to drive ATP synthesis via ATP synthase. Photosynthesis, another major bioenergetic process, is the metabolic pathway used by plants in which solar energy is used to synthesise glucose from carbon dioxide and water. This reaction takes place in the chloroplast. After glucose is synthesised, the plant cell can undergo photophosphorylation to produce ATP.

Cotransport

In August 1960, Robert K. Crane presented for the first time his discovery of the sodium-glucose cotransport as the mechanism for intestinal glucose absorption. Crane's discovery of cotransport was the first ever proposal of flux coupling in biology and was the most important event concerning carbohydrate absorption in the 20th century.

Chemiosmotic Theory

One of the major triumphs of bioenergetics is Peter D. Mitchell's chemiosmotic theory of how protons in aqueous solution function in the production of ATP in cell organelles such as mitochondria. This work earned Mitchell the 1978 Nobel Prize for Chemistry. Other cellular sources of ATP such as glycolysis were understood first, but such processes for direct coupling of enzyme activity to ATP production are not the major source of useful chemical energy in most cells. Chemiosmotic coupling is the major energy producing process in most cells, being utilised in chloroplasts and several single celled organisms in addition to mitochondria. Chemiosmotic Theory is discussed in details in Chapter 12.

ENERGY BALANCE

Energy homeostasis is the homeostatic control of energy balance – the difference between energy obtained through food consumption and energy expenditure – in living systems.

Energy Homeostasis

In biology, energy homeostasis, or the homeostatic control of energy balance, is a biological process that involves the coordinated homeostatic regulation of food intake (energy inflow) and energy expenditure (energy outflow). The human brain, particularly the hypothalamus, plays a central role in regulating energy homeostasis and generating the sense of hunger by integrating a number of biochemical signals that transmit information about energy balance. Fifty percent of the energy from glucose metabolism is immediately converted to heat. Energy homeostasis is an important aspect of bioenergetics.

The first law of thermodynamics states that energy can be neither created nor destroyed. But energy can be converted from one form of energy to another. So, when a calorie of food energy is consumed, one of three particular effects occur within the body: A portion of that calorie may be stored as body fat, triglycerides, or glycogen, transferred to cells and converted to chemical energy in the form of adenosine triphosphate (ATP – a coenzyme) or related compounds, or dissipated as heat.

Energy intake: Energy intake is measured by the amount of calories consumed from food and fluids. Energy intake is modulated by hunger, which is primarily regulated by the hypothalamus, and choice, which is determined by the sets of brain structures that are responsible for stimulus control (i.e. operant conditioning and classical conditioning) and cognitive control of eating behaviour. Hunger is regulated in part by the action of certain peptide hormones and neuropeptides (e.g., insulin, leptin, ghrelin, among others) in the hypothalamus.

Expenditure: Energy expenditure is mainly a sum of internal heat produced and external work. The internal heat produced is, in turn, mainly a sum of basal metabolic rate (BMR) and the thermic effect of food. External work may be estimated by measuring the physical activity level (PAL).

Positive balance: A positive balance is a result of energy intake being higher than what is consumed in external work and other bodily means of energy expenditure.

The main preventable causes are: (i) overeating, resulting in increased energy intake, and (ii) sedentary lifestyle, resulting in decreased energy expenditure through external work.

A positive balance results in energy being stored as fat and/or muscle, causing weight gain. In time, overweight and obesity may develop, with resultant complications.

Negative balance: A negative balance is a result of energy intake being less than what is consumed in external work and other bodily means of energy expenditure.

Homeostasis

Homeostasis is the property of a system within an organism in which a variable, such as the concentration of a substance in solution, is actively regulated to remain very nearly constant. Examples of homeostasis include the regulation of body temperature, the pH of extracellular fluid, or the concentrations of sodium, potassium and calcium ions, as well as that of glucose in the blood plasma, despite changes in the environment, diet, or level of activity. Each of these variables is controlled by a separate regulator or homeostatic mechanism, which, together, maintain life.

Chapter 9

Cell Metabolism

INTRODUCTION

A cell's daily operations are accomplished through the biochemical reactions that take place within the cell. Reactions are turned on and off or sped up and slowed down according to the cell's immediate needs and overall functions. At any given time, the numerous pathways involved in building up and breaking down cellular components must be monitored and balanced in a coordinated fashion. To achieve this goal, cells organise reactions into various enzyme-powered pathways.

Metabolic processes are concerned with all those biological or chemical reactions which can be carried out by the cell. It is essential for the biotechnologist to fully understand these basic metabolic processes, as every present and future biotechnological industry can be economically feasible only if full advantage is taken of the cell's capacity to convert substrate into the desired product.

For the biotechnological evaluation of the usefulness of a microbial process, for example, the stoichiometry of microbial metabolism together with its regulatory mechanisms can be a very useful tool, since stoichiometric equations describing the consumption of a substrate and the formation of biomass and products are always required. With a knowledge of the basic concept of catabolism, it is possible to explore the enormous versatility of the microorganism, plant, algae, mammalian in sustaining and maintaining life under unfavourable conditions. It should always be remembered that organic end product formation is a result of reduced energy and biomass formation. This exchange of energy and biomass for end products leads to major (e.g. primary) or minor (secondary) products.

Metabolism is the intricate interplay between anabolism and catabolism via the regulatory mechanisms to observe the thermodynamic laws of nature. The interconnections between plant cells, animal cells, and microbial cells can be visualised best in the geochemical cycles of matter in nature, the carbon, nitrogen, phosphate, etc. cycles. Without a thorough knowledge of cell metabolism, no improvement in the field of biotechnology is possible. It is essential to fully exploit the genotype , which is only possible through a good understanding of cellular metabolism.

In order to grow, cells have to build up a vast array of chemical substances of which they are composed of. These substances, often quite complex, are synthesised from simpler molecules by processes called anabolism. If the simple molecule is CO_2, one refers to carbon assimilation and the cell is said to be autotrophic (e.g. plants, algae, bacteria). The majority of microbial cells in nature uses simple molecules from the degradation of organic molecules and thus are referred to as heterotrophic. The biosynthetic (anabolic) reactions involved in cellular growth are often energy requiring and ATP formed during photosynthesis or chemosynthesis is used up during these biosynthetic reactions. Chemoheterotrophic cells generate therefore the required energy during the oxidation/utilisation of organic compounds. These reactions involve oxidation-reduction processes accompanied by the release of energy, some of which is conserved in ATP. The particular compound may be oxidised either completely to CO_2 in the case of aerobic respiration or only partially in the case of anaerobic respiration and fermentation to lower molecular carbon compounds.

The processes involved in the oxidation of compounds are collectively called catabolism. Catabolic and anabolic (biosynthetic) reactions are referred to as metabolic reactions. The term metabolism therefore refers to the whole array of oxidative (degradation) and reductive (biosynthetic) reactions taking place within the cell. Although energy is required in certain key biosynthetic reactions, the focus of biosynthesis is not on energy, but rather on carbon and on the intermediates occurring in the build-up of cell constituents from simple starting materials. These intermediates are often formed as a result of catabolism, but also serve as starting materials in biosynthetic reactions. The relationships between catabolism and anabolism occur not only at the common intermediates. Certain pathways play dual roles, as they function in both anabolism and catabolism. For instance, the tricarboxylic acid cycle, as will be demonstrated later, is involved not only in the oxidation of pyruvate and acetyl-CoA to carbon dioxide for energy production, but also in the generation of a number of intermediates such as succinyl-CoA, oxalacetate and keto-glutarate, which serve as starting points for the synthesis of amino acids, porphyrins and other compounds necessary for growth. A pathway that serves the dual function of catabolism and anabolism is called *an amphibolic* pathway. Many pathways are amphibolic.

METABOLIC PATHWAYS

In biochemistry, metabolic pathways are series of chemical reactions occurring within a cell. In each pathway, a principal chemical is modified by chemical reactions. Enzymes catalyse these reactions, and often require dietary minerals, vitamins, and other cofactors in order to function properly. Because of the many chemicals that may be involved, pathways can be quite elaborate. In addition, many pathways can exist within a cell. This collection of pathways is called the metabolic network. Pathways are important to the maintenance of homeostasis within an organism.

Metabolism is a step-by-step modification of the initial molecule to shape it into another product. The result can be used in one of three ways: (i) to be stored by the cell, (ii) to be used immediately, as a metabolic product, and (iii) to initiate another metabolic pathway, called a flux generating step.

A molecule called a substrate enters a metabolic pathway depending on the needs of the cell and the availability of the substrate. An increase in concentration of anabolic and catabolic end-products would slow the metabolic rate for that particular pathway. Each metabolic pathway is composed of a series of biochemical reactions that are connected by their intermediates. The reactants (or substrates) of one reaction are the products of the previous one, and so on. Metabolic pathways are usually considered in one direction (although all reactions are chemically reversible, conditions in the cell are such that it is thermodynamically more favourable for flux to be in one of the directions).

1. Glycolysis was the first metabolic pathway discovered:
   (a) As glucose enters a cell, it is immediately phosphorylated by ATP to glucose 6-phosphate in the irreversible first step. This is to prevent the glucose from leaving the cell.

    (b) In times of excess lipid or protein energy sources, glycolysis may run in reverse (gluconeogenesis) in order to produce glucose 6-phosphate for storage as glycogen or starch.

2. Metabolic pathways are often regulated by feedback inhibition or by a cycle wherein one of the products in the cycle starts the reaction again, such as the Krebs Cycle.

3. Anabolic and catabolic pathways in eukaryotes are separated either by compartmentation or by the use of different enzymes and co-factors.

Major Metabolic Pathways

Cellular respiration: Cellular respiration, also known as 'oxidative metabolism', is one of the key ways a cell gains useful energy. It is the set of the metabolic reactions and processes that take place in organisms' cells to convert biochemical energy from nutrients into adenosine triphosphate (ATP), and then release waste products. The reactions involved in respiration are catabolic reactions that involve the oxidation of one molecule and the reduction of another. Nutrients commonly used by animal and plant cells in respiration include glucose, amino acids and fatty acids, and a common oxidising agent (electron acceptor) is molecular oxygen (O_2). Bacteria and archaea can also be lithotrophs and these organisms may respire using a broad range of inorganic molecules as electron donors and acceptors, such as sulphur, metal ions, methane or hydrogen. Organisms that use oxygen as a final electron acceptor in respiration are described as aerobic, while those that do not are referred to as anaerobic. The energy released in respiration is used to synthesise ATP to store this energy. The energy stored in ATP can then be used to drive processes requiring energy, including biosynthesis, locomotion or transportation of molecules across cell membranes. Several distinct but linked metabolic pathways are used by cells to transfer the energy released by breakdown of fuel molecules to ATP.

These occur within all living organisms in some forms:

1. Glycolysis.

2. Anaerobic respiration.

3. Krebs cycle/Citric acid cycle.

4. Oxidative phosphorylation.

Other pathways occurring in (most or) all living organisms include:

1. Fatty acid oxidation (β-oxidation).

2. Gluconeogenesis.

3. HMG-CoA reductase pathway (isoprene prenylation chains).

4. Pentose phosphate pathway (hexose monophosphate shunt).

5. Porphyrin synthesis (or heme synthesis) pathway.

6. Urea cycle.

Creation of energetic compounds from non-living matter:

1. Photosynthesis (plants, algae, cyanobacteria).

2. Chemosynthesis (some bacteria).

Metabolic Network

A metabolic network is the complete set of metabolic and physical processes that determine the physiological and biochemical properties of a cell. As such, these networks comprise the chemical reactions of metabolism as well as the regulatory interactions that guide these reactions. With the sequencing of complete genomes, it is now possible to reconstruct the network of biochemical reactions in many organisms, from bacteria to human. Several of these networks are available online.

Metabolic Engineering

Metabolic engineering is the practice of optimising genetic and regulatory processes within cells to increase the cells' production of a certain substance. Metabolic engineers commonly work to reduce cellular energy use (i.e. the energetic cost of cell reproduction or proliferation) and to reduce waste production. Producing beer, wine, cheese, pharmaceuticals and other biotechnology products often involves metabolic engineering. Cells are complex systems, genetic and regulatory changes can have drastic effects on the cells' ability to survive. Therefore, trade-offs become apparent during metabolic engineering. Metabolic engineering can be useful in industry. Certain industries use cells to create useful products. Producing the greatest number of those cells is a sought-after goal. The only known method of production, however, may involve oxidising of carbon compounds. The carbon compounds may be in limited supply. Therefore, engineering cells to reproduce or proliferate more rapidly given the same amount of carbon compounds would mean greater industrial efficiency. The role of *Methylophilus methylotrophus* in the animal feed industry is an example. *M. methylotrophus* uses methanol to produce certain proteins used in animal feed. Producing greater masses of proteins using the same mass of methanol would increase efficiency. Windass, accomplished this by silencing genes in *M. methylotrophus* and inserting genes from *E. coli*. This example of metabolic engineering resulted in an organism capable of using a lesser mass of adenosine triphosphate to produce the same mass of glutamate.

ENERGY RELEASED BY CATABOLIC PROCESSES

The free energy released by catabolic processes is conserved through the synthesis of ATP from ADP and phosphate or through the reduction of the coenzyme $NADP^+$ to NADPH. ATP and NADPH are the major free energy sources for anabolic pathways (Fig. 9.1). A striking characteristic of degradative metabolism is that it converts large numbers of diverse substances (carbohydrates, lipids and proteins)

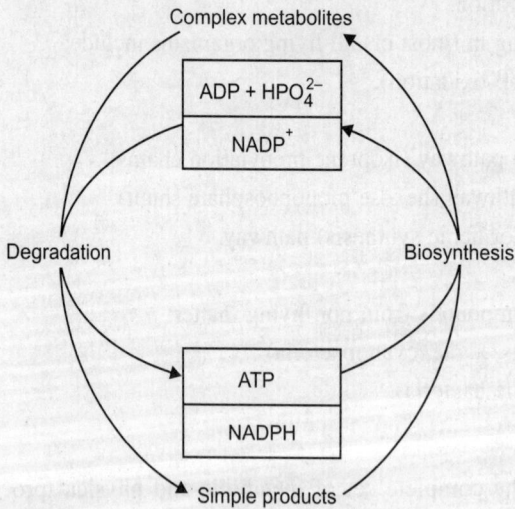

Fig. 9.1: ATP and NADPH are the sources of free energy for biosynthetic reactions. They are generated through the degradation of complex metabolites.

to common intermediates. These intermediates are then further metabolised in a central oxidative pathway that terminates in a few end products. Figure 9.2 outlines the breakdown of various foodstuffs, first to their monomeric units and then to the common intermediate, acetyl-coenzyme A (acetyl-CoA). Biosynthesis carries out the opposite process. Relatively few metabolites, mainly pyruvate, acetyl-CoA and the citric acid cycle intermediates, serve as starting materials or a host of varied biosynthetic products.

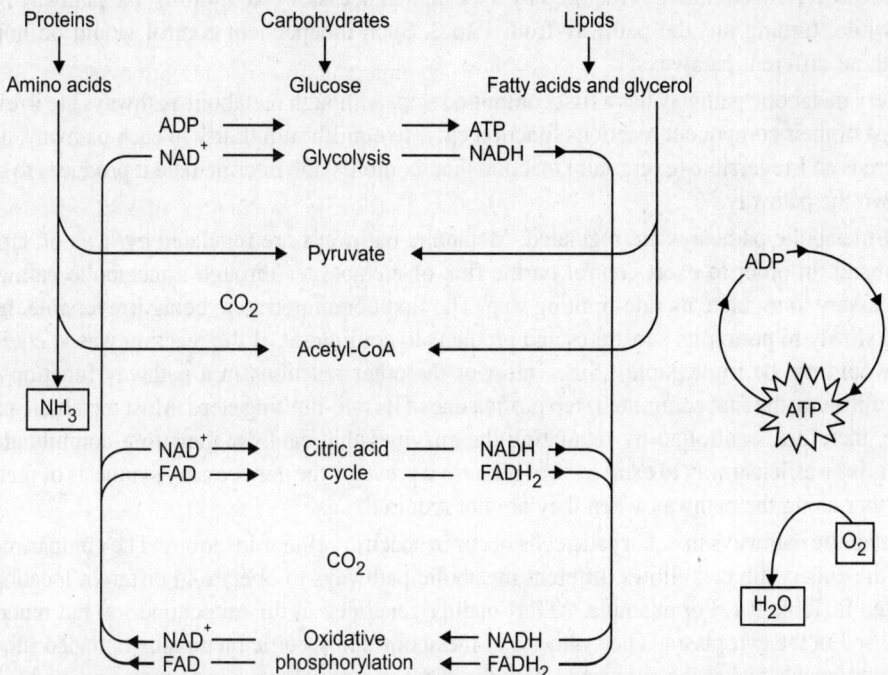

Fig. 9.2: Overview of catabolism: Complex metabolites such as carbohydrates, proteins and lipids are degraded first to their monomeric units, chiefly glucose, amino acids, fatty acids and glycerol and then to the common intermediate, acetyl coenzyme A (acetyl-CoA). The acetyl group is then oxidised to CO_2 via the citric acid cycle with concomitant reduction of NAD^+ and FAD. Re-oxidation of these latter coenzymes by O_2 via the electron-transport chain and oxidative phosphorylation yields H_2O and ATP.

Principal Characteristics of Metabolic Pathways

Five principal characteristics of metabolic pathways stem from their function of generating products for use by the cell.

1. Metabolic pathways are irreversible: A highly exergonic reaction (having a large negative free energy change) is irreversible, that is, it goes to completion. If such a reaction is part of a multistep pathway, it confers directionality on the pathway, that is, it makes the entire pathway irreversible.

2. Catabolic and anabolic pathways must differ: If two metabolites are metabolically interconvertible, the pathway from the first to the second must differ from the pathway from the second back to the first:

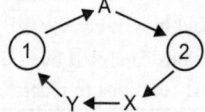

This is because if metabolite 1 is converted to metabolite 2 by an exergonic process, the conversion of metabolite 2 to metabolite 1 requires that free energy be supplied in order to bring this otherwise endergonic process 'back up the hill'. Consequently, the two pathways must differ in at least one of their reaction steps. The existence of independent interconversion routes, as we shall see, is an important property of metabolic pathways because it allows independent control of the two processes. If metabolite 2 is required by the cell, it is necessary to 'turn-off' the pathway from 2 to 1 while 'turning on' the pathway from 1 to 2. Such independent control would be impossible without different pathways.

3. Every metabolic pathway has a first committed step: Although metabolic pathways are irreversible, most of their component reactions function close to equilibrium. Early in each pathway, however, there is an irreversible (exergonic) reaction that 'commits' the intermediate it produces to continue down the pathway.

4. All metabolic pathways are regulated: Metabolic pathways are regulated by laws of supply and demand. In order to exert control on the flux of metabolites through a metabolic pathway, it is necessary to regulate its rate-limiting step. The first committed step, being irreversible, functions too slowly to permit its substrates and products to equilibrate (if the reaction was at equilibrium, it would not be irreversible). Since most of the other reactions in a pathway function close to equilibrium, the first committed step is often one of its rate-limiting steps. Most metabolic pathways are, therefore, controlled by regulating the enzymes that catalyse their first committed step(s). This is an efficient way to exert control because it prevents the unnecessary synthesis of metabolites further along the pathway when they are not required.

5. Metabolic pathways in eukaryotic cells occur in specific cellular locations: The compartmentation of the eukaryotic cell allows different metabolic pathways to operate in different locations, as is listed in Table 9.1. For example, ATP is mainly generated in the mitochondrion but much of it is utilised in the cytoplasm. The synthesis of metabolites in specific membrane-bounded sub-cellular compartments makes their transport between these compartments a vital component of eukaryotic metabolism. Biological membranes are selectively permeable to metabolites because of the presence in membranes of specific transport proteins. The synthesis and utilisation of acetyl-CoA are also compartmentalised.

Table 9.1: Metabolic functions of eukaryotic organelles.

Organelle	Function
Mitochondrion	Citric acid cycle, electron transport and oxidative phosphorylation, fatty acid oxidation, amino acid breakdown
Cytosol	Glycolysis, pentose phosphate pathway, fatty acid biosynthesis, many reactions of gluconeogenesis
Lysosomes	Enzymatic digestion of cell components and ingested matter
Nucleus	DNA replication and transcription, RNA processing
Golgi apparatus	Post-translational processing of membrane and secretory proteins, formation of plasma membrane and secretory vesicles
Rough endoplasmic reticulum	Synthesis of membrane-bound and secretory proteins
Smooth endoplasmic reticulum	Lipid and steroid biosynthesis
Peroxisomes (glyoxisomes in plants)	Oxidative reactions catalysed by amino acid oxidases and catalase: glyoxylate cycle reactions in plants

This metabolic intermediate is utilised in the cytosolic synthesis of fatty acids but is synthesised in mitochondria. Yet there is no transport protein for acetyl-CoA in the mitochondrial membrane. In multicellular organisms, compartmentation is carried a step further to the level of tissues and organs. The mammalian liver, for example, is largely responsible for the synthesis of glucose from non-carbohydrate precursors (gluconeogenesis) so as to maintain a relatively constant level of glucose in the circulation, whereas adipose tissue is specialised for the storage and mobilisation of triacylglycerols.

ORGANIC REACTION MECHANISMS

Almost all of the reactions that occur in metabolic pathways are enzymatically catalysed organic reactions. The various mechanisms enzymes have at their disposal for catalysing reactions: acid-base catalysis, covalent catalysis, metal ion catalysis, electrostatic catalysis, proximity and orientation effects and transition state binding. Few enzymes alter the chemical mechanisms of these reactions, so much can be learned about enzymatic mechanisms from the study of non-enzymatic model reactions. We, therefore, begin our study of metabolic reactions by outlining the types of reactions we shall encounter and the mechanisms by which they have been observed to proceed in non-enzymatic systems.

Christopher Walsh has classified biochemical reactions into four categories: (i) group-transfer reactions, (ii) oxidations and reductions, (iii) eliminations, isomerisations and rearrangements and (iv) reactions that make or break carbon-carbon bonds. Much is known about the mechanisms of these reactions and about the enzymes that catalyse them. In this section, we outline the four reaction categories and discuss how our knowledge of their reaction mechanisms derives from the study of model organic reactions. We begin by briefly reviewing the chemical logic used in analysing these reactions.

Chemical Logic

A covalent bond consists of an electron pair shared between two atoms. In breaking such a bond, the electron pair can either remain with one of the atoms (heterolytic bond cleavage)or separate such that one electron accompanies each of the atoms (homolytic bond cleavage) (Fig. 9.3). Homolytic bond cleavage, which usually produces unstable radicals, occurs mostly in oxidation-reduction reactions.

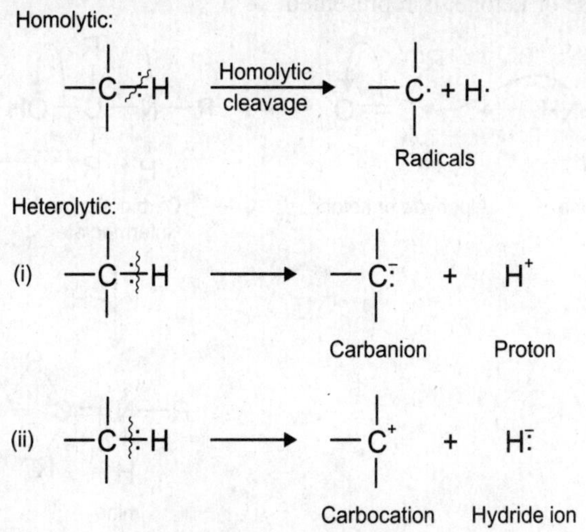

Fig. 9.3: Modes of C—H bond breaking. Homolytic cleavage yields radicals, whereas heterolytic cleavage yields either: (i) a carbanion and a proton and (ii) a carbocation and a hydride ion.

Heterolytic C—H bond cleavage involves either carbanion and proton (H^+) formation or carbocation (carbonium ion) and hydride ion (H^-) formation. Since hydride ions are highly reactive species and carbon atoms are slightly more electronegative than hydrogen atoms, bond cleavage in which the electron pair remains with the carbon atom is the predominant mode of C—H bond breaking in biochemical systems. Hydride ion abstraction occurs only if the hydride is transferred directly to an acceptor such as NAD^+ or $NADP^+$. Compounds participating in reactions involving heterolytic bond cleavage and bond formation are categorised into two broad classes: electron rich and electron deficient. Electron-rich compounds, which are called nucleophiles (nucleus lovers), are negatively charged or contain unshared electron pairs that easily form covalent bonds with electron-deficient centers. Biologically important nucleophilic groups include amino, hydroxyl, imidazole and sulphydryl functions (Fig. 9.4a). The nucleophilic forms of these groups are also their basic forms. Indeed, nucleophilicity and basicity are closely related properties. A compound acts as a base when it forms a covalent bond with H^+, whereas it acts as a nucleophile when it forms a covalent bond with an electron-deficient center other than H^+, usually an electron-deficient carbon atom:

Basic reaction of an amine
$$R\!-\!\ddot{N}H_2 + H^+ \longrightarrow R\!-\!\overset{\overset{\textstyle H}{|}}{\underset{\underset{\textstyle H}{|}}{N}}\!-\!H$$

Nucleophilic reaction of an amine
$$R\!-\!\ddot{N}H_2 + \overset{R'}{\underset{R''}{C}}\!\!=\!\!O \longrightarrow R\!-\!\overset{\overset{\textstyle H}{|}}{N}\!-\!\overset{\overset{\textstyle R'}{|}}{\underset{\underset{\textstyle R''}{|}}{C}}\!-\!OH$$

Electron-deficient compounds are called electrophiles (electron lovers). They may be positively charged, contain an unfilled valence electron shell or contain an electro-negative atom. The most common electrophiles in biochemical systems are H^+, metal ions, the carbon atoms of carbonyl groups and cationic imines (Fig. 9.4b). For example, imine formation, a biochemically important reaction between an amine and an aldehyde or ketone, is represented:

$$R\!-\!\ddot{N}H_2 + \overset{R'}{\underset{R''}{C}}\!\!=\!\!O \longrightarrow R\!-\!\overset{\overset{\textstyle }{|}}{\underset{\underset{\textstyle H}{|}}{\ddot{N}}}\!-\!\overset{\overset{\textstyle R'}{|}}{\underset{\underset{\textstyle R''}{|}}{C}}\!-\!OH$$

Amine   Aldehyde or ketone   Carbinolamine intermediate

$$\downarrow -H^+$$

$$R\!-\!\overset{\overset{\textstyle +}{|}}{\underset{\underset{\textstyle H}{|}}{N}}\!\!=\!\!\overset{R'}{\underset{R''}{C}} + H_2O$$

Imine

Reactions are best understood if the electron pair rearrangements involved in going from reactants to products can be traced. In illustrating these rearrangements we shall use the curved arrow convention in

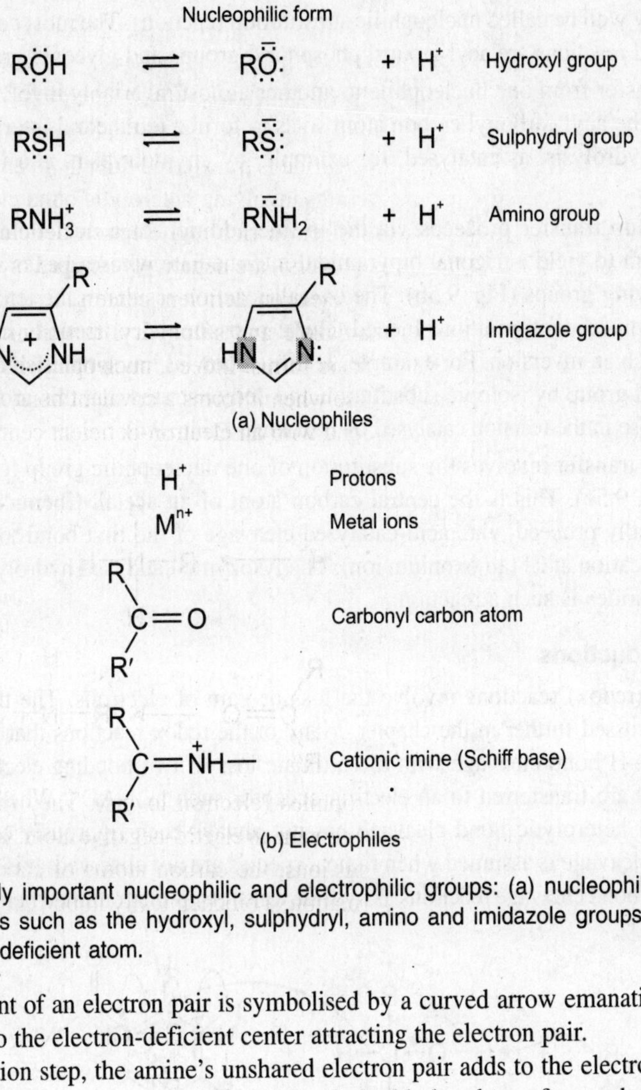

Nucleophilic form

$$R\ddot{O}H \quad \rightleftharpoons \quad R\ddot{\ddot{O}}: \quad + \quad H^+ \quad \text{Hydroxyl group}$$

$$R\ddot{S}H \quad \rightleftharpoons \quad R\ddot{\ddot{S}}: \quad + \quad H^+ \quad \text{Sulphydryl group}$$

$$RNH_3^+ \quad \rightleftharpoons \quad R\ddot{N}H_2 \quad + \quad H^+ \quad \text{Amino group}$$

Imidazole group $+ \quad H^+$

(a) Nucleophiles

H^+ Protons

M^{n+} Metal ions

Carbonyl carbon atom

Cationic imine (Schiff base)

(b) Electrophiles

Fig. 9.4: Biologically important nucleophilic and electrophilic groups: (a) nucleophiles are the conjugate bases of weak acids such as the hydroxyl, sulphydryl, amino and imidazole groups and (b) electrophiles contain an electron-deficient atom.

which the movement of an electron pair is symbolised by a curved arrow emanating from the electron pair and pointing to the electron-deficient center attracting the electron pair.

In the first reaction step, the amine's unshared electron pair adds to the electron-deficient carbonyl carbon atom while one electron pair from its C=O double bond transfers to the oxygen atom. In the second step, the unshared electron pair on the nitrogen atom adds to the electron-deficient carbon atom with the elimination of water. At all times, the rules of chemical reason prevail: For example, there are never five bonds to a carbon atom or two bonds to a hydrogen atom.

Group-Transfer Reactions

The group transfers that occur in biochemical systems involve the transfer of an electrophilic group from one nucleophile to another:

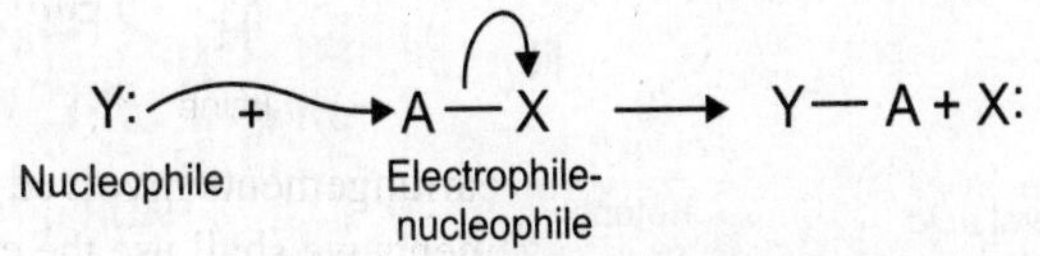

$$Y: \quad + \quad A\!-\!X \quad \longrightarrow \quad Y\!-\!A + X:$$

Nucleophile   Electrophile-nucleophile

They could equally well be called nucleophilic substitution reactions. The most commonly transferred groups in biochemical reactions are acyl groups, phosphoryl groups and glycosyl groups (Fig. 9.5):

1. Acyl group transfer from one nucleophile to another almost invariably involves the addition of a nucleophile to the acyl carbonyl carbon atom so as to form a tetrahedral intermediate (Fig. 9.5a). Peptide bond hydrolysis, as catalysed, for example, by chymotrypsin, is a familiar example of such a reaction.

2. Phosphoryl group transfer proceeds via the in-line addition of a nucleophile to a phosphoryl phosphorus atom to yield a trigonal bipyramidal intermediate whose apexes are occupied by the adding and leaving groups (Fig. 9.5b). The overall reaction results in the tetrahedral phosphoryl group's inversion of configuration. Indeed, chiral phosphoryl compounds have been shown to undergo just such an inversion. For example, Jeremy Knowles has synthesised ATP made chiral at its γ-phosphoryl group by isotopic substitution and demonstrated that this group is inverted on its transfer to glucose in the reaction catalysed by hexokinase (Fig. 9.6).

3. Glycosyl group transfer involves the substitution of one nucleophilic group for another at Cl of a sugar ring (Fig. 9.5c). This is the central carbon atom of an acetal. Chemical models of acetal reactions generally proceed, via., acid-catalysed cleavage of the first bond to form a resonance-stabilised carbocation at Cl (an oxonium ion). The lysozyme-catalysed hydrolysis of bacterial cell wall polysaccharides is such a reaction.

Oxidations and Reductions

Oxidation-reduction (redox) reactions involve the loss or gain of electrons. The thermo-dynamics of these reactions is discussed further in the chapter. Many of the redox reactions that occur in metabolic pathways involve C—H bond cleavage with the ultimate loss of two bonding electrons by the carbon atom. These electrons are transferred to an electron acceptor such as NAD^+. Whether these reactions involve homolytic or heterolytic bond cleavage has not always been rigorously established. In most instances heterolytic cleavage is assumed when radical species are not observed. It is useful, however, to visualise redox C—H bond cleavage reactions as hydride transfers as diagrammed below for the oxidation of an alcohol by NAD^+:

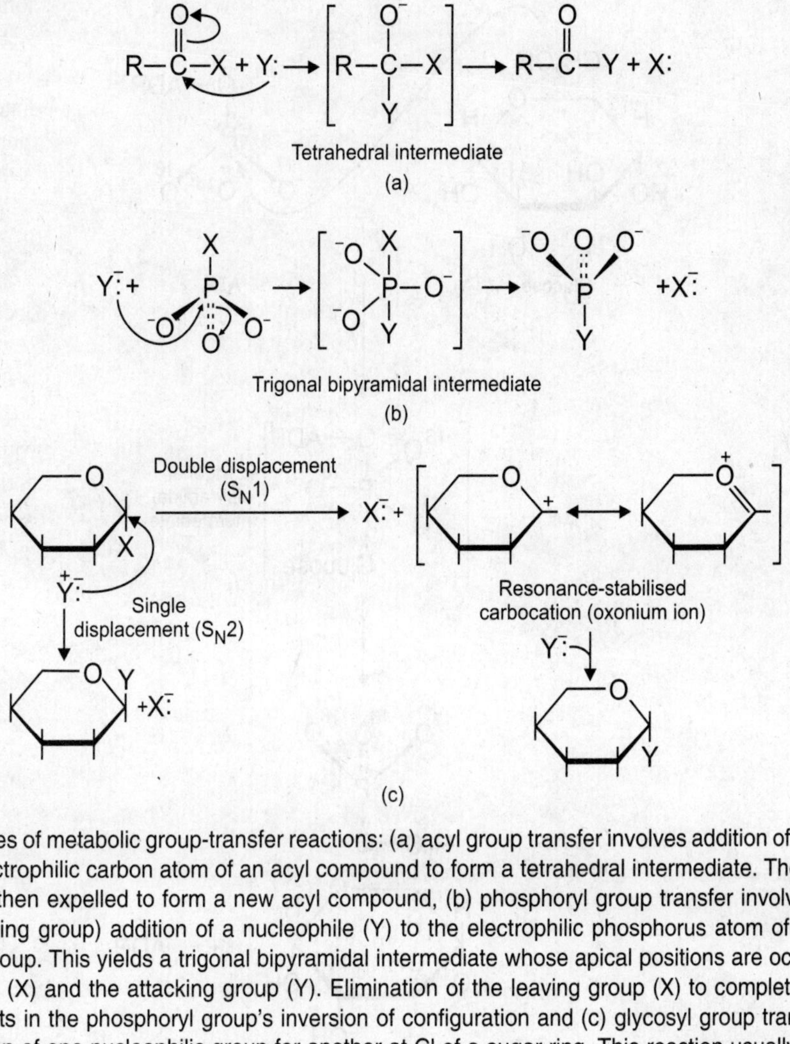

Tetrahedral intermediate
(a)

Trigonal bipyramidal intermediate
(b)

(c)

Fig. 9.5: Types of metabolic group-transfer reactions: (a) acyl group transfer involves addition of a nucleophile (Y) to the electrophilic carbon atom of an acyl compound to form a tetrahedral intermediate. The original acyl carrier (X) is then expelled to form a new acyl compound, (b) phosphoryl group transfer involves the in-line (with the leaving group) addition of a nucleophile (Y) to the electrophilic phosphorus atom of a tetrahedral phosphoryl group. This yields a trigonal bipyramidal intermediate whose apical positions are occupied by the leaving group (X) and the attacking group (Y). Elimination of the leaving group (X) to complete the transfer reaction results in the phosphoryl group's inversion of configuration and (c) glycosyl group transfer involves the substitution of one nucleophilic group for another at Cl of a sugar ring. This reaction usually occurs via a double displacement mechanism in which the elimination of the original glycosyl carrier (X) is accompanied by the intermediate formation of a resonance-stabilised carbocation (oxoniuim ion) followed by the addition of the adding nucleophile (Y). The reaction also may occur, via., a single displacement mechanism in which Y directly displaces X with inversion of configuration.

For aerobic organisms, the terminal acceptor for the electron pairs removed from metabolites by their oxidation is molecular oxygen (O_2).

Recall that this molecule is a ground state diradical species whose unpaired electrons have parallel spins. The rules of electron pairing (the Pauli exclusion principle) therefore dictate that O_2 can only accept unpaired electrons, that is, electrons must be transferred to O_2 one at a time (in contrast to redox processes in which electrons are transferred in pairs). Electrons that are removed from metabolites as pairs must, therefore, be passed to O_2 via the electron-transport chain one at a time. This is accomplished through the use of conjugated coenzymes that have stable radical oxidation states and can, therefore,

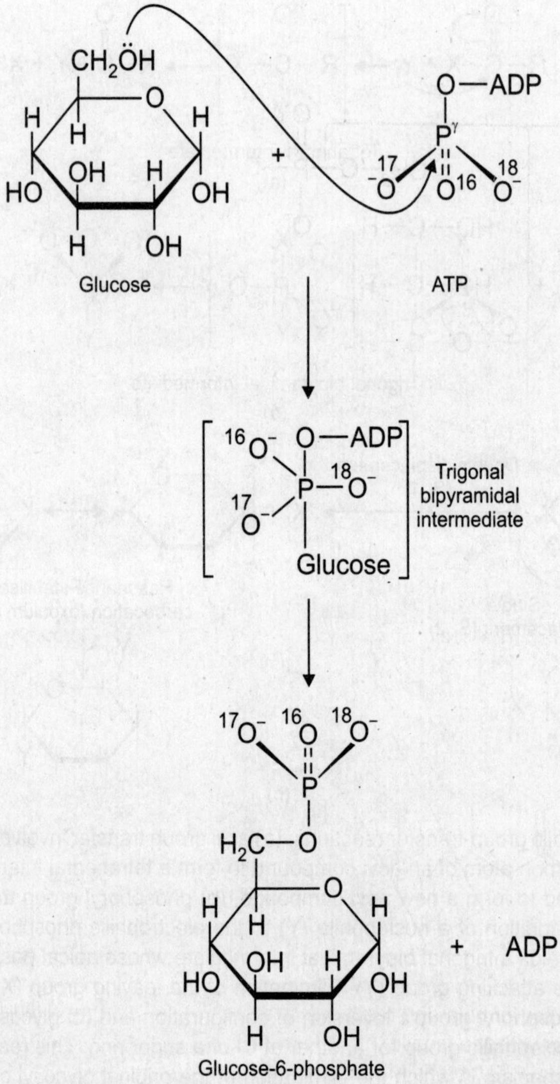

Fig. 9.6: The phosphoryl-transfer reaction catalysed by hexokinase. During its transfer to the 6-OH of glucose, the γ-phosphoryl group of ATP made chiral by isotopic substitution undergoes inversion of configuration, via., a trigonal bipyramidal intermediate.

undergo both $1e^-$ and $2e^-$ redox reactions. One such coenzyme is flavin adenine dinucleotide (FAD, Fig. 9.7). Flavins (substances that contain the isoalloxazine ring) can undergo two sequential one-electron transfers or a simultaneous two-electron transfer that by-passes the semi-quinone state.

Eliminations, Isomerisations and Rearrangements

Elimination reactions form carbon-carbon double bonds: Elimination reactions result in the formation of a double bond between two previously single-bonded saturated centers. The substances eliminated may be H_2O, NH_3, an alcohol (ROH) or a primary amine (RNH_2).

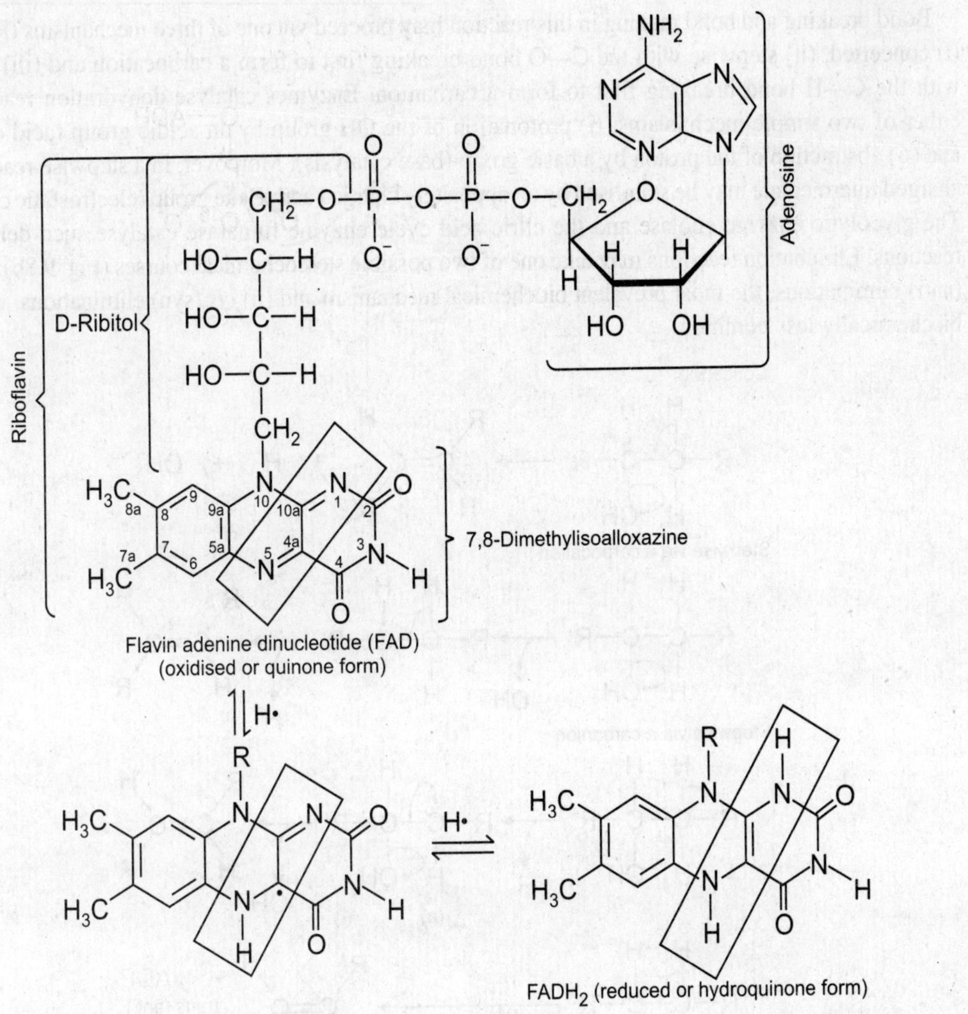

Fig. 9.7: The molecular formula and reactions of the coenzyme flavin adenine dinucleotide (FAD). The term 'flavin' is synonymous with the isoalloxazine system. The D-ribitol residue is derived from the alcohol of the sugar D-ribose. The FAD may be half-reduced to the stable radical FADH• or fully reduced to $FADH_2$ (boxes). Consequently, different FAD-containing enzymes cycle between different oxidation states of FAD. FAD is usually tightly bound to its enzymes, so that this coenzyme is normally a prosthetic group rather than a co-substrate as is, for example, NAD^+. Consequently, although humans and other higher animals are unable to synthesise the isoalloxazine component of flavins and hence must obtain it in their diets [for example, in the form of riboflavin (vitamin B_2)], riboflavin deficiency is quite rare in humans.

The dehydration of an alcohol, for example, is an elimination reaction:

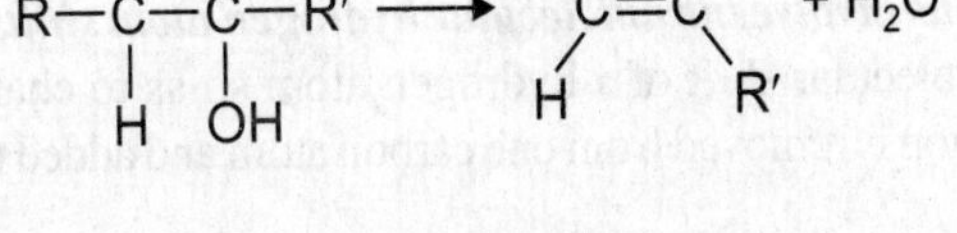

Bond breaking and bond making in this reaction may proceed via one of three mechanisms (Fig. 9.8a): (i) concerted, (ii) stepwise with the C—O bond breaking first to form a carbocation and (iii) stepwise with the C—H bond breaking first to form a carbanion. Enzymes catalyse dehydration reactions by either of two simple mechanisms: (i) protonation of the OH group by an acidic group (acid catalysis) and (ii) abstraction of the proton by a basic group (base catalysis). Moreover, in a stepwise reaction, the charged intermediate may be stabilised by an oppositely charged active site group (electrostatic catalysis). The glycolytic enzyme enolase and the citric acid cycle enzyme fumarase catalyse such dehydration reactions. Elimination reactions may take one of two possible stereochemical courses (Fig. 9.8b): (i) *trans* (anti) eliminations, the most prevalent biochemical mechanism and (ii) *cis* (syn) eliminations, which are biochemically less common.

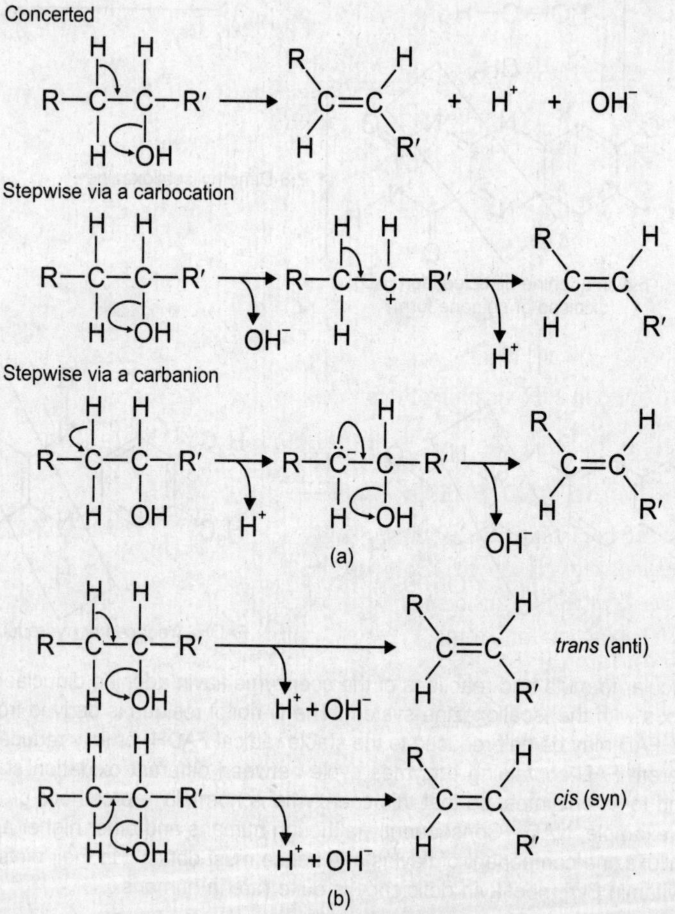

Fig. 9.8: Possible elimination reaction mechanisms using dehydration as an example. Reactions may be: (a) either concerted, stepwise, via., a carbocation intermediate or stepwise, via., a carbanion intermediate and may occur with (b) either *trans* (anti) or *cis* (syn) stereochemistry.

***Biochemical isomerisations involve intramolecular hydrogen atom shifts*:** Biochemical isomerisation reactions involve the intramolecular shift of a hydrogen atom so as to change the location of a double bond. In such a process, a proton is removed from one carbon atom and added to another. The metabolically most prevalent isomerisation reaction is the aldose-ketose interconversion, a base-catalysed reaction that occurs via enediolate anion intermediates. The glycolytic enzyme phosphoglucose isomerase catalyses such a reaction. Racemisation is an isomerisation reaction in which a hydrogen atom shifts its stereochemical position at a molecule's only chiral center so as to invert that chiral center, (e.g. the racemisation of proline by proline racemase). Such an isomerisation is called an epimerisation in a molecule with more than one chiral center.

Rearrangements produce altered carbon skeletons: Rearrangement reactions break and reform C—C bonds so as to rearrange a molecule's carbon skeleton. There are few such metabolic reactions. One is the conversion of L-methylmalonyl-CoA to succinyl-CoA by methylmalonyl-CoA mutase, an enzyme whose prosthetic group is a vitamin B_{12} derivative:

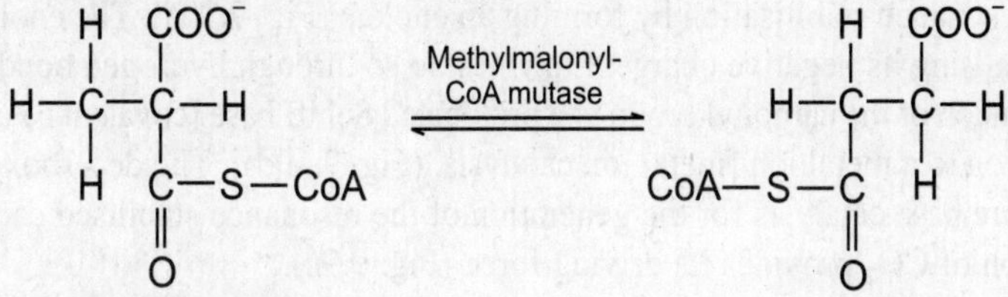

L-Methylmalonyl-CoA   Succinyl-CoA

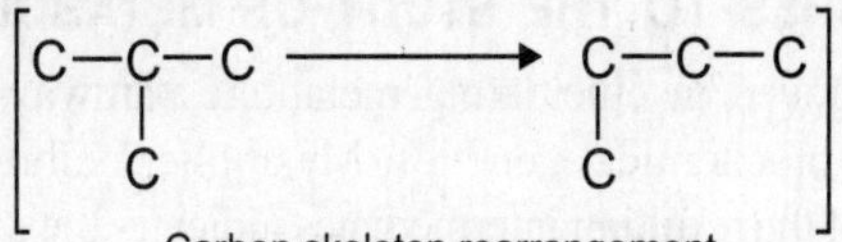

Carbon skeleton rearrangement

This reaction is involved in the oxidation of fatty acids with an odd number of carbon atoms and several amino acids.

REACTIONS THAT MAKE AND BREAK CARBON–CARBON BONDS

Reactions that make and break carbon-carbon bonds form the basis of both degradative and biosynthetic metabolism. The breakdown of glucose to CO_2 involves five such cleavages, whereas its synthesis involves the reverse process. Such reactions, considered from the synthetic direction, involve addition of a nucleophilic carbanion to an electrophilic carbon atom.

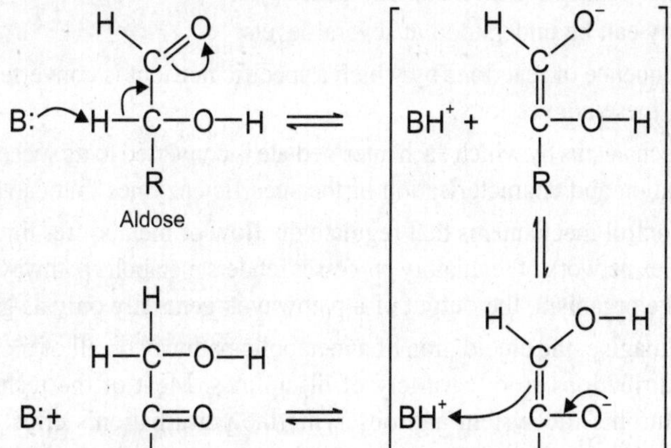

Aldose

Ketose   cis-Enediolate intermediates

The most common electrophilic carbon atoms in such reactions are the sp^2-hybridised carbonyl carbon atoms of aldehydes, ketones, esters and CO_2:

$$-\overset{|}{\underset{|}{C}} \cdot + \quad \overset{\diagup}{\underset{\diagdown}{C}}{=}O \longrightarrow -\overset{|}{\underset{|}{C}}-\overset{|}{\underset{|}{C}}-OH$$

Stabilised carbanions must be generated to add to these electrophilic centers. Three examples are the aldol condensation (catalysed, e.g. by aldolase), Claisen ester condensation (citrate synthase) and the decarboxylation of β-keto acids (isocitrate dehydrogenase) and fatty acid synthase. In non-enzymatic systems, both the aldol condensation and Claisen ester condensation involve the base-catalysed generation of a carbanion α to a carbonyl group Figs 9.9a,b). The carbonyl group is electron withdrawing and thereby provides resonance stabilisation by forming an enolate (Fig. 9.10a). The enolate may be further stabilised by neutralising its negative charge. Enzymes do so through hydrogen bonding or protonation (Fig. 9.10b), conversion of the carbonyl group to a protonated Schiff base [covalent catalysis, (Fig. 9.10c)] or by its coordination to a metal ion [metal ion catalysis, (Fig. 9.10d)]. The decarboxylation of a β-keto acid does not require base catalysis for the generation of the resonance stabilised carbanion, the highly exergonic formation of CO_2 provides its driving force (Fig. 9.9c).

EXPERIMENTAL APPROACHES TO THE STUDY OF METABOLISM

Experimental approaches employed in elucidating metabolic pathways include the use of metabolic inhibitors, growth studies and biochemical genetics. Metabolic inhibitors block pathways at specific enzymatic steps. Identification of the resulting intermediates indicates the course of the pathway. Mutations, which occur naturally in genetic diseases or can be induced by mutagens, X-rays or genetic engineering, may also result in the absence or inactivity of an enzyme. Modern genetic techniques make it possible to express foreign genes in higher organisms (transgenic animals) or eliminate (knock out) a gene and study the effects of these changes on metabolism.

When isotopic labels are incorporated into metabolites and allowed to enter a metabolic system, their paths may be traced from the distribution of label in the intermediates. NMR is a non-invasive technique that may be used to detect and study metabolites *in vivo*.

Studies on isolated organs, tissue slices, cells and sub-cellular organelles have contributed enormously to our knowledge of the localisation of metabolic pathways.

A metabolic pathway can be understood at several levels:

1. In terms of the sequence of reactions by which a specific nutrient is converted to end products and the energetics of these conversions.

2. In terms of the mechanisms by which each intermediate is converted to its successor. Such an analysis requires the isolation and characterisation of the specific enzymes that catalyse each reaction.

3. In terms of the control mechanisms that regulate the flow of metabolites through the pathway. An exquisitely complex network of regulatory processes renders metabolic pathways remarkably sensitive to the needs of the organism, the output of a pathway is generally only as great as required.

As you might well imagine, the elucidation of a metabolic pathway on all of these levels is a complex process, involving contributions from a variety of disciplines. Most of the techniques used to do so involve somehow perturbing the system and observing the perturbation's effect on growth or on the production of metabolic intermediates. One such technique is the use of metabolic inhibitors that block metabolic pathways at specific enzymatic steps. Another is the study of genetic abnormalities that interrupt

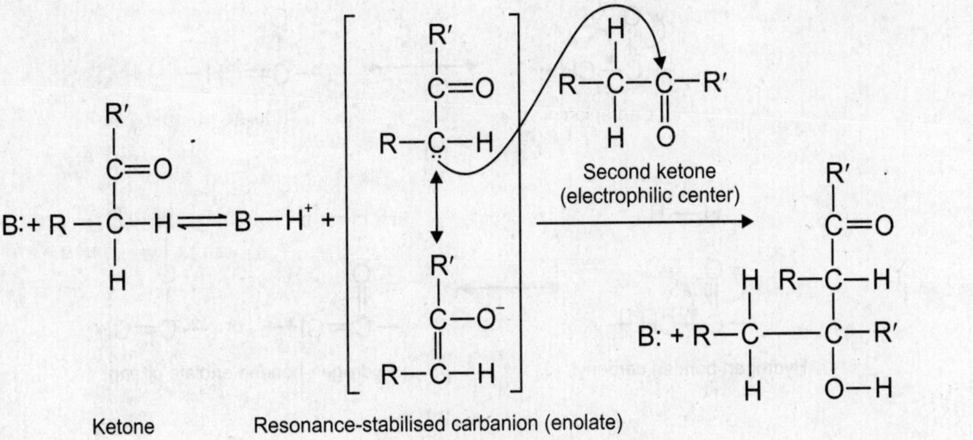

(a) Aldol condensation

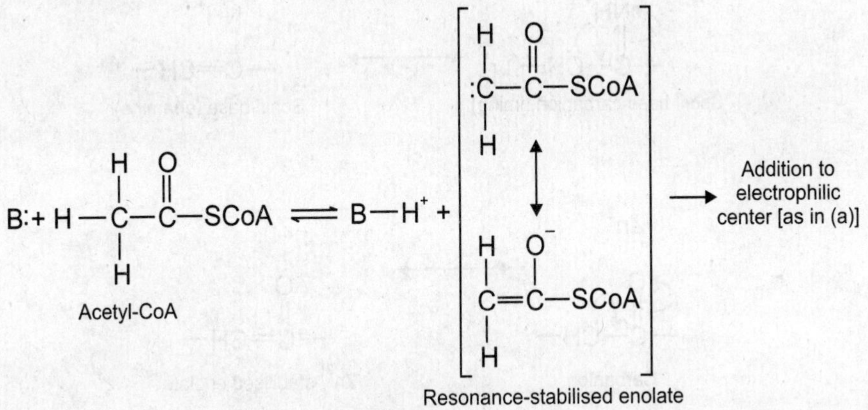

(b) Claisen ester condensation

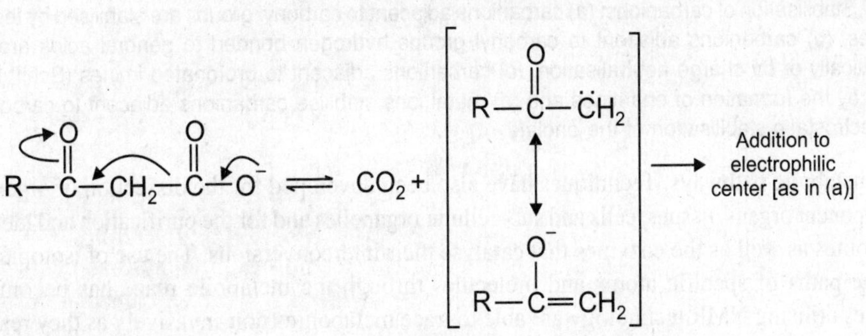

(c) Decarboxylation of a β-keto acid

Fig. 9.9: Example of C—C bond formation and cleavage reactions: (a) Aldol condensation, (b) Claisen ester condensation and (c) decarboxylation of a β-keto acid. All three types of reactions involve generation of a resonance-stabilised carbanion followed by addition of this carbanion to an electrophilic center.

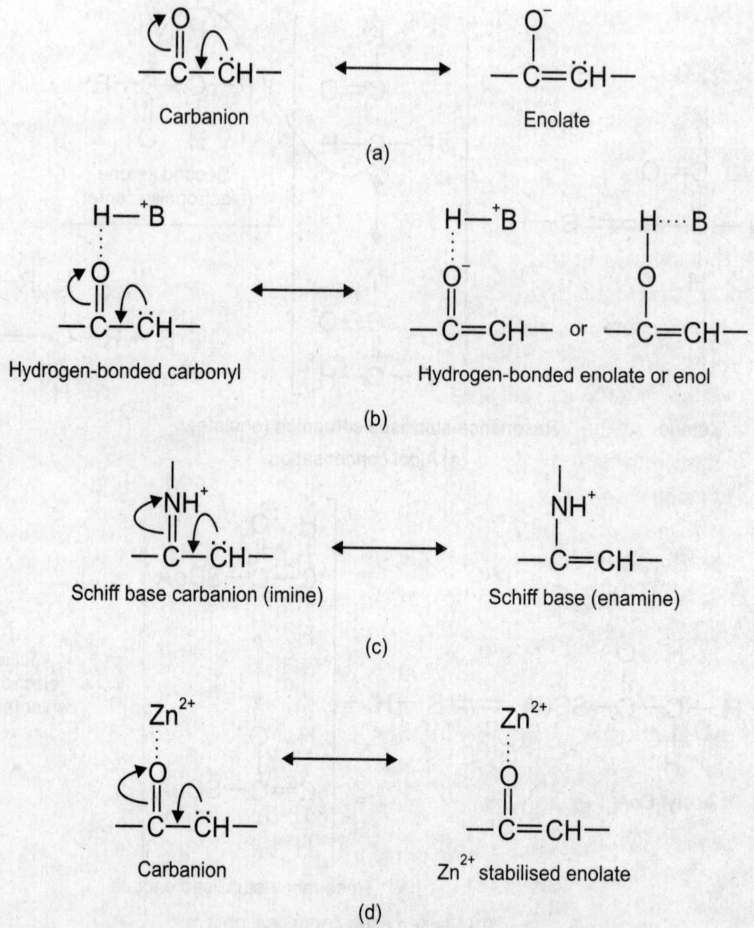

Fig. 9.10: Stabilisation of carbanions: (a) carbanions adjacent to carbonyl groups are stabilised by the formation of enolates, (b) carbanions adjacent to carbonyl groups hydrogen bonded to general acids are stabilised electrostatically or by charge neutralisation, (c) carbanions adjacent to protonated imines (Schiff bases) are stabilised by the formation of enamines and (d) metal ions stabilise carbanions adjacent to carbonyl groups by the electrostatic stabilisation of the enolate.

specific metabolic pathways. Techniques have also been developed for the dissection of organisms into their component organs, tissues, cells and sub-cellular organelles and for the purification and identification of metabolites as well as the enzymes that catalyse their interconversions. The use of isotopic tracers to follow the paths of specific atoms and molecules through the metabolic maze has become routine. Techniques utilising NMR technology are able to trace metabolites non-invasively as they react *in vivo*. This section outlines the use of these various techniques.

Metabolic Inhibitors, Growth Studies and Biochemical Genetics

Pathway intermediates accumulate in the presence of metabolic inhibitors: The first metabolic pathway to be completely traced was the conversion of glucose to ethanol in yeast by a process known as glycolysis. In the course of these studies, certain substances, called metabolic inhibitors, were found to block the pathway at specific points, thereby causing preceding intermediates to build up. For instance, iodoacetate causes yeast extracts to accumulate fructose-1,6-bisphosphate, whereas fluoride causes the build-up of two phosphate esters, 3-phosphoglycerate and 2-phosphoglycerate. The isolation and characterisation of these intermediates was vital to the elucidation of the glycolytic pathway: Chemical intuition combined with this information led to the prediction of the pathway's intervening steps. Each of the proposed reactions was eventually shown to occur *in vitro* as catalysed by a purified enzyme.

Genetic defects also cause metabolic intermediates to accumulate: Archibald Garrod's realisation, in the early 1900s, that human genetic diseases are the consequence of deficiencies in specific enzymes also contributed to the elucidation of metabolic pathways. For example, on the ingestion of either phenylalanine or tyrosine, individuals with the largely harmless inherited condition known as alcaptonuria, but not normal subjects, excrete homogentisic acid in their urine. This is because the liver of alcaptonurics lacks an enzyme that catalyses the breakdown of homogentisic acid. Another genetic disease, phenylketonuria, results in the accumulation of phenylpyruvate in the urine (and which, if untreated, causes severe mental retardation in infants). Ingested phenylalanine and phenylpyruvate appear as phenylpyruvate in the urine of affected subjects, whereas tyrosine is metabolised normally. The effects of these two abnormalities suggested the pathway for phenylalanine metabolism diagrammed in Fig. 9.11. However, the supposition that phenylpyruvate but not tyrosine occurs on the normal pathway of phenylalanine metabolism because phenylpyruvate accumulates in the urine of phenylketonurics has proved incorrect. This indicates the pitfalls of relying solely on metabolic blocks and the consequent build-up of intermediates as indicators of a metabolic pathway. In this case, phenylpyruvate formation was later shown to arise from a normally minor pathway that becomes significant only when the phenylalanine concentration is abnormally high, as it is in phenylketonurics.

Metabolic blocks can be generated by genetic manipulation: Early metabolic studies led to the astounding discovery that the basic metabolic pathway in most organisms are essentially identical. This metabolic uniformity has greatly facilitated the study of metabolic reactions. A mutation that inactivates or deletes an enzyme in a pathway of interest can be readily generated in rapidly reproducing micro-organisms through the use of mutagens (chemical agents that induce genetic changes), X-rays or genetic engineering techniques. Desired mutants are identified by their requirement of the pathway's end product for growth. For example, George Beadle and Edward Tatum proposed a pathway of arginine biosynthesis in the mould *Neurospora crassa* based on their analysis of three arginine-requiring auxotrophic mutants (mutants requiring a specific nutrient for growth), which were isolated after X-irradiation (Fig. 9.12). This landmark study also conclusively demonstrated that enzymes are specified by genes.

Genetic manipulations of higher organisms provide metabolic insights: Transgenic organisms constitute valuable resources for the study of metabolism. They can be used to both create metabolic blocks and to express genes in tissues where they are not normally present. For example, creatine kinase catalyses the formation of phospho-creatine, a substance that functions to generate ATP rapidly when it is in short supply. This enzyme is normally present in many tissues, including brain and muscle, but not in liver.

The introduction of the gene encoding creatinine kinase into the liver of a mouse causes the liver to synthesise phosphocreatine when the mouse is fed creatine, as demonstrated by localised *in vivo* NMR techniques (Fig. 9.13). The presence of phosphocreatine in a transgenic mouse liver protects the animal against the sharp drop in [ATP] ordinarily caused by fructose overload. This genetic manipulation technique is being used to study mechanisms of metabolic control *in vivo*.

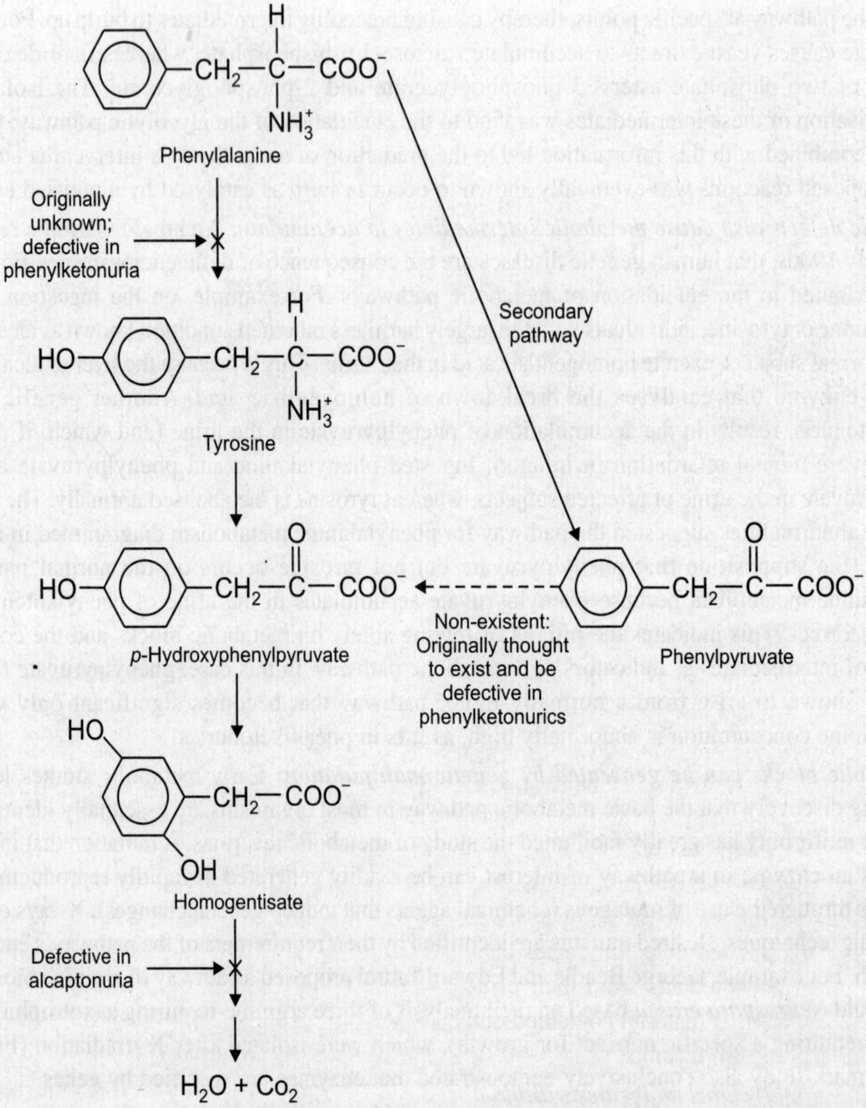

Fig. 9.11: Pathway for phenylalanine degradation: It was originally hypothesised that phenylpyruvate was a pathway intermediate based on the observation that phenylketonurics excrete ingested phenylalanine and phenylpyruvate as phenylpyruvate. Further studies, however, demonstrated that phenylpyruvate is not a homogentisate precursor; rather, phenylpyruvate production is significant only when the phenylalanine concentration is abnormally high. Instead, tyrosine is the normal product of phenylalanine degradation.

Metabolic pathways are regulated both by controlling the activities of regulatory enzymes and by controlling their concentrations at the level of gene expression. The important question of how hormones and diet control metabolic processes at the level of gene expression is being addressed through the use of transgenic animals. Reporter genes (genes whose products are easily detected) are placed under the influence of promoters (genetic elements that regulate transcriptional initiation) that control the expression of specific regulatory enzymes and the resulting composite gene is expressed in animals. The transgenic

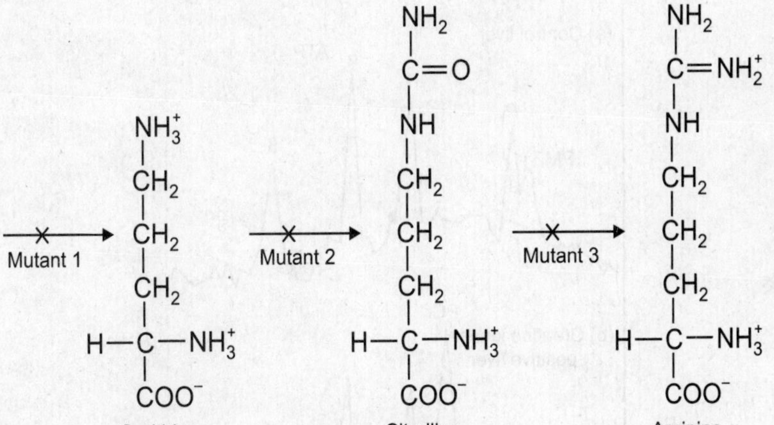

Fig. 9.12: Pathway of arginine biosynthesis indicating the positions of genetic blocks. All of these mutants grow in the presence of arginine, but mutant 1 also grows in the presence of the (non-standard) α-amino acids citrulline or ornithine and mutant 2 grows in the presence of citrulline. This is because in mutant 1, an enzyme leading to the production of ornithine is absent but enzymes farther along the pathway are normal. In mutant 2, the enzyme catalysing citrulline production is defective, whereas in mutant 3 an enzyme involved in the conversion of citrulline to arginine is lacking.

animals can then be treated with specific hormones and/or diets and the production of the reporter gene product measured. Modern techniques also make it possible to insert a mutation that inactivates or deletes an enzyme or control protein in a pathway of interest in higher organisms such as mice. Knockout mice have proved useful for studying metabolic control mechanisms.

Isotopes in Biochemistry

The specific labelling of metabolites such that their interconversions can be traced is an indispensable technique for elucidating metabolic pathways. Franz Knoop formulated this technique in 1904 to study fatty acid oxidation. He fed dogs fatty acids chemically labelled with phenyl groups and isolated the phenyl-substituted end products from their urine. From the differences in these products when the phenyl-substituted starting material contained odd and even numbers of carbon atoms he deduced that fatty acids are degraded in C_2 units.

Isotopes specifically label molecules without altering their chemical properties: Chemical labelling has the disadvantage that the chemical properties of labelled metabolites differ from those of normal metabolites. This problem is eliminated by labelling molecules of interest with isotopes (atoms with the same number of protons but a different number of neutrons in their nuclei). Recall that the chemical properties of an element are a consequence of its electron configuration which, in turn, is determined by its atomic number, not its atomic mass. The metabolic fate of a specific atom in a metabolite can, therefore, be elucidated by isotopically labelling that position and following its progress through the metabolic pathway of interest. The advent of isotopic labelling and tracing techniques in the 1940s, therefore, revolutionised the study of metabolism. Isotope effects, which are changes in reaction rates arising from the mass differences between isotopes, are in most instances negligible. Where they are significant, most noticeably between hydrogen and its isotopes deuterium and tritium, they have been used to gain insight into enzymatic reaction mechanisms.

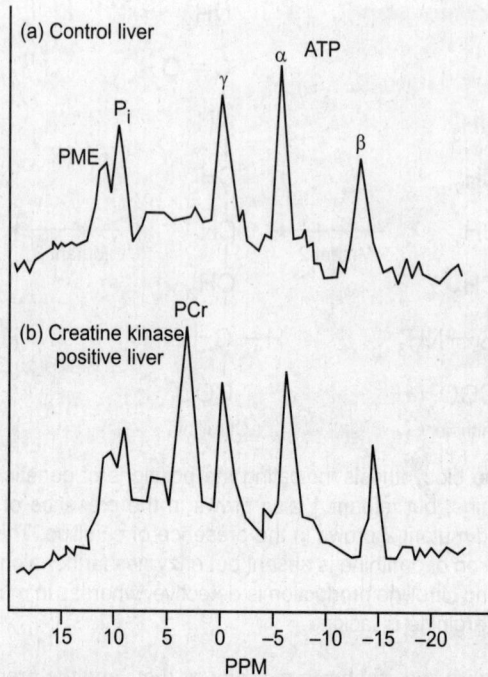

Fig. 9.13: The expression of creatine kinase in transgenic mouse liver as demonstrated by localised *in vivo* ^{31}p NMR: (a) the spectrum of a normal mouse liver after the mouse had been fed a diet supplemented with 2 per cent creatine. The peaks corresponding to inorganic phosphate (P_i), the α, β and γ phosphoryl groups of ATP and phosphomonoesters (PME) are labelled and (b) the spectrum of the liver of a mouse transgenic for creatine kinase that had been fed a diet supplemented with 2 per cent creatine. The phosphocreatine peak is labelled PCr.

NMR can be used to study metabolism in whole animals: Nuclear magnetic resonance (NMR) detects specific isotopes due to their characteristic nuclear spins. Among the isotopes that NMR can detect are ^1H, ^{13}C and ^{31}P. Since the NMR spectrum of a particular nucleus varies with its immediate environment, it is possible to identify the peaks corresponding to specific atoms even in relatively complex mixtures.

The development of magnets large enough to accommodate animals and humans and to localise spectra to specific organs, has made it possible to study metabolic pathways non-invasively by NMR techniques.

Detection of radioactive isotopes: All elements have isotopes. For example, the atomic mass of naturally occurring Cl is 35.45 D because, at least on earth, it is a mixture of 55 per cent ^{35}Cl and 45 per cent ^{36}Cl (other isotopes of Cl are present in only trace amounts). Stable isotopes are generally identified and quantitated by mass spectrometry or NMR techniques. Many isotopes, however, are unstable, they undergo radioactive decay, a process that involves the emission from the radioactive nuclei of sub-atomic particles such as helium nuclei (α particles), electrons (β particles) and/or photons (γ radiation). Radioactive nuclei emit radiation with characteristic energies. Radiation can be detected by a variety of techniques. Those most commonly used in biochemical investigations are proportional counting (known in its simplest form as Geiger counting), liquid scintillation counting and autoradiography. Proportional counters electronically detect the ionisations in a gas caused by the passage of radiation. Moreover, they can also discriminate between particles of different energies and thus simultaneously determine the amounts of two or more different isotopes present.

Radioactive isotopes have characteristic half-lives: Radioactive decay is a random process whose rate for a given isotope depends only on the number of radioactive atoms present.

Isotopes are indispensable for establishing the metabolic origins of complex metabolites and precursor-product relationships: The metabolic origins of complex molecules such as heme, cholesterol and phospholipids may be determined by administering isotopically labelled starting materials to animals and isolating the resulting products. Isotopic tracers are also useful in establishing the order of appearance of metabolic intermediates, their so-called precursor-product relationships. An example of such an analysis concerns the biosynthesis of the complex phospholipids called plasmalogens and alkylacylglycerophospholipids. Alkylacylglycerophospholipids are ethers, whereas the closely related plasmalogens are vinyl ethers. Their similar structures brings up the interesting question of their biosynthetic relationship: Which is the precursor and which is the product?

Two possible modes of synthesis can be envisioned (Fig. 9.14):

1. The staring material is converted to the vinyl ether (plasmalogen), which is then reduced to yield the ether (alkylacylglycerophospholipid). Accordingly, the vinyl ether would be the precursor and the ether the product.

2. The ether is formed first and then oxidised to yield the vinyl ether. The ether would then be the precursor and the vinyl ether the product.

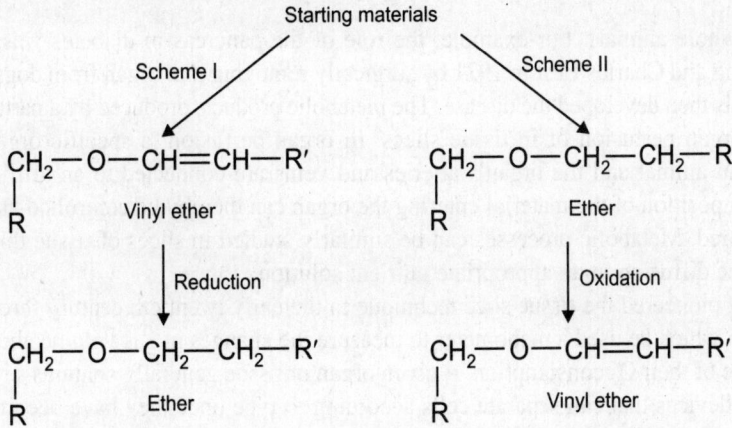

Fig. 9.14: Two possible pathways for the biosynthesis of ether—and vinyl ether-containing phospholipids: (I) the vinyl ether is the precursor and the ether is the product, and (II) the ether is the precursor and the vinyl ether is the product.

Precursor-product relationships can be most easily sorted out through the use of radioactive tracers. A pulse of the labelled starting material is administered to an organism and the specific radioactivities of the resulting metabolic products are followed with time (Fig. 9.15):

$$\text{Starting material*} \rightarrow \text{A*} \rightarrow \text{B*} \rightarrow \text{later products*}$$

(here the * represents the radioactive label).

Isolated Organs, Cells and Sub-cellular Organelles

In addition to understanding the chemistry and catalytic events that occur at each step of a metabolic pathway, it is important to learn where a given pathway occurs within an organism. Early workers studied

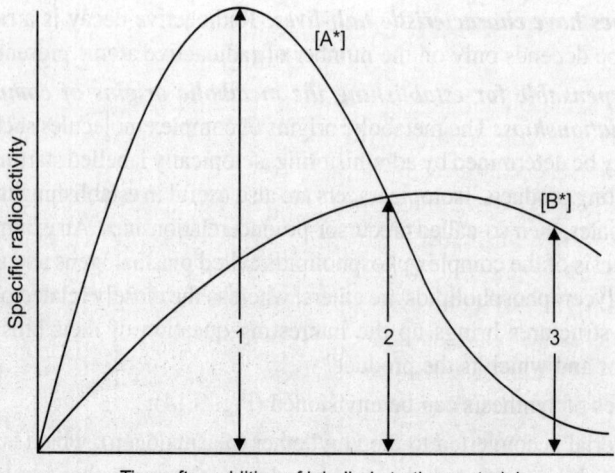

Fig. 9.15: The flow of a pulse of radioactivity from precursor to product. At point 1, product radioactivity (B*, purple) is increasing and is less than that of its precursor (A*, orange), at point 2, product radioactivity is maximal and is equal to that of its precursor and at point 3, product radioactivity is decreasing and is greater than that of its precursor.

metabolism in whole animals. For example, the role of the pancreas in diabetes was established by Frederick Banting and Charles Best in 1921 by surgically removing that organ from dogs and observing that these animals then developed the disease. The metabolic products produced by a particular organ can be studied by organ perfusion or in tissue slices. In organ perfusion, a specific organ is surgically removed from an animal and the organ's arteries and veins are connected to an artificial circulatory system. The composition of the material entering the organ can thereby be controlled and its metabolic products monitored. Metabolic processes can be similarly studied in slices of tissue thin enough to be nourished by free diffusion in an appropriate nutrient solution.

Otto Warburg pioneered the tissue slice technique in the early twentieth century through his studies of respiration, in which he used a manometer to measure the changes in gas volume above tissue slices as a consequence of their O_2 consumption. A given organ or tissue generally contains several cell types. Cell sorters are devices that can separate cells according to type once they have been treated with the enzymes trypsin and collagenase to destroy the intercellular matrix that binds them into a tissue. This technique allows further localisation of metabolic function. A single cell type may also be grown in tissue culture for study. Although culturing cells often results in their loss of differentiated function, techniques have been developed for maintaining several cell types that still express their original characteristics.

As discussed in the beginning of this chapter, metabolic pathways in eukaryotes are compartmentalised in various sub-cellular organelles. For example, oxidative phosphorylation occurs in the mitochondrion, whereas glycolysis and fatty acid biosynthesis occur in the cytosol. Such observations are made by breaking cells open and fractionating their components by differential centrifugation, possibly followed by zonal ultracentrifugation through a sucrose density gradient or by equilibrium density gradient ultracentrifugation in a CsCl density gradient, which, respectively, separate particles according to their size and density. The cell fractions are then analysed for biochemical function.

THERMODYNAMICS OF PHOSPHATE COMPOUNDS

The endergonic processes that maintain the living state are driven by the exergonic reactions of nutrient oxidation. This coupling is most often mediated through the syntheses of a few types of 'high-energy' intermediates whose exergonic consumption drives endergonic processes. These intermediates, therefore, form a sort of universal free energy 'currency' through which free energy-producing reactions 'pay for' the free energy-consuming processes in biological systems. Adenosine triphosphate (ATP, Fig. 9.16), which occurs in all known life-forms, is the 'high-energy' intermediate that constitutes the most common cellular energy currency. Its central role in energy metabolism was first recognised in 1941 by Fritz Lipmann and Herman Kalckar. ATP consists of an adenosine moiety to which three phosphoryl groups ($—PO_3^{2-}$) are sequentially linked via a phosphoester bond followed by two phosphoanhydride bonds. Adenosine diphosphate (ADP) and 5′-adenosine monophosphate (AMP) are similarly constituted but with only two and one phosphoryl units, respectively.

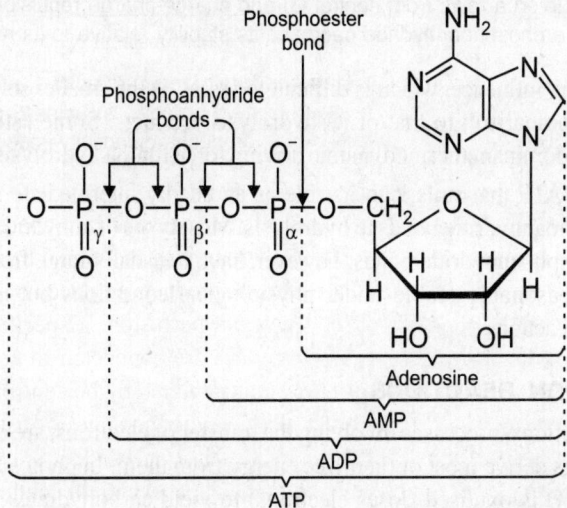

Fig. 9.16: The structure of ATP indicating its relationship to ADP, AMP and adenosine. The phosphoryl groups, starting with that on AMP, are referred to as the α, β and γ phosphates. Note the difference between phosphoester and phosphoanhydride bonds.

Several different factors appear to be responsible for the 'high-energy' character of phosphoanhydride bonds such as those in ATP (Fig. 9.17):

1. The resonance stabilisation of a phosphoanhydride bond is less than that of its hydrolysis products. This is because a phosphoanhydride's two strongly electron-withdrawing phosphoryl groups must compete for the π electrons of its bridging oxygen atom, whereas this competition is absent in the hydrolysis products. In other words, the electronic requirements of the phosphoryl groups are less satisfied in a phosphoanhydride than in its hydrolysis products.

2. Of perhaps greater importance is the destabilising effect of the electrostatic repulsions between the charged groups of a phosphoanhydride in comparison to that of its hydrolysis products. In the physiological pH range, ATP has three to four negative charges whose mutual electrostatic repulsions are partially relieved by ATP hydrolysis.

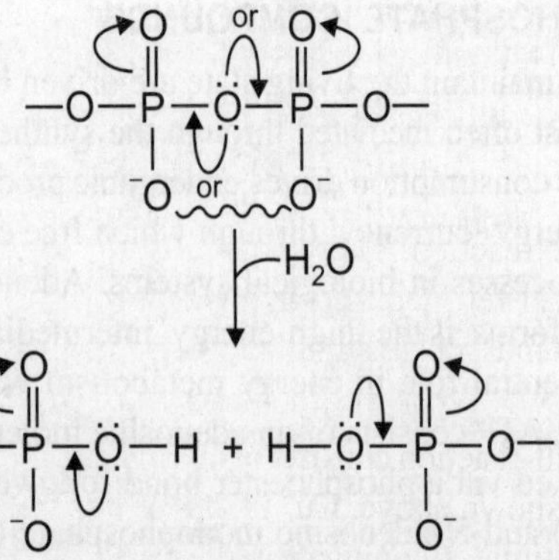

Fig. 9.17: Resonance and electrostatic stabilisation in a phosphoanhydride and its hydrolysis products. The competing resonances (curved arrows from central O) and charge-charge repulsions (zigzag line) between the phosphoryl groups of a phosphoanhydride decrease its stability relative to its hydrolysis products.

3. Another destabilising influence, which is difficult to assess, is the smaller solvation energy of a phosphoanhydride in comparison to that of its hydrolysis products. Some estimates suggest that this factor provides the dominant thermodynamic driving force for the hydrolysis of phosphoanhydrides.

A further property of ATP that suits it to its role as an energy intermediate stems from the relative kinetic stability of phosphoanhydride bonds to hydrolysis. Most types of anhydrides are rapidly hydrolysed in aqueous solution. Phosphoanhydride bonds, however, have unusually large free energies of activation. Consequently, ATP is reasonably stable under physiological conditions but is readily hydrolysed in enzymatically mediated reactions.

OXIDATION-REDUCTION REACTIONS

Oxidation-reduction reactions, processes involving the transfer of electrons, are of immense biochemical significance, living things derive most of their free energy from them. In photosynthesis, CO_2 is reduced (gains electrons) and H_2O is oxidised (loses electrons) to yield carbohydrates and O_2 in an otherwise endergonic process that is powered by light energy. In aerobic metabolism, which is carried out by all eukaryotes and many prokaryotes, the overall photosynthetic reaction is essentially reversed so as to harvest the free energy of oxidation of carbohydrates and other organic compounds in the form of ATP. Anaerobic metabolism generates ATP, although in lower yields, through intramolecular oxidation-reductions of various organic molecules, for example, glycolysis, in certain anaerobic bacteria, ATP is generated through the use of non-O_2 oxidising agents such as sulphate or nitrate. In this section, we outline the thermodynamics of oxidation-reduction reactions in order to understand the quantitative aspects of these crucial biological processes.

Nernst Equation

Oxidation-reduction reactions (also known as redox or oxido-reduction reactions) resemble other type of chemical reactions in that they involve group transfer. For instance, hydrolysis transfers a functional group to water. In oxidation-reduction reactions, the 'groups' transferred are electrons, which are passed from an electron donor (reductant or reducing agent) to an electron acceptor (oxidant or oxidising agent). For example, in the reaction:

$$Fe^{3+} + Cu^+ \rightleftharpoons Fe^{2+} + Cu^{2+}$$

Cu^+, the reductant, is oxidised to Cu^{2+} while Fe^{3+}, the oxidant, is reduced to Fe^{2+}. Redox reactions may be divided into two half-reactions or redox couples, such as:

$$Fe^{3+} + e^- \rightleftharpoons Fe^{2+} \text{ (reduction)}$$

$$Cu^+ \rightleftharpoons Cu^{2+} + e^- \text{ (oxidation)}$$

whose sum is the above whole reaction. These half-reactions occur during oxidative metabolism in the vital mitochondrial electron transfer mediated by cytochrome c oxidase. Note that for electrons to be transferred, both half-reactions must occur simultaneously. In fact, the electrons are the two half-reactions common intermediate.

Electrochemical cells: A half-reaction consists of an electron donor and its conjugate electron acceptor, in the oxidation half-reaction shown above, Cu^+ is the electron donor and Cu^{2+} is its conjugate electron acceptor. Together these constitute a conjugate redox pair analogous to the conjugate acid-base pair (HA and A^-) of a Brønsted acid. An important difference between redox pairs and acid-base pairs, however, is that the two half-reactions of a redox reaction, each consisting of a conjugate redox pair, may be physically separated so as to form an electrochemical cell (Fig. 9.18).

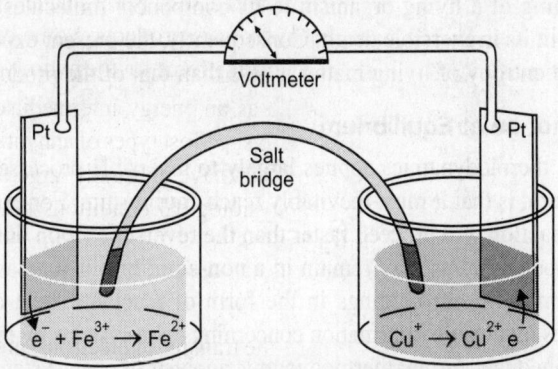

Fig. 9.18: Example of an electrochemical cell. The half-cell undergoing oxidation (here $Cu^+ \rightarrow Cu^{2+} + e^-$) passes the liberated electrons through the wire to the half-cell undergoing reduction (here $e^- + Fe^{3+} \rightarrow Fe^{2+}$). Electroneutrality in the two half-cells is maintained by the transfer of ions through the electrolyte-containing salt bridge.

In such a device, each half-reaction takes place in its separate half-cell, and electrons are passed between half-cells as an electric current in the wire connecting their two electrodes. A salt bridge is necessary to complete the electrical circuit by providing a conduit for ions to migrate in the maintenance of electrical neutrality.

Measurements of Redox Potentials

The free energy change of a redox reaction may be determined, by simply measuring its redox potential with a voltmeter. Consequently, voltage measurements are commonly employed to characterise the sequence of reactions comprising a metabolic electron-transport pathway (such as mediates, e.g. oxidative metabolism).

Electron-transfer reactions are of great biological importance. For example, in the mitochondrial electron-transport chain, the primary source of ATP in eukaryotes, electrons are passed from NADH along a series of electron acceptors of increasing reduction potential to O_2.

Concentration Cells

A concentration gradient has a lower entropy (greater order) than the corresponding uniformly mixed solution and, therefore, requires the input of free energy for its formation. Consequently, discharge of a concentration gradient is an exergonic process that may be harnessed to drive an endergonic reaction. Quantitation of the free energy contained in a concentration gradient is accomplished by use of the concepts of electrochemical cells.

THERMODYNAMICS OF LIFE

One of the last refuges of vitalism, the doctrine that biological processes are not bound by the physical laws that govern inanimate objects, was the belief that living things can somehow evade the laws of thermodynamics. This view was partially refuted by elaborate calorimetric measurements on living animals that are entirely consistent with the energy conservation predictions of the first law of thermodynamics. However, the experimental verification of the second law of thermodynamics in living systems is more difficult. It has not been possible to measure the entropy of living matter because the heat, q_p, of a reaction at a constant T and P is only equal to $T\Delta S$ if the reaction is carried out reversibly. Obviously, the dismantling of a living organism to its component molecules for such a measurement would invariably result in its irreversible death. Consequently, the present experimentally verified state of knowledge is that the entropy of living matter is less than that of the products to which it decays.

Living Systems Cannot be at Equilibrium

Classical or equilibrium thermodynamics applies largely to reversible processes in closed systems. The fate of any isolated system, is that it must inevitably reach equilibrium. For example, if its reactants are in excess, the forward reaction will proceed faster than the reverse reaction until equilibrium is attained ($\Delta G = 0$). In contrast, open systems may remain in a non-equilibrium state as long as they are able to acquire free energy from their surroundings in the form of reactants, heat or work. While classical thermodynamics provides invaluable information concerning open systems by indicating whether a given process can occur spontaneously, further thermodynamic analysis of open systems requires the application of the more recently elucidated principles of non-equilibrium or irreversible thermodynamics. In contrast to classical thermodynamics, this theory explicitly takes time into account.

Living organisms are open systems and, therefore, can never be at equilibrium. As indicated above, they continuously ingest high-enthalpy, low-entropy nutrients, which they convert to low-enthalpy, high-entropy waste products. The free energy resulting from this process is used to do work and to produce the high degree of organisation characteristic of life.

If this process is interrupted, the organism ultimately reaches equilibrium, which for living things is synonymous with death. For example, one theory of ageing holds that senescence results from the random but inevitable accumulation in cells of genetic defects that interfere with and ultimately disrupt the proper functioning of living processes. [The theory does not, however, explain how single-celled organisms or the germ cells of multicellular organisms (sperm and ova), which are in effect immortal, are able to escape this so-called error catastrophe.]

Living systems must maintain a non-equilibrium state for several reasons:

1. Only a non-equilibrium process can perform useful work.
2. The intricate regulatory functions characteristic of life require a non-equilibrium state because a process at equilibrium cannot be directed (similarly, a ship that is dead in the water will not respond to its rudder).

3. The complex cellular and molecular systems that conduct biological processes can be maintained only in the non-equilibrium state. Living systems are inherently unstable because they are degraded by the very biochemical reactions to which they give rise. Their regeneration, which must occur almost simultaneously with their degradation, requires the continuous influx of free energy. Life, therefore, differs in a fundamental way from a complex machine such as a computer. Both require a throughput of free energy to be active. However, the function of the machine is based on a static structure, so that the machine can be repeatedly switched on and off. Life, in contrast, is based on a self-destructing but self-renewing process which, once interrupted, cannot be reinitiated.

Non-equilibrium Thermodynamics and the Steady State

In a non-equilibrium process, something (such as matter, electrical charge or heat) must flow, that is, change its spatial distribution. In classical mechanics, the acceleration of mass occurs in response to force. Similarly, flow in a thermodynamic system occurs in response to a thermodynamic force (driving force), which results from the system's non-equilibrium state. For example, the flow of matter in diffusion is motivated by the thermodynamic force of a concentration gradient, the migration of electrical charge (electric current) occurs in response to a gradient in an electric field (a voltage difference), the transport of heat results from a temperature gradient, and a chemical reaction results from a difference in chemical potential. Such flows are said to be conjugate to their thermodynamic force.

A thermodynamic force may also promote a nonconjugate flow under the proper conditions. For example, a gradient in the concentration of matter can give rise to an electric current (a concentration cell), heat (such as occurs on mixing H_2O and HCl) or a chemical reaction (the mitochondrial production of ATP through the dissipation of a proton gradient). Similarly, a gradient in electrical potential can motivate a flow of matter (electrophoresis), heat (resistive heating) or a chemical reaction (the charging of a battery). When a thermodynamic force stimulates a non-conjugate flow, the process is called energy transduction.

Living things maintain the steady state: Living systems are, for the most part, characterised by being in a steady state. By this it is meant that all flows in the system are constant, so that the system does not change with time. Ilya Prigogine, a pioneer in the development of irreversible thermodynamics, has shown that a steady-state system produces the maximum amount of useful work for a given energy expenditure under the prevailing conditions. The steady state of an open system is, therefore, its state of maximum thermodynamic efficiency. Furthermore, in analogy with Le Châtelier's principle, slight perturbations from the steady state give rise to changes in flows that counteract these perturbations so as to return the system to the steady state. The steady state of an open system is, therefore, analogous to the equilibrium state of an isolated system, both are stable states.

Many biological regulatory mechanisms function to maintain a steady state. For example, the flow of reaction intermediates through a metabolic pathway is often inhibited by an excess of final product and stimulated by an excess of starting material through the allosteric regulation of its key enzymes. Living things have apparently evolved so as to take maximum thermodynamic advantage of their environments.

Thermodynamics of Metabolic Control

Enzymes selectively catalyse required reactions: Biological reactions are highly specific, only reactions that lie on metabolic pathways take place at significant rates despite the many other thermodynamically favourable reactions that are also possible. The free energy barriers of both of the non-enzymatic reactions are far higher than that of the enzyme-catalysed phosphoryl transfer to glucose. Hence enzymatic formation of glucose-6-phosphate is kinetically favoured over the non-enzymatic hydrolysis of ATP. It is the role of an enzyme, in this case hexokinase, to selectively reduce the free energy of activation of a chemically coupled reaction so that it approaches equilibrium faster than the more thermodynamically favoured uncoupled reaction.

Many enzymatic reactions are near equilibrium: Although metabolism as a whole is a non-equilibrium process, many of its component reactions function close to equilibrium. The reaction of ATP and creatine to form phosphocreatine is an example of such a reaction. The ratio [creatine]/[phosphocreatine] depends on [ATP] because creatine kinase, the enzyme catalysing this reaction, has sufficient activity to equilibrate the reaction rapidly. The net rate of such an equilibrium reaction is effectively controlled by varying the concentrations of its reactants and/or products.

Pathway throughput is regulated by controlling enzymes operating far from equilibrium: Other biological reactions function far from equilibrium. Changes in substrate concentrations, therefore, have relatively little effect on the rate of the phospho-fructokinase reaction, the enzyme is close to saturation. Only changes in the activity of the enzyme, through allosteric interactions, for example, can significantly alter this rate. An enzyme such as phosphofructokinase is, therefore, analogous to a dam on a river. Substrate flux (rate of flow) is controlled by varying its activity (allosterically or by other means), much as a dam controls the flow of a river below the dam by varying the opening of its floodgates (when the water levels on the two sides of the dam are different, that is, when they are not at equilibrium).

Understanding of how reactant flux in a metabolic pathway is controlled requires knowledge of which reactions are functioning near equilibrium and which are far from it. Most enzymes in a metabolic pathway operate near equilibrium and, therefore, have net rates that are sensitive only to their substrate concentrations. However, certain enzymes, which are strategically located in a metabolic pathways, operate far from equilibrium. These enzymes, which are targets for metabolic regulation by allosteric interactions and other mechanisms, are responsible for the maintenance of a stable steady-state flux of metabolites through the pathway. This situation, as we have seen, maximises the pathways thermodynamic efficiency.

Chapter 10

Electron Transport and Oxidative Phosphorylation

INTRODUCTION

The electron transport chain is a collection of membrane-embedded proteins and organic molecules, most of them organised into four large complexes labelled I to IV. In eukaryotes, many copies of these molecules are found in the inner mitochondrial membrane. In prokaryotes, the electron transport chain components are found in the plasma membrane.

As the electrons travel through the chain, they go from a higher to a lower energy level, moving from less electron-hungry to more electron-hungry molecules. Energy is released in these 'downhill' electron transfers, and several of the protein complexes use the released energy to pump protons from the mitochondrial matrix to the intermembrane space, forming a proton gradient.

All of the electrons that enter the transport chain come from NADH and $FADH_2$ molecules produced during earlier stages of cellular respiration: glycolysis, pyruvate oxidation, and the citric acid cycle.

- NADH is very good at donating electrons in redox reactions (that is, its electrons are at a high energy level), so it can transfer its electrons directly to complex I, turning back into NAD^+. As electrons move through complex I in a series of redox reactions, energy is released, and the complex uses this energy to pump protons from the matrix into the intermembrane space.

- $FADH_2$ is not as good at donating electrons as NADH (that is, its electrons are at a lower energy level), so it cannot transfer its electrons to complex I. Instead, it feeds them into the transport chain through complex II, which does not pump protons across the membrane.

IN MITOCHONDRIA

Most eukaryotic cells have mitochondria, which produce ATP from products of the citric acid cycle, fatty acid oxidation, and amino acid oxidation. At the mitochondrial inner membrane, electrons from NADH and $FADH_2$ pass through the electron transport chain to oxygen, which is reduced to water. The electron transport chain comprises an enzymatic series of electron donors and acceptors. Each electron donor will pass electrons to a more electronegative acceptor, which in turn donates these electrons to another acceptor, a process that continues down the series until electrons are passed to oxygen, the most electronegative and terminal electron acceptor in the chain. Passage of electrons between donor and acceptor releases energy, which is used to generate a proton gradient across the mitochondrial membrane by actively 'pumping' protons into the intermembrane space, producing a thermodynamic state that has the potential to do work. This entire process is called oxidative phosphorylation, since ADP is phosphorylated to ATP using the energy of hydrogen oxidation in many steps.

A small percentage of electrons do not complete the whole series and instead directly leak to oxygen, resulting in the formation of the free-radical superoxide, a highly reactive molecule that contributes to oxidative stress and has been implicated in a number of diseases and ageing.

Mitochondrial Redox Carriers

Energy obtained through the transfer of electrons down the electron transport chain (ETC) is used to pump protons from the mitochondrial matrix into the intermembrane space, creating an electrochemical proton gradient (ΔpH) across the inner mitochondrial membrane (IMM). This proton gradient is largely but not exclusively responsible for the mitochondrial membrane potential ($\Delta\psi_M$). It allows ATP synthase to use the flow of H^+ through the enzyme back into the matrix to generate ATP from adenosine diphosphate (ADP) and inorganic phosphate. Complex I (NADH coenzyme Q reductase, labeled I) accepts electrons from the Krebs cycle electron carrier nicotinamide adenine dinucleotide (NADH), and passes them to coenzyme Q (ubiquinone, labeled Q), which also receives electrons from complex II (succinate dehydrogenase, labeled II). Q passes electrons to complex III (cytochrome bc1 complex, labeled III), which passes them to cytochrome c (cyt c). Cyt c passes electrons to Complex IV (cytochrome c oxidase, labeled IV), which uses the electrons and hydrogen ions to reduce molecular oxygen to water.

Four membrane-bound complexes have been identified in mitochondria. Each is an extremely complex transmembrane structure that is embedded in the inner membrane. Three of them are proton pumps. The structures are electrically connected by lipid-soluble electron carriers and water-soluble electron carriers. The overall electron transport chain:

$$NADH + H^+ \rightarrow Complex\ I \rightarrow Q \rightarrow Complex\ III \rightarrow Cytochrome\ c \rightarrow Complex\ IV \rightarrow H_2O$$
$$\uparrow$$
$$Complex\ II$$
$$\uparrow$$
$$Succinate$$

Because of this 'bypass,' each $FADH_2$ molecule causes fewer protons to be pumped (and contributes less to the proton gradient) than an NADH.

Complex I: NADH transfers its electrons to complex I. Complex I is quite large, and the part of it that receives the electrons is a flavoprotein, meaning a protein with an attached organic molecule called flavin mononucleotide (FMN). FMN is a prosthetic group, a non-protein molecule tightly bound to a protein and required for its activity, and it's FMN that actually accepts electrons from NADH. FMN passes the electrons to another protein inside complex I, one that has iron and sulphur bound to it (called an Fe-S protein), which in turns transfers the electrons to a small, mobile carrier called ubiquinone (Q).

Complex II: Like NADH, $FADH_2$ deposits its electrons in the electron transport chain, but it does so via complex II, bypassing complex I entirely. As a matter of fact, $FADH_2$ is a part of complex II, as is the enzyme that reduces it during the citric acid cycle, unlike the other enzymes of the cycle, it's embedded in the inner mitochondrial membrane. $FADH_2$ transfers its electrons to iron-sulphur proteins within complex II, which then pass the electrons to ubiquinone (Q), the same mobile carrier that collects electrons from complex I. Beyond the first two complexes, electrons from NADH and $FADH_2$ travel exactly the same route. Both complex I and complex II pass their electrons to a small, mobile electron carrier called ubiquinone (Q), which is reduced to form QH_2 and travels through the membrane, delivering the electrons to complex III. As electrons move through complex III, more H^+ ions are pumped across the membrane, and the electrons are ultimately delivered to another mobile carrier called cytochrome C (cyt C). Cyt C carries the electrons to complex IV, where a final batch of H^+ ions is pumped across the membrane. Complex IV passes the electrons to O_2, which splits into two oxygen atoms and accepts protons from the matrix to form water. Four electrons are required to reduce each molecule of O_2 and two water molecules are formed in the process.

Complex III: Like complex I, complex III includes an iron-sulphur (Fe-S) protein, but it also contains two proteins of another type, known as cytochromes. Cytochromes are a family of related proteins that have heme prosthetic groups containing iron ions. (Have you heard of the protein haemoglobin, which transports oxygen in the blood? Haemoglobin also has heme groups, but they bind oxygen rather than electrons.) In complex III, electrons are passed from one cytochrome to an iron-sulphur protein to a second cytochrome, then finally transferred out of the complex to a mobile electron carrier (cytochrome C). Like complex I, complex III pumps protons from the matrix into the intermembrane space, contributing to the H^+ concentration gradient.

Complex IV: From complex III, cytochrome C delivers electrons to the last complex of the electron transport chain, complex IV. There, the electrons are passed through two more cytochromes, the second of which has a very interesting job: with the help of a nearby copper ion, it transfers electrons to O_2, splitting oxygen to form two molecules of water. The mechanism of the transfer is pretty cool and worth looking up, but basically, the heme group and the copper ion bind tightly to the oxygen molecule and hold it in place until it is fully reduced (has gained electrons and protons to form water). The protons used to form water come from the matrix, contributing to the H^+ gradient, and complex IV also pumps protons from the matrix to the intermembrane space.

Overall, what does the electron transport chain do for the cell? It has two important functions:

- Regenerates electron carriers: NADH and $FADH_2$ pass their electrons to the electron transport chain, turning back into NAD^+ and FAD. This is important because the oxidised forms of these electron carriers are used in glycolysis and the citric acid cycle and must be available to keep these processes running.

- Makes a proton gradient: The transport chain builds a proton gradient across the inner mitochondrial membrane, with a higher concentration of H^+ in the intermembrane space and a lower concentration in the matrix. This gradient represents a stored form of energy, and, as we'll see, it can be used to make ATP.

Chemiosmosis

Complexes I, III, and IV of the electron transport chain are proton pumps. As electrons move energetically downhill, the complexes capture the released energy and use it to pump H^+ ions from the matrix to the intermembrane space. This pumping forms an electrochemical gradient across the inner mitochondrial membrane. The gradient is sometimes called the proton-motive force, and you can think of it as a form of stored energy, kind of like a battery. Like many other ions, protons can't pass directly through the phospholipid bilayer of the membrane because its core is too hydrophobic. Instead, H^+ ions can move down their concentration gradient only with the help of channel proteins that form hydrophilic tunnels across the membrane. In the inner mitochondrial membrane, H^+ ions have just one channel available: a membrane-spanning protein known as ATP synthase. Conceptually, ATP synthase is a lot like a turbine in a hydroelectric power plant. Instead of being turned by water, it's turned by the flow of H^+ ions moving down their electrochemical gradient. As ATP synthase turns, it catalyses the addition of a phosphate to ADP, capturing energy from the proton gradient as ATP.

This process, in which energy from a proton gradient is used to make ATP, is called chemiosmosis. More broadly, chemiosmosis can refer to any process in which energy stored in a proton gradient is used to do work. Although chemiosmosis accounts for over 80% of ATP made during glucose breakdown in cellular respiration, it's not unique to cellular respiration. For instance, chemiosmosis is also involved in the light reactions of photosynthesis.

What would happen to the energy stored in the proton gradient if it weren't used to synthesise ATP or do other cellular work? It would be released as heat, and interestingly enough, some types of cells deliberately use the proton gradient for heat generation rather than ATP synthesis. This might seem wasteful, but it's an important strategy for animals that need to keep warm. For instance, hibernating mammals (such as bears) have specialised cells known as brown fat cells. In the brown fat cells, uncoupling proteins are produced and inserted into the inner mitochondrial membrane. These proteins are simply channels that allow protons to pass from the intermembrane space to the matrix without travelling through ATP synthase. By providing an alternate route for protons to flow back into the matrix, the uncoupling proteins allow the energy of the gradient to be dissipated as heat. Group-translocation processes may also occur during amino acid transport. Chemiosmotic theory is discussed in details in Chapter 12.

Oxidative Phosphorylation

The electron transport chain forms a proton gradient across the inner mitochondrial membrane, which drives the synthesis of ATP via chemiosmosis. Many other organisms, need oxygen to live. As you know if you've ever tried to hold your breath for too long, lack of oxygen can make you feel dizzy or even black out, and prolonged lack of oxygen can even cause death.

As it turns out, the reason you need oxygen is so your cells can use this molecule during oxidative phosphorylation, the final stage of cellular respiration. Oxidative phosphorylation is made up of two closely connected components: the electron transport chain and chemiosmosis. In the electron transport chain, electrons are passed from one molecule to another, and energy released in these electron transfers is used to form an electrochemical gradient. In chemiosmosis, the energy stored in the gradient is used to make ATP.

So, where does oxygen fit into this picture? Oxygen sits at the end of the electron transport chain, where it accepts electrons and picks up protons to form water. If oxygen isn't there to accept electrons (for instance, because a person is not breathing in enough oxygen), the electron transport chain (Fig. 10.1) will stop running, and ATP will no longer be produced by chemiosmosis. Without enough ATP, cells can't carry out the reactions they need to function, and, after a long enough period of time, may even die.

The electron transport chain is a series of proteins and organic molecules found in the inner membrane of the mitochondria. Electrons are passed from one member of the transport chain to another in a series of redox reactions. Energy released in these reactions is captured as a proton gradient, which is then used to make ATP in a process called chemiosmosis. Together, the electron transport chain and chemiosmosis make up oxidative phosphorylation.

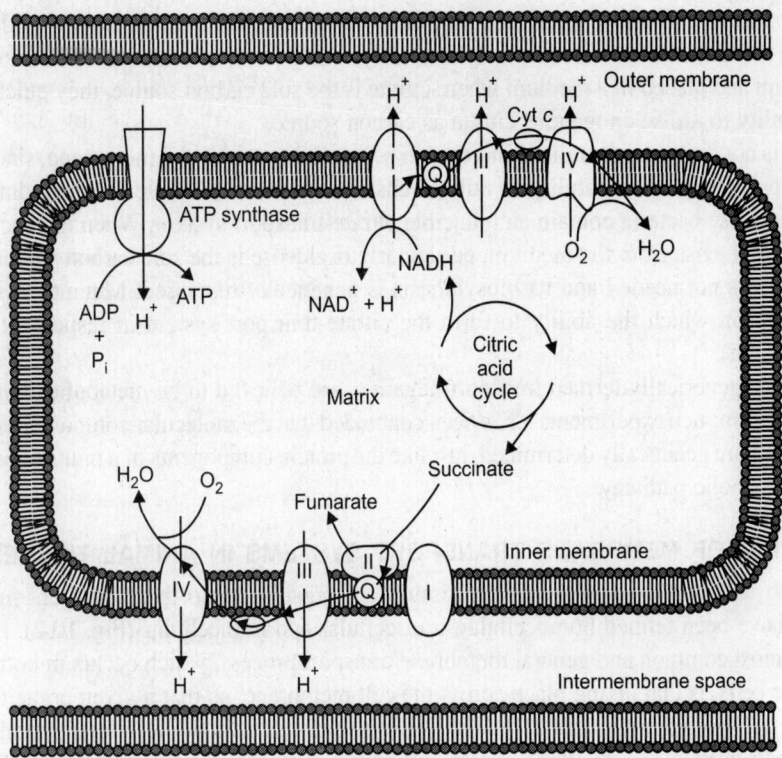

Fig. 10.1: The electron transport chain in the mitochondrion is the site of oxidative phosphorylation in eukaryotes. The NADH and succinate generated in the citric acid cycle is oxidised, providing energy to power ATP synthase.

The key steps of this process, shown in simplified form in the diagram above, include:

- Delivery of electrons by NADH and $FADH_2$: Reduced electron carriers (NADH and $FADH_2$) from other steps of cellular respiration transfer their electrons to molecules near the beginning of the transport chain. In the process, they turn back into NAD^+ and FAD, which can be reused in other steps of cellular respiration.

- Electron transfer and proton pumping: As electrons are passed down the chain, they move from a higher to a lower energy level, releasing energy. Some of the energy is used to pump H^+ ions, moving them out of the matrix and into the intermembrane space. This pumping establishes an electrochemical gradient.

- Splitting of oxygen to form water. At the end of the electron transport chain, electrons are transferred to molecular oxygen, which splits in half and takes up H^+ to form water.

- Gradient-driven synthesis of ATP. As H^+ ions flow down their gradient and back into the matrix, they pass through an enzyme called ATP synthase, which harnesses the flow of protons to synthesise ATP.

GENETIC EVIDENCE FOR TRANSPORT SYSTEMS

Genetic studies have yielded extremely important information on the function and biology of transport systems. An example may be described. When certain bacteria are grown on glucose as the sole carbon source, they are unable to utilise external citrate added to the medium, although they oxidise internally formed citrate at high rates via the tricarboxylic acid cycle. However, if such cells are removed from the glucose medium and placed in a medium where citrate is the sole carbon source, they quickly adapt and acquire the ability to utilise exogenous citrate as carbon source.

This effect is not due to a generalised increase in permeability of the cell membrane, since the citrate-grown cells do not acquire the ability to utilise substrates other than citrate. Such findings led to the conclusion that these bacteria contain an inducible citrate-transport system. When the bacteria have an ample supply of glucose from the medium, particularly if glucose is the sole carbon source, the citrate-transport system is not needed and its biosynthesis is genetically repressed. Mutants of such bacteria have been found in which the ability to form the citrate-transport system in response to exogenous citrate has been lost.

Such mutants, generically termed transport-negative, are believed to be metabolically normal in all other respects. From such experiments it has been concluded that the molecular components of membrane transport systems are genetically determined, just like the protein components of a multi enzyme sequence catalysing a metabolic pathway.

ORGANISATION OF MEMBRANE TRANSPORT SYSTEMS IN ANIMAL TISSUES

The membrane transport systems of animal tissues are organised into three different morphological types, which have been termed homocellular, transcellular and intracellular (Fig. 10.2). Homocellular transport, the most common and general membrane transport process, which occurs in both prokaryotic and eukaryotic cells, is that taking place across the cell membrane, so that a given organic substrate or mineral ion is transported into or out of the cell. All cells possess such homocellular systems for inward transport of their nutrients, particularly sugars and amino acids. Moreover, most types of animal cells contain homocellular transport systems for extruding Na^+ into the medium and maintaining a high intracellular K^+ concentration.

Transcellular transport is a special case of homocellular transport in which the transport system is localised on a specific portion of the cell surface in such a way as to make transport of a substrate through or across the entire cell possible. This arrangement occurs in epithelial cell layers, such as the gastric and intestinal mucosa and the epithelial cells lining kidney tubules. These sheets of epithelial cells promote transport across the cell layer, for example, from the blood to the gastric juice. The transport systems in epithelial cell layers are so organised in the cell membrane that a directional transport across the cell occurs, presumably because the active-transport systems are located on only one side of the cell barrier (Fig. 10.2). The third type of membrane transport in eukaryotic cells is intracellular transport, in which the transport process occurs across the membrane of an intracellular organelle, e.g. mitochondrion, chloroplast or sarcoplasmic reticulum. Such intracellular transport systems serve to transport mineral ions to metabolites between the cytosol and the internal medium of the organelle. This type of membrane transport process is involved in the compartmentation of ATP and many metabolites in mitochondria in the regulation of the contraction-relaxation cycle of muscle by transport of Ca^{2+} between cytosol and sarcoplasmic reticulum and in the transport of Ca^{2+} from the cytosol into the mitochondria.

PASSIVE-TRANSPORT SYSTEMS IN ANIMAL TISSUES

The biochemical characteristics of some representative transport systems in cell of higher animals will now be described. We shall consider passive-transport systems first.

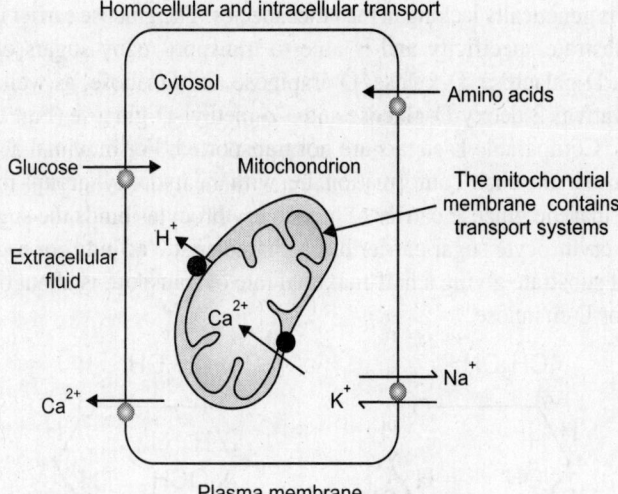

Homocellular and intracellular transport

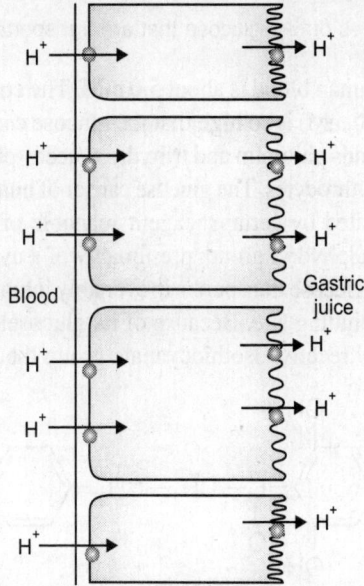

Transcellular transport across an epithelial cell layer to the gastric mucosa.
The direction of net movement is from the blood to the gastric juice

Fig. 10.2: Organisation of membrane transport systems in cells and tissues.

Glucose Carrier of Human Erythrocytes

One of the best known passive-transport systems is the glucose carrier of the human erythrocyte, which promotes net transport of glucose down a concentration gradient of glucose. The rate of entry of D-glucose into human erythrocytes increases with substrate concentration but ultimately approaches a maximum rate, at which the transport system is saturated. However, the rate of entry of glucose into erythrocytes of certain other vertebrate species, such as the cow, does not show a saturation effect, apparently a similar glucose carrier is genetically lacking in the latter species. The glucose carrier in human erythrocytes has a rather broad-substrate specificity and is able to transport many sugars other than D-glucose, including D-mannose, D-galactose, D-xylose, D-arabinose and D-ribose, as well as the unnatural and non-metabolised derivatives 2-deoxy-D-glucose and 3-*o*-methyl-D-glucose (Fig. 10.3), which are often used as test substrates. Comparable L-sugars are not transported. For maximal activity the transported sugar must be a pyranose in the chair conformation, i.e. with the hydroxyl groups in equatorial positions. It has been postulated that the glucose carrier of human erythrocytes binds the sugar at three equatorial hydroxyl groups. The erythrocyte sugar carrier has a characteristic affinity for each sugar. K_M, defined as the concentration of substrate giving a half-maximal rate of transport, is about 6.2 mM for D-glucose and about 18.5 mM for D-mannose.

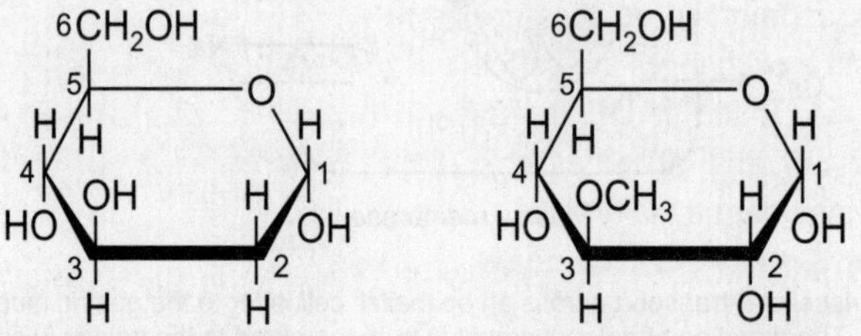

2-Deoxy-α-D-glucose 3-o-Methyl-α-D-glucose

Fig. 10.3: Two derivatives of α-D-glucose that are transported but not metabolised.

The glucose concentration in human blood is about 5.0 mM. The concentration of D-fructose required for half-maximal activity ($K_M > 2000$ mM) is so high that the glucose carrier does not function to transport fructose biologically. The compounds phloretin and trihydroxyaceto-phenone (Fig. 10.4) are competitive inhibitors of glucose transport in erythrocytes. The glucose carrier of human erythrocytes definitely appears to be a protein, since it is inactivated by certain reagents capable of reacting with specific functional groups of amino acid residues. A sulphydryl group, presumably of a cysteine residue and an amino group are required for activity. Moreover, glucose transport is irreversibly inhibited by D-glucosyl isothio-cyanate, which is an affinity label for the binding site. Because of its glucoselike structure this reagent binds to the glucose binding site, its highly reactive isothiocyanate group then reacts covalently with an amino

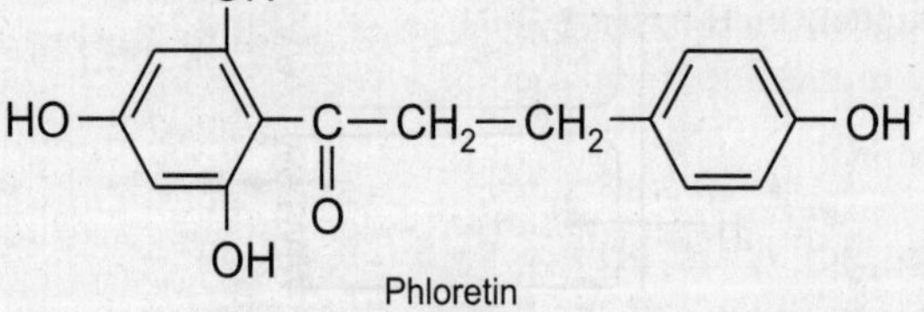

Phloretin

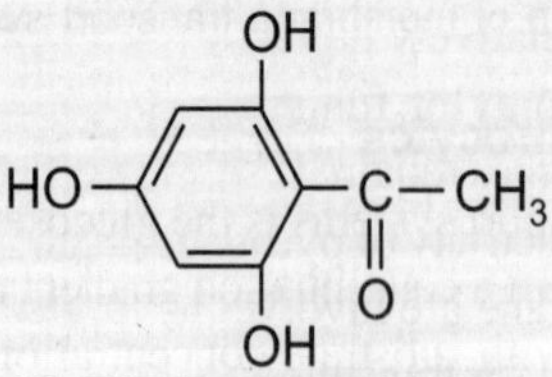

2,4,6,-Trihydroxyacetophenone

Fig. 10.4: Inhibitors of glucose transport by the human erythrocyte.

group on or near the glucose binding site. From experiments with this and other reagents it has been deduced that each erythrocyte contains about 3,00,000 glucose binding sites which function in passive transport of glucose across the membrane.

ATP-ADP Carrier of Mitochondria: Exchange-Diffusion

Several passive exchange-transport or exchange-diffusion systems occur in the mitochondrial inner membrane, such as the dicarboxylate and tricarboxylate carriers described earlier. The best-studied example is the ATP-ADP carrier of the mitochondrial membrane, which normally functions to transport one molecule of ADP into the mitochondrial matrix, where oxidative phosphorylation takes place, in exchange for one molecule of ATP returning to the cytosol from the matrix. The ATP-ADP carrier promotes only an exchange across the membrane, it does not bring about a net transport of nucleotides. Transport systems that promote such exchanges are called antiport systems. The ATP-ADP carrier is specific for ATP and ADP and for dATP and dADP, it will not transport AMP or any other NDPs or NTPs. It is saturable and shows a very high affinity for ADP and ATP. Much evidence indicates that it has two substrate binding sites, one on the inside face and the other on the outside face of the inner membrane. As has been pointed out, the ATP-ADP carrier is strongly and specifically inhibited by atractyloside and bongkrekic acid. The carrier will also exchange ^{14}C-ATP for unlabelled ADP and ^{14}C-ATP for ATP, in either direction.

ACTIVE-TRANSPORT SYSTEMS OF ANIMAL TISSUES

There are three major types of active-transport systems in animal tissues: (i) the Na^+ and K^+ 'pump,' which utilises metabolic energy to transport Na^+ out of the cell and K^+ into it, (ii) active-transport systems for glucose and other sugars and (iii) active-transport systems for amino acids. Of these the Na^+ and K^+ pump appears to be most active and of universal occurrence, it is present in the membrane of nearly all animal cells. Moreover, much evidence suggests that the Na^+ and K^+ pump is also essential for the operation of the pumps for glucose and for amino acids. We shall therefore examine the active transport of Na^+ and K^+ in some detail, particularly since it has been very intensively studied from the biochemical point of view.

Na⁺- and K⁺-Transporting ATPase System

Most animal cells maintain intracellular K^+ at a relatively high and constant concentration, between 120 and 160 mM, whereas the intracellular Na^+ concentration is usually much lower, less than 10 mM. A substantial gradient of K^+ and Na^+ exists across the cell membrane, since the extracellular fluid of mammals contains a relatively high concentration of Na^+, about 150 mM and a very low concentration of K^+, usually less than 4 mM. The constancy of the high internal K^+ concentration is maintained by the energy-requiring extrusion of Na^+ out of the cell and its replacement by K^+, promoted by an active-transport system called the Na^+K^+-ATPase. Relatively high concentrations of internal K^+ are required for several processes vital in the internal economy or function of animals cells. One is protein biosynthesis by ribosomes. Second, a number of enzymes require K^+ for maximum activity. For example, in the glycolytic sequence K^+ is required for maximal activity of pyruvate kinase. Third, metabolically supported gradients of Na^+ and K^+ across the cell membrane are involved in this maintenance of the membrane potential of excitable tissues, which is the vehicle for transmission of impulses in the form of an action potential, i.e. a transient discharge or collapse of the membrane potential caused by an abrupt increase in the permeability of the membrane to Na^+ and K^+ when it is stimulated or excited. In 1957 an important breakthrough opened the molecular basis of Na^+ extrusion and K^+ accumulation to direct biochemical study. In Denmark, J. C. Skou discovered that the hydrolysis of ATP to ADP and phosphate by a fraction of homogenised crab nerve now known to contain cell-membrane fragments requires both K^+ and Na^+ for maximum activity, as well as Mg^{2+} (which is required for most enzymatic reactions involving ATP as substrate). Addition of either Na^+ or K^+ alone produced very little stimulation. This finding was unusual, since most K^+-requiring enzymes are inhibited by Na^+. Most significant, however, was the later observation that the stimulation of the ATPase activity of such cell-membrane preparations by Na^+ and K^+ is inhibited by the glycoside ouabain, long known to inhibit the transport of Na^+ and K^+ by intact cell membranes. Ouabain (Fig. 10.5) is one member of a group of related compounds called cardiac glycosides, which are capable of altering the excitability of heart muscle, a function dependent on the balance of Na^+ and K^+ across the membrane. Skou postulated that this Na^+- and K^+-stimulated ATPase activity of membrane fragments represents the Na^+ and K^+ pump of the nerve cell membrane, which he further postulated requires Na^+ from the inside and K^+ from the outside surface of the membrane for maximal activity and thus maximal rates of ATP hydrolysis. Cell-membrane fractions from many different animal tissues have since been found to contain such a Na^+- and K^+-stimulated ATPase activity. Excitable cells, such as brain, nerve and muscle and the electric organ of electrophorus electricus, the electric eel, are particularly rich in the enzyme. Also very active are Na^+-transporting epithelial tissues such as the kidney cortex, the salivary gland and the salt gland of the seagull. The Na^+-and K^+-stimulated ATPase of cell membranes transports Na^+ and K^+ in a vectorial or directional manner. This was convincingly shown by R. Whittam and his colleagues in classical experiments on the Na^+K^+-ATPase of erythrocytes. When erythrocytes are exposed to distilled water under controlled conditions, they swell and their membranes increase in permeability. As a result, their internal electrolytes, as well as haemoglobin and other cytoplasmic proteins, leak out into the surrounding hypotonic medium.

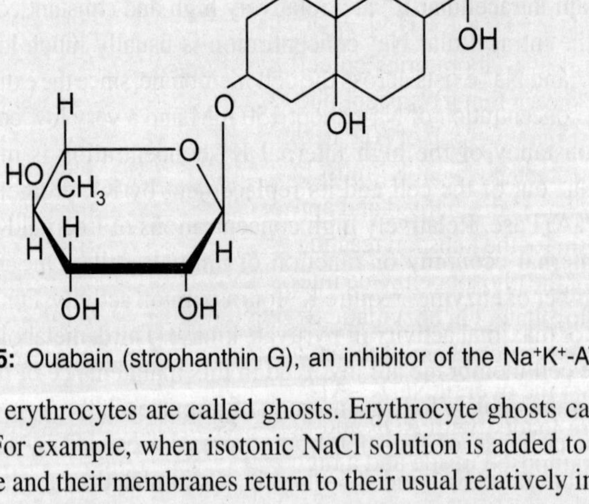

Fig. 10.5: Ouabain (strophanthin G), an inhibitor of the Na^+K^+-ATPase.

These preparations of erythrocytes are called ghosts. Erythrocyte ghosts can now be 'loaded' with different kinds of salts. For example, when isotonic NaCl solution is added to a suspension of ghosts, they shrink to normal size and their membranes return to their usual relatively impermeable state. These preparations are called reconstituted or resealed erythrocytes. During the resealing process the ghosts entrap NaCl in a concentration equivalent to that in the suspending medium. On the other hand, if the reconstitution is carried out in an isotonic KCl solution, they will trap KCl. In this manner, reconstituted erythrocytes can be loaded with varying internal concentrations of KCl or NaCl or various other salts, such as LiCl. Moreover, such erythrocytes can also be loaded with ATP if it is added to the salt medium in which the ghosts are reconstituted.

Whittam prepared reconstituted erythrocytes containing internal ATP and various concentrations of internal NaCl or KCl. He then examined the effect of various internal and external concentrations of Na^+ and K^+ on the rate of the enzymatic hydrolysis of the internal ATP and on the transport of Na^+ and K^+. When the external medium contained a high Na^+ concentration and the internal medium a high K^+ concentration, conditions resembling those existing in normal intact erythrocytes in the blood, the rate of hydrolysis of internal ATP was relatively low. Conversely, when the external medium contained a high concentration of K^+ and the internal medium a high concentration of Na^+, the rate of hydrolysis of internal ATP was high. If both the external and internal media contained only Na^+ (or only K^+), little ATP hydrolysis ensued. The second important observation was that Na^+ and K^+ move across the erythrocyte membrane in the anticipated directions during hydrolysis of internal ATP, as Skou had postulated. If the Na^+ concentration was high on the inside and the K^+ concentration was high on the outside, conditions which evoked maximal ATP hydrolysis, then Na^+ moved out of the cell and K^+ moved in as the internal ATP was hydrolysed. Moreover, it was also found that the reconstituted erythrocyte ghosts utilise only internal ATP, external ATP is not attacked.

Experiments on erythrocyte ghosts have also made it possible to examine the specificity and stoichiometry of the Na^+K^+-ATPase activity. For example, external K^+ can be replaced by Rb^+, NH^+ or certain other monovalent cations, but internal Na^+ is an absolute requirement for the ATPase, which is thus regarded as serving primarily as a Na^+ pump. ATP may be replaced by dATP, CTP and ITP, but these nucleotides are far less active than ATP. It has also been possible to measure the amounts of K^+ and Na^+ transported per molecule of ATP hydrolysed. In erythrocytes three molecules of Na^+ are extruded and two molecules of K^+ are accumulated per molecule of ATP hydrolysed. These ratios are relatively constant and independent of the existing ion-concentration gradient. ATP and its hydrolysis products ADP and P_i remain inside the cell, as does the Mg^{2+}. The Mg^{2+} appears to be required only because it is part of the true substrate, which is the $MgATP^{2-}$ complex. We can then write a vectorial equation for the Na^+K^+-ATPase reaction:

$$3Na^+_{inside} + 2K^+_{outside} + ATP^{4-} + H_2O \rightarrow 3Na^+_{outside} + 2K^+_{inside} + ADP^{3-} + P_i^{2-} + H^+$$

Experiments carried out in the laboratories on cell-membrane vesicles or 'solubilised' preparations of the Na^+K^+-ATPase have shown that a transient phosphoenzyme intermediate is formed by transfer of the ^{32}P-labelled terminal phosphate group of ATP to the ATPase molecule. Transfer of ^{32}P to the enzyme requires the presence of Mg^{2+} and Na^+, but K^+ must be absent. When K^+ is then added to the ^{32}P-labelled ATPase preparation, the isotope is discharged and appears as inorganic phosphate. From these and other findings a two-step mechanism for the transport reaction promoted by the Na^+K^+-ATPase has been postulated (Fig. 10.6). The properties of the phosphoenzyme intermediate resemble those of known acyl phosphates like 3-phosphoglyceroyl phosphate. On enzymatic degradation of the ^{32}P-labelled enzyme, Post and his colleagues found that an aspartyl side chain of the enzyme is phosphorylated at its free β-carboxyl group. It is of particular interest that the overall Na^+K^+-ATPase activity is reversible. M. Glynn has shown that when erythrocyte ghosts are loaded with ADP and phosphate, rather than with ATP and, in addition, a high concentration of K^+ is imposed inside and a high concentration of Na^+ outside the membrane, then

$$ATP + Na^+_{inside} + \textcircled{E} \xrightleftharpoons{\quad Mg^{2+} \quad} Na - \textcircled{E} \sim P + ADP$$

$$Na - \textcircled{E} \sim P \rightleftharpoons Na - \boxed{E} \sim P$$

$$K^+_{outside} + H_2O + Na - \boxed{E} \sim P \rightleftharpoons \textcircled{E} + P_i + Na^+_{outside} + K^+_{inside}$$

Fig. 10.6: A postulated mechanism for transport of Na^+ and K^+ by the Na^+K^+-ATPase. The ATPase molecule is believed to undergo conformational changes between two forms designated $\bigcirc$ and $\square$. Ouabain inhibits the K^+-dependent hydrolysis of Na—$\boxed{E}$~P.

K^+ flows out of the cell, Na^+ flows in and ATP is generated from the ADP and phosphate. Thus an electrochemical gradient of Na^+ and K^+ across the erythrocyte membrane can drive the synthesis of ATP, just as an electrochemical gradient of H^+ across the mitochondrial or chloroplast membrane appears to drive the synthesis of ATP.

The Na^+K^+–ATPase of various tissues, particularly the kidney medulla, brain and electric organ, has been solubilised with detergents and purified over a hundred-fold. It has a molecular weight of about 2,50,000 to 3,00,000 and contains two different types of sub-unit, the larger with a molecular weight of about 1,00,000 to 1,30,000 and the smaller about 50000. The large subunit is the portion of the molecule that is phosphorylated as ATP is hydrolysed. Since it has binding sites for Na^+, K^+, ATP and ouabain, the large sub-unit appears to extend through the entire thickness of the cell membrane with the K^+ and ouabain sites on its outer surface and the Na^+ and ATP sites on its inner surface. The smaller sub-unit of the Na^+K^+-ATPase is a glycoprotein and contains sialic acid, as well as glucose, galactose and other hexose residues. In some tissues the ATPase contains two large and one small sub-unit. The Na^+K^+-ATPase also appears to require or contain certain lipids. The Na^+K^+-ATPase in some cells utilises a very large fraction of their respiratory energy. For example, it has been found that ouabain inhibits the respiration of kidney cells or brain cells by some 70%. Since cells consume oxygen only as fast as needed to regenerate ATP utilised in energy-requiring functions, it has been concluded that kidney and brain cells use some 70% of their ATP output for the purpose of pumping Na^+ and K^+.

Lactin

Lectins are carbohydrate-binding proteins (not to be confused with glycoproteins, which are proteins containing sugar chains or residues) that are highly specific for sugar moieties, particularly, the high specificity of plant lectins for foreign glycoconjugates (e.g. those of fungi, invertebrates and animals). They play a role in the biological recognition phenomena involving cells and proteins. It is hypothesised that some hepatitis C viral glycoproteins attach to C-type lectins on the host cell surface (liver cells) for infection. Lectins may be disabled by specific mono- and oligosaccharides, which bind to ingested lectins from grains, legume, nightshade plants and dairy, binding can prevent their attachment to the carbohydrates within the cell membrane.

Biological functions: Most lectins do not possess enzymatic activity and are not produced naturally by the immune system. Lectins occur ubiquitously in nature. They may bind to a soluble carbohydrate or to a carbohydrate moiety that is a part of a glycoprotein or glycolipid. They typically agglutinate certain animal cells and/or precipitate glycoconjugates.

Functions in animals: Lectins serve many different biological functions in animals, from the regulation of cell adhesion to glycoprotein synthesis and the control of protein levels in the blood. They may also bind soluble extracellular and intercellular glycoproteins. Some lectins are found on the surface of mammalian liver cells that specifically recognise galactose residues. It is believed that these cell-surface receptors are responsible for the removal of certain glycoproteins from the circulatory system. Another lectin is a receptor that recognises hydrolytic enzymes containing mannose-6-phosphate and targets these proteins for delivery to the lysosomes. I-cell disease is one type of defect in this particular system. Lectins are also known to play important roles in the immune system by recognising carbohydrates that are found exclusively on pathogens or that are inaccessible on host cells. Examples are the lectin complement activation pathway and mannose-binding lectin.

Active Transport of Glucose and Amino Acids in Vertebrates

Glucose is transported against concentration gradients across the epithelial cell layer of the small intestine, as part of the process of absorption of sugars into the blood from the intestine. Glucose is also transported against a gradient by the epithelial cell layer of the kidney tubules, from the glomerular filtrate into the blood, thus glucose is not normally excreted in the urine but is salvaged and kept in the bloodstream. Although the substrate specificity of the intestinal and renal glucose-transport systems has been studied, little is known of the molecular mechanism of glucose transport. One significant finding, however, is that glucose transport appears to be coupled to the transport of Na^+, inward glucose transport appears to be optimal when there is a large inward gradient of Na^+ into the cell.

An interesting model for the relationship of glucose transport to Na^+ movements has been postulated (Fig. 10.7). It proposes that glucose enters the cell by binding to a specific carrier molecule, which can also bind Na^+, presumably at a second site on the carrier. The carrier molecule thus facilitates the simultaneous, compulsory transport of both Na^+ and glucose into the cell, such a process is designated cotransport or symport. If the external Na^+ concentration is much higher than the internal concentration, Na^+ bound to this carrier will tend to move inward, down the Na^+ gradient. Since the carrier must also bind glucose in order to function, the inward transport of Na^+ down a gradient can 'drag' glucose into the cell.

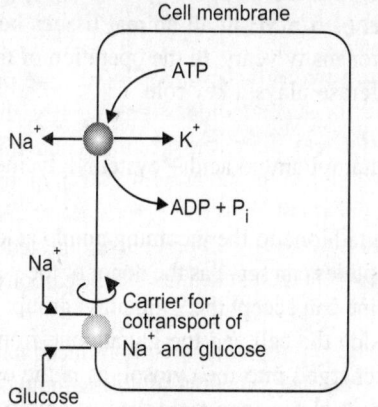

The Na^+K^+-ATPase pumps Na^+ out of the cell to create an inward-directed Na^+ gradient at the expense of ATP.

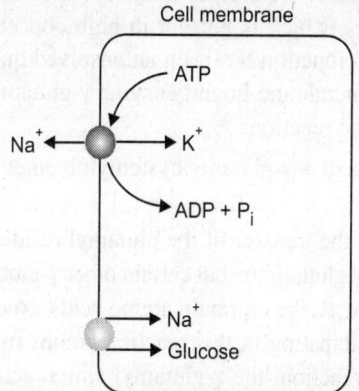

The inward-directed Na^+ gradient so generated rated 'pulls' glucose into the cell by means of a passive carrier which has two binding sites, one for Na^+ and the other for glucose.

Fig. 10.7: Postulated mechanism for the coupling of glucose transport to a Na^+ gradient.

In this manner glucose can be accumulated against a glucose gradient, so long as the inward gradient of Na^+ generated by the Na^+K^+-ATPase exceeds the outward gradient of glucose. The energy required to transport glucose into the cell is furnished by the inward gradient of Na^+ generated by the Na^+K^+-ATPase. Much evidence supports this model of glucose transport in the intestine.

The active transport of amino acids shows a number of similarities with the active transport of glucose. Amino acid transport is particularly pronounced in the intestinal epithelium, where it functions in the intestinal absorption of amino acids into the bloodstream. It also occurs in the kidney tubules, where it functions to salvage amino acids from tubular urine and to retain them in the bloodstream. From the kinetics of transport of the various amino acids and from studies of competition between different amino acids for transport it has been deduced that there are five or more different amino acid transport systems, each of which can transport a group of closely related amino acids. Specific transport systems have been found for: (i) small neutral amino acids, (ii) large neutral amino acids, (iii) basic amino acids, (iv) acidic amino acids and (v) the imino acid proline. Each of these transport systems is characterised by an optimum pH and by specific K_M values for its substrates, they can be inhibited competitively by certain amino acid analogs.

As with glucose transport, external Na^+ is required for inward transport of amino acids in some types of cells. The higher the external Na^+ concentration, the greater the capacity of the amino acid transport system to transport amino acids into the cell. These observations have led to the hypothesis that the energy inherent in a downward gradient of Na^+ into the cell is the immediate driving force for inward transport of amino acids against a gradient, as described above for glucose.

γ-Glutamyl Cycle for Amino Acid Transport

An interesting and novel hypothesis, the γ-glutamyl cycle, has been developed by A. Meister and his colleagues for the mechanism of transport of amino acids into cells of certain animal tissues. It is an example of a group translocation in which the substrate transported appears in a different chemical form inside the cell. The γ-glutamyl cycle involves a sequence of six enzymes, one of which is membrane-bound, the remainder are present in the cytosol. Also involved is the tripeptide glutathione (γ-glutamyl-cysteinylglycine), which is present in high concentrations (~ 5 mM) in all animal tissues but whose major biological function has been an unsolved question for many years. In the operation of this cycle (Fig. 10.8) the membrane-bound enzyme γ-glutamyltransferase plays a key role.

It catalyses the reaction:

$$\text{Amino acid} + \underset{\text{Glutathione}}{\gamma\text{-glutamylcysteinylglycine}} \rightarrow \gamma\text{-glutamyl amino acid} + \text{cysteinylglycine}$$

which results in the transfer of the glutamyl residue of glutathione to the incoming amino acid. In this reaction not only glutathione but certain other γ-glutamylpeptides can serve as the donor of the γ-glutamyl group, moreover, all the common amino acids except proline can accept the γ-glutamyl group. The free amino acid participating in this reaction comes from outside the cell and the glutathione from inside. Following this reaction, the γ-glutamyl amino acid is discharged into the cytosol, as is the cysteinyl-glycine. In the next step the γ-glutamyl amino acid undergoes cleavage to yield the free amino acid and 5-oxoproline, in a reaction catalysed by γ-glutamylcyclotransferase, a cytosol enzyme:

$$\gamma\text{-Glutamyl amino acid} \rightarrow \text{amino acid} + 5\text{-oxoproline}$$

The cysteinylglycine then is postulated to undergo hydrolysis by the action of a peptidase:

$$\text{Cysteinylglycine} + H_2O \rightarrow \text{cysteine} + \text{glycine}$$

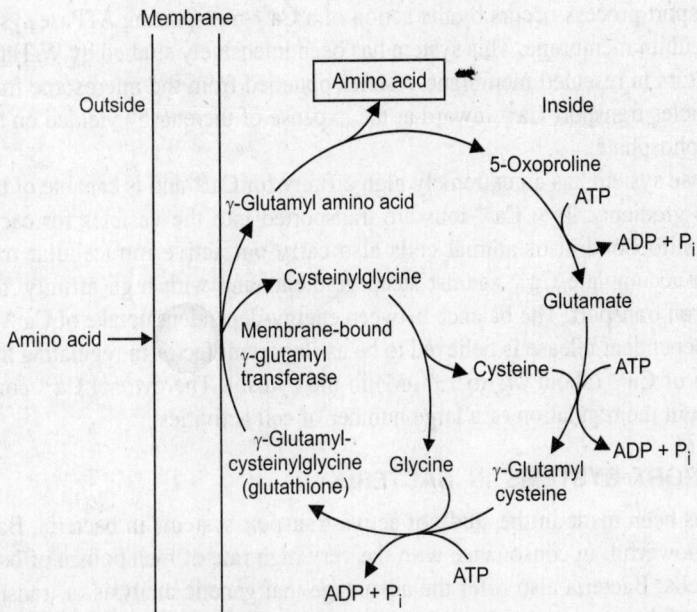

Fig. 10.8: The γ-glutamyl cycle, a postulated group-translocation mechanism for the transport of amino acids.

Thus one molecule of an amino acid has been transported into the cell, at the expense of the energy of hydrolysis of the peptide bonds of glutathione. If this process is to be continuous, the glutathione required must be regenerated from free cysteine, free glycine and 5-oxoproline. Formation of glutathione is brought about by a sequence of three reactions, first discovered by K. Bloch. In the first 5-oxoproline is converted into L-glutamate by the action of 5-oxoprolinase:

$$\text{5-Oxoproline} + \text{ATP} + 2\text{H}_2\text{O} \rightarrow \text{L-glutamate} + \text{ADP} + \text{P}_i$$

In the next step the L-glutamate so formed reacts with L-cysteine by the action of γ-glutamylcysteine synthetase:

$$\text{L-Glutamate} + \text{L-cysteine} + \text{ATP} \rightarrow \gamma\text{-glutamylcysteine} + \text{ADP} + \text{P}_i$$

In the last step glycine is attached to γ-glutamylcysteine to yield glutathione by the action of glutathione synthetase:

$$\gamma\text{-Glutamylcysteine} + \text{glycine} + \text{ATP} \rightarrow \text{glutathione} + \text{ADP} + \text{P}_i$$

The glutathione so formed is now ready to participate in another round of the cycle. Three terminal phosphate bonds of ATP are thus utilised to bring each molecule of an amino acid into the cell by this mechanism. All the enzymes of this cycle are present in high concentrations in a number of tissues active in amino acid transport. Some people have a genetic defect, presumably in the enzyme 5-oxoprolinase, resulting in the excretion of 5-oxoproline in the urine. Such patients also show aberrations in amino acid transport and metabolism. It is of some interest that Na⁺, which is required for amino acid transport, is also necessary for optimal activity of γ-glutamyltransferase.

Intracellular Transport of Ca²⁺ in Animal Cells

An important example of an intracellular active-transport process is the ATP-dependent transport of Ca^{2+} from the sarcoplasm into the sarcoplasmic reticulum, which is responsible for the relaxation of muscle. This transport process occurs by the action of a Ca^{2+}-transporting ATPase system found in the sarcoplasmic reticulum membrane. This system has been intensively studied by W. Hasselbach, as well as other investigators in resealed membrane vesicles obtained from the microsome fraction of skeletal muscle. Such vesicles transport Ca^{2+} inward at the expense of the energy yielded on the hydrolysis of ATP to ADP and phosphate.

The Ca^{2+}-ATPase system has an extremely high affinity for Ca^{2+} and is capable of transporting Ca^{2+} against very high gradients. Two Ca^{2+} ions are transported into the vesicles for each ATP molecule hydrolysed. The mitochondria of animal cells also carry out active intracellular transport of Ca^{2+}. Mitochondria can accumulate Ca^{2+} against steep gradients and with high affinity, the energy being provided by electron transport. The balance between energy-dependent uptake of Ca^{2+} by mitochondria and its energy-independent release is believed to be an important factor in regulating the normally very low concentration of Ca^{2+} (about 0.1 to 1.0 μM) in the cytosol. The cytosol Ca^{2+} concentration is an important element in the regulation of a large number of cell activities.

ACTIVE-TRANSPORT SYSTEMS IN BACTERIA

Much progress has been made in the study of active-transport systems in bacteria. Bacterial transport systems are very powerful, in consonance with the very high rate of metabolism of bacteria compared with eukaryotic cells. Bacteria also offer the advantage that genetic analysis of transport systems can easily be carried out. Moreover, simple methods have been devised to obtain membrane vesicles from bacteria. Particular progress has been made in isolating specific protein components of bacterial systems for group translocation and for active transport of sugars and amino acids.

The first important success in separating transport proteins from bacteria was the extraction by C. F. Fox and E. P. Kennedy of 'M-protein' from the membrane of *E. coli* cells adapted to transport β-galactosides. They showed that this protein (although isolated in inactive form as an *N*-ethylmaleimide derivative) contained the recognition and binding site for β-galactosides.

Another important advance came with the discovery of periplasmic binding proteins of bacteria. Bacterial cells characteristically contain in the periplasmic space one or more specific proteins capable of binding some specific amino acid or sugar. The periplasmic space is the space just outside and surrounding the cell membrane but inside the cell wall. Osmotic shock of certain bacteria placed in a hypotonic medium causes release of the periplasmic proteins. From the released material a large number of specific proteins capable of binding certain amino acids, sugars and inorganic ions have been isolated. The first of the periplasmic binding proteins to be studied, the sulphate-binding protein, has been highly purified and crystallised by A. B. Pardee and his colleagues. It has a molecular weight of 32000 and contains one binding site for sulphate per molecule.

Specific periplasmic binding proteins have been isolated for most of the common amino acids and for glucose, galactose, arabinose, ribose and other sugars. They have molecular weights from 22000 to 42000 and are readily soluble in aqueous systems. Some of them change in conformation on binding their specific ligands. Much evidence suggests that the periplasmic binding proteins are involved in active-transport mechanisms. Release of the binding protein from the bacterial cells is usually accompanied by decrease of transport activity. The substrate specificity of the binding protein is often the same as that of the transport process of the intact cells. Moreover, some mutants that are transport-negative for a given substrate contain a defective binding protein for that substrate. Such evidence has suggested that the periplasmic binding proteins are dissociable components of membrane-bound transport systems that contain the specific substrate-recognition sites for their substrates. They are also believed to be receptor sites in chemotaxis, by which bacteria recognise nutrients and propel themselves by flagellar motion in the direction of increasing nutrient concentration.

Group Translocation of Sugars into Bacteria

Two general types of sugar-transport systems occur in bacteria, sometimes within the same species. One promotes a group translocation of the sugar across the membrane so that it enters the cytoplasm in a different chemical form, whereas the other type promotes active transport of the sugar into the cell, apparently without chemical modification of the sugar molecule.

In a series of important investigations S. Roseman and W. Kundig carried out a biochemical and genetic analysis of sugar transport into certain bacteria via a group-translocation system called the phosphotransferase system (PTS). The system has been studied for the most part in *E. coli*, *Salmonella typhimurium* (Fig. 10.9) and *Staphylococcus aureus* (Fig. 10.10). It is found in many facultative and photosynthetic bacteria but appears to be absent in strictly aerobic bacteria. Its properties vary somewhat with the species. All the basic components of PTS have been isolated and purified. The phosphotransferase system consists of three proteins or protein complexes. Two of these, called enzyme I and HPr, are normally present in the cytoplasm and the third, enzyme II, is located in the cell membrane. Enzyme II contains two separable components, which are possibly different sub-units.

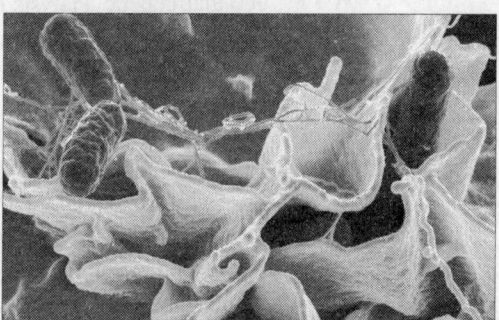

Fig. 10.9: *Salmonella typhimurium.*

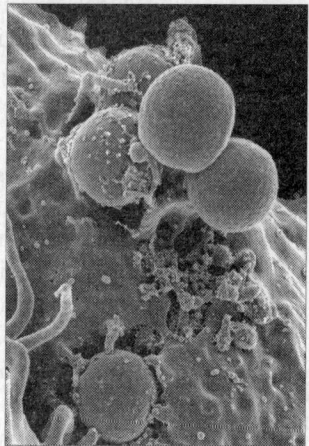

Fig. 10.10: *Staphylococcus aureus.*

The reactions taking place via the action of the phosphotransferase system can be summarised by two equations. In the first, the cytoplasmic protein HPr is phosphorylated at the expense of phosphoenolpyruvate, a reaction that is catalysed by enzyme I:

$$\text{Phosphoenolpyruvate} + \text{HPr} \xrightarrow[\text{Mg}^{2+}]{E_i} \text{pyruvate} + \text{phospho-HPr}$$

This reaction is unusual in two respects. (i) it employs phosphoenolpyruvate as the immediate phosphate donor, whereas most biological phosphorylations require ATP or some other nucleoside triphosphate as phosphate donor and (ii) the HPr protein molecule becomes phosphorylated on nitrogen atom 1 of the imidazole ring of one of its two histidine residues (Fig. 10.11). HPr has been highly purified and has a molecular weight of only 9400. In a second enzymatic reaction, which takes place in the membrane, the phosphorylated HPr donates its phosphate group to the sugar that is being transported, in a reaction catalysed by the membrane-bound enzyme II. With glucose the product of the reaction is glucose 6-phosphate:

$$\text{Phospho-HPr} + \text{glucose} \xrightarrow[\text{Mg}^{2+}]{E_i} \text{HPr} + \text{glucose 6-phosphate}$$

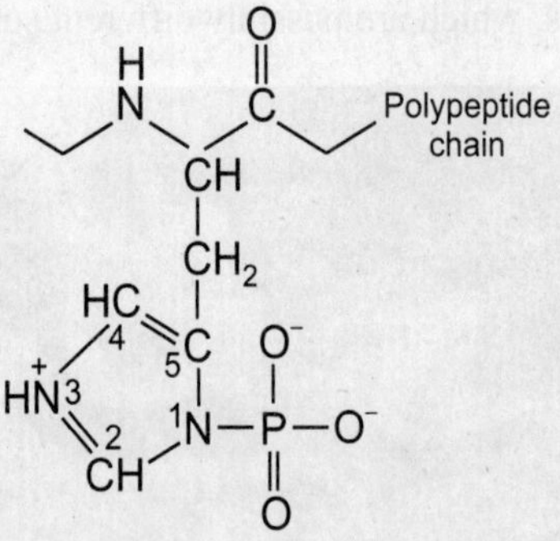

Fig. 10.11: The 1-phosphohistidyl residue of HPr.

In gram-negative bacteria, such as *E. coli*, enzyme II is a complex of two proteins or sub-units, designated IIA and IIB. Protein IIA carries the specificity for the sugar, several different IIA proteins have been isolated, each specific for a given sugar, such as glucose, fructose or mannose. Protein IIB appears to be involved in the catalysis of phosphate transfer from the phosphorylated HPr to the sugar bound to IIA. Protein IIB has a molecular weight of 36000 and makes up nearly 10% of the protein of the bacterial membrane. Many different sugars—including D-glucose and various glucosides, D-galactose and various galactosides, D-fructose, pentoses, pentitols and hexitols—have been identified as phosphate-group acceptors in the phosphotransferase system. The postulated mechanism for sugar transport by the phosphotransferase system is shown in Fig. 10.12.

Much genetic evidence supports this hypothesis. Bacterial mutants that lack enzyme I or HPr cannot accumulate any of the transportable sugars. On the other hand, mutants defective in only one species of enzyme IIA are defective in transporting only that particular sugar. The phosphotransferase system has been reconstituted from purified components. Membrane vesicles isolated from bacterial cells in such a manner that they lack HPr and enzyme I are unable to accumulate sugars as their phosphates. When purified HPr and enzyme I are then added to the vesicles, they became bound to them and the vesicles then gain the ability to accumulate sugar phosphates. *E. coli* cells contain not only the PTS system for

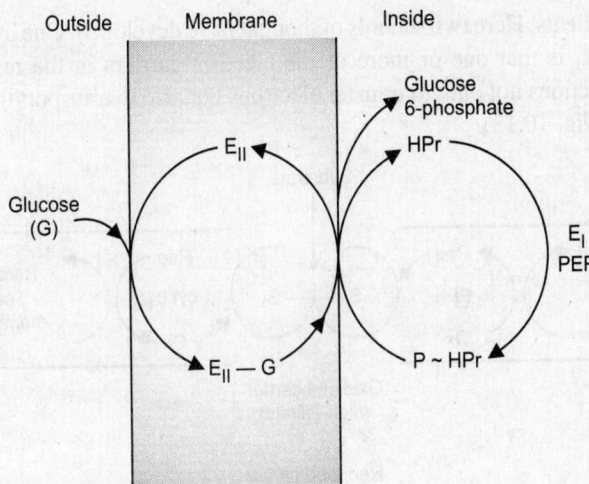

Outside   Membrane   Inside

Fig. 10.12: Energy-coupled group translocation of glucose across the bacterial membrane and accumulation of glucose 6-pyruvate (PEP = phosphoenolpyruvate).

group translocation of sugars, but also, as we shall now see, a system for respiration-coupled active transport of sugars, in which phosphorylation of the sugar does not appear to be involved.

Sugar and Amino Acid Transport Coupled to Electron Transport in Bacteria

H. R. Kaback and his colleagues have made substantial progress in the analysis of the coupling between the energy-requiring active transport of glucose and other sugars into bacteria and the energy-yielding transport of electrons from substrates to oxygen. They have developed a procedure for obtaining membrane vesicles from *E. coli* cells that are nearly devoid of cytoplasmic and cell-wall components. Such vesicles are empty sacs, 0.5 to 1.5 μm in diameter and right side out. They appear to retain full activity of the major active-transport systems and also contain the dehydrogenases and electron carriers of the respiratory chain, all bound to the membrane structure. Such bacterial membrane vesicles promote the active transport of a number of different sugars, including lactose and other β-galactosides, glucose, galactose, arabinose and glucuronic acid providing the vesicles are oxidising certain substrates, such as D-lactate, β-hydroxy-butyrate or succinate to provide the necessary energy. The concentration of sugars attained within such respiring vesicles may exceed by a hundred-fold the external concentration of the sugar in the medium. The accumulated sugar is present in free form and does not appear to be phosphorylated during or after transport into the membrane vesicle. Thus this respiration-dependent transport of sugars differs from the group translocation promoted by the phosphotransferase system.

Because oligomycin, an inhibitor of oxidative phosphorylation, does not prevent sugar transport coupled to D-lactate oxidation, the intermediate formation of ATP is apparently not required for the coupling of the energy of electron transport to the sugar-transport mechanism. This conclusion is supported by the finding that membrane vesicles from certain mutants capable of electron transport but unable to carry out phosphorylation of ADP can still transport sugars. Membrane vesicles from bacteria are capable of accumulating most of the common amino acids in a very similar manner, coupled to electron transport from D-lactate or some other substrate via the electron-transport chain to oxygen.

The key question now concerns the mechanism by which the energy of electron transport is utilised to drive the active transport of sugars and amino acids into the vesicles against (in some cases) rather steep concentration gradients. Here two schools of thought have developed. One hypothesis, vigorously championed by Kaback, is that one or more of the electron carriers in the respiratory chain in the bacterial membrane functions not only to transfer electrons but also to transport the sugar or amino acid across the membrane (Fig. 10.13).

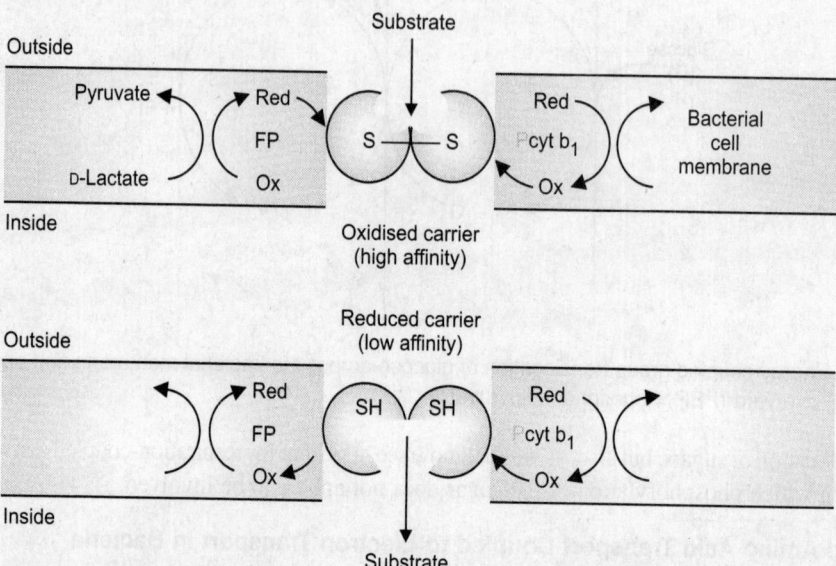

Fig. 10.13: Coupling of the active transport of an external substrate to electron transfer. The respiratory chain of bacteria is in the cell membrane. One of the electron carriers (colour) is postulated to transfer electrons, via its —SH and—S—S— groups and to use the energy of electron transfer to carry the substrate across the membrane. The transport system has a high affinity on its outside face and a much lower affinity on its inside face; interconnection of the two forms is assumed to be responsible for transport against a gradient of concentration.

Kaback has postulated that one of the specific electron carriers in this chain occurs in disulphide (oxidised) and disulphydryl (reduced) forms. These two forms also are capable of binding the substance being transported. The disulphide or oxidised form of this electron carrier is regarded as the high-affinity form capable of binding the transported substrate only on the outside surface of the membrane. The disulphydryl or reduced form of this electron carrier is believed to bind the transported substrate on the inside surface of the membrane with much lower affinity. Thus the oxidised form of the carrier traps the substrate molecule from the external medium with high affinity and the carrier molecule, as it is reduced by electrons coming from the electron donor D-lactate, undergoes a conformational change resulting in a large decrease in affinity and consequent unloading of the transported substrate at the inside surface of the vesicle. A specific role of sulphydryl groups in sugar and amino acid transport is suggested by the fact that reagents capable of blocking—SH groups also block active transport.

The Kaback hypothesis suggests that one substrate molecule should be transported into the vesicle for each pair of electrons being transported from the electron donor to oxygen. However, it has been pointed out that the rate of lactate oxidation is anywhere from 10 to several hundred times greater than the rate of sugar or amino acid transport on a molar basis. An alternative hypothesis for the mechanism of energy coupling between electron transport and the inward transport of sugars and amino acids in bacteria has been proposed by P. Mitchell, F. M. Harold and other investigators, who postulate that bacterial sugar transport is brought about by chemiosmotic coupling, as originally developed for oxidative and photosynthetic phosphorylation.

The chemiosmotic hypothesis proposes that electron transport generates an electro-chemical gradient of H^+ across the membrane, composed of an outside H^+ gradient and an inside negative membrane potential. This gradient, called a proton-motive gradient, has been postulated as the immediate driving force for ATP formation and for other energy-dependent functions of mitochondria and chloroplasts, including ion transport. Several items of evidence support the chemiosmotic hypothesis as the principal means of energy coupling in bacterial membrane vesicles. Electron transport in such vesicles has been shown to generate a membrane potential and to cause extrusion of protons. Moreover, the membrane carrier for galactosides has been found to carry both H^+ and galactosides across the membrane into the cell, apparently in a 1:1 relationship (Fig. 10.14). When membrane vesicles not capable of electron transport are placed in a medium containing a labelled galactoside and then acidified to pH 6.0 to create an inward gradient of H^+, the galactoside is transported into the vesicle, together with H^+. T. H. Wilson and his colleagues have shown ATP hydrolysis also can support galactoside transport, through its capacity to generate a H^+ gradient.

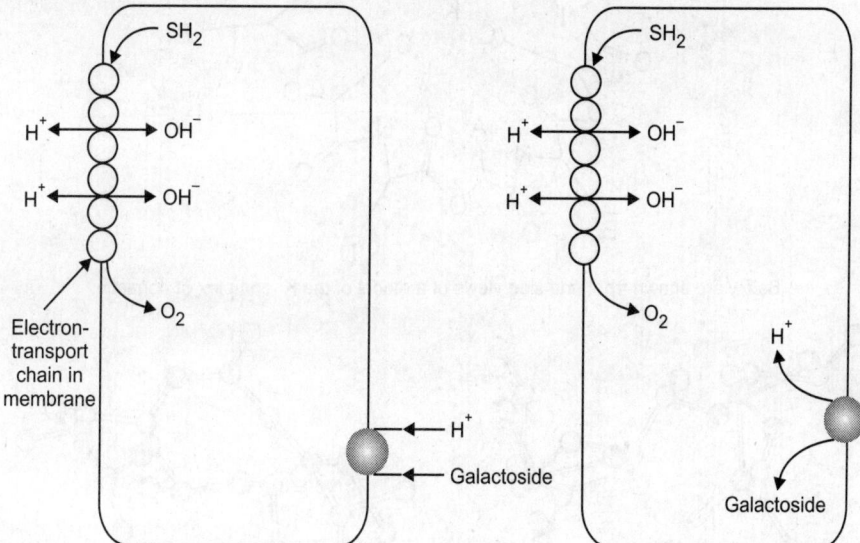

Fig. 10.14: Active transport of galactosides into bacterial cells by obligatory cotransport of H^+ and the galactoside. The electron-transport chain in the cell membrane continuously pumps H^+ outward coupled to electron flow from substrate (SH_2) to oxygen. The galactoside is pulled into the cell by the inward gradient of H^+ via the carrier, which binds both H^+ and galactoside.

IONOPHORES

A large number of antibiotic substances capable of inducing passage of specific ions across biological membranes have been isolated and identified. Among the first in which this property was recognised were gramicidin, which induces the transport of K^+, Na^+ and other monovalent cations across the membranes of mitochondria, erythrocytes and synthetic phospholipid bilayers and valinomycin, which has a high degree of specificity for inducing transport of K^+ across mitochondrial and other membranes.

The mechanism of action of these antibiotics has been intensively investigated by B. C. Pressman, H. A. Lardy, P. Mueller and many other investigators. Valinomycin, like many of the other ionophores, is an annular or ringlike compound with a hydrophobic exterior and hydrophilic interior, within which the K^+ ion precisely fits through coordination bonds. The hydrophobic exterior of valinomycin allows the valinomycin-K^+ complex, which has a single positive charge, to dissolve in and thus pass through the non-polar hydrocarbon layer in the membrane structure (Fig. 10.15). Hence, the generic name ionophore for these antibiotics. Another ionophore antibiotic specific for K^+ is nigericin, which differs from valinomycin in having a single negative charge, the nigericin-K^+ complex thus has no net electric charge. Nigericin promotes exchange of K^+ with H^+, whereas valinomycin promotes passage of K^+ alone.

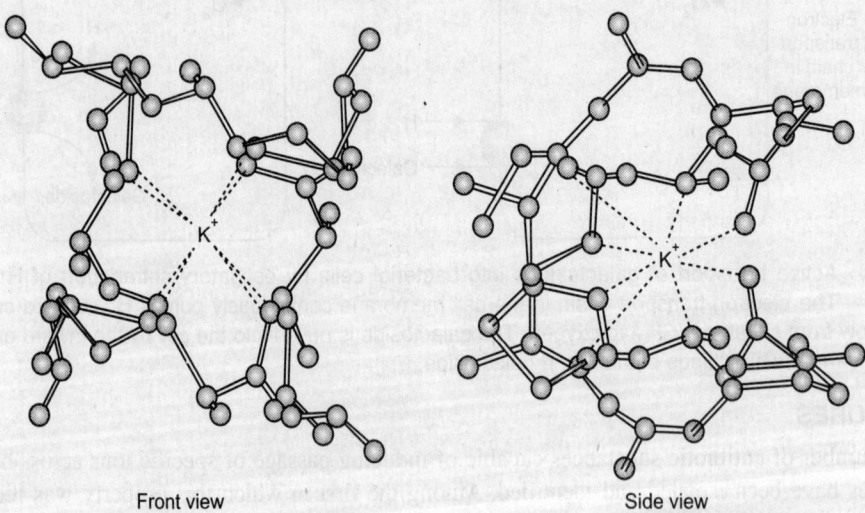

Below are shown front and side views of a model of the K^+ complex of nonactin.

Front view   Side view

Fig. 10.15: Model structures for two K^+-ionophore complexes. The structure of the valinomycin-K^+ complex. A = L-lactate, B = L-valine, C = D-hydroxyisovalerate and D = D-valine.

Certain other ionophores, such as gramicidin, a polypeptide, are linear molecules, however, they are believed to wrap around the monovalent cation to form an annular structure resembling that of valinomycin. Some ionophores are very active in carrying divalent cations, particularly Ca^{2+}. Synthetic ionophores have also been prepared. Ionophores have received intensive study, not only for their characteristic effects on mitochondrial ion transport and oxidative phosphorylation but also as tools in experimental analysis of ion-transport functions of the heart and kidney.

Ionophores enable cations to be transported across synthetic phospholipid bilayers. Study of such artificial transport systems has given important information on the basic physical principles involved in biological transport systems, for which they are important models. For example, the antibiotic alamethicin, when combined with a phospholipid bilayer, enables the system to mimic an action potential when K^+ and Na^+ gradients are imposed and an electric stimulus is applied. Indeed, study of ionophores is giving important clues to the nature of the Na^+ gates of nerve fibers, passive Na^+-transport systems that allow Na^+ to leak out transiently as the action potential passes. Such Na^+ gates, which are few in number but highly active, are vital to nerve activity, they are blocked by tetrodotoxin, the intensely toxic poison of the Japanese puffer fish.

DESMOSOME

A desmosome also known as macula adherens is a cell structure specialised for cell-to-cell adhesion. A type of junctional complex, they are localised spot-like adhesions randomly arranged on the lateral sides of plasma membranes. Desmosomes help to resist shearing forces and are found in simple and stratified squamous epithelium. The intercellular space is very wide (about 30 nm). Desmosomes are also found in muscle tissue where they bind muscle cells to one another.

Desmosomes are molecular complexes of cell adhesion proteins and linking proteins that attach the cell surface adhesion proteins to intracellular keratin cytoskeletal filaments. The cell adhesion proteins of the desmosome, desmoglein and desmocollin, are members of the cadherin family of cell adhesion molecules. They are transmembrane proteins that bridge the space between adjacent epithelial cells by way of homophilic binding of their extracellular domains to other desmosomal cadherins on the adjacent cell. Both have five extracellular domains and have calcium-binding motifs. Cytoplasmic desmosomal components include plakoglobin and plakophilins, which in turn bind intermediate filaments via desmoplakin.

MICROVILLUS

Microvilli are microscopic cellular membrane protrusions that increase the surface area of cells and are involved in a wide variety of functions, including absorption, secretion, cellular adhesion and mechano-transduction. Thousands of microvilli form a structure called the brush border that is found on the apical surface of some epithelial cells, such as the small intestinal. Microvillis (Fig. 10.16) are observed on the plasma surface of eggs, aiding in the anchoring of sperm cells that have penetrated the extracellular coat of egg cells. Clustering of elongated microtubules around a sperm allows for it to be drawn closer and held firmly so fusion can occur. Microvilli are also of importance on the cell surface of white blood cells, as they aid in the migration of white blood cells. Microvilli are covered in plasma membrane, which encloses cytoplasm and microfilaments. Though these are cellular extensions, there are little or no cellular organelles present in the microvilli. Each microvillus has a dense bundle of cross-linked actin filaments, which serves as its structural core. 20 to 30 tightly bundled actin filaments are cross-linked by bundling

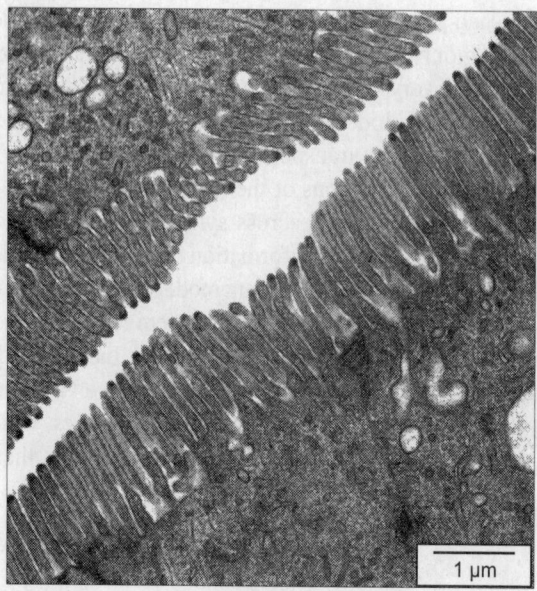

Fig. 10.16: Microvillis.

proteins fimbrin and villin to form the core of the microvilli. In the enterocyte microvillus, the structural core is attached to the plasma membrane along its length by lateral arms made of myosin 1a and Ca^{2+} binding protein calmodulin. Myosin 1a functions through a binding site for filamentous actin on one end and a lipid binding domain on the other. The plus ends of the actin filaments are located at the tip of the microvillus and are capped, possibly by capZ proteins, while the minus ends are anchored in the terminal web composed of a complicated set of proteins including spectrin and myosin II.

Function: Microvilli can act as mechanosensors in kidney proximal tubule. They sense the fluid flow in the tubule lumen and convert this information via biochemical responses into reabsorption. Microvilli are also of importance on the cell surface of white blood cells, as they aid in the migration of white blood cells.

Relationship to cell: As mentioned, microvilli are formed as cell extensions from the plasma membrane surface. Actin filaments, present in the cytosol, are most abundant near the cell surface. These filaments are thought to determine the shape and movement of the plasma membrane. The nucleation of actin fibres occurs as a response to external stimuli, allowing a cell to alter its shape to suit a particular situation. This could account for the uniformity of the microvilli, which are observed to be of equal length and diameter. This nucleation process occurs from the minus end, allowing rapid growth from the plus end. Interestingly, though the length and composition of microvilli is consistent within a certain group of homogenous cells, it can differ slightly in a different part of the same organism. For example, the microvilli in the small and large intestines in mice are slightly different in length and amount of surface coat covering the microvilli of on the cell membrane differs in terms shape

Enzymes: Microvilli function as the primary surface of nutrient absorption in the gastrointestinal tract. Because of this vital function, the microvillar membrane is packed with enzymes that aid in the breakdown of complex nutrients into simpler compounds that are more easily absorbed. For example, enzymes that digest carbohydrates called glycosidases are present at high concentrations on the surface of enterocyte microvilli. Thus, microvilli not only increase the cellular surface area for absorption, they also increase the number of digestive enzymes that can be present on the cell surface.

Glycocalyx: The microvilli are covered with glycocalyx, consisting of peripheral glycoproteins that can attach themselves to a plasma membrane via transmembrane proteins. This layer may be used to aid binding of substances needed for uptake, to adhere nutrients or as protection against harmful elements. It can be another location for functional enzymes to be localised.

Destruction of microvilli: The destruction of microvilli can occur in certain diseases because of the rearrangement of cytoskeleton in host cells. This can lead to malabsorption of nutrients and persistent osmotic diarrhea, often accompanied by fever.

This is seen in infections caused by EPEC subgroup *Escherichia coli*, in Celiac disease and Microvillus Inclusion Disease (an inherited disease characterised by defective microvilli and presence of cytoplasmic inclusions of the cell membrane other than the apical surface). The destruction of microvilli can actually be beneficial sometimes, as in the case of elimination of microvilli on white blood cells which can be used to combat auto immune diseases. Congenital lack of microvilli in the intestinal tract causes microvillous atrophy, a rare, usually fatal condition found in new-born babies.

Chapter 11

Photosynthesis

INTRODUCTION

Plants do need food for their survival and they would not wait or depend on others to provide them with food. There is a particular mechanism in plants with which they prepare their food. This mechanism is known as Photosynthesis. Photosynthesis is a biological process used by plants to prepare food with the help of sunlight water and carbon dioxide. The name photosynthesis is derived from the Greek word 'Photo' meaning light and 'Synthesis' meaning connecting together. This means combining together with the help of light energy. This process is also used by algae and several bacteria to convert solar energy into chemical energy. Oxygen is liberated as a by-product, and light is considered as the major factor to complete the process of photosynthesis. This process occurs usually when plants use light energy to convert carbon dioxide and water into glucose and oxygen gas. Leaves are made up of small cells which have a tiny structure known as chloroplasts. Each chloroplast contains a green coloured pigment called chlorophyll. Light energy is absorbed by chlorophyll molecules whereas carbon dioxide (CO_2) and oxygen (O_2) enter through the tiny pores of stomata located in the epidermis of leaves.

Oxygen is considered one of the most important by-products of this process on which most of the living organism depend upon. Glucose/Sugar is a form of carbohydrates that is processed during the process of photosynthesis. It is commonly used by green plants in the form of an energy source to produce leaves, fruits, flowers, and seeds. The glucose molecules then combine with each other to develop more complex carbohydrates like cellulose and starch. The cellulose is considered as the structural material that is used in plant cell walls. The overall reaction of photosynthesis process is:

$$6CO_2 + 6H_2O \xrightarrow{\text{Light}} C_6H_{12}O_6 + 6O_2 \qquad \text{...(11.1)}$$
$$\text{Glucose}$$

Photosynthesis occurs mainly in leaves of specialised cell structures known as chloroplasts.

- A leaf comprises a petiole, epidermis and a lamina.
- The Lamina is used for absorption of sunlight and carbon dioxide during the process.
- This process that occurs, takes place in chloroplasts that contain a green coloured pigment called chlorophyll which is mainly responsible for green coloured leaves.

- During the process of photosynthesis, chlorophyll absorbs the light energy from the Sun to split water molecules into hydrogen and oxygen.
- The hydrogen from water molecules and carbon dioxide absorbed from the air are used in the production of glucose and the oxygen is liberated into the atmosphere through the leaves.

Glucose is a source of food for plants which provide energy for the growth and development, while the rest is stored in the roots, leaves, or fruits for their later use.

Pigments are other fundamental cellular components of photosynthesis. They are the molecules which impart colour and they absorb light at some specific wavelength and reflect back the unabsorbed light. All green plants mainly contain chlorophyll a, chlorophyll b, and carotenoids which are present in the thylakoids of chloroplasts and help them in capturing the light energy. Chlorophyll a is the main pigment.

We know today that this overall process can be resolved into two phases. The first is the capture of light energy by light absorbing pigments and its conversion into the chemical energy of ATP and certain reducing agents, particularly NADPH. In this process hydrogen atoms are removed from water molecules and used to reduce NADP$^+$, leaving behind molecular oxygen, a by-product of plant photosynthesis, simultaneously, ADP is phosphorylated to ATP. The general equation for the first phase of photosynthesis, which we shall not write in balanced form at this point, is:

$$\text{Water} + \text{NADP}^+ + \text{P}_i + \text{ADP} \xrightarrow{\text{Light}} \text{oxygen} + \text{NADPH} + \text{H}^+ + \text{ATP} \qquad \text{...(11.2)}$$

In the second phase of photosynthesis the energy-rich products of the first phase, NADPH and ATP, are used as the sources of energy to bring about the reduction of carbon dioxide to yield glucose, simultaneously, NADPH is re-oxidised to NADP$^+$ and the ATP is broken down again into ADP and phosphate. This second phase of photosynthesis, which may be represented in general terms as:

$$\text{CO}_2 + \text{NADPH} + \text{H}^+ + \text{ATP} \rightarrow \text{glucose} + \text{NADP}^+ + \text{ADP} + \text{P}_i \qquad \text{...(11.3)}$$

is brought about by conventional enzyme-catalysed reactions which do not require light. Indeed, many of the enzymes catalysing the conversion of carbon dioxide into glucose in the second phase of photosynthesis are also found in animal tissues. The set of reactions in the first phase of photosynthesis, involving the conversion of light energy into the chemical energy of NADPH and ATP, is somewhat loosely referred to as the light reactions or the light phase of photosynthesis. The second stage, in which glucose and other reduced products are formed from CO_2 in plants, is referred to as the dark reactions or dark phase. Although there are other types of photosynthesis in addition to that taking place in higher green plants, we can in all cases distinguish a light phase and a dark phase.

BACTERIAL PHOTOSYNTHESIS

Studies on photosynthetic bacteria provided much useful information and were the basis for a major hypothesis that stimulated research in photosynthesis for many years. The two classes of purple bacteria, sulphur and non-sulphur, have been extensively used. To compare the process of photosynthesis in these organisms, consider writing the overall reaction of photosynthesis as carried out in green plants on the basis of one mole of CO_2 to give:

$$\underset{\text{Reduced}}{\overset{\text{Oxidised}}{CO_2 + H_2O \xrightarrow{\ hv\ } C(H_2O) + O_2}} \qquad \text{...(11.4)}$$

$$\Delta G' = +1,18,000 \text{ cal}$$

We observe that this is an oxidation-reduction reaction in which the oxidising agent CO_2 is reduced to the level of carbohydrate represented by $C(H_2O)$. The reducing agent in this reaction is H_2O that, in turn, is oxidised to O_2. Since the reaction is highly endergonic, it will only proceed when the necessary energy is supplied by light (hv). While this reaction is balanced with regard to the carbon, hydrogen and oxygen atoms involved, we shall see that it is not balanced with regard to the number of electrons used in reducing CO_2.

The purple sulphur bacteria, for example, *Chromatium*, utilise H_2S instead of H_2O as a reducing agent in photosynthesis. Elemental sulphur, S, is produced, but no oxygen is formed:

$$CO_2 + 2H_2S \xrightarrow{\text{hv}} C(H_2O) + 2S + H_2O \qquad \qquad ...(11.5)$$

Note that two moles of H_2S are required to balance the equation, the S^{2-} ions in the H_2S furnishing the total of four electrons required to reduce CO_2 to $C(H_2O)$. Thiosulphate can also serve as the reductant for photosynthesis by purple sulphur bacteria:

$$2CO_2 + Na_2S_2O_3 + 3H_2O \longrightarrow 2C(H_2O) + 2NaHSO_4 \qquad \qquad ...(11.6)$$

In this reaction, the sulphur atoms are oxidised from S^{2+} in $Na_2S_2O_3$ to S^{6+} in $NaHSO_4$.

Thus, each mole of $Na_2S_2O_3$ contributes 2×4 or 8 electrons, sufficient for the reduction of two moles of CO_2 to $C(H_2O)$. This reaction also demonstrates that the reducing agent need not contain hydrogen itself but simply be capable of furnishing electrons. The non-sulphur purple bacteria (e.g. *Rhodospirillum rubrum*) utilise organic reductants such as ethanol, isopropanol or succinate as electron donors. The balanced equation with ethanol, for example, may be written as:

$$CO_2 + 2CH_3CH_2OH \xrightarrow{\text{hv}} C(H_2O) + 2CH_3CHO + H_2O \qquad \qquad ...(11.7)$$

with the four electrons required for reduction of CO_2 being furnished by the oxidation of two moles of ethanol to acetaldehyde.

C. B. Van Niel, a pioneer in the study of photosynthesis, pointed out the similarity of these reactions to the one that occurs in green plants and he suggested that a general reaction for photosynthesis may be represented as:

$$CO_2 + 2H_2A \xrightarrow{\text{hv}} C(H_2O) + 2A + H_2O \qquad \qquad ...(11.8)$$

where, H_2A is a general expression for a reducing agent that, as we have seen, may be a variety of compounds. Since H_2S is a much stronger reducing agent than $Na_2S_2O_3$ or H_2O, it was expected that less light energy would be required for photosynthesis with H_2S as the reducing agent than with $Na_2S_2O_3$ or H_2O.

Experimentally, however, it was observed that the same amount of light energy was required, regardless of the nature of the external reducing agent. This caused van Niel to postulate that the primary reaction is the same in all organisms and that it consists of the splitting of a molecule of H_2O to yield both a reducing agent [H] and an oxidising agent [OH].

$$H_2O \xrightarrow{\text{hv}} [H] + [OH] \qquad \qquad ...(11.9)$$

This productive hypothesis stimulated much experimental work that led to greater understanding of the process of photosynthesis. The realisation that four electrons are required to reduce CO_2 to $C(H_2O)$ meant that Eq. 11.4 had to be re-written to involve two moles of H_2O as reductant, each atom of oxygen in H_2O providing two electrons.

$$CO_2 + 2H_2^{18}O \xrightarrow{\text{hv}} C(H_2O) + H_2O + {}^{18}O_2 \qquad \qquad ...(11.10)$$

Further, this revised equation would indicate that the two oxygen atoms produced in green plant photosynthesis should come only from H_2O. This was confirmed experimentally by Ruben and Kamen in a classical experiment in which H_2O labelled with the isotope ^{18}O was utilised in photosynthesis by algae. The oxygen produced under these conditions contained the same concentration of ^{18}O as the $H_2^{18}O$. Later developments concerning the role of H_2O in photosynthesis made it necessary to abandon van Niel's hypothesis of the photolytic cleavage of H_2O. However, his proposal that the initial photosynthetic act involves the production of an oxidant and a reductant is retained in the current descriptions of the energy-conversion process.

HILL REACTION

In 1937, R. Hill of Cambridge University initiated cell free studies on photosynthesis by working with isolated chloroplasts rather than intact plants. He reasoned that more information might be obtained if grana or chloroplasts, which contain the pigments that absorb the solar energy, were studied separately from the cell. It would have been ideal if the chloroplasts could have carried out both the oxidation of H_2O and the reduction of CO_2 to organic carbon compounds. This was not accomplished at that time. Nevertheless, chloroplasts were able to produce O_2 photochemically in the presence of another oxidising agent, potassium ferric oxalate. In this reaction, the ferric ion substitutes for CO_2 as an oxidant during the photo-oxidation of H_2O:

$$4Fe^{3+} + 2\ H_2O \xrightarrow[\text{Chloroplasts}]{hv} 4Fe^{2+} + 4H^+ + O_2 \qquad ...(11.11)$$

Molecular oxygen is evolved in an amount stoichiometrically equivalent to the oxidising agent added. This observation was of fundamental importance, for it permitted the study of the role of H_2O as a reducing agent in photosynthesis. The reaction is known as the Hill reaction and potassium ferric oxalate is known as a Hill reagent. Other compounds such as benzoquinone were subsequently shown to serve as Hill reagents in studies on isolated chloroplasts.

Benzoquinone   Hydroquinone

Oxidised dyes were later shown to function as Hill reagents by being reduced. Although this approach was criticised because the substances that could serve as Hill reagents were not physiologically important compounds, the properties of these reactions were studied extensively. In 1952, three US laboratories reported that $NADP^+$ (and NAD^+ under certain conditions) could serve as Hill reagents in the presence of spinach grana and light. Thus, for the first time, a physiologically significant compound could function as a Hill reagent. This observation was of prime importance, it constituted a mechanism whereby a reduced nicotinamide nucleotide was produced as the result of a light-dependent reaction:

$$2NADP^+ + 2H_2O \xrightarrow[\text{Chloroplasts}]{hv} 2NADPH + 2H^+ + O_2 \qquad ...(11.12)$$

Numerous examples have been given earlier in this text of the ability of NADPH and NADH to reduce various substrates in the presence of the proper enzyme. Thus, reducing power produced in Eq. 11.12 can be coupled to the biosynthesis of these reduced substrates.

PHOTOPHOSPHORYLATION

Work on the path of carbon during this time had shown that both NADPH and ATP were required to convert CO_2 to carbohydrates in photosynthesis. With the NADPH obtained via a Hill reaction, it was thought that re-oxidation of the reduced nicotinamide nucleotide by oxygen through the cytochrome electron-transport system of plant mitochondria would produce ATP. In the intact plant cell containing chloroplasts and mitochondria, both of these organelles would be required to produce the two co-enzymes NADPH and ATP needed to drive the photosynthetic carbon reduction cycle. In 1954, Arnon and his associates questioned whether ATP is so produced when they discovered that chloroplasts alone, when isolated by special techniques, could convert CO_2 to carbohydrates in the light. Further studies in Arnon's laboratory showed that chloroplasts, in the absence of mitochondria, could synthesise ATP in two types of light-dependent phosphorylation reactions. The first type, cyclic photophosphorylation, yields ATP only and produces no net change in any external electron donor or acceptor.

$$ADP + H_3PO_4 \xrightarrow{hv} ATP + H_2O \qquad \qquad ...(11.13)$$

The second type, noncyclic photophosphorylation, involves a process in which ATP formation is coupled with a light-driven transfer of electrons from water to a terminal electron acceptor such as $NADP^+$ with the resultant evolution of oxygen.

$$2NADP^+ + 2H_2O + 2ADP + 2H_3PO_4 \xrightarrow{hv} 2NADPH + 2H^+ + O_2 + 2ATP + 2H_2O \qquad ...(11.14)$$

This reaction deserves further comment for two reasons:

First, note that the movement of electrons would appear to be the opposite of that encountered in the electron-transport system of mitochondria. In the latter, electrons flow from NADH ($E'_0 = -0.32$) to O_2 ($E'_0 = 0.82$) along a potential gradient that releases energy, some of which is trapped in the form of ATP. According to Eq. 11.9, electrons arising in the oxygen atom of H_2O somehow appear to make their way to $NADP^+$ and reduce it to NADPH. This movement of electrons against the potential gradient clearly requires energy, this is the function of light in photosynthesis. Second, Eq. 11.10 is even more remarkable in that, as electrons are apparently made to flow from H_2O to $NADP^+$, energy is also made available as ATP. These observations will be explained after the photosynthetic apparatus and the photochemistry of photosynthesis are described. Photosynthesis is carried out by both prokaryotic and eukaryotic cells. The prokaryotes include the cyanobacteria (blue-green algae) and the purple and green bacteria, in these organisms, the light-trapping process takes place in small structures called chromatophores. In eukaryotic organisms that photosynthesise (higher green plants, the multicellular red, green and brown algae, dinoflagellates and diatoms), the chloroplast is the site of the photosynthetic process.

FUNDAMENTAL PROCESSES IN PHOTOSYNTHESIS

All photosynthetic organisms except bacteria use water as electron or hydrogen donor to reduce various electron acceptors and from the water they evolve molecular oxygen. The overall equation of photosynthesis for this group of organisms is:

$$H_2O + CO_2 \xrightarrow{Light} (CH_2O) + O_2 \qquad \qquad ...(11.15)$$

in which (CH_2O) designates the carbohydrate formed as the end product of photosynthesis. However, this equation does not apply to all photosynthetic organisms. The photosynthetic bacteria normally neither produce nor use molecular oxygen, in fact, most of them are strict anaerobes and are poisoned by oxygen. Instead of water these organisms use other compounds as electron donors.

The green and purple sulphur bacteria use hydrogen sulphide, according to the equation:

$$2H_2S + CO_2 \xrightarrow{\text{Light}} (CH_2O) + H_2O + 2S \qquad \qquad ...(11.16)$$

The elemental sulphur formed is deposited as globules which either accumulate in the cell or are extruded from it.

Some non-sulphur purple bacteria use an organic hydrogen donor, such as isopropanol, which is oxidised to acetone:

$$\underset{\text{Isopropanol}}{2CH_3CHOHCH_3} + CO_2 \xrightarrow{\text{Light}} (CH_2O) + \underset{\text{Acetone}}{2CH_3COCH_3} + H_2O \qquad ...(11.17)$$

Despite these differences, C. van Niel, a pioneer in the study of the comparative aspects of metabolism and photosynthesis, postulated that plant and bacterial photosynthesis are fundamentally similar, as is evident if the equation of photosynthesis is written in a more general form,

$$2H_2D + CO_2 \xrightarrow{\text{Light}} (CH_2O) + H_2O + 2D \qquad \qquad ...(11.18)$$

in which H_2D symbolises a hydrogen donor and D its oxidised form.

Thus, H_2D may be water, hydrogen sulphide, isopropanol or anyone of a number of different hydrogen donors. The nature of the hydrogen donor that can be used depends on the species of photosynthetic organism van Niel also predicted that the molecular oxygen formed during plant photosynthesis is derived exclusively from the oxygen atoms of water and not from the carbon dioxide, as indicated in the following version of Eq. 11.15:

$$2H_2O + CO_2 \xrightarrow{\text{Light}} (CH_2O) + H_2O + O_2 \qquad \qquad ...(11.19)$$

Photosynthesis taking place in water labelled with an oxygen isotope does in fact yield labelled O_2. Study of the comparative aspects of photosynthesis has also revealed that CO_2 is not the universal electron or hydrogen acceptor in all photosynthetic cells. Carbon dioxide is of course the major electron acceptor in all photosynthetic autotrophs, such as higher plants, which must manufacture all their organic biomolecules from carbon dioxide. However, most higher plants can also use as electron acceptor nitrate, which they reduce to ammonia.

In nitrogen-fixing photosynthetic organisms, molecular nitrogen as well as carbon dioxide may be used as electron acceptors during photo-synthesis, the nitrogen is reduced to ammonia. Moreover, many photosynthetic organisms can use hydrogen ions as the ultimate electron acceptor, from which they form molecular hydrogen, still others can use sulphate as electron acceptor. Typical equations for photosynthesis with different electron acceptors are given below:

Electron donor	Electron acceptor			
$2H_2D$	+	CO_2	$\rightarrow$	$(CH_2O) + H_2O + 2D$ ...(11.20)
$9H_2D$	+	$2NO_3^-$	$\rightarrow$	$2NH_3 + 6H_2O + 9D$ ...(11.21)
$3H_2D$	+	N_2	$\rightarrow$	$2NH_3 + 3D$ ...(11.22)
H_2D	+	$2H^+$	$\rightarrow$	$2H_2 + D$ ...(11.23)

From these considerations, it is clear that photosynthesis may involve different electron donors and different electron acceptors, depending on the species of photosynthetic organism.

Thus we can write a completely general equation for photosynthesis,

$$H_2D + A \xrightarrow{\text{Light}} H_2A + D \qquad \qquad ...(11.24)$$

in which H_2D is the electron or hydrogen donor and A is the electron or hydrogen acceptor. Therefore we should not look upon photosynthesis exclusively as a mechanism for the synthesis of carbohydrates from carbon dioxide. Indeed, even in higher plants the products of the light reactions (ATP and NADPH) are used to carry out the biosynthesis of many cell components other than carbohydrates. We now come to a highly important characteristic of the light reactions of photosynthesis.

In all photosynthetic organisms, regardless of the electron donor and electron acceptor, the light-induced flow of electrons from electron donor to electron acceptor is against the normal gradient of the standard oxidation-reduction potentials of the electron donor and electron-acceptor systems, i.e. the net flow of electrons is in the direction of the system having the lower or more electronegative standard potential.

The direction of flow of electrons in photosynthesis does not violate the thermodynamic laws, since it is the energy of the absorbed light that causes the electrons to flow in reverse, in the direction of a more negative or more energy-rich state, opposite to the direction of flow of electrons in respiration.

LIGHT AND DARK REACTIONS

We have seen that photosynthesis has two phases, the light reactions, which are directly dependent on light energy and the dark reactions, which can occur in the absence of light. This division was first suggested by observations that the rate-limiting step in plant photosynthesis is some step that can take place in the dark. When photosynthetic organisms are subjected to intermittent illumination with very short flashes of light (milliseconds or less) followed by dark intervals of varying duration, the maximum O_2 evolution after a single light flash of 10^{-5}s can be realised only if it is followed by a much longer dark peloid about 0.06 sec or more. This difference in rate is greatly accentuated when the temperature of the cells is lowered.

A more direct experiment proving that there are light and dark phases of photosynthesis was carried out by D. I. Arnon and his colleagues in 1958. They showed that the light and dark phases could be separated temporally. First, they illuminated chloroplasts in the absence of carbon dioxide, which resulted in trapping some of the light energy in a chemical form. They then disrupted the chloroplasts and removed the grana, in which the light-trapping reaction takes place and added radioactive carbon dioxide to the remaining stroma.

They found that the carbon dioxide was converted in the dark into radioactive hexoses at the expense of the chemical energy generated in the preceding light period. These experiments also showed that chloroplasts are capable of the entire photosynthetic process leading to hexose formation, i.e. they are complete photosynthetic units, just as the mitochondria are complete respiratory units.

Today we know that the light reactions of photosynthesis are primarily responsible for converting light energy into chemical energy in the form of ATP and NADPH, whereas the dark reactions involve the utilisation of the chemical energy of ATP and NADPH to bring about the reduction of carbon dioxide to hexose and other products. The term dark reactions should not be taken to mean that they take place only in the dark or at night, in living plants they take place, together with the light reactions, in the daytime. At night green leaf cells respire, utilising oxygen and consuming glucose and other organic fuels generated by photosynthesis in daylight.

Light-Independent Reactions

Calvin cycle

In the light-independent or dark reactions the enzyme RuBisCO captures CO_2 from the atmosphere and in a process that requires the newly formed NADPH, called the Calvin-Benson cycle, releases three-carbon sugars, which are later combined to form sucrose and starch. The overall equation for the light-independent reactions in green plants is:

$$3CO_2 + 9ATP + 6NADPH + 6H^+ \rightarrow C_3H_6O_3\text{-phosphate} + 9ADP + 8P_i + 6NADP^+ + 3H_2O$$

To be more specific, carbon fixation produces an intermediate product, which is then converted to the final carbohydrate products. The carbon skeletons produced by photosynthesis are then variously used to form other organic compounds, such as the building material cellulose, as precursors for lipid and amino acid biosynthesis or as a fuel in cellular respiration. The latter occurs not only in plants but also in animals when the energy from plants gets passed through a food chain (Fig. 11.1).

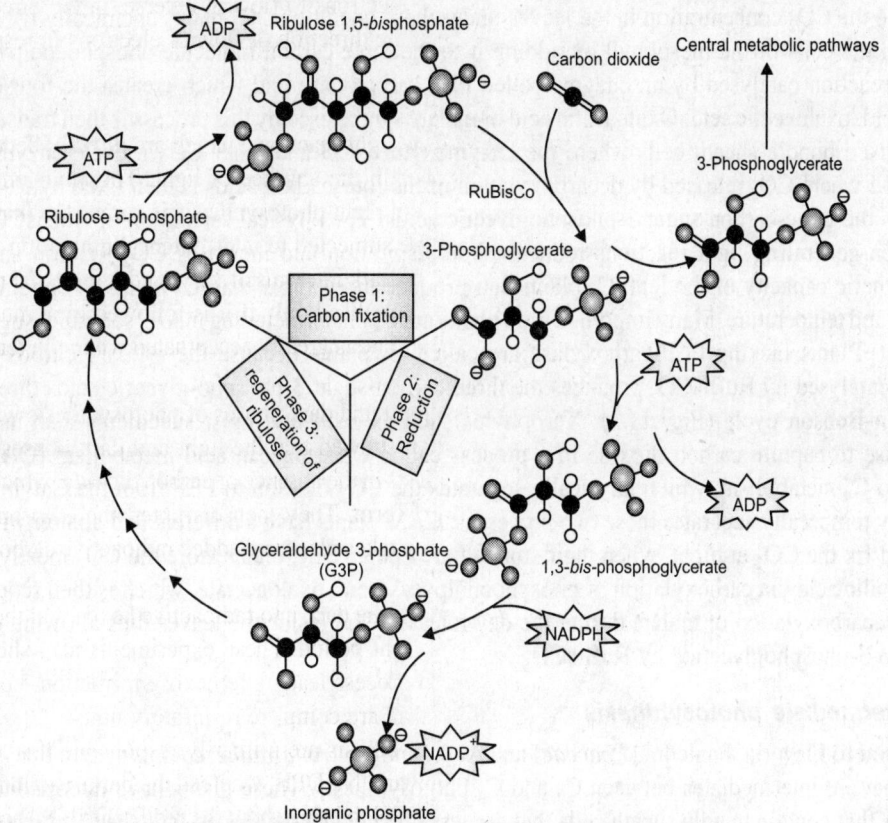

Fig. 11.1: Overview of the Calvin cycle and carbon fixation.

The fixation or reduction of carbon dioxide is a process in which carbon dioxide combines with a five-carbon sugar, ribulose-1,5-bisphosphate (RuBP), to yield two molecules of a three-carbon compound, glycerate 3-phosphate (GP), also known as 3-phosphoglycerate (PGA). GP, in the presence of ATP and NADPH from the light-dependent stages, is reduced to glyceraldehyde 3-phosphate (G3P).

This product is also referred to as 3-phosphoglyceraldehyde (PGAL) or even as triose phosphate. Triose is a 3-carbon sugar. Most (5 out of 6 molecules) of the G3P produced is used to regenerate RuBP so the process can continue. The 1 out of 6 molecules of the triose phosphates not 'recycled' often condense to form hexose phosphates, which ultimately yield sucrose, starch and cellulose. The sugars produced during carbon metabolism yield carbon skeletons that can be used for other metabolic reactions like the production of amino acids and lipids.

C_4 and C_3 photosynthesis and CAM

In hot and dry conditions, plants will close their stomata to prevent loss of water. Under these conditions, CO_2 will decrease and oxygen gas, produced by the light reactions of photosynthesis, will decrease in the stem, not leaves, causing an increase of photorespiration by the oxygenase activity of ribulose-1, 5-*bis*-phosphate carboxylase/oxygenase and decrease in carbon fixation. Some plants have evolved mechanisms to increase the CO_2 concentration in the leaves under these conditions. C_4 plants chemically fix carbon dioxide in the cells of the mesophyll by adding it to the three-carbon molecule phosphoenolpyruvate (PEP), a reaction catalysed by an enzyme called PEP carboxylase and which creates the four-carbon organic acid, oxaloacetic acid. Oxaloacetic acid or malate synthesised by this process is then translocated to specialised bundle sheath cells where the enzyme, RuBisCO and other Calvin cycle enzymes are located and where CO_2 released by decarboxylation of the four-carbon acids is then fixed by RuBisCO activity to the three-carbon sugar 3-phosphoglyceric acids. The physical separation of RuBisCO from the oxygen-generating light reactions reduces photorespiration and increases CO_2 fixation and thus photosynthetic capacity of the leaf. C_4 plants can produce more sugar than C_3 plants in conditions of high light and temperature. Many important crop plants are C_4 plants including maize, sorghum, sugarcane and millet. Plants lacking PEP-carboxylase are called C_3 plants because the primary carboxylation reaction, catalysed by RuBisCO, produces the three-carbon sugar 3-phospho-glyceric acids directly in the Calvin-Benson cycle (Fig. 11.2). Xerophytes such as cacti and most succulents also use PEP carboxylase to capture carbon dioxide in a process called Crassulacean acid metabolism (CAM). In contrast to C_4 metabolism, which physically separates the CO_2 fixation to PEP from the Calvin cycle, CAM only temporally separates these two processes. CAM plants have a different leaf anatomy than C_4 plants and fix the CO_2 at night, when their stomata are open. CAM plants store the CO_2 mostly in the form of malic acid via carboxylation of phosphoenolpyruvate to oxaloacetate, which is then reduced to malate. Decarboxylation of malate during the day releases CO_2 inside the leaves thus allowing carbon fixation to 3-phosphoglycerate by RuBisCO.

C_3-C_4 Intermediate photosynthesis

Moore point to Flaveria, Panicum (*Poaceae*) and Alternanthera (*Amarantheceae*) as genera that contain species that are intermediates between C_3 and C_4 photosynthesis. These plants have intermediate leaf anatomies that contain bundle sheath cells that are less distinct and developed than the C_4 plants. These intermediates are characterised by their resistance to photorespiration so that they can operate in higher temperatures and dryer environments than C_3 plants. The ranges of CO_2 compensation points for the three types of plants are shown in Fig. 11.3. These compensation points are the values at which the plants cease to provide net photosynthesis. The connection to hot and dry conditions comes from the fact that all the plants will close their stomata in hot and dry weather to conserve moisture and the continuing

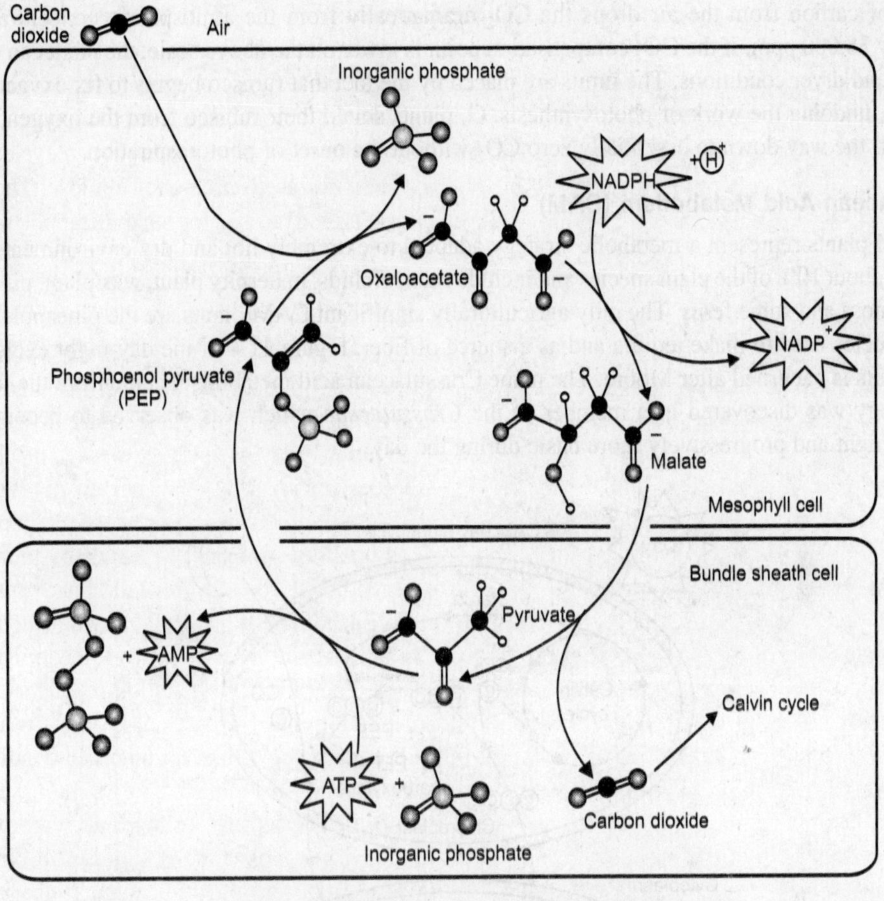

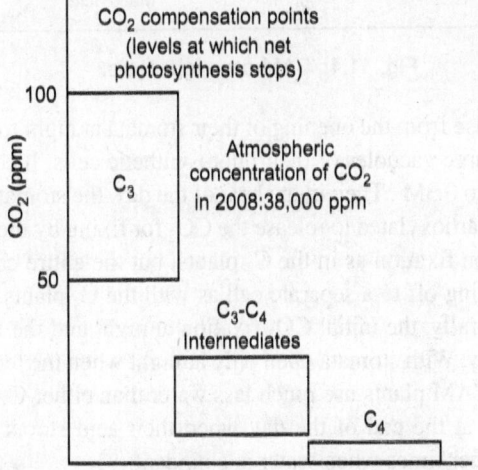

Fig. 11.2: Overview of C₄ carbon fixation.

Fig. 11.3: The ranges of CO₂ compensation points for the three types of plants.

fixation of carbon from the air drops the CO_2 dramatically from the atmospheric concentration of nominally 38,000 ppm. If the CO_2 compensation point is lower on the above scale, the plant can operate in hotter and dryer conditions. The limits are placed by the fact that rubisco begins to fix oxygen rather than CO_2, undoing the work of photosynthesis. C_4 plants shield their rubisco from the oxygen, so can operate all the way down to essentially zero CO_2 without the onset of photorespiration.

Crassulacean Acid Metabolism (CAM)

The CAM plants represent a metabolic strategy adapted to extremely hot and dry environments. They represent about 10% of the plant species and include cacti, orchids, maternity plant, wax plant, pineapple, Spanish moss and some ferns. The only agriculturally significant CAM plants are the pineapple and an Agave species used to make tequila and as a source of fiber. Figure 11.4 of the day-night cycle of the CAM plants is patterned after Moore. The name Crassulacean acid metabolism came from the fact that this strategy was discovered in a member of the *Crassulaceae* which was observed to become very acidic at night and progressively more basic during the day.

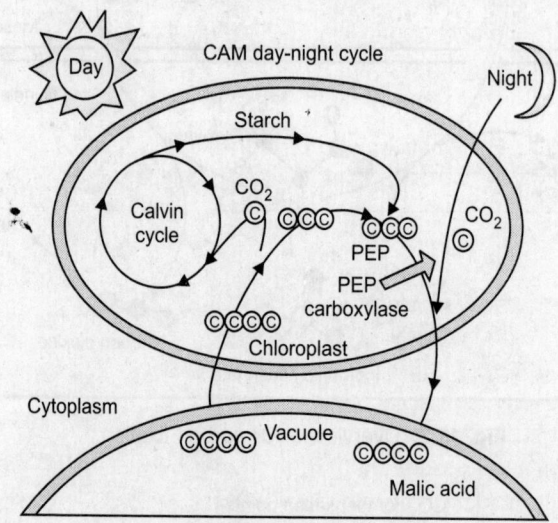

Fig. 11.4: CAM day-night cycle.

The acidity was found to arise from the opening of their stomata at night to take in CO_2 and fix it into malic acid for storage in the large vacuoles of their photosynthetic cells. It could drop the pH to 4 with a malic acid concentration up to 0.3M . Then in the heat of the day, the stomata close tightly to conserve water and the malic acid is decarboxylated to release the CO_2 for fixing by the Calvin cycle. PEP is used for the initial short-term carbon fixation as in the C_4 plants, but the entire chain of reactions occurs in the same cell rather than handing off to a separate cell as with the C_4 plants. In the CAM strategy, the processes are separated temporally, the initial CO_2 fixation at night and the malic acid to Calvin cycle part taking place during the day. With stomata open only at night when the temperature is lower and the relative humidity higher, the CAM plants use much less water than either C_3 plants or C_4 plants. Some varieties convert to C_4 plants at the end of the day when their acid stores are depleted if they have adequate water and even at other times when water is abundant.

EXCITATION OF MOLECULES BY LIGHT

Visible light is a form of electromagnetic radiation of wavelength 400 to 700 nm. Light has properties suggesting that it is propagated in a discontinuous or corpuscular manner, in the form of photons or quanta. The total amount of solar energy falling on the surface of the earth in the form of photons is immense, it is estimated to exceed 2×10^{25} cal/year. Only 12% of this energy is actually available to plant life, the rest is either outside the visible range or is absorbed by the atmosphere or the non-living portion of the earth's surface. The energy content of a photon is represented by hv, in which h is Planck's constant (1.58×10^{-34} cal-s) and v is the frequency of the radiation. E, the energy in kilocalories of 1.0 einstein, that is, 1.0 mol of light, containing 6.023×10^{23} (Avogadro's number) quanta, is most simply given by the formula:

$$E = \frac{28600}{\text{Wavelength (nm)}}$$

In the visible range 1 einstein carries from 40 to 72 kcal of energy, depending on the wavelength of the light (Table 11.1). Photo ns of short wavelength, at the violet end of the spectrum, have the greatest energy content. Note that the energy content of a 'mole' of photons, regardless of wavelength, is considerably greater than the amount of energy required to synthesise 1 mol of ATP from ADP and phosphate, which is 7.3 kcal under standard thermodynamic conditions.

Table 11.1: Energy equivalent of 1 einstein at different wavelengths.

Wavelength, nm	Colour	Kilocalories	Kilo joules
700	Far red	40.9	171
600	Orange	47.7	199
	Yellow		
500	Green	57.2	239
	Blue		
400	Violet	71.5	299

The ability of a compound to absorb photons depends on its atomic structure, particularly on the arrangement of electrons surrounding its atomic nuclei. The absorption spectrum of a compound indicates its capacity to absorb light as a function of wavelength. When a photon strikes an atom or molecule capable of absorbing light at a given wavelength, energy is absorbed by some of the electrons, which are thus boosted to higher energy levels, the atom or molecule is then in an energy rich excited state. Only photons of certain wavelengths can excite a given atom or molecule because the excitation of molecules is not continuous but quantised, i.e. light energy is absorbed only in discrete packets on an all-or-none basis, leading to the term quantum. Excitation of a molecule by light is very rapid, taking less than 10^{-5} s. The excited molecule has two possible fates. It may return to its original low-energy state, the ground state, with simultaneous emission of the energy originally absorbed during excitation, which reappears either as light or as heat or both. The emission of light by excited molecules is called fluorescence. Fluorescent decay of excited molecules, which is complete in less than 10^{-8} s, occurs at a longer wavelength than the exciting wavelength. However, an excited molecule has another possible fate, it may, thanks to its energy rich condition, react more readily with some other molecule. In such a photochemical reaction the excited molecule may lose an electron to the other reacting molecule.

PIGMENTS ABSORB LIGHT USED IN PHOTOSYNTHESIS

In photosynthesis, the Sun energy is converted to chemical energy by photosynthetic organisms. However, the various wavelengths in sunlight are not all used equally in photosynthesis. Instead, photosynthetic organisms contain light-absorbing molecules called pigments that absorb only specific wavelengths of visible light, while reflecting others.

The set of wavelengths absorbed by a pigment is its absorption spectrum. We can see the absorption spectra of three key pigments in photosynthesis: chlorophyll *a*, chlorophyll *b*, and β-carotene. For instance, plants appear green to us because they contain many chlorophyll *a* and *b* molecules, which reflect green light. Most photosynthetic organisms have a variety of different pigments, so they can absorb energy from a wide range of wavelengths.

Chlorophylls

There are five main types of chlorophylls: chlorophylls *a*, *b*, *c* and *d*, plus a related molecule found in prokaryotes called bacteriochlorophyll. In plants, chlorophyll *a* and chlorophyll *b* are the main photosynthetic pigments. Chlorophyll (Fig. 11.5) molecules absorb blue and red wavelengths.

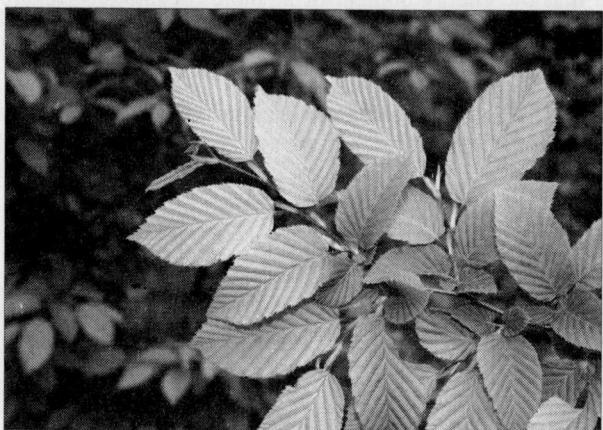

Fig. 11.5: Chlorophylls.

Although both chlorophyll *a* and chlorophyll *b* absorb light, chlorophyll *a* plays a unique and crucial role in converting light energy to chemical energy. All photosynthetic plants, algae, and cyanobacteria contain chlorophyll *a*, whereas only plants and green algae contain chlorophyll *b*, along with a few types of cyanobacteria. Because of the central role of chlorophyll *a* in photosynthesis, all pigments used in addition to chlorophyll *a* are known as accessory pigments—including other chlorophylls, as well as other classes of pigments like the carotenoids. The use of accessory pigments allows a broader range of wavelengths to be absorbed, and thus, more energy to be captured from sunlight.

Carotenoids

Carotenoids are another key group of pigments that absorb violet and blue-green light. The brightly coloured carotenoids (Fig. 11.6) found in fruit—such as the red of tomato (lycopene), the yellow of corn seeds (zeaxanthin), or the orange of an orange peel (β-carotene)—are often used as advertisements to attract animals, which can help disperse the plant's seeds.

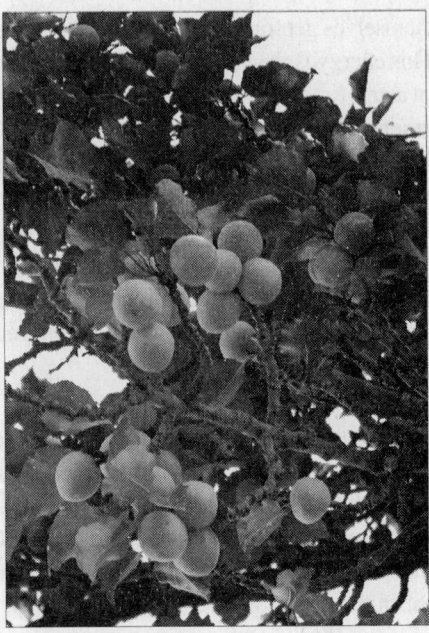

Fig. 11.6: Carotenoids.

In photosynthesis, carotenoids help capture light, but they also have an important role in getting rid of excess light energy. When a leaf is exposed to full Sun, it receives a huge amount of energy, if that energy is not handled properly, it can damage the photosynthetic machinery. Carotenoids in chloroplasts help absorb the excess energy and dissipate it as heat.

When a pigment absorbs a photon of light, it becomes excited, meaning that it has extra energy and is no longer in its normal, or ground, state. At a subatomic level, excitation is when an electron is bumped into a higher-energy orbital that lies further from the nucleus.

Only a photon with just the right amount of energy to bump an electron between orbitals can excite a pigment. In fact, this is why different pigments absorb different wavelengths of light: the 'energy gaps' between the orbitals are different in each pigment, meaning that photons of different wavelengths are needed in each case to provide an energy boost that matches the gap.

When a pigment molecule absorbs light, it is raised from a ground state to an excited state. This means that an electron jumps to a higher-energy orbital. An excited pigment is unstable, and it has various 'options' available for becoming more stable. For instance, it may transfer either its extra energy or its excited electron to a neighboring molecule.

Mechanism of Energy Transfers

The importance of pigment in photosynthesis is that it helps absorb the energy from light. The free electrons at the molecular level in the chemical structure of these photosynthetic pigments revolve at certain energy levels. When light energy (photons of light) falls on these pigments, the electrons absorb this energy and jump to the next energy level. They cannot continue to stay in that energy level, as it is not the state of stability for these electrons, so they must dissipate this energy and come back to their stable energy level. During photosynthesis these high-energy electrons transfer their energy to other molecules, or these electrons themselves get transferred to other molecules. Hence, they release the energy they had captured from light. This energy is then used by other molecules to form sugar and other nutrients by using carbon dioxide and water.

In an ideal situation the pigments must be capable of absorbing light energy of the entire wavelength, so that the maximum energy can be absorbed. To do so, they should appear black, but chlorophylls are actually green or brown in colour and absorb light wavelengths in the visible spectrum. If the pigment starts absorbing wavelength away from the visible light spectrum, such as ultraviolet or infrared rays, the free electrons may gain so much energy that they will either get knocked off their orbit or may soon dissipate energy in the form of heat, thus damaging the pigment molecules. So it is the visible wavelength energy absorbing capability of pigment that is important for photosynthesis to take place.

ENERGETICS OF PHOTOSYNTHESIS

The maximum thermodynamic efficiency of photosynthesis, i.e. its quantum efficiency, has been a celebrated and hotly debated problem. In principle, the problem reduces to the experimental determination of the value of n, the number of light quanta required in the overall equation of photosynthesis. The standard-free-energy change $\Delta G^{o\prime}$ for the synthesis of hexose from CO_2 and H_2O is +686 kcal. If we divide this value by 6, we obtain the energy input, namely, +114 kcal, required to reduce one molecule of CO_2 to (CH_2O), as called for in the equation:

$$H_2O + CO_2 \xrightarrow{\text{Light}} (CH_2O) + O_2 \qquad \qquad ...(11.25)$$

We have seen that the caloric value of a light quantum depends on its wavelength and ranges from 72 kcal einstein^{-1} at 400 nm to about 41 kcal at 700 nm (Fig. 11.7). If we take the smaller of these values, 41 kcal, then the minimum number of quanta n required for equation (11.25) would be 114/41 or about 2.7. Since light quanta are indivisible, the quantum requirement must be an integral number, which is therefore at least 3.0 if all the energy required for hexose formation comes from light.

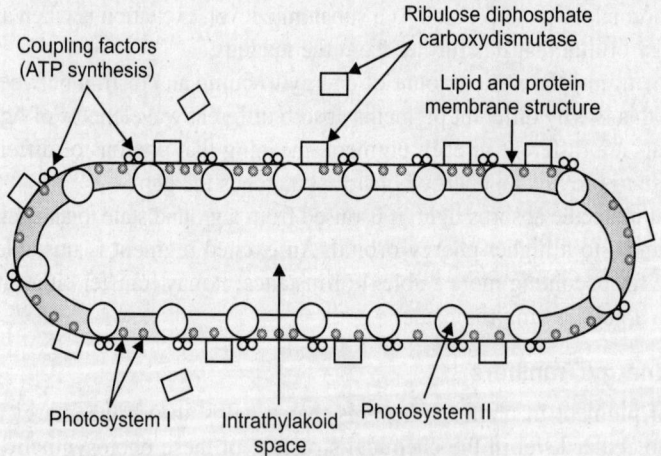

Fig. 11.7: A schematic representation of the ultrastructure of the thylakoid.

The actual quantum requirement of photosynthesis is determined by experimental measurement of the amount of light absorbed by a suspension of photosynthesising cells in relation to the amount of carbon dioxide reduced and/or oxygen evolved. The first systematic measurements of n were carried out by O. Warburg in Germany, in the 1920s. At first he found values of about 5, but many years later, with different techniques, he observed values as low as 3. He postulated that the true value for the quantum yield is actually 1 per molecule of CO_2 reduced. Although 3 quanta are theoretically required, as we have seen, Warburg proposed that the balance of the energy required comes from respiration, a dark process. Warburg's hypothesis has since been found to be inconsistent with a number of other experimental observations. For one thing, most available evidence indicates that all of the energy required for reduction of carbon dioxide to hexose and for oxygen evolution normally comes from light. Moreover, most other investigators, particularly Emerson, have found that in photosynthesis fully supported by light energy the minimum number of quanta required is 8. This value corresponds to a thermodynamic efficiency nearly the same as that of the overall process of respiration, about 38%.

To understand the significance of the quantum yield of 8 we must anticipate a point more fully developed and give the overall equation for the reduction of CO_2 to (CH_2O) during the dark phase of photosynthesis in most green plants, which is:

$$CO_2 + 3ATP + 2NADPH + 2H^+ + 2H_2O \rightarrow (CH_2O) + 3ADP + 3P_i + 2NADP^+ \qquad ...(11.26)$$

To provide the two molecules of NADPH required per molecule of CO_2 reduced in the dark reactions, four electrons are ejected by photosystem I. Correspondingly, four electrons are also ejected by photosystem II, thus yielding one molecule of oxygen (O_2) from water. Since 1 light quantum is required to eject each electron, we require 4 quanta for photosystem I and 4 for photosystem II. Now, if only one photophos-phorylation per pair of electrons occurs during the overall process, as many investigators believe, only two molecules of ATP will be generated by the two pairs of electrons flowing from water to NAD^+, according to the equation:

$$2H_2O + 2NADP^+ + 2ADP + 2P_i \xrightarrow{\text{Light}} O_2 + 2NADPH + 2H^+ + 2ATP + 2H_2O$$

in which coloured type is used to show the formation of ATP. But three molecules of ATP are required to reduce one molecule of CO_2 in the dark phase, as we have seen. However, if two ATPs are formed during light-induced transport of a pair of electrons from water to $NADP^+$, as some investigators have postulated, then four ATPs will be formed per 8 light quanta, which is more than enough to reduce 1 mol of CO_2 to carbohydrate. There is another way in which extra ATP required for dark biosynthetic reactions may be generated, i.e. cyclic photophosphorylation, which may proceed independently of non-cyclic electron flow to generate extra ATP from ADP.

The efficiency of photosynthesis in nature is much lower than the 38% calculated for the basic molecular process. From the amount of carbon fixed by a field of corn in one growing season it has been found that only about 1 to 2% of the solar energy falling on the field is recovered in the form of new photosynthetic products, uncultivated plant life yields far less, perhaps only 0.2%. Cultivated sugarcane is much more efficient, it can yield up to 8% of the captured light energy in the form of organic products. Thus, the process of photorespiration tends to lower the net efficiency of photosynthesis in some plants.

PROPERTIES OF PHOTOSYNTHETIC PHOSPHORYLATION COUPLING FACTORS

The phosphorylation of ADP accompanying photoinduced electron transport in chloroplasts strongly resembles the analogous process of oxidative phosphorylation coupled to electron transport in mitochondria. For example, light-induced non-cyclic electron transport is stimulated by addition of the phosphate acceptor ADP to chloroplasts, which thus shows the phenomenon of acceptor control of photoinduced electron transport, similar to the requirement of ADP for maximal rates of electron transport in mitochondria. Like mitochondrial phosphorylation, photosynthetic phosphorylation can also be uncoupled by certain chemical agents, so that electron flow continues but no phosphorylation takes place. Among the uncoupling agents effective on photosynthetic phosphorylation are NH_4^+ ions and carbonylcyanide phenylhydrazone, the latter is effective against either oxidative or photosynthetic phosphorylation. Ionophores, such as gramicidin, also prevent photophosphorylation. Phloridzin, a toxic glycoside from the bark of pear trees and a synthetic compound called Dio-9 inhibit photophosphorylation by an action resembling that of oligomycin on mitochondrial phosphorylation.

Yet another line of evidence showing the similarity between mitochondrial and photosynthetic phosphorylation is provided by studies of ATPase activity. Chloroplasts normally show no ATPase activity, but after treatment with certain sulphydryl compounds, such as dithiothreitol, a light-dependent ATPase activity is evoked, similar to the ATPase activity of mitochondria evoked by uncoupling agents such as 2,4-dinitrophenol. From corn chloroplasts E. Racker and his colleagues have extracted and purified a protein fraction that acquires the ability to hydrolyse ATP in the presence of Ca^{2+} when exposed to trypsin. The chloroplast ATPase has properties that resemble those of mitochondrial F_1 ATPase functioning in the coupled synthesis of ATP during oxidative phosphorylation. It has about the same molecular weight (3,80,000) and contains five different kinds of sub-units. The chloroplast ATPase, which is designated CF_1, acts as a coupling factor and restores photosynthetic phosphorylation in chloroplasts depleted of CF_1.

A further similarity between chloroplast ATPase and mitochondrial ATPase has been revealed by electron microscopy of the lamellar membranes of corn chloroplasts. These membranes show the presence of 9 nm spheres protruding from the outer surface of the thylakoid membrane, in mitochondria such spheres protrude from the inner surface of the inner membrane. These spheres are lost from chloroplasts when the CF_1 ATPase is extracted from them, the spheres are restored when the CF_1 ATPase is returned to the depleted membranes under appropriate conditions, with restoration of photosynthetic phosphorylation. An electron micrograph of the membrane surfaces of a thylakoid is already shown in Fig. 11.7. The granular bodies are believed to be enzyme complexes, among which are molecules of CF_1 ATPase.

MECHANISM OF PHOTOSYNTHETIC PHOSPHORYLATION

We have seen that currently there are three hypotheses for the mechanism of oxidative phosphorylation, chemical coupling, conformational coupling and chemiosmotic coupling. Because of the striking similarity between oxidative phosphorylation in mitochondria and photophosphorylation in chloroplasts, these three hypotheses for mitochondrial phosphorylation are also applicable to the mechanism of photophos-phorylation. Much evidence is consistent with the chemiosmotic-coupling hypothesis as the basic mechanism of photosynthetic phosphorylation. When chloroplasts are illuminated under conditions in which they exhibit cyclic electron flow, they absorb H^+ ions from the suspending medium, which becomes more alkaline. When the light is turned off and the photoinduced electron flow stops, H^+ ions slowly return from the chloroplasts to the medium. These movements of H^+ ions are remarkably similar to those occurring during electron transport in isolated mitochondria, with one important difference. In mitochondria, H^+ ions are ejected into the medium during electron transport, whereas in chloroplasts H^+ ions are absorbed during electron transport. The sidedness of the chloroplast membrane thus is the reverse of that of the mitochondrial membrane. Another important piece of evidence favouring the chemiosmotic hypothesis is the discovery by A. Jagendorf and his colleagues that a pH gradient artificially imposed across the chloroplast membrane can drive the phosphorylation of ADP in the dark, without the input of light energy (Fig. 11.8). They lowered the internal pH of chloroplasts artificially by soaking

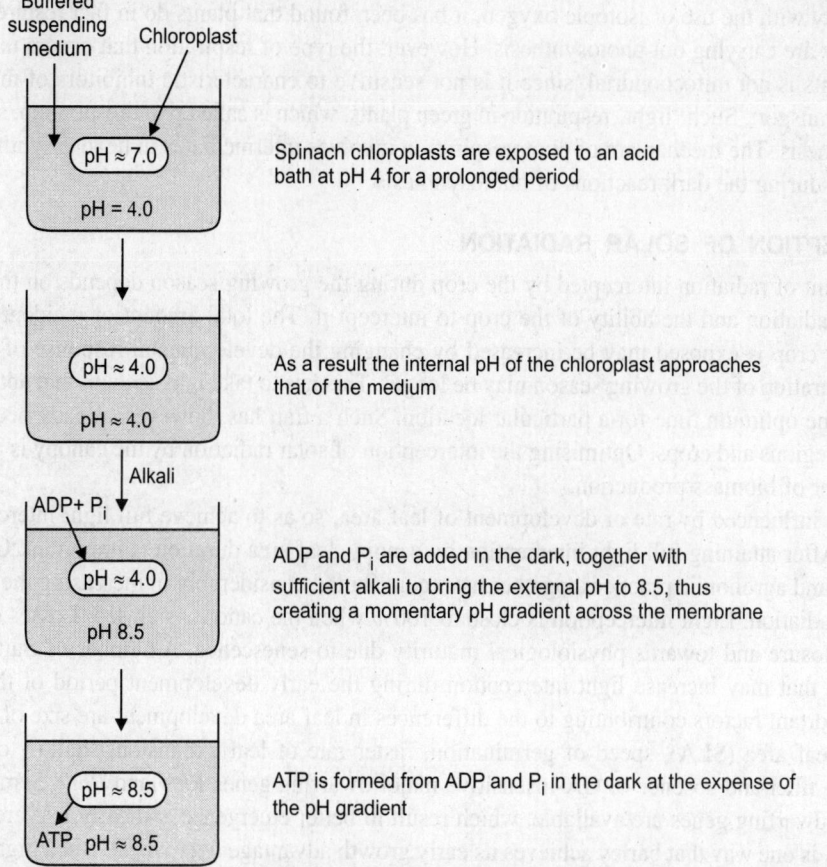

Buffered suspending medium | **Chloroplast**

pH ≈ 7.0
pH = 4.0

Spinach chloroplasts are exposed to an acid bath at pH 4 for a prolonged period

pH ≈ 4.0
pH ≈ 4.0

As a result the internal pH of the chloroplast approaches that of the medium

Alkali

ADP+ P$_i$

pH ≈ 4.0
pH 8.5

ADP and P$_i$ are added in the dark, together with sufficient alkali to bring the external pH to 8.5, thus creating a momentary pH gradient across the membrane

pH ≈ 8.5
ATP pH ≈ 8.5

ATP is formed from ADP and P$_i$ in the dark at the expense of the pH gradient

Fig. 11.8: Light-independent phosphorylation of ADP at the expenses of an artificial pH gradient induced in chloroplasts in the dark.

them in an acid bath, a medium buffered at pH 4.0. The chloroplasts were then quickly mixed in the dark with an alkaline buffer (pH 8.5), in order to impose a momentary pH gradient across the membrane, the alkaline buffer also contained phosphate and ADP. Mixing was followed by a burst of ATP formation, simultaneously, the pH gradient disappeared. When chloroplasts are illuminated with a very short light flash given by a single laser pulse (20 ns), only a single 'turnover' of the electron carriers ensues. This is accompanied by absorption of H$^+$ ions by the chloroplasts. H. Witt and his colleagues in Berlin have used such biophysical methods to establish the quantitative relationships between electron flow, H$^+$ movements and ATP formation. Their observations also support the chemiosmotic hypothesis.

RESPIRATION AND PHOTORESPIRATION IN PLANTS

Green-plant cells contain mitochondria in addition to chloroplasts and it has been established that such cells exhibit mitochondrial respiration and oxidative phosphorylation in the dark, at the expense of substrates generated by photosynthesis in earlier light periods. The question arises whether green-plant cells also respire in the light, during active photosynthesis or whether respiration is turned off. From careful measurements of the rates of oxygen and carbon dioxide exchanges in illuminated plants, particularly with the use of isotopic oxygen, it has been found that plants do in fact respire in the light while they are carrying out photosynthesis. However, the type of respiration that occurs in illuminated green plants is not mitochondrial, since it is not sensitive to characteristic inhibitors of mitochondrial electron transport. Such 'light' respiration in green plants, which is called photorespiration, short-circuits photosynthesis. The mechanism of photorespiration involves intermediates in hexose synthesis that are generated during the dark reactions of photosynthesis.

INTERCEPTION OF SOLAR RADIATION

The amount of radiation intercepted by the crop during the growing season depends on the amount of incident radiation and the ability of the crop to intercept it. The total amount of incident radiation to which the crop is exposed may be increased by changing the developmental response of the crop, so that the duration of the growing season may be longer. This has to take into account that anthesis should occur at the optimum time for a particular location. Such a trait has, however, already been optimised for most regions and crops. Optimising the interception of solar radiation by the canopy is an important component of biomass production.

This is influenced by rate of development of leaf area, so as to achieve full light interception more quickly. After attaining full light interception by canopy, leaf area duration is important. Conventional breeding and agronomic practices together have contributed considerably in increasing the interception of solar radiation. Light interception is close to 100% when the canopy is closed. Losses occur before canopy closure and towards physiological maturity due to senescence. A number of traits have been identified that may increase light interception during the early development period of the crop. The most important factors contributing to the differences in leaf area development are size of the embryo, specific leaf area (SLA), speed of germination, faster rate of leaf expansion, shallow crown depth, coleoptile tiller and absence of GA-insensitive major dwarfing genes *Rht1* and *Rht2*. Semi-dwarf GA-sensitive dwarfing genes are available, which result in better emergence and early leaf area growth. A high SLA is one way that barley achieves its early growth advantage over wheat. But a higher SLA also results in lower assimilation rate, because of a likely reduction in the amount of photosynthetic machinery per unit leaf area associated with a higher SLA. The increase in leaf area, however, more than compensates for this reduction in photosynthesis through greater light interception early in crop development. Thus, for early growth stages of cereals, a high SLA results in higher net assimilation rate (NAR). After canopy closure a high SLA becomes a hindrance to photosynthesis.

Canopy architecture becomes important once the leaf area index (LAI) exceeds 3. An erectophile leaf canopy could theoretically increase crop assimilation rate especially in high-radiation environment. Most of the highest yielding cultivars of maize, rice and wheat already have erect leaf canopies. Simulation work in rice suggests that the benefits of very erect leaf angle in high-radiation environment could only be realised at leaf area indices over 8. In many grain legumes, there is enough scope for improvement of leaf orientation and canopy architecture.

It may, however, be mentioned that LAI beyond the critical value [LAI at which the canopy first reached maximum crop growth rate (CGR)] would be detrimental for a grain crop, because it means that sugars that could have been used to make grain are instead being used to keep useless leaves alive.

The capacity of photosynthesis is dependent on light intensity. It has been shown that leaf metabolism can adapt to different light intensities according to the position in the canopy. The upper leaves in a canopy may show elevated photo-protective responses. On the other hand, the partially shaded lower leaves may have different contents of photosynthetic components from the upper leaves. Consequently, lower leaves have a reduced overall photosynthetic capacity in normal light but equally efficient radiation use efficiency per unit of N at low light intensities. Such canopies would be more efficient. It has been argued that the majority of photosynthesis in field occurs at non saturating light, therefore, it would be more profitable to improve genetically photosynthetic efficiency at low light intensities.

Maintaining green leaf area longer, particularly after anthesis when there is usually a rapid decline in leaf area index, is another important means of increasing total crop photosynthesis and hence biomass production through increased and extended light interception. Indeed, a longer duration of leaf photosynthetic activity has contributed to increased yield in most major crops. In maize, there has been an increase in the duration of photosynthetic activity by the leaves, manifested in their greater 'stay green'. A slower decline in the photosynthetic activity of canopies has been reported in soyabean (*Glycine max* (L.) Merr.) and rice. Improved agronomy and crop protection have made such changes possible.

Moreover, higher N availability also led to selection for increased chlorophyll and rubisco content in wheat. Genetic manipulation of the synthesis of cytokinins has resulted in a delay of leaf senescence and an increase in growth rate of tobacco. In pulses, there is faster senescence of leaves after flowering due to the mobilisation of leaf N and rubisco for development of protein-rich seeds. Mobilisation of leaf nitrogen decreases leaf photosynthesis, induces senescence and restricts the duration of seed-fill period. In chickpea, however, leaf N mobilisation was decreased by irrigation after flowering under north Indian conditions. This resulted in decreased HI, thus indicating the significance of such mobilisation for seed yield in chickpea.

RATE OF PHOTOSYNTHESIS: ENVIRONMENTAL FACTORS

Environmental Factors

Each species is adapted to live in a particular set of conditions. It is said to have an environmental niche. Each species has evolved to suit its own unique niche, which allows it to exist with the minimum amount of competition with other species. According to the competitive exclusion principle, if two species share the same niche, one will be better adapted than the other, out compete it and eventually drive it to extinction. So plants show different adaptations for photosynthesis, according to the conditions to which they are best adapted.

Shade or Sun

Shade-tolerant plants are able to photosynthesis in light of relatively low intensity and can grow in shady places such as woodland floors. Shade-intolerant plants are unable to carry out photosynthesis at a high enough rate to sustain growth in low light conditions. Respiration and photosynthesis are opposites. Aerobic respiration continues all the time in plant cells, using up oxygen and making carbon dioxide. Photosynthesis, in contrast, occurs only in light and uses up carbon dioxide and makes oxygen. There is a light intensity at which respiration and photosynthesis cancel each other out. This is called the compensation point (Fig. 11.9). Below this level carbohydrates are used up and the plant cannot grow.

Shade plants tend to have lower compensation points than Sun plants because they have lower respiration rates and can absorb light more efficiently. To do this they have thinner leaves which spread to catch light over a wider area and have fewer deep cells to reduce the respiration rate. In deep shade, light is more likely to be the limiting factor than carbon dioxide. So shade plants tend to have chloroplasts packed with thylakoids to make maximum use of the limited available light. They have more photosystems to funnel electrons into the same number of electron transport complexes.

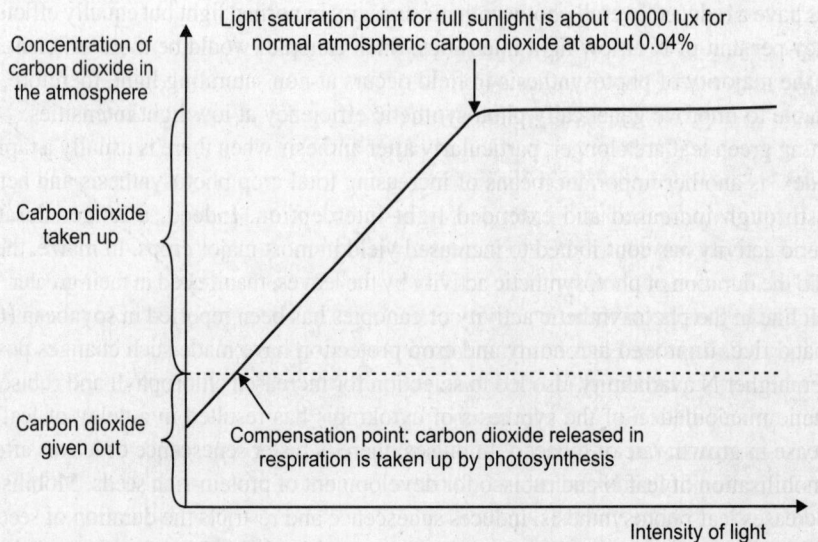

Fig. 11.9: Compensation point: rate of carbon dioxide release = rate of carbon dioxide uptake.

Wavelength of light also affects the rate of photosynthesis. Shade plants most often live in shade created by other plants, especially trees. The leaves of trees absorb red and blue wavelengths, allowing mainly green light through. This is of little use to most plants which have limited ability to survive on woodland floors. However, far red light (long wavelength) passes through the tree canopy more than near red light. PSI absorbs this light better than PSII, so shade plants compensate by having slightly more PSII complexes to restore the balance.

Dry or Wet

Water shortage is greatest in deserts. Here, CAM plants are most abundant. Being able to keep their stomata closed during the day when transpiration losses would be high allows them to survive in areas of extreme water shortage.

Cold or Hot

Plants are able to acclimatise and adapt to cold or hot environments, both by suiting the climates in which they live and by adjusting to changes through the year. Plants from hot climates tend to have higher optimum temperatures for photosynthesis and optimum temperatures tend to be higher in plants during the warmer seasons. As temperatures fall, plants can adjust the composition of membranes to make them more fluid, for example by increasing the polyunsaturated fat content. Some enzymes appear to exist in different forms which have different optimum temperatures.

Hot, Sunny and Wet

In ideal conditions for photosynthesis bright light, high temperatures and plentiful water – photosynthesis tends to reduce carbon dioxide concentration and raise oxygen concentration, favouring photorespiration (high temperatures also help) and greatly reducing the rate of photosynthesis. So many tropical plants use the C_4 pathway to reduce photorespiration.

Water is an essential donor of electrons in photosynthesis, but severe water loss affects most of a plant's metabolism, making it very difficult to establish any direct effects on photosynthesis. However, C_4 also helps in dry conditions where the stomata are partially closed to conserve water, reducing carbon dioxide supply. The increase in photorespiration is much less than would occur in a C_3 plant.

Other Factors Effecting Photosynthesis

Pollutants such as sulphur dioxide inhibit photosynthesis. Some herbicides (weedkillers) inhibit certain enzymes used in photosynthesis. PSII inhibitors such as the triazine herbicides and urea derivatives (like DCMU, dichlorophenyl methyl urea or CMU, *p*-chlorophenyl dimethyl urea) block electron flow to NADPH, causing electrons from water to accumulate on chlorophyll. PSI inhibitors (bipyridyliums like paraquat and diquat) steal electrons from the transfer chains. Both cause excessive oxidation reactions to occur. For example, hydroxyl radicals may form, which disrupt the phospholipids in membranes causing them to become leaky, and prevent the plant from obtaining energy, causing it to die.

A variety of inorganic ions are needed to make chlorophyll pigments. Magnesium and nitrogen are constituents of chlorophyll molecules and chlorophyll cannot be synthesised without the presence of iron. Soils deficient in nitrate, magnesium or iron will give rise to plants that are deficient in chlorophyll, usually with yellow rather than green leaves. The resulting reduction in the rate of photosynthesis causes stunted growth.

Chapter 12

Chemiosmotic Theory

INTRODUCTION

Chemiosmosis is the process of a molecule moving from high to low concentration, based on its charge and concentration inside a cell. This sounds pretty complicated. So, before talking about chemiosmosis, it will be important to understand a basic rule of the word: diffusion.

DIFFUSION

Diffusion is a physical process that refers to the net movement of molecules from a region of high concentration to one of lower concentration. The material that diffuses could be a solid, liquid or gas. Similarly, the medium in which diffusion occurs could also be in one of the three physical states.

One of the main characteristics of diffusion is the movement of molecules along the concentration gradient. While this could be facilitated by other molecules, it does not directly involve high-energy molecules such as adenosine triphosphate (ATP) or guanosine triphosphate (GTP).

The rate of diffusion depends on the nature of interaction between the medium and material. For instance, a gas diffuses very quickly in another gas. An example of this is the way the noxious smell of ammonia gas spreads in air. Similarly, if a canister of liquid nitrogen leaks a little, nitrogen gas that escapes would quickly diffuse into the atmosphere. The same gas would diffuse slightly more slowly in a liquid such as water and slowest in a solid. Similarly, two miscible liquids will also diffuse into each other to form a uniform solution. For instance, when water is mixed with glycerol, over time the two liquids diffuse radially into each other. This can even be observed visually by the addition of different coloured dyes to each of the liquids. However, the same phenomenon is not seen when immiscible liquids like petrol and water are mixed together. Diffusion happens slowly and only across the small surface of interaction between the two fluids.

Examples of Diffusion

Diffusion is an important part of many biological and chemical processes. In biological systems, diffusion occurs at every moment, across membranes in every cell as well as through the body. For example, oxygen is at a higher concentration inside arteries and arterioles, when compared with the oxygen levels in actively respiring cells. By the time blood flows into capillaries in the muscle or liver, for instance, there is only a single layer of cells separating this oxygen from hepatocytes or skeletal muscle fibers. Through a process of passive diffusion, without the active involvement of any other molecule oxygen passes through the capillary membrane and enters cells.

Cells utilise oxygen in the mitochondria for aerobic respiration, which generates carbon dioxide gas as a by-product. Once again, as the concentration of this gas increases within the cell, it diffuses outwards towards capillaries where the force of flowing blood removes the excess gas from the tissue region. This way, the capillaries remain at a low carbon dioxide concentration, allowing the constant movement of the molecule away from cells. This example also shows that the diffusion of any one material is independent of the diffusion of any other substances. When oxygen is moving towards tissues from capillaries, carbon dioxide is entering the bloodstream.

In chemical processes, diffusion is often the central principle driving many reactions. As a simple example, a few crystals of sugar in a glass of water will slowly dissolve over time. This occurs because there is a net movement of sugar molecules into the water medium. Even in large industrial reactions, when two liquids are mixed together, diffusion brings the reactants together and allows the reaction to proceed smoothly. For instance, one of the ways in which polyester is synthesised is by mixing the appropriate organic acid and alcohol in their liquid form. The reaction proceeds as the two reactants diffuse towards each other and undergo a chemical reaction to form esters.

Factors that Affect Diffusion

Diffusion is affected by temperature, area of interaction, steepness of the concentration gradient and particle size. Each of these factors, independently and collectively can alter the rate and extent of diffusion.

Temperature

In any system, molecules are moving with a certain amount of kinetic energy. This is usually not directed in any particular manner, and can appear random. When these molecules collide with one another, there is a change in the direction of movement as well as changes to momentum and velocity. For example, if a block of dry ice (carbon dioxide in solid form) is placed inside a box, carbon dioxide molecules in the center of the block mostly collide with each other and get retained within the solid mass. However, for molecules in the periphery, rapidly moving molecules in the air also influence their movement, allowing them to diffuse into the air. This creates a concentration gradient, with concentration of carbon dioxide gradually decreasing with distance from the lump of dry ice.

With increase in temperature, the kinetic energy of all particles in the system increases. This increases the rate at which solute and solvent molecules move, and increases collisions. This means that the dry ice (or even regular ice) will evaporate faster on a warmer day, simply because each molecule is moving with greater energy and is more likely to quickly escape the confines of a solid state.

Area of interaction

To extend the example given above, if the block of dry ice is broken into multiple pieces, the area that interacts with the atmosphere immediately increases. The number of molecules that only collide with other carbon dioxide particles within dry ice decreases. Therefore, the rate of diffusion of the gas into air also increases. This property can be observed even better if the gas has an odour or colour. For instance, when iodine is sublimated over a hot stove, purple fumes begin to appear and mix with air. If sublimation is carried out in a narrow crucible, the fumes diffuse slowly out towards the mouth of the container and then rapidly disappear. While they are confined to the smaller surface area within the crucible, the rate of diffusion remains low. This is also seen when two liquid reactants are mixed with one another. Stirring increases the area of interaction between the two chemicals and allows these molecules to diffuse towards each other more quickly. The reaction proceeds towards completion at a faster rate. On a similar note, any solute that is broken into small pieces and stirred into the solvent dissolves rapidly – another indicator of molecules diffusing better when the area of interaction increases.

Steepness of the Concentration Gradient

Since diffusion is powered primarily by the probability of molecules moving away from a region of higher saturation, it immediately follows that when the medium (or solvent) has a very low concentration of the solute, the probability of a molecule diffusing away from the central area is higher. For instance, in the example about the diffusion of iodine gas, if the crucible is placed in another closed container and iodine crystals are heated for an extended period of time, the rate at which the purple gas seems to 'disappear' at the mouth of the crucible will reduce. This apparent slowing down is due to the fact that, over time, the larger container begins to have enough iodine gas that some of it will be moving 'backwards' towards the crucible. Even though this is random non-directed movement, with a large bulk, it can create a scenario where there is no net movement of gas from the container.

Particle size

At any given temperature, the diffusion of a smaller particle will be more rapid than that of a larger-sized molecule. This is related to both the mass of the molecule and its surface area. A heavier molecule with a larger surface area will diffuse slowly, while smaller, lighter particles will diffuse more quickly. For example, while oxygen gas will diffuse slightly more quickly than carbon dioxide, both of them will move more quickly than iodine gas.

Functions of diffusion

Diffusion in the human body is necessary for the absorption of digested nutrients, gas exchange, the propagation of nerve impulses, the movement of hormones and other metabolites towards their target organ and for nearly every event in embryonic development.

Types of Diffusion

Diffusion can either be simple diffusion and be facilitated by another molecule

Simple diffusion

Simple diffusion is merely the movement of molecules along their concentration gradient without the direct involvement of any other molecules. It can involve either the spreading of a material through a medium or the transport of a particle across a membrane. All the examples given above were instances of simple diffusion. Simple diffusion is relevant in chemical reactions, in many physical phenomena, and can even influence global weather patterns and geological events. In most biological systems, diffusion occurs across a semi-permeable membrane made of a lipid bilayer. The membrane has pores and openings to allow the passage of specific molecules.

Facilitated diffusion

On the other hand, facilitated diffusion, as the term indicates, requires the presence of another molecule (the facilitator) in order for diffusion to occur. Facilitated diffusion is necessary for the movement of large or polar molecules across the hydrophobic lipid bilayer. Facilitated diffusion is necessary for the biochemical processes of every cell since there is communication between various subcellular organelles. As an example, while gases and small molecules like methane or water can diffuse freely across a plasma membrane, larger charged molecules like carbohydrates or nucleic acids need the help of transmembrane proteins forming pores or channels.

Diffusion is when anything moves from high concentration to low concentration. Think about food colouring in a jar of water. When the food colouring is first added to the water, it is concentrated in the center, but because there is less food colouring in other parts of the water, over time the food colouring spreads out or diffuses. There are many more examples, such as delicious smells wafting from the kitchen during a holiday meal or warm air moving outwards from the house during the winter. The examples are so ubiquitous because diffusion is everywhere! Everything always moves from where there is more to where there is less.

How Does Diffusion Happen in Cells?

There are some special examples of diffusion that occur inside cells. Cells have a plasma membrane, or outer barrier, that only lets certain things in or out. This allows substances to build up on one side of the membrane if there isn't a door to let them through. This creates what we call a gradient. A gradient is a situation in which there is more of a substance on one side than another. Energy can be stored in a gradient over the plasma membrane. If one substance is concentrated on one side of the membrane, it will want to diffuse until the concentrations are even.

Because this process occurs naturally, when it finally does happen, energy is released. The cell can harness this energy to do amasing things. Channel proteins allow substances to diffuse through the plasma membrane.

Chemiosmosis is the movement of ions across a semipermeable membrane, down their electrochemical gradient. An example of this would be the generation of adenosine triphosphate (ATP) by the movement of hydrogen ions (H^+) across a membrane during cellular respiration or photosynthesis.

Hydrogen ions, or protons, will diffuse from an area of high proton concentration to an area of lower proton concentration, and an electrochemical concentration gradient of protons across a membrane can be harnessed to make ATP. This process is related to osmosis, the diffusion of water across a membrane, which is why it is called 'chemiosmosis'. An ion gradient has potential energy and can be used to power chemical reactions when the ions pass through a channel (grey) is shown in Fig. 12.1.

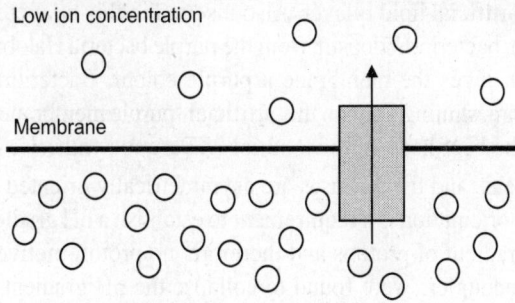

Fig. 12.1: An ion gradient has potential energy and can be used to power chemical reactions when the ions pass through a channel (grey).

HOW DOES CHEMIOSMOSIS WORK?

Chemiosmosis is a special type of diffusion that happens over the plasma membrane. Chemiosmosis not only takes concentration into consideration, but also electrical charge. Thus, chemiosmosis exclusively has to do with the movement of ions (charged atoms) across the plasma membrane. Diffusion not only works to equalise concentration on both sides of the membrane, but also to equalise charge. If there are more positive ions outside compared to inside the cell, positive ions will want to move down their electrical gradient into the cell. However, chemiosmosis also takes into consideration the concentration gradient. The molecule flows based on where there is more of its charge to where there is less and from a higher to lower concentration. The ion is flowing down its electrochemical gradient.

Chemiosmotic Hypothesis

The chemiosmotic hypothesis was proposed by Peter Mitchell. This hypothesis stated that a proton-motive force was responsible for driving the synthesis of ATP. In this hypothesis, protons would be pumped across the inner mitochondrial membrane as electrons went through the electron transfer chain. This would result in a proton gradient with an lower pH in the intermembrane space and a elevated pH in the matrix of the mitochondria. An intact inner mitochondrial membrane, impermeable to protons, is a requirement of such a model. The proton gradient and membrane potential are the proton-motive force that is used to drive ATP synthesis. In effect, the pH gradient acts as a 'battery' which stores energy to produce ATP. Over the past several years, Mitchell's chemiosmotic hypothesis has been widely accepted as the mechanism of coupling of electron transport and ATP synthesis. He was awarded the Nobel Prize in Chemistry in 1978. This acceptance by the scientific community is a result of accumulating experimental evidence supporting the hypothesis.

Some of the evidence supporting Mitchell's chemiosmotic hypothesis is as follows.

1. Electron transport generates a proton gradient. The pH measured on the outside is lower than that measured inside the mitochondria.

2. Only a proton gradient is needed to synthesise ATP. Electron transport is not required as long as there is another mechanism for generating a pH gradient.

3. A reconstitution experiment carried out by Racker and Stoeckenius (J Biol Chem 1974 Jan 25, Reconstitution of purple membrane vesicles catalysing light-driven proton uptake and adenosine triphosphate formation) showed that the generation of a proton gradient can result in ATP synthesis in a totally artificial system. In their experiment, a mitochondrial ATPase complex from beef heart was inserted into an artificial lipid bilayer. Also inserted in this bilayer was a membrane fragment containing the protein, bacteriorhodopsin, from the purple bacteria Halobacterium, so called because the bacteriorhodopsin gives the membrane a purple colour. Bacteriorhodopsin is a light-driven proton pump. Therefore, shining light on this artificial 'purple membrane' formed a proton gradient, which was used by the beef heart mitochondrial ATPase to synthesise ATP.

The electron transfer chains and the ATPases are asymmetrically oriented in the inner mitochondrial membrane. An asymmetric orientation is a requirement to establish a pH gradient. A random arrangement would not result in a net gradient of protons and therefore, no proton-motive force for the synthesis of ATP. Compounds called uncouplers were found to collapse the pH gradient by shuttling protons back across the membrane through the compounds and one such uncoupler is dinitophenol. In the presence of the uncoupler electron transport continues, but no ATP synthesis occurs.

PROTON-MOTIVE FORCE

The movement of ions across the membrane depends on a combination of two factors:

1. Diffusion force caused by a concentration gradient - all particles tend to diffuse from higher concentration to lower.

2. Electrostatic force caused by electrical potential gradient - cations like protons H^+ tend to diffuse down the electrical potential, from the positive (P) side of the membrane to the negative (N) side. Anions diffuse spontaneously in the opposite direction.

Energy conversion by the inner mitochondrial membrane and chemiosmotic coupling between the chemical energy of redox reactions in the respiratory chain and the oxidative phosphorylation catalysed by the ATP synthase (sometimes called as 'mitochondrial mushrooms').

These two gradients taken together can be expressed as an electrochemical gradient.

Lipid bilayers of biological membranes, however, are barriers for ions. This is why energy can be stored as a combination of these two gradients across the membrane. Only special membrane proteins like ion channels can sometimes allow ions to move across the membrane. In chemiosmotic theory transmembrane ATP synthases are very important. They convert energy of spontaneous flow of protons through them into chemical energy of ATP bonds.

Hence researchers created the term proton-motive force (PMF), derived from the electrochemical gradient mentioned earlier. It can be described as the measure of the potential energy stored as a combination of proton and voltage (electrical potential) gradients across a membrane. The electrical gradient is a consequence of the charge separation across the membrane (when the protons H^+ move without a counterion, such as chloride Cl^-).

In most cases the proton-motive force is generated by an electron transport chain which acts as a proton pump, using the Gibbs free energy of redox reactions to pump protons (hydrogen ions) out across the membrane, separating the charge across the membrane. In mitochondria, energy released by the electron transport chain is used to move protons from the mitochondrial matrix (N side) to the stroma (P side). Moving the protons out of the mitochondrion creates a lower concentration of positively charged protons inside it, resulting in excess negative charge on the inside of the membrane. The electrical potential gradient is about -170 mV, negative inside (N). These gradients - charge difference and the proton concentration difference both create a combined electrochemical gradient across the membrane, often expressed as the proton-motive force (PMF). In mitochondria, the PMF is almost entirely made up of the electrical component but in chloroplasts the PMF is made up mostly of the pH gradient because the charge of protons H^+ is neutralised by the movement of Cl^- and other anions. In either case, the PMF needs to be greater than about 460 mV (45 kJ/mol) for the ATP synthase to be able to make ATP.

Thus, the proton-motive force is derived from the Gibbs free energy. Let N denote the inside of a cell, and let P denote the outside. Then:

$$\Delta G = zF\Delta\psi + RT \ln \frac{X^{z+}\ N}{X^{z+}\ P}$$

where,

ΔG is the Gibbs free energy change per unit amount of cations transferred from P to N.

z is the charge number of the cation X^{z+}.

$\Delta\psi$ is the electric potential of N relative to P.

$[X^{z+}]_P$ and $[X^{z+}]_N$ are the cation concentrations at P and N, respectively.

F is the Faraday constant.

R is the gas constant.

T is the temperature.

The molar Gibbs free energy change ΔG is frequently interpreted as a molar electrochemical ion potential $\Delta\mu_{X^{z+}} = \Delta G$.

For an electrochemical proton gradient $z = 1$ and as a consequence:

$$\Delta\mu_{H^+} = F\Delta\psi + RT\ln\frac{[H^+]_N}{[H^+]_P} = F\Delta\psi - (\ln 10)\, RT\Delta pH$$

where,

$$\Delta pH = pH_N - pH_P$$

Mitchell defined the proton-motive force (PMF) as:

$$\Delta p = -\frac{\Delta\mu_{H^+}}{F}$$

For example, $\Delta\mu_{H^+} = 1$ kJ mol^{-1} implies $\Delta p = 10.4$ mV. At 298 K this equation takes the form:

$$\Delta p = -\Delta\psi + (59.1\text{ mV})\,\Delta pH$$

Note that for spontaneous proton import from the P side (relatively more positive and acidic) to the N side (relatively more negative and alkaline), $\Delta\mu_{H+}$ is negative (similar to ΔG) whereas PMF is positive (similar to redox cell potential ΔE).

A diagram of chemiosmotic phosphorylation is shown in Fig. 12.2.

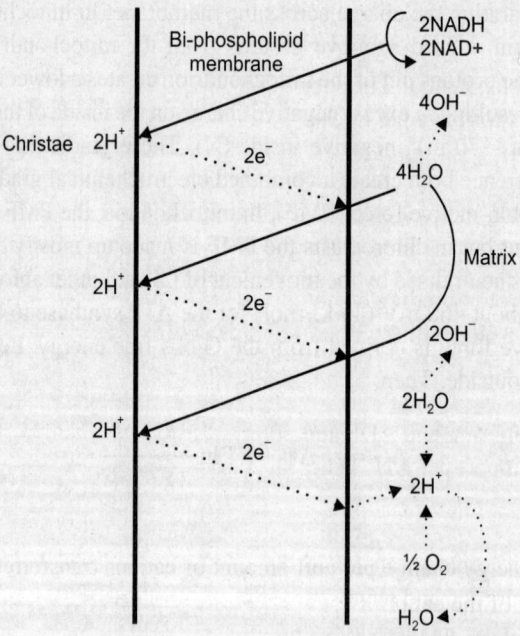

Fig. 12.2: A diagram of chemiosmotic phosphorylation.

It is worth noting that, as with any transmembrane transport process, the PMF is directional. The sign of the transmembrane electric potential difference $\Delta\psi$ is chosen to represent the change in potential energy per unit charge flowing into the cell as above. Furthermore, due to redox-driven proton pumping by coupling sites, the proton gradient is always inside-alkaline. For both of these reasons, protons flow in spontaneously, from the P side to the N side, the available free energy is used to synthesise ATP. For this reason, PMF is defined for proton import, which is spontaneous. PMF for proton export, i.e. proton pumping as catalysed by the coupling sites, is simply the negative of PMF (import).

The spontaneity of proton import (from the P to the N side) is universal in all bioenergetic membranes. This fact was not recognised before the 1990s, because the chloroplast thylakoid lumen was interpreted as an interior phase, but in fact it is topologically equivalent to the exterior of the chloroplast. Azzone and others stressed that the inside phase (N side of the membrane) is the bacterial cytoplasm, mitochondrial matrix, or chloroplast stroma, the outside (P) side is the bacterial periplasmic space, mitochondrial intermembrane space, or chloroplast lumen. Furthermore, 3D tomography of the mitochondrial inner membrane shows its extensive invaginations to be stacked, similar to thylakoid disks, hence the mitochondrial intermembrane space is topologically quite similar to the chloroplast lumen.

The energy expressed here as Gibbs free energy, electrochemical proton gradient, or proton-motive force (PMF), is a combination of two gradients across the membrane:

- The concentration gradient (via ΔpH).
- Electric potential gradient $\Delta\psi$.

When a system reaches equilibrium, $\Delta p = 0$, nevertheless, the concentrations on either side of the membrane need not be equal. Spontaneous movement across the potential membrane is determined by both concentration and electric potential gradients.

The molar Gibbs free energy ΔG_p of ATP synthesis.

$$ADP^{4-} + H^+ + HOPO_3^{2-} \longrightarrow ATP^{4-} + H_2O$$

is also called phosphorylation potential. The equilibrium concentration ratio $[H^+]/[ATP]$ can be calculated by comparing Δp, and ΔG_p, for example in case of the mammalian mitochondrion:

$$H^+/ATP = \Delta G_p/(\Delta p/10.4 \text{ kJ·mol}^{-1}/\text{mV})$$

$$= 40.2 \text{ kJ·mol}^{-1}/(173.5 \text{ mV}/10.4 \text{ kJ·mol}^{-1}/\text{mV})$$

$$= 40.2/16.7 = 2.4.$$

The actual ratio of the proton-binding c-subunit to the ATP-synthesising beta-subunit copy numbers is $8/3 = 2.67$, showing that under these conditions, the mitochondrion functions at 90% (2.4/2.67) efficiency.

In fact, the thermodynamic efficiency is lower in eukaryotic cells because ATP must be exported from the matrix to the cytoplasm, and ADP and phosphate must be imported from the cytoplasm. This 'costs' one 'extra' proton import per ATP, hence the actual efficiency is only 65% (= 2.4/3.67).

In Mitochondria

Directions of chemiosmotic proton transfer in the mitochondrion, chloroplast and in gram-negative bacterial cells (cellular respiration and photosynthesis). The bacterial cell wall is omitted, gram-positive bacterial cells do not have outer membrane is shown in Fig. 12.3. The complete breakdown of glucose in the presence of oxygen is called cellular respiration. The last steps of this process occur in mitochondria.

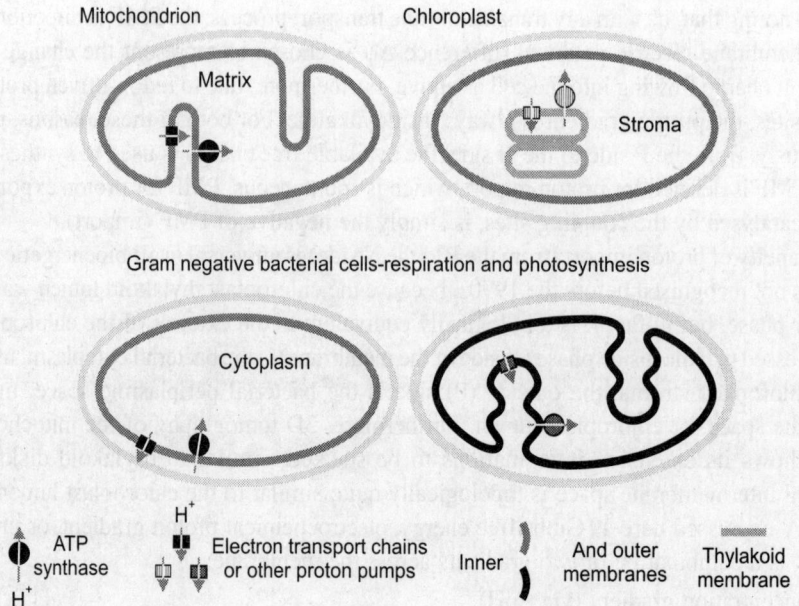

Fig. 12.3: Directions of chemiosmotic proton transfer in the mitochondrion, chloroplast and in gram-negative bacterial cells (cellular respiration and photosynthesis). The bacterial cell wall is omitted, gram-positive bacterial cells do not have outer membrane.

The reduced molecules NADH and $FADH_2$ are generated by the Krebs cycle, glycolysis, and pyruvate processing. These molecules pass electrons to an electron transport chain, which uses the energy released to create a proton gradient across the inner mitochondrial membrane. ATP synthase then uses the energy stored in this gradient to make ATP. This process is called oxidative phosphorylation because it uses energy released by the oxidation of NADH and $FADH_2$ to phospolyrise ADP into ATP.

EXAMPLES OF CHEMIOSMOSIS

Although chemiosmosis is often generally defined as the movement of ions across a membrane, it is really only used in the context of talking about the movement of H^+ ions during the production of ATP. The most common method involving chemiosmosis in the production of ATP is cellular respiration in the mitochondria, the process of which is discussed above. All eukaryotic organisms have mitochondria, so chemiosmosis is involved in ATP production through cellular respiration in the vast majority of different types of organisms, from animals to plants to fungi to protists. However, even though *archaea* and bacteria do not have mitochondria, they also use chemiosmosis to produce ATP through photophosphorylation. This process also involves an electron transport chain, proton gradient, and chemiosmosis of H^+, but it takes place across the inner membrane of the bacterium or *archaeon*, since they have no mitochondria.

In Plants

The light reactions of photosynthesis generate ATP by the action of chemiosmosis. The photons in sunlight are received by the antenna complex of Photosystem II, which excites electrons to a higher energy level. These electrons travel down an electron transport chain, causing protons to be actively pumped across the thylakoid membrane into the thylakoid lumen. These protons then flow down their electrochemical potential gradient through an enzyme called ATP-synthase, creating ATP by the phosphorylation of ADP to ATP. The electrons from the initial light reaction reach Photosystem I, then are raised to a higher energy level by light energy and then received by an electron acceptor and reduce NADP$^+$ to NADPH. The electrons lost from Photosystem II get replaced by the oxidation of water, which is 'split' into protons and oxygen by the oxygen-evolving complex (OEC, also known as WOC, or the water-oxidising complex). To generate one molecule of diatomic oxygen, 10 photons must be absorbed by photosystems I and II, four electrons must move through the two photosystems, and 2 NAPDH are generated (later used for carbon dioxide fixation in the Calvin Cycle).

Plants produce ATP during photosynthesis in the chloroplast in addition to the ATP they generate through cellular respiration in mitochondria. The process is again similar: during photosynthesis, light energy excites electrons, which flow down an electron transport chain, which in turn allows H$^+$ ions to travel through a membrane in the chloroplast. Some bacteria, such as cyanobacteria, also use photosynthesis. The similarities between these ATP production methods are more than just coincidence, both mitochondria and chloroplasts are thought to have evolved from free-living bacteria. This theory is called the endosymbiotic theory. This theory hypothesises that had symbiotic relationships with other cells, aiding them by producing energy in return for a place to live inside the cell. Over time, these bacteria became inextricable from the cells they resided in. The fact that mitochondria and chloroplasts have their own, separate, DNA supports this idea. This is why the chemiosmosis is used in generally the same way whether ATP is being produced in a mitochondrion, chloroplast, or bacterium.

In Prokaryotes

Chemiosmotic coupling between the energy of sunlight, bacteriorhodopsin and phosphorylation (chemical energy) during photosynthesis in halophilic bacteria Halobacterium salinarum (syn. H. halobium). The bacterial cell wall is omitted.

Bacteria and *archaea* also can use chemiosmosis to generate ATP. Cyanobacteria, green sulphur bacteria, and purple bacteria synthesise ATP by a process called photophosphorylation. These bacteria use the energy of light to create a proton gradient using a photosynthetic electron transport chain. Non-photosynthetic bacteria such as *E. coli* also contain ATP synthase. In fact, mitochondria and chloroplasts are the product of endosymbiosis and trace back to incorporated prokaryotes. This process is described in the endosymbiotic theory. The origin of the mitochondrion triggered the origin of eukaryotes, and the origin of the plastid the origin of the *Archaeplastida*, one of the major eukaryotic supergroups.

Chemiosmotic phosphorylation is the third pathway that produces ATP from inorganic phosphate and an ADP molecule. This process is part of oxidative phosphorylation.

CHEMIOSMOTIC COUPLING IN OXIDATIVE PHOSPHORYLATION

Understanding how biological systems convert and store energy is a primary goal of biological research. However, despite the formulation of Mitchell's chemiosmotic theory, which allowed taking fundamental steps forward, we are still far from the complete decryption of basic processes as oxidative phosphorylation (OXPHOS) and photosynthesis. After more than half a century, the chemiosmotic theory appears to need updating, as some of its assumptions have proven incorrect in the light of the latest structural data on respiratory chain complexes, bacteriorhodopsin and proton pumps. Moreover, the existence of an OXPHOS on the plasma membrane of cells casts doubt on the possibility to build up a transversal proton gradient across it, while paving the way for important applications in the field of neurochemistry and oncology. Up-to date biotechnologies, such as fluorescence indicators can follow proton displacement and sinks, and a number of reports have elegantly demonstrated that proton translocation is lateral rather than transversal with respect to the coupling membrane. Furthermore, the definition of the physical species involved in the transfer (proton, hydroxonium ion or proton currents) is still unresolved even though the latest acquisitions support the idea that protonic currents, difficult to measure, are involved. It seems that the concept of diffusion of the proton expressed more than two centuries ago by Theodour von Grotthuss, is decisive for overcoming these issues. All these uncertainties remember us that also in biology it is necessary to take into account the Heisenberg indeterminacy principle, that sets limits to analytical questions.

The 'chemiosmotic theory' formulated by Peter Mitchell, a Researcher with an Anglo-Saxon training in chemistry, dates back to more than 60 years. The theory has universally been accepted since, although it immediately raised several controversies, which they lasted until today. An upgrading of the chemiosmotic theory appears necessary, having the enormous progress. The bioanalytic techniques defined the fine structure of the macromolecular complexes involved in oxidative phosphorylation (OXPHOS). This allows getting further insight into the real proton pathway, a key issue of the theory. In all evidence, it appears that a free proton osmosis would be impossible, as the proton has a huge destructive force and therefore would destroy any biological membrane it passes through. Moreover, in the last years, studies carried out by several laboratories allowed to overcome a basic postulate of the chemiosmotic theory according to which the aerobic synthesis of ATP is characterised by the need of closed compartments. In fact, it was demonstrated that many biological membranes, devoid of closed compartments and of mitochondria, conduct OXPHOS with high efficiency, challenging the idea that it is exclusive of mitochondria, thylakoid and bacteria. Of particular interest are the reports of the ability of plasma membranes to synthesise ATP outside the cell, as they harbour the five complexes of respiration.

The existence of an extra-mitochondrial aerobic ATP synthesis–driven by a machinery very similar to that expressed in mitochondria– challenges the concept of a transversal proton gradient built up across the cell wall with protons gathered on the outer side. New paradigms are needed to explain the basic mechanisms of aerobic metabolism. Scientist and researchers debate the possibility to update the chemiosmotic theory, understanding the ultimate proton role, which could help in developing new strategies for innovative research centered on cellular bioenergetics.

Chemiosmotic Theory and F_1F_o-ATP Synthase

The 1961 basic formulation of Mitchell's theory, where ATP synthase is also indicated, differently from the original formulation where it, necessarily, was not depicted. In the original formulation, ATP synthesis was attributed to the membrane as a whole, as a generic subtraction of H^+ and OH^- 60 to ADP and orthophosphate to form ATP.

The theory is based on three basic postulates:

1. An electron transport chain that transfers H^+ from one side to other side of the membrane.
2. ATP synthase synthesises ATP by translocation H^+ and *vice versa* for ATP hydrolysis.
3. Impermeability of the inner mitochondrial membrane to ionic species thereby including protons.

The experimental data in support of the theory came successively and are reported in literature as a huge amount of contributions. Jagendorf and Uribe, obtained an ATP synthesis inducing a transmembrane leap of pH in chloroplasts *in vitro*. In the same year the Racker and others ascertained that the synthesis of ATP occurred on the so-called 'spheres' referred to as F_1 subunits of the ATP-synthase. Since then the basic contribution of F_1F_o-ATPsynthase to the OXPHOS became clear. Developments in the molecular knowledge regarding F_1F_o-ATP synthase have been comprehensively addressed in many reviews.

The basic requirement for the OXPHOS is a coupling between redox processes, proton translocation and ATP synthesis. The global coupling can arbitrarily be divided in two distinct phases: a coupling between the oxidation-reductive process and the protonic translocation, referred as RedOx.

A delocalised coupling is depicted among proton extruded by the electron transport chain (ETC) and ATP synthesis. The overall process is arbitrarily divided in the two phases: the 'Coupling RedOx', in which the proton movement is operated by the ETC, and the 'Proton Coupling', in which proton movement is coupled with ATP synthesis, by F_1F_o-ATPsynthase. Coupling' and the coupling between protons accumulated on the p-side of the membrane moving to the n-side through the ATP synthase, which determines the synthesis of ATP, here referred as 'Proton Coupling'. About the first coupling, the recent review the mechanism of coupling between oxido-reduction and proton translocation in respiratory chain enzymes evaluated the main characteristics, the recent experimentation and even the controversies around that. Considerable attention was devoted in the 80s and 90s of last century to clarifying the structural-functional details of the respiratory complexes (I, II, III and IV) and F_1F_o-ATPsynthase (Complex V). Important was the study of respiratory complexes organised in supercomplexes with the demonstration that the loss of their aggregation leads to an increase in the production of reactive oxygen species. The possible participation of Complex V has never been demonstrated. The study of super complexes has also benefited from the extraordinary surveys carried out on X-rays.

By contrast, the 'proton coupling' appears to be the most critical passage of the whole OXPHOS process. Literature reports a number of experiments performed with reconstructed systems, i.e. F_1F_o-ATPsynthase incorporated into phospholipid vesicles, carried out about fifteen years after Mitchell's hypothesis. Vesicles obtained from the membranes from the purple Halobacterium salinarium, synthesised ATP as a result of illumination and it was thus demonstrated that illumination moved protons through the membrane supporting the synthesis of ATP. Decisive in 1977 was the reconstitution experiment in artificial membranes of ATP synthase purified by Thermophilic bacterium that synthesised ATP thanks to a transient shift in membrane potential ($\Delta\psi$) induced by valinomycin, allowing rapid passage of K^+ 10^6 ions across a membrane on the sides of which different salt concentrations were set. These experiments demonstrated that proton translocation is the crucial step for the 'Proton Coupling' between protonic movement and ATP synthesis. On this general topic, pivotal is the minireview of Wolfang Junge 10^9, which on one hand enhances the versatility of the F_1F_o-ATPsynthase nano-machine 'unique in converting electrochemical, mechanical and chemical forms of energy' and on the other hand points out that there is still much to be understood about the chemical-physical basis of such process.

CONTROVERSIES ABOUT THE CHEMIOSMOTIC THEORY

A long struggle was necessary for the chemiosmotic theory formulated by Peter Mitchell to be widely accepted. The controversy, central to the history of bioenergetics for more than half a century, appears tackled by more than 200 articles and to have lasted until the most recent years. Giovanni F. Azzone, many years ago published the manuscript 'Oxidative phosphorylation, a history of unsuccessful attempts: is it only an experimental problem?' that already highlighted what did not convince in the theory and that wished for answers from the fine analysis of the macromolecular structures involved in chemiosmosis.

The harshest criticisms came from John Prebble, which emphasised the lack of experimental data in support of the theory. Wolfang Junge effectively described in 2013 the chronicle of the dispute, which even took harsh tones. His review 'Half a century of molecular bioenergetics' examines many issues of bioenergetics, including chemiosmotic theory. Brown and Simcook in their article considered the motivations that have convinced the scientific community to accept the chemiosmotic theory, regardless of great skepticism welcoming it at the beginning. Authors note that: 'science shows tremendous resistance to change and it takes extraordinary perseverance to persuade the community'.

A controversial issue was the correlation between $\Delta\psi$ and the proton motive force, often considered equivalent entities. It was postulated that a $\Delta\psi$ with positive charge on the external p-side of the internal mitochondrial membrane and negative on the n-side in contact with mitochondrial matrix would let protons enter through the rotor F_0 that synthesises ATP in the matrix, thanks to its mechanical connection with the F_1 moiety. Protons would gather across the coupling membrane like chemical ions, creating a driving force for F_1F_0-ATP synthase to synthesise ATP, realising the 'Proton Coupling'. However, the yield in ATP poorly correlates with bulk-to-bulk membrane potential so that the basic chemiosmotic theory appears inadequate.

The awarding of the 1978 Nobel Prize for chemistry to Peter Mitchell cooled the dispute, but not definitively. In fact, in 1979, there was a heated confrontation published by TRENDS between Henry Tedeschi, who disproved the idea that the metabolic activity of mitochondria could contribute to membrane potential and Hagai Rottenberg which instead defended Mitchell's theory. The original theory provides a protonated 'delocalised coupling' while a 'localised coupling' has seen Robert Williams as a great supporter. In the paper 'Proton-Electrostatics Hypothesis for Localised Proton Coupling' J. W. Lee reports a rigorous chemical/physical experiment in favour of localised coupling, demonstrating furthermore that the thylakoid membrane can be a 'proton capacitor'. The putative existence of a proton capacitor is a matter of great importance and later, H. A. Saeed and J. W. Lee showed that protons can actually accumulate on the membrane surface even though they never reside in the aqueous phase. Moreover, concerning the experimental verification of the 'proton coupling', a recent elegant investigation in HeLa cells, bioengineered with green fluorescent protein as pH indicator inserted in respiratory complex III and in F_0 moiety of ATP synthase, points to a localised coupling. A report entitled 'Proton migration along the membrane surface and retarded surface to bulk transfer' by Heberle and others interestingly reconciles the two visions, providing proof that proton transfer from a proton generator (bacteriorhodopsin) to an acceptor, (water-soluble pH indicators) is faster if occurring on the membrane rather than when protons are released in the aqueous bulk. Ferguson emphasised Heberle and others experiments, concluding that the delocalised coupling and lateral proton transfer (localised coupling), between the proton generator and user, occurs very rapidly on the membrane, as compared to the slower and transversal passage through the aqueous bulk. In this context, the recent paper form Von Ballmoos group observed that $\Delta\psi$ and ΔpH are equivalent for the coupling with ATP-synthase. A primary role for membrane buffering on proton mobility in general can be hypothesised. The experimental data showing a close thermodynamic correlation between valinomycin-induced $\Delta\psi$ and ATP synthesis in reconstituted systems are very important, but it seems plausible that they induce a transmembrane protonic flow that probably differs from the path in a native environment. Moreover, the eminent English chemist Robert Williams clearly rejected the hypothesis of the accumulation of protons from p-side: 'the p-phase corresponds to the infinitely extended external space. If protons are extruded into this 'Pacific Ocean', they would be diluted and the entropic component of the pmf would be lost. Williams observed that 'I made it clear that protons in the membrane rather than an osmotic trans-membrane gradient of protons were required to drive ATP formation' based on a series of considerations that excluded the presence of free protons from p-side. An elegant demonstration of Williams's localised coupling hypothesis came in 1976 by an experiment in which purified ATP synthase was added to the octano-water interface. It was observed that protons accumulate in octane, a Brønsted acid, leading to ATP synthesis by ATP synthase. These data have also been recently confirmed. Eighteen years later, it was reported that: 'our results suggest that protons can efficiently diffuse along the membrane surface between a source and a sink (for example H^+-ATP synthase) without dissipation losses into the acqueous bulk'. From all the cited data it can be concluded that protons (or protonic currents) are confined into the membrane, while proton exit from the membrane is to be considered only as a fallback way of escape, mostly *in vitro* reconstituted conditions.

Membrane Potential

A direct measurement of membrane potential of the mitochondrial inner membrane with microelectrodes was only be accomplished by Tedeschi, who showed the existence of a positive inside and negative outside mitochondrial membrane potential ($\Delta\psi$). Such potential (contrary to the canonical) interestingly coincides with that calculated on the basis of the ionic species present on the membrane sides. Clearly, knowledge of the entity and especially the sign of this potential is fundamental for understanding the basic functioning of chemiosmosis, as emerges from the already mentioned historical dispute between Henry Tedeschi and Hagai Rottenberg.

To measure $\Delta\psi$, laboratory tests currently utilise lipophilic fluorescent compounds whose response is considered to be related to $\Delta\psi$. However, tests conducted with rhodamine have cast doubts on such correlation since these indicators inhibited the mitochondrial respiration, so they disturb the system. As such compounds dissolve into the membranes, they may reflect the membrane behaviour, in fact they inhibit a membrane intrinsic process, i.e. the OXPHOS, but do not interfere with $\Delta\psi$. Surely, *in vitro*, proton passage across membranes can be forced with rapid movements of potassium ions by addition of valinomycin.

A laboratory procedure utilising valinomycin and also nigericin has been widely used to create a transient $\Delta\psi$ operating a delocalised coupling linking $\Delta\psi$ and ATP synthesis, but this does not exclude that in the native membranes a localised coupling would operate, independently of $\Delta\psi$.

Crucial Issue: The Membrane Permeability to Protons

In an old study Giovanni Felice Azzone and coll. highlighted the uncertainties of the proton cycle. In the same year Grsesiek and Dencher showed that the phospholipid membranes are intrinsically permeable to protons. Data show that phospholipid membranes, normally impermeant to ionic solutes (transversal or permeability diffusion coefficients varying between 10^{-12} to 10^{-14} cm/sec), exhibit a significant proton permeability, varying from 10^{-3} to 10^{-9} cm/sec. Such variability may be justified by a buffering capacity of the membranes for protons: proton diffusion value could depend on the higher or lower degree of pre-existing protonation.

Recently, the proton leak through lipid bilayers was modelled as a concerted mechanism. Tepper and Voth provided a theoretical interpretation of proton permeability, based on the formation of transient membrane spanning aqueous solvent structure. High proton permeability has also been confirmed in liposomes, independently form their phospholipid composition. It is clear that a high degree of permeability to protons is *per se* in contrast to the third of the aforementioned basic postulates of the chemiosmotic theory. With regard to the relationship between membrane and aqueous phase, many observations confirm the existence of a layer of water molecules on the two sides of the membrane which to some extent isolate it from the aqueous phases present on its two sides.

Proton Solvation

The actual proton path across the membrane, their putative concentration on both sides of the membrane and the consequent membrane potential have been the object of countless studies. A central issue is the knowledge of the actual chemical species of the proton: free, or in the form of H_3O^+. This depends on the phase in which the proton is located. Protons possess peculiar chemical properties, being essentially an atomic nucleus. Free protons do not exist in the aqueous phase, being solvated to H_3O^+, from which the extraction of a proton would be virtually impossible. In fact, in the transition from H_3O^+ to free proton a strong energy barrier higher than 500 meV, must be overcome as specified in the paper: 'Proton in the well and through the desolvation barrier', which corresponds to the enormous amount of 262.4 Cal/mol. An immense literature exists on the subject. An interesting report, not sufficiently taken into account, calculated the number of free protons (actually in the form of H_3O^+) in the volume of a mitochondrion, which is of the femto Liter order of magnitude. This study demonstrated, starting from basic physical chemical data (Avogadro number, ionic water product, mathematical pH expression and mitochondrial volume), that free protons in a mitochondrial periplasmic space are too few (less than ten) to support any process dependent on proton translocation in the aqueous bulk across the membrane and absolutely inadequate to support the thousands of ATP synthase molecules present in a mitochondrion. Moreover, the pH value inside the mitochondrion resulted to differ by 0.5 units from what previously believed. Moreover, the huge energy associated with proton solvation would have a negative consequence: a free membrane proton would quickly be 'sucked' by the near aqueous phase, releasing the huge energy associated with the solvation process, to the detriment of the membrane.

Grotthuss Mechanism and Proton Translocation through the Membranes

A putative mechanism for proton diffusion was hypothesised more than two centuries ago by Theodour von Grotthuss and is synthetically explained by Kreuer: 'Proton diffusion according to the Grotthuss mechanism occurs much faster than molecular diffusion because it is uncoupled from the self-diffusion of its mass'. Protons would not diffuse as a mass, rather as a charge, the latter moving between water molecules or protonable groups of suitable macromolecules of the membranes. The Grotthuss mechanism allows better understanding of the possible ways in which protons or species derived from them move in biological systems. DeCoursey published a review entitled 'Voltage-gated proton channels and other proton transfer pathways', which exhaustively analyses proton movement in water and biological membranes, including HV1 channels which specifically transfer protons in aqueous phase, therefore actual acidity from one side of the membrane to the other. The mechanism of the voltage gated proton channel HV1 is not as yet resolved, as emblematically stated by DeCoursey in the paper entitled 'The voltage-gated proton channel: a riddle, wrapped in a mystery, inside an enigma'. Two mechanisms have been proposed for HV1 as 267 schematically depicted in Fig. 12.4, where on the left side is represented the so-called 'frozen water' mechanism, in which the channel traps one or more molecules of water which allows protons to pass through with Grotthuss-style proton hopping, as in the typical case of Gramicidin. On the right side of Fig. 12.4 is depicted a passage of proton with protonation/deprotonation of ammino acid side-chain, that would realise the so-called 'proton wire', already proposed in the 1978 paper 'Molecular mechanisms for proton transport in membranes' by Nagle and Morowitz. The topic was consolidated successively by Nagle and Nagle. DeCoursey in a debate recently published on the Journal of Physiology supports the mechanism shown in the right part of Fig. 12.4 that provides the action of proton wires through the membrane, while Bennettt and Ramsey support a mechanism of passage through molecule of water as schematised on the left of Fig. 12.4. Interestingly, both mechanisms

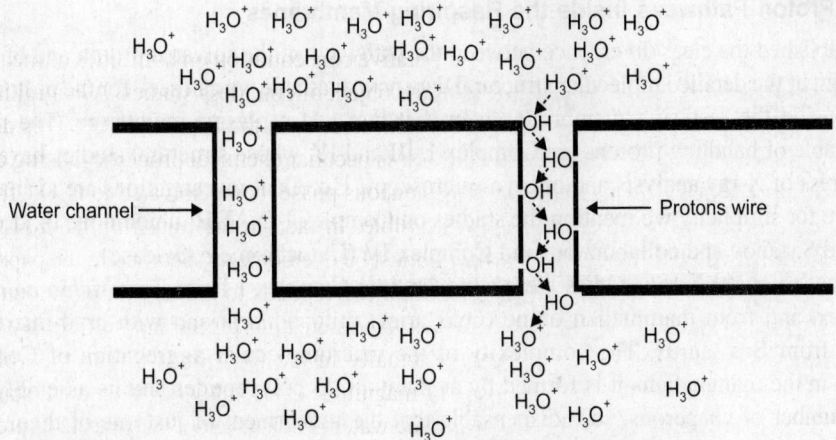

Fig. 12.4: Mechanism for H⁺ transfer through the membrane by HV1. Left, water channel model: the water molecules allow protons to pass through with Grotthuss-style H⁺ hopping. Right, proton wire model: a charge migration occurs (through with Grotthuss-style H⁺ hopping) on polar groups of side chains of amino acids of HV1.

are based on the Grotthuss proton movement between (i) water molecules in the case of the water channel (on the left) and (ii) between side chains of amino acids in the case of protons wires (on the right).

The proton movement in membranes (both biological and artificial) has been analysed by many rigorous chemical/physical studies. The article 'Proton Holes' in Long-Range Proton Transfer Reactions in Solution and Enzymes: A Theoretical Analysis- shows that other compounds in addition to water are involved in the 'proton hopping', and is interesting that a quantum-mechanical approach is applied. The article 'Grotthuss mechanisms: from proton transport in proton wires to bioprotonic devices' presents devices such as proton diodes, transistors, memories and transducers, semiconductor electronic devices that use the Grotthus mechanism.

Notably, HV1 only allows the passage of protons balancing their concentration between two aqueous compartments separated by a membrane. This property does depend on the membrane potential Δψ, similarly to other ion membrane devices abundant in biological membranes (for example the Na⁺ and K⁺ 293 voltage gated channels), acting exclusively on the conformation of the HV1 protein. It appears therefore that to carry protons through the membrane there are adhoc structures that deeply differ from the respiratory complexes, both for the function finality, and for the molecular mechanism. Moreover, the process would be quantitatively linked to an unwanted acidification of a closed compartment. From these and other evidences it can be concluded that the native proton movements in the respiring membranes, when there is no need for acidification of the milieu on one side of a membrane, must take place entirely inside the membrane. As far as the respiratory complexes are concerned, on the other hand, it is theorised that the proton and membrane potential movements are mutually dependent, in that the pumping of protons would generate the membrane potential, which is impossible for thermodynamic considerations that we will elaborate later on.

Moreover this comparison between proton movement in support of the OXPHOS and the actual protonic movement in nature sheds light on the fact that when protons are really transferred through a membrane: (i) they are never in the form of free protons and (ii) are subject to the Grotthuss-style proton hopping. Hence the need for chemiosmotic theory to be revised in the light of all this emerges.

Plausible Proton Pathways inside the Respiring Membranes

Having established the clear divergence between the pathways of the solvated proton and of the proton alone, in light of the detailed molecular structural data now available we can seek for the proton plausible pathways inside the respiring membrane, even if it is a just a plasma-membrane. The respiratory complexes able of handling protons are Complex I, III and IV, whose structural studies have benefited of the progress of X-ray analysis and of cryo-microscopy. Excellent investigations are available on the subject, here for simplicity we mention the studies on Complex I (NADH: ubiquinone oxidoreductase) from Leonid Sazanov and collaborators and Complex IV (Cytochrome *c* Oxidase).

Numerous structural X-ray studies were conducted on Complex I from *Escherichia coli, Thermus thermophiles*, and from mammalian ovine (Ovis aries) mitochondria and with cryo-microscopy on Complex I from Bos taurus. The complexity of the macromolecular aggregation of Complex I is impressive: in the mammalians it is formed by as many as 45 polypeptides and its assembly needs an unknown number of chaperons, so indispensable that the impairment of just one of them (B17.2L) causes of a progressive encephalopathy. Authors state that: 'results demonstrate that B17.2L is a bona fide molecular chaperone that is essential for the assembly of complex I and for the normal function of the nervous system.' As only 5 alpha-helices have been found in the Complex I structure, in order to allow for proton translocation, it was necessary to postulate the existence of two hemi channels: one from the matrix (n) side to the centre of the respiratory complex, referred here to as the 'proton entrance hemi channel' and the other from the centre to the periplasmatic (p) side here indicated as 'proton exit hemi channel'. However, only the latter was well identifiable in Complex I. Instead, the entry pathway has not been identified with certainty so much so that we only can talk about putative pathways labelled with "? ". Furthermore, it clearly emerges from the X-ray studies that there is an obvious proton tunnelling at the centre of the Complex I. Comprehensive studies on the protonic movement inside Complex I have been carried out by the Helsinki Bioenergetic Group of Martin Wikström, which highlighted uncertainty margins on the stoichiometry of protonic extrusion that appears closer to 3 $H^+/2e^-$ instead to the classic 4 $H^+/2e^-$. Also, in the review di Verkhovskaya and Bloch (of Helsinki Bioenergetic Group) four mechanisms for proton translocation are proposed and the 'proton entrance half channel' is not identified with certainty, while the 'proton exit half channel' is clearly identifiable. Emblematically on the website of the Helsinki Bioenergetic Group it is written 'the mechanism of proton transfer in Complex I remains completely enigmatic'.

As far as Complex IV (Cytochrome c-oxidase) is concerned, the proton translocation of has been studied in depth. In their recent review, Martin Wikström and Vivek Sharma talk of an 'anniversary': 'Proton pumping by cytochrome c oxidase - A 40 year anniversary'. Among the many quotations in this review the Chemical Review of the Wikström group stands out. It goes into the details of the possible molecular processes carried out by Complex IV, thereby including proton translocation. The topic is complex and more putative pathway of protons are well developed in the review. For the 'proton entrance half channel' for each molecule of oxygen reduced to water they need 4 H^+ and it is hypothesised that another 4 H^+ for a total of 8 enter through this channel. It seems unlikely that there exists equivalence between protons that exist as mass and link to water molecules, and protons that should move as a charge, according to the Grotthuss mechanism.

Proposal for a Localised Complex I-ATP Synthase Coupling

Taking into account what reported above, it is possible to trace a plausible proton pathway within the respiring membrane. Just in 2006 a direct proton transfer was proposed to couple the Complexes I, III,

IV respiratory pathway with F_oF_1-ATP Synthase. However, in a recent review the concept of transmembrane proton motor force to move the ATP Synthase is reinforced, although it is noted that many aspects of coupling are not yet clarified. Clear cut consideration was proposed some years ago by Akeson and Deamer about speed of proton translocation through putative proton channel as limiting step for ATP synthesis by F_oF_1 ATP-synthase. For the sake of simplicity, we only examine the coupling between the Respiratory Complex I and the F_1F_o-ATP synthase. The existence of a proton pathway at the centre of Complex I is quite clear, and we can hypothesise that the protons are sent to the well-identified four 'exit half channel', as shown in Fig. 12.5. The proton donor at the centre of Complex I has already been tentatively identified in the phospholipid cardiolipin (CL), which appears essential for the OXPHOS.

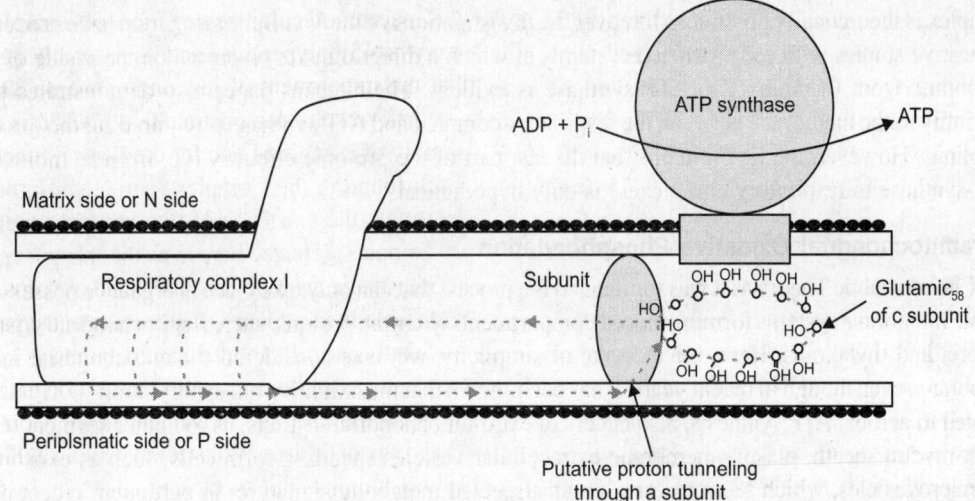

Fig 12.5: A possible H^+ circuit inside respiring membrane. The water insulating shield on both side of the membrane are shown by blue ellipsoids. The image proposes that the H^+ (grey dotted line) are transferred to the Glu 58 (E58) at the centre of subunit c through subunit a of ATP synthase by proton tunnelling. H^+ would flow from the periplasmic side, always bound to phospholipid heads. This can be arranged in each layer of the membrane.

However, for example, phosphatidylethanolamine (PE) is a valid phospholipid for the functioning of the OXPHOS. The experimentation recently carried out by Von Ballmoos group is clear, and also unconventional, on the role played by phospholipids. In fact, pure phosphatidylcholine (PC) is excellent for the coupling, while it increases when the membrane is formed by PC + PE. By contrast, it is dramatically inhibited if the membrane is formed by PC + CL, incredibly diverging from the traditional role assigned to CL.

This research is also important because experiments are performed with a reconstructed system, more adherent to the 'H^+/ATP coupling'. Here, the driving force that feeds ATP synthase was not the rapid transfer of K^+ generated by valinomycin, a widely used method. It emerges that all the membrane phospholipids can act as mobile proton transporters, hindering their relocation in the near aqueous medium, so that protons are never free. The exergonic process of proton solvation would release an impressive amount of energy (262.4 Cal/mol) which, if not transferred on a generic acceptor, would generate heat, devastating not only for the membrane but also for the whole cell integrity. Complex I would transfer protons to the p side of the membrane, but these would not be dispersed in the aqueous bulk. In fact it is well documented the existence of a barrier of water molecules attached to the membrane, determining the lateral displacement of protons on the phosphate heads of phospholipids to meet a sink that is the ATP synthase subunit that through a proton wire would leads the proton to the rotor, accommodating on the central glutamic or aspartic residue (depending on the species) of the c subunit which in variable numbers from 8 to 15 make up the rotor F_0. As F_0 rotates it is conceivable that the proton returns to the centre of Complex I, an highly hydrophobic environment, thus closing the protonic circuit. This last passage, from the rotor exit to the centre of the respiratory complex, appears plausible, for the operativity of the Brownian motion (diffusion) of particles in a highly anisotropic environment that can occurs efficiently and a direct passage of the proton exiting the subunit at the entrance to the Complex is theoretically possible. Moreover the investigations of the Von Ballmoos group have produced exhaustive studies with reconstructed systems, in which a direct transfer of proton on the p-side of the membrane from Complex I to ATP-synthase is evident. Their recent paper also demonstrates that proximity to the membrane between the respiratory complex and ATP synthase is required for the 'proton coupling'. However, the fact remains that the last part of the protonic circuitry (i.e. from F_0 moiety of ATP-synthase to respiratory complexes) is only hypothetical.

Extramitochondrial Oxidative Phosphorylation

The Chemiosmotic Theory as it was formulated is a process that can only take place in organelle possessing double membrane systems forming closed compartments to entrap protons, such as mitochondrial cristae, bacteria and thylakoids. Here, for the sake of simplicity, we have considered the mitochondrial inner membrane, even though in recent years, it has been shown that the oxidative phosphorylation (OXPHOS), coupled to aerobic ATP synthesis, also occurs in extra-mitochondrial districts, as rod outer segment (OS) disks, myelin sheath, plasma membrane extracellular vesicles shedding form cells, such as exosomes and microvesicles, which seem to carry an unsuspected metabolic signature. In particular, recent data indicate an active extramitochondrial OXPHOS in the endoplasmic reticulum of platelets which both have elevated ATP need but possess very little mitochondria. It is worth noting that photoreceptor OS, specialised subcellular compartment that contains lesser molecular system as compared to bulk cytosol, have allowed important discoveries. In fact, Transducin, discovered in the rod OS in 1981, is considered the G protein prototype, in 1986 the OS were proven to contain a considerable amount of the second messenger cyclic GMP and finally in 2009 data emerged accomplishing the discovery of an extra-mitochondrial OXPHOS, coupled to aerobic ATP synthesis in the OS.

Interestingly, the synthesis of extracellular ATP by F_1F_0-ATPsynthase on plasma membrane has been recently demonstrated in human neutrophils confirming data previously obtained. Since the plasma membrane potential is positive on the outside and negative on the inside, it would favor the ATP hydrolysis rather than the synthesis. This datum is in line with the postulated independence of F_1F_0-ATPsynthase activity from the membrane potential and therefore it is plausible that this synthesis of ATP depends on the proton intramembranous coupling.

To sum up, impressive amount of experimental data cited appears globally in contrast with the above cited three assumptions underlying the chemiosmotic theory.

First of all, it excludes that the protons can accumulate on the coupling membrane surface, whose high permeability would dissipate, and essentially since it would correspond to an extreme acidity incompatible with any vital process.

Secondly, since diffusion does occur, it is clear that the membrane potential is irrelevant to translocation.

Thirdly, it can be excluded that the respiratory complexes operate a transmembrane proton transfer from the aqueous bulk, where the proton would exist as hydroxonium ion.

This appears to rule out the actual possibility that ATP synthase can overcome the energy barrier, higher than 500 meV required to extract the proton from water, leaving space for the localised coupling hypothesis as dehydration/hydration reaction from hydroxonium ion to free protons would require 262.4 Cal/mol. Which are the actual processes acting on the $F_o F_1$-ATP synthase? There is no certainty, as highlighted by the emblematic title of an article by John Walker 'The ATP synthase: the understood, the uncertain and the unknown'. In this controversial scenario a decisive contribution is undoubtedly the sophisticated bioengineering experiment that labelled the IV respiratory complex and ATP-Synthase with proteins of the GFP family, to experimentally observe a local ΔpH triggered by the respiratory substrate galactose. Observations were conducted in cultured HeLa cells. The authors conclude: 'the observed lateral variation in the proton-motive force necessitates a modification to Peter Mitchell's chemiosmotic proposal'. The experimentally proven lateral proton motive force is in line with the hypothesis of localised coupling. Indeed, today a constellation of clues leads us to hypothesise the existence of protonic currents internal to the membrane, with the formation of possible circuits travelled by the positive elementary charge, thus realising a localised coupling that excludes an osmotic nature of the process. To trace this circuit, at least for the possible coupling between respiratory Complex I and ATP-synthase it appears realistic that Complex I may transfer protons from its central part to the periplasmatic side, allowing them to travel on the membrane surface thanks to the heads of phospholipids finally entering by tunnelling in the subunit a of the ATP-synthase. Moreover several studies show that the membrane is isolated from the aqueous bulk thanks to a layer of water molecules on both sides of the membrane, which consolidates the idea that the membrane is radically distinct and isolated from the liquid phase. Considering the isolated two phases, the only way evolution could pursue to link proton movement to ATP synthesis was a nanomachine connecting the proton movement inside the membrane to the deformation mechanics of the F_1 sphere immersed in the aqueous phase.

Thus, it can be reasonably assume that the proton movement inside the membranes occurs as a charge, according to the proton hopping Grotthuss mechanism with the establishment of 'protonic currents' inside the membrane. In the non-biological field we find a remarkable adherence to this theory for the development of protonic devices (as proton diodes, transistors, memories and transducers, semiconductor electronic) that could replace devices widely used in electronics. It is surprising that the two areas, the biological and the physical-chemical one, have ignored each other. Since in the history of biology the application of physico-chemical methodologies has led to dramatic advances in biology.

Thus, it is desirable that this fusion of knowledge can be realised in the years to come. Furthermore, the classical mechanical approach cannot be used to approach these currents. In fact, any time there is a movement of charge bound to a mass, the dualism that cannot be assessed by classical mechanics, instead quantum mechanics must be applied, and in this perspective lay the promising recent quantum-mechanical approach by Ivontsin and others. There is the need to take into account the Heisenberg indeterminacy principle as Philip Hunter already highlighted: 'A quantum leap in biology. One inscrutable field helps another, as quantum physics unravels consciousness'.

Chapter 13

Antimetabolites and Chemotherapy

INTRODUCTION

An antimetabolite is a chemical that inhibits the use of a metabolite, which is another chemical that is part of normal metabolism. Such substances are often similar in structure to the metabolite that they interfere with, such as the antifolates that interfere with the use of folic acid; thus, competitive inhibition can occur, and the presence of antimetabolites can have toxic effects on cells, such as halting cell growth and cell division, so these compounds are used as chemotherapy for cancer.

In recent years much study has been directed at the antimetabolites. These compounds have two distinguishing features: (i) they resemble in chemical structure some naturally occurring compound which is essential in living processes, and (ii) they specifically antagonise the biological action of such an essential compound.

The vitally essential compounds have been called 'essential metabolites' and are exemplified by the vitamins, the hormones, and certain other substances. The net result of the interference of the antimetabolite with the essential metabolite is to bring about a deficiency of the essential metabolite. The consequences of such a deficiency may be far reaching for the organism and may bring about its death. These effects can, however, be beneficial, and it is this fact which has led to the use of the antimetabolites in attempts to treat disease. The purpose of this chapter is to give some indication of what the antimetabolites are, and of the sort of thing that is being done with them, both in the elucidation of the mechanisms by means of which living things carry out their physiological reactions, and in the practical applications to the treatment of disease.

ENZYME FUNCTION

To understand what an antimetabolite is, we must recall how an enzyme functions. An enzyme is believed to bring about the specific chemical reaction which it catalyses by combining reversibly with its particular substrate. For many of the enzymes this specific substrate is one of the essential metabolites such as a vitamin, a purine, or an amino acid. The unstable enzyme substrate complex which is thus formed undergoes some sort of molecular rearrangement or fission which yields the products derived from the substrate plus the enzyme. The cycle is then repeated because the enzyme has not been consumed in the process.

The enzyme usually has two substrates instead of one, but this does not alter the mechanism now under discussion, since for the second substrate one conceives of the same basic process, but of a different combining site in the protein. The specificity of the enzyme depends on its ability to combine with a given substrate, and not to combine with unrelated substances. The nature of the combining groups of the enzymes is one of the most fascinating puzzles of biochemistry.

Some beginnings have been made in understanding the chemical structures of such combining groups of a few enzymes, but for none is it yet possible to write an adequate structure. It must be for each enzyme a configuration such as to form a reversible, dissociable union with a specific compound (the substrate) and not with many other substances.

In addition to its substrate, an enzyme usually will combine reversibly with a few structural relatives of the substrate. If the relative is of the same general structure (shape) and has some of the functional groups which are also present in the substrate, the fit is frequently good enough so that the analog will combine with the specific site in the enzyme. This is the first requisite of an antimetabolite. It must 'look like' the substrate to the enzyme, in other words, the enzyme will combine with it in the same fashion as it does with the substrate. The structural analogy with the substrate is the important concern.

When the analog (the antimetabolite) has combined with the active site of the enzyme, this site is occupied so that the normal substrate cannot combine. The result is the exclusion of the substrate from its normal role and the creation of a deficiency of it. If the substrate is a vitamin or a hormone, a characteristic deficiency disease may thus be produced by the antimetabolite.

If the union between analog and enzyme is reversible, then an increase in the concentration of the substrate will allow the analog to be displaced. A deficiency disease induced by an antivitamin can thus be prevented or cured merely by an increase in the amount of vitamin in the food. The ratio between analog and essential metabolite which just allows the metabolite to displace the analog is different for each pair of compounds and each enzyme. What determines the ratio required is the relative combining affinities of substrate and analog for the enzyme. Almost always the enzyme prefers the substrate to the analog, so that much more antimetabolite than essential metabolite is required in order to produce a biological effect of the analog. However, it has been possible to construct antimetabolites which the enzyme prefers to its normal substrate, and these are very potent compounds in biological test systems.

The second essential point about a compound which makes it an antimetabolite, then, is the ability to antagonise some of the biological effects of an essential metabolite. To call forth the characteristic signs of a deficiency disease is thus an important property of a compound if it is to be considered an antimetabolite. If, in addition, the biological effects can be reversed by the essential metabolite, the evidence is considerably strengthened. However, it is not necessary that a demonstration be made of the ability of a metabolite to reverse the effects of an antimetabolite, despite the fact that this is a point about which much argument has raged. Some have maintained that without the demonstration of reversibility a compound cannot be considered to be an antimetabolite. The plain fact is that one can construct an analog of some essential metabolite in such a way that it will be attracted specifically to the combining site of the enzyme and will react with this site irreversibly rather than reversibly. Once this has happened, no amount of extra essential metabolite will dislodge it. As might be expected, such irreversible analogs have frequently proved to be of high potency, since they have such an avidity for the enzyme. Some of the antimetabolites now used in the treatment of certain diseases are such irreversibly acting compounds. Aminopterin (Fig. 13.1), which is used with more or less success in the treatment of childhood leukemia, is such an example. Sometimes the analog combines with the enzyme but, instead of stopping things at this stage, is actually converted into products analogous to those formed from the

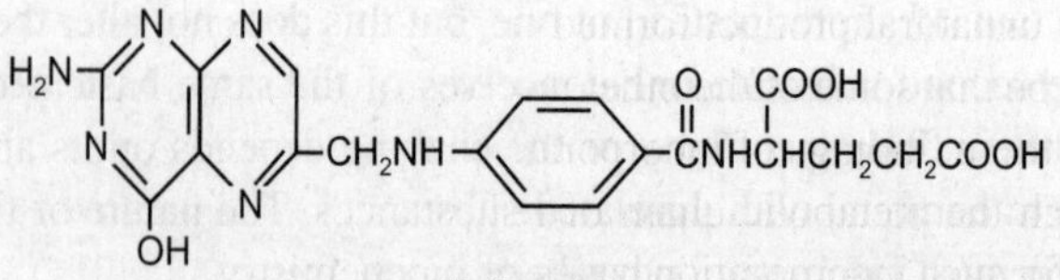

Folic acid

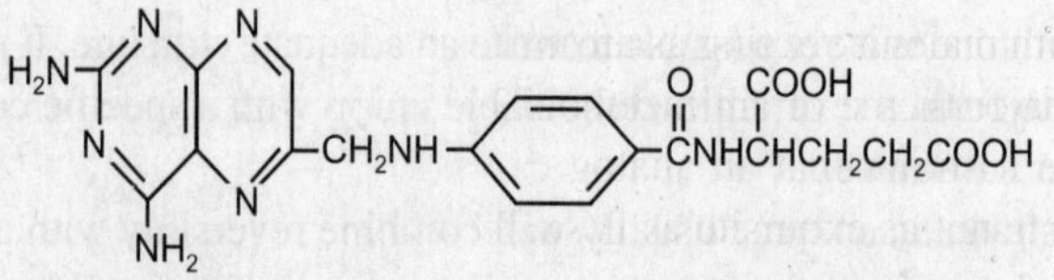

Fig. 13.1: Structures of folic acid and aminopterin.

normal substrate. In other words, the enzyme uses the analog much as it does the natural substrate. The unnatural products formed may now act in the usual way to inhibit the next biological reaction in the physiological pathway. This has been shown to happen with certain analogs of purines and pyrimidines which go into the formation of nucleic acids.

Thus, 8-azaguanine (Fig. 13.2), an analog of guanine, is incorporated into the nucleic acids of bacteria, viruses, and certain other forms of life. The nucleic acids of tobacco mosaic virus can thus be made to contain this unnatural substance. Some evidence suggests that this unnatural virus fails to function normally in the infection of the host plant, although this point is not entirely clear. Similarly, the pyrimidine thymine of the deoxynucleic acid of certain bacteria (*Escherichia coli*) can be partially replaced by the analogous 5-bromouracil (Fig. 13.3). The unnatural nucleic acid is then passed on for generations with each cell division, but the organisms so produced tend to form abnormal (pleomorphic) cell bodies, and to be at other disadvantages.

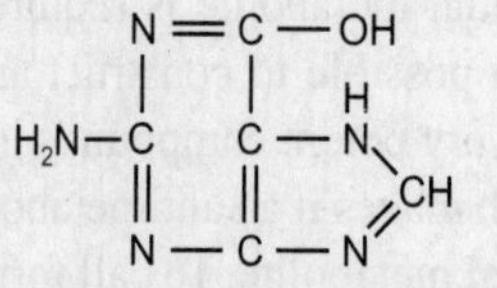

Guanine

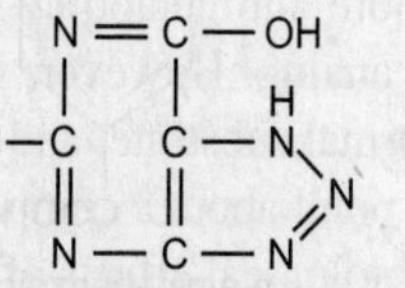

8-Azaguanine

Fig. 13.2: Structures of guanine and 8-azaguanine.

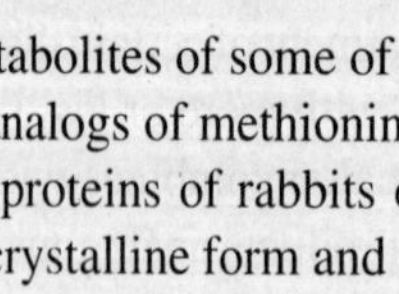

5-Bromouracil

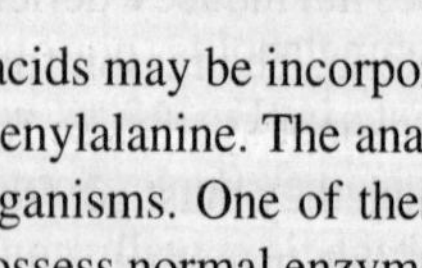

Thymine

Fig. 13.3: Structures of 5-bromouracil and thymine.

In like fashion, antimetabolites of some of the amino acids may be incorporated into proteins, as has been demonstrated with analogs of methionine and of phenylalanine. The analog pfluorophenylalanine is thus incorporated into proteins of rabbits or micro-organisms. One of these unnatural proteins has recently been isolated in crystalline form and shown to possess normal enzymatic activity (aldolase). In this case, therefore, the unnatural product formed from the analog functions in some respects as well as the natural one. It must be that some of the other unnatural products also formed do not function so well. We must not think that these findings of incorporation of analogs mean that all antimetabolites function by being passed through the metabolic chain of reactions usually followed by the substrate. In many instances, no evidence for such incorporation has been found, despite concerted search. In other instances, such incorporation reactions are impossible because of the chemical structures of the analogs. Such, for example, is the case with malonate acting as an antimetabolite of succinate. The incorporation reactions are variations of the major theme of antimetabolite action. However, it is important to remember that they do occur, because it shows that an analog can often function in place of the real substrate. The specificity of enzymes is not as exquisite as is sometimes thought.

Sulfanilamide and Pyrithiamine as Antimetabolites

Two classical examples of antimetabolites can be used to illustrate the basic phenomenon. One of these is sulfanilamide as an antimetabolite of *p*-aminobenzoic acid, and the other is pyrithiamine as an antimetabolite of thiamine. Sulfanilamide, the structure of which is shown in Fig. 13.4, was developed rather empirically as a drug able to control some bacterial infections in man and other animals. Several years after its usefulness had been established, D. D. Woods in 1940 was studying why it inhibited bacterial growth and observed that its harmful effects on micro-organisms could be overcome with small amounts of *p*-aminobenzoic acid. Woods was fully aware of the structural resemblance of sulfanilamide to *p*-aminobenzoic acid, and, in fact, had been led to test *p*-aminobenzoic acid because of the structural resemblance. He predicted that *p*-aminobenzoic acid would be found to be an important compound in the metabolism of bacteria, and this prediction was soon amply substantiated.

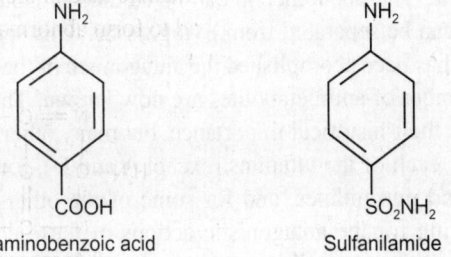

Fig. 13.4: Structure of *p*-aminobenzoic acid and sulfanilamide.

Not only did *p*-aminobenzoic acid prove to be present in many living things in a combined form, but for some it was a dietary essential—that is, it was a vitamin. One of the combined forms into which it was built in living things also proved to be an important substance, namely, the vitamin known as folic acid. It has been demonstrated that in bacteria which are inhibited by sulfanilamide, the formation of folic acid and its derivatives is prevented. The enzyme system which makes this essential metabolite (folic acid) from *p*-aminobenzoic acid seems to be inhibited by sulfanilamide. For this enzyme system, *p*-aminobenzoic acid is the specific substrate, and this competes with the sulfanilamide for the enzyme system. Sulfanilamide does not induce a deficiency of *p*-aminobenzoic acid in higher animals, in contrast to its action on some bacteria. The reason for this is not entirely understood, but seems to be related to the fact that the animals cannot synthesise folic acid, whereas the bacteria can. For the animals, then, folic acid is a vitamin which they must get from their food, but not for the bacteria which can make their own. It is the stoppage of this manufacturing of folic acid which is part of the mechanism of action of this drug. It is also intimately associated with the reason why the drug is selectively toxic and harms the bacteria without poisoning the host animal. The original observation of Woods of the antagonism between sulfanilamide and *p*-aminobenzoic acid in bacterial growth was a landmark in the study of antimetabolites. There had been other prior observations of antagonisms between structurally related compounds, but they had not been widely heeded or understood. Because sulfanilamide was a popular, and, at that time, the best therapeutic agent for the control of several infectious diseases of man, the full impact of Woods demonstration was heeded.

The second example, that of pyrithiamine as an antimetabolite of thiamine (vitamin B_1), is of interest because it was discovered through the use of higher animals. The characteristic signs of dietary lack of thiamine were well known in laboratory animals such as mice, chickens and pigeons, and were thus readily recognisable. This was different from the signs of a deficiency in bacterial cultures, because with the micro-organisms one has principally the failure of growth to indicate disease, and failure of growth may be caused by many things. The induction of characteristic signs of a vitamin deficiency disease in animals thus indicates more clearly what one is dealing with.

In 1943 pyrithiamine was shown to induce the characteristic signs of thiamine deficiency in mice. The structures of antimetabolite and vitamin, where it can be seen that the relationship is close indeed. The deficiency disease caused by the eating of pyrithiamine could be cured or prevented by increasing the thiamine content of the food, so that the antagonism proved to be of the competitive kind. These same kinds of demonstrations were made with many kinds of micro-organisms, as well as with higher animals. Thus, the addition of pyrithiamine to the culture media for several species of bacteria and fungi caused inhibition of growth, and this could be overcome merely by increased thiamine in the solutions. It is not necessary to use living organisms or even organised tissues to observe the antagonism between metabolite and antimetabolite. The phenomenon can be studied in isolated enzyme systems, provided that the enzyme concerned can be separated from living tissue. This separation is not always possible, but in several cases where it has been acomplished the antagonism of the structurally related compounds has been shown. A large number of antimetabolites are now known. The two examples just mentioned were selected principally for their historical importance, but many others could have been used. In fact, there are antimetabolites for each of the vitamins (except A and D), for several hormones, for most of the amino acids, purines, and pyrimidines, and for some of the other essential metabolites of living things. The methods of testing for the antagonistic actions of these compounds are also varied. The variation is as great as is the divergence in methods of assay for biologically active constituents of living matter, because it is the interference in the assay procedure for a given metabolite which is usually used to demonstrate the activity of the antimetabolite.

Importance of Antimetabolites for Theory

The antimetabolites are of importance from a theoretical standpoint for several reasons. Through the use of a suitable antimetabolite, a specific deficiency can be created in a living organism. From the biochemical, anatomical, and functional changes which then arise, much information has been gained about the function of a given essential compound. Furthermore, when the changes induced in an animal in this fashion are seen to resemble the signs of a well recognised but etiologically poorly understood disease, the cause of the disease may be suggested. This is a use of antimetabolites which is being much studied at the present time in the unraveling of the causation of certain mental diseases.

In addition, the demonstrations that some antimetabolites occur naturally, frequently in the same individual in which the metabolite also occurs and functions, has given considerable insight into the regulatory mechanisms at work in a living organism. Some of the 'feedback mechanisms' by means of which cells check certain processes of synthesis, and thus prevent the useless accumulation of excessive amounts of their constituents, have been shown quite recently to be of this general kind. The finished molecule from a series of biochemical reactions frequently, because of its structural resemblance to one of the starting materials, is able to inhibit the enzyme which first directs this starting material through the metabolic pathway. These control mechanisms seem to offer a fertile field for future investigation along these lines

The natural ocurrence of certain antimetabolites also has indicated the nature of some diseases. Thus, for example, a disease of tobacco plants, the socalled wildfire disease, which is the result of infection of the plant by a pathogenic bacterium (Pseudomonas tabaci), is caused by a toxin which this invader liberates. The toxin has been isolated in pure condition and shown to be an antimetabolite of methionine. The disease thus seems to be the expression of a methionine deficiency produced in the host by the invading pathogen.

Finally, the existence of antagonism between structurally related compounds is having a considerable influence on the course of thinking about the active sites of enzymes and hormonal receptors. People are beginning to explore the idea that these may have a structural resemblance to the specific essential metabolites with which they combine. This idea is motivating much of the research in this important and fascinating subject at the present time. The attraction (perhaps due to van der Waals forces) which exists between like groups of atoms may be the binding force which confers the specificity and provides the force of union in these cases. Let us then discuss briefly a few examples (in addition to those just indicated) of these uses of antimetabolites in theoretical science.

The original clues about the reactions by means of which purines are synthesised by living organisms came from the use of antimetabolites. When bacteria such as *Escherichia coli* are grown in an amount of sulfanilamide just sufficient to cause slight inhibition of growth, they form a new compound, which was isolated and characterised as 4-amino 5-carboxamidoimidazole.

Sulfanilamide inhibits the synthesis of folic acid from *p*-aminobenzoic acid, and there was evidence to suggest that folic acid participated in the biosynthesis of the purines. It was therefore not surprising to find that an antimetabolite of folic acid also caused accumulation of this imidazole. All that is required to convert the imidazole to the purine hypoxanthine is the insertion of a carbon atom by means of a reaction with formic acid. It thus became plain that the pathway of purine biosynthesis was to the formation of the imidazole derivative followed by insertion of a formyl group to yield the purine ring. Prior to this work with sulfanilamide, the existence of such a pathway, or even of the imidazole derivative, in living things had not been indicated. More detailed investigation of these reactions with radioisotopes and by classical enzymology has shown that the ribotide of the imidazole is the real precursor, and that inosinic acid (hypoxanthine ribotide), rather than hypoxanthine itself, is the product. Other purines can be derived from inosinic acid by suitable enzymic steps. It is not without interest that the participants in some of these additional steps were also detected partly through the use of antimetabolites of them. The understanding of the biosynthesis of this group of biologically very important compounds was thus discovered to a considerable degree by the use of suitable antimetabolites.

Serotonin

The use of antimetabolites to elucidate the cause of noninfectious diseases could be illustrated by any one of several examples, but the one having to do with schizophrenia will serve to show the way it is done. Serotonin is a recently discovered hormone which causes smooth muscles to contract. It is an essential metabolite which is found in certain tissues such as the argentaflin cells of the stomach and intestines, in the platelets of the blood, in certain portions of the brain, and in some ganglia of the peripheral nervous system. Antimetabolites of serotonin were synthesised recently with the idea in mind that these, when given to animals, would induce specifically a deficiency of serotonin, and that the changes thus incited might reveal some of the purposes for which an animal has this hormone. There was also a practical reason for making these antimetabolites, which will be discussed presently. Some of these antiserotonins were found to call forth in animals and in men a kind of behavior similar to that seen in mentally deranged individuals. Certain other neurological disturbances were also called forth by some of these compounds.

While this work on the synthetic analogs of serotonin was in progress, it was shown that several classes of drugs which had been long known and traditionally obtained from plants were in fact structural analogs of serotonin and were capable of antagonising the actions of this hormone in a reversible fashion on smooth muscles. It was thus clear that these drugs were naturally occurring antimetabolites of serotonin. Harmine and its relatives, yohimbine and its relatives, and the ergot alkaloids were the drugs so studied. It was further noted that at least one member of each of these series of drugs was well known to induce in normal men a temporary condition resembling schizophrenia, with its visual hallucinations and changes in personality.

This ability of naturally occurring as well as of synthetic antimetabolites of serotonin to induce some of the signs of the mental diseases led Woolley and Shaw in 1954 to suggest that the natural disease commonly called schizophrenia was the reflection of a disturbance in the functioning of serotonin in the brain. This suggestion has been much debated recently, but it can be said that a considerable body of supporting evidence has been produced. One such piece of evidence which has received much attention is the finding that a drug which clearly affects the mind, namely, the tranquiliser known as reserpine, is a structural analog of serotonin, being a derivative of yohimbine. It behaves in some respects as an antimetabolite of this hormone.

Just as with the early finding of the antagonism between sulfanilamide and p-aminobenzoic acid, the fact that reserpine (like sulfanilamide) was a drug being widely used in the clinical treatment of a disease counted for more in men's minds than did prior demonstrations of the same fact with chemical compounds which were not being used as fashionable drugs. In the serotonin case, in contrast to the situation with sulfanilamide, the ideas and evidence had been clearly enunciated before the demonstrations with the practical drug. And yet the findings with the practical drug were the ones which seemed to carry more weight in most minds.

The evidence for the participation of serotonin in mental disorders is not yet complete. Work in this direction is going on actively at the present time. If it should prove possible to control adequately the disease as a result of the suggestion that serotonin plays a role in it, then we must say that the causation of this disease, or at least an etiological agent in it, was discovered through the use of antimetabolites.

The work which showed that several kinds of wellknown drugs of plant origin were acting on animals as antimetabolites of serotonin, as outlined above, points to another use of the antimetabolite concept. The mechanism of action of these plant alkaloids, or at least a part of that mechanism, was made clear by these studies. These alkaloids act by creating a deficiency of the hormone serotonin in certain tissues. It must also be added that on some tissues some of these compounds act like serotonin, instead of being antagonistic to it. In these tissues the analog seems to fit the serotonin receptors well enough to function in its stead. It has been earlier in this chapter how an analog may be near enough in structure to the essential metabolite to act as a substitute for that metabolite in some reactions.

ANTIMETABOLITES AND CHEMOTHERAPY

In addition to the uses of antimetabolites in solving questions of theory, uses of a practical kind have been envisioned, and some have been found. These are the uses in chemotherapy of infectious and noninfectious diseases. After the demonstration of the antagonism between sulfanilamide and *p*-aminobenzoic acid there was a wave of enthusiasm, because it was held that the control of infectious diseases by rational rather than chance means was just around the corner. All that would be required would be to make a suitable antimetabolite of some bacterial growth factor.

This proved to be an over simplification. No attention was paid to the question of how to make drugs of this sort which would not poison the host animal as well as the parasite. No attention was paid to many other important considerations. This, and the fact that the empirical approach through the search for antibiotics paid off so well in the discovery of new drugs for the control of infections, made many turn away from the antimetabolites as a practical solution. This was especially so among those looking for drugs with which to control infections.

Despite this, however, some noteworthy results were achieved, principally in the suppression of malaria. Two kinds of antimetabolites were found effective, firstly, some of the antipantothenic acids, and secondly, certain antifolic acids. The antifolic acids are now being used on a rather considerable scale in some equatorial countries. For this purpose, daraprim, shown in Fig. 13.5, is the compound most used. It is not a close structural analog of folic acid but appears to be more closely related to thymine, a pyrimidine which is formed in living things through the participation of folic acid.

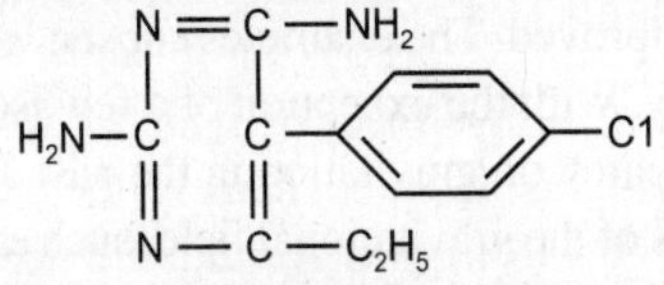

Daraprim

Fig. 13.5: Structure of daraprim.

Nevertheless, existing evidence seems to suggest that daraprim is more of an antifolic acid than an antithymine. Among investigators dealing with noninfectious diseases, the antimetabolite concept has been somewhat more popular as a means to the discovery of therapeutic agents. Among those attempting to control cancers, this has been particularly true, but among students of endocrine disorders there are also those who have had some success in its application. A few of the concepts should concern us here. If a disease arises, as some do, from an excessive amount of a given hormone in the body, it should be possible to control this disorder by administration of a suitable antimetabolite of the hormone. For example, suppose that an excess of serotonin were to arise in the body, either as the result of too great a production or too slow destruction of it. One can measure some of the effects of such an excess merely by injection of some of the hormone. One does not thus see all of the possible effects, but does see some. One feature of injection of serotonin into man is an increase in blood pressure. This is probably the result of the contraction of the smooth muscle of the walls of the arteries and arterioles. Such increases in blood pressure can be prevented by administration of a suitable antimetabolite of serotonin. If, then, some of the cases of human hypertension are related to an excess of serotonin in the body, such an antimetabolite would be expected to bring about a reduction in blood pressure in the disease. It is by no means established that some cases of human hypertension do result from an excess of serotonin, but the reduction of pressure in such patients would be evidence to suggest it as an etiological agent. Especially would this be true if it were found that the antimetabolite did not reduce blood pressure in normal human beings. The antimetabolite of serotonin was synthesised and tested in human hypertension with the idea in mind that the disease in some individuals might be the expression of an excess of serotonin. The compound was found not to reduce the blood pressures of normal animals and men, but did bring about such reduction, and other beneficial effects, in a considerable number of people suffering from high blood pressure. Because of the ability of certain antimetabolites of serotonin to induce mental changes, one may wonder how it was possible to use this antimetabolite safely. The drug was found not to induce the mental changes which are called forth by many other antiserotonins. This resulted, not simply from a lucky chance, but because, in fact, the drug was designed with the intent of keeping it out of the central nervous system. In so far as has been determined, it passes into the brain only with great difficulty, and possibly for this reason it does not cause mental disturbances. We thus see that many factors related to distribution of a drug through the tissues may be of great importance in the designing of therapeutic agents. The antimetabolite concept tells something about the designing of drugs but it does not tell all.

There seem to be many disorders which arise from excesses of this or that hormone. The possibility of controling some of these in the manner indicated seems enticing. Especially is this so when it begins to become clear that several drugs which have been discovered and used empirically for the control of certain disorders are in fact antimetabolites of some hormone or other essential metabolite.

The practical applications of the antimetabolites to attempts at chemotherapy could have been illustrated equally well with a variety of other drugs which have been introduced recently. None of these is completely satisfactory from a practical standpoint, and there are still those who maintain that it is unlikely that this record can be improved. The examples chosen were selected because they indictate the status of the field as it exists today. With the exception of a few isolated experiments, there has been essentially no basic experimental research on gravitation in the past 30 years. There are several reasons for this. First, because of the weakness of the gravitational field, such experiments are invariably difficult, and many of the most important are impossible. Second, because of the successes as well as the basic simplicity and elegance of Einstein's relativistic theory of gravitation, the feeling has been widespread that this theory must be correct. Third, it has been generally believed by physicists that the gravitational interaction is too weak to be important for modern physics. However some researcher do not agree with this diagnosis. First, new experimental techniques now make possible experiments formerly impossible. Second, while Einstein's theory is admittedly elegant, we are not sure that nature has quite the predilection for an elegant theory that man apparently possesses. Third, although gravitation is weak, it may play a crucial role in the structure of a particle. If, as is believed by many physicists, an elementary particle is a complex structure of very small size consisting of a core particle surrounded by a swarm of attendant virtual particles, the gravitational interaction may be one of the dominant forces acting on very high momentum particles found at the core. It has been suggested that it is the failure to take into account such interactions which is the root of the difficulty leading to divergences in quantumfield theories.

Observational Evidence for Theory of General Relativity

The experimental and observational support for Einstein's theory of general relativity consists primarily of facts available before the construction of the theory. These consist of the large body of data on planetary motion, including the anomalous rotation of the perihelion of Mercury's orbit. There is also the accurate experiment of Eotviis (i) and others on the equivalence of inertial and gravitational mass. The only observational facts found subsequently are the gravitational deflection of light by the Sun and the gravitational red shift. Because of the smallness of these effects, both of these checks of the theory of general relativity are inaccurate. The astronomical observations of planetary orbits are very accurate, however, a comparison between the observed orbits and calculated orbits always shows small systematic discrepancies (ii). The discrepancies are believed to be due primarily to computational errors and systematic errors in observation. While this may be true, there is always the possibility that some of the systematic error may be of a more fundamental character. It should also be remembered that the velocities of the planets are so low that gravitational retardation effects are essentially unobservable.

Function of Antimetabolites

Cancer treatment

Antimetabolites can be used in cancer treatment, as they interfere with DNA production and therefore cell division and tumor growth. Because cancer cells spend more time dividing than other cells, inhibiting cell division harms tumor cells more than other cells. Antimetabolite drugs are commonly used to treat leukemia, cancers of the breast, ovary, and the gastrointestinal tract, as well as other types of cancers. In the Anatomical Therapeutic Chemical Classification System antimetabolite cancer drugs are classified under L01B. Antimetabolites generally impair DNA replication machinery, either by incorporation of chemically altered nucleotides or by depleting the supply of deoxynucleotides needed for DNA replication and cell proliferation.

Examples of cancer drug antimetabolites include, but are not limited to the following:
- 5Fluorouracil (5FU)
- 6Mercaptopurine (6MP)
- Capecitabine (Xeloda®)
- Cytarabine (AraC®)
- Floxuridine
- Fludarabine
- Gemcitabine (Gemzar®)
- Hydroxycarbamide
- Methotrexate
- Pemetrexed (Alimta®)

Antimetabolites masquerade as a purine (azathioprine, mercaptopurine) or a pyrimidine, chemicals that become the buildingblocks of DNA. They prevent these substances from becoming incorporated into DNA during the S phase (of the cell cycle), stopping normal development and cell division. Antimetabolites also affect RNA synthesis. However, because thymidine is used in DNA but not in RNA (where uracil is used instead), inhibition of thymidine synthesis via thymidylate synthase selectively inhibits DNA synthesis over RNA synthesis. Due to their efficiency, these drugs are the most widely used cytostatics. Competition for the binding sites of enzymes that participate in essential biosynthetic processes and subsequent incorporation of these biomolecules into nucleic acids, inhibits their normal tumor cell function and triggers apoptosis, or the cell death process. Because of this mode of action, most antimetabolites have high cell cycle specificity and can target arrest of cancer cell DNA replication.

Antibiotics

Antimetabolites may also be antibiotics, such as sulfanilamide drugs, which inhibit dihydrofolate synthesis in bacteria by competing with *para*-aminobenzoic acid (PABA). PABA is needed in enzymatic reactions that produce folic acid, which acts as a coenzyme in the synthesis of purines and pyrimidines, the buildingblocks of DNA. Mammals do not synthesise their own folic acid so they are unaffected by PABA inhibitors, which selectively kill bacteria. Sulfanilamide drugs are not like the antibiotics used to treat infections. Instead, they work by changing the DNA inside cancer cells to keep them from growing and multiplying. Antitumor antibiotics are a class of antimetabolite drugs that are cell cycle nonspecific. They act by binding with DNA molecules and preventing RNA (ribonucleic acid) synthesis, a key step in the creation of proteins, which are necessary for cancer cell survival. Anthracyclines are antitumor antibiotics that interfere with enzymes involved in copying DNA during the cell cycle.

Examples of anthracyclines include:

- Daunorubicin
- Doxorubicin (Adriamycin®)
- Epirubicin
- Idarubicin

Antitumor antibiotics that are not anthracyclines include: actinomycin D, bleomycin, mitomycin C and nitoxantrone.

Other uses of antimetabolites

Antimetabolites, particularly mitomycin C (MMC), are commonly used in America and Japan as an addition to trabeculectomy, a surgical procedure to treat glaucoma. Antimetabolites have been shown to decrease fibrosis of operative sites. Thus, its use following external dacryocystorhinostomy, a procedure for the management of nasolacrimal duct obstruction, is being researched. Intraoperative antimetabolite application, namely mitomycin C (MMC) and 5 Fluorouracil (5FU), is currently being tested for its effectiveness of managing pterygium.

Types of these Drugs

Base analogues (altered nucleobases) – structures that can substitute for a normal nucleobases in nucleic acids. This means that these molecules are structurally similar enough the basic components of DNA that they can be substituted in. However, since they are slightly different that the normal bases after they are incorporated into the DNA, the DNA production is halted and the cell dies.

- Purine analogues – mimic the structure of metabolic purines, the larger bases incorporated into DNA as adenosine and guanosine, e.g. Azathioprine, Thiopurines, and Fludarabine.
- Pyrimidine analogue – mimic the structure of metabolic pyrimidines, the smaller bases incorporated into DNA as cytosine and thymine, e.g. 5 Fluorouracil, Gemcitabine, and Cytarabine.

Nucleoside analogues – nucleosides alternatives which contain a nucleic acid analogue and a sugar. This means these are the same bases as above, but with an added sugar group. For the nucleoside analogues either the base or the sugar component can be altered. They are similar enough to the molecules used to build cellular DNA that they are incorporated by the cell into its DNA, but different enough that after being added the cell's DNA they stop cell growth.

Nucleotide analogues – nucleotides alternatives that contain a nucleic acid, a sugar, and 1–3 phosphates. This means these molecules look exactly like the pieces used to build DNA in a cell and can be incorporated into a growing cell's DNA. However, because they are analogues and therefore slightly different than regular nucleotides, causing the cell's growth to be halted and the cell to die.

Antifolates – chemicals that block the actions of folic acid (vitamin B9) which is needed to build DNA and allow cells to grow.

SECTION IV

Fundamentals of Molecular Biology

Chapter 14

Heredity, Genes and DNA

INTRODUCTION

Heredity, the sum of all biological processes by which particular characteristics are transmitted from parents to their offspring. The concept of heredity encompasses two seemingly paradoxical observations about organisms: the constancy of a species from generation to generation and the variation among individuals within a species. Constancy and variation are actually two sides of the same coin, as becomes clear in the study of genetics. Both aspects of heredity can be explained by genes, the functional units of heritable material that are found within all living cells. Every member of a species has a set of genes specific to that species. It is this set of genes that provides the constancy of the species. Among individuals within a species, however, variations can occur in the form each gene takes, providing the genetic basis for the fact that no two individuals (except identical twins) have exactly the same traits.

The set of genes that an offspring inherits from both parents, a combination of the genetic material of each, is called the organisms genotype. The genotype is contrasted to the phenotype, which is the organisms outward appearance and the developmental outcome of its genes. The phenotype includes an organisms bodily structures, physiological processes, and behaviours. Although the genotype determines the broad limits of the features an organism can develop, the features that actually develop, i.e. the phenotype, depend on complex interactions between genes and their environment. The genotype remains constant throughout an organisms lifetime, however, because the organisms internal and external environments change continuously, so does its phenotype. In conducting genetic studies, it is crucial to discover the degree to which the observable trait is attributable to the pattern of genes in the cells and to what extent it arises from environmental influence.

Because genes are integral to the explanation of hereditary observations, genetics also can be defined as the study of genes. Discoveries into the nature of genes have shown that genes are important determinants of all aspects of an organisms makeup. For this reason, most areas of biological research now have a genetic component, and the study of genetics has a position of central importance in biology. Genetic research also has demonstrated that virtually all organisms on this planet have similar genetic systems, with genes that are built on the same chemical principle and that function according to similar mechanisms. Although species differ in the sets of genes they contain, many similar genes are found across a wide range of species. For example, a large proportion of genes in baker's yeast are also present in humans. This similarity in genetic makeup between organisms that have such disparate phenotypes can be explained by the evolutionary relatedness of virtually all life-forms on Earth. This genetic unity has radically reshaped the understanding of the relationship between humans and all other organisms. Genetics also has had a profound impact on human affairs. Throughout history humans have created or improved many different medicines, foods, and textiles by subjecting plants, animals, and microbes to the ancient techniques of selective breeding and to the modern methods of recombinant DNA technology. In recent years medical researchers have begun to discover the role that genes play in disease. The significance of genetics only promises to become greater as the structure and function of more and more human genes are characterised.

BASIC FEATURES OF HEREDITY

Prescientific Conceptions of Heredity

Heredity was for a long time one of the most puzzling and mysterious phenomena of nature. This was so because the sex cells, which form the bridge across which heredity must pass between the generations, are usually invisible to the naked eye. Only after the invention of the microscope early in the 17th century and the subsequent discovery of the sex cells could the essentials of heredity be grasped. Before that time, ancient Greek philosopher and scientist Aristotle (4th century BC) speculated that the relative contributions of the female and the male parents were very unequal, the female was thought to supply what he called the 'matter' and the male the 'motion.' The Institutes of Manu, composed in India between 100 and 300 AD, consider the role of the female like that of the field and of the male like that of the seed, new bodies are formed 'by the united operation of the seed and the field.' In reality both parents transmit the heredity pattern equally, and, on average, children resemble their mothers as much as they do their fathers. Nevertheless, the female and male sex cells may be very different in size and structure, the mass of an egg cell is sometimes millions of times greater than that of a spermatozoon.

The ancient Babylonians knew that pollen from a male date palm tree must be applied to the pistils of a female tree to produce fruit. German botanist Rudolph Jacob Camerarius showed in 1694 that the same is true in corn (maize). Swedish botanist and explorer Carolus Linnaeus in 1760 and German botanist Josef Gottlieb Kölreuter, in a series of works published from 1761 to 1798, described crosses of varieties and species of plants. They found that these hybrids were, on the whole, intermediate between the parents, although in some characteristics they might be closer to one parent and in others closer to the other parent.

Kölreuter compared the offspring of reciprocal crosses, i.e. of crosses of variety A functioning as a female to variety B as a male and the reverse, variety B as a female to A as a male. The hybrid progenies of these reciprocal crosses were usually alike, indicating that, contrary to the belief of Aristotle, the hereditary endowment of the progeny was derived equally from the female and the male parents. Many more experiments on plant hybrids were made in the 1800s. These investigations also revealed that hybrids were usually intermediate between the parents. They incidentally recorded most of the facts that later led Gregor Mendel to formulate his celebrated rules and to found the theory of the gene. Apparently, none of Mendel's predecessors saw the significance of the data that were being accumulated. The general intermediacy of hybrids seemed to agree best with the belief that heredity was transmitted from parents to offspring by 'blood,' and this belief was accepted by most 19th-century biologists, including English naturalist Charles Darwin.

The blood theory of heredity, if this notion can be dignified with such a name, is really a part of the folklore antedating scientific biology. It is implicit in such popular phrases as 'half blood,' 'new blood,' and 'blue blood.' It does not mean that heredity is actually transmitted through the red liquid in blood vessels, the essential point is the belief that a parent transmits to each child all its characteristics and that the hereditary endowment of a child is an alloy, a blend of the endowments of its parents, grandparents, and more-remote ancestors. This idea appeals to those who pride themselves on having a noble or remarkable 'blood' line. It strikes a snag, however, when one observes that a child has some characteristics that are not present in either parent but are present in some other relatives or were present in more-remote ancestors. Even more often, one sees that brothers and sisters, though showing a family resemblance in some traits, are clearly different in others. How could the same parents transmit different 'bloods' to each of their children?

Mendel disproved the blood theory. He showed: (i) that heredity is transmitted through factors (now called genes) that do not blend but segregate, (ii) that parents transmit only one-half of the genes they have to each child, and they transmit different sets of genes to different children, and (iii) that, although brothers and sisters receive their heredities from the same parents, they do not receive the same heredities (an exception is identical twins). Mendel thus showed that, even if the eminence of some ancestor were entirely the reflection of his genes, it is quite likely that some of his descendants, especially the more remote ones, would not inherit these 'good' genes at all. In sexually reproducing organisms, humans included, every individual has a unique hereditary endowment.

Lamarckism—a school of thought named for the 19th-century pioneer French biologist and evolutionist Jean-Baptiste de Monet, chevalier de Lamarck—assumed that characters acquired during an individual's life are inherited by his progeny, or, to put it in modern terms, that the modifications wrought by the environment in the phenotype are reflected in similar changes in the genotype. If this were so, the results of physical exercise would make exercise much easier or even dispensable in a persons offspring. Not only Lamarck but also other 19th-century biologists, including Darwin, accepted the inheritance of acquired traits. It was questioned by German biologist August Weismann, whose famous experiments in the late 1890s on the amputation of tails in generations of mice showed that such modification resulted neither in disappearance nor even in shortening of the tails of the descendants. Weismann concluded that the hereditary endowment of the organism, which he called the germ plasm, is wholly separate and is protected against the influences emanating from the rest of the body, called the somatoplasm, or soma. The germ plasm–somatoplasm are related to the genotype–phenotype concepts, but they are not identical and should not be confused with them.

The noninheritance of acquired traits does not mean that the genes cannot be changed by environmental influences, X-rays and other mutagens certainly do change them, and the genotype of a population can be altered by selection. It simply means that what is acquired by parents in their physique and intellect is not inherited by their children. Related to these misconceptions are the beliefs in 'prepotency', i.e. that some individuals impress their heredities on their progenies more effectively than others—and in 'prenatal influences' or 'maternal impressions', i.e. that the events experienced by a pregnant female are reflected in the constitution of the child to be born. How ancient these beliefs are is suggested in the Book of Genesis, in which Laban produced spotted or striped progeny in sheep by showing the pregnant ewes striped hazel rods. Another such belief is 'telegony,' which goes back to Aristotle, it alleged that the heredity of an individual is influenced not only by his father but also by males with whom the female may have mated and who have caused previous pregnancies. Even Darwin, as late as 1868, seriously discussed an alleged case of telegony: that of a mare mated to a zebra and subsequently to an

Arabian stallion, by whom the mare produced a foal with faint stripes on his legs. The simple explanation for this result is that such stripes occur naturally in some breeds of horses.

All these beliefs, from inheritance of acquired traits to telegony, must now be classed as superstitions. They do not stand up under experimental investigation and are incompatible with what is known about the mechanisms of heredity and about the remarkable and predictable properties of genetic materials. Nevertheless, some people still cling to these beliefs. Some animal breeders take telegony seriously and do not regard as purebred the individuals whose parents are admittedly 'pure' but whose mothers had mated with males of other breeds. Soviet biologist and agronomist Trofim Denisovich Lysenko was able for close to a quarter of a century, roughly between 1938 and 1963, to make his special brand of Lamarckism the official creed in the Soviet Union and to suppress most of the teaching and research in orthodox genetics. He and his partisans published hundreds of articles and books allegedly proving their contentions, which effectively deny the achievements of biology for at least the preceding century. The Lysenkoists were officially discredited in 1964.

MENDELIAN GENETICS

Discovery and Rediscovery of Mendel's Laws

Gregor Mendel published his work in the proceedings of the local society of naturalists in Brünn, Austria (now Brno, Czech Republic), in 1866, but none of his contemporaries appreciated its significance. It was not until 1900, 16 years after Mendel's death, that his work was rediscovered independently by botanists Hugo de Vries in Holland, Carl Erich Correns in Germany, and Erich Tschermak von Seysenegg in Austria. Like several investigators before him, Mendel experimented on hybrids of different varieties of a plant, he focused on the common pea plant (Pisum sativum). His methods differed in two essential respects from those of his predecessors. First, instead of trying to describe the appearance of whole plants with all their characteristics, Mendel followed the inheritance of single, easily visible and distinguishable traits, such as round versus wrinkled seed, yellow versus green seed, purple versus white flowers, and so on. Second, he made exact counts of the numbers of plants bearing each trait, it was from such quantitative data that he deduced the rules governing inheritance.

Since pea plants reproduce usually by self-pollination of their flowers, the varieties Mendel obtained from seedsmen were pure, i.e. descended for several to many generations from plants with similar traits. Mendel crossed them by deliberately transferring the pollen of one variety to the pistils of another, the resulting first-generation hybrids, denoted by the symbol F_1, usually showed the traits of only one parent. For example, the crossing of yellow-seeded plants with green-seeded ones gave yellow seeds, and the crossing of purple-flowered plants with white-flowered ones gave purple-flowered plants. Traits such as the yellow-seed colour and the purple-flower colour Mendel called dominant, the green-seed colour and the white-flower colour he called recessive. It looked as if the yellow and purple 'bloods' overcame or consumed the green and white bloods.

That this was not so became evident when Mendel allowed the F_1 hybrid plants to self-pollinate and produce the second hybrid generation, F_2. Here, both the dominant and the recessive traits reappeared, as pure and uncontaminated as they were in the original parents (generation P). Moreover, these traits now appeared in constant proportions: about 3/4 of the plants in the second generation showed the dominant trait and 1/4 showed the recessive, a 3 to 1 ratio. It can be seen in the Table 14.1 that Mendel's actual counts were as close to the ideal ratio as one could expect, allowing for the sampling deviations present in all statistical data.

Table 14.1: Pea plants with dominant and recessive characters obtained by Mendel in the second generation of hybrids.

Number	Dominant		Number recessive	Ratio
Round seed	5,474	Wrinkled seed	1,850	2.96:1
Yellow seed	6,022	Green seed	2,001	3.01:1
Purple flowers	705	White flowers	224	3.15:1
Tall plants	787	Short plants	277	2.84:1

Mendel concluded that the sex cells, the gametes, of the purple-flowered plants carried some factor that caused the progeny to develop purple flowers, and the gametes of the white-flowered variety had a variant factor that induced the development of white flowers. In 1909 the Danish biologist Wilhelm Ludvig Johannsen proposed to call these factors genes.

An example of one of Mendel's experiments will illustrate how the genes are transmitted and in what particular ratios. Let R stand for the gene for purple flowers and r for the gene for white flowers (dominant genes are conventionally symbolised by capital letters and recessive genes by lowercase letters). Since each pea plant contains a gene endowment half of whose set is derived from the mother and half from the father, each plant has two genes for flower colour. If the two genes are alike—for instance, both having come from white-flowered parents (rr)—the plant is termed a homozygote. The union of gametes with different genes gives a hybrid plant, termed a heterozygote (Rr). Since the gene R, for purple, is dominant over r, for white, the F_1 generation hybrids will show purple flowers. They are phenotypically purple, but their genotype contains both R and r genes, and these alternative (allelic or allelomorphic) genes do not blend or contaminate each other. Mendel inferred that, when a heterozygote forms its sex cells, the allelic genes segregate and pass to different gametes. This is expressed in the first law of Mendel, the law of segregation of unit genes. Equal numbers of gametes, ovules, or pollen grains are formed that contain the genes R and r. Now, if the gametes unite at random, then the F_2 generation should contain about 1/4 white-flowered and 3/4 purple-flowered plants. The white-flowered plants, which must be recessive homozygotes, bear the genotype rr. About 1/3 of the plants exhibiting the dominant trait of purple flowers must be homozygotes, RR, and 2/3 heterozygotes, Rr. The prediction is tested by obtaining a third generation, F_3, from the purple-flowered plants, though phenotypically all purple-flowered, 2/3 of this group of plants reveal the presence of the recessive gene allele, r, in their genotype by producing about 1/4 white-flowered plants in the F_3 generation.

Mendel also crossbred varieties of peas that differed in two or more easily distinguishable traits. When a variety with yellow round seed was crossed to a green wrinkled-seed variety, the F_1 generation hybrids produced yellow round seed. Evidently, yellow (A) and round (B) are dominant traits, and green (a) and wrinkled (b) are recessive. By allowing the F_1 plants (genotype AaBb) to self-pollinate, Mendel obtained an F_2 generation of 315 yellow round, 101 yellow wrinkled, 108 green round, and 32 green wrinkled seeds, a ratio of approximately 9 : 3 : 3 : 1. The important point here is that the segregation of the colour (A–a) is independent of the segregation of the trait of seed surface (B–b). This is expected if the F_1 generation produces equal numbers of four kinds of gametes, carrying the four possible combinations of the parental genes: AB, Ab, aB, and ab. Random union of these gametes gives, then, the four phenotypes in a ratio 9 dominant–dominant : 3 recessive–dominant : 3 dominant–recessive : 1 recessive–recessive. Among these four phenotypic classes there must be nine different genotypes, a supposition that can be tested experimentally by raising a third hybrid generation. The predicted genotypes are actually found. Another test is by means of a backcross (or testcross), the F_1 hybrid (phenotype yellow round seed, genotype AaBb) is crossed to a double recessive plant (phenotype green wrinkled seed, genotype aabb). If the hybrid gives four kinds of gametes in equal numbers and if all the gametes of the double recessive are alike (ab), the predicted progeny of the backcross are yellow round, yellow wrinkled, green round, and green wrinkled seed in a ratio 1 : 1 : 1 : 1. This prediction is realised in experiments. When the varieties crossed differ in three genes, the F_1 hybrid forms 2^3, or eight, kinds of gametes (2^n = kinds of gametes, n being the number of genes). The second generation of hybrids, the F_2, has 27 (3^3) genotypically distinct kinds of individuals but only eight different phenotypes. From these results and others, Mendel derived his second law: the law of recombination, or independent assortment of genes.

UNIVERSALITY OF MENDEL'S LAWS

Although Mendel experimented with varieties of peas, his laws have been shown to apply to the inheritance of many kinds of characters in almost all organisms. In 1902 Mendelian inheritance was demonstrated in poultry (by English geneticists William Bateson and Reginald Punnett) and in mice. The following year, albinism became the first human trait shown to be a Mendelian recessive, with pigmented skin the corresponding dominant.

In 1902 and 1909, English physician Sir Archibald Garrod initiated the analysis of inborn errors of metabolism in humans in terms of biochemical genetics. Alkaptonuria, inherited as a recessive, is characterised by excretion in the urine of large amounts of the substance called alkapton, or homogentisic acid, which renders the urine black on exposure to air. In normal (i.e. nonalkaptonuric) persons the homogentisic acid is changed to acetoacetic acid, the reaction being facilitated by an enzyme, homogentisic acid oxidase. Garrod advanced the hypothesis that this enzyme is absent or inactive in homozygous carriers of the defective recessive alkaptonuria gene, hence, the homogentisic acid accumulates and is excreted in the urine. Mendelian inheritance of numerous traits in humans has been studied since then.

In analysing Mendelian inheritance, it should be borne in mind that an organism is not an aggregate of independent traits, each determined by one gene. A 'trait' is really an abstraction, a term of convenience in description. One gene may affect many traits (a condition termed pleiotropic). The white gene in *Drosophila* flies is pleiotropic, it affects the colour of the eyes and of the testicular envelope in the males, the fecundity and the shape of the spermatheca in the females, and the longevity of both sexes. In humans many diseases caused by a single defective gene will have a variety of symptoms, all pleiotropic manifestations of the gene.

Allelic Interactions

Dominance relationships

The operation of Mendelian inheritance is frequently more complex than in the case of the traits recorded by Mendel. In the first place, clear-cut dominance and recessiveness are by no means always found. When red- and white-flowered varieties of four-o'clock plants or snapdragons are crossed, for example, the F_1 hybrids have flowers of intermediate pink or rose colour, a situation that seems more explicable by the blending notion of inheritance than by Mendelian concepts. That the inheritance of flower colour is indeed due to Mendelian mechanisms becomes apparent when the F_1 hybrids are allowed to cross, yielding an F_2 generation of red-, pink-, and white-flowered plants in a ratio of 1 red : 2 pink : 1 white. Obviously the hereditary information for the production of red and white flowers had not been blended away in the first hybrid generation, as flowers of these colours were produced in the second generation of hybrids. The apparent blending in the F_1 generation is explained by the fact that the gene alleles that govern flower colour in four-o'clocks show an incomplete dominance relationship. Suppose then that a gene allele R_1 is responsible for red flowers and R_2 for white, the homozygotes R_1R_1 and R_2R_2 are red and white respectively, and the heterozygotes R_1R_2 have pink flowers. A similar pattern of lack of dominance is found in Shorthorn cattle. In diverse organisms, dominance ranges from complete (a heterozygote indistinguishable from one of the homozygotes) to incomplete (heterozygotes exactly intermediate) to excessive or overdominance (a heterozygote more extreme than either homozygote).

Another form of dominance is one in which the heterozygote displays the phenotypic characteristics of both alleles. This is called codominance, an example is seen in the MN blood group system of human beings. MN blood type is governed by two alleles, M and N. Individuals who are homozygous for the M allele have a surface molecule (called the M antigen) on their red blood cells. Similarly, those homozygous for the N allele have the N antigen on the red blood cells. Heterozygotes—those with both alleles— carry both antigens.

Multiple alleles

The traits discussed so far all have been governed by the interaction of two possible alleles. Many genes, however, are represented by multiple allelic forms within a population. (One individual, of course, can possess only two of these multiple alleles.) Human blood groups—in this case, the well-known ABO system—again provide an example. The gene that governs ABO blood types has three alleles: IA, IB, and IO. IA and IB are codominant, but IO is recessive. Because of the multiple alleles and their various dominance relationships, there are four phenotypic ABO blood types: type A (genotypes IAIA and IAIO), type B (genotypes IBIB and IBIO), type AB (genotype IAIB), and type O (genotype IOIO).

Gene Interactions

Many individual traits are affected by more than one gene. For example, the coat colour in many mammals is determined by numerous genes interacting to produce the result. The great variety of colour patterns in cats, dogs, and other domesticated animals is the result of different combinations of complexly interacting genes. The gradual unravelling of their modes of inheritance was one of the active fields of research in the early years of genetics.

Two or more genes may produce similar and cumulative effects on the same trait. In humans the skin-colour difference between so-called blacks and so-called whites is due to several (probably four or more) interacting pairs of genes, each of which increases or decreases the skin pigmentation by a relatively small amount.

Epistatic genes

Some genes mask the expression of other genes just as a fully dominant allele masks the expression of its recessive counterpart. A gene that masks the phenotypic effect of another gene is called an epistatic gene, the gene it subordinates is the hypostatic gene. The gene for albinism (lack of pigment) in humans is an epistatic gene. It is not part of the interacting skin-colour genes described above, rather, its dominant allele is necessary for the development of any skin pigment, and its recessive homozygous state results in the albino condition regardless of how many other pigment genes may be present. Albinism thus occurs in some individuals among dark- or intermediate-pigmented peoples as well as among light-pigmented peoples.

The presence of epistatic genes explains much of the variability seen in the expression of such dominantly inherited human diseases as Marfan syndrome and neurofibromatosis. Because of the effects of an epistatic gene, some individuals who inherit a dominant, disease-causing gene show only partial symptoms of the disease, some in fact may show no expression of the disease-causing gene, a condition referred to as nonpenetrance. The individual in whom such a nonpenetrant mutant gene exists will be phenotypically normal but still capable of passing the deleterious gene on to offspring, who may exhibit the full-blown disease.

Examples of epistasis abound in nonhuman organisms. In mice, as in humans, the gene for albinism has two variants: the allele for nonalbino and the allele for albino. The latter allele is unable to synthesise the pigment melanin. Mice, however, have another pair of alleles involved in melanin placement. These are the agouti allele, which produces dark melanisation of the hair except for a yellow band at the tip, and the black allele, which produces melanisation of the whole hair. If melanin cannot be formed (the situation in the mouse homozygous for the albino gene), neither agouti nor black can be expressed. Hence, homozygosity for the albinism gene is epistatic to the agouti/black alleles and prevents their expression.

Complementation

The phenomenon of complementation is another form of interaction between nonallelic genes. For example, there are mutant genes that in the homozygous state produce profound deafness in humans. One would expect that the children of two persons with such hereditary deafness would be deaf. This is frequently not the case, because the parents' deafness is often caused by different genes. Since the mutant genes are not alleles, the child becomes heterozygous for the two genes and hears normally. In other words, the two mutant genes complement each other in the child. Complementation thus becomes a test for allelism. In the case of congenital deafness cited above, if all the children had been deaf, one could assume that the deafness in each of the parents was owing to mutant genes that were alleles. This would be more likely to occur if the parents were genetically related (consanguineous).

Polygenic inheritance

The greatest difficulties of analysis and interpretation are presented by the inheritance of many quantitative or continuously varying traits. Inheritance of this kind produces variations in degree rather than in kind, in contrast to the inheritance of discontinuous traits resulting from single genes of major effect. The yield of milk in different breeds of cattle, the egg-laying capacity in poultry, and the stature, shape of the head, blood pressure, and intelligence in humans range in continuous series from one extreme to the other and are significantly dependent on environmental conditions. Crosses of two varieties differing in such characters usually give F_1 hybrids intermediate between the parents. At first sight this situation suggests a blending inheritance through 'blood' rather than Mendelian inheritance, in fact, it was probably observations of this kind of inheritance that suggested the folk idea of 'blood theory.'

It has, however, been shown that these characters are polygenic, i.e. determined by several or many genes, each taken separately producing only a slight effect on the phenotype, as small as or smaller than that caused by environmental influences on the same characters. That Mendelian segregation does take place with polygenes, as with the genes having major effects (sometimes called oligogenes), is shown by the variation among F_2 and further-generation hybrids being usually much greater than that in the F_1 generation. By selecting among the segregating progenies the desired variants—for example, individuals with the greatest yield, the best size, or a desirable behaviour—it is possible to produce new breeds or varieties sometimes exceeding the parental forms. Hybridisation and selection are consequently potent methods that have been used for improvement of agricultural plants and animals. Polygenic inheritance also applies to many of the birth defects (congenital malformations) seen in humans. Although expression of the defect itself may be discontinuous (as in clubfoot, for example), susceptibility to the trait is continuously variable and follows the rules of polygenic inheritance. When a developmental threshold produced by a polygenically inherited susceptibility and a variety of environmental factors is exceeded, the birth defect results.

HEREDITY AND ENVIRONMENT

Preformism and Epigenesis

A notion that was widespread among pioneer biologists in the 18th century was that the fetus, and hence the adult organism that develops from it, is preformed in the sex cells. Some early microscopists even imagined that they saw a tiny homunculus, a diminutive human figure, encased in the human spermatozoon. The development of the individual from the sex cells appeared deceptively simple: it was merely an increase in the size and growth of what was already present in the sex cells. The antithesis of the early preformation theories was theories of epigenesis, which claimed that the sex cells were structureless jelly and contained nothing at all in the way of rudiments of future organisms. The naive early versions of preformation and epigenesis had to be given up when embryologists showed that the embryo develops by a series of complex but orderly and gradual transformations. Darwin's 'Provisional Hypothesis of Pangenesis' was distinctly preformistic, Weismann's theory of determinants in the germ plasm, as well as the early ideas about the relations between genes and traits, also tended toward preformism.

Heredity has been defined as a process that results in the progeny's resembling his parents. A further qualification of this definition states that what is inherited is a potential that expresses itself only after interacting with and being modified by environmental factors. In short, all phenotypic expressions have both hereditary and environmental components, the amount of each varying for different traits. Thus, a trait that is primarily hereditary (e.g. skin colour in humans) may be modified by environmental influences (e.g. suntanning). And conversely, a trait sensitive to environmental modifications (e.g. weight in humans) is also genetically conditioned. Organic development is preformistic in so far as a fertilised egg cell contains a genotype that conditions the events that may occur and is epigenetic in so far as a given genotype allows a variety of possible outcomes. These considerations should dispel the reluctance felt by many people to accept the fact that mental as well as physiological and physical traits in humans are genetically conditioned. Genetic conditioning does not mean that heredity is the 'dice of destiny.' At least in principle, but not invariably in practice, the development of a trait may be manipulated by changes in the environment.

Heritability

Although hereditary diseases and malformations are, unfortunately, by no means uncommon in the aggregate, no one of them occurs very frequently. The characteristics by which one person is distinguished from another—such as facial features, stature, shape of the head, skin, eye and hair colours, and voice— are not usually inherited in a clear-cut Mendelian manner, as are some hereditary malformations and diseases. This is not as strange as it may seem. The kinds of gene changes, or mutations, that produce morphological or physiological effects drastic enough to be clearly set apart from the more usual phenotypes are likely to cause diseases or malformations just because they are so drastic.

The variations that occur among healthy persons are, as a general rule, caused by polygenes with individually small effects. The same is true of individual differences among members of various animal and plant species. Even brown-blue eye colour in humans, which in many families behaves as if caused by two forms of a single gene (brown being dominant and blue recessive), is often blurred by minor gene modifiers of the pigmentation. Some apparently blue-eyed persons actually carry the gene for the brown eye colour, but several additional modifier genes decrease the amount of brown pigment in the iris. This type of genetic process can influence susceptibility to many diseases (e.g. diabetes) or birth defects (e.g. cleft lip—with or without cleft palate).

The question geneticists must often attempt to answer is how much of the observed diversity between persons or between individuals of any species is because of hereditary, or genotypic, variations and how much of it is because of environmental influences. Applied to human beings, this is sometimes referred to as the nature-nurture problem. With animals or plants the problem is evidently more easily soluble than it is with people. Two complementary approaches are possible. First, individual organisms or their progenies are raised in environments as uniform as can be provided, with food, temperature, light, humidity, etc. carefully controlled. The differences that persist between such individuals or progenies probably reflect genotypic differences. Second, individuals with similar or identical genotypes are placed in different environments. The phenotypic differences may then be ascribed to environmental induction. Experiments combining both approaches have been carried out on several species of plants that grow naturally at different altitudes, from sea level to the alpine zone of the Sierra Nevada in California. Young yarrow plants (Achillea) were cut into three parts, and the cuttings were replanted in experimental gardens at sea level, at mid-altitude (4,800 feet [1,460 metres]), and at high altitude (10,000 feet [3,050 metres]). It was observed that the plants native at sea level grow best in their native habitat, grow less well at mid-altitudes, and die at high altitudes. On the other hand, the alpine race survives and develops better at the high-altitude transplant station than it does at lower altitudes.

With organisms that cannot survive being cut into pieces and placed in controlled environments, a partitioning of the observed variability into genetic and environmental components may be attempted by other methods. Suppose that in a certain population individuals vary in stature, weight, or some other trait. These characters can be measured in many pairs of parents and in their progenies raised under different environmental conditions. If the variation is owing entirely to environment and not at all to heredity, then the expression of the character in the parents and in the offspring will show no correlation (heritability = zero). On the other hand, if the environment is unimportant and the character is uncomplicated by dominance, then the means of this character in the progenies will be the same as the means of the parents, with differences in the expression in females and in males taken into account, the heritability will equal unity. In reality, most heritabilities are found to lie between zero and one.

It is important to understand clearly the meaning of heritability estimates. They show that, given the range of the environments in which the experimental animals lived, one could predict the average body sizes in the progenies of pigs better than one could predict the average numbers of piglets in a litter. The heritability is, however, not an inherent or unchangeable property of each character. If one could make the environments more uniform, the heritabilities would rise, and with more-diversified environments they would decrease. Similarly, in populations that are more variable genetically, the heritabilities increase, and in genetically uniform ones, they decrease. In humans the situation is even more complex, because the environments of the parents and of their children are in many ways interdependent. Suppose, for example, that one wishes to study the heritability of stature, weight, or susceptibility to tuberculosis. The stature, weight, and liability to contract tuberculosis depend to some extent on the quality of nutrition and generally on the economic well-being of the family. If no allowance is made for this fact, the heritability estimates arrived at may be spurious, such heritabilities have indeed been claimed for such things as administrative, legal, or military talents and for social eminence in general. It is evident that having socially eminent parents makes it easier for the children to achieve such eminence also, biological heredity may have little or nothing to do with this.

A general conclusion from the evidence now available may be stated as follows: diversity in almost any trait—physical, physiological, or behavioural—owes in part to genetic variables and in part to environmental variables. In any array of environments, individuals with more nearly similar genetic endowments are likely to show a greater average resemblance than the carriers of more diverse genetic endowments. It is, however, also true that in different environments the carriers of similar genetic endowments may grow, develop, and behave in different ways.

PHYSICAL BASIS OF HEREDITY

When Gregor Mendel formulated his laws of heredity, he postulated a particulate nature for the units of inheritance. What exactly these particles were he did not know. Today scientists understand not only the physical location of hereditary units (i.e. the genes) but their molecular composition as well. The unravelling of the physical basis of heredity makes up one of the most fascinating chapters in the history of biology.

Chromosomes and Genes

As has been discussed, each individual in a sexually reproducing species inherits two alleles for each gene, one from each parent. Furthermore, when such an individual forms sex cells, each of the resultant gametes receives one member of each allelic pair. The formation of gametes occurs through a process of cell division called meiosis. When gametes unite in fertilisation, the double dose of hereditary material is restored, and a new individual is created. This individual, consisting at first of only one cell, grows via mitosis, a process of repeated cell divisions. Mitosis differs from meiosis in that each daughter cell receives a full copy of all the hereditary material found in the parent cell.

It is apparent that the genes must physically reside in cellular structures that meet two criteria. First, these structures must be replicated and passed on to each generation of daughter cells during mitosis. Second, they must be organised into homologous pairs, one member of which is parcelled out to each gamete formed during meiosis. As early as 1848, biologists had observed that cell nuclei resolve themselves into small rodlike bodies during mitosis, later these structures were found to absorb certain dyes and so came to be called chromosomes (coloured bodies). During the early years of the 20th century, cellular studies using ordinary light microscopes clarified the behaviour of chromosomes during mitosis and meiosis, which led to the conclusion that chromosomes are the carriers of genes.

BEHAVIOUR OF CHROMOSOMES DURING CELL DIVISION

During Mitosis

When the chromosomes condense during cell division, they have already undergone replication. Each chromosome thus consists of two identical replicas, called chromatids, joined at a point called the centromere. During mitosis the sister chromatids separate, one going to each daughter cell. Chromosomes thus meet the first criterion for being the repository of genes: they are replicated, and a full copy is passed to each daughter cell during mitosis.

During Meiosis

It was the behaviour of chromosomes during meiosis, however, that provided the strongest evidence for their being the carriers of genes. In 1902 American scientist Walter S. Sutton reported on his observations of the action of chromosomes during sperm formation in grasshoppers. Sutton had observed that, during meiosis, each chromosome (consisting of two chromatids) becomes paired with a physically similar chromosome. These homologous chromosomes separate during meiosis, with one member of each pair going to a different cell. Assuming that one member of each homologous pair was of maternal origin and the other was paternally derived, here was an event that fulfilled the behaviour of genes postulated in Mendel's first law.

It is now known that the number of chromosomes within the nucleus is usually constant in all individuals of a given species—for example, 46 in the human, 40 in the house mouse, 8 in the vinegar fly (*Drosophila melanogaster*, sometimes called fruit fly), 20 in corn (maize), 24 in the tomato, and 48 in the potato. In sexually reproducing organisms, this number is called the diploid number of chromosomes, as it represents the double dose of chromosomes received from two parents. The nucleus of a gamete, however, contains half this number of chromosomes, or the haploid number. Thus, a human gamete contains 23 chromosomes, while a *Drosophila* gamete contains 4. Meiosis produces the haploid gametes.

At the leptotene stage the chromosomes appear as long, thin threads. At pachytene they pair, the corresponding portions of the two chromosomes lying side by side. The chromosomes then duplicate and contract into paired chromatids. At this stage the pair of chromosomes is known as a tetrad, as it consists of four chromatids. Also at this stage an extremely important event occurs: portions of the maternal and paternal chromosomes are exchanged. This exchange process, called crossing over, results in chromatids that include both paternal and maternal genes and consequently introduces new genetic combinations. The first meiotic division separates the chromosomal tetrads, with the paternal chromosome (whose chromatids now contain some maternal genes) going to one cell and the maternal chromosome (containing some paternal genes) going to another cell. During the second meiotic division the chromatids separate. The original diploid cell has thus given rise to four haploid gametes. Not only has a reduction in chromosome number occurred, but the resulting single member of each homologous chromosome pair may be a new combination (through crossing over) of genes present in the original diploid cell.

Consider the inheritance of two pairs of genes, such as Mendel's factors for seed coloration and seed surface in peas, these genes are located on different pairs of chromosomes. Since maternal and paternal members of different chromosome pairs are assorted independently, so are the genes they contain. This explains, in part, the genetic variety seen among the progeny of the same pair of parents. As stated above, humans have 46 chromosomes in the body cells and in the cells (oogonia and spermatogonia) from which the sex cells arise. At meiosis these 46 chromosomes form 23 pairs, one of the chromosomes of each pair being of maternal and the other of paternal origin. Independent assortment is, then, capable of producing 2^{23}, or 8,388,608, kinds of sex cells with different combinations of the grandmaternal and grandpaternal chromosomes. Since each parent has the potentiality of producing 2^{23} kinds of sex cells, the total number of possible combinations of the grandparental chromosomes is $2^{23} \times 2^{23} = 2^{46}$. The population of the world is now more than 6 billion persons, or approximately 2^{32} persons. It is therefore certain that only a tiny fraction of the potentially possible chromosome and gene combinations can ever be realised. Yet even 2^{46} is an underestimate of the variety potentially possible. The grandmaternal and grandpaternal members of the chromosome pairs are not indivisible units. Each chromosome carries many genes, and the chromosome pairs exchange segments at meiosis through the process of crossing over. This is evidence that the genes rather than the chromosomes are the units of Mendelian segregation.

Linkage of Traits

Simple linkage

As pointed out above, the random assortment of the maternal and paternal chromosomes at meiosis is the physical basis of the independent assortment of genes and of the traits they control. This is the basis of the second law of Mendel. The number of the genes in a sex cell is, however, much greater than that of the chromosomes. When two or more genes are borne on the same chromosome, these genes may not be assorted independently, such genes are said to be linked. When a *Drosophila* fly homozygous for a normal gray body and long wings is crossed with one having a black body and vestigial wings, the F_1 consists of hybrid gray, long-winged flies (see the figure). Gray body (B) is evidently dominant over black body (b), and long wing (V) is dominant over vestigial wing (v). Now consider a backcross of the heterozygous F_1 males to double-recessive black-vestigial females (bbvv). Independent assortment would be expected to give in the progeny of the backcross the following: 1 gray-long : 1 gray-vestigial : 1 black-long : 1 black-vestigial. In reality, only gray-long and black-vestigial flies are produced, in approximately equal numbers, the genes remain linked in the same combinations in which they were found in the parents. The backcross of the heterozygous F_1 females to double-recessive males gives a somewhat different result: 42 per cent each of gray-long and black-vestigial flies and about 8 per cent each of black-long and gray-vestigial classes. In sum, 84 per cent of the progeny have the parental combinations of traits, and 16 per cent have the traits recombined. The interpretation of these results given in 1911 by the American geneticist Thomas Hunt Morgan laid the foundation of the theory of linear arrangement of genes in the chromosomes.

Traits that exhibit linkage in experimental crosses (such as black body and vestigial wings) are determined by genes located in the same chromosome. As more and more genes became known in *Drosophila*, they fell neatly into four linkage groups corresponding to the four pairs of the chromosomes this species possesses. One linkage group consists of sex-linked genes, located in the X chromosome, of the three remaining linkage groups, two have many more genes than the remaining one, which corresponds to the presence of two pairs of large chromosomes and one pair of tiny dotlike chromosomes. The numbers of linkage groups in other organisms are equal to or smaller than the numbers of the chromosomes in the sex cells, e.g. 10 linkage groups and 10 chromosomes in corn, 19 linkage groups and 20 chromosomes in the house mouse, and 23 linkage groups and 23 chromosomes in the human.

As discussed above, the linkage of the genes black and vestigial in *Drosophila* is complete in heterozygous males, while in the progeny of females there appear about 17 per cent of recombination classes. With very rare exceptions, the linkage of all genes belonging to the same linkage group is complete in *Drosophila* males, while in the females different pairs of genes exhibit all degrees of linkage from complete (no recombination) to 50 per cent (random assortment). Morgan's inference was that the degree of linkage depends on physical distance between the genes in the chromosome: the closer the genes, the tighter the linkage and vice versa. Furthermore, Morgan perceived that the chiasmata (crosses that occur in meiotic chromosomes) indicate the mechanism underlying the phenomena of linkage and crossing over.

This realisation opened an opportunity to map the arrangement of the genes and the estimated distances between them in the chromosome by studying the frequencies of recombination of various traits in the progenies of hybrids. In other words, the linkage maps of the chromosomes are really summaries of many statistical observations on the outcomes of hybridisation experiments. In principle at least, such maps could be prepared even if the chromosomes, not to speak of the chiasmata at meiosis, were unknown.

But an interesting and relevant fact is that in *Drosophila* males the linkage of the genes in the same chromosome is complete, and observations under the microscope show that no chiasmata are formed in the chromosomes at meiosis. In most organisms, including humans, chiasmata are seen in the meiotic chromosomes in both sexes, and observations on hybrid progenies show that recombination of linked genes occurs also in both sexes.

Chromosome maps exist for the *Drosophila* fly, corn, the house mouse, the bread mold Neurospora crassa, and some bacteria and bacteriophages (viruses that infect bacteria). Until quite late in the 20th century, the mapping of human chromosomes presented a particularly difficult problem: experimental crosses could not be arranged in humans, and only a few linkages could be determined by analysis of unique family histories. However, the development of recombinant DNA technology provided new understanding of human genetic processes and new methods of research. Using the techniques of recombinant DNA technology, hundreds of genes have been mapped to the human chromosomes and many linkages established.

Sex linkage

The male of many animals has one chromosome pair, the sex chromosomes, consisting of unequal members called X and Y. At meiosis the X and Y chromosomes first pair then disjoin and pass to different cells. One-half of the gametes (spermatozoa) formed contain the X chromosome and the other half the Y. The female has two X chromosomes, all egg cells normally carry a single X. The eggs fertilised by X-bearing spermatozoa give females (XX), and those fertilised by Y-bearing spermatozoa give males (XY).

The genes located in the X chromosomes exhibit what is known as sex-linkage or crisscross inheritance. This is because of a crucial difference between the paired sex chromosomes and the other pairs of chromosomes (called autosomes). The members of the autosome pairs are truly homologous, that is, each member of a pair contains a full complement of the same genes (albeit, perhaps, in different allelic forms). The sex chromosomes, on the other hand, do not constitute a homologous pair, as the X chromosome is much larger and carries far more genes than does the Y. Consequently, many recessive alleles carried on the X chromosome of a male will be expressed just as if they were dominant, for the Y chromosome carries no genes to counteract them. The classic case of sex-linked inheritance, described by Morgan in 1910, is that of the white eyes in *Drosophila*. White-eyed females crossed to males with the normal red eye colour produce red-eyed daughters and white-eyed sons in the F_1 generation and equal numbers of white-eyed and red-eyed females and males in the F_2 generation. The cross of red-eyed females to white-eyed males gives a different result: both sexes are red-eyed in F_1 and the females in the F_2 generation are red-eyed, half the males are red-eyed, and the other half white-eyed. As interpreted by Morgan, the gene that determines the red or white eyes is borne on the X chromosome, and the allele for red eye is dominant over that for white eye. Since a male receives its single X chromosome from his mother, all sons of white-eyed females also have white eyes. A female inherits one X chromosome from her mother and the other X from her father. Red-eyed females may have genes for red eyes in both of their X chromosomes (homozygotes), or they may have one X with the gene for red and the other for white (heterozygotes). In the progeny of heterozygous females, one-half of the sons will receive the X chromosome with the gene for white and will have white eyes, and the other half will receive the X with the gene for red eyes. The daughters of the heterozygous females crossed with white-eyed males will have either two X chromosomes with the gene for white—and hence have white eyes—or one X with the gene for white and the other X with the gene for red and will be red-eyed heterozygotes.

In humans, red-green colour blindness and hemophilia are among many traits showing sex-linked inheritance and are consequently due to genes borne in the X chromosome.

In some animals—birds, butterflies and moths, some fish, and at least some amphibians and reptiles—the chromosomal mechanism of sex determination is a mirror image of that described above. The male has two X chromosomes and the female an X and Y chromosome. Here the spermatozoa all have an X chromosome, the eggs are of two kinds, some with X and others with Y chromosomes, usually in equal numbers. The sex of the offspring is then determined by the egg rather than by the spermatozoon. Sex-linked inheritance is altered correspondingly. A male homozygous for a sex-linked recessive trait crossed to a female with the dominant one gives, in the F_1 generation, daughters with the recessive trait and heterozygous sons with the corresponding dominant trait. The F_2 generation has recessive and dominant females and males in equal numbers. A male with a dominant trait crossed to a female with a recessive trait gives uniformly dominant F_1 and a segregation in a ratio of 2 dominant males : 1 dominant female : 1 recessive female.

Observations on pedigrees or experimental crosses show that certain traits exhibit sex-linked inheritance, the behaviour of the X chromosomes at meiosis is such that the genes they carry may be expected to exhibit sex-linkage. This evidence still failed to convince some skeptics that the genes for the sex-linked traits were in fact borne in certain chromosomes seen under the microscope. An experimental proof was furnished in 1916 by American geneticist Calvin Blackman Bridges. As stated above, white-eyed *Drosophila* females crossed to red-eyed males usually produce red-eyed female and white-eyed male progeny. Among thousands of such 'regular' offspring, there are occasionally found exceptional white-eyed females and red-eyed males. Bridges constructed the following working hypothesis. Suppose that, during meiosis in the female, gametogenesis occasionally goes wrong, and the two X chromosomes fail to disjoin. Exceptional eggs will then be produced, carrying two X chromosomes and eggs carrying none. An egg with two X chromosomes coming from a white-eyed female fertilised by a spermatozoon with a Y chromosome will give an exceptional white-eyed female. An egg with no X chromosome fertilised by a spermatozoon with an X chromosome derived from a red-eyed father will yield an exceptional red-eyed male. This hypothesis can be rigorously tested. The exceptional white-eyed females should have not only the two X chromosomes but also a Y chromosome, which normal females do not have. The exceptional males should, on the other hand, lack a Y chromosome, which normal males do have. Both predictions were verified by examination under a microscope of the chromosomes of exceptional females and males. The hypothesis also predicts that exceptional eggs with two X chromosomes fertilised by X-bearing spermatozoa must give individuals with three X chromosomes, such individuals were later identified by Bridges as poorly viable 'superfemales.' Exceptional eggs with no Xs, fertilised by Y-bearing spermatozoa, will give zygotes without X chromosomes, such zygotes die in early stages of development.

Chromosomal Aberrations

The chromosome set of a species remains relatively stable over long periods of time. However, within populations there can be found abnormalities involving the structure or number of chromosomes. These alterations arise spontaneously from errors in the normal processes of the cell. Their consequences are usually deleterious, giving rise to individuals who are unhealthy or sterile, though in rare cases alterations provide new adaptive opportunities that allow evolutionary change to occur. In fact, the discovery of visible chromosomal differences between species has given rise to the belief that radical restructuring of chromosome architecture has been an important force in evolution.

Changes in chromosome structure

Two important principles dictate the properties of a large proportion of structural chromosomal changes. The first principle is that any deviation from the normal ratio of genetic material in the genome results in genetic imbalance and abnormal function. In the normal nuclei of both diploid and haploid cells, the ratio of the individual chromosomes to one another is 1:1. Any deviation from this ratio by addition or subtraction of either whole chromosomes or parts of chromosomes results in genomic imbalance. The second principle is that homologous chromosomes go to great lengths to pair at meiosis. The tightly paired homologous regions are joined by a ladderlike longitudinal structure called the synaptonemal complex. Homologous regions seem to be able to find each other and form a synaptonemal complex whether or not they are part of normal chromosomes. Therefore, when structural changes occur, not only are the resulting pairing formations highly characteristic of that type of structural change but they also dictate the packaging of normal and abnormal chromosomes into the gametes and subsequently into the progeny.

Deletions

The simplest, but perhaps most damaging, structural change is a deletion—the complete loss of a part of one chromosome. In a haploid cell this is lethal, because part of the essential genome is lost. However, even in diploid cells deletions are generally lethal or have other serious consequences. In a diploid a heterozygous deletion results in a cell that has one normal chromosome set and another set that contains a truncated chromosome. Such cells show genomic imbalance, which increases in severity with the size of the deletion. Another potential source of damage is that any recessive, deleterious, or lethal alleles that are in the normal counterpart of the deleted region will be expressed in the phenotype. In humans, cri-du-chat syndrome is caused by a heterozygous deletion at the tip of the short arm of chromosome 5. Infants are born with this condition as the result of a deletion arising in parental germinal tissues or even in sex cells. The manifestations of this deletion, in addition to the 'cat cry' that gives the syndrome its name, include severe intellectual disability and an abnormally small head.

Duplications

A heterozygous duplication (an extra copy of some chromosome region) also results in a genomic imbalance with deleterious consequences. Small duplications within a gene can arise spontaneously. Larger duplications can be caused by crossovers following asymmetrical chromosome pairing or by meiotic irregularities resulting from other types of altered chromosome structures. If a duplication becomes homozygous, it can provide the organism with an opportunity to acquire new genetic functions through mutations within the duplicate copy.

Inversions

An inversion occurs when a chromosome breaks in two places and the region between the break rotates 180° before rejoining with the two end fragments. If the inverted segment contains the centromere (i.e. the point where the two chromatids are joined), the inversion is said to be pericentric, if not, it is called paracentric. Inversions do not result in a gain or loss of genetic material, and they have deleterious effects only if one of the chromosomal breaks occurs within an essential gene or if the function of a gene is altered by its relocation to a new chromosomal neighbourhood (called the position effect). However, individuals who are heterozygous for inversions produce aberrant meiotic products along with normal products. The only way uninverted and inverted segments can pair is by forming an inversion loop. If no crossovers occur in the loop, half of the gametes will be normal and the other half will contain an inverted chromosome. If a crossover does occur within the loop of a paracentric inversion, a chromosome bridge and an acentric chromosome (i.e. a chromosome without a centromere) will be formed, and this will give rise to abnormal meiotic products carrying deletions, which are inviable. In a pericentric inversion, a crossover within the loop does not result in a bridge or an acentric chromosome, but inviable products are produced carrying a duplication and a deletion.

Translocations

If a chromosome break occurs in each of two nonhomologous chromosomes and the two breaks rejoin in a new arrangement, the new segment is called a translocation. A cell bearing a heterozygous translocation has a full set of genes and will be viable unless one of the breaks causes damage within a gene or if there is a position effect on gene function. However, once again the pairing properties of the chromosomes at meiosis result in aberrant meiotic products. Specifically, half of the products are deleted for one of the chromosome regions that changed positions and half of the products are duplicated for the other. These duplications and deletions usually result in inviability, so translocation heterozygotes are generally semisterile (half-sterile).

Changes in chromosome number

Two types of changes in chromosome numbers can be distinguished: a change in the number of whole chromosome sets (polyploidy) and a change in chromosomes within a set (aneuploidy).

Polyploids

An individual with additional chromosome sets is called a polyploid. Individuals with three sets of chromosomes (triploids, $3n$) or four sets of chromosomes (tetraploids, $4n$) are polyploid derivatives of the basic diploid ($2n$) constitution. Polyploids with odd numbers of sets (e.g. triploids) are sterile, because homologous chromosomes pair only two by two, and the extra chromosome moves randomly to a cell pole, resulting in highly unbalanced, nonfunctional meiotic products. It is for this reason that triploid watermelons are seedless. However, polyploids with even numbers of chromosome sets can be fertile if orderly two-by-two chromosome pairing occurs.

Though two organisms from closely related species frequently hybridise, the chromosomes of the fusing partners are different enough that the two sets do not pair at meiosis, resulting in sterile offspring. However, if by chance the number of chromosome sets in the hybrid accidentally duplicates, a pairing partner for each chromosome will be produced, and the hybrid will be fertile. These chromosomally doubled hybrids are called allotetraploids. Bread wheat, which is hexaploid ($6n$) due to several natural spontaneous hybridisations, is an example of an allotetraploid. Some polyploid plants are able to produce seeds through an asexual type of reproduction called apomixis, in such cases, all progeny are identical to the parent. Polyploidy does arise spontaneously in humans, but all polyploids either abort in utero or die shortly after birth.

Aneuploids

Some cells have an abnormal number of chromosomes that is not a whole multiple of the haploid number. This condition is called aneuploidy. Most aneuploids arise by nondisjunction, a failure of homologous chromosomes to separate at meiosis. When a gamete of this type is fertilised by a normal gamete, the zygotes formed will have an unequal distribution of chromosomes. Such genomic imbalance results in severe abnormalities or death. Only aneuploids involving small chromosomes tend to survive and even then only with an aberrant phenotype.

The most common form of aneuploidy in humans results in Down syndrome, a suite of specific disorders in individuals possessing an extra chromosome 21 (trisomy 21). The symptoms of Down syndrome include intellectual disability, severe disorders of internal organs such as the heart and kidneys, up-slanted eyes, an enlarged tongue, and abnormal dermal ridge patterns on the fingers, palms, and soles. Other forms of aneuploidy in humans result from abnormal numbers of sex chromosomes. Turner syndrome is a condition in which females have only one X chromosome. Symptoms may include short stature, webbed neck, kidney or heart malformations, underdeveloped sex characteristics, or sterility. Klinefelter syndrome is a condition in which males have one extra female sex chromosome, resulting in an XXY pattern. (Other, less frequent, chromosomal patterns include XXXY, XXXXY, XXYY, and XXXYY.) Symptoms of Klinefelter syndrome may include sterility, a tall physique, lack of secondary sex characteristics, breast development, and learning disabilities.

MOLECULAR GENETICS

The data accumulated by scientists of the early 20th century provided compelling evidence that chromosomes are the carriers of genes. But the nature of the genes themselves remained a mystery, as did the mechanism by which they exert their influence. Molecular genetics—the study of the structure and function of genes at the molecular level—provided answers to these fundamental questions.

DNA as the Agent of Heredity

In 1869 Swiss chemist Johann Friedrich Miescher extracted a substance containing nitrogen and phosphorus from cell nuclei. The substance was originally called nuclein, but it is now known as deoxyribonucleic acid, or DNA. DNA is the chemical component of the chromosomes that is chiefly responsible for their staining properties in microscopic preparations. Since the chromosomes of eukaryotes contain a variety of proteins in addition to DNA, the question naturally arose whether the nucleic acids or the proteins, or both together, were the carriers of the genetic information. Until the early 1950s most biologists were inclined to believe that the proteins were the chief carriers of heredity. Nucleic acids contain only four different unitary building blocks, but proteins are made up of 20 different amino acids. Proteins therefore appeared to have a greater diversity of structure, and the diversity of the genes seemed at first likely to rest on the diversity of the proteins.

Evidence that DNA acts as the carrier of the genetic information was first firmly demonstrated by exquisitely simple microbiological studies. In 1928 English bacteriologist Frederick Griffith was studying two strains of the bacterium Streptococcus pneumoniae, one strain was lethal to mice (virulent) and the other was harmless (avirulent). Griffith found that mice inoculated with either the heat-killed virulent bacteria or the living avirulent bacteria remained free of infection, but mice inoculated with a mixture of both became infected and died. It seemed as if some chemical 'transforming principle' had transferred from the dead virulent cells into the avirulent cells and changed them. In 1944 American bacteriologist Oswald T. Avery and his coworkers found that the transforming factor was DNA. Avery and his research team obtained mixtures from heat-killed virulent bacteria and inactivated either the proteins, polysaccharides (sugar subunits), lipids, DNA, or RNA (ribonucleic acid, a close chemical relative of DNA) and added each type of preparation individually to avirulent cells. The only molecular class whose inactivation prevented transformation to virulence was DNA. Therefore, it seemed that DNA, because it could transform, must be the hereditary material.

A similar conclusion was reached from the study of bacteriophages, viruses that attack and kill bacterial cells. From a host cell infected by one bacteriophage, hundreds of bacteriophage progeny are produced. In 1952 American biologists Alfred D. Hershey and Martha Chase prepared two populations of bacteriophage particles. In one population, the outer protein coat of the bacteriophage was labeled with a radioactive isotope, in the other, the DNA was labeled. After allowing both populations to attack bacteria, Hershey and Chase found that only when DNA was labeled did the progeny bacteriophage contain radioactivity. Therefore, they concluded that DNA is injected into the bacterial cell, where it directs the synthesis of numerous complete bacteriophages at the expense of the host. In other words, in bacteriophages DNA is the hereditary material responsible for the fundamental characteristics of the virus. Today the genetic makeup of most organisms can be transformed using externally applied DNA, in a manner similar to that used by Avery for bacteria. Transforming DNA is able to pass through cellular and nuclear membranes and then integrate into the chromosomal DNA of the recipient cell. Furthermore, using modern DNA technology, it is possible to isolate the section of chromosomal DNA that constitutes an individual gene, manipulate its structure, and reintroduce it into a cell to cause changes that show beyond doubt that the DNA is responsible for a large part of the overall characteristics of an organism. For reasons such as these, it is now accepted that, in all living organisms, with the exception of some viruses, genes are composed of DNA.

Structure and composition of DNA

The remarkable properties of the nucleic acids, which qualify these substances to serve as the carriers of genetic information, have claimed the attention of many investigators. The groundwork was laid by pioneer biochemists who found that nucleic acids are long chainlike molecules, the backbones of which consist of repeated sequences of phosphate and sugar linkages—ribose sugar in RNA and deoxyribose sugar in DNA. Attached to the sugar links in the backbone are two kinds of nitrogenous bases: purines and pyrimidines. The purines are adenine (A) and guanine (G) in both DNA and RNA, the pyrimidines are cytosine (C) and thymine (T) in DNA and cytosine (C) and uracil (U) in RNA. A single purine or pyrimidine is attached to each sugar, and the entire phosphate-sugar-base subunit is called a nucleotide. The nucleic acids extracted from different species of animals and plants have different proportions of the four nucleotides. Some are relatively richer in adenine and thymine, while others have more guanine and cytosine. However, it was found by biochemist Erwin Chargaff that the amount of A is always equal to T, and the amount of G is always equal to C.

With the general acceptance of DNA as the chemical basis of heredity in the early 1950s, many scientists turned their attention to determining how the nitrogenous bases fit together to make up a threadlike molecule. The structure of DNA was determined by American geneticist James Watson and British biophysicist Francis Crick in 1953. Watson and Crick based their model largely on the research of British physicists Rosalind Franklin and Maurice Wilkins, who analysed X-ray diffraction patterns to show that DNA is a double helix. The findings of Chargaff suggested to Watson and Crick that adenine was somehow paired with thymine and that guanine was paired with cytosine.

Using this information, Watson and Crick came up with their now-famous model showing DNA as a double helix composed of two intertwined chains of nucleotides, in which the adenines of one chain are linked to the thymines of the other, and the guanines in one chain are linked to the cytosines of the other. The structure resembles a ladder that has been twisted into a spiral shape: the sides of the ladder are composed of sugar and phosphate groups, and the rungs are made up of the paired nitrogenous bases. By making a wire model of the structure, it became clear that the only way the model could conform to the requirements of the molecular dimensions of DNA was if A always paired with T and G with C, in fact, the A-T and G-C pairs showed a satisfying lock-and-key fit. Although most of the bonds in DNA are strong covalent bonds, the A-T and G-C bonds are weak hydrogen bonds. However, multiple hydrogen bonds along the centre of the molecule confer enough stability to hold the two strands together.

The two strands of Watson and Crick's double helix were antiparallel, that is, the nucleotides were arranged in opposite orientation. This can be visualised if the L shape of a nucleotide is imagined to be a sock: the neck of the sock is the nitrogenous base, the toe is the phosphate group, and the heel is the sugar group. The nucleotide chain would then be a string of socks attached heel to toe, with the necks pointing inward toward the centre of the DNA molecule. In one strand the arrangement of the sugar-phosphate backbone would be toe-heel-toe-heel and so on, and in the other strand in the same direction the arrangement would be heel-toe-heel-toe. Chemically, the heel is the 3'-hydroxyl end and the toe is the 5'-phosphate end. (These names are derived from the carbon atoms through which the sugar-phosphate linkage is made.) Therefore, one DNA strand runs from 5' → 3' (five prime to three prime), whereas the other runs from 3' → 5'.

Watson and Crick noted that their proposed DNA structure fulfilled two necessary features of a hereditary molecule. First, a hereditary molecule must be capable of replication so that the information can be passed on to the next generation, therefore, Watson and Crick hypothesised that, if the two halves of the double helix could separate, they could act as templates for the synthesis of two identical double helices. Second, a hereditary molecule must contain information to guide the development of a complete organism, therefore, Watson and Crick speculated that the sequence of nucleotides might represent coded information of this sort. Subsequent research showed that their speculations on both points were correct.

DNA Replication

The Watson-Crick model of the structure of DNA suggested at least three different ways that DNA might self-replicate. The experiments of Matthew Meselson and Franklin Stahl on the bacterium *Escherichia coli* in 1958 suggested that DNA replicates semiconservatively. Meselson and Stahl grew bacterial cells in the presence of 15N, a heavy isotope of nitrogen, so that the DNA of the cells contained ^{15}N. These cells were then transferred to a medium containing the normal isotope of nitrogen, ^{14}N, and allowed to go through cell division. The researchers were able to demonstrate that, in the DNA molecules of the daughter cells, one strand contained only ^{15}N, and the other strand contained ^{14}N. This is precisely what is expected by the semiconservative mode of replication, in which the original DNA molecules should separate into two template strands containing ^{15}N, and the newly aligned nucleotides should all contain ^{14}N.

The hooking together of free nucleotides in the newly synthesised strand takes place one nucleotide at a time in the 5' → 3' direction. An incoming free nucleotide pairs with the complementary nucleotide on the template strand, and then the 5' end of the free nucleotide is covalently joined to the 3' end of a nucleotide already in place.

The process is then repeated. The result is a nucleotide chain, referred to chemically as a nucleotide polymer or a polynucleotide. Of course the polymer is not a random polymer, its nucleotide sequence has been directed by the nucleotide sequence of the template strand. It is this templating process that enables hereditary information to be replicated accurately and passed down through the generations. In a very real way, human DNA has been replicated in a direct line of descent from the first vertebrates that evolved hundreds of millions of years ago.

DNA replication starts at a site on the DNA called the origin of replication. In higher organisms, replication begins at multiple origins of replication and moves along the DNA in both directions outward from each origin, creating two replication 'forks.' The events at both replication forks are identical. In order for DNA to replicate, however, the two strands of the double helix first must be unwound from each other. A class of enzymes called DNA topoisomerases removes helical twists by cutting a DNA strand and then resealing the cut. Enzymes called helicases then separate the two strands of the double helix, exposing two template surfaces for the alignment of free nucleotides. Beginning at the origin of replication, a complex enzyme called DNA polymerase moves along the DNA molecule, pairing nucleotides on each template strand with free complementary nucleotides. Because of the antiparallel nature of the DNA strands, new strand synthesis is different on each template. On the $3' \rightarrow 5'$ template strand, polymerisation proceeds in the $5' \rightarrow 3'$ direction, and this growing strand is called the leading strand. However, polymerisation must be carried out differently on the $5' \rightarrow 3'$ template strand because nucleotides cannot be assembled in the $3' \rightarrow 5'$ direction. Here short sequences of RNA are polymerised on the template. These sequences act as primers to which the DNA polymerase can add nucleotides in the $5' \rightarrow 3'$ direction but in the opposite direction in which synthesis is proceeding on the lagging strand. The DNA polymerase hence makes short segments of DNA called Okazaki fragments in the 'wrong' direction. For this reason the strand synthesised on the $5' \rightarrow 3'$ template strand is called the lagging strand. Later, the RNA primers are removed and the Okazaki fragments are joined. This RNA priming system cannot be used to synthesise the very end of the $3' \rightarrow 5'$ strand, once the last RNA primer is removed, synthesis cannot continue over the remaining gap. To overcome this obstacle, the enzyme telomerase adds multiple copies of a nucleotide sequence to the end of the DNA strand to allow completion of replication. Despite the peculiar events on the lagging strand, the entire DNA strand is eventually polymerised, and the two daughter DNA molecules thus produced are identical.

EXPRESSION OF THE GENETIC CODE: TRANSCRIPTION AND TRANSLATION

DNA represents a type of information that is vital to the shape and form of an organism. It contains instructions in a coded sequence of nucleotides, and this sequence interacts with the environment to produce form—the living organism with all of its complex structures and functions. The form of an organism is largely determined by protein. A large proportion of what we see when we observe the various parts of an organism is protein, for example, hair, muscle, and skin are made up largely of protein. Other chemical compounds that make up the human body, such as carbohydrates, fats, and more-complex chemicals, are either synthesised by catalytic proteins (enzymes) or are deposited at specific times and in specific tissues under the influence of proteins. For example, the black-brown skin pigment melanin is synthesised by enzymes and deposited in special skin cells called melanocytes. Genes exert their effect mainly by determining the structure and function of the many thousands of different proteins, which in turn determine the characteristics of an organism. Generally, it is true to say that each protein is coded for by one gene, bearing in mind that the production of some proteins requires the cooperation of several genes.

Proteins are polymeric molecules, that is, they are made up of chains of monomeric elements, as is DNA. In proteins, the monomers are amino acids. Organisms generally contain 20 different types of amino acids, and the distinguishing factors that make one protein different from another are its length and specific amino acid sequence, which are determined by the number and sequence of nucleotide pairs in DNA. In other words, there is a colinearity (i.e. parallel structure) between the polymer that is DNA and the polymer that is protein.

Hence, genetic information flows from DNA into protein. However, this is not a single-step process. First, the nucleotide sequence of DNA is copied into the nucleotide sequence of single-stranded RNA in a process called transcription. Transcription of any one gene takes place at the chromosomal location of that gene. Whereas the unit of replication is a whole chromosome, the transcriptional unit is a relatively short segment of the chromosome, the gene. The active transcription of a gene depends on the need for the activity of that particular gene in a specific tissue or at a given time.

The nucleotide sequence in RNA faithfully mirrors that of the DNA from which it was transcribed. The uracil in RNA has exactly the same hydrogen-bonding properties as thymine, so there are no changes at the information level. For most RNA molecules, the nucleotide sequence is converted into an amino acid sequence, a process called translation. In prokaryotes, translation begins during the transcription process, before the full RNA transcript is made. In eukaryotes, transcription finishes, and the RNA molecule passes from the nucleus into the cytoplasm, where translation takes place.

The genome of a type of virus called a retrovirus (of which the human immunodeficiency virus, or HIV, is an example) is composed of RNA instead of DNA. In a retrovirus, RNA is reverse transcribed into DNA, which can then integrate into the chromosomal DNA of the host cell that the retrovirus infects. The synthesis of DNA is catalysed by the enzyme reverse transcriptase. The existence of reverse transcriptase shows that genetic information is capable of flowing from RNA to DNA in exceptional cases. Since it is believed that life arose in an RNA world, it is likely that the evolution of reverse transcriptase was an important step in the transition to the present DNA world.

Transcription

A gene is a functional region of a chromosome that is capable of making a transcript in response to appropriate regulatory signals. Therefore, a gene must not only be composed of the DNA sequence that is actually transcribed, but it must also include an adjacent regulatory, or control, region that is necessary for the transcript to be made in the correct developmental context.

The polymerisation of ribonucleotides during transcription is catalysed by the enzyme RNA polymerase. As with DNA replication, the two DNA strands must separate to expose the template. However, transcription differs from replication in that for any gene, only one of the DNA strands, the $3' \rightarrow 5'$ strand, is actually used as a template. Synthesis of RNA is in the $5' \rightarrow 3'$ direction, as with DNA. Hence, the growing point of the RNA chain is the $3'$ end, and polymerisation is continuous as the RNA polymerase moves along the transcribed region. The RNA strand is extruded from the transcription complex like a tail, which grows longer as the transcription process advances. Eventually, a full-length transcript of RNA is produced, and this detaches from the DNA. The process is repeated, and multiple RNA transcripts are produced from one gene.

Prokaryotes possess only one type of RNA polymerase, but in eukaryotes there are several different types. RNA polymerase I synthesises ribosomal RNA (rRNA), and RNA polymerase III synthesises transfer RNA (tRNA) and other small RNAs. The types of RNA transcribed by these two polymerases are never translated into protein. RNA polymerase II transcribes the major type of genes, those genes that code for proteins. Transcription of these genes is considered in detail below.

Transcription of protein-coding genes results in a type of RNA called messenger RNA (mRNA), so named because it carries a genetic message from the gene on a nuclear chromosome into the cytoplasm, where it is acted upon by the protein-synthesising apparatus. The transcription machinery contains many items in addition to the RNA polymerase. The successful binding of the RNA polymerase to the DNA 'upstream' of the transcribed sequence depends upon the cooperation of many additional proteinaceous transcription factors. The region of the gene upstream from the region to be transcribed contains specific DNA sequences that are essential for the binding of transcription factors and a region called the promoter, to which the RNA polymerase binds. These sequences must be a specific distance from the transcriptional start site for successful operation. Various short base sequences in this regulatory region physically bind specific transcription factors by virtue of a lock-and-key fit between the DNA and the protein. As might be expected, a protein binds with the centre of the DNA molecule, which contains the sequence specificity, and not with the outside of the molecule, which is merely a uniform repetition of sugar and phosphate groups.

In eukaryotes, a key segment is the TATA box, a TATA sequence approximately 30 nucleotides upstream from the transcription start site. If this sequence is changed or moved, the rate of transcription drops drastically. The TATA box is bound by a transcription factor called the TATA-binding protein, which, together with RNA polymerase II and numerous other transcription factors, assembles in a precise sequence around the TATA box, binding to each other and to the DNA. Together, RNA polymerase and the transcription factors constitute the transcription complex.

The RNA polymerase is directed by the transcription complex to begin transcription at the proper site. It then moves along the template, synthesising mRNA as it goes. At some position past the coding region, the transcription process stops. Bacteria have well-characterised specific termination sequences, however, in eukaryotes, termination signals are less well understood, and the transcription process stops at variable positions past the end of the coding sequence. A short nucleotide sequence downstream from the coding region acts as a signal for the RNA to be cut at that position, and this becomes the 3' end of the new RNA strand. Subsequently, approximately 200 adenine nucleotides are added to the 3' end to form what is called a poly(A) tail, which is characteristic of all eukaryotic DNA. At the 5' end of the mRNA, a modified guanine nucleotide, called a cap, is added. Noncoding nucleotide sequences called introns are excised from the RNA at this stage in a process called intron splicing. Molecular complexes called spliceosomes, which are composed of proteins and RNA, have RNA sequences that are complementary to the junction between introns and adjacent coding regions called exons. The intron is twisted into a loop and excised, and the exons are linked together. The resulting capped, tailed, and intron-free molecule is now mature mRNA.

Genetic Code

Hereditary information is contained in the nucleotide sequence of DNA in a kind of code. The coded information is copied faithfully into RNA and translated into chains of amino acids. Amino acid chains are folded into helices, zigzags, and other shapes and are sometimes associated with other amino acid chains. The specific amounts of amino acids in a protein and their sequence determine the protein's unique properties, for example, muscle protein and hair protein contain the same 20 amino acids, but the sequences of these amino acids in the two proteins are quite different. If the nucleotide sequence of mRNA is thought of as a written message, it can be said that this message is read by the translation apparatus in 'words' of three nucleotides, starting at one end of the mRNA and proceeding along the length of the molecule. These three-letter words are called codons. Each codon stands for a specific amino acid, so if the message in mRNA is 900 nucleotides long, which corresponds to 300 codons, it will be translated into a chain of 300 amino acids.

Each of the three letters in a codon can be filled by any one of the four nucleotides, therefore, there are 43, or 64, possible codons. Each one of these 64 words in the codon dictionary has meaning. Most codons code for one of the 20 possible amino acids. Two amino acids, methionine and tryptophan, are each coded for by one codon only (AUG and UGG, respectively). The other 18 amino acids are coded for by two to six codons, for example, either of the codons UUU or UUC will cause the insertion of the amino acid phenylalanine into the growing amino acid chain. Three codons—UAG, UGA, and UAA—represent translation-termination signals and are called the stop codons. The first amino acid in an amino acid chain is methionine, encoded by an AUG codon. However, AUG codons are found throughout the coding sequence and are translated into methionines.

One of the surprising findings about the genetic codon dictionary is that, with a few exceptions, it is the same in all organisms. (One exception is mitochondrial DNA, which exhibits several differences from the standard genetic code and also between organisms.) The uniformity of the genetic code has been interpreted as an indication of the evolutionary relatedness of all organisms. For the purpose of genetic research, codon uniformity is convenient because any type of DNA can be translated in any organism.

Translation

The process of translation requires the interaction not only of large numbers of proteinaceous translational factors but also of specific membranes and organelles of the cell. In both prokaryotes and eukaryotes, translation takes place on cytoplasmic organelles called ribosomes. Ribosomes are aggregations of many different types of proteins and ribosomal RNA (rRNA). They can be thought of as cellular anvils on which the links of an amino acid chain are forged. A ribosome is a generic protein-making machine that can be recycled and used to synthesise many different types of proteins. A ribosome attaches to the 5' end of the mRNA, begins translation at the start codon AUG, and translates the message one codon at a time until a stop codon is reached. Any one mRNA is translated many times by several ribosomes along its length, each one at a different stage of translation. In eukaryotes, ribosomes that produce proteins to be used in the same cell are not associated with membranes. However, proteins that must be exported to another location in the organism are synthesised on ribosomes located on the outside of flattened membranous chambers called the endoplasmic reticulum (ER). A completed amino acid chain is extruded into the inner cavity of the ER. Subsequently, the ER transports the proteins via small vesicles to another cytoplasmic organelle called the Golgi apparatus, which in turn buds off more vesicles that eventually fuse with the cell membrane. The protein is then released from the cell.

Another crucial component of the translational process is transfer RNA (tRNA). The function of any one tRNA molecule is to bind to a designated amino acid and carry it to a ribosome, where the amino acid is added to the growing amino acid chain. Each amino acid has its own set of tRNA molecules that will bind only to that specific amino acid. A tRNA molecule is a single nucleotide chain with several helical regions and a loop containing three unpaired nucleotides, called an anticodon. The anticodon of any one tRNA fits perfectly into the mRNA codon that codes for the amino acid attached to that tRNA, for example, the mRNA codon UUU, which codes for the amino acid phenylalanine, will be bound by the anticodon AAA. Thus, any mRNA codon that happens to be on the ribosome at any one time will solicit the binding only of the tRNA with the appropriate anticodon, which will align the correct amino acid for addition to the chain. A tRNA molecule and its attached amino acid must bind to the ribosome as well as to the codon during this amino acid chain-elongation process. A ribosome has two tRNA binding sites, at the first site, one tRNA attaches to the amino acid chain, and at the second site, another tRNA carrying the next amino acid is attached. After attachment, the first tRNA departs and recycles, whereas the second tRNA is now left holding the amino acid chain. At this time the ribosome moves to the next codon, and the whole process is successively repeated along the length of the mRNA until a stop codon is reached, at which time the completed amino acid chain is released from the ribosome. The amino acid chain then spontaneously folds to generate the three-dimensional shape necessary for its function. Each amino acid has its own special shape and pattern of electrical charges on its surface, and ultimately these are what determine the overall shape of the protein. The protein's shape is stabilised by weak bonds that form between different parts of the chain. In some proteins, strong covalent bridges are formed between two cysteines at different sites in the chain. If the protein is composed of two or more amino acid chains, these also associate spontaneously and take on their most stable three-dimensional shape. For enzymes, shape determines the ability to bind to its specific substrate (i.e. the substance on which an enzyme acts). For structural proteins, the amino acid sequence determines whether it will be a filament, a sheet, a globule, or another shape.

Gene Mutation

Given the complexity of DNA and the vast number of cell divisions that take place within the lifetime of a multicellular organism, copying errors are likely to occur. If unrepaired, such errors will change the sequence of the DNA bases and alter the genetic code. Mutation is the random process whereby genes change from one allelic form to another. Scientists who study mutation use the most common genotype found in natural populations, called the wild type, as the standard against which to compare a mutant allele. Mutation can occur in two directions, mutation from wild type to mutant is called a forward mutation, and mutation from mutant to wild type is called a back mutation or reversion.

Mechanisms of mutation

Mutations arise from changes to the DNA of a gene. These changes can be quite small, affecting only one nucleotide pair, or they can be relatively large, affecting hundreds or thousands of nucleotides. Mutations in which one base is changed are called point mutations—for example, substitution of the nucleotide pair AT by GC, CG, or TA. Base substitutions can have different consequences at the protein level. Some base substitutions are 'silent,' meaning that they result in a new codon that codes for the same amino acid as the wild type codon at that position or a codon that codes for a different amino acid that happens to have the same properties as those in the wild type. Substitutions that result in a functionally different amino acid are called 'missense' mutations, these can lead to alteration or loss of protein function. A more severe type of base substitution, called a 'nonsense' mutation, results in a stop codon in a position where there was not one before, which causes the premature termination of protein synthesis and, more than likely, a complete loss of function in the finished protein.

Another type of point mutation that can lead to drastic loss of function is a frameshift mutation, the addition or deletion of one or more DNA bases. In a protein-coding gene, the sequence of codons starting with AUG and ending with a termination codon is called the reading frame. If a nucleotide pair is added to or subtracted from this sequence, the reading frame from that point will be shifted by one nucleotide pair, and all of the codons downstream will be altered. The result will be a protein whose first section (before the mutational site) is that of the wild type amino acid sequence, followed by a tail of functionally meaningless amino acids. Large deletions of many codons will not only remove amino acids from a protein but may also result in a frameshift mutation if the number of nucleotides deleted is not a multiple of three. Likewise, an insertion of a block of nucleotides will add amino acids to a protein and perhaps also have a frameshift effect. A number of human diseases are caused by the expansion of a trinucleotide pair repeat. For example, fragile-X syndrome, the most common type of inherited mental retardation in humans, is caused by the repetition of up to 1,000 copies of a CGG repeat in a gene on the

X chromosome. The impact of a mutation depends upon the type of cell involved. In a haploid cell, any mutant allele will most likely be expressed in the phenotype of that cell. In a diploid cell, a dominant mutation will be expressed over the wild type allele, but a recessive mutation will remain masked by the wild type. If recessive mutations occur in both members of one gene pair in the same cell, the mutant phenotype will be expressed. Mutations in germinal cells (i.e. reproductive cells) may be passed on to successive generations. However, mutations in somatic (body) cells will exert their effect only on that individual and will not be passed on to progeny.

The impact of an expressed somatic mutation depends upon which gene has been mutated. In most cases, the somatic cell with the mutation will die, an event that is generally of little consequence in a multicellular organism. However, mutations in a special class of genes called proto-oncogenes can cause uncontrolled division of that cell, resulting in a group of cells that constitutes a cancerous tumour.

Mutations can affect gene function in several different ways. First, the structure and function of the protein coded by that gene can be affected. For example, enzymes are particularly susceptible to mutations that affect the amino acid sequence at their active site (i.e. the region that allows the enzyme to bind with its specific substrate). This may lead to enzyme inactivity, a protein is made, but it has no enzymatic function. Second, some nonsense or frameshift mutations can lead to the complete absence of a protein. Third, changes to the promoter region of the gene can result in gene malfunction by interfering with transcription. In this situation, protein production is either inhibited or it occurs at an inappropriate time because of alterations somewhere in the regulatory region. Fourth, mutations within introns that affect the specific nucleotide sequences that direct intron splicing may result in an mRNA that still contains an intron. When translated, this extra RNA will almost certainly be meaningless at the protein level, and its extra length will lead to a functionless protein. Any mutation that results in a lack of function for a particular gene is called a 'null' mutation. Less-severe mutations are called 'leaky' mutations because some normal function still 'leaks through' into the phenotype.

Most mutations occur spontaneously and have no known cause. The synthesis of DNA is a cooperative venture of many different interacting cellular components, and occasionally mistakes occur that result in mutations. Like many chemical structures, the bases of DNA are able to exist in several conformations called isomers. The keto form of a DNA base is the normal form that gives the molecule its standard base-pairing properties. However, the keto form occasionally changes spontaneously to the enol form, which has different base-pairing properties. For example, the keto form of cytosine pairs with guanine (its normal pairing partner), but the enol form of cytosine pairs with adenine. During DNA replication, this adenine base will act as the template for thymine in the newly synthesised strand. Therefore, a CG base pair will have mutated to a TA base pair. If this change results in a functionally different amino acid, then a missense mutation may result. Another spontaneous event that can lead to mutation is depurination, the complete loss of a purine base (adenine or guanine) at some location in the DNA. The resulting gap can be filled by any base during subsequent replications.

Researchers have demonstrated that ionising radiation, some chemicals, and certain viruses are capable of acting as mutagens—agents that can increase the rate at which mutations occur. Some mutagens have been implicated as a cause of cancer. For example, ultraviolet (UV) radiation from the Sun is known to cause skin cancer, and cigarette smoke is a primary cause of lung cancer.

Repair of mutation

A variety of mechanisms exists for repairing copying errors caused by DNA damage. One of the best-studied systems is the repair mechanism for damage caused by ultraviolet radiation. Ultraviolet radiation joins adjacent thymines, creating thymine dimers, which, if not repaired, may cause mutations. Special repair enzymes either cut the bond between the thymines or excise the bonded dimer and replace it with two single thymines. If both of these repair methods fail, a third method allows the DNA replication process to bypass the dimer, however, it is this bypass system that causes most mutations because bases are then inserted at random opposite the thymine dimer. Xeroderma pigmentosum, a severe hereditary disease of humans, is caused by a mutation in a gene coding for one of the thymine dimer repair enzymes. Individuals with this disease are highly susceptible to skin cancer.

Reverse mutation from the aberrant state of a gene back to its normal, or wild type, state can result in a number of possible molecular changes at the protein level. True reversion is the reversal of the original nucleotide change. However, phenotypic reversion can result from changes that restore a different amino acid with properties identical to the original. Second-site changes within a protein can also restore normal function. For example, an amino acid change at a site different from that altered by the original mutation can sometimes interact with the amino acid at the first mutant site to restore a normal protein shape. Also, second-site mutations at other genes can act as suppressors, restoring wild type function. For example, mutations in the anticodon region of a tRNA gene can result in a tRNA that sometimes inserts an amino acid at an erroneous stop codon, if the original mutation is caused by a stop codon, which arrests translation at that point, then a tRNA anticodon change can insert an amino acid and allow translation to continue normally to the end of the mRNA. Alternatively, some mutations at separate genes open up a new biochemical pathway that circumvents the block of function caused by the original mutation.

REGULATION OF GENE EXPRESSION

Not all genes in a cell are active in protein production at any given time. Gene action can be switched on or off in response to the cell's stage of development and external environment. In multicellular organisms, different kinds of cells express different parts of the genome. In other words, a skin cell and a muscle cell contain exactly the same genes, but the differences in structure and function of these cells result from the selective expression and repression of certain genes.

In prokaryotes and eukaryotes, most gene-control systems are positive, meaning that a gene will not be transcribed unless it is activated by a regulatory protein. However, some bacterial genes show negative control. In this case the gene is transcribed continuously unless it is switched off by a regulatory protein. An example of negative control in prokaryotes involves three adjacent genes used in the metabolism of the sugar lactose by *E. coli*. The part of the chromosome containing the genes concerned is divided into two regions, one that includes the structural genes (i.e. those genes that together code for protein structure) and another that is a regulatory region. This overall unit is called an operon. If lactose is not present in a cell, transcription of the genes that code for the lactose-processing enzymes—β-galactosidase, permease, and transacetylase—is turned off. This is achieved by a protein called the lac repressor, which is produced by the repressor gene and binds to a region of the operon called the operator. Such binding prevents RNA polymerase, which initially binds at the adjacent promoter, from moving into the coding region. If lactose enters the cell, it binds to the lac repressor and induces a change of shape in the repressor so that it can no longer bind to the DNA at the operon. Consequently, the RNA polymerase is able to travel from the promoter down the three adjacent protein-coding regions, making one continuous transcript. This three-gene transcript is subsequently translated into three separate proteins. Although the operon model (Fig. 14.1) has proved a useful model of gene regulation in bacteria, different regulatory mechanisms are employed in eukaryotes. First, there are no operons in eukaryotes, and each gene is

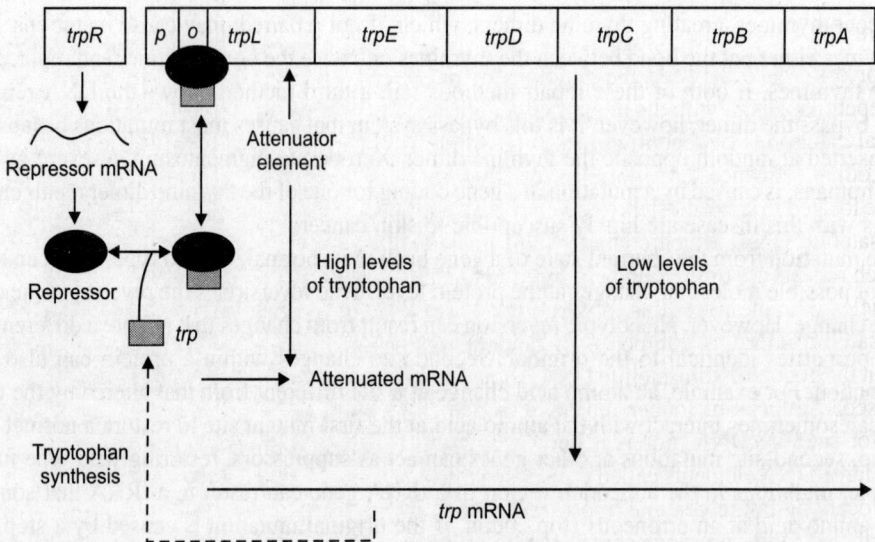

Fig. 14.1: Model of the operon and its relation to the regulator gene.

regulated independently. Furthermore, the series of events associated with gene expression in higher organisms is much more complex than in prokaryotes and involves multiple levels of regulation.

In order for a gene to produce a functional protein, a complex series of steps must occur. Some type of signal must initiate the transcription of the appropriate region along the DNA, and, finally, an active protein must be made and sent to the appropriate location to perform its specific task. Regulation can be exerted at many different places along this pathway. The fundamental level of control is the rate of transcription. Transcription itself is also a complex process with many different components, and each one is a potential point of control. Regulatory proteins called activators or enhancers are needed for the transcription of genes at a specific time or in a certain cell. Thus, control is positive (not negative as in the lac operon) in that these proteins are necessary for the promotion of transcription. Activators bind to specific regions of the DNA in the upstream regulatory region, some very distant from the binding of the initiation complex.

Following the transcription of DNA into RNA, a process of editing and splicing takes place in which noncoding nucleotide sequences called introns are excised from the primary transcript, resulting in functional mRNA. For most genes this is a routine step in the production of mRNA, but in some genes there are alternative ways to splice the primary transcript, resulting in different mRNAs, which in turn result in different proteins. Some genes are controlled at the translational and post-translational levels. One type of translational control is the storage of uncapped mRNA to meet future demands for protein synthesis. In other cases, control is exerted through the stability or instability of mRNA. The rate of translation of some mRNAs can also be regulated. Post-translationally, certain proteins (e.g. insulin) are synthesised in an inactive form and must be chemically modified to become active. Other proteins are targeted to specific locations inside the cell (e.g. mitochondria) by means of highly specific amino acid sequences at their ends, called leader sequences, when the protein reaches its correct site, the leader segment is cut off, and the protein begins to function. Post-translational control is also exerted through mRNA and protein degradation.

Repetitive DNA

One major difference between the genomes of prokaryotes and eukaryotes is that most eukaryotes contain repetitive DNA, with the repeats either clustered or spread out between the unique genes. There are several categories of repetitive DNA: (i) single copy DNA, which contains the structural genes (protein-coding sequences), (ii) families of DNA, in which one gene somehow copies itself, and the repeats are located in small clusters (tandem repeats) or spread throughout the genome (dispersed repeats), and (iii) satellite DNA, which contains short nucleotide sequences repeated as many as thousands of times. Such repeats are often found clustered in tandem near the centromeres (i.e. the attachment points for the nuclear spindle fibres that move chromosomes during cell division).

Microsatellite DNA is composed of tandem repeats of two nucleotide pairs that are dispersed throughout the genome. Minisatellite DNA, sometimes called variable number tandem repeats (VNTRs), is composed of blocks of longer repeats also dispersed throughout the genome. There is no known function for satellite DNA, nor is it known how the repeats are created. There is a special class of relatively large DNA elements called transposons, which can make replicas of themselves that 'jump' to different locations in the genome, most transposons eventually become inactive and no longer move, but, nevertheless, their presence contributes to repetitive DNA.

Extranuclear DNA

All of the genetic information in a cell was initially thought to be confined to the DNA in the chromosomes of the cell nucleus. It is now known that small circular chromosomes, called extranuclear, or cytoplasmic, DNA, are located in two types of organelles found in the cytoplasm of the cell. These organelles are the mitochondria in animal and plant cells and the chloroplasts in plant cells. Chloroplast DNA (cpDNA) contains genes that are involved with aspects of photosynthesis and with components of the special protein-synthesising apparatus that is active within the organelle. Mitochondrial DNA (mtDNA) contains some of the genes that participate in the conversion of the energy of chemical bonds into the energy currency of the cell—a chemical called adenosine triphosphate (ATP)—as well as genes for mitochondrial protein synthesis. The cells of several groups of organisms contain small extra DNA molecules called plasmids. Bacterial plasmids are circular DNA molecules, some carry genes for resistance to various agents in the environment that would be toxic to the bacteria (e.g. antibiotics). Many fungi and some plants possess plasmids in their mitochondria, most of these are linear DNA molecules carrying genes that seem to be relevant only to the propagation of the plasmid and not the host cell.

HEREDITY AND EVOLUTION

At the centre of the theory of evolution as proposed by Charles Darwin and Alfred Russell Wallace were the concepts of variation and natural selection. Hereditary variants were thought to arise naturally in populations, and then these were either selected for or against by the contemporary environmental conditions. In this way, subsequent generations either became enriched or impoverished for specific variant types. Over the long term, the accumulation of such changes in populations could lead to the formation of new species and higher taxonomic categories. However, although hereditary change was basic to the theory, in the 19th-century world of Darwin and Wallace, the fundamental unit of heredity— the gene—was unknown. The birth and proliferation of the science of genetics in the 20th century after the discovery of Mendel's laws made it possible to consider the process of evolution by natural selection in terms of known genetic processes.

Population Genetics

Because the processes of variation and selection take place at the population level, the basic theory of the genetics of evolutionary change is contained in the general area known as population genetics.

A simple way of viewing evolutionary change at the genotypic level would be to invent some hypothetical ancestral genotype, such as AAbbccDDEE, and an 'evolved' derivative, such as aaBBccddee. (For illustrative purposes, only five genes are used, and these are assumed to be all homozygous.) Also, for simplicity it can be assumed that in both the ancestral and the evolved populations all individuals are identical. Clearly for all the genes except cc, a new allele completely replaces the original allele, and the new alleles can be either dominant or recessive. For example, in the case of the first gene, in the ancestral population all alleles are A, and in the evolved population all are a. For a to replace A, the population must go through stages in which there are mixtures of A and a alleles present in the population at the same time. In population genetics, allele frequency is the measurement of the commonness of an allele. The convention is to let the frequency of a dominant allele be p and that of a recessive allele q. Both are generally expressed as decimal fractions. In the above example, p changes from 1 to 0, and q changes from 0 to 1. Since there are only two alleles in this example, p + q must always equal 1. In the intermediate stages, there must be times when there are intermediate allele frequencies, for example when p = 0.4 and q = 0.6.

What can be said about genotype frequencies in the intermediate populations? In the ancestral and derived populations there must have been the following genotypic frequencies:

Ancestral AA = 1, Aa = 0, aa = 0

Evolved AA = 0, Aa = 0, aa = 1

Intuitively it seems that, in the intermediate stages, there must be more-complex proportions, including some heterozygotes. One possible intermediate stage is as follows:

AA = 0.30, Aa = 0.20, aa = 0.50

The allele frequencies at such an intermediate stage can be calculated by 'adding up' the alleles. Hence, the frequency of A will be 0.30 plus 1/2 of 0.20 because the heterozygotes only carry one A allele. This is written

p = 0.30 + 0.20/2 = 0.40

Similarly, q = 0.50 + 0.20/2= 0.60

(Noting these values for p and q, it is possible that this could have been the population discussed earlier, in which these specific values for p and q were hypothesised.)

In general, if D = frequency of homozygous dominants, R = frequency of homozygous recessives, and H = frequency of heterozygotes, then

p = D + H/2 and q = R + H/2

This section has shown the importance of the concepts of allele frequency and genotype frequency in describing the genetic structure of populations. Of these, allele frequency is the simpler descriptor, and it forms the central tool of population genetics. Hence, the genetic basis of evolutionary change at the population level is described in terms of changes of allele frequencies.

Changes in Gene Frequencies

Selection

One assumption behind the calculation of unchanging genotypic frequencies in Hardy-Weinberg equilibrium is that all genotypes have the same fitness. In genetics, fitness does not necessarily have to do with muscles, fitness is a measure of the ability to produce fertile offspring. In reality, the fitnesses of different genotypes are highly variable. The genotype with the greatest fitness is given the fitness value (w) of 1, and the lesser fitnesses are fractions of 1. For example, if snails of genotypes AA and Aa were to have an average of 100 offspring but those of genotype aa only 70, then the fitnesses of these three genotypes would be 1, 1, and 0.7, respectively. The proportional difference from the most fit is called the selection coefficient, s. Hence, s = 1– w.

Alleles carried by less-fit individuals will be gradually lost from the population, and the relevant allele frequency will decline. This is the fundamental way in which natural selection operates in a population. Selection against dominant alleles is relatively efficient, because these are by definition expressed in the phenotype. Selection against recessive alleles is less efficient, because these alleles are sheltered in heterozygotes. Even though populations under selection technically are not in Hardy-Weinberg equilibrium, the proportions of the formula can be used as an approximation to show the relative proportions of homozygous recessives and heterozygotes. If a rare deleterious recessive allele is of frequency 1/50 in the population, then (1/50)2, or 1 out of 2,500, individuals will express the recessive phenotype and be a candidate for negative selection. Heterozygotes will be at a frequency of 2pq = 2 × 49/50 × 1/50, or about 1 in 25. In other words, the heterozygotes are 100 times more common than recessive homozygotes, hence, most of the recessive alleles in a population will escape selection. Because of the sheltering effect of heterozygotes, selection against recessive phenotypes changes the frequency of the recessive allele slowly. Even if the most severe level of selection is imposed, giving the recessive phenotype a fitness of zero (no fertile offspring), the recessive allele frequency (expressed as a fraction of the form 1/x) will increase in denominator by 1 in every generation. Therefore, to halve an allele frequency from 1/50 to 1/100 would proceed slowly from 1/50 to 1/51, 1/52, 1/53, and so on and would take 50 generations to get to 1/100. For lower intensities of selection, the progress would be even slower.

A different type of natural selection occurs when the fitness of a heterozygote exceeds the fitness of both homozygotes. The maintenance in human populations of the severe hereditary disease sickle cell anemia is owing to this form of selection. The disease allele (HbS) produces a specific type of hemoglobin that causes distortion (sickling) of the red blood cells in which the hemoglobin is carried. (Normal hemoglobin is coded by another allele, HbA). Accordingly, the possible genotypes are HbAHbA, HbAHbS, and HbSHbS. The latter individuals are homozygous for the sickle cell allele and will develop severe anemia because the oxygen transporting property of their blood is compromised.

While the condition is not lethal before birth, such individuals rarely survive long enough to reproduce. On these grounds it might be expected that the disease allele would be selected against, driving the allele frequency to very low levels. However, in tropical areas of the world, the allele and the disease are common. The explanation is that the HbAHbS heterozygote is fitter and capable of leaving more offspring than is the homozygous normal HbAHbA in an environment containing the falciparum form of malaria. This extra measure of protection is evidently provided by the sickle cell hemoglobin, which is detrimental to the malaria parasite. In malarial environments, therefore, populations that contain the sickle cell gene have advantages over populations free of this gene. The former populations are in less danger from malaria, although they 'pay' for this advantage by sacrificing in every generation some individuals who die of anemia.

Mutation

Genetics has shown that mutation is the ultimate source of all hereditary variation. At the level of a single gene whose normal functional allele is A, it is known that mutation can change it to a nonfunctional recessive form, a. Such 'forward mutation' is more frequent than 'back mutation' (reversion), which converts a into A. Molecular analysis of specific examples of mutant recessive alleles has shown that they are generally a heterogeneous set of small structural changes in the DNA, located throughout the segment of DNA that constitutes that gene. Hence, in an example from medical genetics, the disease phenylketonuria is inherited as a recessive phenotype and is ascribed to a causative allele that generally can be called k. However, sequencing alleles of many independent cases of phenylketonuria has shown that this k allele is in fact a set of many different kinds of mutational changes, which can be in any of the protein-coding regions of that gene.

Recessive deleterious mutations are relatively rare, generally in the order of 1 per 10^5 or 10^6 mutant gametes per generation. Their constant occurrence over the generations, combined with the even greater rarity of back mutations, leads to a gradual accumulation in the population. This accumulation process is called mutational pressure. Since mutational pressure to a deleterious recessive allele and selection pressure against the homozygous recessives are forces that act in opposite directions, another type of equilibrium is attained that effectively sets the value of q. Mathematically, q is determined by the following expression in which u is the net mutation rate of A to a, and s is the selection coefficient presented above: $q2 = (u/s)$, or $q = $ Square root of $v(u/s)$

Nonrandom Mating

Many species engage in alternatives to random mating as normal parts of their cycle of sexual reproduction. An important exception is sexual selection, in which an individual chooses a mate on the basis of some aspect of the mates phenotype. The selection can be based on some display feature such as bright feathers, or it may be a simple preference for a phenotype identical to the individuals own (positive assortative mating). Two other important exceptions are inbreeding (mating with relatives) and enforced outbreeding. Both can shift the equilibrium proportions expected under Hardy-Weinberg calculations. For example, inbreeding increases the proportions of homozygotes, and the most extreme form of inbreeding, self-fertilisation, eventually eliminates all heterozygotes.

Inbreeding and outbreeding are evolutionary strategies adopted by plants and animals living under certain conditions. Outbreeding brings gametes of different genotypes together, and the resulting individual differs from the parents. Increased levels of variation provide more evolutionary flexibility. All the showy colors and shapes of flowers are to promote this kind of exchange. In contrast, inbreeding maintains uniform genotypes, a strategy successful in stable ecological habitats.

In humans, various degrees of inbreeding have been practiced in different cultures. In most cultures today, matings of first cousins are the maximal form of inbreeding condoned by society. Apart from ethical considerations, a negative outcome of inbreeding is that it increases the likelihood of homozygosity of deleterious recessive alleles originating from common ancestors, called homozygosity by descent. The inbreeding coefficient F is a measure of the likelihood of homozygosity by descent, for example, in first-cousin marriages, $F = 1/16$. A large proportion of recessive hereditary diseases can be traced to first-cousin marriages and other types of inbreeding.

Random Genetic Drift

In populations of finite size, the genetic structure of a new generation is not necessarily that of the previous one. The explanation lies in a sampling effect, based on the fact that a subsample from any large set is not always representative of the larger set. The gametes that form any generation can be thought of as a sample of the alleles from the parental one. By chance the sample might not be random, it could be skewed in either direction. For example, if p = 0.600 and q = 0.400, sampling 'error' might result in the gametes having a p value of 0.601 and a q of 0.399. If by chance this skewed sampling occurs in the same direction from generation to generation, the allele frequency can change radically. This process is known as random genetic drift. As might be expected, the smaller the population, the greater chance of sampling error and hence significant levels of drift in any one generation. In extreme cases, drift over the generations can result in the complete loss of one allele, in these occurrences the other is said to be fixed. Other cases of sampling error occur when new colonies of plants or animals are founded by small numbers of migrants (founder effect) and when there is radical reduction in population size because of a natural catastrophe (population bottleneck). One inevitable effect of these processes is a reduction in the amount of variation in the population after the size reduction. Two species that have gone through drastic bottlenecks with the associated reduction of genetic variation are cheetahs (Africa) and northern elephant seals (North America).

Microevolution

There is ample evidence that the processes described above are at work in natural populations. Together, these changes are called microevolution—in other words, small-scale evolution. Even within the relatively short period of time since Darwin, it has been possible to document such processes. Allelic variation has been found to be common in nature. It is detected as polymorphism, the presence of two or more distinct hereditary forms associated with a gene. Polymorphism can be morphological, such as blue and brown forms of a species of marine mussel, or molecular, detectable only at the DNA or protein level. Although much of this polymorphism is not understood, there are enough examples of selection of polymorphic forms to indicate that it is potentially adaptive. Selection has been observed favouring melanic (dark) forms of peppered moths in industrial areas and favouring resistance to toxic agents such as the insecticide DDT, the rat poison warfarin, and the virus that causes the disease myxomatosis in rabbits.

More-complex genetic changes have been documented, leading to special locally adapted 'ecotypes.' Anoles (a type of lizard) on certain Caribbean islands show convincing examples of adaptations to specific habitats, such as tree trunks, tree branches, or grass. Introductions of lizards onto uncolonised islands result in demonstrable microevolutionary adaptations to the various vacant niches. On the Galapagos Islands, studies over several decades have documented adaptive changes in the beaks of finches. In some studies, documented changes have led to incipient new species. An example is the apple maggot, the larva of a fly in North America that has evolved from a similar fly living on hawthorns—all in the period since the introduction of apples. The formation of new species was a key component of Darwin's original theory. Now it appears that the accumulation of enough small-scale genetic changes can lead to the inability to mate with members of an ancestral population, such reproductive isolation is the key step in species formation. It is reasonable to assume that the continuation of microevolutionary genetic changes over very long periods of time can give rise to new major taxonomic groups, the process of macroevolution. There are few data that bear directly on the processes of macroevolution, but gene analysis does provide a way for charting macroevolutionary relationships indirectly.

DNA Phylogeny

The ability to isolate and sequence specific genes and genomes has been of great significance in deducing trees of evolutionary relatedness. An important discovery that enables this sort of analysis is the considerable evolutionary conservation between organisms at the genetic level. This means that different organisms have a large proportion of their genes in common, particularly those that code for proteins at the central core of the chemical machinery of the cell. For example, most organisms have a gene coding for the energy-producing protein cytochrome C, and furthermore, this gene has a very similar nucleotide sequence in all organisms (that is, the sequence is conserved). However, the sequences of cytochrome C in different organisms do show differences, and the key to phylogeny is that the differences are proportionately fewer between organisms that are closely related. The interpretation of this observation is that organisms that share a common ancestor also share common DNA sequences derived from that ancestor. When one ancestral species splits into two, differences accumulate as a result of mutations, a process called divergence. The greater the amount of divergence, the longer must have been the time since the split occurred. To carry out this sort of analysis, the DNA sequence data are fed into a computer. The computer positions similar species together on short adjacent branches showing a relatively recent split and dissimilar species on long branches from an ancient split. In this way a molecular phylogenetic tree of any number of organisms can be drawn. DNA difference in some cases can be correlated with absolute dates of divergence as deduced from the fossil record. Then it is possible to calculate divergence as a rate. It has been found that divergence is relatively constant in rate, giving rise to the idea that there is a type of 'molecular clock' ticking in the course of evolution. Some ticks of this clock (in the form of mutations) are significant in terms of adaptive changes to the gene, but many are undoubtedly neutral, with no significant effect on fitness. One of the interesting discoveries to emerge from molecular phylogeny is that gene duplication has been common during evolution. If an extra copy of a gene can be made, initially by some cellular accident, then the 'spare' copy is free to mutate and evolve into a separate function. Molecular phylogeny of some genes has also pointed to unexpected cases of, say, a plant gene nested within a tree of animal genes of that type or a bacterial gene nested within a plant phylogenetic tree. The explanation for such anomalies is that there has been horizontal transmission from one group to another. In other words, on rare occasions a gene can hop laterally from one species to another. Although the mechanisms for horizontal transmission are presently not known, one possibility is that bacteria or viruses act as natural vectors for transferring genes.

Synteny

Genomic sequencing and mapping have enabled comparison of the general structures of genomes of many different species. The general finding is that organisms of relatively recent divergence show similar blocks of genes in the same relative positions in the genome. This situation is called synteny, translated roughly as possessing common chromosome sequences. For example, many of the genes of humans are syntenic with those of other mammals—not only apes but also cows, mice, and so on. Study of synteny can show how the genome is cut and pasted in the course of evolution.

Polyploidy

Genomic analysis also has shown that one of the important mechanisms of evolution is multiplication of chromosome sets, resulting in polyploidy (many genomes). In plants and animals, spontaneous doubling of chromosomes can occur. In some plants, the chromosomes of two related species unite via cross-pollination to form a fusion product. This product is sterile because each chromosome needs a pairing partner in order for the plant to be fertile. However, the chromosomes of the fusion product can accidentally double, resulting in a new, fertile species. Wheat is an example of a plant that evolved by this means through a union between wild grasses, but a large proportion of plants went through similar ancestral polyploidisation.

Human Evolution

Many of the techniques of evolutionary genetics can be applied to the evolution of humans. Charles Darwin created a large controversy in Victorian England by suggesting in his book The Descent of Man that humans and apes share a common ancestor. Darwin's assertion was based on the many shared anatomical features of apes and humans. DNA analysis has supported this hypothesis. At the DNA sequence level, the genomes of humans and chimpanzees are 99 per cent identical. Furthermore, when phylogenetic trees are constructed using individual genes, humans and apes cluster together in short terminal branches of the trees, suggesting very recent divergence. Synteny too is impressive, with relatively minor chromosomal rearrangements.

Fossils have been found of various extinct forms considered to be intermediates between apes and humans. Notable is the African genus Australopithecus, generally believed to be one of the earliest hominins and an intermediate on the path of human evolution. The first toolmaker was Homo habilis, followed by Homo erectus and finally Homo sapiens (modern humans). H. habilis fossils have been found only in Africa, whereas fossils of H. erectus and H. sapiens are found throughout the Old World. Phylogenetic trees based on DNA sequencing of all peoples have shown that Africans represent the root of the trees. This is interpreted as evidence that H. sapiens evolved in Africa, spread throughout the globe, and outcompeted H. erectus wherever the two cohabited.

Variations of DNA, either unique alleles of individual genes or larger-sized blocks of variable structure, have been used as markers to trace human migrations across the globe. Hence, it has been possible to trace the movement of H. sapiens out of Africa and into Europe and Asia and, more recently, to the American continents. Also, genetic markers are useful in plotting human migrations that occurred in historical time. For example, the invasion of Europe by various Asian conquerors can be followed using blood-type alleles.

As humans colonised and settled permanently in various parts of the world, they differentiated themselves into distinct groups called races. Undoubtedly, many of the features that distinguish races, such as skin colour or body shape, were adaptive in the local settings, although such adaptiveness is difficult to demonstrate. Nevertheless, genomic analysis has revealed that the concept of race has little meaning at the genetic level. The differences between races are superficial, based on the alleles of a relatively small number of genes that affect external features. Furthermore, while races differ in allele frequencies, these same alleles are found in most races. In other words, at the genetic level there are no significant discontinuities between races. It is paradoxical that race, which has been so important to people throughout the course of human history, is trivial at the genetic level—an important insight to emerge from genetic analysis.

DNA, GENES AND CHROMOSOMES

DNA

DNA stands for deoxyribose nucleic acid. This chemical substance is present in the nucleus of all cells in all living organisms. DNA determines the kind of cell which is formed, (muscle, blood, nerve, etc.) is controlled by DNA. DNA determines the kind of organism which is produced (buttercup, giraffe, herring, human etc) is controlled by DNA. DNA is often called the blueprint of life because it contains the instructions for making proteins within the cell. DNA is a very long *polymer*. The basic shape is like a twisted ladder or zipper. This is called a *double helix*. The DNA double helix has two strands twisted together. DNA (or deoxyribonucleic acid) is the molecule that carries the genetic information in all cellular forms of life and some viruses. It belongs to a class of molecules called the nucleic acids, which are polynucleotides - that is, long chains of nucleotides.

Each nucleotide consists of three components:

1. A nitrogenous base: cytosine (C), guanine (G), adenine (A) or thymine (T).
2. A five-carbon sugar molecule (deoxyribose in the case of DNA).
3. A phosphate molecule.

The backbone of the polynucleotide is a chain of sugar and phosphate molecules. Each of the sugar groups in this sugar-phosphate backbone is linked to one of the four nitrogenous bases.

DNAs ability to store - and transmit - information lies in the fact that it consists of two polynucleotide strands that twist around each other to form a double-stranded helix. The bases link across the two strands in a specific manner using hydrogen bonds: cytosine (C) pairs with guanine (G), and adenine (A) pairs with thymine (T).

The double helix of the complete DNA molecule resembles a spiral staircase, with two sugar phosphate backbones and the paired bases in the centre of the helix. This structure explains two of the most important properties of the molecule. First, it can be copied or 'replicated', as each strand can act as a template for the generation of the complementary strand. Second, it can store information in the linear sequence of the nucleotides along each strand.

It is the order of the bases along a single strand that constitutes the genetic code. The four-letter 'alphabet' of A, T, G and C forms 'words' of three letters called codons. Individual codons code for specific amino acids. A gene is a sequence of nucleotides along a DNA strand - with 'start' and 'stop' codons and other regulatory elements - that specifies a sequence of amino acids that are linked together to form a protein. So, for example, the codon AGC codes for the amino acid serine, and the codon ACC codes for the amino acid threonine.

A	G	C	A	C	C
Serine			Threonine		

There are a two points to note about the genetic code:

1. It is universal. All life on Earth uses the same code (with a few minor exceptions).
2. It is degenerate. Each amino acid can be coded for by more than one codon. For example, AGC and ACC both code for the amino acid serine.

A codon table sets out how the triplet codons code for specific amino acids is shown in Fig. 14.2.

Genes

The gene is the basic physical and functional unit of heredity. It consists of a specific sequence of nucleotides at a given position on a given chromosome that codes for a specific protein (or, in some cases, an RNA molecule).

Genes consist of three types of nucleotide sequence:

• Coding regions, called exons, which specify a sequence of amino acids
• Non-coding regions, called introns, which do not specify amino acids
• Regulatory sequences, which play a role in determining when and where the protein is made (and how much is made)

Second letter

		U	C	A	G	
First letter	U	UUU] Phe UUC] UUA] Leu UUG]	UCU] UCC] Per UCA] UCG]	UAU] Tyr UAC] UAA Stop UAG Stop	UGU] CyS UGC] UGA Stop UGG Stop	U C A G
	C	CUU] CUC] Leu CUA] CUG]	CCU] CCC] Pro CCA] CCG]	CAU] His CAC] CAA] Gln CAG]	CGU] CGC] Arg CGA] CGG]	U C A G
	A	AUU] AUC] Ile AUA] AUG Met	ACU] ACC] Thr ACA] ACG]	AAU] Asn AAC] AAA] Lys AAG]	AGU] Ser AGC] AGA] Arg AGG]	U C A G
	G	GUU] GUC] Val GUA] GUG]	GCU] GCC] Ala GCA] GCG]	GAU] Asp GAC] GAA] Glu GAG]	GGU] GGC] Gly GGA] GGG]	U C A G

Third letter

Fig. 14.2: The triplet codons code for specific amino acids.

A human being has 20,000 to 25,000 genes located on 46 chromosomes (23 pairs). These genes are known, collectively, as the human genome.

Chromosomes

Eukaryotic chromosomes

The label eukaryote is taken from the Greek for 'true nucleus', and eukaryotes (all organisms except viruses, Eubacteria and *Archaea*) are defined by the possession of a nucleus and other membrane-bound cell organelles.

The nucleus of each cell in our bodies contains approximately 1.8 metres of DNA in total, although each strand is less than one millionth of a centimetre thick. This DNA is tightly packed into structures called chromosomes, which consist of long chains of DNA and associated proteins. In eukaryotes, DNA molecules are tightly wound around proteins - called histone proteins - which provide structural support and play a role in controlling the activities of the genes. A strand 150 to 200 nucleotides long is wrapped twice around a core of eight histone proteins to form a structure called a nucleosome. The histone octamer at the centre of the nucleosome is formed from two units each of histones H2A, H2B, H3, and H4. The chains of histones are coiled in turn to form a solenoid, which is stabilised by the histone H1. Further coiling of the solenoids forms the structure of the chromosome proper (Fig. 14.3).

Each chromosome has a p arm and a q arm. The p arm (from the French word 'petit', meaning small) is the short arm, and the q arm is the long arm. In their replicated form, each chromosome consists of two chromatids.

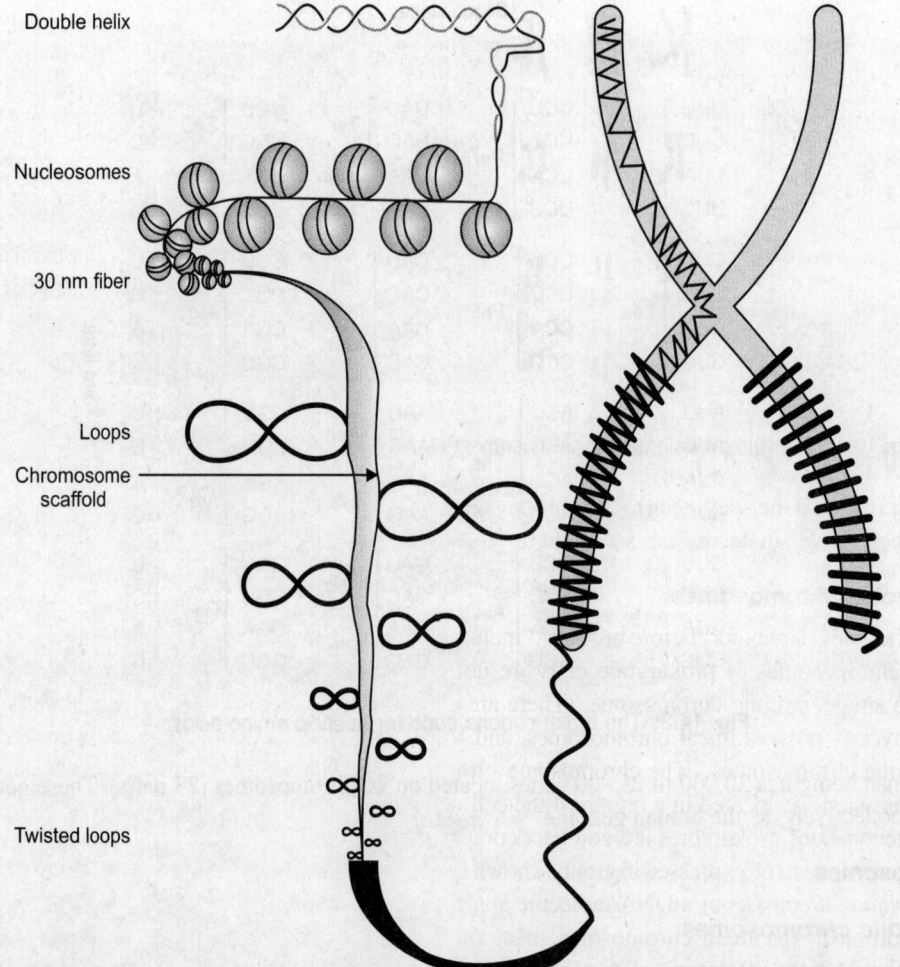

Double helix

Nucleosomes

30 nm fiber

Loops

Chromosome
scaffold

Twisted loops

Fig. 14.3: Chromatin packaging within the chromosome. The length of a DNA molecule is shortened by 10000-fold during the formation of a metaphase chromosome. This is brought about by levels of chromatin packing, built one upon another. The first level of packing is brought about by the wrapping of DNA around nucleosomes to form a structure that has been likened to beads on a string. A folding or coiling of this level of chromatin together with additional chromosomal proteins, such as linker histones, produces the 30-nm diameter chromatin fiber. It is still not certain how chromatin is compacted beyond this stage. The diagram illustrates one particular model, known as the radial loop/scaffold model. In this model it is envisaged that the 30-nm fiber is arranged into loops containing 100 kb of DNA. These loops are anchored at their bases to the chromosome scaffold. Chromatin is finally condensed both by a shortening in length of the chromosome scaffold and by a twisting of lateral loops in toward the chromosome axis/scaffold.

The chromosomes - and the DNA they contain - are copied as part of the cell cycle, and passed to daughter cells through the processes of mitosis and meiosis. Human beings have 46 chromosomes, consisting of 22 pairs of autosomes and a pair of sex chromosomes: two X sex chromosomes for females (XX) and an X and Y sex chromosome for males (XY) is shown in Fig. 14.4. One member of each pair of chromosomes comes from the mother (through the egg cell), one member of each pair comes from

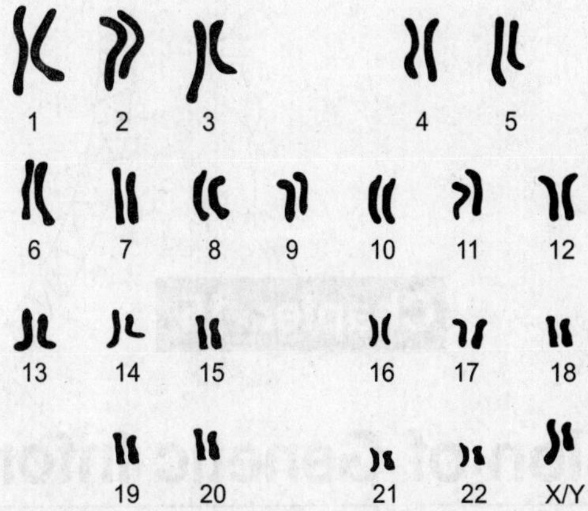

Fig. 14.4: The human beings 46 chromosomes, making up the diploid genome of human male.

the father (through the sperm cell). The chromosomes in a cell is known as a karyotype. The autosomes are numbered 1–22 in decreasing size order.

Prokaryotic Chromosomes

The prokaryotes (Greek for 'before nucleus' - including Eubacteria and *Archaea*) lack a discrete nucleus, and the chromosomes of prokaryotic cells are not enclosed by a separate membrane. Most bacteria contain a single, circular chromosome. (There are exceptions: some bacteria - for example, the genus Streptomyces - possess linear chromosomes, and Vibrio cholerae, the causative agent of cholera, has two circular chromosomes.) The chromosome - together with ribosomes and proteins associated with gene expression - is located in a region of the cell cytoplasm known as the nucleoid.

The genomes of prokaryotes are compact compared with those of eukaryotes, as they lack introns, and the genes tend to be expressed in groups known as operons. The circular chromosome of the bacterium *Escherichia coli* consists of a DNA molecule approximately 4.6 million nucleotides long.

In addition to the main chromosome, bacteria are also characterised by the presence of extra-chromosomal genetic elements called plasmids. These relatively small circular DNA molecules usually contain genes that are not essential to growth or reproduction.

Chapter 15

Expression of Genetic Information

INTRODUCTION

Gene expression is the process by which information from a gene is used in the synthesis of a functional gene product. These products are often proteins, but in non-protein coding genes such as rRNA genes or tRNA genes, the product is a functional RNA. The process of gene expression is used by all known life—eukaryotes (including multicellular organisms), prokaryotes (bacteria and *archaea*) and viruses—to generate the macromolecular machinery for life.

Several steps in the gene expression process may be modulated, including the transcription, RNA splicing, translation, and post-translational modification of a protein. Gene regulation gives the cell control over structure and function, and is the basis for cellular differentiation, morphogenesis and the versatility and adaptability of any organism. Gene regulation may also serve as a substrate for evolutionary change, since control of the timing, location, and amount of gene expression can have a profound effect on the functions (actions) of the gene in a cell or in a multicellular organism. In genetics gene expression is the most fundamental level at which genotype gives rise to the phenotype.

The genetic code is 'interpreted' by gene expression, and the properties of the expression products give rise to the organism's phenotype (Fig. 15.1).

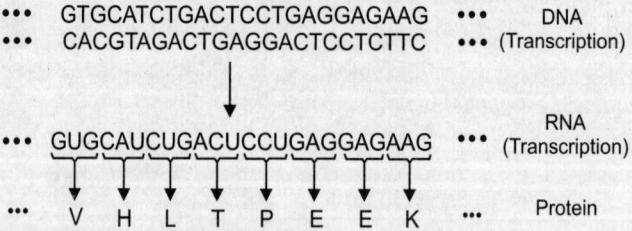

Fig. 15.1: Genes are expressed by being transcribed into RNA and this transcript may then be translated into protein.

Regulation of gene expression ordinarily occurs at the transcriptional, post-transcriptional, translational or post-translational levels. Transcriptional regulation includes all mechanisms that control the information transfer from DNA to RNA by RNA polymerase. Post-transcriptional regulation involves all modifications of the primary RNA transcript before it is translated into proteins. Translational regulation involves those factors that determine the rate of translation of mature mRNA molecules. Post-translational regulation involves mechanisms that control the processing of the primary translation product into the mature protein product. The environmental and metabolic state of the cell has a direct and significant effect on the control of gene expression. Usually, small extracellular or intracellular metabolites trigger the complex mechanisms that result either in stimulation or inhibition of gene expression. The regulation of the expression of genes is absolutely essential for the growth, development, differentiation and the very existence of an organism.

In prokaryotes such as *Escherichia coli* (*E. coli*), regulation of gene expression occurs primarily at the level of transcription and, in general, is mediated by the binding of *trans*-acting proteins to *cis*-acting regulatory elements on their single DNA molecule (chromosome). Prokaryotes are not as structurally complex as eukaryotes, and were once thought not to have any internal structures enclosed by lipid membranes.

The controls that act on gene expression (i.e. the ability of a gene to produce a biologically active protein) are much more complex in eukaryotes than in prokaryotes. A major difference is the presence in eukaryotes of a nuclear membrane, which prevents the simultaneous transcription and translation that occurs in prokaryotes. Whereas, in prokaryotes, control of transcriptional initiation is the major point of regulation, in eukaryotes the regulation of gene expression is controlled nearly equivalently from many different points. In bacteria, genes are clustered into operons: gene clusters that encode the proteins necessary to perform coordinated function, such as biosynthesis of a given amino acid. RNA that is transcribed from prokaryotic operons is polycistronic a term implying that multiple proteins are encoded in a single transcript.

In bacteria, control of the rate of transcriptional initiation is the predominant site for control of gene expression. As with the majority of prokaryotic genes, initiation is controlled by two DNA sequence elements that are approximately 35 bases and 10 bases, respectively, upstream of the site of transcriptional initiation and as such are identified as the −35 and −10 positions. These two sequence elements are termed promoter sequences, because they promote recognition of transcriptional start sites by RNA polymerase. The activity of RNA polymerase at a given promoter is in turn regulated by interaction with accessory proteins, which affect its ability to recognise start sites. These regulatory proteins can act both positively (activators) and negatively (repressors). The accessibility of promoter regions of prokaryotic DNA is in many cases regulated by the interaction of proteins with sequences termed operators. The operator region is adjacent to the promoter elements in most operons and in most cases the sequences of the operator bind a repressor protein. However, there are several operons in *E. coli* that contain overlapping sequence elements, one that binds a repressor and one that binds an activator.

Application of molecular biology techniques can have an important impact on yield and productivity of recombinant bioprocesses. Introduction of a foreign gene whose product is not utilised by the host can perturb cell function at many levels: DNA replication, regulation of transcription, ribosome functions, RNA turnover, activities of regulatory proteins, chaperone and protease levels, membrane energetics, postranslational processing, and energy and intermediary metabolism. Thus, r-protein production processes must be carefully designed to reduce negative effects of host-vector interactions. Recombinant bioprocesses are determined in many ways by the selection of the host and vector. For instance, a prokaryotic host requires totally different production and purification schemes than a mammalian expression system. Several issues must be considered upon vector and host selection, such as intrinsic r-product characteristics (size, postranslational modifications), product performance (stability, activity, authenticity) and even financial considerations (final use, quantity required, cost/added value, time for development, market). Additionally, many production parameters (cultivation mode, medium composition, environmental conditions, and others) have an important relationship with gene expression, plasmid copy number, plasmid stability, etc. In the next two sections a general description of different protein expression systems is presented. Such information is necessary for properly selecting an expression system for industrial r-protein production.

Thus, the process of gene expression simply refers to the events that transfer the information content of the gene into the production of a functional product, usually a protein. Although there are genes whose functional product is an RNA, including the genes encoding the ribosomal RNAs as well as the transfer RNAs and certain other small RNAs, the vast majority of genes within the cell are protein-encoding genes.

TRANSCRIPTION

The initial step in gene expression is the transcription of the DNA molecule into an exact RNA copy. As already discussed, the basic unit of heredity, the gene, is a double stranded DNA molecule and the information in the gene is encoded in the sequence of nucleotides. The transfer of information, to the ultimate synthesis of a protein, is accomplished via an RNA intermediate, the so-called messenger RNA. The mRNA molecule contains the exact same sequence of nucleotides as found in the DNA molecule (with U substituted for T). This occurs through the process known as transcription and is carried out by an enzyme termed DNA-dependent RNA polymerase.

The product of transcription is an RNA molecule that is identical in sequence content to one of the DNA strands (the sense strand) and complementary to the other DNA strand (the template strand). RNA differs from DNA in two respects. First, RNA contains a hydroxyl (OH) residue at the 2' position of the sugar moiety (ribose) whereas DNA contains an H at this position (deoxyribose). This changes some of the chemical properties of the two molecules. Second, RNA replaces the base thymine with uracil. Although they are chemically different, their base pairing properties (complementarity to adenosine) are the same. Thus, in DNA, A pairs with T whereas in RNA, A pairs with U. Transcription always proceeds in a 5' to 3' direction with respect to polarity of the nucleotides in the RNA. Thus, an unmodified primary transcription product would contain a 5' end with a triphosphate and a 3' end with a OH (Fig. 15.2).

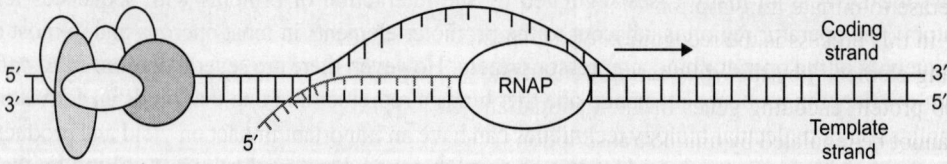

Fig. 15.2: The process of transcription is carried out by RNA polymerase (RNAP), Which uses DNA as a template and produces RNA.

There are actually three distinct forms of RNA polymerase found in eukaryotic cells that are responsible for the transcription of three distinct types of genes: the genes encoding the ribosomal RNAs are transcribed by RNA polymerase I, the protein-encoding genes that produce the messenger RNAs are transcribed by RNA polymerase II, finally, the genes encoding transfer RNAs as well as certain other small RNA molecules are transcribed by RNA polymerase III.

Transcription involves three distinct steps. First, there must be a recognition of the gene by the RNA polymerase. This is accomplished via the interaction of a variety of proteins called transcription factors that provide the recognition step, guiding the polymerase to the correct site. Moreover, the interaction of these transcription factors with their DNA recognition sequences represents a rate-limiting step in the process of transcription initiation. Sequences in the DNA which are recognised by these transcription factors, and which serve as binding sites for the transcription factors, are generally upstream (5') of the start site for transcription and are called promoters. Additional transcription factors can bind to sequence elements called enhancers that may be located further upstream or even downstream of the gene. In either case, the DNA sequences that bind the transcription factors must be located on the same DNA molecule, thus the same chromosome, as the gene which is regulated. As such, these sequences are said to act in *cis*. The promoter is absolutely essential for transcription whereas the enhancer, as its name implies, increases the efficiency of transcription.

In prokaryotes, transcription is carried out by a single type of RNA polymerase, which needs a DNA sequence called a Pribnow box as well as a sigma factor (s factor) to start transcription. In eukaryotes, transcription is performed by three types of RNA polymerases, each of which needs a special DNA sequence called the promoter and a set of DNA-binding proteins—transcription factors—to initiate the process. RNA polymerase I is responsible for transcription of ribosomal RNA (rRNA) genes. RNA polymerase II (Pol II) transcribes all protein-coding genes but also some non-coding RNAs (e.g. snRNAs, snoRNAs or long non-coding RNAs). Pol II includes a C-terminal domain (CTD) that is rich in serine residues. When these residues are phosphorylated, the CTD binds to various protein factors that promote transcript maturation and modification. RNA polymerase III transcribes 5S rRNA, transfer RNA (tRNA) genes, and some small non-coding RNAs (e.g. 7SK). Transcription ends when the polymerase encounters a sequence called the terminator.

Steps Involved in Transcription Initiation

Although variations in any step of gene expression can be regulatory, by far the most frequent form of gene control is the regulation of transcription initiation. Control of transcription involves the regulation of transcription factors that interact with the critical *cis*-acting sequences in the promoter and enhancer that then dictate the frequency of RNA polymerase binding to the gene and subsequent transcription. The process of promoter recognition and utilisation involves a stepwise interaction of a complex series of transcription factors with the promoter to create a stable DNA-protein complex that allows RNA polymerase to initiate transcription.

Key in this process is the recognition of the specific sequences in the promoter DNA sequence (the *cis*-acting elements) by the *trans*-acting transcription factors. Given the fact that there are as many as 100,000 protein-encoding genes in the mammalian genome, it is obvious that the expression of each gene cannot be regulated by unique transcription factors. Rather, it would appear that a limited number of transcription factors are responsible and that the high degree of specificity is generated by specific protein-protein interactions that stabilise otherwise weak interactions on a promoter. Very likely, the ability of specific factors to interact provides the possibility of combinatorial interactions of promoter-specific factors that creates specificity to transcription control.

Although it was initially believed that the three types of eukaryotic genes (Pol I -ribosomal RNA, Pol II -mRNA, Pol III -tRNA) were quite distinct with respect to factors involved in the transcription initiation event, it is now clear that many of the activities involved in promoter recognition are shared. Moreover, although there are distinct RNA polymerases for the three types of genes, many of the subunits of the polymerases are also shared. What distinguishes the classes of genes most clearly is the complexity of regulatory elements and factors necessary for the transcription of the mRNA genes.

As stated before, transcription factors possess two essential properties - the ability to bind to DNA, recognising the *cis*-acting elements, in a sequence specific manner and the ability to stimulate transcription. The fact that these two properties are a function of distinct and separable domains in the proteins has been exploited in a method to detect protein-protein interactions, the so-called yeast two-hybrid assay, in which the DNA sequences encoding the two functional domains of a yeast transcription factor have been separated in two vectors. Sequences are then cloned into these vectors to create chimeric fusion proteins as a method for selecting or assaying for sequences that will bring the two functional domains back together via proteinprotein interaction.

Post-Transcriptional Events of Gene Expression

Whereas the initial transcript of a bacterial gene is the actual messenger RNA, the initial transcript of a eukaryotic gene must be altered in a variety of ways before it can function. Thus, post-transcriptional processing and modification events are critical to the formation of a eukaryotic mRNA.

RNA Processing

While transcription of prokaryotic protein-coding genes creates messenger RNA (mRNA) that is ready for translation into protein, transcription of eukaryotic genes leaves a primary transcript of RNA (pre-mRNA), which first has to undergo a series of modifications to become a mature mRNA.

These include 5′ capping, which is set of enzymatic reactions that add 7-methylguanosine (m^{7}G) to the 5′ end of pre-mRNA and thus protect the RNA from degradation by exonucleases. The m^{7}G cap is then bound by cap binding complex heterodimer (CBC20/CBC80), which aids in mRNA export to cytoplasm and also protect the RNA from decapping.

Another modification is 3′ cleavage and polyadenylation. They occur if polyadenylation signal sequence (5′- AAUAAA-3′) is present in pre-mRNA, which is usually between protein-coding sequence and terminator. The pre-mRNA is first cleaved and then a series of ~200 adenines (A) are added to form poly(A) tail, which protects the RNA from degradation. Poly(A) tail is bound by multiple poly(A)-binding proteins (PABP) necessary for mRNA export and translation re-initiation (Fig. 15.3).

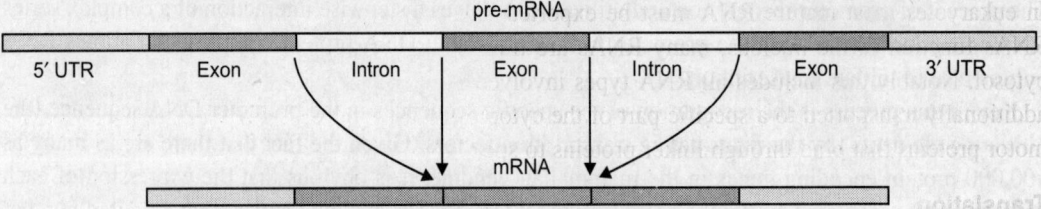

Fig. 15.3: Simple illustration of exons and introns in pre-mRNA and the formation of mature mRNA by splicing. The UTRs are non-coding parts of exons at the ends of the mRNA.

A very important modification of eukaryotic pre-mRNA is RNA splicing. The majority of eukaryotic pre-mRNAs consist of alternating segments called exons and introns. During the process of splicing, an RNA-protein catalytical complex known as spliceosome catalyses two transesterification reactions, which remove an intron and release it in form of lariat structure, and then splice neighbouring exons together. In certain cases, some introns or exons can be either removed or retained in mature mRNA. This so-called alternative splicing creates series of different transcripts originating from a single gene.

Because these transcripts can be potentially translated into different proteins, splicing extends the complexity of eukaryotic gene expression. Extensive RNA processing may be an evolutionary advantage made possible by the nucleus of eukaryotes. In prokaryotes, transcription and translation happen together, whilst in eukaryotes, the nuclear membrane separates the two processes, giving time for RNA processing to occur.

Non-coding RNA Maturation

In most organisms non-coding genes (ncRNA) are transcribed as precursors that undergo further processing. In the case of ribosomal RNAs (rRNA), they are often transcribed as a pre-rRNA that contains one or more rRNAs. The pre-rRNA is cleaved and modified (2'-*o*-methylation and pseudouridine formation) at specific sites by approximately 150 different small nucleolus-restricted RNA species, called snoRNAs. SnoRNAs associate with proteins, forming snoRNPs. While snoRNA part basepair with the target RNA and thus position the modification at a precise site, the protein part performs the catalytical reaction. In eukaryotes, in particular a snoRNP called RNase, MRP cleaves the 45S pre-rRNA into the 28S, 5.8S, and 18S rRNAs. The rRNA and RNA processing factors form large aggregates called the nucleolus.

In the case of transfer RNA (tRNA), for example, the 5' sequence is removed by RNase P, whereas the 3' end is removed by the tRNase Z enzyme and the non-templated 3' CCA tail is added by a nucleotidyl transferase. In the case of micro RNA (miRNA), miRNAs are first transcribed as primary transcripts or pri-miRNA with a cap and poly-A tail and processed to short, 70-nucleotide stem-loop structures known as pre-miRNA in the cell nucleus by the enzymes Drosha and Pasha. After being exported, it is then processed to mature miRNAs in the cytoplasm by interaction with the endonuclease Dicer, which also initiates the formation of the RNA-induced silencing complex (RISC), composed of the Argonaute protein. Even snRNAs and snoRNAs themselves undergo series of modification before they become part of functional RNP complex. This is done either in the nucleoplasm or in the specialised compartments called Cajal bodies. Their bases are methylated or pseudouridinilated by a group of small Cajal body-specific RNAs (scaRNAs), which are structurally similar to snoRNAs.

RNA Export

In eukaryotes most mature RNA must be exported to the cytoplasm from the nucleus. While some RNAs function in the nucleus, many RNAs are transported through the nuclear pores and into the cytosol. Notably this includes all RNA types involved in protein synthesis. In some cases RNAs are additionally transported to a specific part of the cytoplasm, such as a synapse, they are then towed by motor proteins that bind through linker proteins to specific sequences (called 'zipcodes') on the RNA.

Translation

For some RNA (non-coding RNA) the mature RNA is the final gene product. In the case of messenger RNA (mRNA) the RNA is an information carrier coding for the synthesis of one or more proteins. mRNA carrying a single protein sequence (common in eukaryotes) is monocistronic whilst mRNA carrying multiple protein sequences (common in prokaryotes) is known as polycistronic (Fig. 15.4).

Every mRNA consists of three parts: a 5' untranslated region (5'UTR), a protein-coding region or open reading frame (ORF), and a 3' untranslated region (3'UTR). The coding region carries information for protein synthesis encoded by the genetic code to form triplets. Each triplet of nucleotides of the coding region is called a codon and corresponds to a binding site complementary to an anticodon triplet

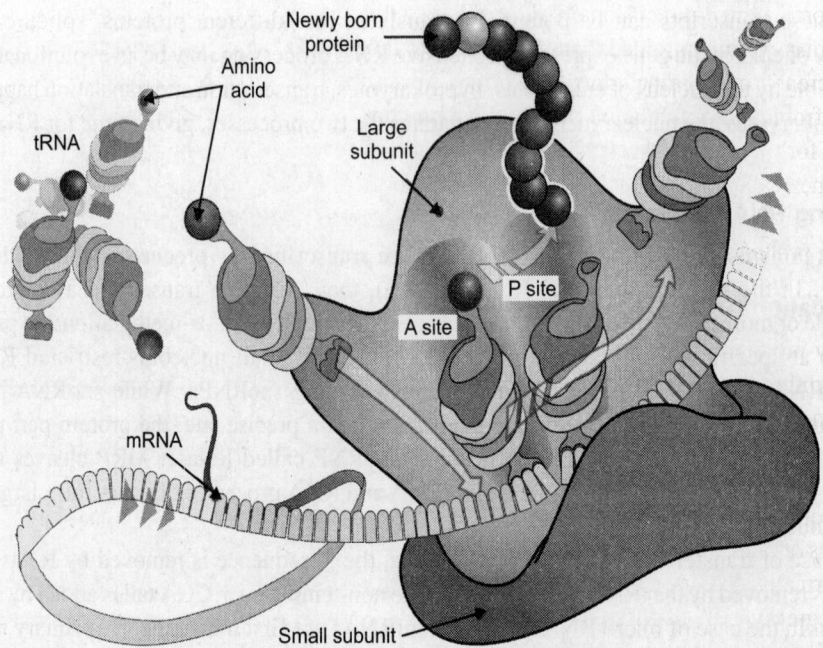

Fig. 15.4: During the translation, tRNA charged with amino acid enters the ribosome and aligns with the correct mRNA triplet. Ribosome then adds amino acid to growing protein chain.

in transfer RNA. Transfer RNAs with the same anticodon sequence always carry an identical type of amino acid. Amino acids are then chained together by the ribosome according to the order of triplets in the coding region. The ribosome helps transfer RNA to bind to messenger RNA and takes the amino acid from each transfer RNA and makes a structure-less protein out of it. Each mRNA molecule is translated into many protein molecules, on average ~2800 in mammals.

In prokaryotes translation generally occurs at the point of transcription (co-transcriptionally), often using a messenger RNA that is still in the process of being created. In eukaryotes translation can occur in a variety of regions of the cell depending on where the protein being written is supposed to be. Major locations are the cytoplasm for soluble cytoplasmic proteins and the membrane of the endoplasmic reticulum for proteins that are for export from the cell or insertion into a cell membrane. Proteins that are supposed to be expressed at the endoplasmic reticulum are recognised part-way through the translation process. This is governed by the signal recognition particle—a protein that binds to the ribosome and directs it to the endoplasmic reticulum when it finds a signal peptide on the growing (nascent) amino acid chain.

Folding

The polypeptide folds into its characteristic and functional three-dimensional structure from a random coil. Each protein exists as an unfolded polypeptide or random coil when translated from a sequence of mRNA into a linear chain of amino acids. This polypeptide lacks any developed three-dimensional structure. Amino acids interact with each other to produce a well-defined three-dimensional structure, the folded protein known as the native state. The resulting three-dimensional structure is determined by the amino acid sequence (Anfinsen's dogma).

The correct three-dimensional structure is essential to function, although some parts of functional proteins may remain unfolded. Failure to fold into the intended shape usually produces inactive proteins with different properties including toxic prions. Several neurodegenerative and other diseases are believed to result from the accumulation of misfolded proteins. Many allergies are caused by the folding of the proteins, for the immune system does not produce antibodies for certain protein structures.

Enzymes called chaperones assist the newly formed protein to attain (fold into) the 3-dimensional structure it needs to function. Similarly, RNA chaperones help RNAs attain their functional shapes. Assisting protein folding is one of the main roles of the endoplasmic reticulum in eukaryotes.

Translocation

Secretory proteins of eukaryotes or prokaryotes must be translocated to enter the secretory pathway. Newly synthesised proteins are directed to the translocation channel by signal peptides. The efficiency of protein secretion in eukaryotes is very dependent on the signal peptide which has been used.

Protein Transport

Many proteins are destined for other parts of the cell than the cytosol and a wide range of signalling sequences or (signal peptides) are used to direct proteins to where they are supposed to be. In prokaryotes this is normally a simple process due to limited compartmentalisation of the cell. However, in eukaryotes there is a great variety of different targeting processes to ensure the protein arrives at the correct organelle.

Not all proteins remain within the cell and many are exported, for example, digestive enzymes, hormones and extracellular matrix proteins. In eukaryotes the export pathway is well developed and the main mechanism for the export of these proteins is translocation to the endoplasmic reticulum, followed by transport via the Golgi apparatus.

GENE REGULATION

The phenotype of a cell as well as the organism as a whole, is the consequence of the regulated expression of a group of genes. Every cell in the organism contains the exact same complement of genes, nevertheless, there are unique proteins produced in the brain that are not produced in the liver, proteins are expressed at a particular time in the cell cycle, proteins are produced in response to hormones, etc. Clearly, an understanding of the molecular basis for the control gene expression is critical to an overall understanding of the basis for cell phenotype.

Regulation of Gene Expression is Responsible for Tissue Differences and Many other Cellular Phenotypes

Since the expression of a gene is ultimately the production of the protein product of the gene, control must be defined as any process that alters the production of the protein. Control of gene expression can be most easily visualised by the pattern of proteins produced in one circumstance versus another. For instance, as schematically depicted in the Fig. 15.5, a two-dimensional gel analysis of proteins (a method that can separate thousands of individual proteins in a sample) in the brain versus in the liver reveals a number of proteins that are common (black spots) but a number of others that are unique to each tissue type.

Thus, even though both tissues possess the exact same complement of genetic information, the expression of this information differs - gene control clearly does exist. The question is - what is the basis for this control? What are the underlying mechanisms?

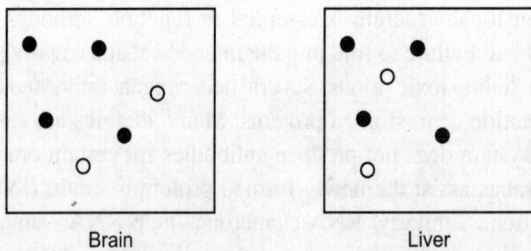

Fig. 15.5: Two-dimensional gel analysis of proteins.

Gene control in prokaryotes and simple unicellular eukaryotes is largely a response to environmental signals - nutrients, etc. In higher eukaryotes (metazoans), the major form of gene control relates to cellular differentiation. Thus, in most cases it is long term and permanent. An example can be seen in the comparison of proteins synthesised in the brain versus in the liver, as analysed by two dimensional gel electrophoresis. Although the majority of proteins that are synthesised are the same in each tissue, one can find examples of species that are unique to one or the other.

Complexity of Eukaryotic Gene Expression Provides Multiple Opportunities for Gene Control

As discussed previously, the events associated with the expression of any given gene in a eukaryotic cell is a very complex process, involving multiple processing events as well as transport from the nuclear to the cytoplasm in order to achieve the final production of afunctional mRNA. Thus, alterations in any of the steps in mRNA biogenesis could alter the final concentration of functional mRNA. Moreover, control of gene expression could also result from an alteration in the translation efficiency of the mRNA or alterations in the stability of the protein product.

Transcription Control

The initial step in gene expression is transcription of the gene and it is now clear from a variety of studies that the control of transcription is a critical regulatory step in the control of gene expression. In considering transcription control, and particularly when carrying out measurements of transcription, one usually defines the transcriptional unit which is that segment of the chromosome (DNA) that specificies the start and the end of transcription. This includes all of the signals necessary for proper transcription.

Transcription regulation could take the form of either initiation control or termination control. Clearly, the control of initiation will determine whether the primary transcript, and thus the funtional mRNA, will be produced and thus represents the most basic form of gene control. Termination can also be a factor if it occurs prior to the completion of the transcript (premature termination). This has in fact been demonstrated to be an important control in the expression of several oncogenes such as the c-myc gene (Fig. 15.6). A similar example of control of transcription elongation can be found in the control of HIV transcription. In the absence of viral regulatory proteins, HIV transcripts initiate properly but fail to efficiently elongate. One of the early viral proteins produced, known as *Tat*, functions to promote elongation and thus increase the efficiency of viral transcript production. Interestingly, the mechanism for the action of *Tat* is unique in that the protein recognises sequences in the 5′ end of the initiated RNA transcript rather than DNA promoter sequences.

How does one measure transcription, and thus determine transcription control? It is important in this regard to distinguish steady state RNA levels from synthesis which requires that the events of transcription

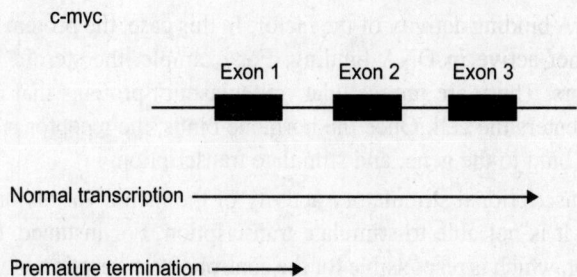

Fig. 15.6: Control in the expression of several oncogenes such as the c-myc gene.

must be separated from subsequent processing steps. Analysis of the RNA in a cellular extract provides a measure of the steady state level - thus, a combination of both transcription and subsequent events. Transcription must be measured by pulse-labeling, usually with a radioactive precursor to RNA, for short time such that no processing has taken place. In short, one is measuring the synthesis of the RNA not the accumulation of the RNA. In actual practice, this is accomplished by incubating cells with radioactive RNA precursors and then measuring the amount of radioactivity incorporated into the RNA, usually by hybridisation to a DNA probe.

Once a gene has been isolated and the promoter/enhancer has been identified, it is also possible to study transcription control, particularly the identification of regulatory sequences, through the use of a reporter gene. The promoter to be studied is fused to a gene that can be easily assayed (a reporter) and then assayed by introduction into appropriate cells, or into animals, scoring for the expression of the reporter. For instance, if a suspected promoter element is placed upstream of a β-galactosidase gene (the reporter), activity of the promoter, and thus transcriptional activity, can be assessed by measuring the production of β-galactosidase activity as shown below:

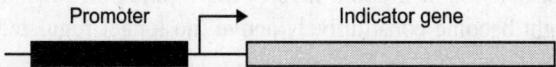

In this way, transcription is being separated from RNA processing contributions by only analysing the role of DNA sequences that contribute to transcription control.

Given the fact that transcription is the key first step in gene expression, and the fact that the binding of *trans*-acting factors to promoter elements is critical for transcription, gene expression can be regulated by controlling the activity of these *trans*-acting factors.

Mechanisms regulating transcription factor activity

1. Control of synthesis of the transcription factor: This is primarily the basis for tissue specific control, i.e. a key regulatory factor or factors is only found in the cell type that the target gene is expressed. For example, the albumin gene is transcribed in the liver but not the brain because the necessary transcription factors are not found in the brain. Another example is the myc transcription factor that functions to regulate the transcription of genes important for cell proliferation. The myc protein is not found in quiescent cells because the myc gene is inactive. Upon stimulation of cell growth, the myc promoter is activated and transcription of the gene is induced. As already discussed, the control of termination of transcription of the myc gene is also a factor in the regulation of myc gene expression.

2. Control of the DNA binding activity of the factor: In this case, the protein (transcription factor) is present but it is not active in DNA binding. For example, the steroid hormone receptors are transcription factors. These are intracellular (cytoplasmic) proteins that bind specifically to the hormone when it enters the cell. Once the hormone binds, the receptor is then activated and can enter the nucleus, bind to the gene, and stimulate transcription.

3. Control of the transcriptional stimulatory activity of the factor: In this instance, the protein can bind to DNA but it is not able to stimulate transcription. For instance, the activity of the E2F transcription factor, which is responsible for the control of transcription of various genes important for DNA replication and cell growth, is regulated by interaction with the retinoblastoma (Rb) tumour suppressor protein. When Rb binds to E2F, the resulting complex can still bind to DNA but it is inactive in stimulating transcription. In fact, the complex can function in just the opposite fashion by serving as a repressor of transcription. The interaction of Rb with E2F is regulated by phosphorylation. That is, unphosphorylated Rb can bind to and regulate E2F but when Rb is phosphorylated by cell cycle regulated protein kinases, it loses the capacity to bind to E2F.

Practical importance of defining transcription control elements

In considering strategies for gene therapy, one must be able to express the protein of interest (for instance, the cystic fibrosis gene product) in the right cell type, at the right time, and in the proper amounts. Thus, an understanding of the mechanisms controlling the expression of the gene to be used is essential in designing the gene therapy vector.

To understand the basis for alterations in transcription control that occur in disease conditions such as cancer, it is critical to know the normal mechanisms of function of the gene. Such alterations can take two general forms:

1. Mutation of *trans*-acting factors: This could involve an inactivation of a factor as the result of a specific mutation or deletion or it could involve the creation of a factor with altered properties. For instance, it might become constitutively active (no longer regulated) or it might acquire an altered specificity.

2. Alteration of *cis*-acting elements of a promoter/enhancer: This could involve mutation of the element resulting in a loss of binding of the transcription factor or it could involve chromosomal alterations that create new elements resulting in a change in the transcription of the gene.

Alterations of transcription regulation in disease

By developing an understanding of normal gene structure, as well as the components of transcription regulation, it has been possible to define the molecular basis for alterations in gene control events that underlie certain disease states. Several such examples are given here. Retrovirus mediated promoter insertion resulting in activation of the c-myc gene As discussed above, transcription of the myc gene, which encodes a transcription factor that controls cell cycle progression, is normally tightly controlled by cell growth regulation.

This normal control can be disrupted as the result of an insertion of a retrovirus (ALV) into the promoter region of the c-myc gene. As a result of this insertion, the myc gene is now controlled by the retrovirus promoter which does not respond to the cell growth regulatory signals. Although this is a rare event, it does raise the potential danger of the use of retrovirus vectors in gene therapy protocols, that is, the inadvertent activation of an oncogene as a result of the retrovirus insertion.

This was a critically important discovery that led directly to the discovery of myc gene rearrangements in human tumours as shown below:

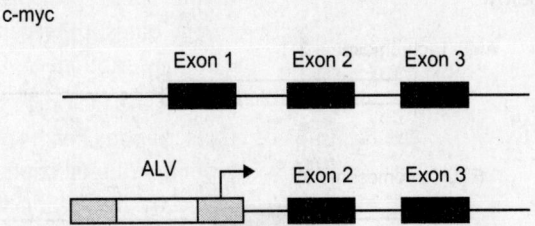

Rearrangement of the c-myc gene in B cell lymphomas

The expression of the c-myc gene is also deregulated in many tumours as the result of chromosome rearrangements, once again resulting from a change in the transcriptional regulatory sequences. For instance, many B cell lymphomas contain a translocation involving chromosome 8 and chromosome 14 that places the c-myc gene in the chromosomal environment of the immunoglobulin heavy chain gene enhancer. In this case, the normal regulation of the myc gene is disrupted with control now being directed by the immunoglobulin enhancer. This then confers a high level of transcription that is B cell-specific and non-cell cycle regulated as shown below:

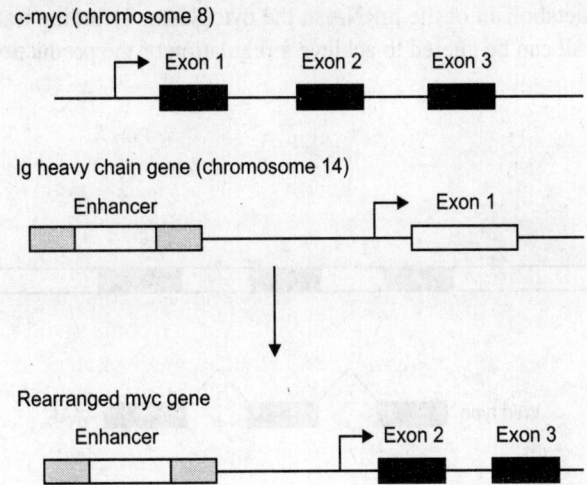

Creation of a chimeric transcription factor in AML by chromosome rearrangments

Whereas the changes detailed above regarding the myc gene result in alterations in regulation of expression of the gene, but still producing the normal protein, another form of transcriptional deregulation can be seen in a chromosomal rearrangement that alters the structure of the encoded protein. The most common chromosomal rearrangment seen in acute myelogenous leukemia is a translocation that fuses a portion of chromosome 8 with a portion of chromosome 21, a socalled 8:21 translocation. The breakpoints involve a gene on chromosome 21 known as AML-1 which encodes a transcription factor and a gene on chromosome 8 known as ETO of unknown function. As a result of the translocation, a new gene is created that encodes a chimeric protein containing sequence from AML-1, including the DNA binding domain, and sequence from ETO. Although the nature of the effect on AML-1 function is unknown, one presumes that some aspect of the specificity or the regulatory properties of the transcription factor has been altered as shown below:

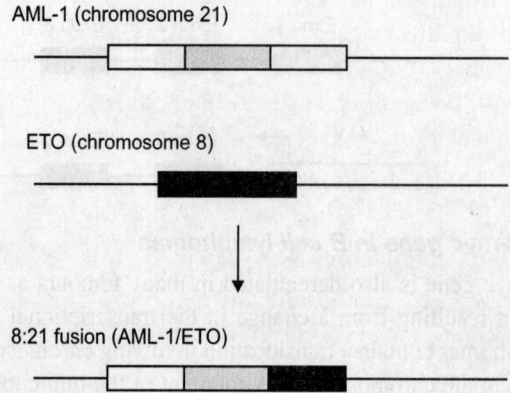

Post-Transcriptional Gene Control

Each one of the steps of mRNA biogenesis following transcription has been demonstrated to participate in gene regulation. Thus, splicing of the primary transcript, 3' end cleavage and polyadenylation, transport to the cytoplasm, and metabolism of the mRNA in the cytoplasm, including translation efficiency and stability of the mRNA, all can be altered to achieve a regulation of the production of the product of the gene as shown below:

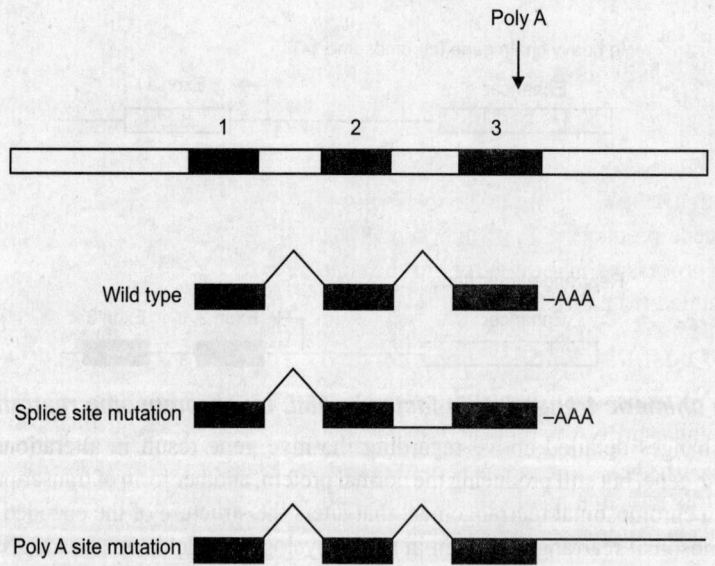

A variety of transcription units have now been shown to possess the potential to produce more than one mRNA as a result of alternative processing. This can include both alternative splicing as well as polyadenylation. A selective use of exons in a primary transcript can thus define a distinct protein product. If this selection is regulated, changing under one circumstance or another, then such changes are defined as events regulating the expression of the gene.

It is also clear that mutation of either critical splice site sequences or poly A site sequences can impair gene expression. Although such mutations would not alter the coding sequences directly, they can result in alterations that do affect the coding capacity. For instance, a splice site mutation that altered the splice donor following exon 2 in the example, would leave the intron sequence in the mRNA which would lead to a frameshift and likely a non-functional protein.

Likewise, a poly A site mutation would prevent processing at the poly A site resulting in an RNA with an extended 3′ terminus and no poly A tail. Such an RNA would not be efficiently transported to the cytoplasm and would be very unstable.

Alternative splicing and polyadenylation as gene control mechanisms

There are a variety of examples of gene control through alternative RNA processing events, both splicing as well as polyadenylation. Perhaps two of the best studies examples include the immunoglobulin heavy chain gene and the calcitonin/CGRP gene. The immunoglobulin heavy is composed of two protein molecules, a heavy chain and a light chain. Antibody diversity is determined by variation in the sequence in both the heavy chain and the light chain as a consequence of gene rearrangement as well as mutation. In addition, the production of the heavy chain is regulated during B cell differentiation. In a mature B cell, the heavy chain, together with the light chain, is inserted into the B cell membrane and serves as an antigen receptor. When antigen binds, the B cell is stimulated to mature to a plasma cell where the immunoglobulin molecule is now secreted as a antibody. This switch in immunoglobulin expression is the result of alternative splicing as well as polyadenylation of the primary transcript of the gene as indicated below. This brings a different set of exon sequences into the 3′ position of the transcript. The Cμ4 exon encodes the secreted form of the protein whereas the M1 and M2 exons encode the membrane bound form of the protein.

Another example can be found in the calcitonin gene which encodes a calcium regulating hormone that is produced in the thyroid. This locus also encodes a distinct separate product known as CGRP (calcitonin gene related peptide), a neuropeptide produced in the brain. Thus, alternative RNA splicing and polyadenylation, that occurs in a tissue specific manner (brain versus thyroid), results in the production of two distinct gene products with distinct function. Finally, one very striking example of the role of alternative RNA processing in the control of gene expression can be seen in the large variety of products that can be generated from the alpha-tropomyosin locus in a tissue-specific fashion.

Other forms of post-transcription gene control

Control of RNA transport: Although there are no clear examples whereby the nuclear/cytoplasmic transport of a cellular mRNA is regulated, there are at least two instances in viral infections in which RNA transport is affected.

First, adenovirus infection results in the inhibition of transport of most cellular mRNAs - a specific viral gene product is required for this to occur and at the same time, this protein facilitates the transport of viral RNA.

Second, as indicated previously, studies of Bryan Cullen and colleagues here at Duke have shown that the product of the HIV rev gene is required for the efficient transport of unspliced viral RNA from the nucleus to the cytoplasm.

Control of mRNA stability: The stability of mRNAs varies over a large range. Some RNAs are quite stable with half lives approaching the cell division time. Other RNAs turn over very rapidly (half lives of a few minutes). As a general rule, RNAs that are expressed in a transient fashion often are short lived. Many RNAs that encode cytokines as well as early responses to mitogens are unstable, dependent on specific sequences in the 3′ untranslated region of the RNA. The unstable nature of the mRNA as a result of recognition of this sequence is associated with shortening of the poly A tail.

Translation control: General control - alterations of translation factors can alter the translation efficiency of mRNAs. For instance, phosphorylation of eIF2 inhibits is action. Translation efficiency is also determined by *cis*-acting sequences in the mRNA - particularly the sequences that surround the AUG initiation codon.

Chapter 16

Recombinant DNA

INTRODUCTION

Recombinant DNA, which is often shortened to rDNA, is an artificially made DNA strand that is formed by the combination of two or more gene sequences. This new combination may or may not occur naturally, but is engineered specifically for a purpose to be used in one of the many applications of recombinant DNA. By combining two or more different strands of DNA, scientists are able to create a new strand of DNA. The most common recombinant process involves combining the DNA of two different organisms. Structure of DNA is given in Fig. 16.1. Recombinant DNA is possible because DNA molecules from all organisms share the same chemical structure. They differ only in the nucleotide sequence within that identical overall structure (Fig. 16.2). Recombinant DNA molecules are sometimes called chimeric DNA, because they are usually made of material from two different species, like the mythical chimera. rDNA technology uses palindromic sequences and leads to the production of sticky and blunt ends. The DNA sequences used in the construction of recombinant DNA molecules can originate from any species. For example, plant DNA may be joined to bacterial DNA, or human DNA may be joined with fungal DNA. In addition, DNA sequences that do not occur any where in nature may be created by the chemical synthesis of DNA and incorporated into recombinant molecules. Using recombinant DNA technology and synthetic DNA, literally any DNA sequence may be created and introduced into any of a very wide range of living organisms. Proteins that can result from the expression of recombinant DNA within living cells are termed recombinant proteins. When recombinant DNA encoding a protein is introduced into a host organism, the recombinant protein is not necessarily produced.

Expression of foreign proteins requires the use of specialised expression vectors and often necessitates significant restructure by foreign coding sequence. Recombinant DNA differs from genetic recombination in that the former results from artificial methods in the test tube, while the latter is a normal biological process that results in the remixing of existing DNA sequences in essentially all organisms.

CREATING RECOMBINANT DNA

Molecular cloning is the laboratory process used to create recombinant DNA. It is one of two widely used methods (along with polymerase chain reaction, abbreviation PCR) used to direct the replication

321

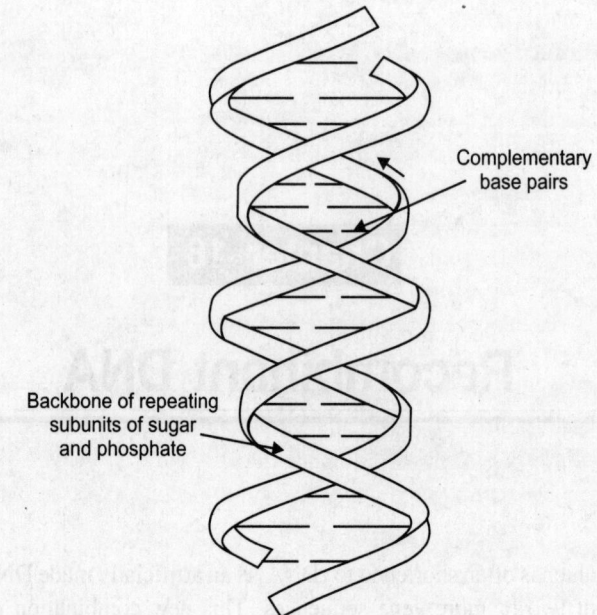

Complementary base pairs

Backbone of repeating subunits of sugar and phosphate

Fig. 16.1: Structure of DNA.

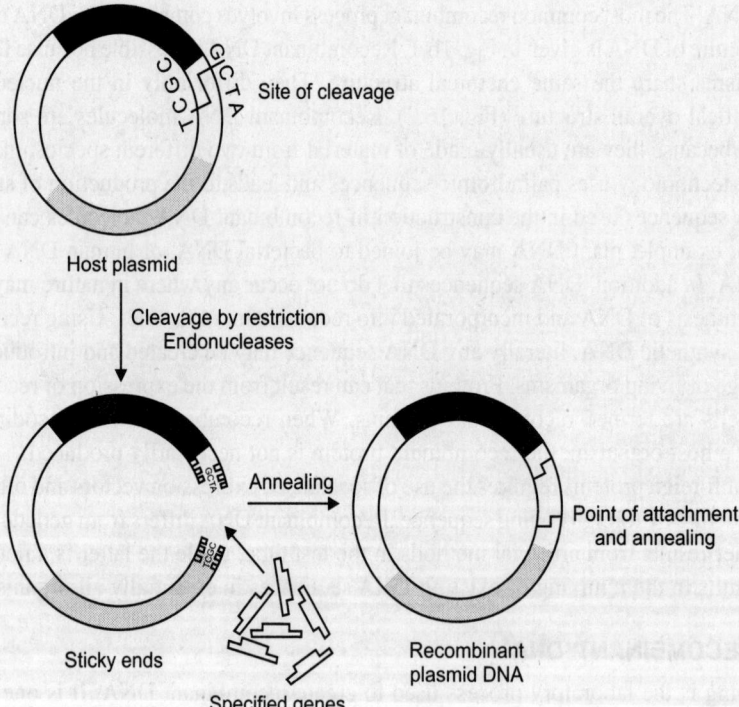

Site of cleavage

Host plasmid

Cleavage by restriction Endonucleases

Annealing

Point of attachment and annealing

Recombinant plasmid DNA

Sticky ends

Specified genes

Fig. 16.2: Construction of recombinant DNA, in which a foreign DNA fragment is inserted into a plasmid vector. In this example, the gene indicated by the white colour is inactivated upon insertion of the foreign DNA fragment.

of any specific DNA sequence chosen by the experimentalist. The fundamental difference between the two methods is that molecular cloning involves replication of the DNA within a living cell, while PCR replicates DNA in the test tube, free of living cells.

Formation of recombinant DNA requires a cloning vector, a DNA molecule that replicates within a living cell. Vectors are generally derived from plasmids or viruses and represent relatively small segments of DNA that contain necessary genetic signals for replication, as well as additional elements for convenience in inserting foreign DNA, identifying cells that contain recombinant DNA, and, where appropriate, expressing the foreign DNA. The choice of vector for molecular cloning depends on the choice of host organism, the size of the DNA to be cloned and whether and how the foreign DNA is to be expressed. The DNA segments can be combined by using a variety of methods, such as restriction enzyme/ligase cloning or Gibson assembly. In standard cloning protocols, the cloning of any DNA fragment essentially involves seven steps: (i) choice of host organism and cloning vector, (ii) preparation of vector DNA, (iii) preparation of DNA to be cloned, (iv) creation of recombinant DNA, (v) introduction of recombinant DNA into the host organism, (vi) selection of organisms containing recombinant DNA and (vii) screening for clones with desired DNA inserts and biological properties.

Expression of Recombinant DNA

Following transplantation into the host organism, the foreign DNA contained within the recombinant DNA construct may or may not be expressed. That is, the DNA may simply be replicated without expression, or it may be transcribed and translated so that a recombinant protein is produced. Generally speaking, expression of a foreign gene requires restructuring the gene to include sequences that are required for producing an mRNA molecule that can be used by the host's translational apparatus (e.g. promoter, translational initiation signal and transcriptional terminator). Specific changes to the host organism may be made to improve expression of the ectopic gene. In addition, changes may be needed to the coding sequences as well, to optimise translation, make the protein soluble, direct the recombinant protein to the proper cellular or extracellular location and stabilise the protein from degradation.

Properties of Organisms Containing Recombinant DNA

In most cases, organisms containing recombinant DNA have apparently normal phenotypes. That is, their appearance, behaviour and metabolism are usually unchanged and the only way to demonstrate the presence of recombinant sequences is to examine the DNA itself, typically using a polymerase chain reaction (PCR) test. Significant exceptions exist and are discussed below.

If the rDNA sequences encode a gene that is expressed, then the presence of RNA and/or protein products of the recombinant gene can be detected, typically using RT-PCR or western hybridisation methods. Gross phenotypic changes are not the norm, unless the recombinant gene has been chosen and modified so as to generate biological activity in the host organism. Additional phenotypes that are encountered include toxicity to the host organism induced by the recombinant gene product, especially if it is over-expressed or expressed within inappropriate cells or tissues. In some cases, recombinant DNA can have deleterious effects even if it is not expressed. One mechanism by which this happens is insertional inactivation, in which the rDNA becomes inserted into a host cell's gene. In some cases, researchers use this phenomenon to 'knock out' genes to determine their biological function and importance. Another mechanism by which rDNA insertion into chromosomal DNA can affect gene expression is by inappropriate activation of previously unexpressed host cell genes. This can happen, for example, when a recombinant DNA fragment containing an active promoter becomes located next to a previously silent host cell gene, or when a host cell gene that functions to restrain gene expression undergoes insertional inactivation by recombinant DNA. There are three different methods by which Recombinant DNA is made. They are transformation, non-bacterial transformation and phage introduction and are described separately below.

Transformation: The first step in transformation is to select a piece of DNA to be inserted into a vector. The second step is to cut that piece of DNA with a restriction enzyme and then ligate the DNA insert into the vector with DNA Ligase. The insert contains a selectable marker which allows for identification of recombinant molecules. An antibiotic marker is often used so a host cell without a vector dies when exposed to a certain antibiotic and the host with the vector will live because it is resistant. The vector is inserted into a host cell, in a process called transformation. One example of a possible host cell is *E..coli*. The host cells must be specially prepared to take up the foreign DNA. Selectable markers can be for antibiotic resistance, colour changes, or any other characteristic which can distinguish transformed hosts from untransformed hosts. Different vectors have different properties to make them suitable to different applications. Some properties can include symmetrical cloning sites, size and high copy number.

Non-bacterial transformation: This is a process very similar to Transformation, which was described above. The only difference between the two is non-bacterial does not use bacteria such as *E. coli* for the host. In microinjection, the DNA is injected directly into the nucleus of the cell being transformed. In biolistics, the host cells are bombarded with high velocity microprojectiles, such as particles of gold or tungsten that have been coated with DNA.

Phage introduction: Phage introduction is the process of transfection, which is equivalent to transformation, except a phage is used instead of bacteria. *In vitro* packagings of a vector is used. This uses lambda or MI3 phages to produce phage plaques which contain recombinants. The recombinants that are created can be identified by differences in the recombinants and non-recombinants using various selection methods.

How does rDNA work?

Recombinant DNA works when the host cell expresses protein from the recombinant genes. A significant amount of recombinant protein will not be produced by the host unless expression factors are added. Protein expression depends upon the gene being surrounded by a collection of signals which provide instructions for the transcription and translation of the gene by the cell. These signals include the promoter, the ribosome binding site and the terminator. Expression vectors, in which the foreign DNA is inserted, contain these signals. Signals are species specific. In the case of *E. coli,* these signals must be *E. coli* signals as *E. coli* is unlikely to understand the signals of human promoters and terminators.

Problems are encountered if the gene contains introns or contains signals which act as terminators to a bacterial host. This results in premature termination and the recombinant protein may not be processed correctly, be folded correctly, or may even be degraded. Production of recombinant proteins in eukaryotic systems generally takes place in yeast and filamentous fungi. The use of animal cells is difficult due to the fact that many need a solid support surface, unlike bacteria and have complex growth needs. However, some proteins are too complex to be produced in bacterium, so eukaryotic cells must be used.

Importance of DNA

Recombinant DNA has been gaining in importance over the last few years and recombinant DNA will only become more important in the 21st century as genetic diseases become more prevelant and agricultural area is reduced.

Below are some of the areas where recombinant DNA will have an impact.

1. Better crops (drought and heat resistance).
2. Recombinant vaccines (i.e. Hepatitis B).
3. Prevention and cure of sickle cell anemia.
4. Prevention and cure of cystic fibrosis.
5. Production of clotting factors.
6. Production of insulin.
7. Production of recombinant pharmaceuticals.
8. Plants that produce their own insecticides.
9. Germ line and somatic gene therapy.

TOOLS AND TECHNIQUES OF RECOMBINANT DNA TECHNOLOGY

Recombinant DNA technology, which is also called gene cloning or molecular cloning, is an umbrella term that encompasses a number of experimental protocols, leading to the transfer of genetic information (DNA fragments, i.e. gene) from one organism to another. There are no single set of methods that can be used to meet this objective; however, a recombinant DNA experiment often follows the following steps.

Step 1: A foreign DNA fragment (gene) from a donor organism is extracted, enzymatically cleaved (cut/digested) and joined (ligated) to another DNA entity (a cloning vector) to form a new, recombinant DNA molecule (cloning vector – insert DNA construct).

Step 2: This cloning vector-insert DNA construct is transferred into and maintained within a host cell by a desired method. This process is called transformation.

Step 3: Those host cells, which have successfully inserted the new DNA fragment in their genome (transformed cells), are identified and selected (separated/isolated), from those who have not been transformed by this effort.

Step 4: The integration of foreign DNA in the host cells are ensured by various methods, e.g. amplification by polymerase chain reaction (PCR), southern blotting of DNA against a known probe, etc. and blotting of the protein product that is encoded by the cloned DNA sequence by the western blotting, etc. It is also confirmed by northern blotting techniques which elucidate synthesis of mRNA to ensure the expression on the introduced foreign genes in the transformed host cells.

Step 5: The modification in the character of the transgenic plant (produced from the transformed cells), which is an outcome of the genetic engineering is verified and steps for the application /use of new product with its commercial, social, environmental health risk assessments and ethical aspects are established.

GENE CLONING

Recombinant DNA technology or gene cloning is a new born discipline of science which aims to alter the heredity apparatus of a living cell. It is also popularly known as genetic engineering which is performed under highly controllable laboratory conditions so that the cell can form completely new functions.

A recombinant DNA molecule is produced in joining together two or more DNA segments usually originating from different organisms. This is achieved by using specific enzymes for cutting the DNA (by the help of restriction enzymes) into suitable fragments and then joining together the appropriate fragments (by, ligase enzyme). It is now possible to isolate a desired piece of DNA (out of millions of nucleotide pairs in a chromosome) and join this isolated piece with another DNA molecule to create a new DNA molecule in test tube (*in vitro*). This molecule is now introduced back into living organisms (such as bacteria) to produce large number of copies (gene cloning). These developments called 'recombinant DNA technique' or 'gene splicing' or 'genetic engineering' have made possible to produce chromosomes with gene combination that is never formed naturally.

Recombinant DNA technology involves several steps in specific sequence such as:

1. Isolation of genetic material.
2. Cutting of DNA at specific locations.
3. Recombinant DNA formation.
4. Cloning of DNA.

Isolation of genetic material (DNA): In majority of organisms deoxynobo-nucleic acid or DNA is the genetic material. It is present in chromosomes within the cell. To isolate DNA, the cell at first is to be broken open by treating cell with enzyme so that DNA with other macromolecules are released. To get pure DNA the other necessary macro molecules such as RNA, protein, polysaccharides are removed by treating with appropriate enzymes. This is often called foreign DNA. It is then incorporated into bacterial plasmid.

Cutting of DNA: To cut DNA at specific location restriction endonuclease enzyme is used. These enzymes are called as molecular scissor or molecular scalpel and found in bacteria. These enzymes can cut the, DNA at any known point. The enzymes can cut DNA of the plasmid as well as foreign DNA at specific sites. These sites or points are mostly 8 palindromic, i.e. the sequences which read the same both backward and forward.

Formation of recombinant DNA: As stated earlier a desired piece of DNA or a gene is first isolated. This is generally called as foreign DNA. It is then incorporated into bacterial plasmid (plasmids are rings of DNA other than main ring shaped DNA of a bacterium which can replicate independent of main DNA). For this DNA of the plasmid is cut open by endonuclease enzyme leaving the sticky ends. The foreign DNA is also cut out (by the same restriction endonuclease) and allowed to join the sticky ends of plasmid DNA. Such a plasmid DNA is now known as recombinant DNA.

Cloning of DNA: The recombinant plasmid DNA obtained above is allowed to multiply to form a clone of recombinant DNA. To achieve this recombinant plasmid DNA is introduced into a rapidly dividing bacterium. Each time the bacterium divides and replicates its DNA, it also copies the introduced recombinant plasmid and also the foreign DNA. This method of introducing plasmid DNA into a bacterium (usually *E. coli*) is known as transformation. In this process bacterial cell takes up pieces of naked DNA from the surrounding medium.

These bacteria with recombinant plasmid DNA are grown in nutrient medium where these double in number in every 20–30 minutes, producing millions of cells. In this way millions of copies of recombinant plasmid DNA are formed.

To recover the foreign DNA from recombinant plasmid DNA, the bacterial cells are broken. The foreign DNA is cut out of the recombinant plasmid DNA by appropriate restriction enzyme and separated by gel electrophoresis.

Important steps in recombinant DNA technology:

1. Isolation of DNA from the selected organism and preparation of DNA fragments (foreign DNA) to be cloned.

2. Insertion of the DNA fragments (foreign DNA) into a suitable vector (such as plasmid DNA) to produce recombinant DNA.

3. Introduction of the recombinant DNA into a suitable organism (such as bacteria) called host. This process is called transformation. Generally *E. coli* is used for cloning.

4. Multiplication of host cells and also multiplication of recombinant DNA and cloning of desired gene.

Molecular Cloning

Through several discoveries in the areas of molecular biology, nucleic acid enzymology and the molecular genetics of bacterial, virus and bacterial extra chromosomal DNA elements (plasmids), as well as of the other eukaryotic organisms, made it possible to develop recombinant DNA technology as such a revolutionary technique in the manipulating living organisms in desired manner. This technology would have not existed without the availability of enzymes (restriction enzyme; restriction endonucleases) that recognise specific double-stranded DNA sequences and cleave the DNA in both strands at these sequences.

Restriction endonucleases

For molecular cloning of a foreign gene into a cloning vector, it is necessary to cut the DNA fragment at a specific site containing the target sequences, both in the source DNA that contain the largest sequences and in the cloning vector. The cut sites in the both kinds of DNA must be consistent for each time into discrete and reproductive fragments. Subjecting isolated DNA to passage through a small-bore needle or to sonication produces double stranded pieces of DNA that may range from 0.3 to 5 kilo basepair (Kb), in length, but these fragments are produced by the random breaking of DNA and each time we may end up with DNA with different sequences. So by these simple procedures we can't cut the DNA at desired site with the targeted sequences.

The discovery of bacterial enzymes, that cut DNA molecules internally at the specific base pair sequences, called type II restriction endonucleases, made it feasible to obtain DNA sequences of desired nature from a source DNA and to insert it in the genome of another organism between the enzymatic cut sizes which can accommodate the new insert/foreign DNA. One of the first of these type II restriction endonucleases characterised from the bacterium *Escherichia coli* and it was designated *Eco* RI.

This enzyme binds to a DNA region with a specific palindromic sequence (the two strands are identical in this region when either is read in the same polarity, i.e. 5′ to 3′) of 6 base pairs (bp) and cuts between the guanine and adenine residues on each strand.

Eco RI enzyme specifically cleaves the internucleotide bond between the oxygen of the 3′ carbon of the sugar of one nucleotide and the phosphate group attached to 5′ carbon of the sugar of the adjacent nucleotide. The symmetrical staggered cleavage of DNA by *Eco* RI produces two single-stranded, complementary cut ends, each with extensions of four nucleotides. Each single-stranded extension, in this case, ends in a 5′-phosphate group and the 3′ – hydroxyl group from the opposite strand is recessed.

Eco RI type enzymes are not the only restriction endonucleases, which have been isolated and used for gene isolation and cloning. Hundred of other type II restriction endonucleases are known which have been isolated from the various bacteria. For naming them, as in *Eco* RI, genus of the source bacteria is the capitalised letter and the first two letters of the species name are in lowercase letters. The strain designation is often omitted from the name and roman numerals are used to designate the order of characterisation of different restriction endonucleases from the same organisms. For example, *Hpa* I and *Hpa* II are the first and second type II restriction endonucleases that were isolated from *Haemophilus parainfluenzae*.

Plant Genomes, Genomic and cDNA Libraries

The genetic information which controls the entire function of a plant is stored in the form of a polymer called deoxyribonucleic acid (DNA), in the cells as in the other eukaryotes. The instructions that control all the activities of a plant are stored in the DNA as genes, which are the DNA sequences making the functional ribonucleic acid (RNA) and proteins. In plants, each gene codes for one protein or functional RNA, so each plant contain a large number of gene which vary species to species and genus to genus. The total amount of DNA in the nucleus of a cell, or in organelles, is called 'the genome'.

In plant cells the genes may be organised in nuclei, mitochondria and chloroplasts. The nuclear genome is contained in large linear DNA molecules called chromosomes, which varies in size and number in different plant species, consequently the size of the genome also varies between the plant species (Table 16.1). The mitochondrial and chloroplast genome are, on the other hand, contained in the circular DNA in multiple copies in each organelle.

Table 16.1: Genome size of various plants.

Plant	Genome size (Mb)	Relative genome size compared with Arabidopsis
Arabidopsis	120–130	1
Rice	389–430	3.0
Maize	2500	20
Barley	5000	38
Wheat	15000–16960	128
Oilseed rape	1200	10
Garden pea	3947	33
Soyabean	1115	9
Potato	840	14
Tomato	950	8

Though the majority of genetic informations in green plants are contained in the nuclear genome, the mitochondria and the chloroplasts also share a significant amount of the genetic information that controls the functional biology of plants.

Significance of Genome Size and Organisation

The size of nuclear genome which represents an unreplicated DNA content (C-value) in the cells of organisms reflects the complexity of the organism. The genome of higher order organisms are generally bigger than those of lower order organism, for example, the C- value vary from $\sim 10^7$ to 10^{11} bp in eukaryotic organisms, having a trend of bigger size of genome in order of fungi, animals and plants as compared to bacteria. However, this simple relationship does not always hold true, a situation known as 'the C value paradox'. We can see that in higher plants, for example, plants of similar size and similar groups can have a genome size that vary by several orders of magnitudes (see rice and wheat in Table 16.1) and many amphibian have C-values much larger than that of humans. Surprisingly only a small percentage of the genome is known to actually encode proteins which lead to the development of a character in terms of function or structure. It means a vast majority of DNA components in a genome in certain organisms are either non-coding and apparently function less or unrevealed yet by the known tools and techniques of plant biology and biotechnology.

CLONING VECTORS

DNA cloning is a technique to produce large quantities of a specific DNA segment. The DNA segment to be cloned is first linked to a vector DNA, which is a vehicle for carrying foreign DNA into a suitable host cell, such as the bacterium *E. coli*. The vector contains sequences that allow it to be replicated within the host cell.

The rDNA technology allows the cloning of random DNA or cDNA segments, often used as probes as well as cloning of the specific genes, which has either been isolated from the genome or synthesised in laboratory or obtained as cDNA from specific mRNA sequences.

Vectors for Genetic Engineering

Genetic engineering become possible because vectors like plasmids and phages reproduce in a host (e.g. *E. coli*) in their usual manner even after insertion of foreign DNA; the inserted DNA also replicate faithfully with the parent DNA (The technique is called gene cloning and the vectors used for this purpose are called cloning vectors). Using a variety of cloning, gene can be isolated, cloned and characterised and new characters can be inserted vector beyond the taxonomic boundaries. The vectors can also manipulate the expression of the inserted genes in the host; expression vactors.

Various kinds of vectors are available, e.g. plasmids, (often used for cloning DNA segments of small size (upto 10 kilobases), phages (20–25 Kbp), cosmids (40–50 Kbp DNA segment), bacteriophage P1 system and F-factor based vectors (BACs = bacterial artificial chromosomes), YACs, MACs, etc. can allow cloning of DNA segments, as large as 100 to 1000 Kbp (or $1 Mp = 10^6$ bp) length (preferred when fragments bigger than 50–100 Kbp are to be cloned), phagemids (combine desirable features of both plasmids and bacteriophases), BACs and PACs (100–300 Kbp), YACs (100–2000 Kbp), MACs (mammalian artificial chromosomes (> 1000 Kbp).

Plasmids and Vectors

Plasmids are self replicating circular (rarely linear) duplex DNA molecules, which are maintained in a bacterial cell, yeast cell or eukaryotic cell organelles, e.g. chloroplasts and mitochondria in a definite number of copies (characteristic to the specific organism or organelle). The number can range from as small as 1 to as large as 1000 copies per cell. Plasmids are a preferable source as cloning vectors, due to their increased yield potential.

The concept of cloning a foreign DNA segment in plasmid is discussed below.

A plasmid (pBR322) confers resistance to both ampicillin and tetracycline. The restriction endonuclease enzyme can cut it at ampicillin site at which a foreign DNA can get inserted.

After insertion this foreign gene ampicillin resistance will be ineffective, whereas the tetracycline resistance will be maintained intact. By the differential resistance capability of the plasmids wild type and recombinant type can be separated.

Plasmid vectors are often used for cloning segments of small size (upto 10 kilobases). Commonly used *E. coli* plasmid vectors are pBR322 and pBR 327 vectors. Some details of *Agrobacterium* plasmid vectors which are most widely used in plant transformation are discussed below.

Lamda phage (λ) vectors

For preparing genomic libraries of the eukaryotes, cloning of larger DNA segments are required. Phase lambda (λ) vectors can permit cloning of 20–25 Kbp lóng segments. Working with phage lambda considered easier and more efficient for making genomic and cDNA libraries.

Cosmids as vectors

Cosmid vectors can also permit cloning of DNA segments upto 45 Kbp long. They are plasmid particles with *cos* sites, allow the packing of DNA into phage particles *in vitro*. Certain specific DNA sequences, those for *cos* sites are inserted easily into cosmids. It is highly efficient vector to produce a complete genomic library of 10^6–10^7 clones from a mere 1 μg of insert DNA.

Mammalian Artificial Chromosomes (MACs)

To clone large DNA segments in mammalian cells MACs, have been produced with the isolation of mammalian telomere and centromere. MACs are designed to be replicate, segregate and express in a mammalian cell like any other mammalian chromosome along with other chromosomes. Since it will be an independent chromosome, with all the functional elements (telomeres, origins of replication, centromere, etc.) MAC will not be integrated with the genome and can be used as a vector maintaining a single copy per cell. It could carry large fragments of DNA (upto 1000 Kbp) representing an intact eukaryotic split gene with exons and introns permitting its normal expression regulated by the associated promoter sequences.

Plant and Animal Viruses as Vectors

Cauliflower mosaic virus (CAMV), Tobacco mosaic virus (TMV) and Gemini viruses are those groups of plant viruses which have been used as vectors for cloning DNA segments. Due to their high potential of fast replication in the appropriate hosts, they can multiply the inserted foreign DNA very fast and in very large numbers of copies. A number of animal viruses are also used as vectors, either for the delivery of DNA into the host genome or for the fast and higher level amplification of foreign genes using the virus based promoters.

Transposons as Vectors

Transposons are mobile DNA segments that are able to move and integrate throughout an organism's genome. Certain transposons of higher plants (e.g. Ac/Ds or Mn1 of maize) and P element of *Drosophila* are the common transposons used as cloning vectors. Transposons possess short terminal reports enclosing along DNA segment containing the gene for transposase enzyme responsible for transposition. Part of this region can be deleted and the transposon can be used for cloning of foreign DNA segments as it occur in other cases.

Genomic and cDNA Libraries

Genomic DNA is the genetic material of an organism stored in its genetic pool, whereas cDNA is DNA sequence derived from mRNA isolated from a specific metabolically active tissue of an organism. A mixture of clones each carrying DNA sequences derived either from the genomic DNA or from cDNA are called as gnomic or cDNA libraries respectively. These libraries are constructed and used for various steps involved in rDNA technology.

Genomic Library

Cloning of a complete genome as library of random genomic clones is also called as a shotgun experiment. In this protocol, genomic DNA is extracted and then broken into fragments of reasonable size by restriction endonucleases and subsequently inserted into a cloning vector to generate a population of chimeric vector molecule. The DNA fragments cloned in this manner are known as genomic library. Once prepared, the clones can be put into the plasmid vector and retrieved whenever required for various purposes, e.g. identification and isolation of genes, source genes for genetic engineering, genetic studies, etc.

Various restriction endonucleases can cut the fragments of varying sizes, which facilitate the fragmentation of genome for library making depending on the genome size and vector type. For a probability level of 99% that all the sequences are present in a genomic library of a species about 1500 cloned fragments are needed for *E. coli*, 4600 for yeast, 48000 for *Drosophila melanogaster* and 8,00,000 for human being.

cDNA Library from mRNAs

cDNA (complementary DNA) libraries are prepared by the help of activated mRNA, isolated from the cells actively synthesising proteins (for example meristems, roots and leaves in plants). The cDNA is obtained as a reverse transcriptase induced copy of mRNA. Though cDNA molecules can be made double stranded (Fig. 16.3) it differ from genomic clones in lacking the introns present in split genes. The advantage of cDNA libraries is being capable to be expressed in bacteria, which do not have the machinery to process the eukaryotic split gene Hn RNA into mRNA. These libraries can be processed with colony hybridisation technique (Fig. 16.4) for isolation of a gene sequence.

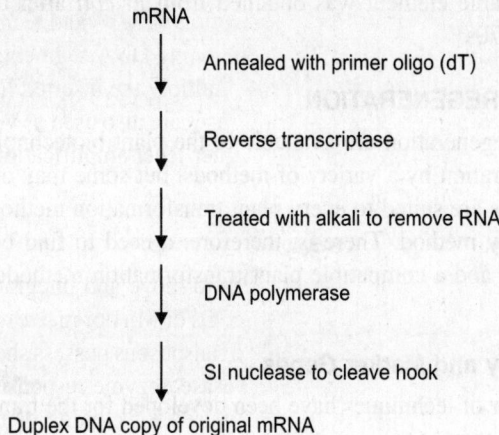

Fig. 16.3: Schematic presentation synthesis of cDNA from mRNA, using reverse transcriptase enzyme.

Transposable Elements and Gene Walking

A transposable element (TE) is a DNA sequence that is able to move and integrate throughout an organism's genome. In contrast to homologous recombination processes that require at least some degree of sequence homology. Thus, the mechanism of integration of TE into chromosomes are considered as non homologous recombination and is highly useful in rDNA technology.

Discovery of transposable elements began in the 1940s with the experimental work of Marcus Roades and Barabara McClintok during their classical work on maize genetics. They indicated that genomes may contain unstable and possibly mobile components as they found the appearance of unexpected phenotypes amongst the progeny of certain strains of maize. Later it was confirmed in bacteria and higher organisms that such unusual genetic results are consequence of the insertion of mobile DNA pieces, known a transposable elements (also called as jumping genes).

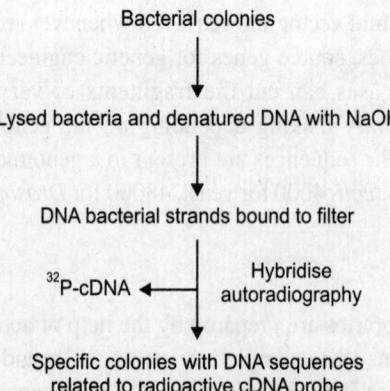

Bacterial colonies

↓

Lysed bacteria and denatured DNA with NaOH

↓

DNA bacterial strands bound to filter

^{32}P-cDNA ←——— Hybridise autoradiography

↓

Specific colonies with DNA sequences
related to radioactive cDNA probe

Fig. 16.4: Colony hybridisation technique for selection and isolation of DNA fragment having sequence complimentary to a radioactively labelled probe.

Though the findings of Roades and McClintock was the first clear indication that movable DNA sequences existed in any genome, the first evidence for occurrence existed in any genome, isolation and characterisation of transposable element was obtained from *E. coli* after development of molecular techniques up to the late 1970s.

VECTORS FOR PLANT REGENERATION

Various methods of plant regeneration are available to the plant biotechnologist. Some plant species may be amenable to regeneration by a variety of methods, but some may only be regenerated by one method. Not all plant tissues are suited to every plant transformation method and not all plant species can be regenerated by every method. There is, therefore, a need to find both a suitable plant tissue culture/regeneration regime and a compatible plant transformation methodology for biotechnological improvement of plants.

Vectors for Gene Delivery and Marker Genes

In last one decade, a number of techniques have been developed for the transfer of genes into plants.

These techniques can be divided into two broad groups:

1. Those employing a vector, such as *agrobacterium* or cauliflower mosaic virus or gemini virus.
2. Non-biological techniques- which employ physical or chemical means of transferring genes into cells/protoplasts or intact plants.

Biology of *agrobacterium*

Agrobacterium are gram negative ubiquitous soil phytopathogen that genetically transforms plant cells. In nature this transformation results in crown gall tumours (cancerous growth) or hairy roots (prolific root formation) at the infection sites in a range the consequence of transfer, integration and expression of a particular segment of DNA, the t-DNA (transfer dNA) from the tumour inducing (*ti*) or root inducing (*ri*) plasmid within the bacterium to plant cell genome. Over the last one decade, the basic principle involved in this transformation process has led to the design of modified non-oncogenic *agrobacterium* strains that can be used to transfer any DNA of interest to plant cells without interfering with their normal growth and regeneration property.

ti plasmid and t-DNA

1. All tumour forming (virulent) strains of *agrobacterium* harbour a large plasmid (140–235 kb) called *ti* or *ri* plasmid. A discrete segment (t-DNA) of this plasmid which is bordered by 25 bp conserved repeats and ranges in size from 14–24 kb (approximately 1/10th of plasmid) is transferred to the plant cell and stably integrated to plant nuclear DNA (Fig. 16.5).

2. Most of the genes that are located within t-dNA do not express in bacteria, but express only after t-dNA is inserted into the plant genome, because these genes possess typical eukaryotic promoter and polyadenylation signals. The products of t-DNA are responsible for oncogenicity (crown gall) formation. The three genes of t-DNA region *tms1 (iaam), tms2 (iaah)* and *tmr (ipt)* direct the constitutive synthesis of the phytohormones, auxin and cytokinins which are responsible for rapid proliferation of plant cells resulting into tumerous growth such as crown gall. The first two genes (*tms1* and *tms2*) encode enzymes that synthesise the plant hormone auxin (indole-3- acetic acid). Specially *tms1* codes for the enzyme tryptophan-2-mono-oxygenase which converts tryptophan to indole-3-acetamide and gene *tms 2* contains the information for indole-3-acetamide hydrolase, which converts indole-3-acetamide to indole-3-acetic acid, in addition, the third gene *tmr* encodes isopentenyl transferase enzyme, which adds 5′-amp to an isoprenoid side chain to form the cytokinin isopentenyl adenine and isopentenyl adenosine.

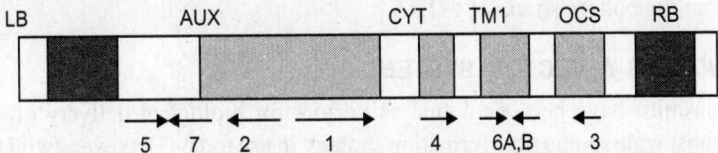

Fig. 16.5: The genetic organisation of the *t1* t-DNA of an octopine-type *ti* plasmid. only the *t1* region is shown as this ha homology with the t-DNA of nopaline-type *ti* plasmids.eight open reading frames (orfs) are indicated (1–7), although orfs 5 and 7 are not discussed in this text. Regions of import are shaded light grey and include the aux genes (which encode enzymes involced in auxin biosynthesis), cyt which encodes isopentyl transferase (an enzyme involved in cytokinin production, *tm1* which is involved in regulating tumour size and ocs (octopine synthase) which encodes opine synthesis.

T-DNA Transfer

Extensive genetic and molecular biology studies have revealed that three genetic components of *agrobacterium* are involved in t-DNA transfer.

Agrobacterium chromosomal genes: The initial step toward gene transfer by *agrobacterium* is the attachment of bacterium to plant cell at wound sites. The nature of plant cell receptors to which *agrobacterium* binds is unknown. Four different bacterial chromosomal virulence loci *chv, cel, psc a* and *att* are involved in the binding of bacteria to plant cells.

Now it is believed that the bacteria respond to certain low molecular weight phenolic compounds such as acetosyringone and hydroxyacetosyringone which are secreted by susceptible wounded plants. These wound -response compounds resemble some of the products of phenylpropanoid metabolism, which is the major plant pathway for the synthesis of plant secondary metabolites such as lignins and flavanoids. These small molecules (i.e. acetosyringone, hydroxyl acetosyringone) act to induce the activity of the virulence (*vir*) genes.

T-DNA BORDER SEQUENCES

The structure and organisation of the integrated t-DNA in tumour cells has been studied in detail. The main conclusions of these studies are listed below.

1. None of the t-DNA encoded genes are required for t-DNA transfer.
2. t-DNA does not influence the site of insertion since t-DNA inserts were found to be at random locations in the genome and present at a range of copy numbers (averaging 2–3) within individual transformed cell lines.
3. t-DNA is a discrete unit which is inserted into the plant genome without modification.
4. t-DNA regions on all *ti* or *ri* plasmids are flanked by almost 25 bp direct repeat or border sequences. These 25 bp repeat sequences particularly those on the right border to t-DNA are absolutely required for t-DNA transfer and that they function in a *cis*-acting and polar fashion. Any DNA sequence placed between these borders can be transferred into plant cell.
5. Detection of the first 6 bp or the last 10 bp of the 25 bp sequence blocks t-DNA transfer.

T-DNA Transfer Process

Two proteins encoded by the *vird* operon, *vird1* and *vird2*, act as a site specific endonuclease which produce nicks between 3 or 4 base pairs on the bottom strand of each 25 bp repeat. The *vird2* protein attaches to the 5' terminus of the nicked right border t-DNA and replicative process synthesises a single stranded DNA from the bottom strand of t-DNA.

AGROBACTERIUM AS A VECTOR SYSTEM

Agrobacterium plasmids have been exploited as vectors for biological delivery of foreign DNA to plants, this is the most wide spread transformation strategy in use today. However, (wild type *ti* plasmids) have several serious limitations as routine cloning vector.

The phytohormone biosynthetic genes encoded on t-DNA of wild-type *ti* plasmids interfere with the regeneration of transformed cells growing in culture. Therefore, the phytohormone (auxin and cytokinin) genes completely removed (disarmed plasmid) for t-DNA to regenerate complete plants from transformed plant cells. A gene encoding opine synthesis is not useful to a transgenic plant and may lower the final plant yield by diverting plant resources into opine production. Therefore, the opine synthesis gene should be removed. For recombinant DNA experiments, however, a much smaller version is preferred, so large segments of DNA that are not essential for a cloning vector must be removed. Because *ti* plasmid does not replicate in *E. coli*, the convenience of perpetuating and manipulating *ti* plasmids carrying inserted DNA sequences in this bacterium does not exist. Therefore, in developing *ti* plasmid - based vectors, an origin of replication that can be used in *E. coli* must be added.

To overcome these constraints, many non-oncogenic transformation vectors with different features have been constructed. They fall into two broad categories, the *cis* and the *trans* vectors.

cis vectors contain both the border sequences and the *vir* region on the same replicon (co-integration) whereas in *trans* vectors both the border and *vir* functions are on two replicons (binary vectors).

Co-integrate Vectors and Other Vectors for Gene Transfer to Plants

The co-integrating system involves two independent plasmids. (i) a non-oncogenic (disarmed) *ti* plasmid (in which majority of t-DNA is removed and replaced by a section of DNA homologous to small *E. coli* cloning vector) in *agrobacterium* and (ii) an intermediate vector which can't replicate in *agrobacterium*, is used for cloning and manipulation of the gene which are to be introduced in *E. coli*. Since both the plasmids have a region of homology which undergoes recombination to form a large, co-integrated plasmid after conjugation between *agrobacterium* and *E. coli*.

The main advantage of the co-integrate vectors is their high stability in *agrobacterium*. However, two disadvantages are the detailed knowledge required of the *ti* plasmid before it can be manipulated and, the relatively low rates of co-integrate formation (about 10^{-5}).

Binary Vector

The binary vectors are based on the principle that *vir* gene products can function in trans configuration. These vectors (binary vectors) contain t-DNA border repeats as well as both *E. coli* and *agrobacterium* origin of replication but no *vir* genes, it is actually an *E. coli agrobacterium* shuttle vector. All the cloning steps are carried out in *E. coli* before the vector conjugatively transferred into *agrobacterium* which contains a disarmed *ti* plasmid lacking the entire t-DNA region, but an intact *vir* region (helper *ti* plasmid, e.g. *pal4404*).

Many binary vectors have been developed which differ in size, source of 25 bp repeat sequence, plant selection marker, bacterial selection marker and cloning sites for the insertion of DNA for transfer to plants. Unlike co-integrative vectors, binary vectors need not have any homology with the resident *ti* plasmid and are capable of autonomous replication, usually in multiple copies within *agrobacterium*. This gives the binary a considerable advantage over the co-integrative system since any binary can be used in conjunction with any *vir* helper strain even with wild type oncogenic strains of *agrobacterium*.

The presence of genes encoded in the t-DNA of a binary plasmid in *agrobacterium* is confirmed easily by plasmid restriction digests, rather than by southern hybridisation or PCR, which is required to detect large co-integrated plasmids. As a result of these features, binary vectors have virtually excluded co-integrate vectors.

CAMV as Vector

One feature of CAMV which makes it attractive as a vector is that viruses spread systematically throughout the plant. In order for CAMV to be transmitted through the vascular system of plant, the DNA must be assembled within virion. The strategy for delivering foreign genes using CAMV has to replace a small section of genome, not required for virus propagation, with foreign DNA small enough not to interfere with packing of genome into the virion particle.

Direct Gene Transfer Methods

Table 16.2 in addition to the vector mediated gene transfer methods, these are certain direct gene transfer methods has been used for genetic transformation a brief account of these methods.

Table 16.2: Direct gene transfer method.

Direct gene transfer method	Comments
Particle bombardment	Very successful method. Risk of gene rearrangements and high copy number. Useful for transient expression assays
Electroporation	Transgenic plants obtained from a range of cereal crops low efficiency. Requires careful optimisation
DNA uptake into protoplasts	Used for all major cereal crops. Requires optimisation with a regenerable cell suspension that may not be available
Silicon carbide fibres	Requires regenerable cell suspensions. Transgenic plants obtained from a number of species

Promoters and terminators

An obvious requirement for any gene that is to be expressed as transgene in plants is that it is expressed correctly (or at least in a predictable fashion). It is known that the major determinant of gene expression (level, location and timing) is the region upstream of the coding region. This region, termed 'the promoter', is therefore of vital importance. Any gene, that is to be expressed in the transformed plant must has to possess an eukaryotic promoter that will function in plants. This is an important consideration as many of the genes that are to be expressed in plants, *Bt* gene, reporter genes and selectable marker genes, etc. are bacterial in origin. They, therefore, have to be cloned with a promoter that will drive their expression in plants. Transgenes also need to have suitable terminator sequences at their 3′ terminus to ensure that transcription ceases at the correct position. Failure to stop transcription can lead to the production of aberrant transcripts and can result in a range of deleterious effects, including inactivation of gene products and increased gene silencing. In additions to the basic need for the promoter to be capable of driving expression of the gene in plants, there are other considerations that need to be taken into account, such as promoter strength, tissue specificity and developmental regulations, etc.

Agrobacterium derived promoter and terminator sequences: The genes from the *ti* plasmid of *Agrobacterium* that code for opine synthesis and in particular the nopaline synthase (*nos*) gene, are widely used as a source of both promoters and terminators in plant transformation vectors. Although derived from bacterial genes, their presence on the T-DNA means they are adapted to function in plants. The *nos* promoter is usually considered to be constitutive.

The 35 S promoter

The most widely used promoter used to drive expression of genes in plant transformation vectors is the promoter of the cauliflower mosaic virus 35 S RNA gene (35 S promoter). This promoter is considered to be expressed in all tissues of transgenic plants (though not necessarily in all cell types). In dicots it drives expression at high levels, although in monocots the level of expression is not so high. This makes the 35 S promoter ideal for driving the expression of selectable marker genes and in some cases of reporter genes, as expression is more or less guaranteed. In monocots, alternatives, such as the maize *ubiquitin I* promoter or the rice actin promoter/first intron sequence, are often used to drive the high level expression of transgenes.

Tissue specific promoters

Considerable effort has been made in isolating promoters that can be used to drive expression in a tissue specific manner. The expression of any potentially harmful substances can be limited to tissues that are not consumed by animals or humans and genes involved in specific processes can be limited to tissues in which that process occurs. In certain cases the promoters have been found not to function, or not to drive expression in the predicted pattern, in heterologous systems. Therefore considerable care has been taken with the use of promoters.

Inducible promoters

Inducible expression systems can be divided into three categories: (i) non-plant-derived systems, (ii) plant derived systems, (iii) plant-derived systems based on developmental control of gene expression.

Non-plant-derived systems are independent of the normal plant processes, requiring use of inducers on agricultural scale. While the plant derived systems do not have the advantage of independence from normal plant processes. This makes their use potentially simpler as the application of an inducer is not required.

Marker genes

During the genetic transformation of plants, often the success in integration of introduced foreign gene(s) is a very-low frequency event. It will be, otherwise wastage of time, energy and resources to maintain a large number of regenerants (shoots or somatic embryos) obtained from the initial transformation efforts. Therefore it is vital that some means for selecting the transformed tissue/plantlets at initial stages should be deviced. To achieve the above target some marker genes are also cloned along with the 'gene of interest' in the cloning vectors. The marker genes are broadly of two types: (i) selectable markers and (ii) reporter genes.

Selectable markers

The selectable marker gene cloned within the vector confers resistance that is toxic to plants. The selection in such cases is based on the inclusion of a substance toxic to the plants in the culture media. The transformed cells/tissues/plants expressing the bacterial genes showing resistance to such toxic substances are survived onto such culture media, whereas other normal (wild type) non transformed cells/tissues/plants get die. Table 16.3 list certain selectable markers often used in plant genetic engineering.

Table 16.3: Selectable markers used in plant transformation.

Selectable marker gene	Abbreviation	Source of gene	Selection mechanism	Selective agent
Hygromycin phosphotransferase	hpt/aphiv/byg	E. coli	Antibiotic resistance	Hygromycin
Neomycin phosphotransferase II	nptII/neo	E. coli	Antibiotic resistance	Kanamycin Geneticin (G 418)
Neomycin phosphotransferase III	nptII	Streptococcus faecalis	Antibiotic resistance	Kanamycin Geneticin (G 418)
Glyphosphate oxidoreductase	gox	Achromobacter	LBAA resistance	Herbicide Glyphosate
Phophinothricin acetyltransferase	bar/pat	Streptomyces hygroscopicus	Herbicide resistance	Bialophos Glufosinate
Mannose-6-phosphate isomerase	bmi/man A	E. coli	Alternative carbon source	Mannose
Betaine aldehyde dehydrogenase	badh	Spinach	Detoxication	Betain aldehyde

Reporter genes

In addition to the selectable markers or as an alternative to them, reporter genes (Table 16.4) are used as markers in many plant transformation vectors. At present, only a small number of reporter genes in widespread use in plant transformation vectors the reporter genes should be, ideally, easy to assay, preferably with a non-destructive assay system and there should be little or no endogenous activity in the plant to be transformed.

MONITORING PLANT DIVERSITY THROUGH DNA

The living world is a complex combination of different levels of organisms. The key components of life are at one extreme and communities of species at the other extreme.

Table 16.4: Reporter genes used in plant transformation.

Reporter gene	Abbreviation	Source of gene	Detection/assay
β-glucuronidase	gus/uid A	E. coli	Fluorimetric (quantitative) or historical (*in situ*), non-radioactive
Green fluorescent protein	gfp	Aequorea victoria (jelly fish)	Fluorescence, non-destructive
Chloromphenicol	cat	E. coli	Radioactive assay of plant extract, sensitive, acetyltransferase semi-quantitative
Luciferase	luc	Photinus pyralis (firefly)	Luminscence
Luciferase	Lux A, Lux B	Vibrio barveyi	Luminscence

The manifestations of all types of diversities are found at all these levels of organisms. Biodiversity is the shorter form of word biological diversity which means diversity in the biological world. Thus one can define biodiversity as the degree of variety in nature with regards to biological species.

TYPES OF BIODIVERSITY

Genetic Diversity

It is the variation of genes within the species. This results distinct population of one, even same species. It gives genetic variation within a population or varieties within one species. There are two reasons for differences between individual organisms. One is variation in the gene which all organisms possess which is passed from one to its offsprings. The other is the influence of environment on each individual organism. The variation in the sequence of four base pairs in DNA chain forms the genetic variation in the organism. The recombination of genetic material during cell division makes it an imperative for genetic diversity within a species. Loss of genetic diversity within a species is called genetic erosion.

The whole area of agricultural productivity and development depend on genetic diversity. The plant as well as animal genetic resources play important role in the economy of a country. Genetic diversity is the whole basis for a sustainable life system in the earth.

Assessment of Genetic Diversity in Crop Plants

The assessment of genetic diversity within and between plant populations is routinely performed using various techniques such as: (i) morphological, (ii) biochemical characterisation/evaluation (allozyme), in the pregenomic era and (iii) DNA (or molecular) marker analysis especially single nucleotide polymorphism (SNPs) in postgenomic era.

Markers can exhibit similar modes of inheritance, as we observe for any other traits, that is, dominant/recessive or codominant. If the genetic pattern of homozygotes can be distinguished from that of heterozygotes, then a marker is said to be codominant. Generally codominant markers are more informative than the dominant markers. Morphological markers are based on visually accessible traits such as flower colour, seed shape, growth habits and pigmentation and it does not require expensive technology but large tracts of land area are often required for these field experiments, making it possibly more expensive than molecular assessment in western (developed) countries and equally expensive in Asian and Middle East (developing) countries considering the labour cost and availability. These marker traits are often susceptible to phenotypic plasticity; conversely, this allows assessment of diversity in the presence of environmental variation which cannot be neglected from the genotypic variation. These types of markers are still having advantage and they are mandatory for distinguishing the adult plants from their genetic contamination in the field, for example, spiny seeds, bristled panicle and flower/leaf colour variants. Second type of genetic marker is called biochemical markers, allelic variants of enzymes called isozymes that are detected by electrophoresis and specific staining. Isozyme markers are codominant in nature. They detect diversity at functional gene level and have simple inheritance. It requires only small amounts of plant material for its detection. However, only a limited number of enzymes markers are available and these enzymes are not alone but it has complex structural and special problems; thus, the resolution of genetic diversity is limited to explore. The third and most widely used genetic marker type is molecular markers, comprising a large variety of DNA molecular markers, which can be employed for analysis of genetic and molecular variation. These markers can detect the variation that arises from deletion, duplication, inversion and/or insertion in the chromosomes. Such markers themselves do not affect the phenotype of the traits of interest because they are located only near or linked to genes controlling the traits. These markers are inherited both in dominant and codominant patterns. Different markers have different genetic qualities (they can be dominant or codominant, can amplify anonymous or characterised loci, can contain expressed or nonexpressed sequences, etc.).

A molecular marker can be defined as a genomic locus, detected through probe or specific starter (primer) which, in virtue of its presence, distinguishes unequivocally the chromosomic trait which it represents as well as the flanking regions at the 3' and 5' extremity. Molecular markers (MM) may or may not correlate with phenotypic expression of a genomic trait. They offer numerous advantages over conventional, phenotype-based alternatives as they are stable and detectable in all tissues regardless of growth, differentiation, development, or defense status of the cell. Additionally, they are not confounded by environmental, pleiotropic and epistatic effects.

Species Diversity

Species diversity is defined as the number of species and abundance of each species that live in a particular location. The number of species that live in a certain location is called species richness. If you were to measure the species richness of a forest, you might find 20 bird species, 50 plant species and 10 mammal species. Abundance is the number of individuals of each species. This refers to the variety of species within a particular region. The number of species in a region is a measure for such diversity. The richness of species in a given region provides a yard stick for species diversity. Species diversity depends as much on the genetic diversity as on the environmental condition. Colder regions support less than the warmer regions for species diversity. The good climate with good physical geography supports a better species diversity. Species richness is a term which is used to measure the biodiversity of a given site. In addition to species richness, species endemism is a term used to measure biodiversity by way of assessing the magnitude of differences between species. In the taxonomic system similar species are grouped together in general, similar genera in families, families in orders and so on till in the level of kingdom. This process is a genuine attempt to find relationships between organisms. The higher taxa have thousands of species. Species that are very different from one another contributes more to overall biodiversity.

Importance of Species Diversity

There are numerous reasons why species diversity is essential. Each species has a role in the ecosystem. For example, bees are primary pollinators. Imagine what would happen if bees went extinct. Fruits and vegetables could be next and subsequently the animals that feed off them - this chain links all the way to humans. Various species provide us not only with food but also contribute to clean water, breathable air, fertile soils, climate stability, pollution absorption, building materials for our homes, prevention of disease outbreaks, medicinal resources and more. Species diversity contributes to ecosystem health. Each species is like a thread holding together an ecosystem. If a species disappears, an entire ecosystem can start to unravel. Species diversity is crucial for ecosystem health. For example, in the Pacific Northwest, salmon holds together the entire ecosystem. Salmon carry rich nutrients from the ocean back to the stream environment. When salmon die, those nutrients are gobbled up by insects, plants, mammals and birds. If salmon were to disappear, the impacts would be felt through the entire food chain.

Species diversity also contributes to medicine. Scientists have discovered that over 3000 plants have cancer-fighting properties. For example, a plant called rosy periwinkle has natural chemicals that help treat childhood leukemia. Also, the fruit of a tree called the Chinese star anise is an ingredient in flu vaccines. The list goes on: aspirin, codeine and pseudoephedrine all are sourced from plants. There are medicinal treasures still yet to be discovered. Perhaps hidden in some forest is the cure to cancer.

Ecological Diversity

Ecological diversity relates to the different forms of life which are present in a particular site; in a more precise sense, it concerns the different species of a particular genus which are present in an ecological community. The measures, or indices, of ecological diversity, are statistical summaries of the abundance vector, that is, the frequencies or proportions of each species in the community. As a concept, diversity relates both to the number of species (richness) and to their apportionment within the community (evenness or equitability); other things being equal, there is greater diversity when the number of species grows and when all the species are fairly represented.

In other words ecological diversity is the number of species in a community of organisms. Maintaining both types of diversity is fundamental to the functioning of ecosystems and hence to human welfare. Relationships between plant diversity and ecosystem properties can be explored by classifying component species into three categories – dominants, subordinates and transients. Dominants recur in particular vegetation types, are relatively large, exhibit coarse-grained foraging for resources and, as individual species, make a substantial contribution to the plant biomass. Subordinates also show high fidelity of association with particular vegetation types but they are smaller in stature, forage on a more restricted scale and tend to occupy microhabitats delimited by the architecture and phenology of their associated dominants. Transients comprise a heterogeneous assortment of species of low abundance and persistence; a high proportion are juveniles of species that occur as dominants or subordinates in neighbouring ecosystems.

Components of Biodiversity

Thus, while discussing biodiversity as a whole these three components are tackled together. Genetic diversity is the first step in the process where a base mutation, in a suitable locus, could lead to a new species. Continuous inbreeding often unbalances the genetic make-up of a species by promoting admixture of genes. Accumulated knowledge by population genetics indicates that each species has its own inherent gene diversity that diverges through natural selection. The species diversity and ecosystem diversity then follow. In ecosystem, even soil microbes can determine diversity within plants and animals—by their interactions with them. So, biodiversity is the total gene pool or genetic polymorphism in an area and ecosystems have the collection of all organisms within a particular area each differing in physical structure, genome composition and gene function. Along a latitudinal gradient, species diversity tends to increase toward tropical areas. Within tropical areas, species diversity increases along a longitudinal gradient. Availability of nutrients is also another main factor for species diversity. The picture is the same on land, rivers and delta. Therein sunlight, nutrients and biotic interferences determine diversity. It ultimately leads to evolution.

Land and aquatic ecosystems are highly dynamic—though they are often disturbed by biotic interferences. Coral reef though has an entirely different ecosystem, it is also subjected to outside interferences. On the other hand, deep-sea ecosystem has less outside interferences. It may be noted that a minimum amount of genetic diversity within a population is essential for a species survival. Healthy ecosystem supports high biological diversity, on the other hand, stressed, unhealthy, or highly disturbed ecosystems do not. By recent DNA techniques these can be monitored.

CONSEQUENCES OF THREATENED ECOSYSTEM

The factors which threat biodiversity would change the environment and humans would be in danger, because humans (a small segment of earth's germplasm) exploit the majority of Earth's, resources. At present, scientists, media, public and governmental agencies worldwide have begun to recognise the danger from large-scale human interferences that lead to species extinctions.

The rate of this extinction on this globe—particularly in developing and under-developed countries—is occurring on an enormous scale—at a rate that had rivalled or even surpassed those of the Cretaceous period when many species including the dinosaurs became extinct.

At present, every nation is conscious about its natural resources and is trying to catalogue local flora and fauna, especially endemic species by looking at their DNA profiles because unlike other characters DNA is less susceptible to environment and biotic factors.

However, the change at species level first comes at DNA level of an individual. That change is manifested in the phenotypic appearance and adaptability of that individual within a population. Better forms diverge quickly. Even within highly diverse ecosystems, species elements can differ widely—bringing the incompatibility barrier between two or more populations.

SUSTAINABLE USE OF PLANT DIVERSITY

At present, it is of paramount importance to note the threats to plant biodiversity and to device methodology to counteract them, because plants provide medicine, food and materials for the industries. The situation will remain unchanged, as long Homo sapiens would survive. If the species richness vanishes from this globe, the very survival of Homo sapiens would be problematical.

Moreover, maintenance of the biological diversity of marine and estuarine systems is largely overlooked, all over the world even though it is generally accepted that marine systems are far more species rich and have greater ecosystem diversity than terrestrial systems.

So, maintenance or sustainability of plant resources on land, ponds, lakes, river and oceans is essential. Sustainable use of plant biodiversity (of course entire biodiversity) is the need of today's world because bio-prospecting is the new terminology for the use of microbes, wild flora and fauna.

MONITORING DNA-DIVERSITY

The best way to measure the degree of genetic diversity and measuring genome polymorphism, within a population, species, genus, or higher-level taxon, is a resolution by molecular markers, particularly the DNA and protein marker. The advantage of a molecular marker over morphological markers is its superior quality and environment has no effect on these markers during the growth and differentiation of an organism.

DNA MARKERS

The important properties of a good marker are given below:

1. Easy recognition of all phenotypes (homo-or heterozygotes).
2. Early expression during plant development.
3. No effect on alternate alleles on plant morphology.
4. No or low interaction among markers, etc.

Unlike morphological markers, genetic (molecular) markers can fulfill these criteria because rate of evolution could be measured by looking into genetic molecules of related or unrelated taxa. Amongst the two types of molecular markers (DNA and proteins), DNA is superior over protein markers as they are least affected by the environmental fluctuations. Gene sequences are useful to develop molecular markers. Often arbitrary sequences are also used successfully to measure genetic diversity. Works of many scientists, who are currently using DNA markers in plant genetics and plant evolution, was timely from the standpoint that this is a rapidly developing technology that can be compared with the nuclear science in mid-twentieth century. Moreover, repetitive DNAs often may be highly mobile (transposon). So, often they control gene function. By doing so, repetitive DNAs provide tools to mother nature to play—to evolve different life forms. So, for an attempt to measure biological diversity, the best bet would be to look into gene-control elements sequence-diversity.

The absolute amount of single copy appears to remain meagre in large plant genome where genome replication is the rule rather than an exception. In maize, broad bean, lily and in many other plants, no more than a very small percentage of genome appears to consist of single-copy DNA sequences.

It is important to note that many kinetic measurements, with single-copy DNAs, are overestimates because the re-association kinetics was performed at criteria where extensively diverged 'fossil' repeats displayed single-copy kinetics. An additional complication is that extensive short-repeat sequence interspersion makes it difficult to find single-copy sequences much larger than several kbp (kilo basepairs) in all but small genomes, e.g. *Arabidopsis*.

At present, any genome structure can be investigated with DNA markers. Restriction fragment length polymorphism analysis is the first technique widely used to detect variation even at the gene sequence level. It is a DNA-DNA hybridisation technique where a labelled DNA probe is used to identify the level of base sequence diversity by hybridising that probe with template DNA strand. Another aspect of RFLP is the use of restriction endonucleases that could detect sequence diversity in allied genomes. A probe (marker)-enzyme combination is used to resolute the differences between individual genomes.

The application of RFLP as molecular markers has proven to be a powerful tool for studies in both basic and applied plant genetics and also to study genome evolution. The principal difficulty with RFLP is its reliance on cloning (to produce marker), Southern blotting and Southern hybridisation. For this, one must aim at the development, optimisation and validation of methodologies with special emphasis on high-throughput procedures right from the beginning (e.g. homogenisation of material and DNA extraction). Methods thus developed are to use the probes (markers) to detect the presence or absence of a gene, pedigree analysis, expression of a particular trait, etc. Therefore it is not only time-consuming but costly too.

PCR-based techniques: DNA replication protocol that is known as polymerase chain reaction (PCR). This protocol can be recognised as 'Photocopying of a DNA molecule' by repeated DNA polymerisation reactions. It could replace the requirement of cloning for multiplying DNA probes (DNA fragments, marker). In recent years, use of PCR-based markers could solve some of the limitations of earlier RFLP protocols.

Chapter 17

Detection of Nucleic Acid and Proteins

INTRODUCTION

A major portion of most biochemical investigations involves the purification of the materials under consideration because these substances must be relatively free of contaminants if they are to be properly characterised. This is often a formidable task because a typical cell contains thousands of different substances, many of which closely resemble other cellular constituents in their physical and chemical properties. Furthermore, the material of interest may be unstable and exist in vanishingly small amounts. Typically, a substance that comprises < 0.1% of a tissues dry weight must be brought to ~98% purity. Purification problems of this magnitude would be considered unreasonably difficult by most synthetic chemists. It is therefore hardly surprising that our understanding of biochemical processes has by and large paralleled our ability to purify biological materials.

This chapter presents an overview of the most commonly used techniques for the isolation, the purification and to some extent, the characterisation of proteins and nucleic acids, as well as other types of biological molecules. These methods are the basic tools of biochemistry whose operation dominates the day-to-day efforts of the practicing biochemist.

Furthermore, many of these techniques are routinely used in clinical applications. Indeed, a basic comprehension of the methods described here is necessary for an appreciation of the significance and the limitations of much of the information presented in this text. Many of the techniques used for protein and nucleic acid fractionation are similar.

In the sections that follow we consider how various characteristic properties of globular proteins in solution can be exploited to separate mixtures of proteins, based on their: (i) molecular size, (ii) solubility, (iii) electric charge, (iv) differences in adsorption characteristics and (v) biological affinity for other molecules.

SEPARATION PROCEDURES BASED ON MOLECULAR SIZE

The most striking characteristic of proteins is their large size, which makes possible simple methods for separation of proteins from small molecules, as well as methods for resolving mixtures of proteins.

Dialysis and Ultrafiltration

Globular proteins in solution can easily be separated from low-molecular-weight solutes by dialysis (Fig. 17.1), which utilises a semi-permeable membrane to retain protein molecules and allow small solute molecules and water to pass through. Another way of separating proteins from small molecules is by ultrafiltration (Fig. 17.2), in which pressure or centrifugal force is used to filter the aqueous medium and small solute molecules through a semi-permeable membrane, which retains the protein molecules. Cellophane and other synthetic materials are commonly used as the membrane in such procedures.

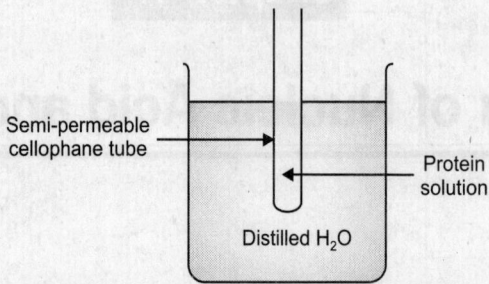

Fig. 17.1: Dialysis: Since the membrane enclosing the protein solution is semi-permeable, water and small solutes, such as glucose or ammonium sulphate, pass through the membrane freely but proteins do not. By replacing the outer aqueous phase with distilled H_2O several times, the concentration of small solute molecules in the protein solution can be decreased to a vanishingly small amount.

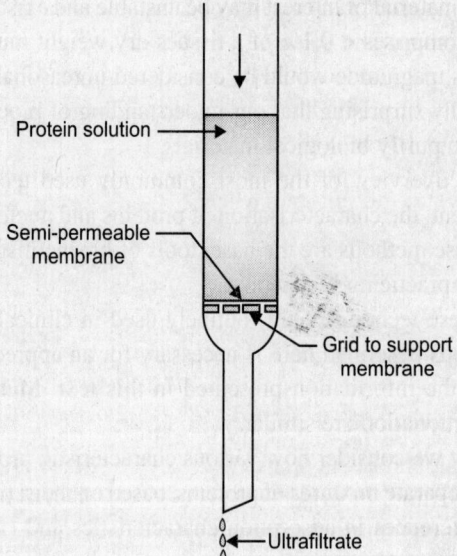

Fig. 17.2: Ultrafiltration of a protein solution. By applying positive pressure above (or a vacuum below) the membrane the protein can be concentrated by filtration of water and dissolved salts.

Density-Gradient (Zonal) Centrifugation

Because proteins in solution tend to sediment at high centrifugal fields, thus overcoming the opposing tendency of diffusion, it is possible to separate mixtures of proteins by centrifugal methods. Density-gradient or zonal centrifugation is a widely used and versatile procedure for separating not only proteins and other types of macromolecules but also organelles and viruses. In the most common procedure (Fig. 17.3) a continuous density gradient of sucrose is first prepared in a plastic centrifuge tube by a device that mixes concentrated sucrose solution and water in decreasing ratio as the tube is filled, so that the density of the medium is greatest at the bottom of the tube. The mixture of macromolecules to be resolved is layered on top of the gradient.

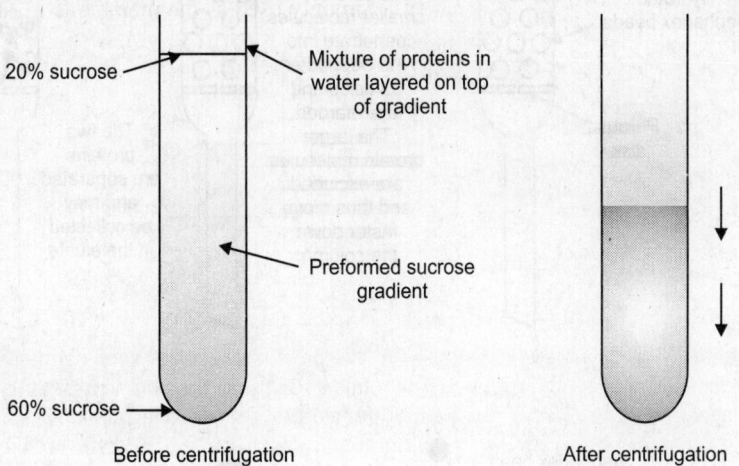

20% sucrose

Mixture of proteins in water layered on top of gradient

Preformed sucrose gradient

60% sucrose

Before centrifugation   After centrifugation

Fig. 17.3: Separation of proteins by centrifugation in a sucrose density gradient. The individual proteins band according to their size, shape and density.

Centrifugation of the tube in a horizontal position in a rotor at a high speed causes each type of macromolecule to sediment down the density gradient at its own rate, determined primarily by its particle weight but also by its density and shape, in the form of separate bands or zones. Usually centrifugation is stopped before equilibrium is reached. The positions of the protein bands can be located optically or by draining off the contents of the tube carefully through a pinhole in the bottom and analysing successive small samples. Alternatively, the plastic tube can be frozen solid and then cut into thin slices for analysis.

Molecular-Exclusion Chromatography

One of the most useful and powerful tools for separating proteins from each other on the basis of size is molecular-exclusion chromatography, also known as gel-filtration or molecular-sieve chromatography. It differs from ion-exchange chromatography, which separates solutes on the basis of their electric charge and acid-base properties. In molecular-exclusion chromatography the mixture of proteins, dissolved in a suitable buffer, is allowed to flow by gravity down a column packed with beads of an inert, highly hydrated polymeric material that has previously been washed and equilibrated with the buffer alone. Common column materials are Sephadex, the commercial name of a polysaccharide derivative, Bio-Gel, a commercial polyacrylamide derivative, and agarose, another polysaccharide—all of which can be prepared with different degrees of internal porosity. In the column proteins of different molecular size penetrate into the internal pores of the beads to different degrees and thus travel down the column at different rates (Fig. 17.4). Very large protein molecules cannot enter the pores of the beads, they are said to be excluded and thus remain in the excluded volume of the column, defined

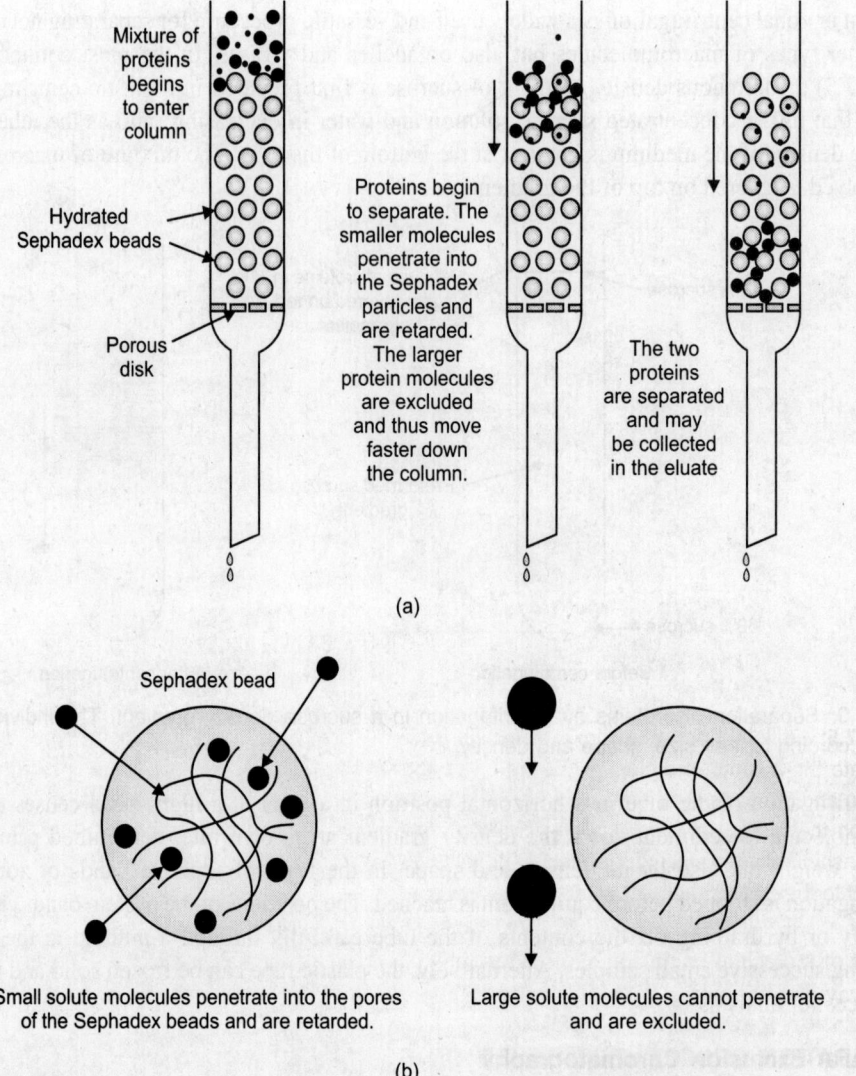

Mixture of
proteins
begins
to enter
column

Hydrated
Sephadex beads

Porous
disk

Proteins begin
to separate. The
smaller molecules
penetrate into
the Sephadex
particles and
are retarded.
The larger
protein molecules
are excluded
and thus move
faster down
the column.

The two
proteins
are separated
and may
be collected
in the eluate

(a)

Sephadex bead

Small solute molecules penetrate into the pores
of the Sephadex beads and are retarded.

Large solute molecules cannot penetrate
and are excluded.

(b)

Fig. 17.4: (a) Separation of two proteins of different size on a Sephadex column and (b) magnification showing the exclusion process.

as the volume of the aqueous phase outside the beads. On the other hand, very small proteins can enter the pores of the beads freely (Fig. 17.4).

Small proteins are retarded by the column while large proteins pass through rapidly, since they cannot enter the hydrated polymer particles. Proteins of intermediate size will be excluded from the beads to a degree that depends on their size, hence the term exclusion chromatography. From measurements of the protein concentration in small fractions of the eluate an elution curve can be constructed (Fig. 17.5). Molecular-exclusion chromatography can also be used to separate mixtures of other kinds of macromolecules, as well as very large biostructures, e.g. viruses, ribosomes, cell nuclei or even bacteria, simply by using beads or gels with different degrees of internal porosity. The resolving

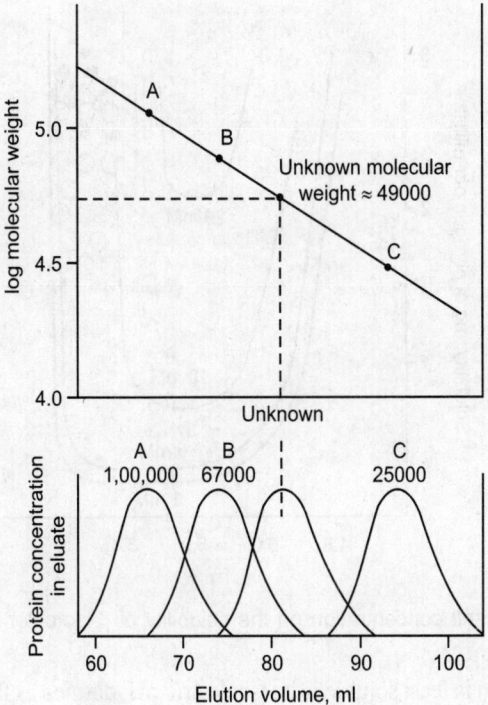

Fig. 17.5: Elution of proteins from a molecular-exclusion column and determination of molecular weight. To calibrate the column, proteins (A, B and C) of known molecular weight are allowed to pass through the column and their peak elution volumes are plotted against the logarithm of the molecular weight. From such a graph the molecular weight of an unknown protein can be extrapolated, given its elution volume. This relationship holds true only for spherical proteins. For non-spherical particles, the elution volume is directly related to the Stokes radius, i.e. the radius of a spherical particle of equivalent hydrodynamic properties.

power of molecular-exclusion chromatography is so great that this simple method is now widely used as a way of determining the molecular weight of proteins (Fig. 17.5).

SEPARATION PROCEDURES BASED ON SOLUBILITY DIFFERENCES

Proteins in solution show profound changes in solubility as a function of: (i) pH, (ii) ionic strength, (iii) the dielectric properties of the solvent and (iv) temperature. These variables—reflections of the fact that proteins are electrolytes of very large molecular weight—can be used to separate mixtures of proteins, since each protein has a characteristic amino acid composition, which determines its behaviour as an electrolyte.

Isoelectric Precipitation

The solubility of most globular proteins is profoundly influenced by the pH of the system. Figure 17.6 shows that the solubility of β-lactoglobulin, a milk protein, is at a minimum at pH 5.2 to 5.3, regardless of the concentration of sodium chloride present. On either side of this critical pH, the solubility rises very sharply. Nearly all globular proteins show a solubility minimum, although the pH at which it occurs varies from one protein to another.

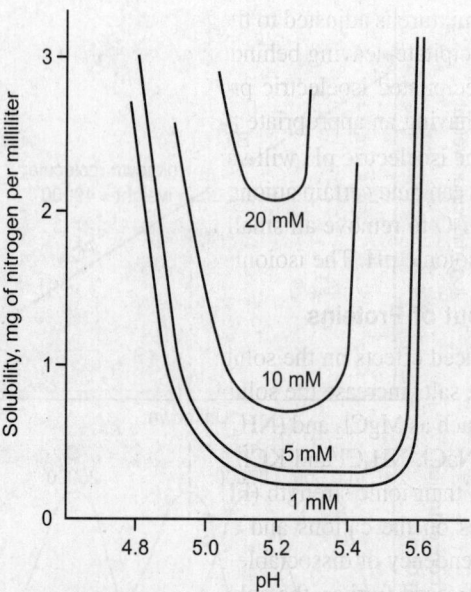

Fig. 17.6: Effect of pH and salt concentration on the solubility of β-lactoglobulin at 25°C. Figure gives the concentration of NaCl.

The pH at which a protein is least soluble is its isoelectric pH, defined as that pH at which the molecule has no net electric charge and fails to move in an electric field (Table 17.1). Under these conditions there is no electrostatic repulsion between neighbouring protein molecules and they tend to coalesce and precipitate. However, at pH values above or below the isoelectric point, all the protein molecules have a net charge of the same sign. They therefore repel each other, preventing coalescence of single molecules into insoluble aggregates. Some proteins are virtually insoluble at their isoelectric pH.

Table 17.1: Isoelectric point of some proteins.

Proteins	*Isoelectric pH*
Pepsin	~1.0
Egg albumin	4.6
Serum albumin	4.9
Urease	5.0
β-Lactoglobulin	5.2
γ₁-Globulin	6.6
Haemoglobin	6.8
Myoglobin	7.0
Ribonuclease	9.6
Chymotrypsinogen	9.5
Cytochrome *c*	10.6
Lysozyme	11.0

Since different proteins have different isoelectric pH values, because their content of amino acids with ionisable R groups differs, they can often be separated from each other by isoelectric precipitation.

When the pH of a protein mixture is adjusted to the isoelectric pH of one of its components, much or all of that component will precipitate, leaving behind in solution proteins with isoelectric pH values above or below that pH. The precipitated isoelectric protein remains in its native conformation and can be re-dissolved in a medium having an appropriate pH and salt concentration.

For any given protein the isoelectric pH will vary somewhat, depending on the ionic composition of the medium, since proteins can bind certain anions and/or cations. When a protein solution is thoroughly dialysed against distilled H_2O to remove all small ions other than H^+ and OH^-, the pH of the resulting solution is known as the isoionic pH. The isoionic pH is a constant for any given protein.

Salting-in and Salting-out of Proteins

Neutral salts have pronounced effects on the solubility of globular proteins, as shown in Figs 17.6 and 17.7. In low concentration, salts increase the solubility of many proteins, a phenomenon called salting-in. Salts of divalent ions, such as $MgCl_2$ and $(NH_4)_2SO_4$, are far more effective at salting-in than salts of monovalent ions, such as NaCl, NH_4Cl and KCl. The ability of neutral salts to influence the solubility of proteins is a function of their ionic strength (Fig. 17.7), a measure of both the concentration and the number of electric charges on the cations and anions contributed by the salt. Salting-in effects are caused by changes in the tendency of dissociable R groups on the protein to ionise. On the other hand, as the ionic strength is increased further, the solubility of a protein begins to decrease (Fig. 17.7). At sufficiently high ionic strength a protein may be almost completely precipitated from solution, an effect called salting-out. The physico-chemical basis of salting-out is rather complex, one factor is that the high concentration of salt may remove water of hydration from the protein molecules, thus reducing their solubility, but other factors are also involved. Whatever their physical basis, salting-in and salting-out are important procedures in the separation of protein mixtures, since different proteins vary in their response to the concentration of neutral salts.

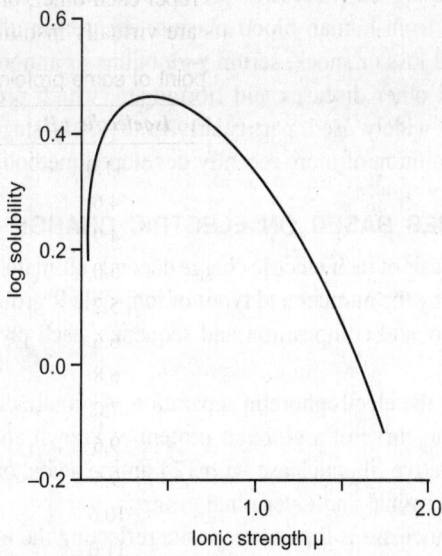

Fig. 17.7: Effect of a neutral salt (K_2SO_4) on the solubility of carbon monoxide haemoglobin at its isoelectric pH. The ionic strength of a solution μ is given by $1/2 \, Sc_i z_i^2$, in which c is the concentration and z is the charge. At low ionic strength, the protein is salted-in, i.e. increases in solubility. At high salt con-centration, it is salted-out.

Proteins precipitated by salting-out retain their native conformation and can be dissolved again, usually without denaturation. Ammonium sulphate is preferred for salting-out proteins because it is so soluble in water that very high ionic strengths can be attained.

Solvent Fractionation

The addition of water-miscible neutral organic solvents, particularly ethanol or acetone, decreases the solubility of most globular proteins in water to such an extent that they precipitate out of solution. Quantitative study of this effect shows that protein solubility at a fixed pH and ionic strength is a function of the dielectric constant of the medium. Since ethanol has a lower dielectric constant than water, its addition to an aqueous protein solution increases the attractive force between opposite charges, thus decreasing the degree of ionisation of the R groups of the protein. As a result, the protein molecules tend to aggregate and precipitate. Mixtures of proteins can be separated on the basis of quantitative differences in their solubility in cold ethanol-water or acetone-water mixtures. A disadvantage of this method is that since such solvents can denature proteins at higher temperatures, the temperature must be kept rather low.

Effect of Temperature on Solubility of Proteins

Within a limited range, from about 0 to about 40°C, most globular proteins increase in solubility with increasing temperature, although there are some exceptions, as there are for simple electrolytes. Above 40 to 50°C, most proteins become increasingly unstable and begin to denature, ordinarily with a loss of solubility at the neutral pH zone. Protein-fractionation procedures are usually carried out at 0°C or refrigerator temperatures, since most proteins are stable at low temperatures, however, there are exceptions. Some proteins are most stable and maximally soluble at room temperature or the temperature of their normal cellular surroundings. Utilising these four basic parameters of protein solubility, namely, pH, ionic strength, dielectric constant and temperature, E. J. Cohn and J. T. Edsall and their colleagues at Harvard Medical School designed successful procedures during World War II for the large-scale isolation of various proteins from human blood plasma, e.g. serum albumin, used to restore blood volume in patients with blood loss or shock, serum γ-globulins or antibodies, useful for immunisation against measles, mumps and other diseases and fibrinogen, which promotes blood clotting. These solubility parameters are still widely used, particularly in the early stages of protein purification, but they cannot give the high resolution of more recently developed methods.

SEPARATION PROCEDURES BASED ON ELECTRIC CHARGE

Separation of proteins on the basis of their electric charge depends ultimately on their acid-base properties, which are largely determined by the number and types of ionisable R groups in their polypeptide chains. Since proteins differ in amino acid composition and sequence, each protein has distinctive acid-base properties.

The principles involved in the electrophoretic separation of proteins are best understood if we first consider the acid-base titration curve of a globular protein of known amino acid content. Figure 17.8 shows the titration curve of native ribonuclease with 124 amino acids, of which 34 possess ionising R groups, in addition to the N-terminal and C-terminal groups.

The titration curve of ribonuclease is thus a composite reflecting the ionisation of many groups. The approximate contribution of each type of ionising R group can be determined (Table 17.2). These data show that the average pK' values for some types of R groups in ribonuclease may vary somewhat from the pK's of these groups in free amino acids, due to the effects of neighbouring charges.

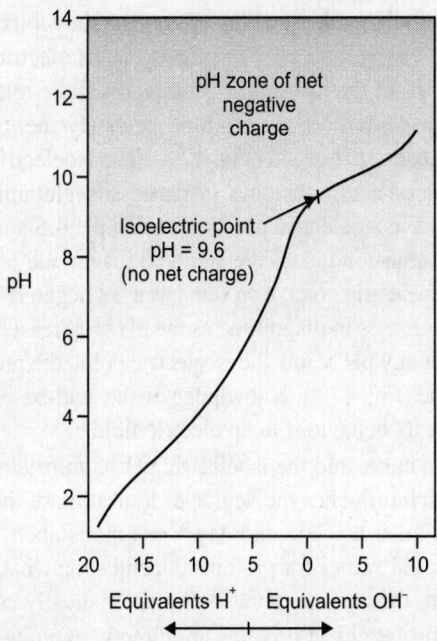

Fig. 17.8: Titration of ribonuclease: It is assumed that the titratian is begun from the isoelectric point of ribonuclease (pH 9.6) and proceeds (to the left) by addition of acid or (to the right) by addition of base. The addition of H+ brings the protein into the pH zone where it has a net positive charge; the addition of base brings it into the zone of net negative charge. The shape of the titration curve reflects the number and type of ionising groups (see Table 17.2).

Table 17.2: Titratable groups of ribonuclease*.

Group	Number per molecule From amino acid composition	From titration curve	Approximate pK′	pK′ of group in free amino acid
α-COOH	1		4.7	2.3
R—COOH (Glu, Asp)	10		4.7	4.0
Imidazole (His)	4	5	6.5	6.0
α-Amino	1	5	7.8	9.7
Phenolic OH (Tyr)	6	16	9.95	10.0
ε-Amino (Lys)	10	16	10.2	10.5
Guanidinyl (Arg)	4	4	12	12.5

*For titration curve see Fig. 17.8.

All the R groups of ribonuclease are accessible to acid-base titration, in agreement with the generalisation from X-ray studies that nearly all the ionising R groups of native globular proteins are on the outer surface of the molecule. Some native proteins, however, possess one or more ionising groups that are not accessible to titration, presumably because they are hidden or participate in hydrogen bonding. On denaturation of the native protein such as hidden R groups become accessible. For example, in myoglobin, the R groups of 5 of the 11 histidine residues are inaccessible to titration until the protein is denatured. The titration curve of ribonuclease (Fig. 17.8) also shows its isoelectric pH, at which the molecule carries no net electric charge and fails to migrate in an electric field. The isoelectric pH is determined by the number and pK' of the ionising R groups. It will be relatively high, above pH 7.0, if the protein has a relatively high content of basic amino acids (lysine, arginine), as is the case with ribonuclease, which has an isoelectric pH of 9.6 (Fig. 17.8). The isoelectric pH will be relatively low if the protein has a preponderance of acidic residues (aspartic and glutamic acids), as is the case with pepsin. Most globular proteins have isoelectric points between pH 4.5 and 17.5 (Table 17.1).

The titration curve of a protein also indicates the sign and magnitude of its net electric charge at any given pH. At any pH above the isoelectric point, a protein has a net negative charge and will move toward the anode. Its negative charge increases in magnitude as the pH is increased in accordance with the shape of the titration curve. Similarly, at any pH below the isoelectric point, the protein has a net positive charge and will move toward the cathode (Fig. 17.8). Knowledge of the acid-base properties of a given protein thus makes it possible to predict its behaviour in an electric field.

Both the shape of the titration curve and the isoelectric pH of a protein may change significantly in the presence of neutral salts, which influence the degree of ionisation of the different types of R groups. Proteins also may bind cations such as Ca^{2+} and Mg^{2+} or anions such as Cl^- or HPO_4^{2-}. For these reasons, the observed isoelectric pH values for proteins depend somewhat on the nature of the medium in which the protein is dissolved, the isoionic point is characteristically constant for each protein.

The characteristic acid-base properties of proteins are directly exploited in two widely used general methods for separating and analysing protein mixtures, electrophoresis and ion-exchange chromatography.

Electrophoretic Methods

There are a number of different forms of electrophoresis, also called ionophoresis, useful for analysing and separating mixtures of proteins. The prototype of all modern methods is free or moving boundary, electrophoresis, first developed by A. Tiselius in Sweden in the 1930s. The mobility μ in square centimeters per volt-second of a molecule in an electric field is given by the ratio of the velocity of migration v, in centimeters per second, to electric field strength E, in volts per centimeter:

$$\mu = \frac{v}{E}$$

For small ions, such as chloride, μ is between 4 and 9×10^{-4} cm^2 V^{-1} s^{-1} (25°C), for proteins, it is about 0.1 to 1.0×10^{-4} cm^2 V^{-1} s^{-1}. Proteins thus migrate much more slowly in an electric field than small ions such as Na^+ or Cl^-, simply because they have a much smaller ratio of charge to mass. In free electrophoresis a buffered solution of the protein mixture is placed in a U-shaped observation cell, with pure buffer layered over the protein solution (Fig. 17.9). The cell is immersed in a constant-temperature bath insulated from vibrations and an electric field is generated between the electrodes, negatively charged proteins move toward the anode and positively charged proteins toward the cathode. In order to get a complete picture of all the proteins in a mixture the pH is usually chosen so that most or all of the proteins will have the same charge but different mobilities. As the negatively charged protein molecules move toward the anode, they migrate from the protein solution into the zone of protein-free buffer and form a front or boundary. The refractive index of the solution changes sharply at this boundary because the index of refraction of the protein molecules is different from that of the pure buffer. Optical measurements of the refractive-index changes along the electrophoresis cell yield electrophoretic patterns (called schlieren patterns) that show the direction and relative rate of migration of the major proteins in

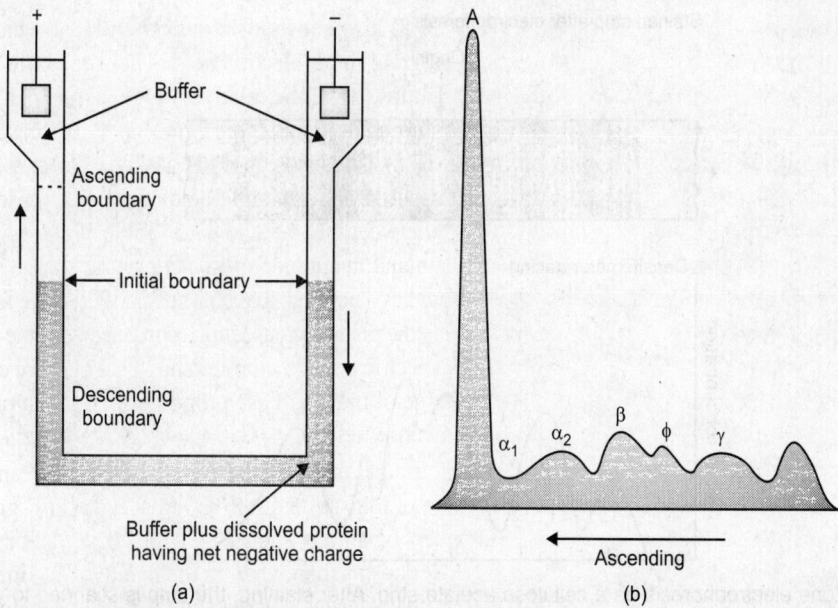

Fig. 17.9: Free electrophoresis: (a) schematic view of Tiselius moving-boundary electro-phoresis apparatus and (b) electrophoretic pattern of human blood plasma protein (pH 8.6). A = serum albumin, ϕ = fibrinogen, α_1, α_2, β and γ are various globulins.

the mixture. Figure 17.9 shows such a pattern, each peak in the pattern corresponds to the position of the moving boundary of a specific protein (it does not represent the peak of protein concentration). If the electrophoretic mobility of a given protein is determined at several different pH values, the isoelectric pH of the protein can be extrapolated. Actually, the titration curve of a protein is an approximate measure of its electrophoretic mobility as a function of pH. For many years moving-boundary electrophoresis was the most valuable method for quantitative analysis of complex mixtures of proteins, e.g. those in blood plasma. Free electrophoresis has been largely supplanted by various forms of zone electrophoresis, which are much simpler, have much greater resolving power and require smaller samples. In zone electrophoresis the aqueous protein solution is immobilised in a solid matrix or support, a hydrated porous material that has mechanical rigidity, eliminating convection and vibration disturbance. The most widely used supports are filter paper or cellulose acetate strips, relatively inert materials that do not interact with migrating proteins or retard them. The electrophoretic process is allowed to continue until the major protein components separate into discrete zones, hence the name zone electrophoresis. The position and amount of the proteins in the separated zones are determined by applying a protein stain, the density of staining, which is proportional to the amount of protein, can be estimated with a scanning densitometer (Fig. 17.10). Zone electrophoresis is capable of significantly higher resolution than free electrophoresis. This method is often used in hospital laboratories to measure the amounts of the major proteins in blood plasma. Much higher electrophoretic resolution, is possible when the support or matrix material can retard or exclude protein molecules on the basis of molecular size, like the materials used in molecular-exclusion chromatography. This form of zone electrophoresis can separate a protein mixture on the basis of both electric charge and molecular size. For this purpose, gels of potato starch or polyacrylamide are commonly used. By this technique the protein components of blood plasma

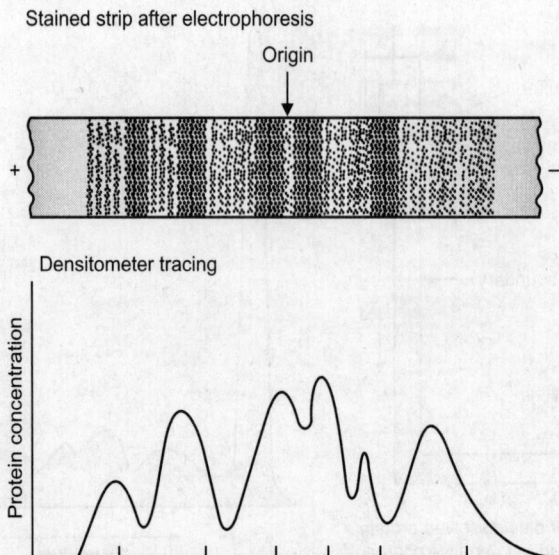

Stained strip after electrophoresis

Origin

+   –

Densitometer tracing

Protein concentration

Fig. 17.10: Zone electrophoresis on a cellulose acetate strip. After staining, the strip is scanned to yield the tracing of the protein peaks.

can be resolved into 15 or more bands, compared with about 5 or 6 observed with free or zone electrophoresis of the simple kind outlined above. Polyacrylamide gel electrophoresis can be scaled up to carry out isolation of larger quantities of purified proteins.

In yet another variation of zone electrophoresis, called disc electrophoresis, the protein mixture to be analysed is subjected to an electric field in a retarding gel support that is separated into two sections differing in porosity and buffered at different pHs. The protein mixture migrates from the more porous into the less porous gel, a process accompanied by a change in pH. As a result, each protein species becomes concentrated into a very thin, sharp band, producing much higher resolution than can be achieved in a continuous buffer. This form of zone electrophoresis is called disc (not disk) electro-phoresis because of the discontinuous buffer employed and the discoid appearance of the protein zones (Fig. 17.11).

Perhaps the most ingenious and effective electrophoretic method for separating proteins is isoelectric focusing or electrofocusing, invented by H. Svensson in Sweden, in which the mixture of proteins is subjected to an electric field in a gel support in which a pH gradient has first been generated. Each protein then migrates toward and is 'focused' at that portion of the pH gradient where the pH is equal to its isoelectric pH and forms a sharp stationary band there (Fig. 17.12). The power of isoelectric focusing is extraordinary: it can resolve the proteins of human blood plasma into 40 or more bands. Isoelectric focusing is normally used as an analytical tool but can also be used on a large scale to prepare purified proteins.

Ion-Exchange Chromatography

A second general way of utilising the acid-base behaviour of proteins as a basis for separation is ion-exchange chromatography, which also has a number of variations. The same basic principles that make the separation and analysis of amino acid or peptide mixtures on columns of ion-exchange resins feasible were first successfully applied to the separation of protein mixtures by H. Sober and E. Peterson in the United States in the 1950s. The most commonly used materials for chromatography of proteins are

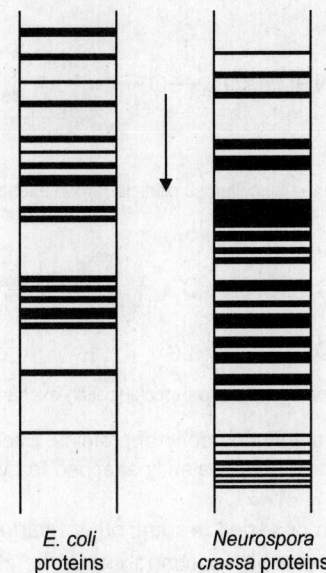

E. coli
proteins

Neurospora
crassa proteins

Fig. 17.11: Separated zones of proteins revealed by staining of the gel after disc electro-phoresis.

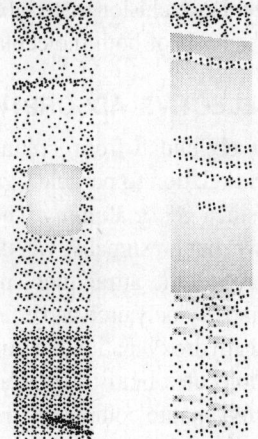

Fig. 17.12: Resolution of the isozymes (different molecular forms) of crystalline L-amino acid oxidase from rattlesnake venom by electrofocusing. Disc gel electrophoresis (left) separates the isozymes into only three bands, whereas electrofocusing (right) resolves 18 different molecular forms of the enzyme.

synthetically prepared derivatives of cellulose. Diethylaminoethylcellulose (abbreviated DEAE-cellulose) contains positively charged groups at pH 7.0 and is therefore an anion exchanger (Fig. 17.13). Carboxymethyl cellulose (abbreviated CM-cellulose) contains negatively charged groups at neutral pHs and is a cation exchanger. Protein mixtures are resolved and the individual components successively eluted from DEAE-cellulose columns by passing a series of buffers of decreasing pH or a series of salt solutions of increasing ionic strength, which have the effect of decreasing the binding of anionic proteins. The composition of the eluting solution may also be varied gradually and continuously during chromatography, this process is called gradient elution. Gradients used for this purpose may be linear

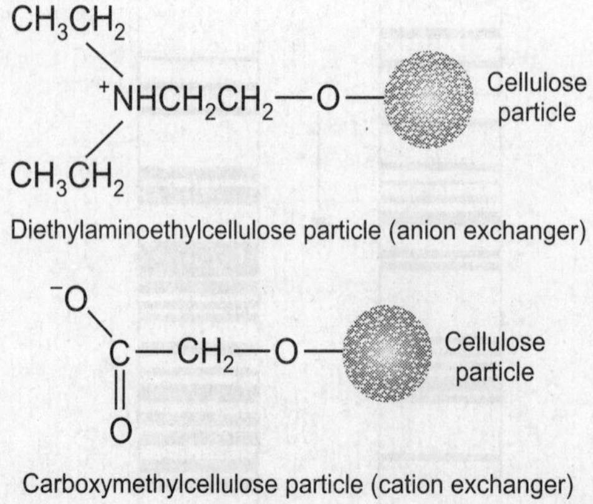

Fig. 17.13: Ion-exchange materials for chromatography of proteins. Each cellulose particle contains a large number of the ion-exchange groups, which are covalently attached to hydroxyl groups of the cellulose.

with the volume of the eluting solution or varied in some other relationship by using devices capable of mixing liquids in varying ratios. The protein concentration in the eluate, which is collected in small fractions, is estimated optically by its capacity to absorb light in the ultraviolet region. In an important variation of this method the ion-exchange and molecular-exclusion principles have been combined. The diethyl-aminoethyl derivative of the molecular-exclusion material Sephadex (DEAE-Sephadex) is widely used for resolving protein mixtures on the basis of both molecular size and electric charge.

SEPARATION OF PROTEINS BY SELECTIVE ADSORPTION

Proteins can be adsorbed to and selectively eluted from, columns of finely divided, relatively inert materials with a very large surface area in relation to particle size. They include non-polar substances, e.g. charcoal and polar substances, e.g. silica gel or alumina. The precise nature of the forces binding the protein to such adsorbents is not known, but presumably van der Waals and hydrophobic interactions prevail with non-polar adsorbents, whereas ionic attractions and/or hydrogen bonding are the main forces with polar adsorbents. Perhaps the most widely used and effective adsorbent for protein purification is a form of crystalline calcium phosphate, hydroxyapatite, the same mineral found in bone. Presumably negatively charged groups in protein molecules bind to the Ca^{2+} ions in the hydroxyapatite crystal lattice. Proteins can be eluted from hydroxyapatite columns with phosphate buffers.

SEPARATIONS BASED ON LIGAND SPECIFICITY: AFFINITY CHROMATOGRAPHY

Some proteins can be isolated from a very complex mixture and brought to a high degree of purification, often in a single step, by affinity chromotography. This method is based on a biological property of some proteins, namely, their capacity for specific, non-covalent binding of another molecule, called the ligand. For example, some enzymes bind their specific co-enzymes very thightly through non-covalent forces. In order to separate such an enzyme from other proteins by affinity chromatography, its specific co-enzyme is covalently attached, by means of an appropriate chemical reaction, to a functional group on the surface of large hydrated particles of a porous column material, e.g. the polysaccharide agarose, which otherwise allows protein molecules to pass freely (Fig. 17.14). When a mixture of proteins containing the enzyme to be isolated is added to such a column, the enzyme molecule, which is capable of binding tightly and specifically to the immobilised ligand molecule, adheres to the ligand-derivatised

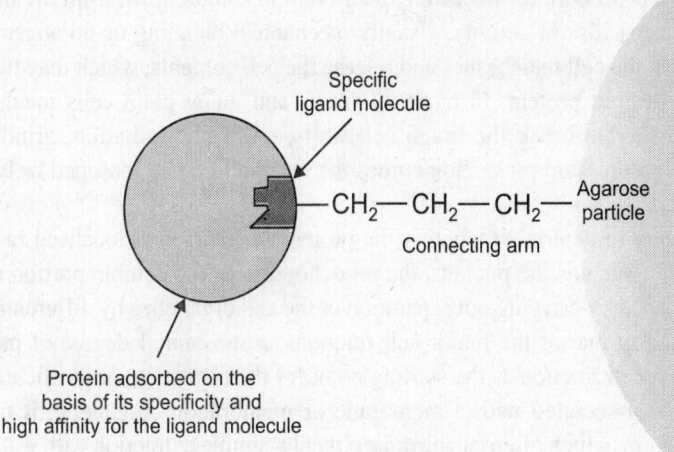

Specific
ligand molecule

$$CH_2—CH_2—CH_2—$$

Connecting arm

Agarose
particle

Protein adsorbed on the
basis of its specificity and
high affinity for the ligand molecule

Fig. 17.14: Principle of affinity chromatography.

agarose particles, whereas all the other proteins, which lack a specific binding site for that particular ligand molecule, will pass through. Similarly, one might use a substrate or a competitive inhibitor of an enzyme as the specific ligand derivatised to the column material. This method thus depends on the biological affinity of the protein for its characteristic ligand. The protein specifically bound to the column particles in this manner can then be eluted, often with a solution of the free ligand molecule.

Affinity chromatography is used to isolate not only enzymes but also the receptor molecules in cell membranes that bind specific hormones. For example, the insulin receptor protein of the plasma membrane of certain animal cells has been separated and greatly purified by affinity chromatography on a column material to which insulin molecules had been covalently attached.

EXTRACTION AND PURIFICATION OF PROTEINS

The great number of different proteins, their great variety of biological activities and the chemical difference between homologous proteins of different organisms make the extraction, purification and characterisation of proteins central to all research in biochemistry. Over a thousand different enzymes have been at least partially purified and 200 or more have been obtained in pure crystalline form. In addition, hundreds of proteins other than enzymes have been isolated with a high degree of purity.

Early methods for isolation of proteins were empirical, slow and very labourious. However, with the new methods now available, some of which were described above, protein isolation has become a fine art. There is no single procedure or set of procedures by which any and every protein can be isolated, but for any protein it is usually possible to choose a sequence of separation steps that will result in a high degree of purification and a high yield. The general objective is to increase the purity or biological activity of the desired protein per unit weight, by ridding it of inactive or unwanted proteins while at the same time maximising the yield. The first requirement is a specific and sensitive method to distinguish and measure quantitatively the particular protein to be isolated. If it is an enzyme, a quantitative assay system capable of estimating its catalytic activity is required. If the protein is a hormone, a suitable bioassay must be available. If the protein has a distinctive chemical component, e.g. a trace metal such as copper, a sensitive analytical method for that component can be utilised.

Also necessary is a procedure for liberating the protein in soluble form from the intact cell or tissue structure without causing loss of activity. Usually mechanical blending or homogenisation of animal tissues is used to break the cell membranes and release the cell contents, which may then be assayed for their content of the desired protein. In bacteria, yeasts and many plant cells much more vigourous procedures are necessary to break the tough cell walls, e.g. sonic radiation, grinding with sand or fragmentation in a high-pressure press. Sometimes the cell wall can be loosened or lysed by treatment with certain enzymes.

Next, it is customary to determine whether the protein in question is localised in one of the major sub-cellular organelles, such as the nucleus, the mitochondria or the soluble portion of the cytoplasm. This can be accomplished by carrying out separation of the cell organelles by differential centrifugation. If the protein is found in one of the major cell fractions, a substantial degree of purification can be achieved by using that cell fraction as the starting point for the next stage of purification. If the desired protein happens to be associated with a membrane or membranous organelle, it must be extracted therefrom in soluble form, which often can be done either by simple extraction with water, by mechanical or sonic disruption of the membranes or by use of detergents to disaggregate membrane structure.

Once the desired protein has been obtained in soluble form, the fractionation methods described earlier in this chapter can be applied to separate it from contaminating proteins. By direct assay it can be determined in which fraction the desired protein appears and whether it has been selectively enriched with an increase in its specific activity. Since the starting cell or tissue extract may contain hundreds of different proteins, the purification of a given protein may require many steps, in order to remove a large number of other proteins from that to be purified. Variety of procedures are used in an empirically chosen sequence.

Among the separation procedures used as early steps are isoelectric precipitation, fractionation by salting-out or solvent precipitation. At each fractionation step the enrichment factor and the yield of the desired protein are determined. These early steps, which do not have much resolving power, are usually followed by chromatographic procedures. Often molecular-exclusion chromatography and ion-exchange chromatography are used, in either sequence, to obtain fractions enriched in the desired protein on the basis of molecular size and electric charge respectively. When affinity chromatography is possible, it is a very powerful method and may be used after or instead of other forms of chromatography. Sometimes, as a last purification step, usually carried out on a small scale, the protein is subjected to one or another form of zone electrophoresis, disc electrophoresis or isoelectric focusing, to bring about high-resolution separation of the protein from the remaining impurities.

If the overall yield of the purified protein following a sequence of such purification steps has been sufficiently high, it is often possible to crystallise the protein. One procedure is very slowly to approach the salt concentration or pH required for salting-out or isoelectric precipitation, respectively. Another method is to reverse this procedure, the protein, is salted-out and diluted just enough to re-dissolve it and the solution is allowed to stand to lose water by evaporation. However, crystallisation is not necessarily a sign of complete purity, since protein crystals often contain trapped contaminants. Throughout procedures of the kind described, the pH must be carefully controlled with appropriate buffers and the temperature held at its optimal level, which for most proteins is near 0°C.

Table 17.3 shows the published procedure for the isolation of the enzyme acetylcholinesterase from the electric tissue of the electric eel, Electrophorus electricus.

Table 17.3: Purification of acetylcholinesterase by standard procedures.

Step	Specific activity $\mu mol\ min^{-1}\ mg^{-1}$	Yield, %
Fresh tissue homogenate	16.7	–
Extraction and ammonium sulphate precipitation	520	100
DEAE-cellulose	2330	52
Concentration and dialysis	2420	50
Sephadex G-200	4170	43
Cellex-P (a cation exchanger)	6830	25
DEAE-cellulose	7910	16
DEAE-Sephadex	8330	12

This enzyme, which catalyses the reaction:

$$\text{Acetylcholine} + H_2O \rightarrow \text{acetic acid} + \text{choline}$$

was quantitatively assayed by measuring the increase in acidity (decrease in pH) as the substrate acetylcholine is hydrolysed with formation of acetic acid. The specific activity of each enzyme fraction is shown in micromoles of acetylcholine hydrolysed per minute per milligram of protein. At each purification step the specific activity increases, from a specific activity of 16.7 μmol mg^{-1} in the first tissue homogenate to 8330 μmol mg^{-1} in the final product. Simultaneously, there were losses in the activity recovered after each step, at the end of the procedure only 12% of the starting activity was recovered. This is not an unusually low yield, considering the large number of steps involved.

To show the great power of affinity chromatography, Table 17.4 gives the specific activity and yield of acetylcholinesterase when affinity chromatography was used to purify the enzyme from the starting material. In only a single step this procedure yielded a product with a significantly higher specific activity than the sequence of procedures in Table 17.3 and in a much higher yield.

Table 17.4: Purification of acetylcholinesterase by affinity chromatography.

Step	Specific activity $\mu mol\ min^{-1}\ mg^{-1}$	Yield, %
Ammonium sulphate precipitate (see Table 17.3)	470	(100)
Affinity chromatography (see Fig. 17.15)	9750	70

The structure of the specific ligand attached to the column material in order to bind acetylcholinesterase molecules selectively is shown in Fig. 17.15. It is a very specific competitive inhibitor of acetylcholinesterase, which resembles the natural substrate in structure but is not cleaved by the enzyme.

CHARACTERISATION OF PROTEIN MOLECULES

After a given protein has been isolated in highly purified form, its homogeneity must be established. For this purpose free electrophoresis and sedimentation analysis in the ultracentrifuge were once common, but these expensive and relatively insensitive methods have been largely supplanted by simpler methods, e.g. molecular-exclusion chromatography, electrophoresis on polyacrylamide gels and isoelectric focusing, which have much higher resolving power and can easily detect the presence of minor protein

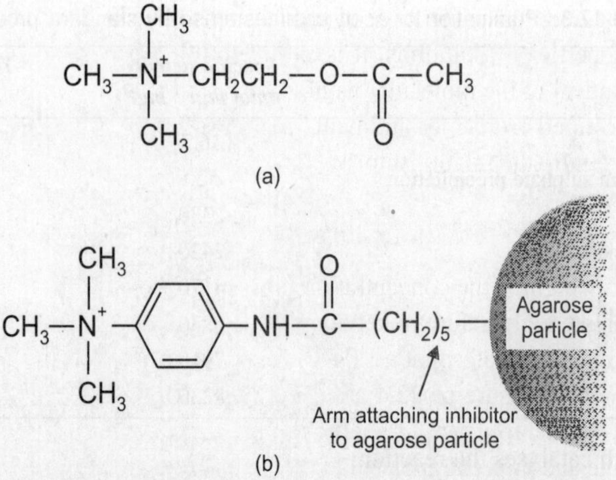

(a)

(b)

Fig. 17.15: Affinity chromatography of acetylcholinesterase: (a) structure of acetylcholine, the normal substrate and (b) inhibitor of acetylcholinesterase covalently attached to agarose particle.

impurities. Once the homogeneity of the protein is established, it can be characterised in a succession of approaches to ascertain: (i) its molecular weight, (ii) whether it contains a single or multiple polypeptide chains, (iii) the molecular weight of the polypeptide chains, (iv) their amino acid composition and (v) their amino acid sequence. We have already seen how amino acid composition and sequence can be ascertained. Here we shall consider briefly the principles of different methods commonly used to establish the molecular weight and sub-unit composition of globular proteins.

Determination of Minimum Molecular Weight from Chemical Composition

Since each molecule of a given protein must contain at least one molecule of its prosthetic group or at least one residue of any of its component amino acids, the mass of the protein in daltons containing one such residue is equal to the minimum molecular weight. For example, myoglobin contains 0.335% iron. The minimum molecular weight can be calculated as:

$$\text{Minimum molecular weight} = \frac{\text{Atomic weight of iron}}{\% \text{ iron}} \times 100$$

$$= \frac{55.8}{0.335} \times 100 = 16700$$

The true molecular weight is n times the minimum molecular weight where n is the number of iron atoms per molecule. Since $n = 1$ in myoglobin, its true molecular weight is 16700. Haemoglobin also contains iron, but it has four iron atoms per molecule. Thus, $n = 4$ and the true molecular weight is 4 times the minimum molecular weight calculated from the iron content. Such calculations are most accurate if the residue or element used as the basis for calculation has a small value for n.

Determination of the Molecular Weight from Osmotic-Pressure Measurements

When a semi-permeable membrane separates a solution of a protein from pure water, the water moves across the membrane into the compartment containing the solute, a process called osmosis. Osmosis is a reflection of the tendency of the water to move in whatever direction will make its thermodynamic activity uniform throughout all parts of the system available to it. The osmotic pressure is the force that must be applied to counterbalance the force of such osmotic flow (Fig. 17.16). Osmotic pressure is one of the colligative properties of solutions, it is a function of the number of solute particles per unit volume but is independent of the molecular nature of the solute or its shape. The molecular weight of a protein can be determined from measurements of the osmotic pressure of a solution of a known concentration of protein by the relationship:

$$M = \frac{c}{\pi} RT$$

where M is molecular weight, c the concentration in grams per liter, R the gas constant (0.082 liter-atm mol^{-1} K^{-1}), T the absolute temperature in kelvins and π the osmotic pressure in atmospheres. Expressed another way, this relationship states that a 1.0 M solution of an ideal non-dissociating solute in an ideal solvent gives an osmotic pressure of 22.4 atmosphere at 0°C. However, in practice, this relationship holds only for very dilute solutions. Usually osmotic-pressure measurements are made at several concentrations of solute and then extrapolated to zero protein concentration.

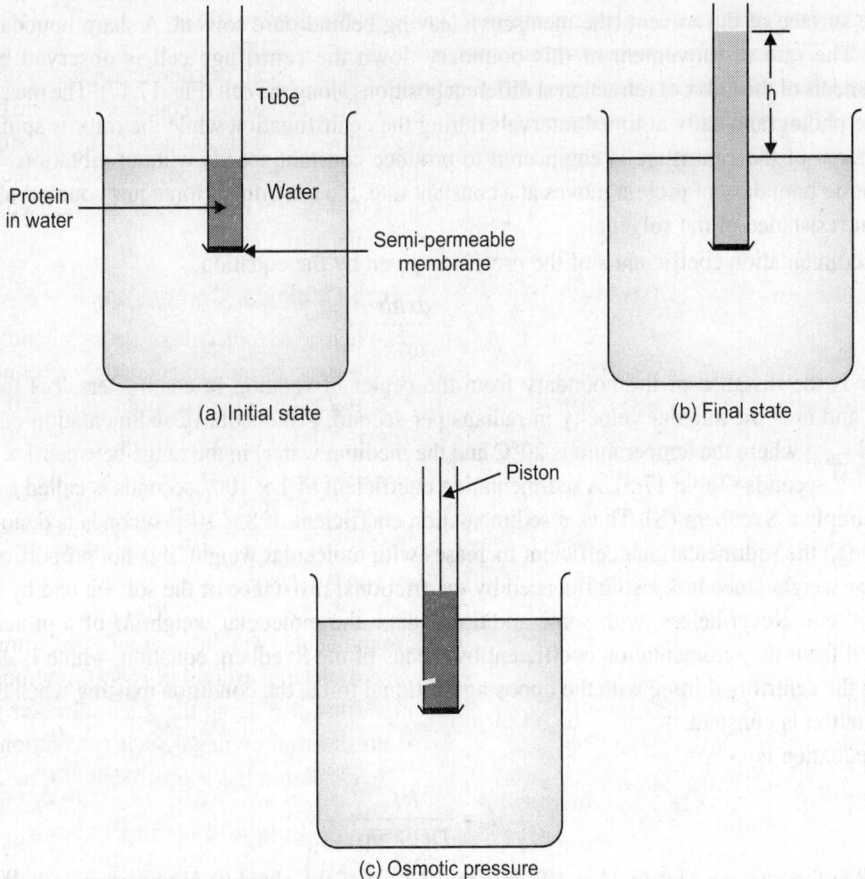

(a) Initial state (b) Final state

(c) Osmotic pressure

Fig. 17.16: Osmosis and osmotic pressure: (a) initial stage, (b) final stage in which water has moved into the protein solution. At equilibrium, the hydrostatic pressure h of the column of protein solution just counter-balances the osmotic flow of water and (c) the osmotic pressure is equal to the hydrostatic pressure of head h.

The osmotic pressure method has important theoretical advantages, e.g. it requires no knowledge of the shape of the protein. However, since the osmotic pressure depends on the number of molecules in solution, an impermeant molecule of small mass has the same effect as a molecule of large mass. The method is therefore highly susceptible to errors caused by low-molecular-weight impurities and is seldom used today.

Determination of Molecular Weight by Sedimentation Analysis

The ultracentrifuge, invented by Svedberg in 1925, can yield centrifugal fields exceeding 2,50,000 times the force of gravity. Such a high centrifugal field causes protein molecules to sediment from solution, opposing the force of diffusion, which normally keeps them evenly dispersed in solution. Three types of sedimentation measurements are used to determine the molecular weight of proteins: sedimentation velocity, sedimentation equilibrium and approach to equilibrium.

Sedimentation-velocity method

First, we shall consider the sedimentation-velocity method. If the centrifugal force exerted on protein molecules in a solution greatly exceeds the opposing diffusion force, the molecules will sediment down from the surface of the solvent (the meniscus), leaving behind pure solvent. A sharp boundary is thus formed. The rate of movement of this boundary down the centrifuge cell is observed by optical measurements of the index of refraction at different positions along the cell (Fig. 17.17). The measurements are made photographically at timed intervals during the centrifugation while the rotor is spinning. The drive system of the centrifuge is engineered to produce constant speeds without vibration. When the sedimenting boundary of protein moves at a constant rate, the centrifugal force just counterbalances the frictional resistance of the solvent.

The sedimentation coefficient s of the protein is given by the equation:

$$s = \frac{dx/dt}{\omega^2 x}$$

where, x is the distance of the boundary from the center of rotation in centimeters, t is the time in seconds and ω is the angular velocity in radians per second. Proteins have sedimentation coefficients (denoted $s_{20,w}$, where the temperature is 20°C and the medium water) in the range between 1×10^{-13} and 200×10^{-13} seconds (Table 17.5). A sedimentation coefficient of 1×10^{-13} seconds is called a Svedberg unit or simply a Svedberg (S). Thus, a sedimentation coefficient of 8×10^{-13} seconds is denoted 8S.

Although the sedimentation coefficient increases with molecular weight, it is not proportional to the molecular weight since it is also influenced by the frictional resistance of the solvent and by the shape of the protein. Nevertheless, with some additional data, the molecular weight M of a protein can be calculated from the sedimentation coefficient by means of the Svedberg equation, which is derived by equating the centrifugal force with the opposing frictional force, the condition existing when the rate of sedimentation is constant.

This equation is:

$$M = \frac{RTs}{D(1 - \overline{v}\rho)}$$

where, R is the gas constant (8.31×10^7 ergs mol^{-1} K^{-1}), T the absolute temperature in kelvins, s the sedimentation coefficient, $\overline{v}$ the partial specific volume of the protein, ρ the density of the solvent and D the diffusion coefficient.

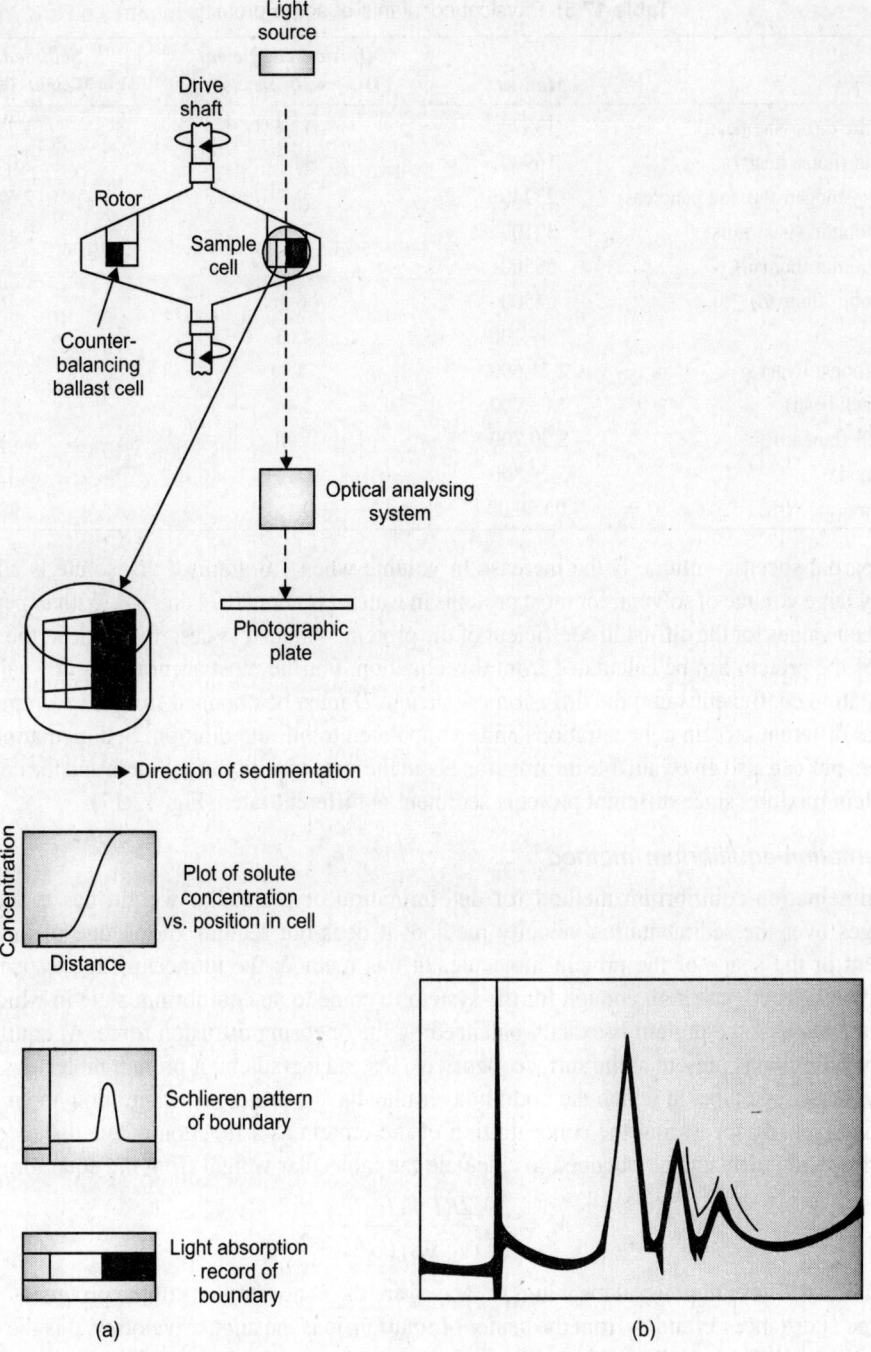

Fig. 17.17: (a) Principle of the ultracentrifuge, showing how opitcal meansurements are made while sample is undergoing sedimentation and (b) a schlieran pattern for a mixture of three sedimenting proteins, each peak indicating the position of a boundary.

Table 17.5: Physical constants of some proteins.

Protein	Mol. wt.	Diffusion coefficient $D_{20,w} \times 10^7 \, cms^2 \, s^{-1}$	Sedimentation coefficient $S_{20,w} \times 10^{13} \, s$
Cytochrome c (bovine heart)	13370	11.4	1.71
Myoglobin (horse heart)	16900	11.3	2.04
Chymotrypsinogen (bovine pancreas)	23240	9.5	2.54
β-Lactoglobulin (goat milk)	37100	7.48	2.85
Serum albumin (human)	68500	6.1	4.6
Haemoglobin (human)	64500	6.9	4.46
Aldolase	1,49,100	4.63	7.35
Catalase (horse liver)	2,21,600	4.3	11.2
Urease (jack bean)	4,82,700	3.46	18.6
Fibrinogen (human)	3,39,700	1.98	7.63
Myosin (cod)	5,24,800	1.10	6.43
Tobacco mosaic virus	4,05,90,000	0.46	198

The partial specific volume is the increase in volume when 1.0 gram of dry solute is added to an infinitely large volume of solvent, for most proteins in water it is about 0.74 cm^3 g^{-1}. With experimentally determined values for the diffusion coefficient of the protein, obtained as described below, the molecular weight of the protein can be calculated from this equation. For the most accurate results, values of the sedimentation coefficient s and the diffusion coefficient D must be obtained from measurements made at several different protein concentrations and extrapolated to infinite dilution. Sedimentation-velocity measurements can also give valuable information about the state of purity of a protein and the composition of a protein mixture, since different proteins sediment at different rates (Fig. 17.17).

Sedimentation-equilibrium method

The sedimentation-equilibrium method for determination of molecular weight has two important advantages over the sedimentation-velocity method: it does not require knowledge of the diffusion coefficient or the shape of the protein molecule. In this method, the ultracentrifuge is operated at a relatively low speed, just high enough for the system to come to an equilibrium state in which the rate of sedimentation of the protein is exactly balanced by the opposing diffusion force. At equilibrium no pure solvent region is present at the surface meniscus, instead a gradient of protein molecules is formed down the centrifuge tube, in which the bottom layer may have a protein concentration about twice that of the top layer. By measuring the concentration of the protein as a function of the distance from the center of rotation, data can be obtained to calculate the molecular weight from the equation:

$$M = \frac{2RT \ln (c_2/c_1)}{\omega^2 (1 - \overline{v}\rho) (x_2^2 - x_1^2)}$$

in which R and T have their usual meanings, c_1 and c_2 are the concentrations of the protein at two points in the tube at distances x_1 and x_2 from the center of rotation, ω is the angular velocity, ρ is the density of solvent and $\overline{v}$ is the partial specific volume of the protein. Although the sedimentation-equilibrium method is the most accurate of the sedimentation methods, it may require several days of centrifugation to attain equilibrium, a difficulty solved in part by using cells with only a very short column of protein solution (1 to 2 mm). Further, the protein must be quite pure and homogeneous.

Approach-to-equilibrium method

The approach-to-equilibrium method represents a compromise, in which some of the accuracy of the equilibrium method is sacrificed to make a more rapid measurement of molecular weight possible. In the approach-to-equilibrium method, the rotor speed is brought to approximately the equilibrium speed over a 1 to 2 h period by a series of adjustments. Each time, measurements of protein concentration are made near the bottom of the tube. From these, the molecular weight can be extrapolated.

Diffusion and the Diffusion Coefficient

The sedimentation-velocity method for determination of the molecular weight of a protein requires knowledge of its diffusion coefficient. Since diffusion has broad biological significance, a brief discussion of diffusion and the diffusion coefficient is warranted. In a solution of a protein at equilibrium the distribution of the solute is statistically uniform throughout the solution, although the protein molecules are in constant thermal motion. If a concentration gradient of the protein is formed, e.g. by carefully layering pure water over a solution of the protein in water, the protein molecules will tend to move from the region of high concentration in the lower layer to the region of low concentration in the upper layer. At equilibrium the protein molecules will be uniformly randomised throughout the system. Such a net movement of solute molecules in response to a concentration gradient is called diffusion.

The rate of diffusion is given by Fick's first law of diffusion: the amount of solute ds diffusing across the area A in a period of time dt is proportional to the concentration gradient dc/dx at that point:

$$\frac{ds}{dt} = -DA\frac{dc}{dx}$$

The proportionality constant D is the diffusion coefficient, it is defined as the quantity of solute diffusing per second across a surface area of 1.0 cm^2 when there is a concentration gradient of unity. Since diffusion is in the direction of the lower concentration, the sign of the expression is negative. The diffusion coefficient is a function of the size and shape of the molecule and the frictional resistance offered by the viscosity of the solvent. For spherical macromolecules the diffusion coefficient is inversely proportional to the cube root of the molecular weight.

The diffusion coefficient of a protein can be determined by measuring its upward-migration rate after pure solvent is layered over a protein solution of known concentration. The change with time in the concentration of the protein at a specific point in the cell (Fig. 17.18) is followed optically. The diffusion coefficient of proteins decreases with increasing molecular weight (Table 17.5). However, it will be noted that serum albumin, which has the same shape but twice the molecular weight of β-lactoglobulin, has a diffusion coefficient that is only 23% less, in agreement with the fact that the diffusion coefficient is inversely proportional to the cube root of the molecular weight.

Diffusion is opposed by the frictional resistance of the solvent, a very sensitive function of the radius of the particle. For this reason, the diffusion coefficient alone is not a useful measure of the molecular weight of a protein, but combined with sedimentation-rate measurements, it can yield quite accurate values for spherical proteins. Diffusion is a fundamental process in all cellular transport activities. The rate of diffusion and the diffusion-path length of various metabolites and enzymes are believed to set physical limits on the size and volume of the metabolising mass of living cells and their organelles.

Determining Molecular Weight by Light Scattering

When a beam of light is passed through a protein solution in a darkened room, the path of the beam can be seen because the light is scattered by the protein molecules. This is called the Tyndall effect. From

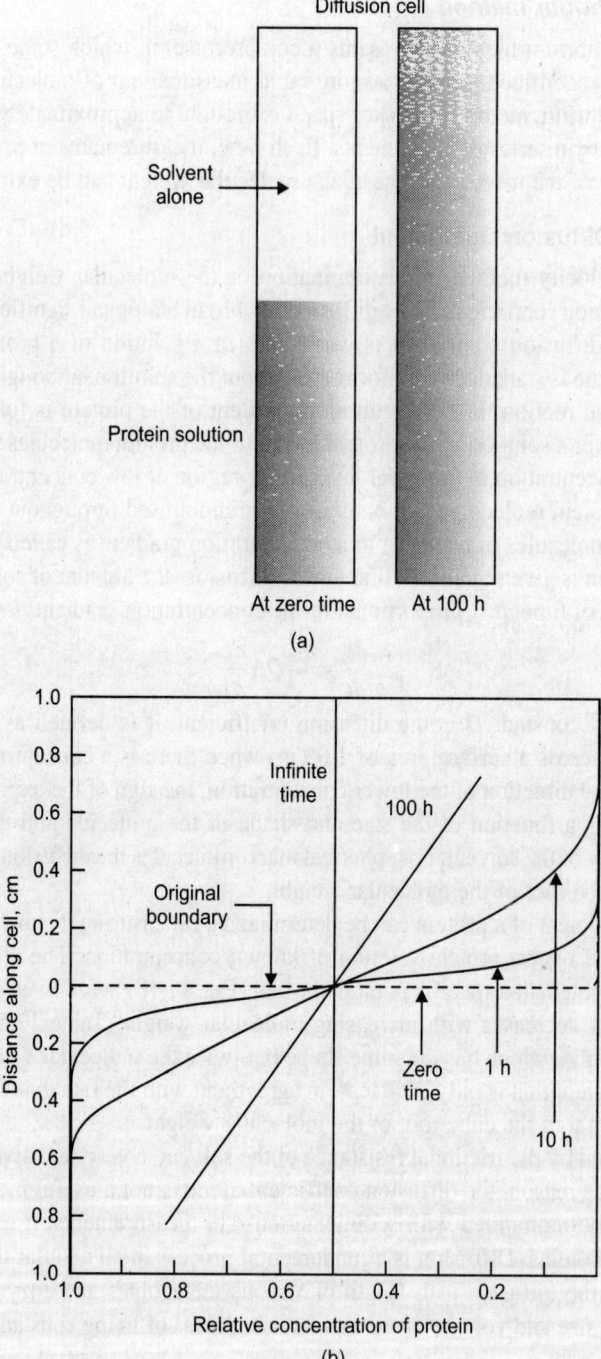

Fig. 17.18: (a) The protein distribution in the diffusion cell at zero time and at 100 h and (b) graphical representation showing the concentration of protein in the cell at different time intervals.

the wavelength of the incident radiation, the intensity of the scattered light, the refractive index of the solvent and solute and the concentration of the solute, the molecular weight of the protein can be calculated. Since the measurements can be made instantaneously and recorded with time, the method can be used to study rapid changes in molecular weight, like those occurring during dissociation or polymerisation of a protein. No other method for measuring molecular weight permits such continuous measurements, however, extraneous dust particles produce very large errors and must be removed by careful filtration.

Determining Molecular Weight by Molecular-Exclusion Chromatography

We have seen that protein mixtures can be sorted out on the basis of molecular weight by molecular-exclusion chromatography. This simple method, which requires no complex equipment, can yield surprisingly accurate determinations of the molecular weight of a protein. Molecular-exclusion columns measure not the true molecular weight of an unknown protein but its Stokes radius which is most simply defined as the radius of a perfect unhydrated sphere having the same rate of passage through the column as the unknown protein in question. If the unknown and marker proteins are spherical, the method yield the molecular weight directly.

Molecular-exclusion chromatography has another unique advantage: it can yield the Stokes radius or approximate molecular weight of a given protein even in very complex mixtures, providing the protein has a characteristic biological activity or property that can be measured. For example, although a crude cell extract may contain hundred of different enzymes, it is often possible to determine the approximate molecular weight of a single type of enzymes this extra without isolating it, simply by passing the extra through a Sephadex column and determining the position the peak of the enzyme's catalytic activity in the eluates. The presence of other proteins is irrelevant since each protein passes through the column independent of the others, at a rate determined by its Stokes radius. Molecular-exclusion columns are also extremely useful for measuring association and dissociation of protein molecules.

DETERMINING THE NUMBER AND MOLECULAR WEIGHT OF SUB-UNITS: SDS-GEL ELECTROPHORESIS

Many proteins are oligomeric and contain more than one polypeptide chain. By a variation of zone electrophoresis called SDS-gel electrophoresis, an oligomeric protein can be dissociated into its subunits and the molecular weight of the sub-units determined. The method also can be used to determine the molecular weight of single-chain proteins. The purified protein is treated with the detergent sodium dodecyl sulphate (SDS), which dissociates the protein into subunits and completely unfolds each polypeptide chain to form a long, rodlike SDS-polypeptide complex. In this complex the polypeptide chain is coated with a layer of SDS molecules in such a way that their hydrocarbon chains are in tight hydrophobic association with the polypeptide chain and the charged sulphate groups of the detergent are exposed to the aqueous medium. Such complexes contain a constant ratio of SDS to protein (about 1.4:1 by weight) and differ only in mass.

When an SDS-treated single-chain protein is subjected to electrophoresis in a molecular-sieve gel containing SDS, its rate of migration is determined primarily by the mass of the SDS-polypeptide particle, through the molecular-exclusion principle. The electric field simply supplies the driving force for the molecular sieving. To calibrate a given gel system, marker proteins of known molecular weight are run for comparison.

Many other specialised procedures are available for characterisation of protein molecules according to molecular weight, shape and conformation.

Thus, proteins can be separated from each other on the basis of differences in: (i) size, (ii) solubility properties, (iii) electric charge, (iv) adsorption behaviour and (v) the biological affinity of a protein for a specific ligand. Separation of proteins on the basis of molecular size can be carried out by different forms of density-gradient centrifugation and by molecular-exclusion chromatography. Proteins can also be separated on the basis of differential solubility, depending on the four variables of pH, ionic strength, dielectric constant of the medium and temperature. Salting-out and isoelectric precipitation are especially useful. Separation of proteins on the basis of electric charge depends on their acid-base properties, which are a reflection of the ionisable R groups of the polypeptide chain(s). Each protein possesses a characteristic isoelectric pH, at which it will not move in an electric field. Above the isoelectric pH, it has a net negative charge, below it, a net positive charge. Mixtures of proteins can be separated on the basis of their relative rates of movement in an electric field, either by free electrophoresis in aqueous solution or by zone electrophoresis in a gel or semi-solid support. Disc electrophoresis and isoelectric focusing provide especially great resolving power. Proteins can also be separated by ion-exchange chromatography.

Protein purification involves: (i) availability of a specific assay method, (ii) a method to release the protein from the cell, either in solution or associated with a sub-cellular organelle, (iii) extraction of the protein from the organelle, if needed and (iv) use of a sequence of different fractionation procedures until maximum and constant specific activity of the protein is attained and homogeneity is established by physico-chemical criteria, such as gel electrophoresis or isoelectric focusing. The molecular weight of a protein can be determined from knowledge of its chemical composition, from osmotic-pressure measurements, from measurement of sedimentation velocity or equilibrium or by means of gel-exclusion chromatography. The sub-unit polypeptide chains of proteins can be separated and their molecular weight determined by gel electrophoresis in the presence of detergents such as sodium dodecyl sulphate.

Chapter 18

Gene Function in Eukaryotes

INTRODUCTION

Gene is a part of DNA that specifies a protein/RNA. All the proteins/RNA are not required by the cell all the time. Some proteins are required at some time and yet other proteins are required at another time. Moreover these proteins are required in lesser quantities at one time, yet at other times they may be required in higher quantities. There are yet another class of proteins which are constantly (always) present in the cell, like the enzymes of the TCA cycle.

Therefore genes can be conveniently grouped under two classes:

1. Constitutive genes: Those genes whose products are constantly present in the cell are called constitutive genes or housekeeping genes.

2. Inducible genes: Those genes whose products vary with time and need, both in their presence and concentration are called inducible genes or those genes whose products (proteins/RNA) are induced by some inducer molecule. The activity of the constitutive genes is not regulated as their products don't vary much with time, whereas the activity of inducible genes is always regulated. The regulation is primarily at the level of transcription. The gene or a set of related genes are switched on or off as per the need of the cell. These changes are brought about by some proteins or modulator.

If a particular protein/compound puts a gene into operation then that protein is called stimulatory protein/compound and the process is called positive regulation. If a protein/compound stops the operation of a gene then it is called the repressor protein/compound and this process is referred to as negative regulation. The steroid hormone acts as a positive modulator, wherein its presence enhances the rate of gene expression. As soon as the hormone is destroyed the gene expression diminishes. The mechanism of regulation, though similar in the prokaryotes and eukaryotes, it differs in some aspects. Hence regulation of gene expression in prokaryotes and eukaryotes will be taken separately.

Regulation of gene expression in prokaryotes: Many prokaryotic genes are regulated in units called operons. Operon is unit of genetic expression consisting of one or more related genes and sequences (gene) controlling them, which includes the operator and promoter sequences that regulate their transcription.

The lac operon: It is the operon for utilisation and metabolism of lactose in bacteria.

It consists of the following set of genes:

PI = The promoter gene for regulatory genes.

I = The gene for regulatory protein (repressor protein).

P = The promoter sequence for the related genes.

O = Operator sequence for these genes.

Z = The first gene for utilisation of lactose, which forms the enzyme beta-galactosidase.

Y = The second gene for the membrane protein galactoside permease.

A = The third gene for the enzyme thiogalactoside transacetylase.

This complete set of sequences (i.e. the operon) helps in switching on/off, the machinery for the utilisation of the carbohydrate-lactose by the bacteria *E. coli*. When glucose is present in the media where the cell is growing, then the *lac operon* is switched off and when the medium is devoid of glucose and instead lactose is present as the sole source of carbon, then the *lac operon* becomes operational.

The transcription by RNA polymerase begins at the promoter site, i.e. the enzyme binds to the promoter and moves along the DNA towards the structural genes of the operon to transcribe the mRNA for these genes and in this process it passes through the operator region of the operon.

Under all circumstances, i.e. whether glucose or lactose is to be utilised by the cell, the I gene of the *lac operon* synthesises a protein called repressor protein. This protein binds to the operator site in the DNA and thus prevents the movement of the RNA polymerase beyond this point (site), which results in the inhibition of the synthesis of the structural genes Z, Y and A. *Lac operon* in repressed state is shown in Fig. 18.1.

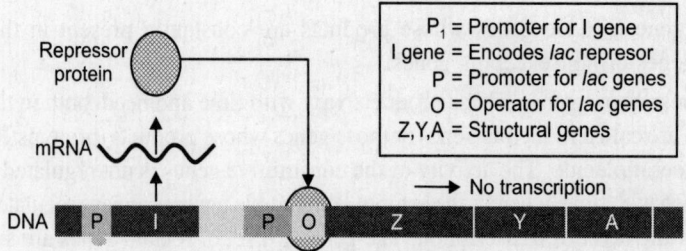

Fig. 18.1: *Lac operon* in repressed state.

The activity of the *lac operon* is not only dependent upon the binding and release of repressor molecule (with modulator) but it is also cAMP dependent. When glucose is low in the media/cell, then the cellular cAMP concentration increases. This increased amount of cAMP results in its binding at a particular site (sequences) on the promoter.

The promoter site can be divided into two parts:

1. The site for the binding of RNA polymerase.

2. The site for a protein called catabolite gene activator protein (CAP).

The RNA polymerase can bind to the promoter site only if the CAP is bound to the promoter sequence and CAP can bind to the promoter only if cAMP is bound to it and cAMP binds to CAP only when its cellular concentration increases, which occurs when the cell is devoid of glucose and hence this facilitates the utilisation of these sugars and the presence of lactose converts it to allolactose. This acts as a positive modulator for switching on the *lac operon* genes by releasing the repressor protein from the operator site and producing the products of the three structural genes which produces:

1. The membrane protein β-galactoside permease, that enhances the uptake of lactose by the cells.

2. β-galactosidase which hydrolysis lactose to allolactose and then to glucose and galactose.

3. The enzyme thiogalacatosidase-transacetylase, whose function is unknown.

When glucose is again available to the cell the cAMP concentration decreases in the cytosol, resulting in its release from the CAP, this in turn results in the release of CAP from promoter site, which in turn results in release of the enzyme RNA polymerase from the promoter site and further prevents its binding to promoter. This again results in the diminished synthesis of the structural genes, one of which is beta-galactosidase, that results in low production of allolactose (or no synthesis of allolactose), this is turn results in the repressor protein (formed from I gene) being devoid of the modulator and thus is free to bind at the operator site thereby prevent the movement of RNA polymerase and thus resulting in the inhibition of *lac operon* (Fig. 18.2). Each and every metabolite has got its own operon, with different number of structural genes and when-ever the genes for that metabolite are required it is switched on by a similar mechanism as that of the *lac operon* and switched off whenever not required.

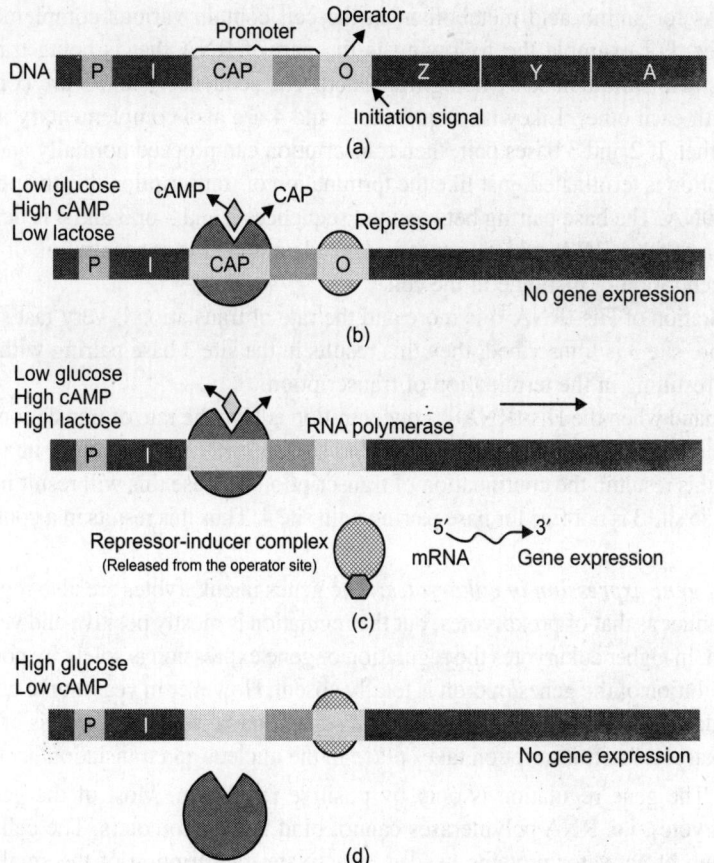

Fig. 18.2: Combined effect of glucose and lactose on expression of the *lac opertion.*

The other operons and their details are as under:

Operon for	No. of structural genes	Function
His operon	9	Enzymes required in synthesis of histidine
Leu operon	4	Conversion of alpha-keto-isovalerate to leucine
Ara operon	4	Transport and utilisation of the carbohydrate arabinose

All of the operons found in the bacteria do not function only by completely switching on or off their genes. Some operons function at differential rates depending upon the need of the cell by a mechanism called the transcription attenuation, i.e. slowing down of the rate of synthesis of enzymes and these enzymes involved in the synthesis of amino acids (His).

Attenuation: Transcription attenuation is a process in which transcription is initiated normally but is abruptly halted before the complete operon genes are transcribed. The frequency with which transcription is attenuated depends upon the cellular concentration of that particular amino acid for which the operon is meant for.

Attenuation of His operon: In bacteria, transcription and translation are closely coupled. The rate at which RNA is transcribed and the rate at which that protein is translated is almost the same. Most of the transcribed RNAs for amino acid metabolism in the cell contain various complementary intra base pairing sequences. For example the following is the part of RNA that is being transcribed for His operon, which is also simultaneously being translated. The sequence 2 and 3 are complementary and can base pair with each other. Likewise sequences 3 and 4 are also complementary and can also base pair with each other. If 2 and 3 bases pair, then transcription can proceed normally and if 3 and 4 bases pair the transcription is terminated, just like the termination of transcription due to appearance of a hair pin structure in DNA. The base pairing between the sequences 2 and 3 or 3 and 4 is dependent upon the rate of translation of the mRNA, which in turn is dependent upon the concentration of His-tRNA^{His} that reflects the concentration of histidine in the cell.

If the concentration of His-tRNA^{His} is more and the rate of translation is very fast such that it passes the 2nd site before site 3 is transcribed, then this results in the site 3 base pairing with site 4 as soon as it is transcribed resulting in the termination of transcription.

On the other hand when the His-tRNA^{His} concentration is low, the rate of translation is very slow and thus the process of translation does not pass the 2nd site on mRNA by the time site (sequences) 3rd is transcribed then this result in the continuation of transcription because this will result in the 2 and 3 sites base pairing and so site 3 is not free for base pairing with site 4. Thus this results in a continuous operation of His operon.

Regulation of gene expression in eukaryotes: The genes in eukaryotes are also regulated in more or less the same manner as that of prokaryotes, but the regulation is mostly positive and very rarely negative regulation is seen. In higher eukaryotes the regulation of gene expression is solely by positive modulation and negative inhibition of the genes/operon is totally absent. However in yeast some genes are regulated by negative modulation. Further, there is a physical separation between the process of transcription and translation is eukaryotes as transcription takes place in the nucleus and translation occurs in the cytosol.

Mechanism: The gene regulation is only by positive regulation. Most of the genes are normally inactive in eukaryotes, i.e. RNA polymerases cannot bind to the promoters. The cells synthesise only the selected group of activator proteins needed to activate transcription of the small subset of genes required in that cell.

There are at least five regulatory sites for RNA polymerase promoter sites in higher eukaryotes designated as: (i) TATA box, (ii) GC box and (iii) CAT box. In yeast there are two types of promoter sequences, i.e. TATA box and UAS, i.e. upstream activator sequence. Regulation of gene expression is shown in Fig. 18.3. These sequences are the binding sites for the transcription factors called TF-II-D that is required for RNA polymerase binding. Each of these sequences are recognised and bound specifically by one or more regulatory proteins called transcription factors. These regulatory sequences are about 1000 bases away form the main gene, thus to activate the main gene a protein-protein interaction is required which can reach the main gene sequence.

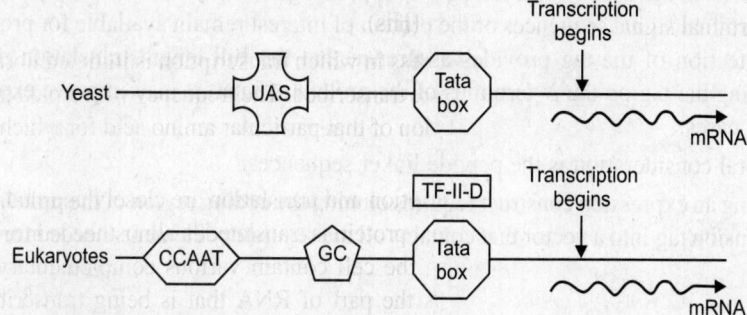

Fig. 18.3: Regulation of gene expression.

FUSION PROTEINS

Fusion proteins are used to understand protein function. They facilitate protein expression and purification, study of protein:protein and protein:nucleic acid interactions and protein labelling *in vivo* for localisation. Standard methods require use of different tags for different applications, necessitating the creation of multiple fusion constructs.

Fusion proteins or chimeric proteins (literally, made of parts from different sources) are proteins created through the joining of two or more genes that originally coded for separate proteins. Translation of this fusion gene results in a single or multiple polypeptides with functional properties derived from each of the original proteins. Recombinant fusion proteins are created artificially by recombinant DNA technology for use in biological research or therapeutics. Chimeric or chimera usually designate hybrid proteins made of polypeptides having different functions or physico-chemical patterns.

Chimeric mutant proteins occur naturally when a complex mutation, such as a chromosomal translocation, tandem duplication, or retrotransposition creates a novel coding sequence containing parts of the coding sequences from two different genes. Naturally occurring fusion proteins are commonly found in cancer cells, where they may function as on coproteins. The bcr-abl fusion protein is a well-known example of an oncogenic fusion protein and is considered to be the primary oncogenic driver of chronic myelogenous leukemia.

Some fusion proteins combine whole peptides and therefore contains all functional domains of the original proteins. However, other fusion proteins, especially those that are naturally occurring, combine only portions of coding sequences and therefore do not maintain the original functions of the parental genes that formed them.

Many whole gene fusions are fully functional and can still act to replace the original peptides. Some, however, experience interactions between the two proteins that can modify their functions. Beyond these effects, some gene fusions may cause regulatory changes that alter when and where these genes act. For partial gene fusions, the shuffling of different active sites and binding domains have potential to result in new proteins with novel functions.

Expression systems: Fusion proteins may be expressed in cell-based and cell-free systems. Downstream applications will dictate the choice and the chosen systems will determine the regulatory elements that must be present in the expression vector.

Structural considerations: The position of the tag on the fusion protein can affect protein functionality and expression level. The optimal configuration must be determined empirically.

For *in vivo* expression, there are two advantages of appending the tag on the C-terminus of the protein of interest: (i) *N*-terminal signal sequences of the protein of interest remain available for processing and (ii) subsequent detection of the tag provides assurance that the full-length translation product was produced. Appending the tag on the *N*-terminus of the protein of interest may improve expression and solubility, in some cases.

Another structural consideration is the peptide linker sequences.

Cloning: Creating an expression construct requires cloning the coding region of the protein of interest, the linker and the fusion tag into a vector that contains all the regulatory elements needed for expression.

BIOFILMS

A biofilm is any group of micro-organisms in which cells stick to each other on a surface. These adherent cells are frequently embedded within a self-produced matrix of extracellular polymeric substance (EPS). Biofilm extracellular polymeric substance, which is also referred to as slime (although not everything described as slime is a biofilm), is a polymeric conglomeration generally composed of extracellular DNA, proteins and polysaccharides. Biofilms may form on living or non-living surfaces and can be prevalent in natural, industrial and hospital settings. The microbial cells growing in a biofilm are physiologically distinct from planktonic cells of the same organism, which, by contrast, are single-cells that may float or swim in a liquid medium.

Microbes form a biofilm in response to many factors, which may include cellular recognition of specific or non-specific attachment sites on a surface, nutritional cues, or in some cases, by exposure of planktonic cells to sub-inhibitory concentrations of antibiotics. When a cell switches to the biofilm mode of growth, it undergoes a phenotypic shift in behaviour in which large suites of genes are differentially regulated. Knowing the types of organisms that can grow in a distribution system biofilm and their requirements for survival can help facility operators provide safe drinking water by anticipating biofilms and taking precautions to prevent their occurrence.

Formation of Biofilms

Biofilms are formed in distribution system pipelines when microbial cells attach to pipe surfaces and multiply to form a film or slime layer on the pipe. Probably within seconds of entering the piping system, large particles, including micro-organisms, adsorb to the clean pipe surface. Some micro-organisms can adhere directly to the pipe surface, via., appendages that extend from the cell membrane, other bacteria form a capsular material of extracellular polysaccharides (EPS), sometimes called a glycocalyx, that anchors the bacteria to the pipe surface. The organisms take advantage of the macro-molecules attached to the pipe surface for protection and nourishment. The water flowing past carries nutrients (carbon-containing molecules, as well as other elements) that are essential for the organisms' survival and growth.

Biofilms are dynamic micro environments, encompassing processes such as metabolism, growth and product formation and finally detachment, erosion, or 'sloughing' of the biofilm from the surface. The rate of biofilm formation depends on the physico-chemical (chemical, thermodynamic) properties of the interface, the physical roughness of the surface and physiological factors of the attached micro-organisms. Sheer forces generated by fluid velocity and possible effects of disinfectants on EPS may be important in the release of biofilms from surfaces. The biofilm may grow until the surface layers begin to slough off into the water. The pieces of biofilm released into the water may continue to provide protection for the organisms until they can colonise a new section of the distribution system.

The ability of bacteria to attach to surfaces in flowing, generally nutrient-deficient environments (such as drinking water) demonstrates several important ecological observations:

1. Macro-molecules tend to accumulate at solid-liquid interfaces, creating a favourable environment in an otherwise nutrient-deficient situation.

2. A high flow rate in the system can transport tremendous quantities of nutrients to fixed micro-organisms, even when the nutrient concentration in the water is low.

3. Production of EPS helps to anchor attached bacteria, EPS also may be a factor in nutrient capture.

4. Bacteria embedded in EPS matrices are protected from disinfectants by a combination of physical and transport phenomena.

These factors and others have led microbiologists to conclude that most bacteria in aquatic environments can exist at solid-liquid interfaces, as long as sufficient nutrients are available. Scanning electron photomicrographs of pipe 'coupons' (small pieces of pipe material) that have been submerged in distribution water flow provide a picture of the biofilm micro environment.

The photomicrographs reveal a hard but porous surface, a complex of crystals beneath the surface and microcolonies of similarly shaped organisms, suggesting growth, at the biofilm surface. They also show that microcolonies of cells tend to form at rough surfaces, such as cracks, crevices and pits in old and corroding pipes. Such corrosion provides an increased surface area and greater protection from the shear force of the flowing water.

Kinds of Micro-organisms that make up the Biofilm

Knowing the types of organisms likely to survive in the distribution system and their requirements for growth will aid in controlling biofilm organisms or preventing them from becoming established. *In situ* studies of biofilm communities in the pipe are difficult to perform, but analyses of samples scraped from the pipe walls and growth on pipe coupons have revealed large variations in the number and types of micro-organisms. Few organisms living in distribution system biofilms pose a threat to the average consumer. The following survey of the organisms found in biofilms shows that, although water treatment is intended to remove all pathogenic (disease-causing) bacteria, systems should be aware that treatment does not produce water free of all micro-organisms (that is, it is not sterile). In fact, some otherwise harmless organisms may survive the treatment process and cause disease in children, the elderly, or others with weakened resistance to infection. (These types of organisms are called *opporlunistic pathogens*).

Bacteria

Bacteria comprise the largest portion of the biofilm population. Heterotrophic bacteria (those requiring organic compounds as sources of carbon and energy) are often measured by the Heterotrophic Plate Count (HPC) method. These bacteria are the most common and their source normally is not known.

These organisms may survive the disinfection process to colonise the distribution system at the time of installation, or they may be introduced through cross connections, backflow events, line breaks, or repair operations. The public health risk from these organisms is not known, although a study by Smith describes a correlation between heterotrophic bacteria growing in home water filtration devices and gastrointestinal illness. Among the heterotrophic bacteria are a group of closely related micro-organisms, the total coliforms. Coliforms are usually present at high densities in water contaminated with human and/or animal feces, but may also grow in nonfecal environments such as water, soil and vegetation. Although they do not cause disease as a group, they are usually present when enteric pathogens are present. This is one reason coliforms are used as the primary microbial indicator of drinking water quality.

Fecal coliforms are a subgroup of the total coliform group. The predominant fecal coliform is *Escherichia coli,* a bacterium closely associated with the gut of warmblooded animals. Because *E. coli* usually do not survive long in the aquatic environment, their presence in drinking water indicates that fresh fecal contamination is present and consequently, that an urgent public health problem probably exists, since human pathogens usually coexist with fecal coliforms.

The types of coliform bacteria found in distribution system biofilms may vary according to location and the procedures used to analyse samples, but the predominant coliform species (spp.) generally include *Enterobacter cloacae, Klebsiella* spp., *Citrobacter freundii* and *Enterobacter agglomerans. E. coli,* most often used as an indicator of fecal contamination, has been found in distribution system biofilms, but only rarely. More often, when *E. coli* is found it is evidence of recent fecal contamination. Coliforms of both fecal and nonfecal origin may enter the drinking water distribution systems and grow in biofilms even in the presence of excess chlorine remaining after treatment (called the chlorine residual). Although biofilms may represent the greatest concentration of biological material (biomass) in the distribution system, health surveys conducted in systems experiencing biofilm growth problems have revealed no increase in illnesses due to contaminated drinking water. However, coliform bacteria that do not themselves necessarily pose a health threat can interfere with the system's ability to detect the presence of bacteria that do cause diseases (those that enter the water system because of loss of integrity of the treatment or distribution systems).

Opportunistic pathogens: An opportunistic pathogen is an organism that can cause disease in individuals with compromised immune systems, but that a healthy person's immune system can resist. Elderly people, infants, cancer patients receiving chemotherapy or mdiation, people with AIDS and burn or transplant patients in hospitals are especially susceptible to infection by opportunistic pathogens.

Antibiotic-resistant bacteria: Some bacteria have developed or acquired resistance to antibiotics as a result of previous exposure to the antibiotics (for example, in farm animals treated with drugs), heavy metals, or genetic transfer. This may create a public health problem if the resistant bacteria are also pathogens.

Disinfectant-resistant bacteria: Most bacteria survive in disinfected drinking water by finding or creating environments where they are protected from the disinfectant residual. Factors related to increased survival of bacteria in chlorinated water include attachment to surfaces, encapsulation, aggregation, lownutrient growth conditions and strain variation.

Pigmented bacteria and actinomycetes: Some heterotrophic bacteria that live in biofilms may cause esthetic problems with water quality, including offtastes, odours and coloured water problems. Biofilm organisms that fall into this nuisance category include *Actinomyces, Streptomyces*, *Nocardia* and *Arthrobacter*. Complaints about taste and odour have resulted from *Streptomyces* and *Nocardia* spp., at concentrations greater than 10 organisms per 100 mL of water. For pigmented bacteria, the degree of pigment formation observed in cultured cells will depend on the media used for isolating the bacteria in the water sample. Many HPC bacteria isolated from distribution system biofilms will produce yellow, orange, or pink colonies when grown on R_2A agar. These organisms may occur at high levels, colouring the treated water.

Fungi: Fungi, which include yeasts (single-celled spherical fungi) and molds (multibranched, filamentous fungi), can be found in finished water and can colonise and multiply in the pipe system. Fungi have been found on pipe surfaces in densities ranging from 0.0 to 5.6×10^4 cells/l00 cm^2 for yeast and 0.0 to 2.0×10^3 colony-forming units (cfu)/100 cm^2 for filamentous fungi. Yeast are more resistant to disinfection than bacteria, probably due to their thick cell walls. The primary concerns for fungi in drinking water are taste and odour complaints, although some strains may cause allergies and toxic reactions when inhaled in vapours or through contact while bathing. Drinking water, however, is not a major source of fungal infection. Food, soil and even air contain far more fungi and are probably more important factors in human infection.

Protozoa and other invertebrates: Biofilms in potable water systems may contain a variety of nonpathogenic protozoa and other invertebrates including amoebae, nematodes, amphipods, copepods and fly larvae. There is no evidence that these organisms present any health risk themselves, although recent research has shown that *Legionella* may grow and survive inside certain amoebae.

Factors that Favour Biofilm Growth

For years researchers have investigated the factors that lead to biofilm growth. Geldreich and Hutchinson and Ridgway concluded that in general, growth occurs when organic materials and sediment accumulate in distribution pipes, disinfectant residuals dissipate and water temperatures increase. Environmental factors (e.g. pH, temperature and rainfall), nutrient availability, the presence and effectiveness of disinfectant residuals, internal corrosion and sediment accumulation and hydraulic effects have been related to growth of coliform bacteria in drinking water. These results can help you develop an investigative protocol to determine whether and when your system is susceptible to biofilm growth. They also can suggest ways to manipulate the environmental variables to control bacterial growth in the system.

Environmental factors

Water temperature is perhaps the most important rate controlling factor regulating microbial growth. Directly or indirectly, temperature affects all of the factors that govern microbial growth. Temperature influences treatment plant efficiency, microbial growth rate, disinfection efficiency, dissipation of disinfectant residuals, corrosion rates and distribution system hydraulics and water velocity through customer demand (i.e. watering lawns, filling swimming pools, washing cars). Unfortunately, most water utilities can do little to change water temperature. Therefore, efforts should focus on controlling the parameters that contribute to temperature's influence. For example, if changes in temperature affect the effectiveness of disinfection residuals, the system should monitor the temperature and adjust the residual concentration accordingly.

Most investigators have observed significant microbial activity in water at temperatures of 15°C or higher. *E. coli* and other enteric bacteria (bacteria that normally live in animals' intestines) are known as mesophiles, growing in temperatures ranging from 5 to 45°C. Fransolet found that growth of *E. coli* and *fnterobacter aerogenes* was very slow (growth rates divisions per hour) at temperatures lower than 20°C.

In temperate climates, seasonal phases of coliform growth often are observed in distribution systems. Smith observed seasonal coliform occurrence trends in 81 water distribution systems, with highest coliform levels occurring during summer months. The researchers also found that the species of coliform bacteria present varied with water temperature. However, in warm climates, or in large buildings where the plumbing is kept at room temperature, seasonal variations in temperature are less pronounced and therefore seasonal variations in coliform presence will be less dramatic as well.

In a careful study by Fransolet, the investigators found that water temperature influenced not only the growth rate, but the lag time (the length of time after entering the system before cell division starts) and cell yield as well. The length of the lag time was found to be quite important to the organisms survival in the distribution system. For *Pseudomonas pufida* the lag in the growth phase was about 3 days at 7.5°C, but only 10 hr at 17.5°C. These results show that at low temperatures, cells are washed out of the distribution system before significant growth is achieved.

Rainfall is another environmental factor that influences the bacterial quality of drinking water. Some investigators have suggested that rainfall is a catalyst for coliform growth. Lowther and Moser found that raw water organic nutrient levels were highest when turbidity increased after rainfall events. LeChevallier observed that coliform bacteria routinely appeared in distribution system waters 7 days after rainfall events. The authors speculated that rainfall washed nutrients into the watershed resulting in increased bacterial densities after a transit pariod and growth lag. For some systems, however, rainfall events can lead to breakthrough of bacteria from the treatment system directly into the distribution system. The increased turbidity caused by runoff may provide bacteria with particles for attachment and protect the organisms from disinfection and the high load of bacteria and particles can overwhelm the treatment system capacity. For example, in Rochester, New York, coliform occurrences were preceded by heavy rainfalls that increased turbidity in the system's open surface water reservoirs. Several New England water systems have experienced increased coliform densities after heavy rainfall as well.

Nutrient availability

To grow, organisms must derive from the environment all the substances that they require to synthesise cell material and generate energy. For coliform and heterotrophic bacteria, the principal nutrient sources are phosphorus, nitrogen and organic carbon. Trace nutrients also are required, but these compounds have not been investigated in drinking water.

Carbon: Organic carbon is utilised by heterotrophic bacteria for production of new cellular material (assimilation) and as an energy source (dissimilation). Because heterotrophic bacteria require carbon, nitrogen and phosphorus in a ratio of approximately 100:10:1 (C:N:P), organic carbon is often a growth-limiting nutrient. Most organic carbon compounds in water supplies are natural in origin, derived from living and decaying vegetation. These compounds may include humic and fulvic acids, polymeric carbohydrates, proteins and carboxylic acids.

Carbon in drinking water is measured in three ways, as total organic carbon (TOC), which is the total amount of soluble and insoluble organic carbon compounds present in the water, dissolved organic carbon (DOC), which is the soluble fraction of TOC and assimilable organic carbon (AOC), which is the fraction of DOC that can be readily digested and used for growth by aquatic organisms.

Nitrogen and phosphorus: Nitrogen is used by micro-organisms to build amino acids and genetic material. The exact role of nitrogen in growth of coliform bacteria is unclear, especially because some strains of *Klebsiella* can fix molecular nitrogen. Nitrogen is often present in raw water supplies due to vegetation decay, runoff containing agricultural fertilisers, leachate from landfills, or wastewater discharges.

Phosphorus in the environment occurs almost exclusively as orthophosphate (PO_4^{3-}). Phosphates are sometimes added to the water supply to control corrosion. Rosenzweig found that phosphate-based corrosion inhibitors did not significantly influence the growth of several strains of coliform bacteria.

Other sources of nutrients: Certain construction materials, including rubber, silicon, polyvinyl chloride (PVC), polyethylene and bituminous coatings, have been reported to stimulate bacterial growth.

Disinfection residual concentrations

An inability to maintain a disinfectant residual may allow bacterial growth in drinking water supplies. If disinfectant levels are too low (e.g. if more than 5% of monitoring samples do not contain a detectable disinfectant residual), then the utility should increase disinfectant doses, install 'booster' stations that add disinfectant at various points in the distribution system, or use a more stable disinfectant (e.g. chloramines). The inability of the disinfectant to penetrate distribution system biofilms can account for the occurrence of coliform bacteria in highly chlorinated waters. A better understanding of the interaction of disinfectants with distribution system interfaces is necessary to formulate appropriate strategies for biofilm control.

Corrosion

Corrosion provides a protective surface for micro-organisms, slows water flow and contributes to backflow occurrences where iron pipe walls corrode. Corrosion of distribution system pipes can be due to chemical, physical, or biological action.

Sediment accumulation

Sediments and debris in pipe systems can provide habitats for microbial growth and protection from disinfection. Carryover of aluminum floc from primary treatment or improper formation of calcium carbonate scale (used in the distribution system to protect pipes against corrosion) may form uneven deposits on pipe walls, increasing the concentration of organic compounds available for assimilation and protecting bacteria from disinfection. Organic and inorganic sediments can transport micro-organisms into the distribution system and provide protection from disinfection. Carbon fines from application of powdered activated carbon and granular activated carbon filters in the treatment system can break through the treatment process and enter the distribution system.

Occurrence of Biofilm

Pathogens may occur in drinking water supplies due to breakthrough of contamination into the distribution system from the treatment facility, disruption of the integrity of the distribution system (e.g. cross connections or pipe breaks), or growth of bacteria in distribution system biofilms. It is usually difficult to distinguish with reasonable certainty between coliforms associated with biofilms and those from other sources. For example, low-level breakthrough contamination may subsequently result in growth in the distribution system. It is important, therefore, to thoroughly examine treatment practices and distribution system maintenance procedures (which can detect and control contamination events) before deciding that growth of biofilm bacteria is the cause of excess total bacteria and/or coliform levels.

This decision is no trivial matter because contamination may be intermittent or not detectable by traditional monitoring methods. The conclusion that bacteria are growing in the distribution system often is based on negative findings, i.e. an inability to find an alternative cause, such as a problem in the treatment system. However, once the available information supports the consistent reliability of the treatment procedures and integrity of the distribution system, the water system should turn its attention to locating and controlling the growth of biofilm bacteria, particularly fecal coliform bacteria.

Detection of breakthrough contamination

Characteristic of breakthrough and regrowth events is a large initial episode of coliform organism occurrence followed by a gradual decline in bacterial levels over time, possibly as long as several months. If a system experiences occurrences of coliform bacteria, the first priority is to determine whether fecal contamination has occurred. Although *E. coli* is generally harmless and may be found in distribution system biofilms not associated with pathogens, its presence may be an indication of recent fecal contamination and immediate steps should be taken to protect public health. If coliform bacteria, spikes of turbidity, or periods of low chlorine residual are detected, then treatment efficiency is suspect. Other indicators of treatment deficiency may include increases in particle counts, heterotrophic bacteria, or changes in the number of non-coliform background bacteria in the membrane filter (MF) total coliform test. Treatment plant monitoring should include not only the treatment plant effluent but also individual filter effluents. It is possible for the faulty performance of one filter in a series (or in parallel) to be masked, or averaged, by the good performance of the other filters. Particulates and micro-organisms from the faulty filter can enter the distribution system and be responsible for bacterial problems.

Breakthrough of coliform organisms in treatment plants may occur even when effluents are apparently of good microbiological quality. Incomplete disinfection may only injure bacteria, which may not be detected using standard coliform media. Observations made by McFeters and Kippen indicate that injured coliform bacteria in treatment plant effluents may be recoverable on conventional media after spending some time in the distribution system. Watters and McFeters showed that injured bacteria can repair cellular lesion and resuscitate in biofilms.

Several reports describe situations in which the detection of injured coliforms in treatment plant effluents has helped plant operators detect and correct microbiological problems.

Bacteria also may break through treatment barriers by attachment to organic or inorganic particles. Because turbidity interferes with detection of coliform bacteria by the membrane filter method, particle-associated bacteria may not be detected in plant effluent samples. The solution to solving breakthrough and subsequent growth problems is to eliminate the source of contamination. A thorough sanitary survey can help detect treatment deficiencies and distribution system problems (e.g. cross connections, breaks in pipes, backsiphonage). Application of microbiological media that will support and allow identification of injured coliforms (e.g. m-T7 agar), an intensive sampling regime, large volume analysis, or desorption of particle associated bacteria, however, may be necessary to identify sources of contamination.

Detection of biofilms

In systems with biofilm problems, the phenomenon of bacterial growth is best characterised by the persistent occurrence of coliforms in the treated drinking water.

Several factors distinguish chronic coliform growth in distribution systems:

1. No coliform organisms (or extremely low counts) are detected in treatment plant effluents even when sensitive methodologies (m-T7 agar, high-volume sample analysis) are employed.
2. High densities of coliform bacteria are routinely detected in distribution system samples.
3. The duration of the coliform episode is prolonged (several years).
4. Coliform bacteria persist in distribution system samples despite the maintenance of a disinfectant residual.

5. Proper operations and maintenance practices have been carried out, including:
   (a) Consistently maintaining positive pressure in the distribution system.
   (b) Implementing an aggressive cross connection control programme.
   (c) Thoroughly flushing pipes after repairs and new construction.

When coliform growth occurs, the increased bacterial levels typically occur as randomised patterns in different types of pipes, valves and fittings throughout the distribution system. In severe cases, the occurrence can be nearly continuous, even though coliform counts for water entering the distribution system are below 1 per 100 mL. In less severe cases, coliform occurrence may be sporadic, random throughout the system and last for short periods of time (although these short episodes may occur repeatedly over several years).

Such occurrences often are not associated with treatment disturbances. Often, no other water quality parameters (e.g. HPC and chlorine levels, water temperature) indicate any deterioration in water quality, the only deviation from normal water quality is the coliform level in the sample. Coliform occurrence due to the presence of a biofilm first may appear to be the result of laboratory contamination, especially if identification of the coliform isolates is not performed. Any utility experiencing possible biofilm problems must take extra measures to establish quality control in the bacteriological laboratory. The laboratory must record the order of analysis of the samples and the equipment used (e.g. numbering the funnels) to verify that randomness of the coliform occurrence is not due to contamination of laboratory equipment.

Characteristics of biofilm problems

Several characteristics of the bacterial population in the distribution system may point to the development of a biofilm: Seasonality, density, types and diversity of bacteria and the persistence of coliforms inspite of a disinfectant residual.

Biofilm Control Strategies

After determining that a biofilm problem exists, the system manager should not assume that all coliforms are due to the biofilm. Coliforms in the water could indicate an important treatment or distribution system deficiency and therefore a potential public health threat. If potable water samples are positive for total coliforms, particularly if the system has had no problems in the past, the possibility of a treatment breakthrough or cross connection should be investigated. The system should take precautions to ensure that public health is protected at all times through careful monitoring and follow-up testing.

When a biofilm problem occurs, drinking water systems should take immediate steps to limit the factors that favour bacterial growth. Sometimes a task force can be formed to deal with coliform occurrences. The best way to avoid coliform biofilm problems is to anticipate their occurrence. Knowing the factors that contribute to biofilm growth gives the system a head start in ensuring that biofilm growth is limited in the distribution system. The system may consider instituting a coliform biofilm control plan before positive tests for coliforms appear.

Biofilm control plan

Comprehensive maintenance programme: A maintenance programme for the distribution system is central to controlling and preventing biofilm growth. However, routine systematic flushing, a primary component of distribution system maintenance, is frequently neglected due to a need to cut costs or lack of personnel. Regular flushing helps to distribute the disinfectant residual to all portions of the system and scour existing biofilms. More aggressive cleaning, using cabledrawn or water-propelled devices (pigging), may be necessary when corrosion tuberculation is severe. Flushing and mechanically cleaning distribution system lines can be effective preventive procedures, but may not be sufficient to resolve biological growth once the problem has become severe. Increased chlorination and flushing of the New Haven distribution system actually increased coliform levels in drinking water, presumably by releasing biofilms from the pipe surface through changes in shear forces or oxidative processes.

Maintenance of reservoirs: Reservoirs used to store finished water are constructed below ground, above ground, or at ground level. All are subject to bacterial growth from a variety of factors. Above-ground tanks, usually constructed of steel with a corrosion-resistant liner, can suffer from bacterial growth on the liners. These problems may be severe within the first several months of service as organic compounds leach from the liner surface. These reservoirs should be rinsed prior to use, retention times should be limited and adequate disinfection residuals should be maintained. Frequent monitoring of the reservoirs, especially immediately after placement into service, can help detect problems before they become severe.

Corrosion control: Limiting corrosion in distribution system pipes inherently limits biofilm growth by reducing the numbers of places available for attachment by micro-organisms. Corrosion can be monitored by direct or indirect methods. Direct methods involve sampling scale from the inside of the pipes or immersing coupons in the distribution water for a period of time and determining the amount of weight loss. Electropotential devices can provide immediate readouts of water corrosivity. These instruments are useful because they can provide immediate information on changes in treatment practices. In this way, utilities can operate at a target corrosion level. The presence of iron and sulphur bacteria in the water samples also may provide an indication that corrosion is taking place. Because corrosion can be very slow, indirect monitoring methods require a data base gathered over a long time period.

Since corrosion occurs at the pipe surface and involves chemical reactions between the pipe material and the water, the primary methods for controlling corrosion serve to separate the water and pipe, or change the corrosive characteristics of either one. These methods include:

1. Modifying the water quality (e.g. changing the pH and/or reducing oxygen content) to make it less corrosive.
2. Providing a protective barrier between the water and pipe, such as corrosion-resistant linings, coatings, or paints.
3. Using corrosion inhibitors (e.g. sodium silicate or phosphate-based inhibitors) that form a molecular layer on the pipe surface, protecting it from the water.

Appropriate disinfection practices

One of the first steps that utilities usually take to control bacterial problems is to increase disinfectant residuals. The disinfectant chosen to control bacteria originating from distribution system pipe surfaces must be evaluated carefully, however. The problem requires a disinfectant capable of penetrating the biofilm and inactivating attached micro-organisms. The disinfectant also must be relatively stable to be able to persist in the distribution system. In addition, it must be potable and not produce hazardous by-products. Removal of compounds that use up the disinfectant through selection of appropriate treatment practices, pipe relining, or main replacement-or all three-can help maintain a disinfectant residual. In the end, a more stable alternative to free chlorine residual (e.g. chloramines) may be needed to help control bacterial growths. Note, however, that for first-stage disinfection of pathogenic organisms in the treatment system, chloramines are not recommended unless the utility can demonstrate adequate inactivation of Giardia and viruses. Many in the water industry have found that applying a second disinfectant such as a combined chlorine residual just before the water enters the distribution system can effectively control bacterial levels in the distribution system. Although there is no perfect disinfectant, recent research has suggested that mono-chloramine may be more effective for biofilm control than free chlorine.

Controlling nutrient levels

Controlling the levels of nutrients available for bacterial growth is the most direct means of resolving biofilm problems. Unfortunately, it is also the most difficult. To control bacterial nutrients, utilities must adopt new monitoring and treatment techniques. One way to reduce AOC levels in water is through the use of activated carbon filters. Granulated activated carbon (GAC) and powdered activated carbon (PAC) are porous particles that adsorb and hold organic contaminants.

They are commonly used to remove contaminants that cause taste and odour problems in drinking water. In the context of biofilm control, they are agents for removing dissolved organics from the source water, discouraging bacterial growth.

Mixed filters of GAC and sand can be more effective for reducing AOC levels than are filters made of sand alone (monomedia filters). This is probably because GAC has a greater surface area to support biological growth and adsorb organic substrates. Although the dual media filter was not as effective for AOC removal as systems using sand filters followed by a GAC filter, Smith concluded that mixed GAC/sand filters are an economical and practical alternative to two filters in series.

Other issues related to biofilm control

Training/upgrading personnel: The technical ability and level of understanding of the water treatment plant operator is crucial to the success of the treatment and monitoring required under the Safe Drinking Water Act (SDWA). The Surface Water Treatment Rule, for example, states that the operator must meet qualifications set by the primacy state. Most states have operator license certification programmes. Not only do system operators need to have an under-standing of the regulations and requirements under SDWA, but they must be familiar with the day-to-day operations of the plant.

Operators also should participate in continuing education programmes to learn new treatment and distribution system maintenance techniques. With experienced and knowledgeable operations staff, utilities have greater latitude in choosing treatment options, maintenance and analytical procedures and equipment.

CHROMOSOME

In the nucleus of each cell, the DNA molecule is packaged into thread-like structures called chromosomes. Each chromosome is made up of DNA tightly coiled many times around proteins called histones that support its structure.

Chromosomes are not visible in the cell's nucleus—not even under a microscope—when the cell is not dividing. However, the DNA that makes up chromosomes becomes more tightly packed during cell division and is then visible under a microscope. Most of what researchers know about chromosomes was learned by observing chromosomes during cell division.

Chromosomes vary both in number and structure among organisms (Table 18.1) and the number of chromosomes is characteristic of every species.

Table 18.1: Number of chromosomes in different organisms.

Organism	No. of chromosomes
Arabidopsis thaliana (diploid)	10
Maize (diploid)	20
Wheat (hexaploid)	42
Common fruit fly (diploid)	8
Earthworm (diploid)	36
Mouse (diploid)	40
Human (diploid)	46
Elephants (diploid)	56
Donkey (diploid)	62
Dog (diploid)	78
Gold fish (diploid)	100–104
Tobacco(tetraloid)	48
Oat (hexaploid)	42

Chromosomes are tightly coiled DNA around basic histone proteins, which help in the tight packing of DNA. During interphase, the DNA is not tightly coiled into chromosomes, but exists as chromatin. The structure of a chromosome is given in Fig. 18.4. In eukaryotes to fit the entire length of DNA in the nucleus it undergoes condensation and the degree to which DNA is condensed is expressed as its packing ratio which is the length of DNA divided by the length into which it is packaged into chromatin along with proteins. The shortest human chromosome contains 4.6×10^7 bp of DNA. This is equivalent to 14000 μm of extended DNA. In its most condensed state during mitosis, the chromosome is about 2 μm long. This gives a packing ratio of 7000 (14000/2). The DNA is packaged stepwise into the higher order chromatin structure and this is known as 'hierarchies of chromosomal organisation'.

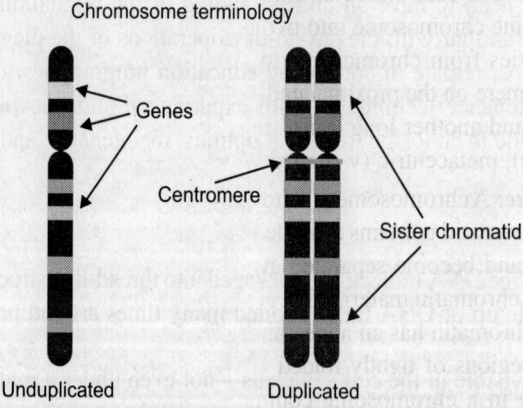

Chromosome terminology

Genes

Centromere

Sister chromatid

Unduplicated

Duplicated

Fig. 18.4: Eukaryotic chromosome.

Chromosome Number

There are normally two copies of each chromosome present in every somatic cell. The number of unique chromosomes (N) in such a cell is known as its haploid number and the total number of chromosomes

(2N) is its diploid number. The suffix 'ploid' refers to chromosome 'sets'. The haploid set of the chromosome is also known as the genome. Structurally, eukaryotes possess large linear chromosomes unlike prokaryotes which have circular chromosomes. In eukaryotes other than the nucleus chromosomes are present in mitochondria and chloroplast too.

The number of chromosomes in each somatic cell is same for all members of a given species. The organism with lowest number of chromosome is the nematode, *Ascaris megalocephalusunivalens* which has only two chromosomes in the somatic cells (2n = 2).

Autosomes and Sex Chromosomes

In a diploid cell, there are two of each kind of chromosome (termed homologus chromosomes) except the sex chromosomes. In humans one of the sex has two of the same kind of sex chromosomes and the other has one of each kind. In humans there are 23 pairs of homologous chromosomes (2n = 46). The human female has 44 non sex chromosomes, termed autosomes and one pair of homomorphic sex chromosomes given the designation XX. The human male has 44 autosomes and one pair of heteromorphic sex chromosomes, one X and one Y chromosome.

Morphology

Size: The size of chromosome is normally measured at mitotic metaphase and may be as short as 0.25 μm in fungi and birds to as long as 30 μm in some plants such as Trillium. However, most mitotic chromosome falls in the range of 3 μm in *Drosophila* to 5μm in man and 8–12 μm in maize. The monocots contain large sized chromosomes as compared to dicots. Organisms with less number of chromosomes contain comparatively large sized chromosomes. The chromosomes in set vary in size.

Shape: The shape of the chromosome changes from phase to phase in the continuous process of cell growth and cell division. During the resting/interphase stage of the cell, the chromosomes occur in the form of thin, coiled, elastic and contractile, thread like stainable structures, the chromatin threads. In the metaphase and the anaphase, the chromosome becomes thick and filamentous. Each chromosome contains a clear zone, known as centromere or kinetochore, along their length.

The centromere divides the chromosome into two parts and each part is called chromosome arm. The position of centromere varies from chromosome to chromosome providing it a different shape. They could be telocentric (centromere on the proximal end of the chromosome), acrocentric (centromere at one end giving it a very short and another long arm), submetacentric (J or L shaped chromosome with the centromere near the centre), metacentric (v shaped with centromere at the centre).

Structure of chromosome: A chromosome at mitotic metaphase consists of two symmetrical structures called chromatids. Each chromatid contains a single DNA molecule and both chromatids are attached to each other by centromere and become separated at the beginning of anaphase. The chromomeres are bead like accumulations of chromatin material that are sometimes visible along interphase chromosomes. The chromomere bearing chromatin has an appearance of a necklace in which several beads occur on a string. Chromomeres are regions of tightly folded DNA and become especially prominent in polytene chromosomes. Centromere in a chromosome contain specific DNA sequences with special proteins bound to them, forming a disc shaped structure, called kinetochore. In electron microscope the kinetochore appears as a plate or cup like disc, 0.20–0.25 nm, in diameter situated upon the primary constriction or centromere. The chromosomes of most organisms contain only one centromere and are known as monocentric chromosomes. Some species have diffused centromeres, with microtubules attached along the length of the chromosomes and are termed holocentric chromosomes.

Chromosomes of *Ascaris megalocephala* are examples of diffused centromeric chromosomes. Telomere is the chromosomal ends which prevents other chromosomal segments to be fused with it. Besides the primary constrictions or centromeres, chromosomes also posses secondary constriction at any point of the chromosome and are constant in their position and extent. These constrictions are helpful in identifying particular chromosomes in a set. Chromosomes also contain nucleolar organisers which are certain secondary constrictions that contain the genes coding for 5.8S, 18S and 28S ribosomal RNA and induce the formation of nucleoli. Sometimes the chromosomes bear round, elongated or knob like appendages known as satellites. The satellite remains connected with the rest of the chromosomes by a thin chromatin filament.

CHROMATIN

Chemical Composition of Chromatin

Chromatin consists of DNA, RNA and protein. The protein of chromatin could be of two types: histones and non histones.

DNA: DNA is the most important chemical component of chromatin, since it plays central role of controlling heredity and is most conveniently measured in picograms. In addition to describing the genome of an organism by its number of chromosomes, it is also described by the amount of DNA in a haploid cell. This is usually expressed as the amount of DNA per haploid cell (usually expressed as picograms) or the number of kilobases per haploid cell and is called the C-value. This is constant for all cells of a species. For diploid cells it is 2C. Extending the C-value we reach the C-value paradox. One immediate feature of eukaryotic organisms highlights a specific anomaly that was detected early in molecular research. Even though eukaryotic organisms appear to have 2–10 times as many genes as prokaryotes, they have many orders of magnitude more DNA in the cell. Furthermore, the amount of DNA per genome is correlated not with the presumed evolutionary complexity of a species. This is stated as the C-value paradox: the amount of DNA in the haploid cell of an organism is not related to its evolutionary complexity. Lower eukaryotes in general have less DNA, such as nematode *Caenorhabditis elegans* which has 20 times more DNA than *E. coli*. Vertebrates have greaer DNA content about 3pg, in general about 700 times more than *E. coli*. Salamander *Amphiuma* has a very high DNA content of about 84pg. Man has about 3pg of DNA per haploid genome.

Histones: Histones are basic proteins as they are enriched with basic proteins arginine and lysine. At physiological pH they are cationic and can interact with anionic nucleic acids. They form a highly condensed structure. The histones are of five types called H1, H2A H2B, H3 and H4-which are very similar among different species of eukaryotes and have been highly conserved during evolution. H1 is the least conserved among all and is also loosely bound with DNA. H1 histone is absent in *Sacharomyces cerevisiae*.

Non-histones: In addition to histones the chromatin comprise of many different types of non-histone proteins, which are involved in a range of activities, including DNA replication and gene expression. They display more diversity or are not conserved. They may also differ between different tissues of same organism.

Euchromatin: The lightly-stained regions in chromosome when stained with basic dyes are called euchromatin and contain single-copy of genetically-active DNA. The extent of chromatin condensation varies during the life cycle of the cell and plays an important role in regulating gene expression. In the interphase of cell cycle the chromatin are decondensed and known as euchromatin leading to gene transcription and DNA replication.

Heterochromatin: The word heterochromatin was coined by Emil Heitz based on cytological observations. They are highly condensed and ordered areas in nucleosomal arrays. About 10% of interphase chromatin is called heterochromatin and is in a very highly condensed state that resembles the chromatin of cells undergoing mitosis. They contain a high density of repetitive DNA found at centromeres and telomeres form heterochromatin. Heterochromatin are of two types, the constitutive and facultative heterochromatin. The regions that remain condensed throughout the cell cycle are called constitutive heterochromatin whereas the regions where heterochromatin condensation state can change are known as facultative. Constitutive heterochromatin is found in the region that flanks the telomeres and centromere of each chromosome and in the distal arm of the Y chromosome in mammals.

Constitutive heterochromatin possesses very few genes and they also lead to transcriptional inactivation of nearby genes. This phenomenon of gene silencing is known as 'position effect'. Constitutive hetero-chromatin also inhibits genetic recombination between homologous repetitive sequences circumventing DNA duplications and deletion. Whereas facultative heterochromatin is chromatin that has been specifically inactivated during certain phases of an organism's life or in certain types of differentiated cells. Dosage compensation of X-chromosome or X-chromosome inactivation in mammals is an example of such heterochromatin. Hetero-chromatin spreads from a specific nucleation site, causing silencing of most of the X-chromosome, thereby regulating gene dosage.

Centromeres: Centromeres are those condensed regions within the chromosome that are responsible for the accurate segregation of the replicated chromosome during mitosis and meiosis. When chromosomes are stained they typically show a dark-stained region that is the centromere. The actual location where the attachments of spindle fibres occur is called the kinetochore and is composed of both DNA and protein. The DNA sequence within these regions is called CEN DNA. Because CEN DNA can be moved from one chromosome to another and still provide the chromosome with the ability to segregate, these sequences must not provide any other function. Typically CEN DNA is about 120 base pairs long and consists of several sub-domains, CDE-I, CDE-II and CDE-III (Fig. 18.5). Mutations in the first two sub-domains have no effect upon segregation, but a point mutation in the CDE-III sub-domain completely eliminates the ability of the centromere to function during chromosome segregation. Therefore CDE-III must be actively involved in the binding of the spindle fibres to the centromere. The protein component of the kinetochore is only now being characterised. A complex of three proteins called Cbf-III binds to normal CDE-III regions but cannot bind to a CDE-III region with a point mutation that prevents mitotic segregation. Furthermore, mutants of the genes encoding the Cbf-III proteins also eliminates the ability for chromosomes to segregate during mitosis. Additional analyses of the DNA and protein components of the centromere are necessary to fully understand the mechanics of chromosome segregation.

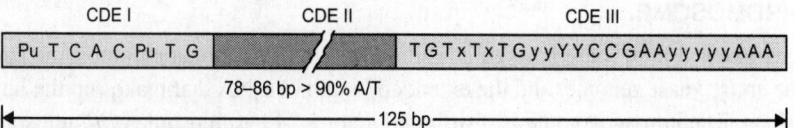

Fig. 18.5: The *S. cerevisiae* centrosome. The *S. cerevisae* centromere (CEN) sequences consist of two short conserved sequences (CDE I and CDE III) separated by 78 to 86 base pairs (bp) of ATrich DNA (CDE II). The sequences shown are consensus sequences derived from analysis of the centromere sequences of individual yeast chromosomes. Pu = A or G, x =A or T, y = any base.

Telomeres: Telomeres are the region of DNA at the end of the linear eukaryotic chromosome that are required for the replication and stability of the chromosome. McClintock recognised their special features when she noticed, that if two chromosomes were broken in a cell, the ends were sticky and end of one could attach to the other and vice versa. However she never observed the attachment of the broken end to the end of an unbroken chromosome suggesting that the end of chromosomes have unique features. Telomere sequences remain conserved throughout vertebrates and they form caps that protect the chromosomes from nucleases and other destabilising influences, and they prevent the ends of chromosomes from fusing with one another. The telomeric DNA contains direct tandemly repeated sequences of the form (T/A)xGy where x is between 1 and 4 and y is greater than 1. Human telomeres contain the sequence TTAGGG repeated from about 500 to 5000 times. Certain bacteria possess telomeres in their linear genetic material which are of two types, one of the types is called a hairpin telomere. As its name implies, the telomeres bend around from the end of one DNA strand to the end of the complimentary strand. The other type of telomere is known as an invertron telomere. This type acts to allow an overlap between the ends of the complimentary DNA strands.

Telomere replication: Telomere replication is an important aspect in DNA replication. The primary difficulty with telomeres is the replication of the lagging strand. Because DNA synthesis requires a RNA template (that provides the free 3′-OH group) to prime DNA replication and this template is eventually degraded, a short single-stranded region would be left at the end of the chromosome. This region would be susceptible to enzymes that degrade single-stranded DNA. The result would be that the length of the chromosome would be shortened after each division. This is known as the end replication problem which is not observed. The action of the telomerase enzymes ensure that the ends of the lagging strands are replicated correctly. Telomerase was discovered in 1984 by Elizabeth Blackburn and Carol Greider of the University of California, Berkeley. It is a reverse transcriptase that synthesises DNA using an RNA template. Unlike most reverse transcriptases, the enzyme itself contains the RNA that serves as its template, i.e. telomerase can add new repeat units to the 3′ end of the overhanging strand. A well-studied system involves the *Tetrahymena* protozoa organism. The telomeres of this organism end in the sequence 5′-TTGGGG-3′. The telomerase adds a series of 5′-TTGGGG-3′ repeats to the ends of the lagging strand. A hairpin occurs when unusual base pairs between guanine residues in the repeat form. Next the RNA primer is removed and the 5′ end of the lagging strand can be used for DNA synthesis. Ligation occurs between the finished lagging strand and the hairpin. Finally, the hairpin is removed at the 5′-TTGGGG-3′ repeat. Telomerase activity is retained in germ cells and zygote and somatic cells after few cell division cycles do not show such activities because otherwise they would divide indefinitely and lead to cancer. Thus telomeres shrink causing chromosome shortening to a critical point when the cell ceases to grow and divide. An inherited disease called the Werner's syndrome that causes patients to age much more rapidly than normal is characterised by abnormal telomere maintenance.

HUMAN CHROMOSOME

The human genome is 3×10^9 base pairs of DNA and the smallest human chromosome is several times larger than the entire yeast genome, and the extended length of DNA that makes up the human genome is about 1 m long. The human genome is distributed among 24 chromosomes (22 autosomes and the 2 sex chromosomes), each containing between 45 and 280 Mb of DNA. The sex chromosomes are denoted by X and Y and they contain genes which determine the sex of an individual, i.e. XX for female and XY for male. The rest are known as autosomes. The haploid human genome contains about 23000 protein-coding genes, which are far fewer than had been expected before sequencing. In fact, only about 1.5% of the genome codes for proteins, while the rest consists of non-coding genes, regulatory sequences, introns and non-coding DNA. Chromosomes are stained with A-T (G bands) and G-C (R bands) base pair specific dyes. When they are stained, the mitotic chromosomes have a banded structure that unambiguously identifies each chromosome of a karyotype. Each band contains millions of DNA nucleotide pairs which do not correspond to any functional structure. G-banding is obtained with Giemsa stain yielding a series of lightly and darkly stained bands. The dark regions tend to be heterochromatic and AT rich. The light regions tend to be euchromatic and GC rich. R-banding is the reverse of G-banding where the dark regions are euchromatic and the bright regions are heterochromatic.

Types of Human Chromosomes

There are four types of chromosomes based upon the position of the centromere in humans (Fig. 18.6).

1. Metacentric: In this type of chromosome the centromere occurs in the centre and all the four chromatids are of equal length.
2. Submetacentric: In this type of chromosome the centromere is a little away from the centre and therefore chromatids of one side are slightly longer than the other side.
3. Acrocentric: In this type of chromosome the centromere is located closer to one end of chromatid therefore the chromatids on opposite side are very long. A small round structure, attached by a very thin thread is observed on the side of shorter chromatid. The small round structure that is a part of the chromatid is termed as satellite. The thin strands at the satellite region are termed as nucleolar organiser region.
4. Telocentric: In this type of chromosome the centromere is placed at one end of the chromatid and hence only one arm. Such telocentric chromosomes are not seen in human cells.

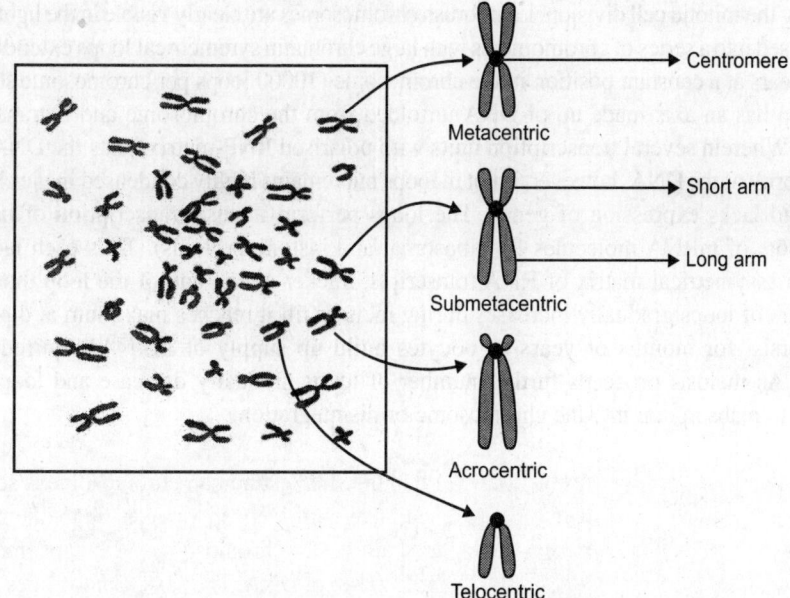

Fig. 18.6: Types of human chromosomes.

GIANT CHROMOSOMES

Some cells at certain particular stage of their life cycle contain large nuclei with giant or large sized chromosomes. Polytene and lampbrush chromosomes are examples of giant chromosomes.

Polytene Chromosome

Giant chromosomes were first time observed by E.G. Balbiani in the year 1881 in nuclei of certain secretory cells (salivary glands) of Chironomas larvae (Diptera). However he could not conclude them to be chromosomes. They were conclusively reported for the first time in insect cells (*Drosophila*) by Theophilus Painter of the University of Texas in the year 1933. Since they were discovered in the salivary glands of insects they were termed as salivary gland chromosomes. The anme polytene chromosome was proposed by Kollar due to the occurrence of many chromonemata (DNA) in them. Cells in the larval salivary gland of *Drosophila*, mosquito and *Chironema* contain chromosomes with high DNA content.

However they may also occur in malphigian tubules, rectum, gut, foot pads, fat bodies, ovarian nurse cells, etc. Polyteney of giant chromosomes happens by replication of the chromosomal DNA several times without nuclear division (endomitosis) and the resulting daughter chromatids do not separate but remain aligned side by side. During endomitosis the nuclear envelope does not rupture and no spindle formation takes place. The polytene chromosomes are visible during interphase and prophase of mitosis.

Lampbrush Chromosome

Lampbrush chromosomes are functional for studying chromosome organisation and genome function during meiotic prophase. Additionally lampbrush chromosomes are widely used for construction of detail cytological maps of individual chromosomes.

They are of exceptionally large sizes and present in bivalent form. They are formed due to the active synthesis of mRNA molecules for future use by the egg cells, when no synthesis of mRNA molecule is possible during the mitotic cell division. Lampbrush chromosomes are clearly visible in the light microscope they are organised into a series of chromomeres with large chromatin symmetrical loops extending laterally. Each loop appears at a constant position in the chromosome (10000 loops per chromosome set or haploid set). Each loop has an axis made up of DNA unfolded from the chromosome and is transcriptionally highly active. Wherein several transcription units with polarised RNP-matrix coats the DNA axis of the loop. The majority of the DNA, however, is not in loops but remains highly condensed in the chromomeres on the axis and lacks expression of genes. The loops perform intense transcription of heterogenous RNA (precursors of mRNA molecules for ribosomal and histone proteins). Thus each lateral loop is covered by an assymetrical matrix of RNA transcripts, thicker at one end of the loop than other. The number of pairs of loops gradually increases during meiosis till it reaches maximum at diplotene. This stage may persist for months or years as oocytes build up supply of mRNA required for further development. As meiosis proceeds further number of loops gradually decrease and loops ultimately disappear due to reabsorption into the chromosome or disintegration.

Chapter 19

DNA Provirus Hypothesis

INTRODUCTION

A provirus is a virus genome that is integrated into the DNA of a host cell. In the case of bacterial viruses (bacteriophages), proviruses are often referred to as prophages. This state can be a stage of virus replication, or a state that persists over longer periods of time as either inactive viral infections or an endogenous viral element. In inactive viral infections the virus will not replicate itself except through replication of its host cell. This state can last over many host cell generations.

Endogenous retroviruses are always in the state of a provirus. When a (nonendogenous) retrovirus invades a cell, the RNA of the retrovirus is reverse-transcribed into DNA by reverse transcriptase, then inserted into the host genome by an integrase.

A provirus does not directly make new DNA copies of itself while integrated into a host genome in this way. Instead, it is passively replicated along with the host genome and passed on to the original cell's offspring, all descendants of the infected cell will also bear proviruses in their genomes. This is known as lysogenic viral reproduction. Integration can result in a latent infection or a productive infection. In a productive infection, the provirus is transcribed into messenger RNA which directly produces new virus, which in turn will infect other cells via the lytic cycle. A latent infection results when the provirus is transcriptionally silent rather than active.

A latent infection may become productive in response to changes in the hosts environmental conditions or health, the provirus may be activated and begin transcription of its viral genome. This can result in the destruction of its host cell because the cell's protein synthesis machinery is hijacked to produce more viruses. Proviruses may account for approximately 8% of the human genome in the form of inherited endogenous retroviruses.

A provirus not only refers to a retrovirus but is also used to describe other viruses that can integrate into the host chromosomes, another example being adeno-associated virus. Not only eukaryotic viruses integrate into the genomes of their hosts, many bacterial and archaeal viruses also employ this strategy of propagation. All families of bacterial viruses with circular (single-stranded or double-stranded) DNA genomes or replicating their genomes through a circular intermediate (e.g. tailed dsDNA viruses) have temperate members.

The genetic information in RNA is transferred to DNA during the replication of some viruses, including some that cause cancer. This transfer of information from the messenger molecule, RNA, to the genome molecule, DNA, apparently contradicted the 'central dogma of molecular biology', formulated in the late 1950's. This mode of information transfer was first postulated and established for the replication of Rous sarcoma virus, a strongly transforming avian C-type ribodeoxyvirus. (Ribodeoxyviruses are RNA viruses that replicate through a DNA intermediate.)

This chapter discusses the experiments that led to the formulation of the DNA provirus hypothesis, the experiments that established the DNA provirus hypothesis and, therefore, the existence of RNA-directed DNA synthesis, some aspects of the present status of our knowledge of the mechanism of formation of the DNA provirus, and, finally, some implications of this work for the questions of the origin of animal viruses, how cancers may be caused by viruses, and how the majority of cancers, which do not involve infectious viruses, are caused.

The majority of the ideas discuss today came from experiments with Rous sarcoma virus (RSV), the prototype RNA tumour virus. Rous sarcoma virus was originally described by Peyton Rous in 1911. He stated, A transmissible sarcoma of the chicken has been under observation in this laboratory for the past fourteen months, and it has assumed of late a special interest because of its extreme malignancy and a tendency to wide-spread metastasis. In a careful study of the growth, tests have been made to determine whether it can be transmitted by a filtrate free of the tumour cells. Small quantities of a cell-free filtrate have sufficed to transmit the growth to susceptible fowl. Although Rous and his associates carried out many experiments with RSV, as the virus is now called, and had many prophetic insights into its behaviour, they and other biologists of that time did not have the scientific concepts or the technical tools to exploit his discovery. And in about 1915 Rous himself stopped work with RSV.

The major scientific concepts required to understand the behaviour of RSV were that genetic information was contained in and transferred from nucleic acids, developed especially by Avery, MacLeod and McCarthy, and by Watson and Crick, as well as the concept that viral genomes could become part of cell genomes, developed especially by Lwoff. The major technical tools required were those of quantitative virology and of the study of animal viruses in cell culture, developed especially by Delbrück, Enders, Robbins, and Weller, and Dulbecco.

ASSAY FOR ROUS SARCOMA VIRUS

It was found that addition of RSV to cultures of chicken embryo cells in a sparse layer, rather than in a crowded monolayer as then used for the assay of other animal viruses, led to the appearance of foci of transformed cells (Fig. 19.1). The number of these foci was proportional to the concentration of virus, and the foci resulted from altered morphology and altered control of multiplication of the infected cells. The foci were cell culture analogs of tumours in chickens.

This assay allowed RSV to be studied like other viruses, leading to the demonstration that RSV-infected cells could produce virus and divide and to the demonstration by Crawford and Crawford that the genome of RSV was RNA. The assay for RSV was also a model for the assay of other transforming viruses, such as polyoma virus, as discussed by Dr. Dulbecco.

Further observation of RSV-induced foci revealed that some of the foci contained long fusiform cells rather than the rounded cells seen in the focus in Fig. 19.1. Virus produced by these fusiform foci caused the formation of further foci of long fusiform cells, that is, the virus from these foci was a genetic variant. These and other observations indicated that viral genes controlled the morphology of transformed cells and led to the hypothesis that transformation is the result of the action of viral genes,

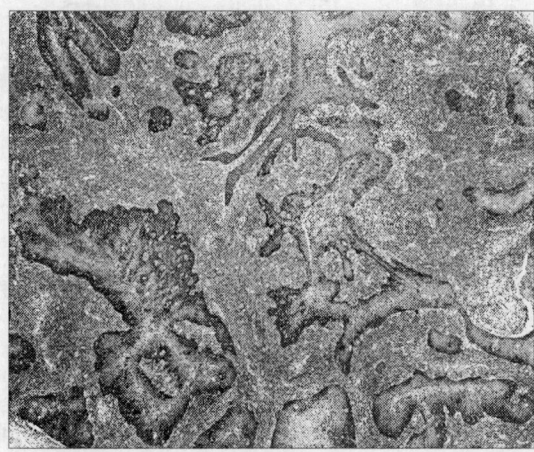

Fig. 19.1: Focus induced by Rous sarcoma virus in chicken cells. A sparse monolayer of chicken embryo fibroblasts was exposed to Bryan standard Rous sarcoma virus. The cells were overlaid with tissue culture medium and incubated at 38° C for ten days. This photograph of one focus was taken with an inverted microscope at a magnification of 25.

that is, transformation is a conversion analogous to lysogenic conversion. This hypothesis has been amply confirmed for RSV by the isolation of variant viruses temperature-sensitive for transformation or defective for transformation.

These observations also led to the study of differences between transformed and normal cells. At least two important results came from these studies: (i) the concept of an altered requirement of transformed cells for specific multiplication-stimulating factors in serum, and (ii) the discovery by Reich and coworkers of increased production by transformed cells of an activator of a serum protease.

PROVIRUS HYPOTHESIS

Smith and others studied the kinetics of mutation of the viral genes controlling cell and focus morphology, the effects of mutation in these viral genes on the morphology of infected cells, and the inheritance of these genes in cells infected with two different Rous sarcoma viruses. These studies demonstrated that these viral genes mutated at a high rate, that mutation in a viral gene present in an infected cell often led to change in the morphology of that infected cell, that two different viruses infecting one cell were stably inherited, and that the intracellular viral genomes were probably located at only one or two sites in the cell genome.

These observations led to the provirus hypothesis (Fig. 19.2) infection of chicken cells by RSV leads to the formation of one or two copies of a regularly inherited structure with the information for progeny virus and for cell morphology from studies of RSV-infected rat cells independently postulated the existence of a provirus in RSV-infected cells.

The provirus hypothesis was a genetic hypothesis and contained no statement about the molecular nature of the provirus. However, the regular inheritance of the provirus led to postulate that the provirus was integrated with the cell genome.

The provirus hypothesis was further supported by the behaviour of converted RSV-infected chicken cells that were not producing infectious virus. Analysis of similar cells by others led to the concept of defectiveness of some strongly transforming RNA tumour viruses

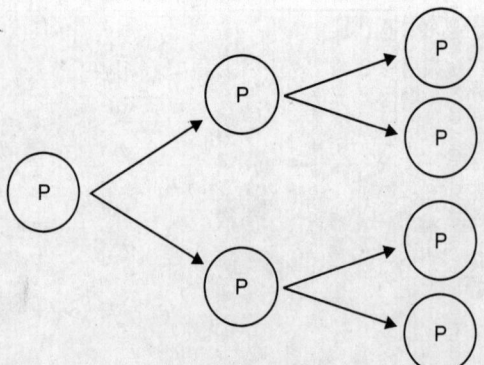

Fig. 19.2: The provirus hypothesis. Virus information (P) is contained in infected cells in one or two copies of a regularly inherited structure with the information for progeny virus and for cell morphology.

DNA PROVIRUS HYPOTHESIS

At the time of formulation of the provirus hypothesis in 1960, the general rules for information transfer in living systems were being clearly established in what was called 'the central dogma of molecular biology', that is, genetic information is transferred from DNA to RNA to protein. RNA viruses were an apparent exception to this 'dogma'. Studies with the newly discovered RNA bacteriophage and with animal RNA viruses, especially using the antibiotic actinomycin D, indicated that RNA viruses transferred their information from RNA to RNA and from RNA to protein and that DNA was not directly involved in the replication of these RNA viruses.

Wisconsin-Madison, used actinomycin D to isolate the provirus of Rous sarcoma virus, just as David Baltimore and others were using actinomycin to study the intermediates in the replication of other animal RNA viruses. However, when actinomycin D was added to Rous sarcoma virus-producing cells, it inhibited virus production (Fig. 19.3). Control experiments demonstrated that this inhibition was neither of early events in infection (as was found by Barry, Ives, and Cruickshank with influenza virus) nor of the ability of the treated cells to support replication of other animal RNA viruses. These results indicated to me that the provirus was DNA.

Smith and others carried out further experiments that indicated that new DNA synthesis was required for RSV infection and that new RSV-specific DNA was found in infected chicken cells. Based on the results of these experiments, Smith proposed the DNA provirus hypothesis at a meeting in the Spring of 1964 - the RNA of infecting RSV acts as a template for the synthesis of viral DNA, the provirus, which acts as a template for the synthesis of progeny RSV RNA (Fig. 19.4).

Smith and others tried to obtain direct molecular evidence for the DNA provirus by looking for RNA-directed DNA polymerase activity in cells soon after infection, for infectious DNA in infected cells, and for better systems of nucleic acid hybridisation. These initial efforts were unsuccessful. Smith then developed systems with better controlled cells to study RSV infection - at first, synchronised cells, and later stationary cells. Experiments with these cells indicated that a normal replicative cell cycle was needed for initiation of RSV production.

Thus, the experiments performed that demonstrated more clearly a requirement for new non-S phase DNA synthesis for RSV infection, and Smith demonstrated that this new DNA synthesis was virus-specific. Finally, using infection of stationary cells, it was demonstrated that the newly synthesised viral DNA could be labelled with 5-bromodeoxyuridine and inactivated by light (Fig. 19.5).

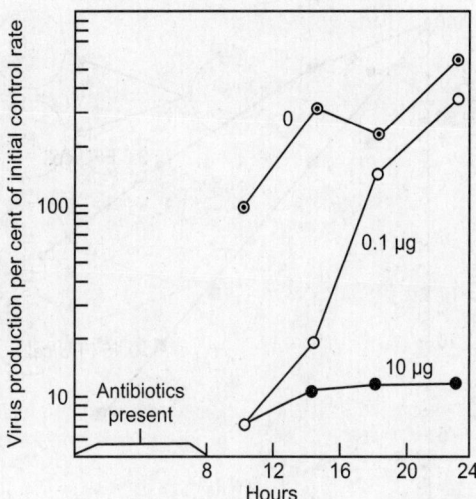

Fig. 19.3: Effects of actinomycin D on production of Rous sarcoma virus. Chicken cells producing RSV were exposed to 0, 0.1 or 10 μg (g)/m l of actinomycin D. After 8 hr, the medium was removed, the cells were washed, and fresh medium was added. At the indicated times, the medium was harvested and assayed for focus forming units of RSV.

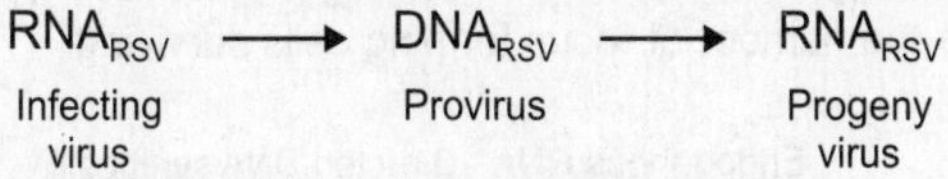

$$RNA_{RSV} \longrightarrow DNA_{RSV} \longrightarrow RNA_{RSV}$$

| Infecting virus | Provirus | Progeny virus |

Fig. 19.4: DNA provirus hypothesis.

RSV VIRION DNA POLYMERASE

Paoletti, and Grace had found a DNA-directed RNA polymerase in poxvirus virions, and in 1968 Borsa and Graham, and Shatkin and Sipe had found an RNA-directed RNA polymerase in virions of reovirus. The conclusion that RSV virions contain a DNA polymerase could have been deduced in 1967 or 1968 from the DNA provirus hypothesis and the existence of these virion polymerases, but it was not RSV virions contain an endogenous DNA polymerase activity with the following characteristics (Fig. 19.6). The virion polymerase activity incorporates deoxyribonucleoside monophosphates into DNA and requires all four deoxyribonucleoside triphosphates, a divalent cation, and a detergent to disrupt the virion envelope. Furthermore, the polymerase activity is inactivated by heat, which denatures the polymerase, and by ribonuclease, which destroys the template, and it is partially resistant to actinomycin D.

The avian RNA tumour virus DNA polymerases are stable and easy to solubilise and study. Numerous workers have purified these enzymes, especially from avian myeloblastosis virus, and this DNA polymerase has become a standard reagent for molecular biologists. It is especially useful because it has no deoxyribonuclease activity, but it does have ribonuclease H activity. (Ribonuclease H activity degrades the RNA strand of an RNA . DNA hybrid molecule, but not single-stranded RNA.)

ESTABLISHMENT OF THE DNA PROVIRUS HYPOTHESIS

Although the discovery of the RSV virion DNA polymerase immediately provided convincing evidence for the DNA provirus hypothesis, actual proof of the existence of a DNA provirus depended upon later

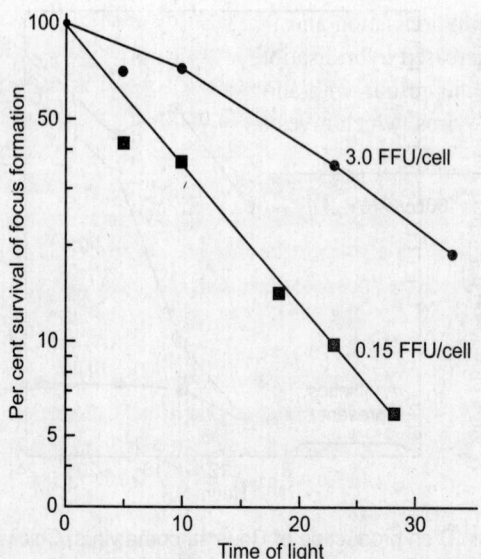

Fig. 19.5: Light inactivation of focus formation by chicken cells infected with RSV in the presence of 5-bromo-deoxyuridine. Stationary chicken cells were exposed to RSV at two multiplicities of infection (0.15 or 3.0 focus forming units per cell), incubated in medium containing 5-bromodeoxyuridine, exposed to light, and plated on rat cells to determine the number of focus forming cells surviving.

Endogenous RNA - Directed DNA synthesis

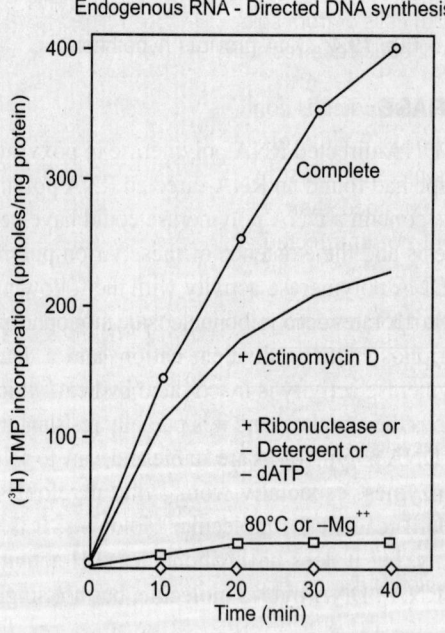

Fig. 19.6: Endogenous RNA-directed DNA synthesis by avian leukosis virus virions. Purified virions (2 µg protein) of an avian leukosis virus were incubated in a complete system with the indicated pretreatments, additions, or subtractions, and the incorporation of label was measured.

work involving nucleic acid hybridisation and infectious DNA experiments. Neiman was the first to demonstrate convincingly increased hybridisation of labelled RSV RNA to DNA of infected chicken cells. It was latter confirmed his results with another avian RNA virus that replicates through a DNA intermediate, spleen necrosis virus, which gives a clearer and cleaner result (Fig. 19.7).

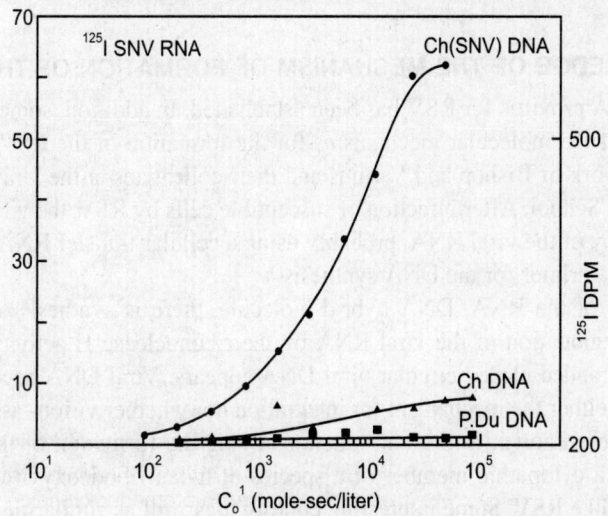

Fig. 19.7: Hybridisation of labelled viral RNA to DNA from infected and uninfected cells. ^{125}I-labelled RNA from spleen necrosis virus (SNV) was incubated for different times with a large excess of DNA from uninfected chicken (Ch) or Peking duck (P. Du) cells or from spleen necrosis virus-infected chicken (Ch(SNV)) cells, and the percentage of RNA that was ribonuclease-resistant was determined.

The DNA of ribodeoxyvirus-infected cells contains new nucleotide sequences complementary to the RNA of the infecting ribodeoxyvirus. To a virologist an even more satisfying proof for the existence of the DNA provirus was the demonstration, first by Hill and Hillova, of infectious DNA for RSV. Smith and others, have repeated and extended their work, making it more quantitative (Table 19.1). Rous sarcoma virus-infected cells, but not uninfected cells, contain a nucleic acid with the information for RSV (the provirus).

Table 19.1: Infectious Rous sarcoma virus DNA[a].

DNA	Infectious dose 50 (ID$_{60}$) (µg)
RSV-infected chicken cell	0.1
RSV-infected chicken cell, deoxyribonuclease	>10
RSV-infected chicken cell, alkali	1.0
RSV-infected chicken cell, ribonuclease	0.1
RSV-infected chicken cell, pronase	0.31
RSV-infected chicken cell, cesium chloride density gradient centrifugation	0.1
RSV-infected rat cell	0.1

[a] DNA was isolated from RSA-infected chicken or rat cells, treated as indicated, and assayed for infectivity in chicken fibroblasts. Infectivity is presented as the amount of DNA required to infect half of the assay culture. The lower the amount of DNA required for infection, the more infectious the DNA was.

This information is contained in DNA as shown by its inactivation by deoxyribonuclease, its resistance to alkali, ribonuclease, and Pronase, and its density in equilibrium cesium chloride density gradient centrifugation. A single molecule of about 6×10^6 daltons of doublestranded DNA is sufficient to cause infection, and the efficiency of infection is similar to that of the DNA isolated from animal small DNA viruses.

STATUS OF KNOWLEDGE OF THE MECHANISM OF FORMATION OF THE DNA PROVIRUS

The existence of a DNA provirus for RSV has been established. In addition, some knowledge has been gained of the details of the molecular mechanisms for the formation of the RSV provirus. Especially notable has been the work of Bishop and Varmus and their colleagues at the University of California-San Francisco Medical School. After infection of susceptible cells by RSV, the virion DNA polymerase synthesises a DNA copy of the viral RNA, probably using a cellular transfer RNA molecule associated with the viral RNA as a primer for the DNA synthesis.

After the formation of the RNA, DNA hybrid molecule, there is synthesis of a second strand of DNA, perhaps after degradation of the viral RNA by the ribonuclease H activity of the virion DNA polymearse. Double-stranded closed circular viral DNA appears. Viral DNA becomes integrated with host DNA. However, neither the mechanism for integration nor whether virion- associated enzymes are involved in integration is known. Smith and others studying the formation of the provirus of spleen necrosis virus (SNV), a cytopathic member of a species of avian ribodeoxyviruses distinct from the avian leukosis viruses like RSV. Some interesting contrasts, as well as similarities, have been found.

Instead of using only a pre-formed primer for DNA synthesis, spleen necrosis virus may at times synthesise an RNA primer *de novo*. The virions of spleen necrosis virus contain an RNA polymerase activity as well as a DNA polymerase activity. This RNA polymerase activity can initiate synthesis of new RNA chains, and its product RNA, a small molecule, is hydrogen-bonded to viral RNA. Thus, SNV virions contain both DNA polymerase and RNA polymerase activities-the only virions so far reported to contain both of these enzyme activities.

Smith and others studied the kinetics of formation of infectious SNV DNA. After infection of chicken cells by SNV, infectious viral DNA appeared in an unintegrated form, found in the supernatant of a Hirt extract, shortly before it appeared in an integrated form, found in the pellet of a Hirt extract. Surprisingly there were large further increases in the amounts of both unintegrated and integrated viral DNAs, and some unintegrated viral DNA persisted for over a week after infection. In contrast to these results with dividing cells, little infectious viral DNA was formed in stationary cells exposed to SNV. This result indicates that a normal replicative cell cycle is required for formation of infectious viral DNA.

The forms of unintegrated infectious viral DNA were analysed by agarose gel electrophoresis. Three forms were found, reminiscent of the three forms of DNA in papovavirus virions. The majority of the infectious viral DNA was in linear molecules, but there were minor components of closed circular and nicked infectious SNV DNA. Thus, the early events in ribodeoxyvirus infection are complex, and much remains to be learned before we can describe the formation of the provirus in molecular detail.

ORIGIN OF RIBODEOXYVIRUSES

Avian RNA tumor viruses undergo a great amount of genetic variation. This variation is the result of both mutation and recombination. Recombination takes place not only between viruses, but also between viruses and cells. The recombination between viruses and cells does not appear to be random, but is primarily with specific cellular genes. These genes are called endogenous ribodeoxyvirus-related genes and are, of course, part of the normal cellular DNA. Endogenous avian leukosis virus-related genes were first recognised about 10 years ago by the presence and Mendelian inheritance of a Rous sarcoma virus virion antigen in some uninfected chicken cells. Later an avian leukosis virus virion envelope protein was found in some uninfected chicken cells, and, finally, nucleotide sequences of avian leukosis virus RNA were found in the DNA of all uninfected chicken cells. (Similar results have been found with mammalian leukemia viruses and cells.)

Study of the phylogenetic distribution of the endogenous avian leukosis virus-related nucleotide sequences revealed a relationship between the amount of these sequences in cell DNA from a particular species of bird and the closeness of the relationship of that species to chickens, for example, more avian leukosis virus nucleotide sequences were found in pheasant DNA than in duck DNA.

This distribution is consistent with an hypothesis (the protovirus hypothesis) which was originally proposed in 1970 to explain the origin of ribodeoxyviruses evolved from normal cellular components. The normal cellular components are the endogenous ribodeoxyvirusrelated genes. These genes are involved in normal DNA to RNA to DNA in formation transfer. This normal process of information transfer in cells could not exist only for its ability to give rise to viruses. It must exist as a result of its role in normal cellular processes, for example, cell differentiation, antibody formation, and memory.

One prediction of this protovirus hypothesis is that there are relationships between ribodeoxyvirus and cell DNA polymerases. Smith and others demonstrated such relationships by an antibody blocking test. In this test, for example, the activity of an antibody against avian leukosis virus DNA polymerases was blocked by incubation with chicken cell DNA polymerases or a DNA polymerase from an otherwise unrelated avian ribodeoxyvirus. Therefore, certain predictions of the protovirus hypothesis for the origin of ribodeoxyviruses have been verified. But, obviously, much further work must be done to establish or disprove this hypothesis.

FURTHER IMPLICATIONS OF PROTOVIRUS HYPOTHESIS

The protovirus hypothesis can explain the origin of ribodeoxyviruses, but it does not help in understanding the origin of other animal viruses. The presence of an RNA polymerase activity in virions of spleen necrosis virus might, however, present a clue to the origin of the other animal enveloped RNA viruses. As Dr. Baltimore has described, many animal enveloped RNA viruses contain an RNA polymerase activity. If there were genetic changes so that the SNV RNA polymerase activity synthesised a complete copy of SNV RNA rather than only a small molecule, the first step in the synthesis of a viral RNA intermediate would occur (Fig. 19.8). Further genetic changes leading to copying of the newly synthesised RNA strand would complete the replication of the viral RNA. Therefore, it was proposed that other animal enveloped RNA viruses evolved from ribodeoxyviruses. (The recent reports of DNA intermediates in carrier cultures of some animal enveloped RNA viruses could indicate a vestige of the origin of these viruses from ribodeoxyviruses.) Animal small DNA viruses might also have originated from ribodeoxyviruses. As discussed above, the unintegrated infectious DNA in SNV-infected cells exists in several forms, and the amount of the unintegrated DNA in creases for several days after infection.

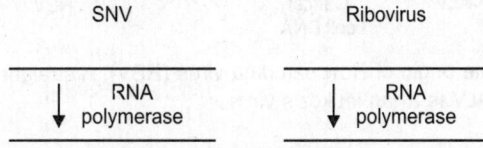

Fig. 19.8: Initial RNA synthesis by SNV and by other RNA viruses.

This unintegrated ribodeoxyvirus DNA could represent a precursor of animal small DNA viruses. Continued replication of unintegrated viral DNA and encapsidation in viral proteins would also be required. Therefore, it was summarised that animal small DNA viruses also evolved from ribodeoxyviruses.

In most of this discussions of virus replication and virus origins, the aspect of cancer is not mentioned. In fact, the absence of such discussion makes an important point: RNA tumor virus replication is not sufficient for cancer formation by RNA tumor viruses. Strongly transforming RNA tumor viruses like RSV cause cancer by introducing genes for cancer into cells. But there are viruses that replicate in much the same way as RSV, for example, SNV or Rous-associated virus-O, that do not cause cancer because they do not contain genes for cancer.

In addition, the majority of human cancers are not caused primarily by infectious viruses like RSV, but by other types of carcinogens, for example, the chemicals in cigarette smoke. These nonviral carcinogens probably act to mutate a special target in the cell DNA to genes for cancer (Fig. 19.9).

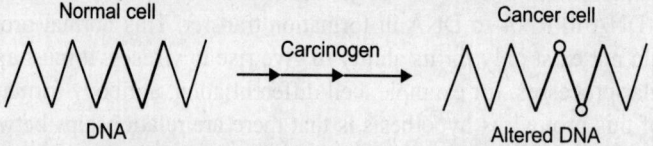

Fig. 19.9: The protovirus hypothesis for the origin of the genes for cancer. The heavy lines indicate DNA involved in DNA to RNA to DNA information transfer.

To relate this hypothesis to the existence of animal RNA viruses like RSV, which do cause cancer efficiently, it is suggested that the targets for the non-viral carcinogens are the genes involved in information transfer from DNA to RNA to DNA. Under this hypothesis, genes for cancer would be formed in a process involving RNA-directed DNA synthesis in both RNA virus-induced and non-viral carcinogen-induced cancers. Finally it began with Peyton Rous and RSV, we can speculate on the origin of RSV. As it was quoted in beginning. Rous noted a change with transplantation in the behaviour of the chicken tumor. This change, propose, was the result of the formation of RSV, that is, the Rous sarcoma appeared before the Rous sarcoma virus. More specifically, other events not involving a virus led to the formation of genes for cancer and the chicken sarcoma. This sarcoma was infected by an avian leukosis virus, and RSV was formed by a rare recombination (Fig. 19.10).

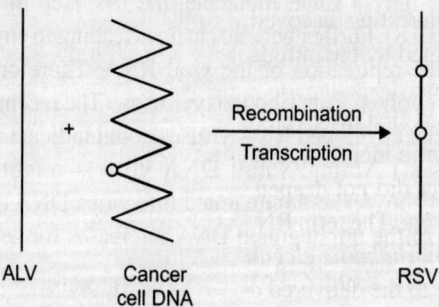

Fig. 19.10: A hypothesis for the origin of Row sarcoma virus (RSV). A straight line represents RNA, and a zig-zag line represents DNA. ALV is avian leukosis virus.

Chapter 20

RNA Interference

INTRODUCTION

RNA interference (RNAi) is a post-transcriptional, highly conserved process in eukaryotes that leads to specific gene silencing through degradation of the target mRNA. This mechanism is mediated by double-stranded RNA (dsRNA) that is homologous in sequence to the silenced gene. The dsRNA is processed into small interfering RNA (siRNA) by an enzyme called Dicer, and the siRNAs are then incorporated into a multi-component RNA-induced silencing complex, which finds and cleaves the target mRNA. In plants and worms, amplification of the silencing signal and cell-to-cell RNAi spreading is observed. The proposed biological roles of RNAi include resistance to viruses, transposons (mainly in plants), and the silencing and regulation of gene expression, particularly during development. In developmental gene control, specific small RNAs (micro RNA and small temporal RNA) are involved, which are processed in the same way as dsRNAs but act at the level of translation. RNAi technology has become a powerful tool in functional genomic analyses and may prove to be a useful method to develop highly specific gene-silencing therapeutics against viral infections and cancer in the future. In recent years many RNA-based silencing mechanisms, e.g. post-transcriptional gene silencing, cosuppression, quelling, and RNA interference (RNAi), have been discovered among species of different kingdoms (fungi, plants, and animals). One of the most interesting discoveries was RNAi, a post-transcriptional sequence-specific gene-silencing mechanism initiated by the introduction of double-stranded RNA (dsRNA) homologous in sequence to the silenced gene.

The phenomenon of RNAi was first discovered in plants during experiments connected with changes in pigmentation in the petunia. Introducing supernumerary copies of a pigment gene designed to increase the colour intensity in the flower did not deepen flower colour as expected: the flowers became even less colourful than the wild flowers. The term RNAi was first coined after the discovery that injection of dsRNA into the nematode *Caenorhabditis elegans* (Fig. 20.1) leads to the specific silencing of genes highly homologous in sequence to the delivered dsRNA. RNAi has also been observed in a wide range of other species, including plants, fungi, nematodes, protozoa, insects (*Drosophila melanogaster*), and vertebrates. This suggests an ancient evolutionary origin of this phenomenon. The conservation of RNAi by eukaryotes clearly suggests that this adaptive response means a lot to these organisms: RNAi

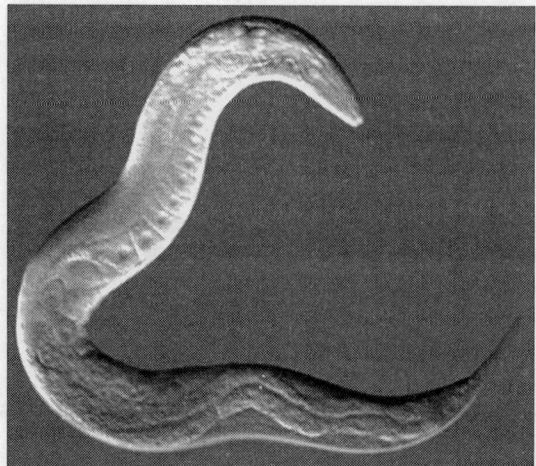

Fig. 20.1: *Caenorhabditis elegans.*

protects the most sensitive part of a species, its genetic code. RNAi has not been found in prokaryotes, so it is probably a eukaryotic innovation.

MECHANISM OF RNAi

A combination of genetic and biochemical studies suggests that RNAi has a very similar mechanism in many organisms and that the enzymes involved in this process exhibit high homology across species. The initial step of RNAi is connected with the appearance of dsRNA in the cell which is perfectly homologous in sequence to the silenced gene. dsRNA can either be intracellularly synthesised or exogenously introduced directly into cells. The minimal length of dsRNA to induce RNAi is 26 nucleotides, although long dsRNAs are more effective. That is why nucleotides about a few hundred nucleotides long are often used. On the other hand, transfection of long dsRNA (hundreds of nucleotides) into cultured mammalian cells induces the interferon response, whereas short dsRNAs (about 20 nucleotides) only induce RNAi. The interferon response protects neighbouring cells from infection and blocks viral replication. Long dsRNAs activate a dsRNA-dependent kinase, protein kinase R (PKR), which phosphporylates and inactivates the translation factor eIF2α. This activation leads to a generalised inhibition of translation and can dramatically alter cellular metabolism and often activates apoptotic and nonapoptotic pathways. PKR may be one of several kinases in mammalian cells that can mediate this response. A second dsRNA-response pathway activates 2′–5′ oligoadenylate polymerase, the product of which is an essential cofactor for a sequence-non-specific ribonuclease, RnaseL. To overcome these difficulties, short dsRNAs are used in many cases to trigger RNAi in mammalian cells (dsRNAs less than 30 nucleotides long are unable to activate PKR, and full activation requires ~80 nucleotides).

The dsRNAs are recognised by the Dicer enzyme, which is an Rnase III ribonuclease family member (Fig. 20.2). Dicer enzymes are evolutionarily conserved and these proteins have been found in *Drosophila melanogaster, C. elegans,* tobacco, and mammals. Humans and *C. elegans* have only one Dicer, but *Drosophila* has two (Dicer-2 is the major small inteferin RNA – siRNA – producer in RNAi, and Dicer-1 probably binds micro RNA – miRNA) and *Arabidopsis* four Dicer enzymes. Dicer is ATP dependent and contains several characteristic domains: an *N*-terminal helicase domain, a PAZ (a conservative domain found in proteins in *Drosophila* and *Arabidopsis*, involved in developmental control), dual

Rnase III domains, and a dsRNA-binding domain. Dicer acts as a dimeric enzyme, although one of the active sites in each Dicer enzyme is defective. Dicer processes dsRNA into double-stranded siRNA 21–25 nucleotides in length, depending on the species (Fig. 20.2), although plants produce two distinct classes of siRNAs: short (21–23 nuclotides) and long (24–25 nucleotides). These molecules contain 3′ hydroxyl termini and additional characteristic 2-nucleotide 3′ overhangs and 5′ phosphorylated termini. It was shown that the described structural features of siRNAs are crucial for the next stages of the RNAi pathway. For example, modification of the 5′ end of the antisense strand inhibits siRNA activity, and blunt-ended siRNAs become inefficient intermediates in the further steps. The siRNAs produced by Dicer are incorporated into a multicomponent nuclease complex, RNA-induced silencing complex (RISC) (Fig. 20.2), which must be converted from a latent form, containing a double-stranded siRNA, to an active form by unwinding the siRNA by a helicase in an ATP-dependent process (an ATP-dependent RNA helicase). The RISC also contains an endoribonuclease which, using the sequence encoded by the antisense siRNA strand, finds and destroys the complementary sequence of mRNA (Fig. 20.2). During studies on the biochemistry of RNAi, some other proteins in the RISC have been identified and characterised. For example, in human RISC two proteins were found: eIF2C1 (Argonaute1, a translation factor) and eIF2C2/GERp95 (a translation factor, component of the Golgi apparatus or endoplasmic reticulum, and a component of the survival of motor neurons complex). The argonaute protein has two characteristic domains: PAZ, also found in Dicer, and PIWI. The PAZ domain probably acts as an RNA binding module for Argonautes, recognising and binding the characteristic 2-nuleotide 3′ overhang of siRNAs. The 3′ end recognition by PAZ may be important for only two protein families which contain these domains, Dicers and Argonautes, to distinguish between siRNAs and other RNA molecules. In *Drosophila* there is also the RISC loading complex that contains Dicer-2 and R2D2 (Dicer-2-associated protein). The exact role of these proteins in RISC is still unclear, and the identification of other RISC components is still being awaited. The target mRNA is cleaved for fragments of about 22 nucleotides (21–23 nucleotide intervals) long. When the cleavage is completed, the RISC departs and the siRNA can be used in a new cycle of mRNA recognition and cleavage, which protects this molecule from rapid degradation, the normal fate of small single-stranded RNA in cells.

The described processes probably take place in the cytoplasm. There are two indications of this: first, RISC has been found to copurify with ribosomes and, secondly, it was also reported that dsRNAs targeted against intronic and promoter sequences are not effective as inductors of RNAi. In plants and worms, amplification of the silencing signal and cell-to-cell RNAi spreading have been observed. As yet this 'systemic' spreading has not been noticed in mammalian cells. In both plants and *C. elegans*, enzyme RNA-dependent RNA polymerase (RdRp) has been found. It is responsible for the generation and amplification of siRNA into dsRNA1 (Fig. 20.2). These siRNAs are used as primers for the generation of new dsRNAs by RdRp, which can subsequently serve as targets for the Dicer enzyme and be processed into new siRNAs1, (Fig. 20.2). Thanks to this system in plant and worm cells, specific numbers of dsRNA molecules are able to inactivate more copies of endogenous transcripts. RdRps are also encoded by a wide variety of RNA viruses for genome replication, mRNA synthesis, RNA recombination, and other processes. Many if not most eukaryotes also encode RdRps whose roles are still being uncovered.

Besides the signal amplification system, there is also a system of cell-to-cell signal transmission throughout most tissues of the organism. This effect is termed systemic suppression. In plants, the movement of dsRNA or siRNA between cells can take place through cytoplasmic bridges (plasmodesmata) and/or via the vascular system. It is still unclear how this process proceeds in worms, but recent experiments show that products of the *sid-1*, *sid-2*, and *sid-3* genes are required for systemic spreading in the worm

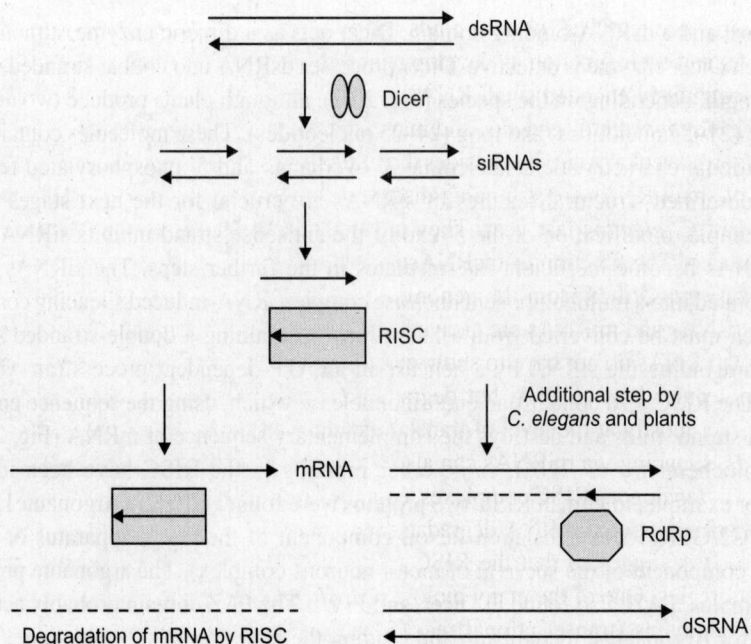

Fig. 20.2: Schematic model of the RNAi mechanism. The cellular enzyme Dicer cleaves intracellularly synthesised or exogenously administered dsRNA into 21-25 nucleotide siRNAs. The siRNAs are incorporated into the RNA-induced silencing complex (RISC), which uses the antisense strand of the siRNA to find and destroy the target mRNA. The siRNAs can also be used as primers for the generation of new dsRNA by RNA-dependent RNA polymerase (RdRp). This step has only been found in plants and *C. elegans*.

body. It is possible that the SID-1 membrane protein can act as a channel for importing the silencing signal. Such transfer could involve a sequence-specific component, probably nucleic acid. SID-1 has homologues in the mouse as well as in humans, and these proteins share significant aminoacid identify and have strikingly similar transmembrane profiles.

SIGNIFICANCE OF RNAi

In plants and invertebrates, RNAi is a system of defense against mobile genetic elements such as transposons and viruses. It is clear that RNAi protects and controls viral infections in plants. For a lot of viruses, a mutation in the RNAi system can cause an increase in the severity of viral pathogenesis. In addition, many plant viruses encode proteins which are able to inactivate essential genes in the RNAi machinery. These viruses promote in this way their replication in the host genome. For example, the tombusvirus p19 protein blocks RNAi in plants by binding RNA duplexes, thereby blocking their assembly into the RISC. There is no evidence that RNAi is an antiviral system in vertebrates, and its specific function in these organisms is unclear. In plants, dsRNA induces genomic methylation at sites of sequences homology. This methylation is asymmetric and is not restricted to CpG sequences. If methylation occurs in promoter sequences, it can cause transcriptional gene silencing before the proper mRNA transcript arises. In worms and vertebrates, RNAi is probably involved in developmental gene control. For this process, specific small RNAs, miRNAs or small temporal RNAs (stRNAs such as lin4 and let7), are probably very important. In plants, miRNAs can be the targets for a viral silencing suppressor such as p19 tombusvirus protein. This protein binds miRNAs in a double-stranded state, preventing maturation of miRNAs and their function as developmental regulators.

The family of endogenously encoded small RNAs is very large, and over 100 of these RNAs have been identified in *D. melanogaster, C. elegans*, and mammals. It is still not known how many functions these small RNAs perform in eukaryotic cells besides their functions in gene silencing and developmental timing. New classes of small RNAs are still being discovered. Tiny non-coding RNAs (tncRNAs), for instance, were found in *C. elegans* last year. They are not evolutionarily conserved, but some are developmentally regulated. The function of tncRNAs is still unknown.

The small RNAs are transcribed from the genome as hairpin precursors 21–22 nucleotides long. Similar to dsRNAs, stRNAs and miRNAs are cleaved by Dicer and only one strand is then used in the further stages. The small RNAs do not have to show perfect complementarity to their target, in contrast to dsRNAs. These molecules bind mRNA, but degradation of the transcript is not initiated because miRNAs and stRNAs act mostly at the level of translation and inhibit protein chain elongation (plants and animals). In plants, silencing via miRNAs can also occur via destruction of the target mRNA. It is possible that there are two analogous RISC complexes, containing either siRNAs or stRNAs and miRNAs. In the first case, post-transcriptional mRNA degradation is induced and in the second case, ribosomal elongation is blocked. It is suggested that the RISC may be a flexible enzyme complex involved in different regulatory strategies. One of the many biological functions of the RNAi machinery may be to form heterochromatic domains (transcriptional inactive chromatin) in the nucleus, which is a very important process for genome organisation and stability. RNAi can affect gene expression at the level of chromatin structure in *D. melanogaster, C. elegans*, and fungi. There are interconnections between RNAi and other metabolic pathways. In *C. elegans*, seven genes, *smg*, are responsible for nonsense-mediated mRNA decay. Three of these genes are also required for persistence of RNAi. It is clear that gene silencing is connected with other cellular processes, but it is not known how these metabolic pathways interplay and influence each other.

CELLULAR MECHANISM

RNAi is RNA-dependent gene silencing process that is controlled by the RNA-induced silencing complex (RISC) and is initiated by short double-stranded RNA molecules in a cell's cytoplasm, where they interact with the catalytic RISC component argonaute. When the dsRNA is exogenous (coming from infection by a virus with an RNA genome or laboratory manipulations), the RNA is imported directly into the cytoplasm and cleaved to short fragments by Dicer. The initiating dsRNA can also be endogenous (originating in the cell), as in pre-microRNAs expressed from RNA-coding genes in the genome. The primary transcripts from such genes are first processed to form the characteristic stem-loop structure of pre-miRNA in the nucleus, then exported to the cytoplasm. Thus, the two dsRNA pathways, exogenous and endogenous, converge at the RISC.

Exogenous dsRNA initiates RNAi by activating the ribonuclease protein Dicer, which binds and cleaves double-stranded RNAs (dsRNAs) in plants, or short hairpin RNAs (shRNAs) in humans, to produce double-stranded fragments of 20–25 base pairs with a 2-nucleotide overhang at the 3' end. Bioinformatics studies on the genomes of multiple organisms suggest this length maximises target-gene specificity and minimises non-specific effects. These short double-stranded fragments are called small interfering RNAs (siRNAs). These siRNAs are then separated into single strands and integrated into an active RISC, by RISC-Loading Complex (RLC). RLC includes Dicer-2 and R2D2, and is crucial to unite Ago2 and RISC. TATA-binding protein-associated factor 11 (TAF11) assembles the RLC by facilitating Dcr-2-R2D2 tetramerisation, which increases the binding affinity to siRNA by 10-fold. Association with TAF11 would convert the R2-D2-Initiator (RDI) complex into the RLC. R2D2 carries tandem double-stranded RNA-binding domains to recognise the thermodynamically stable terminus of siRNA duplexes, whereas Dicer-2 the other less stable extremity. Loading is asymmetric: the MID domain of Ago2 recognises the thermodynamically stable end of the siRNA. Therefore, the 'passenger' (sense) strand whose 5′ end is discarded by MID is ejected, while the saved 'guide' (antisense) strand cooperates with AGO to form the RISC.

After integration into the RISC, siRNAs base-pair to their target mRNA and cleave it, thereby preventing it from being used as a translation template. Differently from siRNA, a miRNA-loaded RISC complex scans cytoplasmic mRNAs for potential complementarity. Instead of destructive cleavage (by Ago2), miRNAs rather target the 3′ untranslated region (UTR) regions of mRNAs where they typically bind with imperfect complementarity, thus blocking the access of ribosomes for translation.

Exogenous dsRNA is detected and bound by an effector protein, known as RDE-4 in *C. elegans* and R2D2 in *Drosophila*, that stimulates dicer activity. The mechanism producing this length specificity is unknown and this protein only binds long dsRNAs.

In *C. elegans* this initiation response is amplified through the synthesis of a population of 'secondary' siRNAs during which the dicer-produced initiating or 'primary' siRNAs are used as templates. These 'secondary' siRNAs are structurally distinct from dicer-produced siRNAs and appear to be produced by an RNA-dependent RNA polymerase (RdRP).

MicroRNA

MicroRNAs (miRNAs) are genomically encoded non-coding RNAs that help regulate gene expression, particularly during development. The phenomenon of RNA interference, broadly defined, includes the endogenously induced gene silencing effects of miRNAs as well as silencing triggered by foreign dsRNA. Mature miRNAs are structurally similar to siRNAs produced from exogenous dsRNA, but before reaching maturity, miRNAs must first undergo extensive post-transcriptional modification. A miRNA is expressed from a much longer RNA-coding gene as a primary transcript known as a pri-miRNA which is processed, in the cell nucleus, to a 70-nucleotide stem-loop structure called a pre-miRNA by the microprocessor complex. This complex consists of an RNase III enzyme called Drosha and a dsRNA-binding protein DGCR8. The dsRNA portion of this pre-miRNA is bound and cleaved by Dicer to produce the mature miRNA molecule that can be integrated into the RISC complex, thus, miRNA and siRNA share the same downstream cellular machinery. First, viral encoded miRNA was described in EBV. Thereafter, an increasing number of microRNAs have been described in viruses. VIRmiRNA is a comprehensive catalogue covering viral microRNA, their targets and anti-viral miRNAs.

siRNAs derived from long dsRNA precursors differ from miRNAs in that miRNAs, especially those in animals, typically have incomplete base pairing to a target and inhibit the translation of many different mRNAs with similar sequences. In contrast, siRNAs typically base-pair perfectly and induce mRNA cleavage only in a single, specific target. In *Drosophila* and *C. elegans*, miRNA and siRNA are processed by distinct argonaute proteins and dicer enzymes.

Three Prime Untranslated Regions and microRNAs

Three prime untranslated regions (3′UTRs) of messenger RNAs (mRNAs) often contain regulatory sequences that post-transcriptionally cause RNA interference. Such 3′-UTRs often contain both binding sites for microRNAs (miRNAs) as well as for regulatory proteins. By binding to specific sites within the 3'-UTR, miRNAs can decrease gene expression of various mRNAs by either inhibiting translation or directly causing degradation of the transcript. The 3'-UTR also may have silencer regions that bind repressor proteins that inhibit the expression of a mRNA. The 3'-UTR often contains microRNA response elements (MREs). MREs are sequences to which miRNAs bind. These are prevalent motifs within 3'-UTRs. Among all regulatory motifs within the 3'-UTRs (e.g. including silencer regions), MREs make up about half of the motifs.

As of 2014, the miRBase web site, an archive of miRNA sequences and annotations, listed 28,645 entries in 233 biologic species. Of these, 1,881 miRNAs were in annotated human miRNA loci. miRNAs were predicted to have an average of about four hundred target mRNAs (affecting expression of several hundred genes). Friedman and others estimate that >45,000 miRNA target sites within human mRNA 3'UTRs are conserved above background levels, and >60% of human protein-coding genes have been under selective pressure to maintain pairing to miRNAs.

Direct experiments show that a single miRNA can reduce the stability of hundreds of unique mRNAs. Other experiments show that a single miRNA may repress the production of hundreds of proteins, but that this repression often is relatively mild (less than 2-fold).

The effects of miRNA dysregulation of gene expression seem to be important in cancer. For instance, in gastrointestinal cancers, nine miRNAs have been identified as epigenetically altered and effective in down regulating DNA repair enzymes. The effects of miRNA dysregulation of gene expression also seem to be important in neuropsychiatric disorders, such as schizophrenia, bipolar disorder, major depression, Parkinson's disease, Alzheimer's disease and autism spectrum disorders.

RISC Activation and Catalysis

Exogenous dsRNA is detected and bound by an effector protein, known as RDE-4 in *C. elegans* and R2D2 in *Drosophila*, that stimulates dicer activity. This protein only binds long dsRNAs, but the mechanism producing this length specificity is unknown. This RNA-binding protein then facilitates the transfer of cleaved siRNAs to the RISC complex. In *C. elegans* this initiation response is amplified through the synthesis of a population of 'secondary' siRNAs during which the dicer-produced initiating or 'primary' siRNAs are used as templates. These 'secondary' siRNAs are structurally distinct from dicer-produced siRNAs and appear to be produced by an RNA-dependent RNA polymerase (RdRP).

The active components of an RNA-induced silencing complex (RISC) are endonucleases called argonaute proteins, which cleave the target mRNA strand complementary to their bound siRNA. As the fragments produced by dicer are double-stranded, they could each in theory produce a functional siRNA. However, only one of the two strands, which is known as the guide strand, binds the argonaute protein and directs gene silencing. The other anti-guide strand or passenger strand is degraded during RISC activation. Although it was first believed that an ATP-dependent helicase separated these two strands, the process proved to be ATP-independent and performed directly by the protein components of RISC. However, an *in vitro* kinetic analysis of RNAi in the presence and absence of ATP showed that ATP may be required to unwind and remove the cleaved mRNA strand from the RISC complex after catalysis. The guide strand tends to be the one whose 5' end is less stably paired to its complement, but strand selection is unaffected by the direction in which dicer cleaves the dsRNA before RISC incorporation. Instead, the R2D2 protein may serve as the differentiating factor by binding the more-stable 5' end of the passenger strand.

The structural basis for binding of RNA to the argonaute protein was examined by X-ray crystallography of the binding domain of an RNA-bound argonaute protein. Here, the phosphorylated

5' end of the RNA strand enters a conserved basic surface pocket and makes contacts through a divalent cation (an atom with two positive charges) such as magnesium and by aromatic stacking (a process that allows more than one atom to share an electron by passing it back and forth) between the 5' nucleotide in the siRNA and a conserved tyrosine residue. This site is thought to form a nucleation site for the binding of the siRNA to its mRNA target. Analysis of the inhibitory effect of mismatches in either the 5' or 3' end of the guide strand has demonstrated that the 5' end of the guide strand is likely responsible for matching and binding the target mRNA, while the 3' end is responsible for physically arranging target mRNA into a cleavage-favorable RISC region.

It is not understood how the activated RISC complex locates complementary mRNAs within the cell. Although the cleavage process has been proposed to be linked to translation, translation of the mRNA target is not essential for RNAi-mediated degradation. Indeed, RNAi may be more effective against mRNA targets that are not translated. Argonaute proteins are localised to specific regions in the cytoplasm called P-bodies (also cytoplasmic bodies or GW bodies), which are regions with high rates of mRNA decay, miRNA activity is also clustered in P-bodies. Disruption of P-bodies decreases the efficiency of RNA interference, suggesting that they are a critical site in the RNAi process.

Transcriptional Silencing

Components of the RNAi pathway are used in many eukaryotes in the maintenance of the organisation and structure of their genomes. Modification of histones and associated induction of heterochromatin formation serves to downregulate genes pre-transcriptionally, this process is referred to as RNA-induced transcriptional silencing (RITS), and is carried out by a complex of proteins called the RITS complex. In fission yeast this complex contains argonaute, a chromodomain protein Chp1, and a protein called Tas3 of unknown function. As a consequence, the induction and spread of heterochromatic regions requires the argonaute and RdRP proteins. Indeed, deletion of these genes in the fission yeast *S. pombe* disrupts histone methylation and centromere formation, causing slow or stalled anaphase during cell division. In some cases, similar processes associated with histone modification have been observed to transcriptionally upregulate genes.

The mechanism by which the RITS complex induces heterochromatin formation and organisation is not well understood. Most studies have focused on the mating-type region in fission yeast, which may not be representative of activities in other genomic regions/organisms. In maintenance of existing heterochromatin regions, RITS forms a complex with siRNAs complementary to the local genes and stably binds local methylated histones, acting co-transcriptionally to degrade any nascent pre-mRNA transcripts that are initiated by RNA polymerase. The formation of such a heterochromatin region, though not its maintenance, is dicer-dependent, presumably because dicer is required to generate the initial complement of siRNAs that target subsequent transcripts. Heterochromatin maintenance has been suggested to function as a self-reinforcing feedback loop, as new siRNAs are formed from the occasional nascent transcripts by RdRP for incorporation into local RITS complexes. The relevance of observations from fission yeast mating-type regions and centromeres to mammals is not clear, as heterochromatin maintenance in mammalian cells may be independent of the components of the RNAi pathway.

Crosstalk with RNA Editing

The type of RNA editing that is most prevalent in higher eukaryotes converts adenosine nucleotides into inosine in dsRNAs via the enzyme adenosine deaminase (ADAR). It was originally proposed in 2000 that the RNAi and A→I RNA editing pathways might compete for a common dsRNA substrate.

Some pre-miRNAs do undergo A→I RNA editing and this mechanism may regulate the processing and expression of mature miRNAs. Furthermore, at least one mammalian ADAR can sequester siRNAs from RNAi pathway components. Further support for this model comes from studies on ADAR-null *C. elegans* strains indicating that A→I RNA editing may counteract RNAi silencing of endogenous genes and transgenes.

Variation among Organisms

Organisms vary in their ability to take up foreign dsRNA and use it in the RNAi pathway. The effects of RNA interference can be both systemic and heritable in plants and *C. elegans*, although not in *Drosophila* or mammals. In plants, RNAi is thought to propagate by the transfer of siRNAs between cells through plasmodesmata (channels in the cell walls that enable communication and transport). Heritability comes from methylation of promoters targeted by RNAi, the new methylation pattern is copied in each new generation of the cell. A broad general distinction between plants and animals lies in the targeting of endogenously produced miRNAs, in plants, miRNAs are usually perfectly or nearly perfectly complementary to their target genes and induce direct mRNA cleavage by RISC, while animals miRNAs tend to be more divergent in sequence and induce translational repression. This translational effect may be produced by inhibiting the interactions of translation initiation factors with the messenger RNAs polyadenine tail.

Some eukaryotic protozoa such as Leishmania major and Trypanosoma cruzi lack the RNAi pathway entirely. Most or all of the components are also missing in some fungi, most notably the model organism *Saccharomyces cerevisiae*. The presence of RNAi in other budding yeast species such as *Saccharomyces castellii* and Candida albicans, further demonstrates that inducing two RNAi-related proteins from *S. castellii* facilitates RNAi in *S. cerevisiae*. That certain ascomycetes and basidiomycetes are missing RNA interference pathways indicates that proteins required for RNA silencing have been lost independently from many fungal lineages, possibly due to the evolution of a novel pathway with similar function, or to the lack of selective advantage in certain niches.

Related Prokaryotic Systems

Gene expression in prokaryotes is influenced by an RNA-based system similar in some respects to RNAi. Here, RNA-encoding genes control mRNA abundance or translation by producing a complementary RNA that anneals to an mRNA. However these regulatory RNAs are not generally considered to be analogous to miRNAs because the dicer enzyme is not involved. It has been suggested that CRISPR interference systems in prokaryotes are analogous to eukaryotic RNA interference systems, although none of the protein components are orthologous.

Biological Functions of RNA Interference

Immunity

RNA interference is a vital part of the immune response to viruses and other foreign genetic material, especially in plants where it may also prevent the self-propagation of transposons. Plants such as *Arabidopsis thaliana* (Fig. 20.3) express multiple dicer homologs that are specialised to react differently when the plant is exposed to different viruses. Even before the RNAi pathway was fully understood, it was known that induced gene silencing in plants could spread throughout the plant in a systemic effect and could be transferred from stock to scion plants via grafting. This phenomenon has since been recognised as a feature of the plant adaptive immune system and allows the entire plant to respond to a

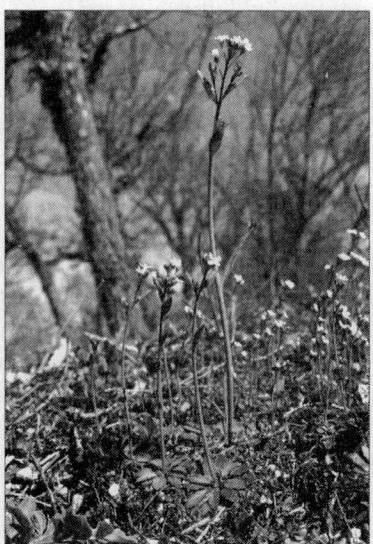

Fig. 20.3: *Arabidopsis thaliana.*

virus after an initial localised encounter. In response, many plant viruses have evolved elaborate mechanisms to suppress the RNAi response. These include viral proteins that bind short double-stranded RNA fragments with single-stranded overhang ends, such as those produced by dicer. Some plant genomes also express endogenous siRNAs in response to infection by specific types of bacteria. These effects may be part of a generalised response to pathogens that downregulates any metabolic process in the host that aids the infection process.

Although animals generally express fewer variants of the dicer enzyme than plants, RNAi in some animals produces an antiviral response. In both juvenile and adult *Drosophila*, RNA interference is important in antiviral innate immunity and is active against pathogens such as *Drosophila* X virus. A similar role in immunity may operate in *C. elegans*, as argonaute proteins are upregulated in response to viruses and worms that overexpress components of the RNAi pathway are resistant to viral infection.

The role of RNA interference in mammalian innate immunity is poorly understood, and relatively little data is available. However, the existence of viruses that encode genes able to suppress the RNAi response in mammalian cells may be evidence in favour of an RNAi-dependent mammalian immune response, although this hypothesis has been challenged as poorly substantiated. Evidence for the existence of a functional antiviral RNAi pathway in mammalian cells has been presented. Other functions for RNAi in mammalian viruses also exist, such as miRNAs expressed by the herpes virus that may act as heterochromatin organisation triggers to mediate viral latency.

Downregulation of genes

Endogenously expressed miRNAs, including both intronic and intergenic miRNAs, are most important in translational repression and in the regulation of development, especially on the timing of morphogenesis and the maintenance of undifferentiated or incompletely differentiated cell types such as stem cells. The role of endogenously expressed miRNA in downregulating gene expression was first described in *C. elegans* in 1993. In plants this function was discovered when the 'JAW microRNA' of Arabidopsis was shown to be involved in the regulation of several genes that control plant shape. In plants, the majority of genes regulated by miRNAs are transcription factors, thus miRNA activity is particularly wide-ranging and regulates entire gene networks during development by modulating the expression of key regulatory genes, including transcription factors as well as F-box proteins. In many organisms, including humans, miRNAs are linked to the formation of tumors and dysregulation of the cell cycle. Here, miRNAs can function as both oncogenes and tumor suppressors.

Upregulation of genes

RNA sequences (siRNA and miRNA) that are complementary to parts of a promoter can increase gene transcription, a phenomenon dubbed RNA activation. Part of the mechanism for how these RNA upregulate genes is known: dicer and argonaute are involved, possibly via histone demethylation. miRNAs have been proposed to upregulate their target genes upon cell cycle arrest, via unknown mechanisms.

Evolution

Based on parsimony-based phylogenetic analysis, the most recent common ancestor of all eukaryotes most likely already possessed an early RNA interference pathway, the absence of the pathway in certain eukaryotes is thought to be a derived characteristic. This ancestral RNAi system probably contained at least one dicer-like protein, one argonaute, one PIWI protein, and an RNA-dependent RNA polymerase that may also have played other cellular roles. A large-scale comparative genomics study likewise indicates that the eukaryotic crown group already possessed these components, which may then have had closer functional associations with generalised RNA degradation systems such as the exosome. This study also suggests that the RNA-binding argonaute protein family, which is shared among eukaryotes, most archaea, and at least some bacteria (such as Aquifex aeolicus), is homologous to and originally evolved from components of the translation initiation system.

The ancestral function of the RNAi system is generally agreed to have been immune defense against exogenous genetic elements such as transposons and viral genomes. Related functions such as histone modification may have already been present in the ancestor of modern eukaryotes, although other functions such as regulation of development by miRNA are thought to have evolved later.

RNA interference genes, as components of the antiviral innate immune system in many eukaryotes, are involved in an evolutionary arms race with viral genes. Some viruses have evolved mechanisms for suppressing the RNAi response in their host cells, particularly for plant viruses. Studies of evolutionary rates in *Drosophila* have shown that genes in the RNAi pathway are subject to strong directional selection and are among the fastest-evolving genes in the *Drosophila* genome.

Applications of RNA Interference

Gene knockdown

The RNA interference pathway is often exploited in experimental biology to study the function of genes in cell culture and *in vivo* in model organisms. Double-stranded RNA is synthesised with a sequence complementary to a gene of interest and introduced into a cell or organism, where it is recognised as exogenous genetic material and activates the RNAi pathway. Using this mechanism, researchers can cause a drastic decrease in the expression of a targeted gene. Studying the effects of this decrease can show the physiological role of the gene product. Since RNAi may not totally abolish expression of the gene, this technique is sometimes referred as a 'knockdown', to distinguish it from 'knockout' procedures in which expression of a gene is entirely eliminated. In a recent study validation of RNAi silencing efficiency using gene array data showed 18.5% failure rate across 429 independent experiments.

Extensive efforts in computational biology have been directed toward the design of successful dsRNA reagents that maximise gene knockdown but minimise 'off-target' effects. Off-target effects arise when an introduced RNA has a base sequence that can pair with and thus reduce the expression of multiple genes. Such problems occur more frequently when the dsRNA contains repetitive sequences. It has been estimated from studying the genomes of humans, *C. elegans* and *S. pombe* that about 10% of possible siRNAs have substantial off-target effects. A multitude of software tools have been developed implementing algorithms for the design of general mammal-specific, and virus-specific siRNAs that are automatically checked for possible cross-reactivity.

Depending on the organism and experimental system, the exogenous RNA may be a long strand designed to be cleaved by dicer, or short RNAs designed to serve as siRNA substrates. In most mammalian cells, shorter RNAs are used because long double-stranded RNA molecules induce the mammalian interferon response, a form of innate immunity that reacts nonspecifically to foreign genetic material. Mouse oocytes and cells from early mouse embryos lack this reaction to exogenous dsRNA and are therefore a common model system for studying mammalian gene-knockdown effects.

Specialised laboratory techniques have also been developed to improve the utility of RNAi in mammalian systems by avoiding the direct introduction of siRNA, for example, by stable transfection with a plasmid encoding the appropriate sequence from which siRNAs can be transcribed, or by more elaborate lentiviral vector systems allowing the inducible activation or deactivation of transcription, known as conditional RNAi.

Functional Genomics

Most functional genomics applications of RNAi in animals have used *C. elegans* and *Drosophila*, as these are the common model organisms in which RNAi is most effective. *C. elegans* is particularly useful for RNAi research for two reasons: firstly, the effects of gene silencing are generally heritable, and secondly because delivery of the dsRNA is extremely simple. Through a mechanism whose details are poorly understood, bacteria such as *E. coli* that carry the desired dsRNA can be fed to the worms and will transfer their RNA payload to the worm via the intestinal tract. This 'delivery by feeding' is just as effective at inducing gene silencing as more costly and time-consuming delivery methods, such as soaking the worms in dsRNA solution and injecting dsRNA into the gonads. Although delivery is more difficult in most other organisms, efforts are also underway to undertake large-scale genomic screening applications in cell culture with mammalian cells.

Approaches to the design of genome-wide RNAi libraries can require more sophistication than the design of a single siRNA for a defined set of experimental conditions. Artificial neural networks are frequently used to design siRNA libraries and to predict their likely efficiency at gene knockdown. Mass genomic screening is widely seen as a promising method for genome annotation and has triggered the development of high-throughput screening methods based on microarrays. However, the utility of these screens and the ability of techniques developed on model organisms to generalise to even closely related species has been questioned, for example from *C. elegans* to related parasitic nematodes.

Functional genomics using RNAi is a particularly attractive technique for genomic mapping and annotation in plants because many plants are polyploid, which presents substantial challenges for more traditional genetic engineering methods. For example, RNAi has been successfully used for functional genomics studies in bread wheat (which is hexaploid) as well as more common plant model systems Arabidopsis and maize.

Medicine

The first instance of RNA silencing in animals was documented in 1996, when Guo and Kemphues observed that, by introducing sense and antisense RNA to par-1 mRNA in Caenorhabditis elegans caused degradation of the par-1 message. It was thought that this degradation was triggered by single stranded RNA (ssRNA), but two years later, in 1998, Fire and Mello discovered that this ability to silence the par-1 gene expression was actually triggered by double-stranded RNA (dsRNA). They would eventually share the Nobel Prize in Physiology or Medicine for this discovery. Just after Fire and Mello's groundbreaking discovery, Elbashir and others discovered, by using synthetically made small interfering RNA (siRNA), it was possible to target the silencing of specific sequences in a gene, rather than silencing the entire gene. Only a year later, McCaffrey and colleagues demonstrated that this sequence specific silencing had therapeutic applications by targeting a sequence from the Hepatitis C virus in transgenic mice. Since then, multiple researchers have been attempting to expand the therapeutic applications of RNAi, specifically looking to target genes that cause various types of cancer.

Finally, in 2004, this new gene silencing technology entered a Phase I clinical trial in humans for wet age-related macular degeneration. Six years later the first-in-human Phase I clinical trial was started, using a nanoparticle delivery system to target solid tumors. Although most research is currently looking into the applications of RNAi in cancer treatment, the list of possible applications is extensive. RNAi could potentially be used to treat viruses, bacterial diseases, parasites, maladaptive genetic mutations, control drug consumption, provide pain relief, and even modulate sleep.

Therapeutic applications

Viral infection: Antiviral treatment is one of the earliest proposed RNAi-based medical applications, and two different types have been developed. The first type is to target viral RNAs. Many studies have shown that targeting viral RNAs can suppress the replication of numerous viruses, including HIV, HPV, hepatitis A, hepatitis B, Influenza virus, Respiratory syncytial virus (RSV), SARS coronavirus (SARS-CoV), Adenovirus and Measles virus. The other strategy is to block the initial viral entries by targeting the host cell genes. For example, suppression of chemokine receptors (CXCR4 and CCR5)on host cells can prevent HIV viral entry.

Cancer: While traditional chemotherapy can effectively kill cancer cells, lack of specificity for discriminating normal cells and cancer cells in these treatments usually cause severe side effects. Numerous studies have demonstrated that RNAi can provide a more specific approach to inhibit tumor growth by targeting cancer-related genes (i.e. oncogene). It has also been proposed that RNAi can enhance the sensitivity of cancer cells to chemotherapeutic agents, providing a combinatorial therapeutic approach with chemotherapy. Another potential RNAi-based treatment is to inhibit cell invasion and migration.

Neurological diseases: RNAi strategies also show potential for treating neurodegenerative diseases. Studies in cells and in mouse have shown that specifically targeting Amyloid beta-producing genes (e.g. BACE1 and APP) by RNAi can significantly reduced the amount of Aβ peptide which is correlated with the cause of Alzheimers disease. In addition, this silencing-based approaches also provide promising results in treatment of Parkinsons disease and Polyglutamine disease.

Difficulties in therapeutic application

To achieve the clinical potential of RNAi, siRNA must be efficiently transported to the cells of target tissues. However, there are various barriers that must be fixed before it can be used clinically. For example,

'Naked' siRNA is susceptible to several obstacles that reduce its therapeutic efficacy. Additionally, once siRNA has entered the bloodstream, naked RNA can be degraded by serum nucleases and can stimulate the innate immune system. Due to its size and highly polyanionic (containing negative charges at several sites) nature, unmodified siRNA molecules cannot readily enter the cells through the cell membrane. Therefore, artificial or nanoparticle encapsulated siRNA must be used. However, transporting siRNA across the cell membrane still has its own unique challenges. If siRNA is transferred across the cell membrane, unintended toxicities can occur if therapeutic doses are not optimised, and siRNAs can exhibit off-target effects (e.g. unintended downregulation of genes with partial sequence complementarity). Even after entering the cells, repeated dosing is required since their effects are diluted at each cell division.

Safety and uses in cancer treatment

Compared with chemotherapy or other anti-cancer drugs, there are a lot of advantages of siRNA drug. SiRNA acts on the post-translational stage of gene expression, so it doesn't modify or change DNA in a deleterious effect. SiRNA can also be used to produced a specific response in a certain type of way, such as by downgrading suppression of gene expression. In a single cancer cell, siRNA can cause dramatic suppression of gene expression with just several copies. This happens by silencing cancer-promoting genes with RNAi, as well as targeting an mRNA sequence.

RNAi drugs treat cancer by silencing certain cancer promoting genes. This is done by complementing the cancer genes with the RNAi, such as keeping the mRNA sequences in accordance with the RNAi drug. Ideally, RNAi is should be injected and/or chemically modified so the RNAi can reach cancer cells more efficiently. RNAi uptake and regulation is monitored by the kidneys.

Stimulation of immune response

The human immune system is divided into two separate branches: the innate immune system and the adaptive immune system. The innate immune system is the first defense against infection and responds to pathogens in a generic fashion. On the other hand, the adaptive immune system, a system that was evolved later than the innate, is composed mainly of highly specialised B and T cells that are trained to react to specific portions of pathogenic molecules.

The challenge between old pathogens and new has helped create a system of guarded cells and particles that are called safe framework. This framework has given humans an army systems that search out and destroy invader particles, such as pathogens, microscopic organisms, parasites, and infections. The mammalian safe framework has developed to incorporate siRNA as a tool to indicate viral contamination, which has allowed siRNA is create an intense innate immune response.

siRNA is controlled by the innate immune system, which can be divided into the acute inflammatory responses and antiviral responses. The inflammatory response is created with signals from small signaling molecules, or cytokines. These include interleukin-1 (IL-1), interleukin-6 (IL-6), interleukin-12 (IL-12) and tumor necrosis factor a (TNF-α). The innate immune system generates inflammation and antiviral responses, which cause the release pattern recognition receptors (PRRs). These receptors help in labeling which pathogens are viruses, fungi, or bacteria. Moreover, the importance of siRNA and the innate immune system is to include more PRRs to help recognise different RNA structures. This makes it more likely for the siRNA to cause an immunostimulant response in the event of the pathogen.

Prospects as a therapeutic technique

Clinical Phase I and II studies of siRNA therapies conducted between 2015 and 2017 have demonstrated potent and durable gene knockdown in the liver, with some signs of clinical improvement and without unacceptable toxicity. Two Phase III studies are in progress to treat familial neurodegenerative and cardiac syndromes caused by mutations in transthyretin (TTR). Numerous publications have shown that *in vivo* delivery systems are very promising and are diverse in characteristics, allowing numerous applications. The nanoparticle delivery system shows the most promise yet this method presents additional challenges in the scale-up of the manufacturing process, such as the need for tightly controlled mixing processes to achieve consistent quality of the drug product.

Biotechnology

RNA interference has been used for applications in biotechnology and is nearing commercialisation in other fields. RNAi has resulted in the invention of novel crops such as nicotine-free tobacco, decaffeinated coffee, nutrient fortified vegetation, and hypoallergenic crops. The genetically-engineered Arctic apples received FDA approval in 2015. The apples were produced by RNAi suppression of the PPO (polyphenol oxidase) gene, making apple varieties that will not undergo browning after being sliced. PPO-silenced apples are unable to convert chlorogenic acid into the standard quinone product.

There are several opportunities for the applications of RNAi in crop science for its improvement such as stress tolerance and enhanced nutritional level. RNAi will prove its potential for inhibition of photorespiration to enhance the productivity of C3 plants. This knockdown technology may be useful in inducing early flowering, delayed ripening, delayed senescence, breaking dormancy, stress-free plants, overcoming self-sterility, etc.

Foods: RNAi has been used to genetically engineer plants to produce lower levels of natural plant toxins. Such techniques take advantage of the stable and heritable RNAi phenotype in plant stocks. Cotton seeds are rich in dietary protein but naturally contain the toxic terpenoid product gossypol, making them unsuitable for human consumption. RNAi has been used to produce cotton stocks whose seeds contain reduced levels of delta-cadinene synthase, a key enzyme in gossypol production, without affecting the enzymes production in other parts of the plant, where gossypol is itself important in preventing damage from plant pests. Similar efforts have been directed toward the reduction of the cyanogenic natural product linamarin in cassava plants.

No plant products that use RNAi-based genetic engineering have yet exited the experimental stage. Development efforts have successfully reduced the levels of allergens in tomato plants and fortification of plants such as tomatoes with dietary antioxidants. Previous commercial products, including the Flavr Savr tomato and two cultivars of ringspot-resistant papaya, were originally developed using antisense technology but likely exploited the RNAi pathway. RNAi silencing of alpha-amylase have also been used to decrease *Aspergillus flavus* fungal growth in maize which would have otherwise contaminated the kernels with dangerous aflatoxins. Silencing lachrymatory factor synthase in onions have produced tearless onions and RNAi has been used in BP1 genes in rapeseeds to improve photosynthesis. SBEIIa and SBEIIb genes in wheat have been targeted in wheat in order to produce higher levels of amylose in order to improve bowel function.

Other crops: Another effort decreased the precursors of likely carcinogens in tobacco plants. Other plant traits that have been engineered in the laboratory include the production of non-narcotic natural products by the opium poppy and resistance to common plant viruses.

Insecticide: RNAi is under development as an insecticide, employing multiple approaches, including genetic engineering and topical application. Cells in the midgut of some insects take up the dsRNA molecules in the process referred to as environmental RNAi. In some insects the effect is systemic as the signal spreads throughout the insects body (referred to as systemic RNAi).

Animals exposed to RNAi at doses millions of times higher than anticipated human exposure levels show no adverse effects. RNAi has varying effects in different species of Lepidoptera (butterflies and moths). Possibly because their saliva and gut juice is better at breaking down RNA, the cotton bollworm, the beet armyworm and the Asiatic rice borer have so far not been proven susceptible to RNAi by feeding. To develop resistance to RNAi, the western corn rootworm would have to change the genetic sequence of its Snf7 gene at multiple sites. Combining multiple strategies, such as engineering the protein Cry, derived from a bacterium called *Bacillus thuringiensis* (*Bt*), and RNAi in one plant delay the onset of resistance.

Transgenic plants: Transgenic crops have been made to express dsRNA, carefully chosen to silence crucial genes in target pests. These dsRNAs are designed to affect only insects that express specific gene sequences. As a proof of principle, in 2009 a study showed RNAs that could kill any one of four fruit fly species while not harming the other three.

In 2012 Syngenta bought Belgian RNAi firm Devgen for $522 million and Monsanto paid $29.2 million for the exclusive rights to intellectual property from Alnylam Pharmaceuticals. The International Potato Center in Lima, Peru is looking for genes to target in the sweet potato weevil, a beetle whose larvae ravage sweet potatoes globally. Other researchers are trying to silence genes in ants, caterpillars and pollen beetles. Monsanto was the first to market, with a transgenic corn seed that expresses dsRNA based on gene Snf7 from the western corn rootworm, a beetle whose larvae annually cause one billion dollars in damage in the United States alone. A 2012 paper showed that silencing Snf7 stunts larval growth, killing them within days. In 2013 the same team showed that the RNA affects very few other species.

Topical: Alternatively dsRNA can be supplied without genetic engineering. One approach is to add them to irrigation water. The molecules are absorbed into the plants' vascular system and poison insects feeding on them. Another approach involves spraying dsRNA like a conventional pesticide. This would allow faster adaptation to resistance. Such approaches would require low cost sources of dsRNAs that do not currently exist

Genome-scale screening: Genome-scale RNAi research relies on high-throughput screening (HTS) technology. RNAi HTS technology allows genome-wide loss-of-function screening and is broadly used in the identification of genes associated with specific phenotypes. This technology has been hailed as a potential second genomics wave, following the first genomics wave of gene expression microarray and single nucleotide polymorphism discovery platforms. One major advantage of genome-scale RNAi screening is its ability to simultaneously interrogate thousands of genes. With the ability to generate a large amount of data per experiment, genome-scale RNAi screening has led to an explosion of data generation rates. Exploiting such large data sets is a fundamental challenge, requiring suitable statistics/bioinformatics methods. The basic process of cell-based RNAi screening includes the choice of an RNAi library, robust and stable cell types, transfection with RNAi agents, treatment/incubation, signal detection, analysis and identification of important genes or therapeutical targets.

RNAI – PERSPECTIVES FOR THE FUTURE

RNAi is a potentially powerful research tool for a wide variety of gene-silencing applications. Possible repercussions of RNAi in mammals are its use in the fight against certain diseases, such as cancer or virus and parasite infections, as well as in the analysis of problems in cell and developmental biology: there are, for example, many efficient human and murine siRNA sequences against members of apoptotic pathways, such as caspase-1, -2, -3, -8, and Fas. RNAi can also be used to study the functions and interactions of genes. siRNAs are easily synthesised and used to silence genes in cell cultures, and it is possible that silencing cell lines will be obtained. One of the earliest uses of RNAi technology in drug development has been its application in functional genomic analyses. During these studies many components of complex pathways have been identified and isolated and their relevance to various drug discovery applications has been assessed. RNAi can be used as a tool to identify possible novel targets in drug discovery. This approach has several advantages: it permits rapid target identification and processing and does not depend on preexisting knowledge of target biology. Using bioinformatics, libraries of designed siRNAs (several different siRNAs oligos per gene) can be used to elucidate novel targets for any biological pathway. This method allows for the functional analysis of thousands of genes simultaneously, is highly reproducible, and requires small amounts of siRNA oligos. This procedure allows for high-throughput testing of potential targets without compromising high specificity and sensitivity. siRNAs could also represent the next generation of antiviral therapeutics, and DNAs encoding siRNAs should be useful in various forms of gene therapy. The activation of siRNAs appears to be short-lived in mammals. They are sequence-specific natural cellular products, do not produce toxic metabolites, have a long life-span in cell culture and calf serum, and are efficient even in low concentrations.

Introducing siRNAs reduces the immune response against newly introduced agents, which may be a problem in gene therapy. Delivering of siRNAs to the appropriate cells is a major challenge. Effective strategies to deliver siRNAs to target cells in a cell culture include physical (electroporation, injection) or chemical (lipid-mediated gene delivery or a new designed method: the peptide-based gene delivery system MPG) transfection (Table 20.1). Chemical synthesis of siRNA is the most commonly used method to generate RNAi. T7-transcribed siRNAs as well as siRNAs isolated from *D. melanogaster* embryo protein extracts were also shown to be effective (Table 20.1). It may be difficult to introduce short dsRNAs directly into cells. An alternative strategy uses the endogenous expression of siRNAs by various RNA polymerase III promoter systems (mouse U6, human H1, tRNA promoters) that allow transcription of functional siRNAs or their precursors.

Table 20.1: siRNA delivery strategies.

Physical methods	Chemical methods	
Electroporation	Lipid-mediated gene delivery	
Injection	Peptide-mediated gene delivery	
	siRNA	
Isolated from *Drosophila* embryo	Synthetic RNAs	Plasmid generated RNAs
	siRNAs, dsRNA	siRNas pol III promoters-mouse U6, human H1, tRNA promoter
		dsRNAs pol II and T7 promoters

This way the produced siRNAs could be expressed for longer periods than exogenously introduced siRNAs, particularly in cells where the expression unit will integrate with the host genome. Zheng and others have developed a dual-promoter siRNA expression system (pDual) in which a synthetic DNA encoding a gene-specific siRNA sequence is inserted between two different opposing polymerase III promoters, the mouse U6 and human H1 promoters. Upon transfection into mammalian cells, the sense and antisense strands of the duplex are transcribed by these two promoters from the same template, resulting in an siRNA duplex with a uridine overhang on each 3′ terminus, similar to the siRNA generated by Dicer. These siRNAs can be incorporated into the RISC without any further modifications and specifically and efficiently suppress gene functions. Furthermore, they have developed a single-step PCR protocol that allows the production of siRNA expression cassettes in a high-throughput manner and they have constructed an arrayed siRNA expression cassette library that targets about 8000 genes with two sequences per gene. Injection of plasmid DNA expressing long cytoplasmic dsRNA induces efficient RNAi in nonembryonic mammalian cells without stress response pathways. This approach may prove to be the best method of inducing RNAi in mammals. In this case there will be simultaneous expression of a large number of siRNAs from a single precursor dsRNA, and longer dsRNA could include more than one message in a single construct. Liver cells seem to be particularly receptive to exogenous RNA. Neurons seem to be more resistant to RNAi than other cell types, perhaps because of differences related to RNA transport across the cell membrane or the RNAi pathway in these cells. It has been claimed that very high concentrations of dsRNAs (15 μg/ml) can induce inhibition of target gene expression in proliferating and differentiating cells in a nematode neuronal culture. Better delivery methods are required before siRNAs can be used as therapeutics, especially to suppress gene expression in tissues other than liver. Recently, vectors have been investigated which contain a cytomegalovirus (CMV) promoter and express long (about 500 nucleotides) dsRNAs, but these dsRNAs are not transported into cytoplasm and do not induce the interferon response. These dsRNAs are cleaved into siRNAs in the nucleus and are then transported to the cytosol, where they silence the target mRNA. This system is based on the polymerase II promoter and, although the CMV promoter is active in most cell types, these findings are a first step toward the use of tissue-specific polymerase II promoters. The potential advantage of this method is that there are numerous tissue-specific polymerase II promoters available.

RNAi is a good candidate for an antiviral drug. Recently some studies have shown the capacity of chemically synthesised siRNAs to specifically inhibit some viruses. Pre-treatment of human and mouse cells with siRNAs to a virus genome reduced the titer of virus progeny and promoted clearance of the virus from most infected cells. For example, RNAi can inhibit HIV-1 replication in mammalian cells at multiple steps of the HIV life cycle. SiRNAs may induce the cleavage of pre-integrated RNA or interfere with post-integration HIV-1 RNA transcripts and block progeny virus production. SiRNAs targeting CD4, CXCR4, or CCR5 RNA transcripts inhibit virus attachment to the CD4 receptor (the main receptor for HIV on the cell surface) or chemokine receptors (coreceptors for HIV) mediating HIV-1 fusion and entry. Effective blockade of receptors or coreceptors which are expressed on the cell surface represents a new strategy in therapy.

Good examples are chemokine receptors involved in inflammatory, allergic, and immunoregulatory disorders. Overexpression of CXCR4 has been associated with a number of malignant disorders, such as metastasis of breast carcinoma cells, angiogenesis of normal and tumor tissue, or B cell chronic lymphocytic leukemia. Thus, CXCR4 may be an important therapeutic target. The involvement of CCR5 in inflammatory processes and rheumatoid arthritis has been documented. Selective viral vectors containing siRNAs directed to CXCR4 and CCR5 in specifically targeted cells or after *ex vivo* manipulation of stem cells could be used to alter the role of chemokine receptors in various diseases.

Another receptor involved in the development of some disorders is the Fas receptor. Fas-mediated apoptosis is implicated in a broad spectrum of liver diseases, where inhibition of hepatocyte death would be a live-saving measure. Song and others investigated the *in vivo* silencing effect of siRNAs targeting the Fas gene encoding the Fas receptor to protect mice from liver failure and fibrosis in two models of autoimmune hepatitis. Intravenous injection of Fas siRNA specifically reduced Fas mRNA levels in mouse hepatocytes. Hepatocytes isolated from mice treated with Fas siRNAs were resistant to apoptosis, which is a sign that silencing expression with RNAi could be used in therapy to prevent liver injury by protecting hepatocytes from cytotoxicity. In another investigation siRNA was used against caspase-8 to prevent not only Fas-specific liver injury, but also acute liver failure induced by the wild-type adenovirus. The RNAi methodology has also been used as a tool against severe acute respiratory syndrome-associated coronavirus (SARS-CoV), which is responsible for SARS. The siRNA used specifically and effectively inhibited Spike protein from SARS-CoV. This protein is probably important in the interaction with the host cell surface receptors and the fusion event between the viral envelope and cellular membrane. Therefore, thanks to RNAi technology it is possible to block viron entrance into host cells and inhibit SARS-CoV infection. RNAi also blocks poliovirus, respiratory syncytial virus, and human papilloma virus infections and could be easily extended to other human viruses.

To sum up, the use of genetic modelling systems such as RNAi has been the key to understanding gene structure and function, the biology of cells and organisms and, ultimately, the molecular aspects of human disease. Libraries of short RNAs or of DNA vectors encoding short RNAs have been generated to target a few thousand human genes to determine their functions. Unlike classical antisense techniques, dsRNAs act as powerful gene silencers, which influences their therapeutic potential. As an ideal therapeutic, RNAi should also act selectively, long-term, and be able to systemically modulate gene targets distal from the inoculation area. A major problem in therapeutic gene silencing is still the delivery problem. The improvement of *in vivo* nucleic acid delivery technologies is the most important obstacle to overcome for scientists in the coming years. These small RNA molecules will probably have several applications in biology and in medicine in the future.

SECTION V

Genomes, Proteomics and System Biology

Chapter 21

Genomes and Transcriptomes

INTRODUCTION

Genomics focuses on the dynamic aspects such as gene transcription, translation and protein – protein interactions, as opposed to the static aspects of the genomic information such as DNA sequence or structures. Functional genomics attempts to answer questions about the function of DNA at the levels of genes, RNA transcripts and protein products. A key characteristic of functional genomics studies is their genome-wide approach to these questions, generally involving high-throughput methods rather than a more traditional 'gene-by-gene' approach.

Functional genomics is a field of molecular biology that attempts to make use of the vast wealth of data produced by genomic projects (such as genome sequencing projects) to describe gene (and protein) functions and interactions. Unlike genomics, functional genomics focuses on the dynamic aspects such as gene transcription, translation, and protein–protein interactions, as opposed to the static aspects of the genomic information such as DNA sequence or structures. Functional genomics attempts to answer questions about the function of DNA at the levels of genes, RNA transcripts, and protein products. A key characteristic of functional genomics studies is their genome-wide approach to these questions, generally involving high-throughput methods rather than a more traditional 'gene-by-gene' approach.

GOALS OF FUNCTIONAL GENOMICS

The goal of functional genomics is to understand the relationship between an organisms genome and its phenotype. The term functional genomics is often used broadly to refer to the many possible approaches to understanding the properties and function of the entirety of an organisms genes and gene products. This definition is somewhat variable, Gibson and Muse define it as 'approaches under development to ascertain the biochemical, cellular, and/or physiological properties of each and every gene product', while Pevsner includes the study of nongenic elements in his definition: 'the genome-wide study of the function of DNA (including genes and nongenic elements), as well as the nucleic acid and protein products encoded by DNA'. Functional genomics involves studies of natural variation in genes, RNA, and proteins over time (such as an organisms development) or space (such as its body regions), as well as studies of natural or experimental functional disruptions affecting genes, chromosomes, RNA, or proteins.

The promise of functional genomics is to expand and synthesise genomic and proteomic knowledge into an understanding of the dynamic properties of an organism at cellular and/or organismal levels. This would provide a more complete picture of how biological function arises from the information encoded in an organisms genome. The possibility of understanding how a particular mutation leads to a given phenotype has important implications for human genetic diseases, as answering these questions could point scientists in the direction of a treatment or cure.

TECHNIQUES AND APPLICATIONS OF GENOMICS

Functional genomics includes function-related aspects of the genome itself such as mutation and polymorphism (such as single nucleotide polymorphism (SNP) analysis), as well as measurement of molecular activities. The latter comprise a number of '-omics' such as transcriptomics (gene expression), proteomics (protein expression), and metabolomics. Functional genomics uses mostly multiplex techniques to measure the abundance of many or all gene products such as mRNAs or proteins within a biological sample. Together these measurement modalities endeavor to quantitate the various biological processes and improve our understanding of gene and protein functions and interactions.

At the DNA Level

Genetic interaction mapping

Systematic pairwise deletion of genes or inhibition of gene expression can be used to identify genes with related function, even if they do not interact physically. Epistasis refers to the fact that effects for two different gene knockouts may not be additive, that is, the phenotype that results when two genes are inhibited may be different from the sum of the effects of single knockouts.

The ENCODE project

The ENCODE (Encyclopedia of DNA elements) project is an in-depth analysis of the human genome whose goal is to identify all the functional elements of genomic DNA, in both coding and noncoding regions. To this point, only the pilot phase of the study has been completed, involving hundreds of assays performed on 44 regions of known or unknown function comprising 1% of the human genome. Important results include evidence from genomic tiling arrays that most nucleotides are transcribed as coding transcripts, noncoding RNAs, or random transcripts, the discovery of additional transcriptional regulatory sites, further elucidation of chromatin-modifying mechanisms.

At the RNA Level: Transcriptome Profiling

Microarrays

Microarrays measure the amount of mRNA in a sample that corresponds to a given gene or probe DNA sequence. Probe sequences are immobilised on a solid surface and allowed to hybridise with fluorescently labelled 'target' mRNA. The intensity of fluorescence of a spot is proportional to the amount of target sequence that has hybridised to that spot, and therefore to the abundance of that mRNA sequence in the sample. Microarrays allow for identification of candidate genes involved in a given process based on variation between transcript levels for different conditions and shared expression patterns with genes of known function.

SAGE

SAGE (serial analysis of gene expression) is an alternate method of gene expression analysis based on RNA sequencing rather than hybridisation. SAGE relies on the sequencing of 10–17 base pair tags which are unique to each gene.

These tags are produced from poly-A mRNA and ligated end-to-end before sequencing. SAGE gives an unbiased measurement of the number of transcripts per cell, since it does not depend on prior knowledge of what transcripts to study (as microarrays do).

At the Protein Level: Protein–Protein Interactions

Yeast two-hybrid system

A yeast two-hybrid (Y2H) screen tests a 'bait' protein against many potential interacting proteins ('prey') to identify physical protein–protein interactions. This system is based on a transcription factor, originally GAL4, whose separate DNA-binding and transcription activation domains are both required in order for the protein to cause transcription of a reporter gene. In a Y2H screen, the 'bait protein is fused to the binding domain of GAL4, and a library of potential 'prey' (interacting) proteins is recombinantly expressed in a vector with the activation domain. *In vivo* interaction of bait and prey proteins in a yeast cell brings the activation and binding domains of GAL4 close enough together to result in expression of a reporter gene. It is also possible to systematically test a library of bait proteins against a library of prey proteins to identify all possible interactions in a cell.

Affinity purification and mass spectrometry (AP/MS)

Affinity purification and mass spectrometry (AP/MS) is able to identify proteins that interact with one another in complexes. Complexes of proteins are allowed to form around a particular 'bait' protein. The bait protein is identified using an antibody or a recombinant tag which allows it to be extracted along with any proteins that have formed a complex with it. The proteins are then digested into short peptide fragments and mass spectrometry is used to identify the proteins based on the mass-to-charge ratios of those fragments.

Loss-of-function Techniques

Mutagenesis

Gene function can be investigated by systematically 'knocking out' genes one by one. This is done by either deletion or disruption of function (such as by insertional mutagenesis) and the resulting organisms are screened for phenotypes that provide clues to the function of the disrupted gene.

RNAi

RNA interference (RNAi) methods can be used to transiently silence or knock down gene expression using ~20 base-pair double-stranded RNA typically delivered by transfection of synthetic ~20-mer short-interfering RNA molecules (siRNAs) or by virally encoded short-hairpin RNAs (shRNAs). RNAi screens, typically performed in cell culture-based assays or experimental organisms (such as *C. elegans*) can be used to systematically disrupt nearly every gene in a genome or subsets of genes (sub-genomes), possible functions of disrupted genes can be assigned based on observed phenotypes.

Functional Annotations for Genes

Genome annotation

Putative genes can be identified by scanning a genome for regions likely to encode proteins, based on characteristics such as long open reading frames, transcriptional initiation sequences, and polyadenylation sites. A sequence identified as a putative gene must be confirmed by further evidence, such as similarity to cDNA or EST sequences from the same organism, similarity of the predicted protein sequence to known proteins, association with promoter sequences, or evidence that mutating the sequence produces an observable phenotype.

Rosetta stone approach

The Rosetta stone approach is a computation method of *de novo* protein function prediction, based on the hypothesis that some proteins involved in a given physiological process may exist as two separate genes in one organism and as a single gene in another. Genomes are scanned for sequences that are independent in one organism and in a single open reading frame in another. If two genes have fused, it is predicted that they have similar biological functions that make such coregulation advantageous.

Functional Genomics and Bioinformatics

Because of the large quantity of data produced by these techniques and the desire to find biologically meaningful patterns, bioinformatics is crucial to analysis of functional genomics data. Examples of techniques in this class are data clustering or principal component analysis for unsupervised machine learning (class detection) as well as artificial neural networks or support vector machines for supervised machine learning (class prediction, classification). Functional enrichment analysis is used to determine the extent of over- or under-expression (positive- or negative- regulators in case of RNAi screens) of functional categories relative to a background sets. Gene ontology based enrichment analysis are provided by DAVID and Gene Set Enrichment Analysis (GSEA), pathway based analysis by Ingenuity and Pathway studio and protein complex based analysis by COMPLEAT.

STRUCTURAL GENOMICS

Structural genomics seeks to describe the 3-dimensional structure of every protein encoded by a given genome. This genome-based approach allows for a high-throughput method of structure determination by a combination of experimental and modelling approaches. The principal difference between structural genomics and traditional structural prediction is that structural genomics attempts to determine the structure of every protein encoded by the genome, rather than focusing on one particular protein. With full-genome sequences available, structure prediction can be done more quickly through a combination of experimental and modelling approaches, especially because the availability of large number of sequenced genomes and previously solved protein structures allows scientists to model protein structure on the structures of previously solved homologs. Because protein structure is closely linked with protein function, the structural genomics has the potential to inform knowledge of protein function. In addition to elucidating protein functions, structural genomics can be used to identify novel protein folds and potential targets for drug discovery. Structural genomics involves taking a large number of approaches to structure determination, including experimental methods using genomic sequences or modelling-based approaches based on sequence or structural homology to a protein of known structure or based on chemical and physical principles for a protein with no homology to any known structure.

As opposed to traditional structural biology, the determination of a protein structure through a structural genomics effort often (but not always) comes before anything is known regarding the protein function. This raises new challenges in structural bioinformatics, i.e. determining protein function from its 3D structure. Structural genomics emphasises high throughput determination of protein structures. This is performed in dedicated centers of structural genomics.

While most structural biologists pursue structures of individual proteins or protein groups, specialists in structural genomics pursue structures of proteins on a genome wide scale. This implies large-scale cloning, expression and purification. One main advantage of this approach is economy of scale. On the other hand, the scientific value of some resultant structures is at times questioned. One advantage of structural genomics, such as the Protein Structure Initiative, is that the scientific community gets immediate access to new structures, as well as to reagents such as clones and protein. A disadvantage is that many of these structures are of proteins of unknown function and do not have corresponding publications. This requires new ways of communicating this structural information to the broader research community. The Bioinformatics core of the Joint center for structural genomics (JCSG) has recently developed a wiki-based approach namely Open protein structure annotation network (TOPSAN) (link) for annotating protein structures emerging from high-throughput structural genomics centers.

Goals of Structural Genomics

One goal of structural genomics is to identify novel protein folds. Experimental methods of protein structure determination require proteins that express and/or crystallise well, which may inherently bias the kinds of proteins folds that this experimental data elucidate. A genomic, modelling-based approach such as *ab initio* modelling may be better able to identify novel protein folds than the experimental approaches because they are not limited by experimental constraints.

Protein function depends on 3-D structure and these 3-D structures are more highly conserved than sequences. Thus, the high-throughput structure determination methods of structural genomics have the potential to inform our understanding of protein functions. This also has potential implications for drug discovery and protein engineering. Furthermore, every protein that is added to the structural database increases the likelihood that the database will include homologous sequences of other unknown proteins. The Protein Structure Initiative (PSI) is a multifaceted effort funded by the National Institutes of Health with various academic and industrial partners that aims to increase knowledge of protein structure using a structural genomics approach and to improve structure-determination methodology.

Methods

Structural genomics takes advantage of completed genome sequences in several ways in order to determine protein structures. The gene sequence of the target protein can also be compared to a known sequence and structural information can then be inferred from the known protein's structure. Structural genomics can be used to predict novel protein folds based on other structural data. Structural genomics can also take modelling-based approach that relies on homology between the unknown protein and a solved protein structure.

de novo methods

Completed genome sequences allow every open reading frame (ORF), the part of a gene that is likely to contain the sequence for the mRNA and protein, to be cloned and expressed as protein. These proteins are then purified and crystallised, and then subjected to one of two types of structure determination: X-ray crystallography and Nuclear Magnetic Resonance (NMR). The whole genome sequence allows for the design of every primer required in order to amplify all of the ORFs, clone them into bacteria, and then express them. By using a whole-genome approach to this traditional method of protein structure determination, all of the proteins encoded by the genome can be expressed at once. This approach allows for the structural determination of every protein that is encoded by the genome.

Modelling-based methods

ab initio modelling: This approach uses protein sequence data and the chemical and physical interactions of the encoded amino acids to predict the 3-D structures of proteins with no homology to solved protein structures. One highly successful method for *ab initio* modelling is the Rosetta programme, which divides the protein into short segments and arranges short polypeptide chain into a low-energy local conformation. Rosetta is available for commercial use and for non-commercial use through its public programme, Robetta.

Sequence-based modelling: This modelling technique compares the gene sequence of an unknown protein with sequences of proteins with known structures. Depending on the degree of similarity between the sequences, the structure of the known protein can be used as a model for solving the structure of the unknown protein. Highly accurate modelling is considered to require at least 50% amino acid sequence identity between the unknown protein and the solved structure. 30–50% sequence identity gives a model of intermediate-accuracy, and sequence identity below 30% gives low-accuracy models. It has been predicted that at least 16,000 protein structures will need to be determined in order for all structural motifs to be represented at least once and thus allowing the structure of any unknown protein to be solved accurately through modelling. One disadvantage of this method, however, is that structure is more conserved than sequence and thus sequence-based modelling may not be the most accurate way to predict protein structures.

Threading: Threading bases structural modelling on fold similarities rather than sequence identity. This method may help identify distantly related proteins and can be used to infer molecular functions.

Examples of Structural Genomics

There are currently a number of ongoing efforts to solve the structures for every protein in a given proteome.

Thermotogo maritima proteome

One current goal of the Joint Center for Structural Genomics (JCSG), a part of the Protein Structure Initiative (PSI) is to solve the structures for all the proteins in Thermotogo maritima, a thermophillic bacterium. *T. maritima* was selected as a structural genomics target based on its relatively small genome consisting of 1877 genes and the hypothesis that the proteins expressed by a thermophilic bacterium would be easier to crystallise. Lesley and other used *Escherichia coli* to express all the open-reading frames (ORFs) of *T. martima*. These proteins were then crystallised and structures were determined for successfully crystallised proteins using X-ray crystallography. Among other structures, this structural genomics approach allowed for the determination of the structure of the TM0449 protein, which was found to exhibit a novel fold as it did not share structural homology with any known protein.

Mycobacterium tuberculosis proteome

The goal of the TB Structural Genomics Consortium is to determine the structures of potential drug targets in *Mycobacterium tuberculosis*, the bacterium that causes tuberculosis. The development of novel drug therapies against tuberculosis are particularly important given the growing problem of multi-drug-resistant tuberculosis.

The fully sequenced genome of *M. tuberculosis* has allowed scientists to clone many of these protein targets into expression vectors for purification and structure determination by X-ray crystallography. Studies have identified a number of target proteins for structure determination, including extracellular proteins that may be involved in pathogenesis, iron-regulatory proteins, current drug targets, and proteins predicted to have novel folds. So far, structures have been determined for 708 of the proteins encoded by *M. tuberculosis*.

Protein Structure Databases and Classifications

Protein Data Bank (PDB): repository for protein sequence and structural information
    UniProt: Provides sequence and functional information.
    Structural Classification of Proteins (SCOP classifications): Hierarchical-based approach.
    Class, Architecture, Topology and Homologous superfamily (CATH): Hierarchical-based approach.

PHARMACOGENOMICS

Pharmacogenomics (a portmanteau of pharmacology and genomics) is the study of the role of genetics in drug response. It deals with the influence of genetic variation on drug response in patients by correlating gene expression or single-nucleotide polymorphisms with drug absorption, distribution, metabolism and elimination, as well as drug receptor target effects. Pharmacogenomics may be used interchangeably with the term pharmacogenetics, which focuses on the effects of candidate genes in drug response. Pharmacogenomics aims to develop rational means to optimise drug therapy, with respect to the patients genotype, to ensure maximum efficacy with minimal adverse effects. Such approaches promise the advent of 'personalised medicine', in which drugs and drug combinations are optimised for each individuals unique genetic makeup. In order to provide pharmacogenomic based recommendations for a given drug, two possible types of input can be used: genotyping or exome or whole genome sequencing. Sequencing provides many more data points, including detection of mutations that prematurely terminate the synthesised protein.

Drug Metabolism

There are several known genes which are largely responsible for variances in drug metabolism and response. The most common are the cytochrome P450 (CYP) genes, which encode enzymes that influence the metabolism of more than 80 per cent of current prescription drugs. Codeine, clopidogrel, tamoxifen, and warfarin are examples of medications that follow this metabolic pathway.

Patient genotypes are usually categorised into predicted phenotypes. For example, if a person receives one 1 allele each from mother and father to code for the CYP2D6 gene, then that person is considered to have an extensive metaboliser (EM) phenotype. An extensive metaboliser is considered normal. Other CYP metabolism phenotypes include: intermediate, ultra-rapid, and poor. In theory, each phenotype is based upon the allelic variation within the individual genotype. However, several genetic events can influence a same phenotypic trait, and establishing genotype-to-phenotype relationships can thus be far from consensual with many enzymatic patterns.

For instance, the influence of the CYP2D61/4 allelic variant on the clinical outcome in patients treated with Tamoxifen remains debated today. In oncology, genes coding for DPD, UGT1A1, TPMT, CDA involved in the pharmacokinetics of 5-FU/capecitabine, irinotecan, 6-mercaptopurine and gemcitabine/cytarabine, respectively, have all been described as being highly polymorphic. A strong body of evidence suggests that patients affected by these genetic polymorphisms will experience severe/lethal toxicities upon drug intake, and that pre-therapeutic screening does help to reduce the risk of treatment-related toxicities through adaptive dosing strategies.

Identification of the genetic basis for polymorphic expression of a gene is done through intronic or exomic SNPs which abolishes the need for different mechanisms for explaining the variability in drug metabolism. The SNPs based variations in membrane receptors lead to multidrug resistance (MDR) and the drug–drug interactions. Even drug induced toxicity and many adverse effects can be explained by genome-wide association studies (GWAS).

Applications

Pharmacogenomics has applications in illnesses like cancer, cardiovascular disorders, depression, bipolar disorder, attention deficit disorders, HIV, tuberculosis, asthma, and diabetes. In cancer treatment, pharmacogenomics tests are used to identify which patients are most likely to respond to certain cancer drugs. In behavioural health, pharmacogenomic tests provide tools for physicians and care givers to better manage medication selection and side effect amelioration. Pharmacogenomics is also known as companion diagnostics, meaning tests being bundled with drugs. Examples include KRAS test with cetuximab and EGFR test with gefitinib. Beside efficacy, germline pharmacogenetics can help to identify patients likely to undergo severe toxicities when given cytotoxics showing impaired detoxification in relation with genetic polymorphism, such as canonical 5-FU. In cardio vascular disorders, the main concern is response to drugs including warfarin, clopidogrel, beta blockers, and statins.

EPIGENETICS

Epigenetics is the study of changes in gene expression caused by certain base pairs in DNA, or RNA, being 'turned off' or 'turned on' again, through chemical reactions. In biology, and specifically genetics, epigenetics is mostly the study of heritable changes that are not caused by changes in the DNA sequence, to a lesser extent, epigenetics also describes the study of stable, long-term alterations in the transcriptional potential of a cell that are not necessarily heritable. Unlike simple genetics based on changes to the DNA sequence (the genotype), the changes in gene expression or cellular phenotype of epigenetics have other causes, thus use of the term epi-genetics.

The term also refers to the changes themselves: functionally relevant changes to the genome that do not involve a change in the nucleotide sequence. Examples of mechanisms that produce such changes are DNA methylation and histone modification, each of which alters how genes are expressed without altering the underlying DNA sequence. Gene expression can be controlled through the action of repressor proteins that attach to silencer regions of the DNA. These epigenetic changes may last through cell divisions for the duration of the cell's life, and may also last for multiple generations even though they do not involve changes in the underlying DNA sequence of the organism, instead, non-genetic factors cause the organisms genes to behave (or 'express themselves') differently. (There are objections to the use of the term epigenetic to describe chemical modification of histone, since it remains unclear whether or not histone modifications are heritable.)

One example of an epigenetic change in eukaryotic biology is the process of cellular differentiation. During morphogenesis, totipotent stem cells become the various pluripotent cell lines of the embryo, which in turn become fully differentiated cells. In other words, as a single fertilised egg cell–the zygote–continues to divide, the resulting daughter cells change into all the different cell types in an organism, including neurons, muscle cells, epithelium, endothelium of blood vessels, etc. by activating some genes while inhibiting the expression of others. The methylation of mRNA plays a critical role in human energy homeostasis. The obesity-associated FTO gene is shown to be able to demethylate N6-methyladenosine in RNA.

The term 'epigenetics', however, has been used to describe processes which have not been demonstrated to be heritable such as histone modification, there are therefore attempts to redefine it in broader terms that would avoid the constraints of requiring heritability. For example, Sir Adrian Bird defined epigenetics as 'the structural adaptation of chromosomal regions so as to register, signal or perpetuate altered activity states.' This definition would be inclusive of transient modifications associated with DNA repair or cell-cycle phases as well as stable changes maintained across multiple cell generations, but exclude others such as templating of membrane architecture and prions unless they impinge on chromosome function. 'Epigenetics is an emerging frontier of science that involves the study of changes in the regulation of gene activity and expression that are not dependent on gene sequence. For purposes of this programme, epigenetics refers to both heritable changes in gene activity and expression (in the progeny of cells or of individuals) and also stable, long-term alterations in the transcriptional potential of a cell that are not necessarily heritable. While epigenetics refers to the study of single genes or sets of genes, epigenomics refers to more global analyses of epigenetic changes across the entire genome.'

Molecular Basis

Epigenetic changes can modify the activation of certain genes, but not the sequence of DNA. Additionally, the chromatin proteins associated with DNA may be activated or silenced. This is why the differentiated cells in a multicellular organism express only the genes that are necessary for their own activity. Epigenetic changes are preserved when cells divide. Most epigenetic changes only occur within the course of one individual organisms lifetime, but, if gene inactivation occurs in a sperm or egg cell that results in fertilisation, then some epigenetic changes can be transferred to the next generation. This raises the question of whether or not epigenetic changes in an organism can alter the basic structure of its DNA, a form of Lamarckism.

Specific epigenetic processes include paramutation, bookmarking, imprinting, gene silencing, X chromosome inactivation, position effect, reprogramming, transvection, maternal effects, the progress of carcinogenesis, many effects of teratogens, regulation of histone modifications and heterochromatin, and technical limitations affecting parthenogenesis and cloning.

DNA damage can also cause epigenetic changes. DNA damages are very frequent, occurring on average about 10,000 times a day per cell of the human body. These damages are largely repaired, but at the site of a DNA repair, epigenetic changes can remain. In particular, a double strand break in DNA can initiate unprogrammed epigenetic gene silencing both by causing DNA methylation as well as by promoting silencing types of histone modifications (chromatin remodelling). In addition, the enzyme Parp1 (poly(ADP)-ribose polymerase) and its product poly(ADP)-ribose (PAR) accumulate at sites of DNA damage as part of a repair process. This accumulation, in turn, directs recruitment and activation of the chromatin remodelling protein ALC1 that can cause nucleosome remodelling. Nucleosome remodelling has been found to cause, for instance, epigenetic silencing of DNA repair gene MLH1. DNA damaging chemicals, such as benzene, hydroquinone, styrene, carbon tetrachloride and trichloroethylene, cause considerable hypomethylation of DNA, some through the activation of oxidative stress pathways. Foods are known to alter the epigenetics of rats on different diets. Some food components epigenetically increase the levels of DNA repair enzymes such as MGMT and MLH1 and p53. Other food components can reduce DNA damage, such as soya isoflavones and bilberry anthocyanins. Epigenetic research uses a wide range of molecular biologic techniques to further our understanding of epigenetic phenomena, including chromatin immunoprecipitation (together with its large-scale variants ChIP-on-chip and ChIP-Seq), fluorescent *in situ* hybridisation, methylation-sensitive restriction enzymes, DNA adenine methyltransferase identification (DamID) and bisulphite sequencing. Furthermore, the use of bioinformatic methods is playing an increasing role. Computer simulations and molecular dynamics approaches revealed the atomistic motions associated with the molecular recognition of the histone tail through an allosteric mechanism.

Mechanisms of Epigenetics

Several types of epigenetic inheritance systems may play a role in what has become known as cell memory, note however that not all of these are universally accepted to be examples of epigenetics.

DNA methylation and chromatin remodelling

Because DNA methylation and chromatin remodelling play such a central role in many types of epigenic inheritance, the word 'epigenetics' is sometimes used as a synonym for these processes. However, this can be misleading. Chromatin remodelling is not always inherited, and not all epigenetic inheritance involves chromatin remodelling. Because the phenotype of a cell or individual is affected by which of its genes are transcribed, heritable transcription states can give rise to epigenetic effects. There are several layers of regulation of gene expression. One way that genes are regulated is through the remodelling of chromatin.

Chromatin is the complex of DNA and the histone proteins with which it associates. If the way that DNA is wrapped around the histones changes, gene expression can change as well. Chromatin remodelling is accomplished through two main mechanisms:

1. The first way is post translational modification of the amino acids that make up histone proteins. Histone proteins are made up of long chains of amino acids. If the amino acids that are in the chain are changed, the shape of the histone might be modified. DNA is not completely unwound during replication. It is possible, then, that the modified histones may be carried into each new copy of the DNA. Once there, these histones may act as templates, initiating the surrounding new histones to be shaped in the new manner. By altering the shape of the histones around them, these modified histones would ensure that a lineage-specific transcription programme is maintained after cell division.

2. The second way is the addition of methyl groups to the DNA, mostly at CpG sites, to convert cytosine to 5-methylcytosine. 5-Methylcytosine performs much like a regular cytosine, pairing with a guanine in double-stranded DNA. However, some areas of the genome are methylated more heavily than others, and highly methylated areas tend to be less transcriptionally active, through a mechanism not fully understood. Methylation of cytosines can also persist from the germ line of one of the parents into the zygote, marking the chromosome as being inherited from one parent or the other.

Mechanisms of heritability of histone state are not well understood, however, much is known about the mechanism of heritability of DNA methylation state during cell division and differentiation. Heritability of methylation state depends on certain enzymes (such as DNMT1) that have a higher affinity for 5-methylcytosine than for cytosine. If this enzyme reaches a 'hemimethylated' portion of DNA (where 5-methylcytosine is in only one of the two DNA strands) the enzyme will methylate the other half. Although histone modifications occur throughout the entire sequence, the unstructured *N*-termini of histones (called histone tails) are particularly highly modified. These modifications include acetylation, methylation, ubiquitylation, phosphorylation, sumoylation, ribosylation and citrullination. Acetylation is the most highly studied of these modifications. For example, acetylation of the K14 and K9 lysines of the tail of histone H3 by histone acetyltransferase enzymes (HATs) is generally related to transcriptional competence.

One mode of thinking is that this tendency of acetylation to be associated with 'active' transcription is biophysical in nature. Because it normally has a positively charged nitrogen at its end, lysine can bind the negatively charged phosphates of the DNA backbone. The acetylation event converts the positively charged amine group on the side chain into a neutral amide linkage. This removes the positive charge, thus loosening the DNA from the histone. When this occurs, complexes like SWI/SNF and other transcriptional factors can bind to the DNA and allow transcription to occur. This is the '*cis*' model of epigenetic function. In other words, changes to the histone tails have a direct effect on the DNA itself.

Another model of epigenetic function is the '*trans*' model. In this model, changes to the histone tails act indirectly on the DNA. For example, lysine acetylation may create a binding site for chromatin-modifying enzymes (or transcription machinery as well). This chromatin remodeler can then cause changes to the state of the chromatin. Indeed, a bromodomain—a protein domain that specifically binds acetyl-lysine—is found in many enzymes that help activate transcription, including the SWI/SNF complex. It may be that acetylation acts in this and the previous way to aid in transcriptional activation.

The idea that modifications act as docking modules for related factors is borne out by histone methylation as well. Methylation of lysine 9 of histone H3 has long been associated with constitutively transcriptionally silent chromatin (constitutive heterochromatin). It has been determined that a chromodomain (a domain that specifically binds methyl-lysine) in the transcriptionally repressive protein HP1 recruits HP1 to K9 methylated regions. One example that seems to refute this biophysical model for methylation is that tri-methylation of histone H3 at lysine 4 is strongly associated with (and required for full) transcriptional activation. Tri-methylation in this case would introduce a fixed positive charge on the tail.

It has been shown that the histone lysine methyltransferase (KMT) is responsible for this methylation activity in the pattern of histones H3 & H4. This enzyme utilises a catalytically active site called the SET domain (Suppressor of variegation, Enhancer of zeste, Trithorax). The SET domain is a 130-amino acid sequence involved in modulating gene activities. This domain has been demonstrated to bind to the histone tail and causes the methylation of the histone.

Differing histone modifications are likely to function in differing ways, acetylation at one position is likely to function differently from acetylation at another position. Also, multiple modifications may occur at the same time, and these modifications may work together to change the behaviour of the nucleosome. The idea that multiple dynamic modifications regulate gene transcription in a systematic and reproducible way is called the histone code, although the idea that histone state can be read linearly as a digital information carrier has been largely debunked. One of the best-understood systems that orchestrates chromatin-based silencing is the SIR protein based silencing of the yeast hidden mating type loci HML and HMR. DNA methylation frequently occurs in repeated sequences, and helps to suppress the expression and mobility of 'transposable elements': Because 5-methylcytosine can be spontaneously deaminated (replacing nitrogen by oxygen) to thymidine, CpG sites are frequently mutated and become rare in the genome, except at CpG islands where they remain unmethylated. Epigenetic changes of this type thus have the potential to direct increased frequencies of permanent genetic mutation. DNA methylation patterns are known to be established and modified in response to environmental factors by a complex interplay of at least three independent DNA methyltransferases, DNMT1, DNMT3A, and DNMT3B, the loss of any of which is lethal in mice. DNMT1 is the most abundant methyltransferase in somatic cells, localises to replication foci, has a 10–40-fold preference for hemimethylated DNA and interacts with the proliferating cell nuclear antigen (PCNA). By preferentially modifying hemimethylated DNA, DNMT1 transfers patterns of methylation to a newly synthesised strand after DNA replication, and therefore is often referred to as the 'maintenance' methyltransferase. DNMT1 is essential for proper embryonic development, imprinting and X-inactivation. To emphasise the difference of this molecular mechanism of inheritance from the canonical Watson-Crick base-pairing mechanism of transmission of genetic information, the term 'Epigenetic templating' was introduced. Furthermore, in addition to the maintenance and transmission of methylated DNA states, the same principle could work in the maintenance and transmission of histone modifications and even cytoplasmic heritable states.

Histones H3 and H4 can also be manipulated through demethylation using histone lysine demethylase (KDM). This recently identified enzyme has a catalytically active site called the Jumonji domain (JmjC). The demethylation occurs when JmjC utilises multiple cofactors to hydroxylate the methyl group, thereby removing it. JmjC is capable of demethylating mono-, di-, and tri-methylated substrates.

Chromosomal regions can adopt stable and heritable alternative states resulting in bistable gene expression without changes to the DNA sequence. Epigenetic control is often associated with alternative covalent modifications of histones. The stability and heritability of states of larger chromosomal regions are suggested to involve positive feedback where modified nucleosomes recruit enzymes that similarly modify nearby nucleosomes. A simplified stochastic model for this type of epigenetics is found here.

It has been suggested that chromatin-based transcriptional regulation could be mediated by the effect of small RNAs. Small interfering RNAs can modulate transcriptional gene expression via epigenetic modulation of targeted promoters.

RNA transcripts and their encoded proteins

Sometimes a gene, after being turned on, transcribes a product that (directly or indirectly) maintains the activity of that gene. For example, Hnf4 and MyoD enhance the transcription of many liver- and muscle-specific genes, respectively, including their own, through the transcription factor activity of the proteins they encode. RNA signalling includes differential recruitment of a hierarchy of generic chromatin modifying complexes and DNA methyltransferases to specific loci by RNAs during differentiation and development. Other epigenetic changes are mediated by the production of different splice forms of RNA, or by formation of double-stranded RNA (RNAi). Descendants of the cell in which the gene was turned on will inherit this activity, even if the original stimulus for gene-activation is no longer present. These genes are often turned on or off by signal transduction, although in some systems where syncytia or gap junctions are important, RNA may spread directly to other cells or nuclei by diffusion. A large amount of RNA and protein is contributed to the zygote by the mother during oogenesis or via nurse cells, resulting in maternal effect phenotypes. A smaller quantity of sperm RNA is transmitted from the father, but there is recent evidence that this epigenetic information can lead to visible changes in several generations of offspring.

MicroRNAs

MicroRNAs (miRNAs) are members of non-coding RNAs that range in size from 17 to 25 nucleotides. As indicated by Wang, miRNAs regulate a large variety of biological functions in plants and animals. So far, in 2013, about 2000 miRNAs have been discovered in humans and these can be found online in an miRNA database. Each miRNA expressed in a cell may target about 100 to 200 messenger RNAs that it downregulates. Most of the downregulation of mRNAs occurs by causing the decay of the targeted mRNA, while some downregulation occurs at the level of translation into protein. It appears that about 60% of human protein coding genes are regulated by miRNAs. Many miRNAs are epigenetically regulated. About 50% of miRNA genes are associated with CpG islands, that may be repressed by epigenetic methylation. Transcription from methylated CpG islands is strongly and heritably repressed. Other miRNAs are epigenetically regulated by either histone modifications or by combined DNA methylation and histone modification.

sRNAs

sRNAs are small (50–250 nucleotides), highly structured, non-coding RNA fragments found in bacteria. They control gene expression including virulence genes in pathogens and are viewed as new targets in the fight against drug-resistant bacteria. They play an important role in many biological processes, binding to mRNA and protein targets in prokaryotes. Their phylogenetic analyses, for example through sRNA–mRNA target interactions or protein binding properties, are used to build comprehensive databases. sRNA-gene maps based on their targets in microbial genomes are also constructed.

Prions

Prions are infectious forms of proteins. In general, proteins fold into discrete units that perform distinct cellular functions, but some proteins are also capable of forming an infectious conformational state known as a prion. Although often viewed in the context of infectious disease, prions are more loosely defined by their ability to catalytically convert other native state versions of the same protein to an infectious conformational state. It is in this latter sense that they can be viewed as epigenetic agents capable of inducing a phenotypic change without a modification of the genome.

Fungal prions are considered by some to be epigenetic because the infectious phenotype caused by the prion can be inherited without modification of the genome. PSI+ and URE3, discovered in yeast in 1965 and 1971, are the two best studied of this type of prion. Prions can have a phenotypic effect through the sequestration of protein in aggregates, thereby reducing that proteins activity. In PSI+ cells, the loss of the Sup35 protein (which is involved in termination of translation) causes ribosomes to have a higher rate of read-through of stop codons, an effect that results in suppression of nonsense mutations in other genes. The ability of Sup35 to form prions may be a conserved trait. It could confer an adaptive advantage by giving cells the ability to switch into a PSI+ state and express dormant genetic features normally terminated by stop codon mutations.

Structural inheritance systems

In ciliates such as Tetrahymena and Paramecium, genetically identical cells show heritable differences in the patterns of ciliary rows on their cell surface. Experimentally altered patterns can be transmitted to daughter cells. It seems existing structures act as templates for new structures. The mechanisms of such inheritance are unclear, but reasons exist to assume that multicellular organisms also use existing cell structures to assemble new ones.

Functions and Consequences of Epigenetics

Development

Somatic epigenetic inheritance through epigenetic modifications, particularly through DNA methylation and chromatin remodelling, is very important in the development of multicellular eukaryotic organisms.

The genome sequence is static (with some notable exceptions), but cells differentiate into many different types, which perform different functions, and respond differently to the environment and intercellular signalling. Thus, as individuals develop, morphogens activate or silence genes in an epigenetically heritable fashion, giving cells a 'memory'. In mammals, most cells terminally differentiate, with only stem cells retaining the ability to differentiate into several cell types ('totipotency' and 'multipotency'). In mammals, some stem cells continue producing new differentiated cells throughout life, such as in neurogenesis, but mammals are not able to respond to loss of some tissues, for example, the inability to regenerate limbs, which some other animals are capable of. Unlike animals, plant cells do not terminally differentiate, remaining totipotent with the ability to give rise to a new individual plant. While plants do utilise many of the same epigenetic mechanisms as animals, such as chromatin remodelling, it has been hypothesised that some kinds of plant cells do not use or require 'cellular memories', resetting their gene expression patterns using positional information from the environment and surrounding cells to determine their fate.

Epigenetics can be divided into predetermined and probabilistic epigenesis. Predetermined epigenesis is a unidirectional movement from structural development in DNA to the functional maturation of the protein. 'Predetermined' here means that development is scripted and predictable. Probabilistic epigenesis on the other hand is a bidirectional structure-function development with experiences and external molding development.

Medicine

Epigenetics has many and varied potential medical applications as it tends to be multidimensional in nature. Congenital genetic disease is well understood, and it is also clear that epigenetics can play a role, for example, in the case of Angelman syndrome and Prader-Willi syndrome. These are normal genetic diseases caused by gene deletions or inactivation of the genes, but are unusually common because individuals are essentially hemizygous because of genomic imprinting, and therefore a single gene knock out is sufficient to cause the disease, where most cases would require both copies to be knocked out.

Evolution

Epigenetics can impact evolution when epigenetic changes are heritable. A sequestered germ line or Weismann barrier is specific to animals, and epigenetic inheritance is more common in plants and microbes. Eva Jablonka and Marion Lamb have argued that these effects may require enhancements to the standard conceptual framework of the modern evolutionary synthesis. Other evolutionary biologists have incorporated epigenetic inheritance into population genetics models or are openly skeptical.

Two important ways in which epigenetic inheritance can be different from traditional genetic inheritance, with important consequences for evolution, are that rates of epimutation can be much faster than rates of mutation and the epimutations are more easily reversible.

An epigenetically inherited element such as the PSI+ system can act as a 'stop-gap', good enough for short-term adaptation that allows the lineage to survive for long enough for mutation and/or recombination to genetically assimilate the adaptive phenotypic change. The existence of this possibility increases the evolvability of a species.

Current research findings and examples of effects

Epigenetic changes have been observed to occur in response to environmental exposure—for example, mice given some dietary supplements have epigenetic changes affecting expression of the agouti gene, which affects their fur colour, weight, and propensity to develop cancer.

One study indicates that traumatic experiences can produce fearful memories which are passed to future generations via epigenetics. A study carried out on mice in 2013 found that mice could produce offspring which had an aversion to certain items which had been the source of negative experiences for their ancestors. In the case of humans with different environmental exposures, Fraga and others studied young monozygotic (identical) twins and older monozygotic twins. They found that although such twins were epigenetically indistinguishable during their early years, older twins had remarkable differences in the overall content and genomic distribution of 5-methylcytosine DNA and histone acetylation. The twin pairs who had spent less of their lifetime together and/or had greater differences in their medical histories were those who showed the largest differences in their levels of 5methylcytosine DNA and acetylation of histones H3 and H4.

More than 100 cases of transgenerational epigenetic inheritance phenomena have been reported in a wide range of organisms, including prokaryotes, plants, and animals. For instance, Mourning Cloak butterflies will change colour through hormone changes in response to experimentation of varying temperatures. Recent analyses have suggested that members of the APOBEC/AID family of cytosine deaminases are capable of simultaneously mediating genetic and epigenetic inheritance using similar molecular mechanisms.

Epigenetic Effects in Humans

Genomic imprinting and related disorders

Some human disorders are associated with genomic imprinting, a phenomenon in mammals where the father and mother contribute different epigenetic patterns for specific genomic loci in their germ cells. The best-known case of imprinting in human disorders is that of Angelman syndrome and Prader-Willi syndrome—both can be produced by the same genetic mutation, chromosome 15q partial deletion, and the particular syndrome that will develop depends on whether the mutation is inherited from the child's mother or from their father. This is due to the presence of genomic imprinting in the region. Beckwith-Wiedemann syndrome is also associated with genomic imprinting, often caused by abnormalities in maternal genomic imprinting of a region on chromosome 11.

Cancer and developmental abnormalities

A variety of compounds are considered as epigenetic carcinogens—they result in an increased incidence of tumors, but they do not show mutagen activity (toxic compounds or pathogens that cause tumors incident to increased regeneration should also be excluded). Examples include diethylstilbestrol, arsenite, hexachlorobenzene, and nickel compounds.

Many teratogens exert specific effects on the fetus by epigenetic mechanisms. While epigenetic effects may preserve the effect of a teratogen such as diethylstilbestrol throughout the life of an affected child, the possibility of birth defects resulting from exposure of fathers or in second and succeeding generations of offspring has generally been rejected on theoretical grounds and for lack of evidence. However, a range of male-mediated abnormalities have been demonstrated, and more are likely to exist.

Recent studies have shown that the mixed-lineage leukemia (MLL) gene causes leukemia by rearranging and fusing with other genes in different chromosomes, which is a process under epigenetic control. Other investigations have concluded that alterations in histone acetylation and DNA methylation occur in various genes influencing prostate cancer. Gene expression in the prostate can be modulated by nutrition and lifestyle changes.

DNA methylation in cancer

DNA methylation is an important regulator of gene transcription and a large body of evidence has demonstrated that aberrant DNA methylation is associated with unscheduled gene silencing, and the genes with high levels of 5-methylcytosine in their promoter region are transcriptionally silent. DNA methylation is essential during embryonic development, and in somatic cells, patterns of DNA methylation are in general transmitted to daughter cells with a high fidelity. Aberrant DNA methylation patterns have been associated with a large number of human malignancies and found in two distinct forms: hypermethylation and hypomethylation compared to normal tissue. Hypermethylation is one of the major epigenetic modifications that repress transcription via promoter region of tumour suppressor genes. Hypermethylation typically occurs at CpG islands in the promoter region and is associated with gene inactivation. Global hypomethylation has also been implicated in the development and progression of cancer through different mechanisms.

DNA repair epigenetics in cancer

Germ line (familial) mutations have been identified in 34 different DNA repair genes that cause a high risk of cancer, including, for example BRCA1 and ATM. These are listed in the article DNA repair-deficiency disorder. However, cancers caused by such germ line mutations make up only a very small proportion of cancers. For instance, germ line mutations cause only 2 to 5% of colon cancer cases.

Epigenetic reductions in expression of DNA repair genes, however, are very frequent in sporadic (non-germ line) cancers, while mutations in DNA repair genes in sporadic cancer are very rare.

DNA MICROARRAY

A DNA microarray (also commonly known as DNA chip or biochip) is a collection of microscopic DNA spots attached to a solid surface. Scientists use DNA microarrays to measure the expression levels of large numbers of genes simultaneously or to genotype multiple regions of a genome. Each DNA spot contains picomoles (10^{-12} moles) of a specific DNA sequence, known as probes (or reporters or oligos). These can be a short section of a gene or other DNA element that are used to hybridise a cDNA or cRNA (also called anti-sense RNA) sample (called target) under high-stringency conditions. Probe-target hybridisation is usually detected and quantified by detection of fluorophore-, silver-, or chemilumine-scence-labelled targets to determine relative abundance of nucleic acid sequences in the target.

Basic Microarray

Since an array can contain tens of thousands of probes, a microarray experiment can accomplish many genetic tests in parallel. Therefore arrays have dramatically accelerated many types of investigation. In standard microarrays, the probes are synthesised and then attached via surface engineering to a solid surface by a covalent bond to a chemical matrix (via epoxy-silane, amino-silane, lysine, polyacrylamide or others). The solid surface can be glass or a silicon chip, in which case they are colloquially known as an Affy chip when an Affymetrix chip is used. Other microarray platforms, such as Illumina, use microscopic beads, instead of the large solid support. Alternatively, microarrays can be constructed by the direct synthesis of oligonucleotide probes on solid surfaces. DNA arrays are different from other types of microarray only in that they either measure DNA or use DNA as part of its detection system.

DNA microarrays can be used to measure changes in expression levels, to detect single nucleotide polymorphisms (SNPs), or to genotype or targeted resequencing.

Microarrays also differ in fabrication, workings, accuracy, efficiency, and cost. Additional factors for microarray experiments are the experimental design and the methods of analysing the data.

Principle

The core principle behind microarrays is hybridisation between two DNA strands, the property of complementary nucleic acid sequences to specifically pair with each other by forming hydrogen bonds between complementary nucleotide base pairs. A high number of complementary base pairs in a nucleotide sequence means tighter non-covalent bonding between the two strands. After washing off non-specific bonding sequences, only strongly paired strands will remain hybridised. Fluorescently labelled target sequences that bind to a probe sequence generate a signal that depends on the hybridisation conditions (such as temperature), and washing after hybridisation. Total strength of the signal, from a spot, depends upon the amount of target sample binding to the probes present on that spot. Microarrays use relative quantitation in which the intensity of a feature is compared to the intensity of the same feature under a different condition, and the identity of the feature is known by its position.

Uses and Types

Many types of arrays exist and the broadest distinction is whether they are spatially arranged on a surface or on coded beads: The traditional solid-phase array is a collection of orderly microscopic 'spots', called features, each with thousands of identical and specific probes attached to a solid surface, such as glass, plastic or silicon biochip (commonly known as a genome chip, DNA chip or gene array). Thousands of these features can be placed in known locations on a single DNA microarray. The alternative bead array is a collection of microscopic polystyrene beads, each with a specific probe and a ratio of two or more dyes, which do not interfere with the fluorescent dyes used on the target sequence. DNA microarrays can be used to detect DNA (as in comparative genomic hybridisation), or detect RNA (most commonly as cDNA after reverse transcription) that may or may not be translated into proteins. The process of measuring gene expression via cDNA is called expression analysis or expression profiling.

Applications of DNA microarray

- Gene expression profiling.
- Comparative genomic hybridisation.
- GeneID.
- Chromatin immunoprecipitation on Chip.
- DamID.
- SNP detection.
- Alternative splicing detection.
- Fusion genes microarray.
- Tiling array.

Fabrication

Microarrays can be manufactured in different ways, depending on the number of probes under examination, costs, customisation requirements, and the type of scientific question being asked. Arrays may have as few as 10 probes or up to 2.1 million micrometre-scale probes from commercial vendors.

Spotted vs in situ synthesised arrays

Microarrays can be fabricated using a variety of technologies, including printing with fine-pointed pins onto glass slides, photolithography using pre-made masks, photo-lithography using dynamic micromirror devices, ink-jet printing, or electrochemistry on microelectrode arrays.

In spotted microarrays, the probes are oligonucleotides, cDNA or small fragments of PCR products that correspond to mRNAs. The probes are synthesised prior to deposition on the array surface and are then 'spotted' onto glass. A common approach utilises an array of fine pins or needles controlled by a robotic arm that is dipped into wells containing DNA probes and then depositing each probe at designated locations on the array surface. The resulting 'grid' of probes represents the nucleic acid profiles of the prepared probes and is ready to receive complementary cDNA or cRNA 'targets' derived from experimental or clinical samples. This technique is used by research scientists around the world to produce 'in-house' printed microarrays from their own labs. These arrays may be easily customised for each experiment, because researchers can choose the probes and printing locations on the arrays, synthesise the probes in their own lab (or collaborating facility), and spot the arrays. They can then generate their own labelled samples for hybridisation, hybridise the samples to the array, and finally scan the arrays with their own equipment. This provides a relatively low-cost microarray that may be customised for each study, and avoids the costs of purchasing often more expensive commercial arrays that may represent vast numbers of genes that are not of interest to the investigator.

In oligonucleotide microarrays, the probes are short sequences designed to match parts of the sequence of known or predicted open reading frames. Although oligonucleotide probes are often used in 'spotted' microarrays, the term 'oligonucleotide array' most often refers to a specific technique of manufacturing. Oligonucleotide arrays are produced by printing short oligonucleotide sequences designed to represent a single gene or family of gene splice-variants by synthesising this sequence directly onto the array surface instead of depositing intact sequences.

Sequences may be longer (60-mer probes such as the Agilent design) or shorter (25-mer probes produced by Affymetrix) depending on the desired purpose, longer probes are more specific to individual target genes, shorter probes may be spotted in higher density across the array and are cheaper to manufacture. One technique used to produce oligonucleotide arrays include photolithographic synthesis (Affymetrix) on a silica substrate where light and light-sensitive masking agents are used to 'build' a sequence one nucleotide at a time across the entire array. Each applicable probe is selectively 'unmasked' prior to bathing the array in a solution of a single nucleotide, then a masking reaction takes place and the next set of probes are unmasked in preparation for a different nucleotide exposure. After many repetitions, the sequences of every probe become fully constructed. More recently, Maskless Array Synthesis from NimbleGen Systems has combined flexibility with large numbers of probes.

Two-channel vs one-channel detection

Two-colour microarrays or two-channel microarrays are typically hybridised with cDNA prepared from two samples to be compared (e.g. diseased tissue versus healthy tissue) and that are labelled with two different fluorophores. Fluorescent dyes commonly used for cDNA labelling include Cy3, which has a fluorescence emission wavelength of 570 nm (corresponding to the green part of the light spectrum), and Cy5 with a fluorescence emission wavelength of 670 nm (corresponding to the red part of the light spectrum). The two Cy-labelled cDNA samples are mixed and hybridised to a single microarray that is then scanned in a microarray scanner to visualise fluorescence of the two fluorophores after excitation with a laser beam of a defined wavelength. Relative intensities of each fluorophore may then be used in ratio-based analysis to identify up-regulated and down-regulated genes. Oligonucleotide microarrays often carry control probes designed to hybridise with RNA spike-ins. The degree of hybridisation between the spike-ins and the control probes is used to normalise the hybridisation measurements for the target probes. Although absolute levels of gene expression may be determined in the two-colour array in rare instances, the relative differences in expression among different spots within a sample and between samples is the preferred method of data analysis for the two-colour system. Examples of providers for such microarrays includes Agilent with their Dual-Mode platform, Eppendorf with their DualChip platform for colorimetric Silverquant labelling, and TeleChem International with Arrayit.

In single-channel microarrays or one-colour microarrays, the arrays provide intensity data for each probe or probe set indicating a relative level of hybridisation with the labelled target. However, they do not truly indicate abundance levels of a gene but rather relative abundance when compared to other samples or conditions when processed in the same experiment. Each RNA molecule encounters protocol and batch-specific bias during amplification, labelling, and hybridisation phases of the experiment making comparisons between genes for the same microarray uninformative. The comparison of two conditions for the same gene requires two separate single-dye hybridisations. Several popular single-channel systems are the Affymetrix 'Gene Chip', Illumina 'Bead Chip', Agilent single-channel arrays, the Applied Microarrays 'CodeLink' arrays, and the Eppendorf 'DualChip & Silverquant'. One strength of the single-dye system lies in the fact that an aberrant sample cannot affect the raw data derived from other samples, because each array chip is exposed to only one sample. Another benefit is that data are more easily compared to arrays from different experiments so long as batch effects have been accounted for. A drawback to the one-colour system is that, when compared to the two-colour system, twice as many microarrays are needed to compare samples within an experiment.

BIOINFORMATICS: MICROARRAYS ANALYSES

We have witnessed in the past years the rapid progresses in the human genome project and biotechnologies. These advances result in many complex datasets associated with indepth scientific knowledge, e.g. genome sequences of many species, microarray expression profiles of different cell lines, single nucleotide polymorphisms (SNPs) in the human genome, etc. These data together with their underlying scientific challenges spawn the new field of Bioinformatics, which sprawls many academic disciplines as well as the pharmaceutical industry, and create one of the most exciting times for all quantitative researchers. There is no doubt that statistics will be pivotal in this new field, but it remains a challenge to us statisticians whether we can play a leading role in this biology and informatics revolution. This is not just a challenge, in fact, but also a golden opportunity for our discipline.

The recent developments of two high throughput biological data generation technologies help foster the bioinformatics hype in statistics: the genome sequencing technology and the DNA chip technology. The word 'genome' refers to the collection of all the chromosomes (chains of DNA bases, human has 23 pairs of these) in a cell. Certain segments of the genome, called 'genes' (or coding regions), encode the information needed to make proteins, which are action molecules of the cell, responsible for nearly all cellular processes. It is estimated that the human genome has about 30,000 genes, which, surprisingly, only account for ~3% of the genome. The expression of these genes, i.e. the amount of protein products to be made in a cell, is tightly regulated so as to meet the requirements of specific cells and for cells to respond to changes in their environment. A central goal of molecular biology is to understand the regulation of protein synthesis. In order to make a protein molecule, a gene is first *transcribed* to messenger RNA (mRNA), an easily degradable molecule, which then carries the information to a cellular machinery (ribosome) for protein production. While there are several levels of gene regulation, the dominant form is transcriptional regulation. Specific sequence signals upstream of each gene provide a target, called the promoters, for *RNA polymerase* (a machinery for transcription) to bind so as to initiate the transcription. When transcription factors (TFs, proteins specialised in regulating gene expressions) bind near the promoter region of a gene, they interfere with the function of RNA polymerase, thus, either repressing or enhancing the production of mRNA. The amount of a certain mRNA copies in a cell reflect, albeit imperfectly, the expression level of the corresponding gene.

By orderly arranging samples, the microarray provides a large-scale medium for matching known and unknown DNA segments based on base-pairing rules. There are two classes of microarrays. The cDNA arrays apply to glass slides (or nylon membranes) spots of *complimentary DNAs* (cDNAs), which are generated in biological labs by reverse transcription (so that they only include the protein-coding part of the genome). The oligonucleotide arrays (often referred to as the Affymetrix arrays) place many thousands of gene-specific oligonucleotides (called probes) synthesised directly on a silicon chip. The probes are about 25 base pairs long, and 20 probe-pairs (one perfect fact and one mismatch) are often used to represent each gene (like a 20 digit barcode).

In order to compare two types of cells (e.g. a cancer cell versus a normal cell), for example, the biologist first extracts the DNA materials from all the cells and labels those from one cell type by fluorescence cy5 (red) and the other cell type by cy3 (green). The microarray is then exposed to the mixture of the two DNA samples for hybridisation. When mRNA for a gene is more abundant in the cancer cell than in the normal cell, for example, the array spot corresponding to that gene will show a red colour. Numerically, a vector of length G is reported, where G is the number of spots (genes) in the array, and each entry of the vector records the ratios of the fluorescence intensities (cy5/cy3). Thus, through the use of DNA microarrays, one can monitor simultaneously the expression levels of thousands of genes in different types of cells.

Role of Statistics

The amount of data produced by microarray experiments is daunting even to statisticians. An important pre-processing step, often termed as 'low-level' analysis, involves the so called 'normalisation', which removes systematic biases due to imperfect experimental conditions, and quality filtering, which picks out 'bad spots' and removes artifacts. For example, due to hybridisation bias and other reasons the mRNA levels labelled by Cy5 may be systematically higher than that labelled by Cy3. The first normalisation method is to subtract a constant from the expression measurements of all the genes. But as demonstrated by Li and Wong, such an approach can be problematic due to certain expression intensitydependent biases. More sophisticated statistical approaches using 'rank invariant' genes or robust curve estimation (e.g. 'LOESS') are often more appropriate.

A central task intended for the microarray experiment is to find genes that are differentially expressed in the two samples (or types of cells). Suppose that the identical microarray experiment is repeated p times (e.g. leukemia cells from p patients compared with p wild types). Then, we obtain a dataset $(m_{ij}, i = 1,... ,G, j = 1,...,p)$, in which m_{ij} is the expression ratio of gene i in jth experiment. The number G ranges from thousands to tens of thousands, while the number of replications p can be as low as a few. The statement 'differentially expressed (DF)' simply means that, mathematically, $E(m_{ij}) \neq 0$.

Although biologists can discover DF genes even with $p = 1$, it has been realised lately that making independent replications is a good practice. The standard *t*-test is an obvious first attempt for recognising DF genes and has been implemented in all commercial microarray analysis packages. But the distributional assumption and the problem of multiple testing make the statisticians wonder how reliable the *t*-tests are in and what the 'false discovery rate' is. Recently, empirical Bayes and parametric Bayes methods have been suggested to tackle these questions.

Another set of important and related tasks, often termed as unsupervised learning, is to find genes that behave similarly in various conditions (i.e. clustering the row vectors), and to find subgroups of samples (or patients' tissues) that similar to each other (i.e. clustering the column vectors). While the first task can lead the biologists to novel discovery of genes in related biological pathways or having related functions, the second task can be result in clinically important subgroups of patients.

Due to the influential article Eisen and its associated software, the clustering method of choice for biologists has been hierarchical clustering. Other methods such as the *k*-means method, self-organised maps, Gaussian mixture models, plaid models, etc. have later been applied to microarrays, although none of them become as prominent as 'Eisen clustering.' There is also no definitive conclusion as to which method is the optimal choice. With gene clusters available, one may be able to use motif-searching tools to help infer groups of co-regulated genes. A further and much more difficult challenge is to infer gene regulatory pathways (i.e. the cascade of genes that lead to cellular function). Closely related to clustering is the classification or supervised learning problem. For example, Golub were interested in predicting the two subtypes of leukemia based on the gene expression profile of each sample. In such problems, one has a 'training dataset' (usually of very small size) in which the class indicator for each sample is known, and wants to generate a good 'rule' for predicting a future sample. This is where various 'statistical learning' techniques come into the play. For example, Fisher's linear discriminate analysis, the nearest neighbour classification, support vector machines. Bayesian networks, classification and regression trees, boosting, bagging, logistic regressions, independent component analysis, etc. have all been applied to the array data. New techniques are still being developed.

Since typically thousands to tens of thousands of genes are surveyed in a microarray study, it is of interest to select a small subset of genes that can best characterise the two groups. This is of great value to the pharmaceutical industry because of their need to find effective biomarkers for monitoring treatments and for defining a subpopulation that response to a certain drug.

Integration with other Array Data

More biological data of similar nature to DNA microarrays are becoming available. Among the many array technologies, Chromatin Immunoprecipitation (ChIP) combined with microarrays, the so-called 'ChIP-chip' data, has recently become popular for studying *in vivo* interactions between transcription factors (TFs) and their target binding sites in the genome. In this procedure, the expressions of those DNA segments that are bound by the TF of interest are enhanced. Thus, when mixed with a normal cell extract and hybridised to microarrays, the spots corresponding to those TF binding sites will light up. By combining ChIP-chip data with the gene expression data, scientists can often gain more insights on how the regulatory network should be mapped out. The ChIP-chip data can also be combined with the genome sequence information for discovering the exact regulatory motif sites and patterns.

Many important cellular tasks are achieved by interactions between proteins—they may interact to pass on signals (part of a signal transduction pathway) or to form a complex for tackling a difficult job (e.g. transcription or translation). In conjunction with high throughput expression and purification of recombinant proteins, biologists can prepare microarrays of functionally active proteins on glass slides. These arrays can then be used to identify protein-protein interactions, to identify the substrates of protein kinases, or to identify the targets of biologically active small molecules. Another technology, the yeast two-hybrid system, has also been used successfully to investigate protein-protein interactions. The integration of the protein interaction data with the DNA microarray data has revealed some interesting connections between expression profiles of the genes and the interactions among their protein products. Other promising array technologies are also under development. For example, the small molecule microarrays can be used to screen large libraries of compounds to identify new ligands for proteins of interest, antibody arrays can be used to study regulation at the protein level, and SNP arrays can be used to sample molecular variability in natural populations, diagnose genetic defects, and genotype rapidly a large number of SNP markers). It is desirable, yet challenging, to develop a systematic approach to integrate these different types of data.

Broader Array of Bioinformatics Problems

Microarray analysis provides for statisticians an excellent entry point to bioinformatics/computational biology. Here other bioinformatics challenges that await statisticians' contributions are discussed.

The protein folding problem, i.e. the prediction of the three-dimensional fold of a protein molecule based only on its primary sequence information, is often regarded as the crown jewel of the biopolymer research. Knowledge on the structures of target proteins and on how they interact with ligands is of paramount importance to drug designers. Although the 3-D structures of many proteins have been worked out by X-ray crystallographers, these structures only account for a small part of the protein universe and scientists are still not capable of predicting protein tertiary structures *ab initio*. Recently, theoreticians have turned their attentions to much simpler black-white bead model for understanding the design principles of protein structures. Practitioners have opted to use more statistically based threading method. This method 'threads' the given protein sequence into a set of known structural templates and finds the most suitable sequence-template fit. Many structural templates are constructed by combining the known protein structures with statistical model-based protein sequence analysis.

Multiple sequence alignment is still the main tool for protein sequence analysis, which has been at the center of computational biology for about 30 years. With the completion of the human genome and genomes of many other species, the task of organising and understanding the generated sequence and structural data becomes even more pressing and challenging. Many statistical and computational methods for sequence alignment has been proposed over the years, among which the most popular ones include Clustal W., PSI-BLAST, SAM, and HMMER, etc. In particular, the application of hidden Markov models and the Gibbs sampler to biopolymer sequence analysis has revolutionised the field. Pfam database contains a large collection of annotated protein family profiles built based on hidden Markov models and is becoming very influential in protein research. An emerging challenge is the analysis of aligned protein sequences in order to gain further insights on protein functions.

There have been some recent interests in incorporating gene ontology (GO) in microarray analyses. Gene ontology refers to a dynamically controlled vocabulary that can be applied to (the genes of) all organisms. Each gene product can be described by its molecular function (e.g. transcription factor), its involvement in biological processes (e.g. mitosis), and its cellular location (e.g. nucleus). Bringing GO into the analysis of high throughput biological data such as microarrays can be extremely insightful.

Recently, in the analysis of circadian gene regulation, Storch mapped various clusters of genes based on their microarray experiments to GO hierarchies and found that clock-regulated genes in heart and liver participate in many related processes even though the two sets of genes have almost no overlap.

TFs identify the genes they are intended to regulate by recognising via weak energetic interactions specific binding sites, often located upstream of the genes. It has been realised early on that these sites are often conserved. For example, the binding sites of STE12 of yeast look lik3 'TGAAACA.' If the genome were indeed a 'novel', then these patterns are like key words (with typos) in the novel. Thus, techniques for discovering new 'words' in a text have been developed and applied to discover the TF motif sites and pattern.

Some other important bioinformatics problems in which statistics is likely to play an important role include rational drug designs, evolutionary analysis, and the analyses of SNPs in the human genome. As the great evolutionist *T. Dobzhansky* pointed out: nothing in biology made sense except in the context of evolution. Evolution study cannot only help us understand where and how we come from, but also shed light on protein functions and cellular processes. The SNPs have recently attracted much attention from scientists because of the SNPs' great potential in mapping genes responsible for complex diseases and the availability of high throughout SNP detection and analysis tools. Statistical modelling and computation are crucial to these developments. To sum up the advent of inexpensive microarray experiments created several specific bioinformatics challenges:

- The multiple levels of replication in experimental design (Experimental design).
- The number of platforms and independent groups and data format (Standardisation).
- The treatment of the data (Statistical analysis).
- Accuracy and precision (Relation between probe and gene).
- The sheer volume of data and the ability to share it (Data warehousing).

TRANSCRIPTOME

The transcriptome is the set of all RNA molecules in one cell or a population of cells. It is sometimes used to refer to all RNAs, or just mRNA, depending on the particular experiment (Fig. 21.1). It differs from the exome in that it includes only those RNA molecules found in a specified cell population, and usually includes the amount or concentration of each RNA molecule in addition to the molecular identities.

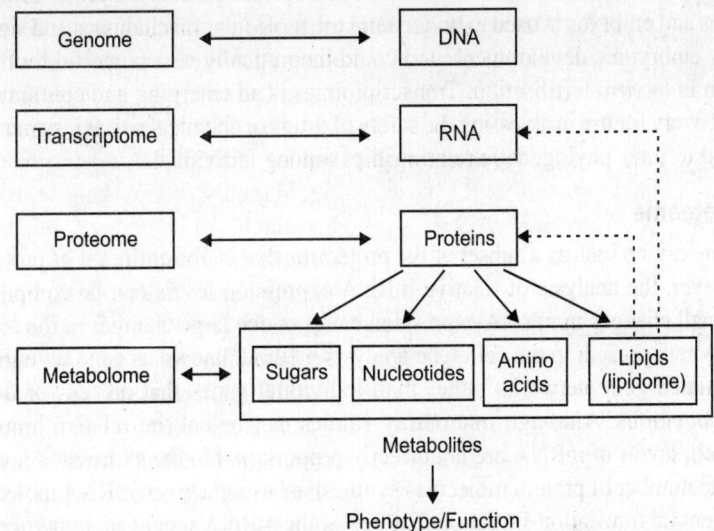

Fig. 21.1: General scheme showing the relationships of the genome, transcriptome, proteome, and metabolome (lipidome).

Scope

The term can be applied to the total set of transcripts in a given organism, or to the specific subset of transcripts present in a particular cell type. Unlike the genome, which is roughly fixed for a given cell line (excluding mutations), the transcriptome can vary with external environmental conditions. Because it includes all mRNA transcripts in the cell, the transcriptome reflects the genes that are being actively expressed at any given time, with the exception of mRNA degradation phenomena such as transcriptional attenuation. The study of transcriptomics, examines the expression level of RNAs in a given cell population, often focusing on mRNA, but sometimes including others such as tRNAs, sRNAs.

Methods of Construction

Transcriptomics techniques include DNA microarrays and next-generation sequencing technologies called RNA-Seq. Transcription can also be studied at the level of individual cells by single-cell transcriptomics. There are two general methods of inferring transcriptome sequences. One approach maps sequence reads onto a reference genome, either of the organism itself (whose transcriptome is being studied) or of a closely related species. The other approach, *de novo* transcriptome assembly, uses software to infer transcripts directly from short sequence reads.

Analysis

A number of organism specific transcriptome databases have been constructed and annotated to aid in the identification of genes that are differentially expressed in distinct cell populations. RNA-seq is emerging as the method of choice for measuring transcriptomes of organisms, though the older technique of DNA microarrays is still used.

Applications

The transcriptomes of stem cells and cancer cells are of particular interest to researchers who seek to understand the processes of cellular differentiation and carcinogenesis. Analysis of the transcriptomes of human oocytes and embryos is used to understand the molecular mechanisms and signalling pathways controlling early embryonic development, and could theoretically be a powerful tool in making proper embryo selection in *in vitro* fertilisation. Transcriptomics is an emerging and continually growing field in biomarker discovery for use in assessing the safety of drugs or chemical risk assessment. Transcriptomes may also be used to infer phylogenetic relationships among individuals.

Relation to Proteome

The transcriptome can be seen as a subset of the proteome, that is, the entire set of proteins expressed by a genome. However, the analysis of relative mRNA expression levels can be complicated by the fact that relatively small changes in mRNA expression can produce large changes in the total amount of the corresponding protein present in the cell. One analysis method, known as gene set enrichment analysis, identifies coregulated gene networks rather than individual genes that are up- or down-regulated in different cell populations. Although microarray studies can reveal the relative amounts of different mRNAs in the cell, levels of mRNA are not directly proportional to the expression level of the proteins they code for. The number of protein molecules synthesised using a given mRNA molecule as a template is highly dependent on translation-initiation features of the mRNA sequence, in particular, the ability of the translation initiation sequence is a key determinant in the recruiting of ribosomes for protein translation. The complete protein complement of a cell or organism is known as the proteome.

Chapter 22

Proteomics

INTRODUCTION

Proteomics is the large-scale study of proteins, particularly their structures and functions. Proteins are vital parts of living organisms, as they are the main components of the physiological metabolic pathways of cells. The proteome is the entire set of proteins, produced or modified by an organism or system. This varies with time and distinct requirements, or stresses, that a cell or organism undergoes. Proteomics is an interdisciplinary domain formed on the basis of the research and development of the Human Genome Project, it is also emerging scientific research and exploration of proteomes from the overall level of intracellular protein composition, structure, and its own unique activity patterns. It is an important component of functional genomics.

While proteomics generally refers to the large-scale experimental analysis of proteins, it is often specifically used for protein purification and mass spectrometry.

PROTEOMICS AND BIOLOGICAL SYSTEMS

After genomics and transcriptomics, proteomics is the next step in the study of biological systems. It is more complicated than genomics because an organisms genome is more or less constant, whereas the proteome differs from cell to cell and from time to time. Distinct genes are expressed in different cell types, which means that even the basic set of proteins that are produced in a cell needs to be identified. In the past this phenomenon was done by mRNA analysis, but it was found not to correlate with protein content. It is now known that mRNA is not always translated into protein, and the amount of protein produced for a given amount of mRNA depends on the gene it is transcribed from and on the current physiological state of the cell. Proteomics confirms the presence of the protein and provides a direct measure of the quantity present.

Post-translational Modifications

Not only does the translation from mRNA cause differences, but many proteins are also subjected to a wide variety of chemical modifications after translation. Many of these post-translational modifications are critical to the proteins function.

Phosphorylation

One such modification is phosphorylation, which happens to many enzymes and structural proteins in the process of cell signalling. The addition of a phosphate to particular amino acids—most commonly serine and threonine mediated by serine/threonine kinases, or more rarely tyrosine mediated by tyrosine kinases—causes a protein to become a target for binding or interacting with a distinct set of other proteins that recognise the phosphorylated domain. Because protein phosphorylation is one of the most-studied protein modifications, many 'proteomic' efforts are geared to determining the set of phosphorylated proteins in a particular cell or tissue-type under particular circumstances. This alerts the scientist to the signalling pathways that may be active in that instance.

Ubiquitination

Ubiquitin is a small protein that can be affixed to certain protein substrates by enzymes called E3 ubiquitin ligases. Determining which proteins are poly-ubiquitinated helps understand how protein pathways are regulated. This is, therefore, an additional legitimate 'proteomic' study. Similarly, once a researcher determines which substrates are ubiquitinated by each ligase, determining the set of ligases expressed in a particular cell type is helpful.

Additional modifications

Listing all the protein modifications that might be studied in a 'proteomics' project would require a discussion of most of biochemistry. Therefore, a short list illustrates the complexity of the problem. In addition to phosphorylation and ubiquitination, proteins can be subjected to (among others) methylation, acetylation, glycosylation, oxidation and nitrosylation. Some proteins undergo all these modifications, often in time-dependent combinations. This illustrates the potential complexity of studying protein structure and function.

Distinct Proteins are made under Distinct Settings

Even studying a particular cell type, that cell may make different sets of proteins at different times, or under different conditions. Furthermore, as mentioned, any one protein can undergo a wide range of post-translational modifications.

Therefore a 'proteomics' study can become complex, even if the topic of the study is restricted. In more ambitious settings, such as when a biomarker for a tumour is sought–when the proteomics scientist is obliged to study sera samples from multiple cancer patients–the amount of complexity that must be dealt with is as great as in any modern biological project.

Proteomics is the large scale of study of proteins, particularly their function and structure. Proteomics is an excellent approach for studying changes in metabolism in response to different stress conditions.

Protein, highly complex substance that is present in all living organisms. Proteins are the polymers of amino acids. Proteins play an important role in metabolic activities. Primary structure of protein is determined by the sequence of specific amino acids, encoded by the mRNA, which directs the proper folding of the polypeptide chain into the secondary structure. One type of secondary structure is the alpha helix, a region of the polypeptide that folds into a corkscrew shape. Beta strands are linear structures of polypeptides, bonding together to form a flat beta sheet. Turns and coils interact chemically with each other to form the unique three dimensional shape of the proper three dimensional structure creates the final protein. Many proteins, however, have several different polypeptide subunits that make the final active protein. For these proteins, the interactions between the different subunits form the quaternary structure. One of the most promising developments to come from the study of human genes and proteins has been the identification of potential new drugs for the treatments of disease. This relies on genome and proteome information to identify proteins associated with a disease. The term 'proteomics' was first coined in 1995 and was defined as the large-scale characterisation of the entire protein complement of a cell line, tissue, or organism. Proteomics is the large-scale study of proteins particularly their composition, structures, functions, and interactions of the proteins directing the activities of cell. The main theme of interest proteomics it gives a much better understanding of an organism than genomics. Genomics can give a rough estimation of expression of a protein. Most of the proteins function in collaboration with other proteins, and the main goal of proteomics are to identify which proteins interact. After genomics, proteomics is often considered as the advanced step in the study of biological systems. It is much more complicated than genomics, mostly because while an organism's genome is more or less constant, the total protein expression profile always changes with time, micro and macro environmental conditions.

Mass spectrometry (MS) has been widely used in forensic science in the identification of compounds, particularly illicit drugs. MS is a technique that allows the detection of compounds by separating ions by their unique mass (mass-to-charge ratios) using a mass spectrometer. The method relies on the fact that every compound has a unique fragmentation pattern (mass spectrum). The sample is ionised, the sample ions are separated based on their differing masses and relative abundance.

TYPES OF PROTEOMICS

Based on the protein response under stress conditions proteomics are classified into different groups.

Expression Proteomics

Expression proteomics is used to study the qualitative and quantitative expression of total proteins under two different conditions. Like the normal cell and treated or diseased cell can be compared to understand the protein that is responsible for the stress or diseased state or the protein that is expressed due to disease. Typically, expression proteomics studies are addressed to the investigation of the expression protein patterns in abnormal cells. For example, compare tumour tissue sample and the normal tissue can be analysed for differential protein expression. 2-D gel electrophoresis, mass spectrometry technique were used to observed the protein expressional changes, which is present and absent in tumour tissue, when compared with normal tissue. These are over expressed and under expressed can be identified and characterised protein activities multi-protein complexes, and signalling pathways. Identification of these proteins will give valuable information about molecular biology of tumour formation and disease-specific manner for use as diagnostic markers or therapeutic targets.

Structural Proteomics

Structural proteomics helps to understand three dimensional shape and structural complexities of functional proteins. Structural prediction of a protein when its amino acid sequence is determined directly by sequencing or from the gene with a method called homology modelling. Structural proteomics can give detailed information about the structure and function of protein complexes present in a specific cellular organelle. It is possible to identify all the proteins present in a complex system such as membranes, ribosomes, and cell organelles and to characterise all the protein interactions that can be possible between these proteins and protein complexes. Different technologies such as X-ray crystallography and NMR spectroscopy were mainly used for structure determination.

Functional Proteomics

Functional proteomics explains understanding the protein functions as well as unravelling molecular mechanisms within the cell then depend on the identification of the interacting protein partners. The association of an unknown protein with partners belonging to a specific protein complex involved in a particular mechanism would in fact, be strongly suggestive of its biological function. Furthermore detailed description of the cellular signalling pathways might greatly benefit from the elucidation of protein-protein interactions *in vivo*.

Techniques Involved in Proteomics

In proteomic analysis both analytical and bioinformatics tools were used to characterise protein structure and functions. Analytical techniques 2-D gel electrophoresis, MALDI-TOF MS were used. In case of bioinformatics numbers of software tools were used.

2-D Gel Electrophoresis

In 2-D gel electrophoresis, protein samples are resolved based on charge, in a step called isoelectric focusing, and then based on molecular weight in second step 13. The result is an image in thousands of small spots, each representing a protein. A good 2-D gel can resolve one thousand to two thousand protein spots, which appear after staining, as dots in the gel. 2-D gel electrophoresis technique is mainly used to compare two similar samples to find specific protein differences.

2-D Electrophoresis Workflow Chart

2-D Electrophoresis workflow chart are shown in Fig. 22.1. Prepare the protein at a concentration and in a solution suitable for IEF. Choose a method that maintains the native charge, solubility, and relative abundance of proteins of interest. Separate proteins according to pI by IEF. Select the appropriate IPG strip length and pH gradient for the desired resolution and sample load. Select appropriate sample loading and separation conditions.

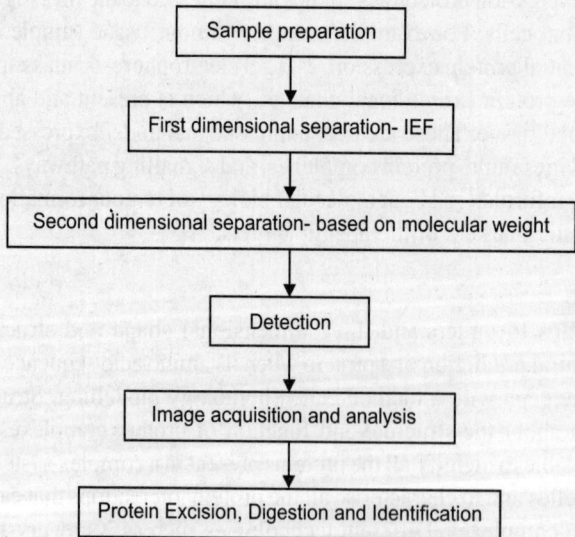

Fig. 22.1: 2-D Electrophoresis workflow chart.

Separate proteins according to size by SDS-PAGE. Select the appropriate gel size and composition and separation conditions. Visualise proteins using either a total protein stain or fluorescent protein tags. Select a staining technique that matches sensitivity requirements and available imaging equipment. Capture digital images of the 2-D patterns using appropriate imaging equipment and software. Then analyse the patterns using 2-D software. Excise protein spots of interest from the gel digest the proteins, and the digests by MS.

MS Analysis

Mass spectrometry is an analytical technique that produces spectra of the masses of the atoms or molecules comprising a sample of material. The spectra are used to determine the elemental or isotopic signature of a sample, the masses of particles and of molecules, and to elucidate the chemical structures of molecules, such as peptides and other chemical compounds. Mass spectrometry works by ionising chemical compounds to generate charged molecules or molecule fragments and measuring their mass to charge ratios. MALDI-TOF is the most useful technique for protein identification.

MALDI-TOF-MS

Matrix Assisted Laser Desorption/Ionisation is a soft ionisation technique used in spectrometry, allowing to analysis the biomolecules like DNA, protein, peptides. Biomolecules and synthetic polymers have low volatility and are thermally unstable, which has limited the use of MS as a means of characterisation. These problems have been minimised through the development of MALDI-TOF MS (Fig. 22.2), which allows for the mass determination of biomolecules by ionisation and vaporisation without degradation, a Laser beam used to ionise the sample.

Protein sample have been characterised by HPLC or SDS PAGE by generating peptide maps. These peptide maps have been used as fingerprints of protein or as a tool to know the purity of a known protein in a known sample. Mass spectrometry gives a peptide map when proteins are digested with proteolytic enzymes like trypsin. This peptide map can be used to search a sequence database to find a good match from the existing database.

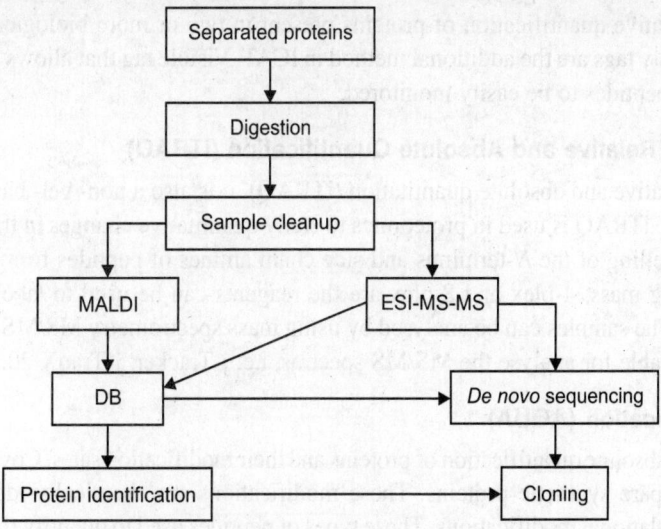

Fig. 22.2: MALDI-TOF MS analysis representing image.

Sample Preparation

MALDI-TOF MS is used to characterise, biomolecules like proteins, peptides and polymers of organic compounds. Sample preparation for MALDI-TOF is very interesting and important step. Purify the protein sample before going MALDI-TOF analysis because it is more tolerant to sample contaminants but contaminants can seriously disturb incorporation of sample molecules with growing matrix crystals. Sample can mix with matrix in 1:2 ratio. Different types of matrices are used based on sample, some of matrix are 2-(4-hydroxy phenylazo benzoic acid, 2,4,6-trihydroxyacetophenone, 3-aminoquinolone, cinnamic acid, etc.). Dried droplet technique is predominantly applied for MALDI-TOF analysis, protein sample, mixed with matrix on a metal plate. The combination of matrices yielded slightly performance. Small volumes should be used for standard metal plates. On the other hand, hydrophilic sample anchors are efficient for the generation of small spots.

Matrix

A good matrix consist the following properties i.e. Matrix must be able to absorb UV wavelength of usually 237 nm, being easily exited and ability to transfer of proton to the sample molecules. Main role of the matrix is adsorption of energy from laser pulse, and then transfer to sample this energy can causes the vaporisation of the sample. For protein samples typical MALDI matrix consist of hydroxylated benzoic acid and cinnamic acid derivatives.

ADVANCED METHODS IN PROTEOMICS

Isotope-coded Affinity Tags (ICAT)

It is a gel- free method for quantitative proteomics that relies on chemical labelling reagents. These chemical probes consist of three general elements i.e. defined amino acid side chain, an isotopically coded linker, and a tag for the affinity isolation of labelled proteins/peptides. For quantitative comparison of two proteomes, sample labelled with isotopically light, and other one is heavy version. Both samples combined with isotope-coded tagging reagents. These peptides are analysed by LC-MS. The technique mainly used the relative quantification of proteins present in two or more biological samples. Visible isotope-coded affinity tags are the additional method in ICAT- Visible tag that allows the electrophoresis position of tagged peptides to be easily monitored.

Isobaric Tags for Relative and Absolute Quantification (iTRAQ)

Isobaric tags for relative and absolute quantitation (iTRAQ), it is also a non- gel- based technique used to quantify proteins. iTRAQ is used in proteomics to study quantitative changes in the proteome. Based on the covalent labelling of the N-terminus and side chain amines of peptides from protein digestions with tags of varying mass, 4-plex and 8-plex are the reagents can be used to label all peptides from different samples. The samples can be analysed by using mass spectrometry MS/MS. Different types of software's are available for analyse the MS/MS spectras, i.e. j-Tracker, j-TraqX 20.

Absolute Quantification (AQUA)

AQUA, studies the absolute quantification of proteins and their modification sates. Covalent modifications can be used to prepare synthetic proteins. These modifications are chemically identical to naturally occurring post-translational modifications. These types of peptides used to quantify the post translational modified proteins after proteolysis with the help of tandem mass spectrometer.

ESI-Q-IT-MS

Micro electrospray ionisation (ESI)-Quadrupole ion trap (QIT) Time of flight (TOF) mass spectrometer (MS) has a very good resolution. In ESI ionisation proteins are ionised in solution and carry multiple charge state. The advantage of using ESI-QTOF analysis for protein mass determination is that due to the high charge state of proteins their m/z measurements is typically less than 2000 and the TOF detector has a very good mass accuracy in this scan range. This result is more accurate mass measurements for proteins in ESI-QTOF.

SELDI-TOF-MS

The technique Surface-enhanced laser desorption/ionisation (SELDI) is used for the analysis of protein mixtures, it is an ionisation method in mass spectrometry. SELDI is typically used with time-of-flight mass spectrometers and is used to detect proteins in clinical samples, to compare protein levels with and without a disease can be used for biomarker discovery.

APPLICATIONS OF PROTEOMICS

Proteomics is widely used technique in biological fields, mainly applied in Oncology (Tumour biology), Bio-medicine, Agriculture and Food Microbiology.

Oncology

Oncology refers study of Tumour cell, Tumour metastasis, is the process spread of cancer from one organ to another non-adjacent organ cause death in patients. The major challenge in medicine to describe the molecular and cellular mechanisms underlying tumour metastasis. Analyse the protein expressions correlated to the metastatic process which help to understand the mechanism of metastasis and thus facilitate the development of strategies for the therapeutic interventions and clinical management of cancer. Proteomics is a systematic research, the main aim of this research is to characterise the protein expressions, functions of tumour cells and widely used in biomarker discovery.

Bio-medical Applications

The study of interactions between microbial pathogens and their hosts is called 'infectomics'. It is very interesting area in proteomics. It deals with the fundamentals of the infections origin and their effect on organs. The main aim of this research is to prevent or cure disease at starting level. Advanced diagnostic issues related to emerging infections, increasing of fastidious bacteria, and generation of patient- tailored phenotypes.

Agricultural Applications

The applications of plant proteomics scientific research is still in budding stage. Proteomics is also used to know plant-insect interactions that help identify candidate genes involved in the defensive response of plants to herbivore. Population growth and effect of global climate changes imposing severe limits on the sustainability of agricultural crop production.

Food Microbiology

The use of proteomics in food technology is presented especially for characterisation and standardisation of raw materials, process development, and detection of batch-to batch variations and quality control of the final product. Further attention is paid to the aspects of food safety, especially regarding biological and microbial safety and the use of genetically modified foods.

Based on the above findings the present review was concluded that the applications for proteomics are relevant to all of the biological process and provides a means to utilise the expressed protein data in a more effective way.

LIMITATIONS OF GENOMICS AND PROTEOMICS STUDIES

Proteomics gives a different level of understanding than genomics for many reasons:

- The level of transcription of a gene gives only a rough estimate of its level of translation into a protein. An mRNA produced in abundance may be degraded rapidly or translated inefficiently, resulting in a small amount of protein.

- As mentioned above many proteins experience post-translational modifications that profoundly affect their activities, for example some proteins are not active until they become phosphorylated. Methods such as phosphoproteomics and glycoproteomics are used to study post-translational modifications.

- Many transcripts give rise to more than one protein, through alternative splicing or alternative post-translational modifications.

- Many proteins form complexes with other proteins or RNA molecules, and only function in the presence of these other molecules.

- Protein degradation rate plays an important role in protein content.

Reproducibility: Proteomics experiments conducted in one laboratory are not easily reproduced in another. For instance, Peng and others have identified 1504 yeast proteins in a proteomics experiment of which only 858 were found in a similar previous study. Further, the previous study identified 607 proteins that were not found by Peng and others. This translates to a reproducibility of 57 to 59%.

Chapter 23

System Biology

INTRODUCTION

Biochemical systems biology augments more traditional disciplines, such as genomics, biochemistry and molecular biology, by championing: (i) mathematical and computational modelling, (ii) the application of traditional engineering practices in the analysis of biochemical systems, and in the past decade increasingly (iii) the use of near-comprehensive data sets derived from 'omics platform technologies, in particular 'downstream' technologies relative to genome sequencing, including transcriptomics, proteomics and metabolomics. The future progress in understanding biological principles will increasingly depend on the development of temporal and spatial analytical techniques that will provide high-resolution data for systems analyses. To date, particularly successful were strategies involving: (i) quantitative measurements of cellular components at the mRNA, protein and metabolite levels, as well as *in vivo* metabolic reaction rates, (ii) development of mathematical models that integrate biochemical knowledge with the information generated by high-throughput experiments, and (iii) applications to microbial organisms. The inevitable role bioinformatics plays in modern systems biology puts mathematical and computational sciences as an equal partner to analytical and experimental biology. Furthermore, mathematical and computational models are expected to become increasingly prevalent representations of our knowledge about specific biochemical systems.

The term 'systems biology' has emerged recently to describe the frontier of cross-disciplinary research in biology. This term was propelled into the mainstream merely ten years ago, coinciding with the completion of the Human Genome Project (HGP) and the concomitant emergence of 'omics technologies, namely transcriptomics, proteomics, and metabolomics. However, the origins of modern systems biology can be traced back to the middle of last century, with history that is both conceptually complex and institutionally convoluted. For example, a general systems theory was developed and applied to biology in late 1960's. Independently, the theory of metabolic control was developed, and metabolic flux was recognised as a 'systemic property'. Here, we focus on the re-emergence of 'systems thinking' linked to the post-genomic era and the development of global molecular profiling methods collectively known as 'omics technologies'. Interest in systems biology has increased rapidly in the past decade, as evidenced by the number of referencing publications. Systems biology has fuzzy boundaries and overlaps with several emerging, post-genomic fields, such as synthetic biology, systems microbiology, systems biotechnology, integrative biology, systems biomedicine, and metagenomics. Numerous definitions of systems bioloy have been proposed, but to date, there is no universally accepted definition—reflecting the difficulty in defining a heterogeneous school of thought by a comprehensive yet concise definition. Each of the proposed definitions, however, revolves around a fundamental understanding of biological systems based on the underlying component interactions (molecular interactions, in the case of biochemical systems biology). In a broad sense, the same is the goal of more traditional disciplines, such as molecular biology, genomics, and biochemistry. Hence, the question 'what is new in systems biology?' has been extensively discussed. Furthermore, it has been argued that systems biology is an approach, rather than a scientific discipline in the traditional sense. While the room for future debate on these questions remains, it is clear that systems biology fundamentally depends on the applications of mathematical and computational modelling. As the computational applications in biology are most often associated with the province of bioinformatics, another relevant question is: 'what is the relationship between systems biology and bioinformatics?'. Here, we address this question by focusing on the recent, post-HGP history, and the reemergence of biochemical systems biology.

GENOMICS TO SYSTEMS BIOLOGY

The term 'genomics' was coined by Thomas Roderick in 1986, and soon after was adopted as the name of the new journal aimed to support the new discipline of genome mapping and sequencing. This was a time of great excitement and profound transformation in biology brought about by the development of increasingly efficient methods for DNA sequencing. At the time, the call for the sequencing of the human genome was gaining momentum, and in 1988, the National Research Council of the US Academy of Sciences recommended the initiation of the Human Genome Project (HGP). The HGP, completed a decade later, was an enormous success, thus validating the new discipline of genomics. It rallied the scientific community in unprecedented ways, from being a global collaboration of 20 sequencing centers from six countries to opening new horizons in large-scale biology. The momentum of the HGP has spurred a plethora of genome-sequencing projects of other organisms, including plants, animals, and micro-organisms. In the early phases, the sequencing projects focused mainly on mapping, sequencing, and identifying genes. As the various genome-sequencing projects gathered momentum, it has become clear that collected genome sequences were only revealing more of hidden complexity, and are opening new and deeper biological questions. As a result, an increasing emphasis was placed upon the relationship between the sequence and function, and the field of genomics started to differentiate into 'sequence genomics' and 'functional genomics'.

The early view underpinning genomics was that the genome, the ultimate sequence map of the organisms DNA, is 'a rosetta stone from which the complexities of gene expression in development can be translated and the genetic mechanisms of disease interpreted'. This simplistic view rested on the deterministic concept of a gene and its role in determining biological function and organism's phenotype, the notion of which was tacitly extended to the entire genome. The degree of elusiveness of the gene concept has become fully apparent only in the last decade, based on the analysis of sequenced genomes, and extensive studies of the transcriptome with new techniques (such is cap-analysis gene expression (CAGE) and tiling arrays).

Several facts highlight the complexity of the relationship between the organisms phenotype and its genome: (i) less than 2% of human DNA directly encodes proteins, (ii) the genomes of eukaryotic organisms are nearly entirely transcribed, (iii) a massive amount of noncoding RNA transcripts identified in higher organisms is thought to have an important regulatory role, and (iv) a critical importance of post-transcriptional and post-translational regulation in the control of the function of gene products, which is both spatially and temporally regulated. As a result, in the past five years, the concept of the gene has been subject of substantial revisions.

Only temporarily overshadowed with the excitement about generating genome sequences, the true complexity of the relationship between an organisms genome and phenotype was recognised early. Even in the initial development of genomics we can recognise the elements of 'systems' thinking. In 1997, Hieter and Boguski wrote 'Functional genomics will supplement the detailed understanding of gene function provided by traditional approaches with a powerful new perspective on the holistic operation of biological systems'.

In the next few years, the idea of a 'holistic understanding' was further articulated in terms of mathematical models, whole-genome data sets, and the experience accumulated in studies of complex systems. Almost simultaneously, the need for an engineering mindset in molecular biology was suggested in an influential (and humorous) article written by a prominent biologist. An aspect of systems thinking is the recognition that biological systems are 'complex' in the mathematical sense. Such complex systems have long been of interest in physics and mathematics, and the direct relevance of the knowledge accumulated in these disciplines to biology was realised. It is now widely recognised that the availability of fully sequenced genomes and high-throughput ('omics) data sets makes the aspirations of "systems" thinking in biology an achievable goal.

SYSTEM-LEVEL DESCRIPTION, SYSTEM-LEVEL UNDERSTANDING, AND THE SYSTEM ITSELF

There are two frequently quoted approaches to systems biology, namely, 'top-down' and 'bottom-up'. Furthermore, systems biology practitioners can be arbitrarily divided into two (not mutually exclusive) camps: 'pragmatic' and 'systems oriented'. O'Malley and Dupre suggested that both camps of systems biologists lack a clear definition of what constitutes a 'system'. Indeed, the literature abounds with different definitions and calls for 'system-level description' and 'system-level understanding'. This only confounds the matter since the universally accepted definition of 'system' is lacking. While confusing at first sight, the meaning of 'system' in systems biology depends on the problem at hand, the objectives of the study, and the choices made in the art of mathematical modelling.

Mathematical modelling is often used in genomics and molecular biology, but in systems biology, it takes center stage, as 'no more, but no less, than a way of thinking clearly'. Biological systems consist of a large number of functionally diverse components, which interact highly selectively and often nonlinearly to produce coherent behaviours. These components may be individual molecules (such as in signaling or metabolic networks), assemblies of interacting complexes, sets of physical factors that guide the development of an organism (genes, mRNA, associated proteins and protein complexes), cells in tissues or organs, and even entire organisms in ecological communities. What is common to all these examples is the sheer number of components, and their selective, non-linear interactions that render the behaviours of these systems beyond the intuitive grasp.

Take, for example, the cell cycle in the yeast *Schizosaccharomyces pombe* (Fig. 23.1) the model of its cellcycle regulatory network involves about twenty components, whose interactions can be approximately described with a dozen differential equations and about 30 kinetic parameters. The dynamic behaviour of this network of interactions is possible to grasp only with the help of computer simulations and dynamical systems theory. Another example is the cellular response of yeast to hyperosmotic shock: it is only with

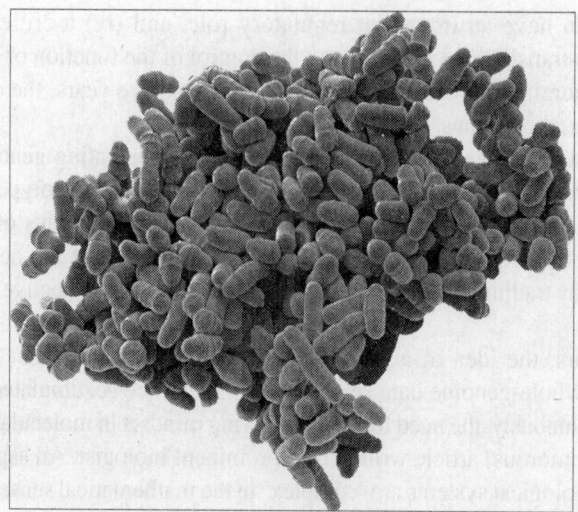

Fig. 23.1: *Schizosaccharomyces pombe.*

mathematical modelling that a coherent picture emerges, connecting various known components of the system with the observed properties.

There are other reasons why the concept of 'system' is so elusive. The role of mathematical models, particularly in generating experimentally testable hypotheses, has been discussed extensively. Perhaps less widely appreciated is that mathematical models of biological systems are increasingly being used to represent our knowledge about these systems. For example, the *i*AF1260 model of *Escherichia coli*'s metabolic network not only predicts experimentally observed behaviour of *E. coli* under genetic perturbations, but also in itself is a representation of the *E. coli* metabolic network. Similarly, the kinetic model of glycolysis in the bloodstream form of *Trypanosoma brucei* (Fig. 23.2) is the state-ofthe-art representation of glycolysis in this organism. There is no alternative way of quantitative thinking about these complex systems but through models that rely on precise mathematical descriptions.

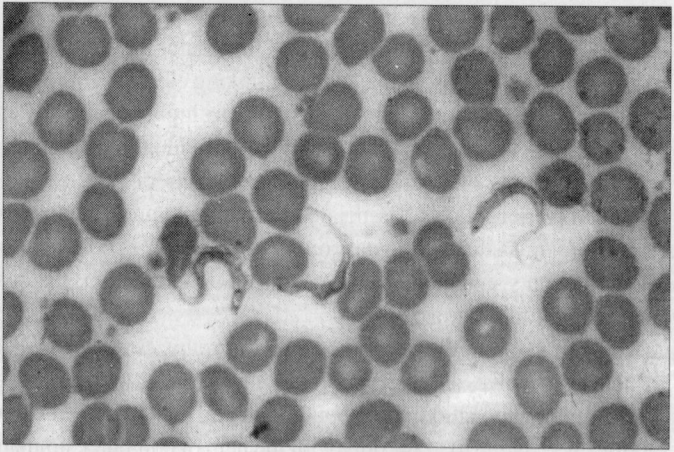

Fig. 23.2: *Trypanosoma brucei.*

These mathematical or computational models are essentially beyond a simple intuitive grasp, and represent concise summaries of our current knowledge of respective systems. There may be significant differences in scope and scale between different models used in systems biology. Consider, for example, the model of the yeast genome-scale metabolic network and the model of glycolysis in yeast. It is not that one model is better than the other, rather the twomodels have different motivations, objectives, scales, and capabilities: the first is the genome-scale model of the entire metabolic network, while the second is a model of a single metabolic pathway which includes detailed descriptions of kinetics of individual enzyme catalysed reactions. This illustrates an important general principle of mathematical modelling, highly relevant to systems biology: every mathematical model aims for a certain level of description, which depends on the objective of the study, limitations in our knowledge about the system of interest, and our ability to experimentally observe the system/phenomena of interest (necessary for testing the models predictions).

Genome-scale metabolic models typically ignore kinetic parameters of individual reactions because such models aim to be comprehensive, and the kinetic parameters for most reactions are unknown. In contrast, kineticmodels are much more detailed but less comprehensive, however, they can provide not only the information about the steady state but also the time course given some initial conditions. Choosing the correct 'level of description' is one of the more difficult aspects in mathematical modelling and is a pervasive challenge in systems biology. Another challenge is choosing the boundaries of the model (note: this amounts to defining the 'system'). This usually requires exquisite familiarity with the phenomena of interest, and a considerable experience in mathematical modelling. Complex dynamical systems form structures, and nature often provides modular designs. This modularity must be both understood and exploited correctly for optimal modelling. In genome-scale studies of microbial organisms, a convenient system boundary is the cell boundary, in most other cases, the question of the appropriate systems boundary is more opaque and must be addressed based on the prior knowledge of components and the coupling between these components. Trivial examples of this include tissue structure in a multicellular organism or subcellular compartmentalisation of metabolites. Hence all the difficulties in defining the 'system' in systems biology.

Modern systems biology is a rapidly evolving discipline. In the past, systems thinking was invoked in the context of a variety of systems and processes: from humans to micro-organisms, animals, and plants, and in regards to different levels of biological organisation, from molecular subnetworks, to cellular interaction networks, cells, entire organs, organisms, and even communities of organisms. Areas that have proven particularly fruitful for systems biology include studies of biochemical networks and applications to micro-organisms.

BIOCHEMICAL NETWORKS INMICRO-ORGANISMS

We are only beginning to appreciate the full complexity and the multidimensional nature of biochemical networks operating in all living organisms. Studies of metabolic networks, gene regulatory networks, and protein-protein interaction networks in microbial organisms have significantly contributed to this, and indeed to the identity of systems biology. Micro-organisms are convenient models for systems studies for several reasons: (i) decades of genetic and biochemical work have generated deep biological insights, and resulted in sophisticated molecular biology techniques for experimental manipulation, (ii) they can be readily and rapidly cultured in inexpensive media, providing ample material for controlled experiments, (iii) many are pathogens of humans, plants, and domestic animals, and therefore are of medical or environmental interest, and (iv) many are important in industrial processes and therefore are relevant for biotechnology. Furthermore, microbial organisms are unicellular, and the cell membrane provides a convenient boundary that delineates the 'system' for genome-wide studies. In the past, microbes have been used in numerous systems studies, including that of genetic networks, protein-protein interactions, metabolic networks, cell cycle regulation, and signal transduction networks.

Three types of biochemical networks, roughly corresponding to three different levels or 'omes', have been mostly studied in the past: gene regulatory networks, protein interaction networks and metabolic networks.When prior knowledge of modularity allowed the assumption of decoupling, systems studies on biochemical subnetworks or cross-networks were possible. Examples of this include modelling of the cell cycle in yeast, specific metabolic pathways, and signal transduction pathways. Several pioneering studies integrated responses across individual 'omes'. Examples of this include studies of transcriptome and proteome responses to perturbations in metabolic pathways, the effects of a transcriptional regulator on central carbon metabolism in *Bacillus subtilis*, and coordinated analysis of the minimal bacterium *Mycoplasma pneumoniae*, including analysis of its mRNA, protein complexes, and the metabolic network.

What are these studies telling us? Integrating the information from different biological levels reveals complex and unanticipated global behaviours in what were thought to be 'simple' organisms and biochemical systems. For example, the metabolic network in *E. coli* appears remarkably stable with respect to various types of perturbations, but the mechanism for how this stability is achieved appears profoundly different for environmental and genetic perturbations.

Surprisingly, the flux through the *E. coli* pentose phosphate pathway is reversed in response to a blocking mutation, and yet, this is achieved with only subtle changes in the enzyme levels. Another telling example is the smallest self-replicating organism, the bacterium *M. pneumoniae* whose genome encodes merely 689 proteins. Compared to more complex bacteria (*E. coli* encodes ~4,200 proteins), *M. pneumoniae* lacks most transcription factors and other regulators, yet this organism shows a highly complex, intrinsically structured transcriptional response, with many alternative transcripts and multiple regulators per gene. In spite of its minimal genome, the proteome of *M. pneumoniae* exhibits modularity and extensive reuse of functional components, with a substantial crosstalk between different cellular processes. Furthermore, *M. pneumoniae* shows highly coordinated changes in gene expression, specific responses to metabolic perturbations, and adaptability to carbon sources similar to that observed in *E. coli*. It is unlikely that *M. pneumoniae* is a fundamentally unusual organism, rather, these observations suggest a host of unknown regulatory mechanisms that operate across the levels of transcriptome, proteome, and metabolome.

As a result of decades of detailed biochemical work, metabolic networks are the best understood of all biochemical networks We have near-complete collections of components and topologies of metabolic networks in modelmicro-organisms such as *E. coli* and *Saccharomyces cerevisiae*. For the model organism *E. coli*, the majority of metabolic reactions, enzymes, cofactors, substrates, and products are known. This, however, represents only the first step towards understanding how these components function in spatial and temporal integration, and precisely what are the controls exerted on them. While the topologies of metabolic networks are well understood, we are only beginning to understand interactions that control metabolism. Metabolite equilibrium concentrations are accessible experimentally through quantitative metabolomic approaches, which is directly comparable to the measurement of mRNA and protein levels in transcriptomics and proteomics, respectively. In contrast to all other types of biochemical networks, experimental approaches for assessing *in vivo* reaction rates (fluxes) are also well developed for metabolic networks. This is of great importance, as metabolic fluxes are the key determinants of cellular physiology and cannot be predicted from mRNA, protein, or even metabolite levels. Thus, measurement of metabolic flux is equivalent to the measurement of information flow through a signaling pathway, or the information flow between genes residing on the same control circuit. New theoretical frameworks for more efficient extraction of information from experimental data continue to be proposed, and a considerable progress has been made in the analysis of metabolic fluxes under isotopic nonstationary conditions. Since nonstationary flux analysis relies on shorter, transient experiments, this opens an array of new possibilities for flux analysis in higher organisms, improving the scope of systems biology studies of metabolic networks.

BIOINFORMATIC TOOLS FOR SYSTEMS BIOLOGY

While many systems biology approaches involve mathematical and computational modelling, the development, maintenance, and dissemination of tools for systems biology is in itself a significant challenge. Examples of this include development of data repositories, data standards and software tools for simulation, analysis and visualisation of system components such as biochemical networks. Another example are applications of high-throughput molecular profiling technologies which often require sophisticated data processing and analysis, and typically involve elements of signal processing and statistical analysis. As the resulting quantitative measurements are transferred to formal mathematical models for the purpose of modelling, the endeavor becomes perhaps more systems biology and less bioinformatics. However, that is only a matter of a degree, with often no clear boundary between bioinformatics and systems biology.

The need for effective exchange of formal, quantitative systems biology models has driven the development of the Systems Biology Markup Language (SBML). The SBML project aims for the development of the computerreadable format for the representation of biological processes. SBML provides a well-defined format which different software tools can use for the exchange of biological models with high fidelity. A testimony to the importance of SBML is its adoption by software tools concerned with biological modelling (at the time of this writing, over 180 software tools support SBML). The graphical notation for the representation of biological processes has been proposed recently (Systems Biology Graphical Notation, SBGN). The current SBGN specification consists of three complementary languages which aim to describe biological processes and relationships between biological entities.

Since studies of biochemical networks are particularly successful aspect of systems biology, it is not surprising that a plethora of computational tools that address different needs in the analysis of biochemical networks have been reported, and in many cases, these tools are freely accessible. Without attempting to be comprehensive, we highlight some of the widely used research and training tools. Systems Biology Workbench (SWB) is a framework that allows different components for systems biology to communicate, exchange models via SBML, and reuse capabilities without understanding all the details of the each component implementation. From the users perspective, SWB is a collection of tools for systems biology that includes programmes for building, viewing, and editing of biochemical networks, tools for simulation, and tools for import and translation of models. Another highly useful tool is cell designer, a Javabased programme for constructing and editing of biochemical networks. Recent versions of cell designer are able to import models in SBML and support display of biochemical networks based on process diagram language specified by SBGN. In cell designer models can be simulated either with a built-in simulator, or alternatively cell designer can connect to external simulators, such as those provided by SWB.

An independent simulator of models encoded in SBML is COPASI. COPASI can simulate models based on ordinary differential equations (ODEs) as well as stochastic models by using the Gillespie's algorithm. COPASI provides tools for visual analysis of simulation results, and can also perform steady-state and metabolic control analyses. As biological research accelerates through the development of new technologies and instrumentation, biological databases have become an indispensable partner in such research. Building and maintaining of primary databases such as GenBank or Protein Data Bank have long been recognised as important bioinformatics work. Primary biological databases serve both as repositories of experimentally derived information and are the basis for the development of secondary databases that capture higherlevel knowledge. An example of such secondary database is Pfam database of proteins families and domains. Concomitantly with the development of the biochemical systems biology, an important niche of secondary biological databases has emerged: the databases that capture the properties and processes in biochemical networks. The ecosystem of such databases and associated tools is rapidly growing and includes metabolic pathways databases organised around the BioCyc project, database of human biological pathways, database of interactions between small molecules and proteins, and databases of protein-protein interactions. As these databases attempt to reconstruct and organise information about interactions between cellular components, they also attempt to build higher-level knowledge and theories about the biological processes they are concerned with. Such *in silico* knowledge is much needed, as the integral complexity ofmost biological processes is beyond what is comprehensible to the human mind. Therefore, these 'systems biology databases' often represent important foundations for quantitative modelling of biological systems. In some cases, these databases allow a direct export of mathematical models. Also, the first collections of mathematical models of biological processes have been developed (databases of models), concerned solely with archiving and curating the models in SBML for future reuse and refinement. Much needed bioinformatics tools for systems biology research are the tools for visualisation of network structures and network overlay of simulated and experimental data. These tools include yEd graph editor for editing networks, and tools for visualisation of 'omics data in the context of biochemical networks, such as Cytoscape and Pathway Tools Omics Viewer.

FUTURE PERSPECTIVES OF SYSTEMS BIOLOGY

Systems biology is rapidly gaining momentum, as evidenced by the number of publications referencing the term. To understand the relevance of 'systems' thinking for future biochemical research, one needs only to remember that we know most of the components in many biochemical systems, often in exquisite detail, yet understand very little about how these components interact to produce coherent temporal and spatial behaviours that are the hallmark of biological systems. On the other hand, bioinformatics has originally grown from the need to provide tools and handle increasingly large amounts of biological data. As a discipline bioinformatics continues to grow in this important role, but is also increasingly merging and contributing to systems approaches to provide tools necessary for perhaps the most exciting phase in the development of biological sciences.

One of the defining features of systems biology is the use of mathematical and computational models, which are essential to rigorously account for the inherent complexity of biological systems. This complexity arises from the diversity of components (genes, proteins, and metabolites), the high selectivity of their interactions, and a non-linear nature of these interactions. These properties together render the behaviour of biological systems intractable to pure intuition. The computational models used in biochemical systems biology typically require iterative building and stepwise improvements based on the comparison with experiments. Once sufficiently refined, such models have the ability to predict the behaviour of the biochemical system under different perturbations, or hypothetical conditions that may be of interest but are not feasible in experimental settings (e.g. when they are too expensive for practical implementation, or when the analysis of many different conditions is desirable). However, in the new era of systems biology, mathematical models are more than just tools for integrating observations, making testable predictions, or for high throughput *in silico* experimentation. Highly refined mathematical models also serve as the embodiments of our current knowledge about specific biochemical systems.

Mathematical and computational models that underpin biochemical studies may involve different levels of detail and scale, depending on the objectives of the study, what is known *a priori*, and what additional information is accessible experimentally. For example, protein complexes may be studied comprehensively, or the focus may be on a subset of proteins responsible for a specific function, such as protein import into mitochondria. Most of the so-called bottom-up approaches, which start from the descriptions of interactions, focus on a part of the biological system because we lack a comprehensive information about the system of interest. Nevertheless, bottom-up approaches provide highly useful frameworks for the integration of diverse knowledge, for example, the principles established from decades of biochemical work with the information accessible only with the latest experiments. In contrast, top-down approaches are largely data driven, with the caveat that their comprehensiveness is limited by the limitations in experimental approaches. For example, in one of the most comprehensive metabolomic studies to date, 198 out of an expected 453 primary metabolites were quantified simultaneously in cells grown in minimal medium. Therefore, in such applications advances in technology drive the level of 'comprehensiveness' that can be achieved. Many biochemical processes can be conceptualised as complex dynamic networks on the molecular level, and studies of biochemical networks are assuming centre stage in systems biology. Measurements on different 'omics levels provide different, often complementary views of the functions of molecular networks. Recently scientists are interested in the crosstalk between the genes, transcripts, proteins, and metabolites that the gene's expression impacts upon. Increasingly sophisticated models will be required to account for increasingly accurate and comprehensive experimental measurements. Systems approaches have already provided a deeper understanding of diverse biochemical processes, from individual metabolic pathways, to signaling networks, to genome-scale metabolic networks. Therefore, we can safely predict that systems thinking will become even more pervasive in future. The role of formal mathematical and computational models in systems approaches renders the role of bioinformatics increasingly important for systems biology research.

SUMMARY OF THE STEP FOLLOWED IN SYSTEMS BIOLOGY

Characteristics of Biological Systems

Emergence - most complex systems are assumed to be composed of large no. of simple components emerge to exhibit complex behaviours. In many cases, components of the system are assumed to be homogeneous. But biological systems (cells, proteins, genes) are heterogeneous, hence more complex. Thus, biological systems are best char by: (i) heterogeneity of components, (ii) complexity of components, and (iii) selectivity of interactions.

Design Patterns and Control Principles

Structures of biological systems are formed through evolution. Evolution selects circuits that are more likely to be functional. But there is no guarantee they are optimally designed for their function. Hence we should - identify patterns of design, create a library, develop methods to identify which is used in a specific biological system. Many biological circuits have common control mechanisms. Robustness and stability are commonly achieved by using:

- Feedback loops: (i) sophisticated control system, (ii) closes loop of signal circuits, (iii) attains desired control of system, e.g. negative feedback.

- Redundancy: (i) Improve a systems robustness against damages to its components, (ii) Multiple pathways to accomplish function, e.g. MAP Kinase pathway, futile cycle.
- Modular design: (i) Prevents damage from spreading without limit, (ii) Eases evolutionary upgrading of some of the system components.

System Structure Identification

To understand a biological system, we have to first identify its structure (components, their functions, interactions). Difficulty – structure of system cannot be inferred from experimental data based on some principles or universal rules, because systems evolved via a stochastic process. There can be multiple solutions to one given problem.

Example: Stripe-pattern formation:

- *Pomacanthus* (Fig. 23.3) (turing wave), marine angel fish.
- *Drosophila melanogaster* [even-skipped (eve) gene], fruit fly.
- Same phenotype, different mechanisms.

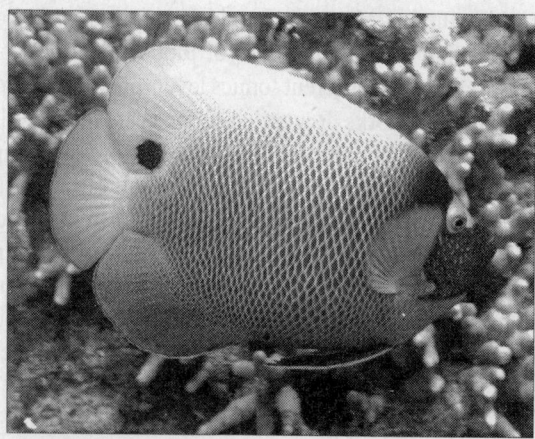

Fig. 23.3: *Pomacanthus.*

Approaches for structure identification: Bottom-up approach:

- Construct a gene regulatory network from independent experimental data.
- Suitable when most of the genes and regulatory relationships are relatively well understood.
- Aim: To build a precise simulation model so that dynamical properties of system can be analysed by changing parameters.

Approaches for structure identification: Top-down approach:

- Infer gene regulatory network from high-throughput DNA microarray data and other new measurement technologies.
- Clustering methods are suitable for handling largescale data but do not directly provide network structures.
- Hence some heuristics must be imposed.

Approaches for structure identification: Hybrid approach:

- It is likely that some knowledge should be assumed in the process of gene network inference.

- Use of trustworthy knowledge can significantly reduce the kinds of network structures feasible.
- Hybrid approach appears to be a promising and practical method.

Computational challenges: 'Given a set of noisy expression profiles, experimental data, and partially correct networks, find a set of plausible gene regulatory network topologies and their associated parameters.'

- Parameters are important, for experimental validation.
- GA and simulated annealing are common parameter optimisation methods.
- Caution: Multiple parameter sets may generate simulation results equally well fitted to experimental data.

System Behaviour Analysis

To have system-level understanding, we need to understand the robustness and stability of the system. In engineering systems, increasing complexity increases stability and robustness of a system. *Mycoplasma* has 400 genes, live under narrowly specific conditions, vulnerable to environmental fluctuations. *E. coli* has 4000 genes, live in varying environments. Evolved genetic and biochemical circuits (–ve feedback) for stress responses and basic behavioural strategies. Feedback in biological systems. Redundancy in biological systems.

Software Platform

Systems biology research requires software systems for data collection, simulators, parameter optimisation, data visualisation, analytical tools. Simulation is important for understanding the behaviour of existing systems. Hence, we need highly functional, accurate, user-friendly simulator systems. Simulator needs to be coupled with parameter optimisation tools, a hypothesis generator, and a group of analysis tools. Algorithms underlying these softwares need to be designed

To sum up, systems biology is an emerging field in biology aiming at system-level understanding of biological systems. It requires a range of new analysis techniques, measurements techniques, experimental methods, software tools, and concepts for looking at biological systems. There is still a long way to go before deep understanding of biological systems can be achieved.for biological research.

Chapter 24

Human Genomes

INTRODUCTION

Human genome, all of the approximately three billion base pairs of deoxyribonucleic acid (DNA) that make up the entire set of chromosomes of the human organism. The human genome includes the coding regions of DNA, which encode all the genes (between 20,000 and 25,000) of the human organism, as well as the noncoding regions of DNA, which do not encode any genes. By 2003 the DNA sequence of the entire human genome was known. The human genome, like the genomes of all other living animals, is a collection of long polymers of DNA. These polymers are maintained in duplicate copy in the form of chromosomes in every human cell and encode in their sequence of constituent bases [guanine (G), adenine (A), thymine (T), and cytosine (C)] the details of the molecular and physical characteristics that form the corresponding organism. The sequence of these polymers, their organisation and structure, and the chemical modifications they contain not only provide the machinery needed to express the information held within the genome but also provide the genome with the capability to replicate, repair, package, and otherwise maintain itself.

In addition, the genome is essential for the survival of the human organism, without it no cell or tissue could live beyond a short period of time. For example, red blood cells (erythrocytes), which live for only about 120 days, and skin cells, which on average live for only about 17 days, must be renewed to maintain the viability of the human body, and it is within the genome that the fundamental information for the renewal of these cells, and many other types of cells, is found.

The human genome is not uniform. Excepting identical (monozygous) twins, no two humans on Earth share exactly the same genomic sequence. Further, the human genome is not static. Subtle and sometimes not so subtle changes arise with startling frequency. Some of these changes are neutral or even advantageous, these are passed from parent to child and eventually become common place in the population. Other changes may be detrimental, resulting in reduced survival or decreased fertility of those individuals who harbour them, these changes tend to be rare in the population. The genome of modern humans, therefore, is a record of the trials and successes of the generations that have come before. Reflected in the variation of the modern genome is the range of diversity that underlies what are typical traits of the human species.

There is also evidence in the human genome of the continuing burden of detrimental variations that sometimes lead to disease. Knowledge of the human genome provides an understanding of the origin of the human species, the relationships between subpopulations of humans, and the health tendencies or disease risks of individual humans. Indeed, in the past 20 years knowledge of the sequence and structure of the human genome has revolutionised many fields of study, including medicine, anthropology, and forensics. With technological advances that enable inexpensive and expanded access to genomic information, the amount of and the potential applications for the information that is extracted from the human genome is extraordinary.

Human genetic engineering relies heavily on science and technology. It was developed to help end the spread of diseases. With the advent of genetic engineering, scientists can now change the way genomes are constructed to terminate certain diseases that occur as a result of genetic mutation. Today genetic engineering is used in fighting problems such as cystic fibrosis, diabetes, and several other diseases. Another deadly disease now being treated with genetic engineering is the 'bubble boy' disease (Severe Combined Immunodeficiency). This is a clear indication that genetic engineering has the potential to improve the quality of life and allow for longer life span. Clearly, one of the greatest benefits of this field is the prospect of helping cure illness and diseases in unborn children. Having a genetic screening with a fetus can allow for treatment of the unborn. Overtime this can impact the growing spread of diseases in future generations.

ROLE OF THE HUMAN GENOME IN RESEARCH

Since the 1980s there has been an explosion in genetic and genomic research. The combination of the discovery of the polymerase chain reaction, improvements in DNA sequencing technologies, advances in bioinformatics (mathematical biological analysis), and increased availability of faster, cheaper computing power has given scientists the ability to discern and interpret vast amounts of genetic information from tiny samples of biological material. Further, methodologies such as fluorescence *in situ* hybridisation (FISH) and comparative genomic hybridisation (CGH) have enabled the detection of the organisation and copy number of specific sequences in a given genome.

Understanding the origin of the human genome is of particular interest to many researchers since the genome is indicative of the evolution of humans. The public availability of full or almost full genomic sequence databases for humans and a multitude of other species has allowed researchers to compare and contrast genomic information between individuals, populations, and species. From the similarities and differences observed, it is possible to track the origins of the human genome and to see evidence of how the human species has expanded and migrated to occupy the planet.

ORIGINS OF THE HUMAN GENOME

Comparisons of specific DNA sequences between humans and their closest living relative, the chimpanzee, reveal 99 per cent identity, although the homology drops to 96 per cent if insertions and deletions in the organisation of those sequences are taken into account. This degree of sequence variation between humans and chimpanzees is only about 10-fold greater than that seen between two unrelated humans. From comparisons of the human genome with the genomes of other species, it is clear that the genome of modern humans shares common ancestry with the genomes of all other animals on the planet and that the modern human genome arose between 150000 and 300000 years ago.

Ongoing collaboration between archaeologists, anthropologists, and molecular geneticists at the Max Planck Institute in Germany and the Lawrence Berkeley National Laboratory and the Joint Genome

Institute in the United States has enabled sequence comparisons between modern humans (Homo sapiens) and Neanderthals (*H. neanderthalensis*). The data obtained so far demonstrate that modern humans and Neanderthals share about 99.5 per cent genome sequence identity, some scientists have claimed that sequence identity may actually be as high as 99.9 per cent.

Research suggests that populations of *H. sapiens* split from *H. neanderthalensis* ancestral populations perhaps as recently as 370,000 years ago and likely shared a common ancestor some 500,000–700,000 years ago. Genomic studies have indicated that there was almost no interbreeding between *H. sapiens* and *H. neanderthalensis*. This suggests that when Neanderthals, the last of the Homo relatives of modern humans, became extinct about 30,000 years ago, only modern humans were left to populate Earth. However, other research has revealed that modern *H. sapiens* in Eurasia, specifically peoples in Europe, China, and Papua New Guinea, have genomes that are more similar to the Neanderthal genome than they are to the genomes of modern *H. sapiens* in Africa. Scientists estimate that 1 to 4 per cent of DNA of modern Eurasians is shared with Neanderthals, a level of similarity that is not found between Neanderthals and modern Africans. These findings indicate that limited interbreeding and gene flow took place between Neanderthals and ancestral *H. sapiens* populations after the latter migrated out of Africa but before they dispersed to other parts of the world.

Comparing the DNA sequences of groups of modern humans from different continents also allows scientists to define the relationships and even the ages of these different populations. By combining these genetic data with archeological and linguistic information, anthropologists have been able to discern the origins of Homo sapiens in Africa and to track the timing and location of the waves of human migration out of Africa that led to the eventual spread of humans to other continents of the globe. For example, genetic evidence indicates that the first humans migrated out of Africa approximately 60,000 years ago, settling in southern Europe, the Middle East, southern Asia, and Australia. From there, subsequent and sequential migrations brought humans to northern Eurasia and across what was then a land bridge to North America and finally to South America.

As humans migrated across the continents, sequence variations arose that became differentially fixed in different populations. Some variations likely reflect what are called founder effects, changes in gene frequency that occur in small populations. Founder effects are generally characterised by genes that are expressed with increasing frequency from one generation to the next and can be traced back to the original founders of the population. Other variations reflect differential selective pressures at work. For example, populations living in equatorial climates were under strong selective pressure that favoured dark skin colour to protect against extreme Sun exposure, thereby decreasing the deleterious health effects caused by sunburn and skin cancer. In contrast, populations migrating to more polar latitudes, where levels of Sun exposure are relatively low, experienced strong selective pressure that favoured light skin colour, thereby facilitating the absorption of sunlight by the skin for the synthesis of vitamin D. In northern Europe and Scandinavia, therefore, individuals with genetic variations leading to lighter skin colour were less likely to become vitamin D deficient and suffer from the bone disease known as rickets.

SOCIAL REGULATION OF HUMAN GENE EXPRESSION

Recent analyses have discovered broad alterations in the expression of human genes across different social environments. The emerging field of social genomics has begun to identify the types of genes sensitive to social regulation, the biological signalling pathways mediating these effects, and the genetic polymorphisms that modify their individual impact. The human genome appears to have evolved specific 'social programmes' to adapt molecular physiology to the changing patterns of threat and opportunity ancestrally associated with changing social conditions. In the context of the immune system, this programming now fosters many of the diseases that dominate public health. The embedding of individual genomes within a broader metagenomic network provides a framework for integrating molecular, physiologic, and social perspectives on human health.

The conceptual relationship between genes and the social world has shifted significantly during the past 35 years. As genes have come to be understood in concrete molecular terms, rather than as abstract heritability constructs, it has become clear that social factors can play a significant role in regulating the activity of the human genome. DNA encodes the potential for cellular behaviour, but that potential is only realised if the gene is expressed—if its DNA is transcribed into RNA (Fig. 24.1). RNA and its translated proteins are what mediate cellular behaviours such as movement, metabolism, and biochemical response to external stimuli (e.g. neurotransmission or immune response). Absent their expression in the form of RNA, DNA genes have no effect on health or behavioural phenotypes. The development of DNA microarray and high-throughput RNA sequencing technologies now allows researchers to survey the expression of all human genes simultaneously and map the specific subset of genes that are active in a given cell at a given point in time—the RNA 'transcriptome'. 'Functional genomics' studies surveying RNA transcriptomes have shown that cells are highly selective about which genes they express, and humans' DNA encodes a great deal more genetic potential than is actually realised in RNA. Even more striking has been the discovery that the social world outside one's body can markedly influence these gene expression profiles.

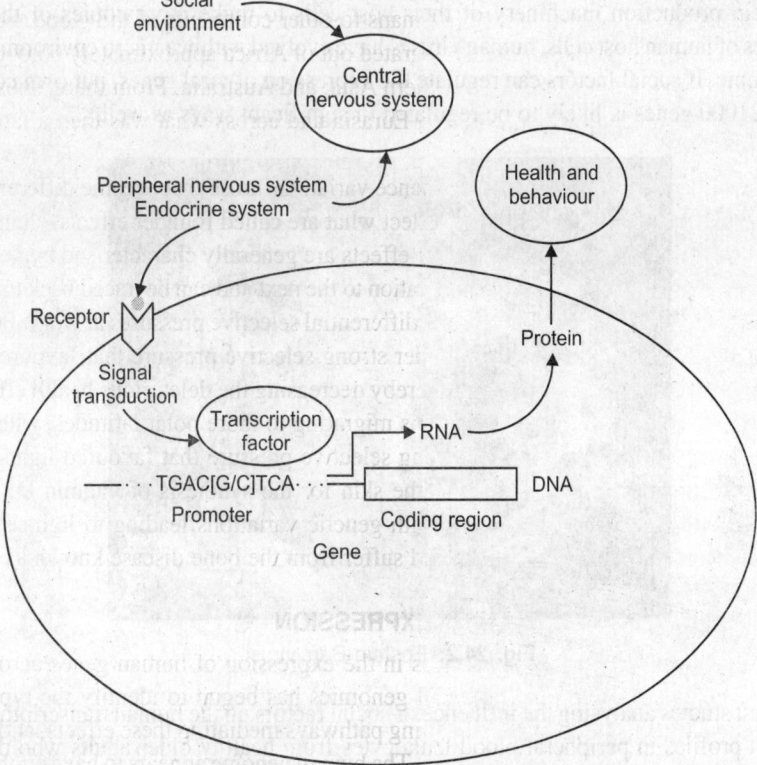

Fig 24.1: Social signal transduction.

This chapter reviews the emerging field of human social genomics, including its recent scientific development, some developing themes regarding the number and nature of 'socially sensitive' genes, and emerging data on the psychological, neural, and endocrine signalling pathways that mediate social influences on gene expression. The presentation also considers some evolutionary theories regarding the teleology of such 'social signal transduction' and the implications of these dynamics for environmental programming of human development and life-span health trajectories. The role of gene polymorphisms (genetics) in modulating individual genomic sensitivity to socio-environmental influences is considered, as are implications of social genomic relationships for public health and policy, including optimal intervention strategies, new opportunities for integrating social genomics into epidemiology, and implications of a public health perspective for understanding how individual human genomes cross-regulate one another in the context of social networks (i.e. social regulation of the human 'metagenome,' or the collective system of individual human genomes). Social genomics research provides a concrete molecular framework for understanding the long-observed relationship between social conditions and the distribution of human health and disease.

SOCIAL REGULATION OF GENE EXPRESSION

The possibility that social factors might regulate gene expression first emerged in the context of studies analysing the effects of stress and social isolation on viral gene expression (e.g. in herpes simplex viruses, HIV-1, Epstein-Barr virus (Fig. 24.2), cytomegalovirus (Fig. 24.3), and the Kaposi's sarcoma—associated human herpesvirus 818). Viruses are little more than small packages of 10 to 100 genes that hijack the protein production machinery of their host cells to make more copies of themselves. As obligate parasites of human host cells, human viruses have evolved within a micro environment structured by our own genome. If social factors can regulate the expression of viral genes, our own complement of approximately 21000 genes is likely to be regulated in significant ways as well.

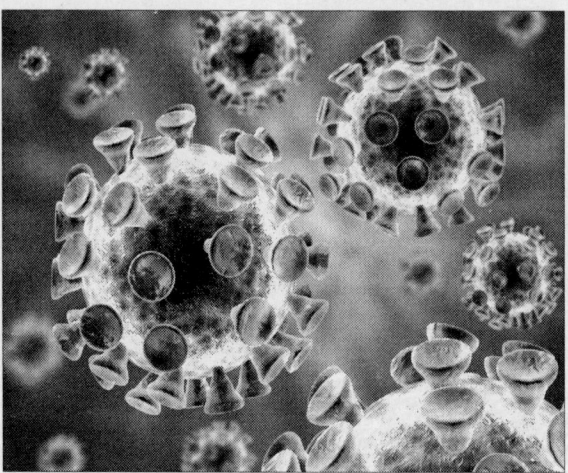

Fig. 24.2: Epstein-Barr virus.

One of the first studies analysing the influence of social factors on the human transcriptome compared gene expression profiles in peripheral blood leukocytes from healthy older adults who differed in the extent to which they felt socially connected to others. Among the 22 283 transcripts assayed, 209 showed

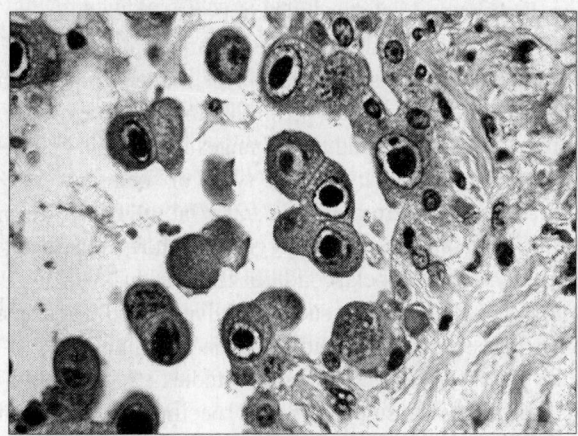

Fig. 24.3: Cytomegalovirus.

systematically different levels of expression in people who consistently reported feeling lonely and distant from others over the course of 4 years. These effects did not involve a random smattering of all human genes but instead had a focal impact on 3 functionally related groups of genes, or 'gene programmes.' Genes supporting the early 'accelerator' phase of the immune response—inflammation—were selectively up-regulated. Down-regulated were genes involved in innate antiviral responses (particularly type I interferons) and genes and Implications for Public Health involved in the production of specific antibody isotypes by B lymphocytes (particularly immunoglobulin G). This complementary up-regulation of pro-inflammatory genes and down-regulation of antiviral and antibodyrelated genes provided a molecular framework for understanding the previously puzzling epidemiological observations that social isolation is associated with diseases that involve both up-regulated immune function (inflammation-related diseases such as heart disease, neurodegenerative diseases, and some types of cancer) and down-regulated immune function (reduced responses to vaccines and viral infections in particular). This specific proinflammatory/ anti-antiviral shift in the basal leukocyte transcriptome showed that social adversity is not broadly immunosuppressive, as had previously been hypothesised, but instead selectively suppresses some groups of immune-response genes (e.g. type I interferons and specific immunoglobulin genes) while simultaneously activating others (e.g. proinflammatory cytokines).

A similar pattern of pro-inflammatory/antiantiviral transcriptome skewing has since been observed in leukocytes sampled from people exposed to a diverse array of adverse life circumstances such as imminent bereavement, traumatic stress, social isolation, low socio-economic status (SES), and cancer diagnosis. Similar dynamics have also been observed in experimental animal models of social instability, low social rank, and repeated social defeat. The mammalian immune system appears to have developed a conserved transcriptional response to adversity (CTRA) that induces a pro-inflammatory/anti-antiviral skew in the circulating leukocyte transcriptome whenever environmental conditions are experienced as threatening, stressful, or uncertain for an extended period of time. Although different types of social adversity can activate a common CTRA, their transcriptional effects are by no means identical because each context generally activates some distinctive transcriptional responses as well.

Laboratory gene regulation analyses have suggested that the common transcriptional components of the CTRA likely stem from the fact that diverse types of social risk factors can induce common neural and hormonal stress responses. For example, catecholamine neurotransmitters released during fight-or-flight stress responses can directly modulate the transcription of several key master regulator genes that orchestrate the activity of broad sets of inflammatory and antiviral genes (e.g. IL1B, IL6, and IFNB). Randomised controlled studies have also shown that stress reducing interventions can reverse CTRA related transcriptional dynamics to down regulate pro-inflammatory genes and upregulate genes involved in type I interferon responses. These stress-induced changes in immune-cell gene expression provide a molecular framework for understanding why diverse types of social adversity come to be associated with a common set of diseases ranging from asthma and viral infections to cancer and cardiovascular disease. Transcriptome profiling of other tissues and organs has shown that social influences can penetrate remarkably deeply into the body. Adverse social conditions have been linked to gene expression alterations in the central nervous system, peripheral organs such as the lymph nodes and spleen, and diseased tissues such as ovarian carcinomas, prostate cancers, and ischemic brain injuries.

Given the much smaller number of social genomics studies targeting solid tissues and the relative difficulty in ascertaining the functional significance of specific transcriptional alterations outside the well-charted territories of the immune response, it is not yet clear what basic gene programmes are being activated in these other tissue contexts (e.g. are they defense responses analogous to the leukocyte CTRA). However, the widespread penetrance of social conditions into gene regulatory dynamics in diverse tissue sites raises the question of how such external social stimuli are physically transduced into biochemical dynamics that can proximally regulate gene transcription within the nuclei of diverse cell types distributed widely throughout the body. New insights into this question have come from bioinformatic analyses of social signal transduction.

SOCIAL SIGNAL TRANSDUCTION

Biologists have traditionally construed signal transduction as the biochemical processes that translate extracellular signals, such as hormones or neurotransmitters, into changes in gene expression through the activation of protein transcription factors that bind to DNA and flag it for transcription into RNA. Social signal transduction extends this analysis to include the upstream neural dynamics that translate social conditions into systemically distributed signalling molecules (e.g. release of norepinephrine during fight-or-flight stress responses) and to include the specific downstream gene modules that are activated by a given transcription factor. For example, when norepinephrine is released from the sympathetic nervous system during fight-or-flight stress responses, cells bearing β-adrenergic receptors translate that signal into activation of the transcription factor cyclic adenosine monophosphate response element-binding protein (CREB). Activated CREB proteins can upregulate the transcription of hundreds of cellular genes. Which genes can be activated by CREB is determined by the nucleotide sequence of the genes promoter—the stretch of DNA lying upstream of the coding region of the gene that is transcribed into RNA. For example, CREB binds to the nucleotide motif TGACGTCA, whereas the microbe-responsive transcription factor nuclear factor kappa-lightchain-enhancer of activated B cells (NF-jB) targets the motif GGGACTTTCC. These 2 transcription factors are activated by different receptor-mediated signal transduction pathways, providing distinct molecular channels through which specific extracellular signalling molecules and, by extension, their specific upstream environmental triggers, can regulate intracellular genomic response. The distribution of transcription factor-binding motifs across humans' approximately 21000 gene promoters constitutes a 'wiring diagram' that maps specific types of environmental processes (e.g. infection vs a fight-or-flight stress response) onto a specific pattern of genome-wide transcriptional response (e.g. CREB vs NF-jB target genes). In that sense, each transcription factor can be said to represent some type of evolutionarily significant characteristic of the environment outside the cell (e.g. CREB = threat or stress, NF-jB = microbe or damaged cell), and the distribution of specific transcription factor-binding DNA motifs across the promoters of humans' approximately 21000 genes can be understood as an evolved 'wisdom of the genome' regarding which genes should be activated to optimally adapt to that environment.

Biological signal transduction research has generally emphasised the role of the physico-chemical or microbial stimuli in transcription factor activation, but studies of social signal transduction have suggested that subjective psychological interpretations of the external environment can also play a significant role in regulating gene expression profiles. For example, activation of the leukocyte CTRA is often more strongly linked to subjective perceptions of the environment than it is to objective environmental conditions, and CTRA transcriptome skewing can be reversed by psychological interventions that target those subjective psychological experiences. In studies of social connection, for example, the subjective experience of loneliness is associated with twice as many differentially expressed genes as is the objective frequency of social contacts, and psychological interventions that reduce subjective loneliness are associated with concomitant reductions in pro-inflammatory gene expression. In women with early-stage breast cancer, CTRA transcriptional profiles are also more strongly associated with the subjective degree of life threat women experience than with objective measures of disease severity such as tumour grade or stage, and cognitive—behavioural stress management interventions can reverse that threat-related transcriptome skewing. In children with asthma, SES-related perceptions of the social world as hostile or threatening are more strongly linked to leukocyte transcriptional alterations than are objective measures of SES such as household income. Objective features of the environment such as the number of interpersonal contacts are, of course, associated with variations in gene expression.

However, subjective social experience also plays a significant role, and the effects of subjective and objective conditions are often transduced into gene expression via different molecular signalling pathways. The combination of genome-wide transcriptional profiling with promoter-based bioinformatic analyses has greatly accelerated the identification of the specific transcription factors that translate subjective social experience into the activation of specific gene programmes.

This approach first identifies the subset of genes that is differentially expressed in response to an environmental risk factor (e.g. social isolation) and then scans the promoters of those differentially expressed genes for transcription factor—binding motifs that are substantially over represented relative to their prevalence across the genome as a whole and might thus reveal which specific transcription factors induced the observed transcriptional alterations. For example, the subset of genes up-regulated in tissues from people experiencing significant social adversity often show a higher prevalence of CREB—target promoter sequences than is found across the population of all human genes, implying that CREB may have played a role in activating that specific gene programme. That inference is consistent with CREB's known role in mediating the gene transcriptional effects of β-adrenergic receptor signalling in response to catecholamines produced during fight-or-flight stress responses. In the context of the leukocyte CTRA, promoter-based bioinformatics analyses have repeatedly implicated increased NF-κB transcription factor activity in the pro-inflammatory gene responses and decreased signalling by interferon regulatory factor family transcription factors in the decreased antiviral gene component.

Promoter-based bioinformatics have also revealed some more surprising differences between the hormonal signals sent by the brain and the transcriptional signals heard by the human genome. In studies of chronic social isolation, impending bereavement, post-traumatic stress disorder, and low SES, promoter bioinformatics have indicated decreased activity of the anti-inflammatory glucocorticoid receptor (GR) in association with the leukocyte CTRA. Under normal circumstances, activation of the

GR by cortisol from the hypothalamic—pituitary—adrenal (HPA) axis would both stimulate the expression of anti-inflammatory GR target genes and cross-inhibit the pro-inflammatory NF-κB transcription factors. However, in people experiencing chronic stress, both of those dynamics appear to be blunted, resulting in a net pro-inflammatory skew in the leukocyte transcriptome. None of these studies found decreases in HPA axis output of cortisol that might explain the reduced levels of GR activity. Instead, the explanation appears to involve a stress-induced reduction in the GRs sensitivity to cortisol— rendering the leukocyte transcriptome partially deaf to the HPA axis request to down-regulate pro-inflammatory genes via glucocorticoid output. A similar glucocorticoid desensitisation dynamic has been observed in mice repeatedly exposed to social stress. In addition to clarifying the molecular origin of the leukocyte CTRA, these findings also highlight a broader possibility that measuring blood levels of hormones, neurotransmitters, and other extracellular signalling molecules may miss some important receptor-level influences on the transcriptional mediators of health and disease. Transcriptome-based bioinformatic assessment of social signal transduction provides an integrated measure of both pre- and post-receptor dynamics at the level that matters most for the molecular biology of disease—gene expression.

Epigenetic dynamics provide another pathway by which social environments might potentially regulate gene expression. Epigenetic influences involve biochemical modifications of DNA such as methylation or histone protein engagement that block gene transcription without altering a gene's DNA sequence. Research with experimental animal models has linked favourable social conditions (e.g. maternal licking of rat pups, high social rank in monkeys) to altered patterns of DNA methylation and gene expression in immune cells and brain structures such as the hippocampus. Correlational human studies have documented associations between DNA methylation profiles and socio-environmental risk factors such as low SES and childhood stress exposure. Although environmental factors clearly influence epigenetic dynamics in human immune cells, much remains to be learned about the signalling pathways that mediate such dynamics and their functional role in social regulation of human gene expression.

EVOLUTION OF SOCIAL PROGRAMMING

As social genomics studies map the particular gene programmes that are empirically sensitive to social conditions, new theoretical analyses are emerging to explain why such connections may have evolved in the first place (i.e. the teleological basis for social programming of the human genome). In the context of the leukocyte CTRA, for example, social adversity redeploys the leukocyte's basal transcriptional resources away from antiviral defenses and toward pro-inflammatory gene products that protect the body against bacterial infections. This shift in the leukocyte's basal transcriptional stance may have been adaptive under Pleistocene hunter—gatherer conditions in which the social ecology outside the body played a major role in shaping the pathogen ecology within the body. Homo sapiens is a distinctively social organism, and its highly social life history strategy has conferred substantial adaptive advantages at the price of increased vulnerability to socially transmitted infectious diseases. Viral infections, for example, are predominately transmitted through extended periods of close social contact, so it would be highly adaptive for an intrinsically social organism to evolve a strong antiviral bias as its default immune response bias. However, when the social world turns hostile and individuals either are isolated or confront conspecific aggression (i.e. feel threatened), the risk of wound mediated bacterial infection increases dramatically, and it would be adaptive to temporarily redeploy leukocyte transcriptional resources toward inflammatory defenses against bacterial infection by linking pro-inflammatory gene expression to β-adrenergic fight-or-flight signalling. RNA as a molecular medium of recursive development are shown in Fig. 24.4.

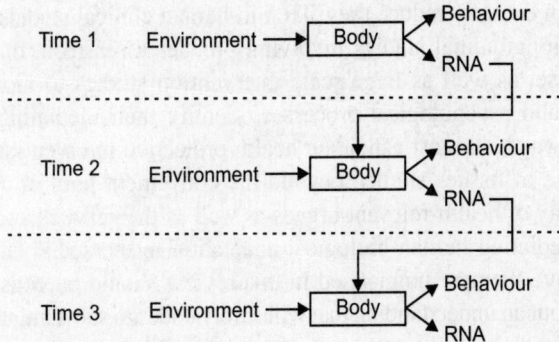

Fig. 24.4: RNA as a molecular medium of recursive development.

Such social programming of immune response biases may well have been adaptive during humans hunter—gatherer prehistory, but in the context of more complex and unstable contemporary social systems the connection of experienced threat, stress, or uncertainty to pro-inflammatory/anti-antiviral transcriptional skewing primes the human in Fig. 24.4, and that molecular composition is itself subject to remodelling by socio-environmental influences, gene expression constitutes both a cause and a consequence of behaviour. RNA can be construed as the physical medium of a recursive developmental system in which social, behavioural, and health outcomes at one point in time also constitute inputs that shape one's future responses to the environment (e.g. as in Heckman's model of human capability development, which analyses how capacities developed at Time 1 have an impact on one's ability to capitalise on environmental opportunities at Time 2). Viewed from another perspective, the evolution of the RNA transcriptomes within the body provides a kind of molecular record of an individual body's cumulative adaptation to the history of environmental exposures that it has encountered, in much the same way as the evolution of a species DNA genome records the history of its adaptation to the environmental exposures it has encountered over the course of its evolutionary history.

LIMITATIONS AND OPPORTUNITIES OF HUMAN GENOMES

The first generation of social genomics studies has opened new vistas on the connection between the human genome and its social environment, but a great deal remains to be clarified, and the existing literature needs to strengthen in several ways. Because of the substantial expense and technical demands of early microarray assays, first-generation social genomics studies involved small cross-sectional analyses with limited assessment of the socio-environmental confounders, rendering the causal relationships unclear. As second generation technologies have lowered cost and technical burden, studies of larger samples and experimental studies have become available. Results of these second-generation studies have broadly replicated the pattern of results from first generation studies (e.g. compare social isolation CTRA dynamics in Cole and others at $n = 14$ with Cole and others at $n = 93$ or rural- and urbanrelated differences in Idaghdour and others at $n = 46$ with Idaghdour and others at $n = 194$). The surprising precision of genomic analyses in small samples stems in part from the statistical advantages of treating thousands of individual genes as multiple noisy indicators of shared higher order 'themes' regarding common biochemical functions, transcription factor targets, and cellular origins of gene expression. Second-generation studies have also included randomised intervention studies showing that adverse social conditions can causally activate the CTRA in animal models and that psychologically targeted interventions can causally reduce the CTRA in human clinical studies. However, a great need remains for large-scale longitudinal studies involving broader assessment of the social environment throughout the life course, as well as large-scale intervention studies to more decisively define the causal effects of social and psychological processes, identify their mediating neural, endocrine, and transcription factor pathways, and test candidate health-protective interventions. There is also a great need to expand the range of tissues studied beyond the convenient pool of circulating leukocytes to encompass a broader array of health-relevant organs as well as the nervous and endocrine systems that play a central role in mediating human biological adaptation to the social environment. Given these limitations, the substantive themes summarised in this review should be considered researchers' best available understanding, but an understanding that will surely undergo substantial revision as the empirical literature deepens over time.

IMPLICATIONS FOR PUBLIC HEALTH

Social regulation of human gene expression implies that many aspects of individual health actually constitute a form of public health in the sense that they emerge as properties of an interconnected system of human beings. Some of one's genes operate differently depending on the presence of other people and their (subjectively perceived) implications for one's own fitness outcomes such as survival and reproduction. As a result, some of the regulatory architecture of the human genome lies outside of the cell in the constraints and affordances present in the social ecology and in people's subjective perceptions and interpretations of those ecologies. From this perspective, individual genomes constitute elements of a broader human metagenomic network (i.e. an interconnected system of related genomes) in which some gene regulatory dynamics represent emergent properties of the system as a whole. Public health can thus be understood as a metagenomic dynamic in which fast-evolving cultural systems interact with slowly evolving (but very long-memoried) human genomes and more rapidly evolving pathogen genomes to produce a pattern of RNA transcriptional responses across a network of elements whose individual properties vary as a function of both genetic and environmental polymorphism.

This conception of public health raises a host of new conceptual questions, such as, Which types of genes are subject to network-level regulation? How are network transcriptional dynamics affected by individual genetic characteristics, by historical—developmental influences, or by network structural characteristics such as linkage patterns, community blocks, and individual linkage characteristics such as centrality, density, or redundancy? Which parts of the central nervous system transduce social signals into gene expression changes? What role does human culture play in metagenomic dynamics and individual social signal transduction? How has a socially networked human genome shaped the development of human social systems and gene—culture coevolution? Do individual transcriptional alterations affect network structure (e.g. via behavioural or biological homophily or heterophily)? How do physico-chemical or microbial features of the environment interact with human social systems to regulate metagenomic systems?

Are these physical environmental influences transmitted through different networks and transduction pathways than are subjective or symbolic social influences? How do positive, supportive, or playful social interactions influence human gene expression (e.g. do they simply abate the adversity-related dynamics, as recently suggested for the leukocyte CTRA, or does there exist a distinct set of prosocial genes involved in the positive neurobiological effects of social interaction)?

As the next generation of social genomics research begins to address these questions, the integration of social network analyses with individual social signal transduction and the evolved social programming of the human genome will open up an array of new opportunities for synthesising molecular, organismic, and population-level analyses into a coherent overall understanding of human health.

In addition to these conceptual advances, new technological developments in gene expression profiling now offer new opportunities to integrate genomics-based perspectives into large-scale field epidemiology. First- and second-generation social genomics studies relied on laboratory-centered research paradigms involving venipuncture blood samples and technically intensive, time-sensitive RNA extraction procedures. However, new developments in RNA stabilisation chemistry and enzymatic amplification of small RNA samples now allow genome-wide transcriptome profiling from more field-friendly sampling modes such as saliva collection tubes, finger-stick dried blood spots, and venipuncture blood samples that can be mailed or stored for months before processing. These technical innovations should allow widespread and economical collection of transcriptome data from epidemiological-scale samples (i.e. n = 1000–10 000) collected in their natural environments. Coupled with ongoing 10- to 100-fold reductions in the cost of transcriptome profiling and the emergence of automated data analytic and bioinformatic interpretation systems, these developments should allow public health research to begin routinely integrating the deep physiological, evolutionary, and molecular genetic perspectives that were formerly the province of basic laboratory research into mainstream epidemiological analyses of human host resistance and disease distribution. The new substantive insights that emerge from these field studies of the human genome will also greatly enrich laboratory and clinical studies by more clearly mapping the basic functional relationships between human social conditions and the activity of individual gene programmes.

As studies more definitively link specific gene expression profiles to disease vulnerability, field-based transcriptome profiling may also provide a new form of molecular surveillance that could potentially identify both overt disease states and host vulnerability conditions that have not yet been converted into disease (i.e. up-regulated inflammatory signalling or impaired antiviral gene expression, as in the CTRA). Such a molecular window into the body could help guide public health interventions and social policies to more proactively address the general host resistance factors that seem to precipitate multiple diseases rather than responding reactively to specific diseases only after they clinically emerge. It might be possible, for example, to use a CTRA profile as an indicator of generalised host resistance or vulnerability (i.e. a latent liability to disease) that is assessed in parallel with realised disease to help gauge the toxicity of various social or geographic environments or the success of public policies and interventions. In combination with the conceptual advances of a network-level metagenomic approach to human health, researchers' growing technical capacity to gauge host resistance at a molecular level before the onset of disease and within the normal social ecology will help accelerate the ongoing transformation of public health from a disease-reactive model to a more proactive and health-centered approach that also accounts for human vitality and physiological resilience.

BIOINFORMATICS AND HUMAN GENOMES

Massive quantities of genomic data and high throughput technologies are now enabling studies on a vastly larger scale than ever before. Examples include simultaneously monitoring and comparing the activity of tens of thousands of genes in cancerous and noncancerous tissue. Advanced computational tools and interdisciplinary experts are needed to capture, represent, store, integrate, distribute, and analyse the data. Gene Gateway was created as a companion to the Human Genome Landmarks wall poster.

Bioinformatics is the term coined for the new field that merges biology, computer science, and information technology to manage and analyse the data, with the ultimate goal of understanding and modelling living systems. Computing and information demands will continue to rise with the explosive torrent of data from large-scale studies at the molecular, cellular, and whole-organism levels.

CHARACTERISTIC OF HUMAN GENOMES

Some of the important characteristic of human genomes are given below:

- The human genome contains 3.2 billion chemical nucleotide base pairs (A, C, T, and G).
- The average gene consists of 3000 base pairs, but sizes vary greatly, with the largest known human gene being dystrophin at 2.4 million base pairs.
- Functions are unknown for more than 50% of discovered genes.
- The human genome sequence is almost exactly the same (99.9%) in all people.
- About 2% of the genome encodes instructions for the synthesis of proteins.
- Repeat sequences that do not code for proteins make up at least 50% of the human genome.
- Repeat sequences are thought to have no direct functions, but they shed light on chromosome structure and dynamics. Over time, these repeats reshape the genome by rearranging it, thereby creating entirely new genes or modifying and reshuffling existing genes.
- The human genome has a much greater portion (50%) of repeat sequences than the mustard weed (11%), the worm (7%), and the fly (3%).
- Over 40% of predicted human proteins share similarity with fruit-fly or worm proteins.
- Genes appear to be concentrated in random areas along the genome, with vast expanses of noncoding DNA between.
- Chromosome 1 (the largest human chromosome) has the most genes (3,168), and Y chromosome has the fewest (344).
- Particular gene sequences have been associated with numerous diseases and disorders, including breast cancer, muscle disease, deafness, and blindness.
- Scientists have identified millions of locations where single-base DNA differences occur in humans. This information promises to revolutionise the processes of finding DNA sequences associated with such common diseases as cardiovascular disease, diabetes, arthritis, and cancers.

How does the human genome stack up is shown in Table 24.1.

Table 24.1: How does the human genome stack up?

Organism	Genome size (bases pairs)	Estimated genes
Human (*Homo sapiens*)	3.2 billion	25000
Laboratory mouse (*M. musculus*)	2.6 billion	25000
Mustard weed (*A. thaliana*)	100 million	25,000
Roundworm (*C. elegans*)	97 million	19,000
Fruit fly (*D. melanogaster*)	137 million	13,000
Yeast (*S. cerevisiae*)	12.1 million	6,000
Bacterium (*E. coli*)	4.6 million	3,200
Human immunodeficiency virus (HIV)	9700	9

Chapter 25

Synthetic Biology

INTRODUCTION

There is no agreed definition of synthetic biology, but it is best understood as the deliberate design of biological systems and living organisms using engineering principles.

The technological manipulation of life was first advocated at the turn of the last century and was instrumental in shaping the rise of molecular biology. However, the widespread use of the term has only occurred since the mid-2000s, as the field has emerged owing to the falling cost of gene sequencing and synthesis. The aims of synthetic biology include: (i) the production of minimal living genomes, (ii) the design of interchangeable parts that can be assembled into pathways for the fabrication of novel components, (iii) the construction of entirely artificial cells, and (iv) the creation of synthetic biomolecules.

One of the main aims of synthetic biology is the creation of novel genetically modified organisms (GMOs), which may have utility in the production of energy and bioremediation. However, such a prospect raises concerns about their accidental release into the environment, as by their very nature such biological machines could evolve, proliferate and produce unexpected interactions that might alter the ecosystem. A number of measures are being proposed or adopted to ensure adequate biological control, including: engineering bacteria to be dependent on nutrients with limited availability, and integration of self-destruct mechanisms that are triggered should the population density become too great. The ability of synthetic biology to produce known, modified or new micro-organisms designed to be hostile to humans is a major concern, and has been demonstrated by the synthesis of the polio virus and the pandemic Spanish Flu virus of 1918. A major issue in this respect is the ready availability and poor control over commercial DNA synthesis. Furthermore, in the future 'garage biology' (synthetic biology at home) may be established as a hobby. However, most concern arises from state-level biological warfare programmes. A number of proposals have been made by both scientific groups and government agencies to address the dual use (military/civilian) nature of synthetic genomics, including: controls over commercial DNA synthesis and public research, and considering the impact of synthetic biology on international bioweapons conventions. As yet there is no policy consensus on these issues. Furthermore, there is an ongoing debate about whether improved biosecurity measures should be achieved through professional self-regulation or formal statutory oversight.

Patenting and the creation of monopolies: The drive to create a micro-organism that can turn biomass into fuels such as ethanol or hydrogen is a major focus of research, which has prompted a concern that patenting may lead to the creation of commercial monopolies or inhibit basic research. In response, there have been moves to develop an open-source movement (based on so called BioBricks) involving creation of a 'commons' that will facilitate open scientific research.

Trade and global justice: Perhaps the biggest success in synthetic biology to date has been in the production of terpenoids for the manufacture of the antimalarial medicine artemisin in, a drug that holds significant promise for worldwide malaria victims. However, there are concerns that synthetic artemisinin would ensure that no local production of natural *Artemisia* could be sustained in developing countries, thereby maintaining the discrepancy of wealth and health between rich and poor nations.

Creating artificial life: One of the most potent promises of synthetic biology is the creation of 'artificial life'. This has provoked fears about scientists 'playing God' and raises philosophical and religious concerns about the nature of life and the process of creation. It has been suggested that a stable definition of 'life' is impossible and that synthetic biologists are confused over what life is, where it begins and particularly, how complex it must be. In response a number of scientists have proposed a modified version of Turing's test for life imitation. However, it is unclear whether these moves to undermine lay concepts of life will ameliorate deeper fears about the blurring of the boundary between the artificial and the natural world.

IMPORTANCE OF SYNTHETIC BIOLOGY

Synthetic biology should be understood in terms of both well established traditions within molecular biology and as an emerging field in its own right. Whilst concerns should be contextualised in this historical approach, it is important to recognise that something new and important is happening. In part this represents a growing confidence in the scientific community to undertake the project of engineering life, but it also marks the maturity of a series of powerful technologies, which may be converging with other developments in computing, materials science and nanotechnology. However, whilst rapid scientific progress is possible, it must be recognised that translating this knowledge into real world applications is often a slow process requiring significant investment.

It is vital to recognise the importance of maintaining public legitimacy and support. In order to achieve this, scientific research must not get too far ahead of public attitudes and potential applications should demonstrate clear social benefits. Furthermore, the potential benefits of the technology must not be overhyped for this risks both creating excessive public anxiety and unrealistic hopes.

The scientific community must take, and be seen to be taking, a lead in debating the implications of their research and engaging with broader society around the issues raised by synthetic biology.

Partnership with civil society groups, social scientists and ethicists should be pursued as a highly effective way of understanding critical issues, engaging with publics and winning support for emerging scientific fields. Experiments in upstream engagement and public consultation should be undertaken to provide a valuable channel for helping negotiate the boundaries of what is socially acceptable science.

A robust governance framework must be in place before the applications of synthetic biology are realised. This will require a thorough review of existing controls and regulations, and the development of new measures, particularly relating to biosafety, environmental release and biosecurity.

Research agencies, such as the Biotechnology and Biological Sciences Research Council (BBSRC), have an important role, not only in terms of funding the best science, but also in steering and shaping the field. Thus research can be undertaken in a way that ensures ongoing public support and realises the potential social and economic benefits of these powerful technologies, whilst controlling risks in a way that reassures both the public and the scientific community.

Synthetic biology is an exciting multidisciplinary field that promises many benefits, whilst at the same time raising important social and ethical issues. Yet although it is a rapidly emerging field, it must be stressed that work on synthetic biology is still at a very early stage.

This chapter aims to briefly review the main social and ethical issues raised in public debates about synthetic biology. In particular, it draws on media reports, academic publications and grey literature mostly published in the last five years. The first two sections provide some definitions of synthetic biology and summarise the central areas of scientific research. This is followed by a description of how the science and technology has developed in recent years, the emergence of public debate about its implications and the policy response to these concerns in a number of key areas. Finally, some reflections on the lessons that might be learnt from the earlier debates over genetic engineering and recommendations for policy are offered in the chapter.

DEFINITION OF SYNTHETIC BIOLOGY

Synthetic biology is a new interdisciplinary area that involves the application of engineering principles to biology. It aims at the redesign and fabrication of biological components and systems that do not already exist in the natural world. Synthetic biology combines chemical synthesis of DNA with growing knowledge of genomics to enable researchers to quickly manufacture catalogued DNA sequences and assemble them into new genomes. Improvements in the speed and cost of DNA synthesis are enabling scientists to design and synthesise modified bacterial chromosomes that can be used in the production of advanced biofuels, bio-products, renewable chemicals, bio-based specialty chemicals (pharmaceutical intermediates, fine chemicals, food ingredients), and in the health care sector as well.

Synthetic biologists have been debating their neologism for years. Rob Carlson, an early advocate of the subject, recalls the various appellations of 'Intentional Biology', 'Constructive Biology', 'Natural Engineering', 'Synthetic Genomics' and 'Biological Engineering'. Quoting 'Making Sense of Life' by Evelyn Fox Keller in his forthcoming book 'Learning to Fly: the past, present and future of Biological Technology' Carlson suggests that the term 'Synthetic Biology' has been in use for over a century and as such its continued employ is somewhat inevitable. Though some of these varied terms are deployed simultaneously, it does appear from reviews of the literature that 'Synthetic Biology' is becoming the dominant term describing this new field.

What seems to be at stake in this struggle for nomenclature is not only the establishment of a disjunction, the drawing up of boundaries for a new field, but also the weight of social implications and public misunderstandings of what it promises to achieve. Indeed, due to internal fears over possible incitement of anti-recombinant-DNA riots the proposed title of Steven Benner's 1988 conference in Switzerland, 'Redesigning Life', had to be renamed. There seems to be a fear that the single word synthetic connotes negative images of monstrous life forms let loose by maniacal scientists. However, it is certain that whilst terminology plays a role in perception, the fears for and about synthetic biology will not be allayed by simply changing its name.

Whatever umbrella term is placed over the research the goals are broadly similar and can be summarised thus: synthetic biology attempts to recreate in unnatural chemical systems the emergent properties of living systems the engineering community has given further meaning to the title to extract from living systems interchangeable parts that might be tested, validated as construction units, and reassembled to create devices that might (or might not) have analogues in living systems.

SOMETHING OLD, SOMETHING NEW

The scientifically compelling idea of the technological manipulation of life was first advocated by Jacques Loeb at the turn of the last century. In particular, he elaborated a materialistic and mechanistic view of living things which would allow them to be engineered. This 'engineering principle' in biology directly influenced many of the early leaders in genetics, including both Morgan and Muller, the latter testifying that after he read Loeb's work in 1911, his major scientific goal was to control evolution. This objective played a key role in Muller's search for a means of artificially creating mutations and eventually led him to successfully experiment with X-rays. Muller's work was fundamentally important as it was the first demonstration that heredity could be artificially manipulated by means other than selective breeding.

The aim of engineering life was also instrumental in shaping the development of what became known as molecular biology during the 1930s. A key factor in the emergence of this new science and the realisation of what Kay has called the 'molecular vision of life' was the role of the Rockefeller Foundation in sponsoring a very large programme of research into the physical and chemical basis of life. Before the war the Foundation was the largest source of funding for basic research in biology, with Federal government support only becoming significant after 1945.

The concept of living things as having machine-like properties that can be deliberately altered became institutionalised in the rise of post-war molecular biology and was clearly articulated by pioneer researchers such as Monod, Rostand and Tatum. Despite this, it was only in 1974 that the Polish geneticist Waclaw Szybalski introduced the term 'synthetic biology' at the birth of the recombinant DNA era.

However, the widespread use of the term synthetic biology has only occurred since the mid-2000s. The reasons for this are complex, but the resurgence of interest in the idea of using engineering principles to create artificial life is largely down to the falling cost of gene sequencing and synthesis following the completion of the human genome project and the development of high speed automation. In this sense, advances in the speed and scale of existing technologies, rather than the arrival of new ones, have enabled the realisation of one of the longest held promises of modern biology.

Scope of Synthetic Biology

Research within synthetic biology can be explored through one of two approaches: top-down, or bottom-up. The top-down approach attempts to eliminate the problem of natural complexity by removing it, e.g. by stripping a genome of all genetic material that is not absolutely essential for replication and functionality. The bottom-up approach uses naturally occurring organisms that appear to have little complexity and adds the required functions by engineering them into the existing genome. There are a number of major areas of research that constitute the field of synthetic biology. These can crudely be broken down under the following headings: making minimal genomes, designing modular components, pathway engineering, expanding the genetic pool, production of artificial cells, and creation of synthetic biomolecules.

Minimal genomes

The production of minimal genome microbes entails experiments designed to determine the smallest number of genes required for a bacterium to survive and follows the top-down approach to synthetic biology. Craig Venter's team at the Institute for Genomic Research began to experiment with the bacterium *Mycoplasma genitalium* (Fig. 25.1) in the 1990s. This research built on a survey of the *M. genitalium* genome using random sequencing and resulted in the estimation of a gene complement of 470 coding regions for such things as DNA repair, energy metabolism and other essential processes. This figure was reduced to 386 essential genes by 2005. The production of minimal living genomes is undertaken

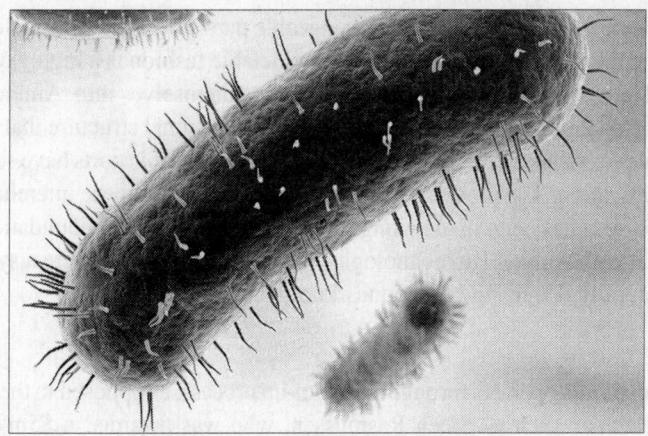

Fig. 25.1: *Mycoplasma genitalium.*

to produce a 'chassis' that can have other synthetic pathways added, thereby enabling various products to be made from the same basic organism. It is hoped that these basic cells could be utilised for such things as producing efficient fuel alternatives or as a means to slow climate change. Though the basic science involved in the production of these minimal genomes, predominantly gene knockout technology, has been utilised for some time, the outcome of such experimentation in the production of minimal genomes is relatively new. Furthermore, the development of those minimal genome microbes into working systems for the production of fuels or clean up of environmental contaminants is still at a very early stage.

Modular components, pathway engineering and the expanded gene pool

Whereas other disciplines in biology are seen to struggle with modelling and describing the complexity of systems, the engineering perspective strips the system to its bare bones and then develops a 'limited number of well characterised, standardised objects', which can be modelled using present computing capacity. These standardised objects, or interchangeable parts, represent a top-down approach to synthetic biology and can be built from first principles, in a hierarchical manner, into complex systems, in which each component and its interactions are known. This predictability means that at every level in the hierarchy in a system the details of how the components are constructed from parts is irrelevant. Thereby the abstraction of design and fabrication can be accomplished, meaning that complex machines can be developed from a small number of basic modular elements.

To achieve this engineering abstraction research is intensively focused both on the standardisation of these interchangeable parts and the decoupling of complex systems into more manageable components. This allows for researchers dispersed across the world to collaborate independently.

Benner and Sismour outline the two types of interchangeable parts being developed by the synthetic biology community: DNA and proteins. Deoxyribonucleic acid has proven to be an excellent structure for modification since the backbone that supports the base pairs is relatively stable, even when entirely synthetic nucleic acids are added to the sequence. Slight modifications to the DNA polymerase enzyme allow for normal 'reading' of a DNA sequence that contains nucleotides other than AGCT. The two artificial nucleotides produced by Benner's team are K and X, forming what he calls AEGIS (An Expanded Genetic Information System).

In contrast, the search for protein-based interchangeable parts has proven more difficult. Engineering proteins by modifying the amino acid sequence in a predictable fashion is a highly complex process due to the secondary and tertiary structures that proteins arrange themselves into. Amino acids interact with each other causing the chain to fold and bend into a three dimensional structure that is hard to anticipate from sequence data alone. As such, attempts to engineer interchangeable parts have so far been successful mostly by DNA modification. The production of pathways made up of these interchangeable parts is the ultimate goal and progress has been made along those lines by the Gate's Foundation-backed Berkeley team. In collaboration with Amyris Biotechnologies they have been developing a synthetic pathway for the production of naturally occurring compounds known as isoprenoids.

Artificial cells

The creation of artificial cells operates through a bottom-up process, as opposed to the top-down strategies so far described. Scientists such as Steen Rasmussen, who was awarded a $5m grant from the Los Alamos National Laboratory, are attempting to build life-like cells from scratch. They place three components at the centre of that project: a system of metabolism, an information-storing molecule, and a membrane to hold it together. Rasmussen's team is developing a 'protocell'. The protocell is different from naturally occurring cells, or minimal living organisms, perhaps most evidently in the use of Peptide Nucleic Acid (PNA) in place of DNA. PNA uses peptides in place of the DNA sugar-phosphate backbone. Rasmussen's lab is just one of the 13 partners in the PACE (Programmable Artificial Cell Evolution) consortium. This research network aims to produce self-organising, evolvable, life-like systems to make the next generation of self-repairing computer and robotics technologies and to 'direct all kinds of complex production and remediation on the nanoscale'.

Synthetic biomolecules

As earlier indicated the search for interchangeable parts through protein modification has proven complex due to the secondary and tertiary structural features of these molecules. The modification of amino acid sequences after they have been transcribed from genes in the cell can greatly alter the functionality of the sequence, offering some explanation for the observed discrepancy between low gene number and increased complexity in the higher animals. British scientists have recently developed a chemical tagging system that utilises established GM techniques (the LacZ reporter enzyme scaffold) to attach post-translation modifications to amino acid sequences, thereby producing proteins that have functions such as detecting mammalian brain inflammation and disease. Other examples of protein modification are detailed in a Science perspectives article, and include such things as the construction of a synthetic mimic of erythropoietin that has a prolonged circulation time in the body.

Application of Synthetic Biology

1. Biomedicine
   (a) Complex molecular devices for tissue repair/regeneration.
   (b) Smart drugs.
   (c) Biological delivery systems.
   (d) Vectors for therapy.
   (e) Personalised medicine.
   (f) Cells with new properties that improve human health.

2. Synthesis of biopharmaceuticals:

 (a) Complex natural products.

3. Sustainable chemical industry

 (a) Environmentally friendly production of chemicals.

4. Environment and energy:

 (a) Bioremediation.

 (b) Production of energy.

 (c) GMO safety.

5. Production of smart materials and biomaterials.

6. Security/counter-terrorism.

SYNTHETHICS, OR SYNBIOETHICS: THE RISE OF CONCERNS ABOUT SYNTHETIC BIOLOGY

The scientific community hasn't shied away from acknowledging the potential dangers of synthetic life forms, with ethics playing a role in international conferences and with almost every review of synthetic biology indicating a need for ethical debate, internal regulation and safe practice. Indeed a declaration made by members at the Second International Meeting on Synthetic Biology (Synthetic Biology 2.0) supports the adoption of policies to ensure safe practice in the scientific community. There is feeling that ethics and standards guidelines should be followed. A code of ethics and standards should emerge for biological engineering as it has done for other engineering disciplines. A particular theme that crops up in the discussion on the ethics of this emergent science is the comparison to the situation faced by genetic engineering in the 1970s and 1980s. Synthetic Biology needs to establish itself as a community effort that is safe and nurtures responsible practices and attitudes. For this, a code of ethics and standards need to be developed for biological engineering. Learning from gene therapy, we should imagine worst-case scenarios and protect against them.

In part, the readiness of the scientific community to discuss ethical issues stems from concerns within the profession and there have been calls for greater self-regulation. However, it also acknowledges the fact that a number of NGOs and civil society groups have raised social, safety and ethical concerns about the development of this new field. These include environmental organisations such as the action group on Erosion, Technology and Concentration (ETC) and Friends of the Earth, as well as peace and security groups such as the Bulletin of Atomic Scientists.

In thinking about the ethical, social and legal issues raised by synthetic biology a number of areas of concern can be identified: uncontrolled release into the environment, bioterrorism, patenting and the creation of monopolies, trade and global justice, and the creation of artificial life.

UNCONTROLLED RELEASE

Scientific/Technical Development

An example of how synthetic organisms may be deliberately released into the environment is for the bioremediation of soil (e.g. for removal of environmental pollutants), something Venter's various research teams are interested in. Whilst genetically engineered micro-organisms have been developed for such purposes they have only once been tested in the field and there are none in the regulatory pipeline.

Social and Ethical Issues Raised

The main concerns in this area are centred on the development of synthetic organisms that are either intentionally or accidentally released into the environment. The ETC Group raises this as a major issue that parallels the debates about GM crops. Their report was spurred by the widely publicised patent application for a minimal bacterial genome, a list of genes, submitted by the Venter Institute, detailing the least number of genes that the bacterium *M. genitalium* requires for survival and reproduction. Further concerns were expressed following the announcement of Venter's bacterial genome swap. Generally the media reports quickly dismiss certain concerns, celebrate the research, and present a rather balanced approach.

A major issue raised by the critics of this technology is that by their very nature biological machines are evolutionary machines, they are subject to natural selection and potentially gene flow. This means that mutations in the genome of the synthetic organisms could produce unexpected interactions with the environment and other living, natural organisms. Considering the myriad unusual functions enabled by BioBricks that could be integrated in synthetic genomes, a concern is that functions upon which nature has never operated may provide advantages over natural organisms leading to unexpected proliferation of a synthetic biology product, thereby radically altering the ecosystem. Micro-organisms intended for clean up of one particular chemical may interact with others, potentially passing synthetic genes to natural species thereby 'contaminating' the gene pool. It's also claimed that even without such evolutionary intervention the released species may interact with naturally existing substances and cause unexpected side-effects. These fears are reminiscent of the concerns voiced by anti-nano groups and individuals such as Prince Charles, who famously envisaged a world reduced to 'grey goo' by out of control nano machines.

In this context questions have been asked about the adequacy of existing regulatory regimes for the control of GMOs, which are based on assessing relatively simple genetic changes to bacteria. In particular, established risk assessment methods may not be adequate to deal with the much more complex changes brought about by synthetic biology, which involves the engineering of entire biochemical pathways. This challenge may require important changes to the methods and procedures used to assess the environmental risks posed by the novel organisms created by synthetic biology.

Scientific and Policy Response

These concerns are quite similar to those raised about the 'old' genetic engineering. A number of commentators have suggested that none of the more pressing fears about recombinant DNA has yet emerged as real threats due to early, strict regulation that was eased over the course of the field's maturation. Furthermore, in addition to working within the established regulatory regime, a number of technical measures have been adopted to tackle this issue. Specifically, the threat of escape and proliferation has been offset by engineering bacteria dependent on particular nutrients that don't readily occur in the natural environment, thereby significantly reducing their competitive capacity. Similar proposals are being made with regards to using synthetic components of the DNA structure (e.g. synthetic amino acids) such that the organism cannot replicate in an environment devoid of them. Other strategies involve utilising some of the naturally-inspired BioBricks that monitor the size of the population as it divides. These could be connected to a 'self-destruct' mechanism that is triggered should a population spurt occur or should the population density become too great. It has also been suggested that engineering biological systems to reduce their viability outside the lab should become common practice. Tucker and Zilinskas advocate the precautionary principle, 'treat synthetic micro-organisms as dangerous until proven harmless.' Using the NIH guidelines for genetically engineered micro-organisms they suggest that any synthetic DNA containing BioBricks would have to be studied under high levels of physical containment. A report, produced by Drew Endy of MIT, several of the J. Craig Venter Institute team and G.L Epstein from the Center for Strategic and International Studies proposes numerous 'options for governance' of synthetic genomics. The authors attribute the current biosafety framework to the 'foresight of the scientists who invented recombinant DNA' and argue that any proposed framework for synthetic genomics should be based upon this existent scheme, since it has 'enabled the demonstrably safe development and application of recombinant DNA technology over the past three decades'.

They identify six policy options to improve the safety of benign/beneficial synthetic genomics:

1. Education about the risks of, and guidance on best practice for, synthetic genomic experiments at the undergraduate and postgraduate levels.
2. Production of a safety manual specifically tailored for synthetic biology labs.
3. Development of a clearing house mechanism to dispense advice on best practice and emergency procedures.
4. Broadening of the Institutional Biosafety Committees' (IBC) remit.
5. Creation of a National Advisory Group for extra-risky/novel experiments.
6. Broader IBC review and enhanced enforcement of compliance with biosafety guidelines.

The first two options form part of a 'modest' portfolio of options, these two combined with 4 and 5 may indirectly produce a more effective portfolio, but at greater expense. Implementation of all six options would, according to the report, represent an 'aggressive' policy towards biosafety.

BIOTERRORISM

Scientific/Technical Development

The development of biological weapons has a long history, with military programmes using advances in basic biology, including recombinant DNA techniques, to try to create new forms of offensive weapons. In this context, it is notable that a CIA Report from 2003 painted a dark picture of the bioweapons future suggesting that some 'engineered biological agents could be worse than any disease known to man' and that the genomic revolution had made such rapid progress that the traditional methods of monitoring weapons of mass destruction could prove inadequate. To ensure that the intelligence services remained knowledgeable on the potential applications of bioengineering the report suggests a closer working relationship with the biological science community. In the UK similar concerns have arisen about synthetic biology with the Ministry of Defence highlighting the field as one that may impact future military capabilities and in 2006 the Defence Science Advisory Council agreed to examine the military opportunities and threats arising from the field.

The major issues about synthetic biology's ability to be misused centre around the production of known, modified or new micro-organisms designed to be hostile to humans either directly or indirectly. The development, production and stockpiling of bioweapons is restricted under the 1972 Biological and Toxin Weapons Convention. Tucker and Zilinskas point out that synthetic biology not only allows for production of new forms of life, but also the synthesis of those that exist already. By reproducing known pathogens in the lab, such as influenza, one might be able to obfuscate the controls imposed on the movement of such organic substances.

Researchers funded by DARPA at Stonybrook University successfully synthesised polio virus from scratch. The lead scientist, Dr. E. Wimmer, under criticism from the media and fellow scientists defended the research suggesting that it would not fuel bioterrorism since they created the virus from readily available components and that it underscored the need to continue vaccination against the disease. Three years later another team of scientists published a paper in Science announcing they had sequenced and built the pandemic Spanish Flu virus of 1918, which killed an estimated 20–50 million people worldwide. This research was undertaken to understand the virus in more depth, since much that was known about it was largely speculative. It was also hoped that the research would help scientists understand virulent flu viruses more generally. An editorial of the same issue of the journal Science defends its production and publication. Craig Venter described this as the 'the first true Jurassic Park scenario.

SOCIAL AND ETHICAL ISSUES

Though researchers in the field are quick to point out the potential ethical dilemmas and social implications, or at least acknowledge that they need to be investigated , the media has continued to see this as a major issue. In 2006 a Guardian reporter ordered part of the DNA sequence of the smallpox virus and had it sent to his home, which raised questions about the regulation of DNA sequence supply. An article in the New Scientist on the sequence suppliers found that, 'of the 12 companies that replied, just five said they screen every sequence received. Four said they screen some sequences, and three admitted not screening sequences at all'. The Guardian article also found that of three UK sequencing companies, 'one did not screen customers or sequences, one carried out checks on customers only and a third checked customers and had carried out a pilot study on screening DNA orders but is not currently doing so.' The major question raised by these reports is that if a Guardian or New Scientist journalist can order and be supplied with genetic sequences from dangerous pathogens then who else may have, or may be able to do so?

Whilst the academic community continues debating regulation and ethics, biohacking or 'garage biology' is, according to some media reports, being established as a home hobby. As DNA sequencing becomes cheaper and quicker and second hand equipment becomes available on eBay the power to create synthetic sequences may be dispersed to many individuals and groups. Biohackers have also become known by the portmanteau 'biopunk' (biotech punk), that has its origins as a science fiction genre. The most recent, and significant addition to this movement has been the online publication of a 'Primer for Synthetic Biology', a manual, written in simple, non-technical language, for those wishing to engage themselves in some bio hacking. Interestingly Mohr, a student at Boston University at the time of writing, includes in his 72 page draft a notice of intent to provide an outline of the key ethical issues facing synthetic biology titled 'ethics for everyone'. Though biohacking is beginning to develop a web presence, and is certainly becoming quite prominent in the blogosphere there is little evidence, as yet, that it has any active/practising following. Tucker and Zilinskas identify two potential terrorist categories: the 'lone operator' and 'the biohacker'. The lone operator is a rogue synthetic biologist and the biohacker is, as above, a college kid eager to demonstrate their technological prowess. If indeed second hand tools for genome assembly are becoming available to the public at affordable costs then this would seem to add weight to the concerns over possible terrorist use of synthetic biology research.

However, Tucker and Zilinskas argue that 'At present, the primary threat of misuse appears to come from state-level biological warfare programmes'. They suggest that the construction of an entirely new pathogen using synthetic sequences is unlikely given the present state of the art and that the more likely threat is from the creation of already known pathogens, such as polio, as discussed above. The technological obstacles to producing either pathogen are seen as a limiting factor that renders synthetic biology no more concerning that previous debates about genetic engineering. Furthermore, even if such organisms could be produced, they are hard to 'weaponise' – something which would be essential for their role as offensive weapons or instruments of terror. Whilst the prospects for the creation of biological weapons based on synthetic biology remain contentious and uncertain, a more fundamental problem has been raised about the level of awareness within the scientific community of the potential military uses of the technology. Most proposals for governance and oversight depend on scientists being aware of and reporting potential misuses. However, this in turn will critically depend on researchers being aware of the possible applications and risks of synthetic biology. A recent study carried out by Alexander Kelle found a low level of awareness of the key policy documents and debates about biosecurity amongst synthetic biology researchers in Europe. This raises major questions about how easy it will be to implement any such measures in this area.

Scientific and Policy Response

The US policy agency, the National Science Advisory Board (NSABB) Working Group on Synthetic Genomics produced a report that addresses itself to the dual use nature of synthetic genomics – meaning that technology and knowledge from the field can be both used and misused for and against the public health and national security. The working group sought to establish whether the existing regulatory framework for Select Agents was sufficient to cover the generation of synthetic organisms *de novo*. They highlighted a potential difficulty with the present regulatory framework with regards to identifying whether or not a synthetic organism is a Select Agent due to problems with screening sequences that may not exactly resemble those covered under SAR. Following consultation with various groups the NSABB considered and rejected a number of proposals, including:

- Restricting access to new sequence information about select agents.
- Monitoring the sale of chemicals and lab equipment used to synthesise DNA.
- Voluntary/involuntary surveillance/tracking of researchers/students using or trained to use synthetic genomics.
- Modifying the SAR so that all select agent genomes are covered.
- Modifying the SAR or issuing new regulations defining Select Agents in terms of their sequence.

The Sunshine Project, an anti-bioweapons NGO, argued that there was a conflict of interest at the NSABB. In particular, the Project claimed that the NSABB has set up a working group to ostensibly make recommendations for the safe government of synthetic biology, but that it 'will instead assault regulation of a wide range of biodefense and biotech risks'. This, they argued, came from pressure exerted by powerful scientists on the NSABB and the working group. The Sunshine Project identified a competition for funding between two scientific camps: synthetic biologists and infectious disease researchers. Whilst the two compete for funding they have a shared common goal, 'to take down what they perceive as a threat: biosecurity legislation designed to protect the public'.

The Sunshine Project has been very sceptical about the report and suggests that the findings and recommendations are not logically coherent. They go even further and argue that the report is a preemptive attack on the regulation of synthetic biology and the SA rule to free up regulatory space for the development of synthetic applications.

Where the Sunshine Project, along with many other civil society organisations, advocate external regulation, the majority of the scientific community seek to establish self-regulatory practices. In preparation for debate on self governance at the Synthetic Biology 2.0 conference, Maurer, Lucas and Terrell produced a report on safety and security. Their document argues that self regulation is important, but that it shouldn't 'necessarily displace traditional interventions based on regulation, legislation, and treaties'. They argued that the difference between the ethical problems associated with more traditional biotechnological developments and synthetic biology are minor and suggested the risk posed by synthetic biology is relatively small.

The four main areas of concern in the paper are: (i) sequence screening, (ii) community norms, (iii) continuing debate, (iv) technological solutions.

1. The practice of screening genetic sequences by oligo companies is mixed. The paper suggests enforcing screening practices at the commercial side and a community pledge not to place orders with any company that fails to adequately screen from Jan 1st 2007. Furthermore, companies should interconnect to ensure that dangerous sequences are not split over multiple orders. Software for such screening should also be improved.

2. Synthetic biologists have a responsibility to ensure their work isn't making terrorism easier. An ethics advisory committee should be developed. Advice should be freely available and confidential, perhaps via an Ethics Hotline.

3. The ethics of synthetic biology are not fully clear and may change over time and as such debate must continue. An ethics 'clearing house' website where members could report potential accidents and biosecurity threats should be established. Creation of professional entities such as formal standards, codes of ethics, advisory bodies, and a professional society seem reasonable.

4. Synthetic biologists may be perfectly poised to develop solutions to ethical problems at the design level. Barcodes that identify the creator of a synthetic organism could be implemented and should be explored. Inherently safe organisms can be developed that do not survive and propagate in nature.

PATENTING AND THE CREATION OF MONOPOLIES

Scientific/Technical Development

A major aspiration of synthetic biology is the alteration of micro-organisms by genomic intervention for production of living machines that can turn biomass into fuels such as ethanol or hydrogen. Venter's team hopes to produce a synthetic form of *Clostridium* (Fig. 25.2) by amalgamating the genomes of two separate species, *Clostridium cellulolyticum* and *Clostridium acetobutylicum*, that together could do just that. This application is garnering a lot of funding from multiple sources with the Joint BioEnergy Institute, a team of national US laboratories, expecting $125m over the next five years from the US Department of Energy. As huge amounts of money are being invested in synthetic biology groups it is clear that there are high expectations of a significant commercial return.

Social and Ethical Issues Raised

One of the main issued raised is that synthetic biology falls into US intellectual property 'at the confluence of biotechnology and computing'. Rai and Boyle highlight that patenting appeals have proven a rather problematic case for the Federal Circuit Court of Appeals, which has consistently ignored the 'obviousness' clause of patent legitimacy, relying instead on *per se* rules developed for 20th century chemical inventions. Coupled to this are the problems that software caused by neither fitting into the intellectual property regime of patents or copyrights, an issue that was hardly resolved by forcing it under both. Rai and Boyle suggest that difficulty with the way in which the law handles software and biotechnology individually could come together to form 'a perfect storm'.

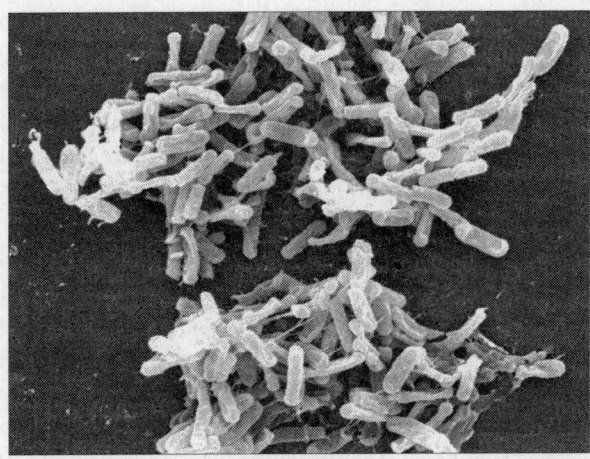

Fig. 25.2: *Clostridium.*

There are two major concerns about the intellectual property puzzle of synthetic biology, namely patents that are too broad and those that are too narrow. The difficulty is that broad patents may restrict collaboration and stifle development in the field, and narrow patents may over-complicate the process, meaning that hundreds of patents have to be negotiated to produce a system from standardised parts.

The spur for debate on the IP problems surrounding synthetic biology has come from Venter's patenting of Synthia. He hasn't only sought a patent for the minimal living cell in the US, but also at the international level through the World Intellectual Property Organisation. More recently Venter has filed patent applications for making synthetic genomes (UPSTO no. 20070264688) and putting them into cells (20070269862). The ETC Group claims that Venter's 'enterprises are positioning themselves to be the Microsoft of synthetic biology', or what they called Microbesoft. ETC argues that the landmark ruling of Diamond vs. Chakrabarty opened the door to patent all biological products and processes, and that synthetic biology easily fits into its scope. Other than the detraction to potential research on synthetic biology the ETC Group doesn't expand on why such a monopoly on synthetic life forms should be avoided.

Scientific and Policy Response

MIT's BioBricks project has been setup as a way round the restrictions placed on innovators by broad patent claims and hopes to replicate the open-source software movement. Since 2004 the registry has increased from around 100 available parts to approximately 2000 in 2008. The BioBricks Foundation (BBF) is a non-profit organisation established to ensure that the parts produced for the registry remain freely available to the public. As part of that goal the BBF has trademarked 'BioBrick' and 'BioBricks'. This project has been referred to as a 'Synthetic Biology Commons'. Rai and Boyle suggest that copyright backing for the commons might not be easily attainable and patents may prove far too expensive for a not-forprofit organisation. A possible solution may lie in their analysis of recent movements in statements of non-assertion, whereby those that hold patents on parts may make a statement to the effect that they promise not to assert their right over academic researchers. Another possibility they identify is the 'Clickwrap' license, as used in the International HapMap project that disables those purchasing the license from patenting products utilising the SNP data and from distributing it to anyone who has not also signed the license.

Henkel and Maurer point out that the development of registries of standardised parts is likely to stimulate the emergence of competing libraries that may seek to license the entire library rather than individual components: 'Suppose that Company Y owns 70% of the most popular parts and Company Z owns the remaining 30%. Then, Company Y can get 100% of the business by offering a complete suite of whatever parts that the users need, that is, turning the contest into a competition between libraries instead of individual parts.' This potential problem of monopoly stems from what economists call a network effect, wherein the competition between parts is mediated by reducing costs as some parts are used more frequently than others. Costs reduce as experience increases. Thus a part may become 'locked in' by being used more initially: those in the network benefit by using the same parts over and over, whilst other competing parts become used less frequently and may ultimately fall out of use. This is known as a 'tipping dynamic'. Henkel and Maurer go on to argue that the challenge to the open-source synthetic biology movement is to foster the design of institutions that encourage appropriate decision making as regards patents. They cite research that they say indicates companies can earn more by sharing information rather than hoarding it. They provide a further alternative to Rai and Boyle's versions of the patenting puzzle by suggesting that the registry be open only to those who agree to make the parts they develop similarly available, perhaps after a specified number of years of royalty returns. In a presentation given at SB 3.0 Henkel and Maurer indicated that parts of the MIT registry were already patented and that the registry may benefit from making it clear which these are so that researchers can avoid using them. They conclude that synthetic biology will require a mixture of IP and open-source.

Whereas Rai and Boyle fear the intellectual property 'perfect storm', a Nature editorial considered this conjunction to be more a 'tempest in a test-tube'. The editors claim that Venter's patent looks unlikely to be awarded on the basis that: (i) it doesn't give sufficient information to enable an expert in the field to make or use it, and (ii) many of the non-essential genes described are already in the public domain. However, if Venter's patent application for the minimal genome is successful then he could monopolise the market for biofuel production. Henkel and Maurer, as paraphrased above, indicate that via the 'tipping dynamic' early leaders in a field may become steadily entrenched over time and come to dominate. Indeed Venter's plans do sound grand, he told the Sunday Times, 'Obviously, if we made an organism that produced fuel, that could be the first billion or trillion-dollar organism' and according to the Guardian he plans to do it within a decade.

TRADE AND GLOBAL JUSTICE

Scientific and Technical Developments

Perhaps the biggest success and at least the most applied research in synthetic biology to date has been in the production of terpenoids. These natural products are often isolated from plants and are used 'as commercial flavour and fragrance compounds and antimalarial and anticancer drugs'. It is for the purpose of producing antimalarial drugs that the Gate's Foundation has funded a collaboration between UC Berkeley scientists, Amyris Biotechnology and the Institute for OneWorld Health. The particular compound, artemisinin, commonly known as wormwood, has found limited use because of the cost of extracting it from plant sources. At present, farmers in East Asia and some parts of Africa are growing wormwood for medicinal production. Thanks to synthetic biology the gene responsible, amorpha-4, 11-diene synthase, and the mevalonate isoprenoid pathway from *Saccharomyces cerevisiae* have been engineered into an *E. coli* for mass production. Due to increasing resistance to other drugs the synthetic artemisinin holds significant promise for malaria victims worldwide.

Social and Ethical Issues Raised

The ETC Group claims that the development of artemisinin has 'become the *raison d'être* of synthetic biology and given the field a philanthropic sheen'. They draw a comparison to the poster child of the agricultural biotech industry 'Golden Rice' which was designed to feed the poor and tackle vitamin deficiencies. The ETC group suggests that the scale of the success has been drastically inflated to ensure continued funding of Keasling's lab and that ongoing research on synthetic biology for such social and economic problems diverts resources from other more effective approaches. It is recommended by the WHO that artemisinin should be mixed with other malaria drugs, Artemisinin Combination Therapies (ACTs), to ensure that resistance does not build up. However, ETC argues that Novartis has a virtual monopoly on ACTs and quote the Royal Tropical Institute of the Netherlands 'This monopoly-like situation has created an imperfect market defined by scarcity of raw materials, speculation and extremely high retail prices'. Critics contend that synthetic artemisinin would ensure that no local production of natural *Artemisia* could be stimulated or sustained, thereby maintaining the discrepancy of wealth and health.

The Gates foundation has been applauded for its charitable and practical aim, but it is not clear that producing a drug of this sort in developed countries is the best way of either eradicating malaria in the long term or supporting sustainable development in the poorest countries. As with many other advanced technologies, such as GM crops, when applied to issues of economic development, public health and global justice, a number of important questions are raised about the extent to which these innovations help tackle these problems or make them worse.

CREATING ARTIFICIAL LIFE

Scientific and Technical Developments

One of the core ideas in synthetic biology is the notion of creating 'artificial life'. This has simultaneously provoked fears about scientists 'playing God' and raises deeper philosophical and religious concerns about the nature of life itself and the process of creation. The principle area of synthetic biology to raise these issues is the production of life-like cells, which has been outlined above. Venter's team calls these minimal genome micro-organisms, synthetic biologists more broadly may refer to them as chassis, those in the UK synthetic chemistry field have named them chells. Whichever term is utilised in this discussion, the significant feature of their controversy is that they may be alive through human invention. Indeed, a recent media furore was related to this project of life creation following the announcement of the synthesis of the first bacterial genome at the J. Craig Venter Institute.

A number of research teams have the creation of life-like cells as a major objective. For example, a consortium of 13 partner institutions has been formed under the banner 'PACE' (Programmable Artificial Cell Evolution) and has, as its mission statement, the goal of bringing the binary and living worlds closer together.

Social and Ethical Issues Raised

The NEST high-level expert report indicates that the discussion of artificial life is likely to be prompted by public concerns over scientists 'playing God'. The same report welcomes the discussion on synthetic life, but cautions 'that it will be productive only if we can develop a more sophisticated appreciation of what is meant by 'life' than is current in popular discourse'. As witnessed by a number of media reports, there is a feeling that the science of synthetic biology may have outstripped our ethical reference points.

On the moral front, Mooney (of the ETC Group) says of Venter: 'God has competition.' To argue that the making of life should remain the province of a divine creator is no argument at all. Fears have been raised about the dangers of tinkering with life and releasing malignant bugs. 'We don't yet know what are the social, ethical and even bioweapons implications of this research,' said Hope Shand of the ETC technology pressure group. The most ominous note was struck by a scientist at MIT: 'The genetic code is 3.6 billion years old. It's time for a rewrite.'

Scientists are a step closer to creating artificial life after transforming one type of bacteria into another. But the announcement has also triggered unease, with some critics warning that the scientists were 'playing god'.

Synthetic biology has been touted as the discipline geared towards 'engineering life'. It is the notion of artificiality, the unknown quality, of synthetic biology's products that seems to underlie many of the aforementioned ethical concerns. Furthermore, the living, breeding nature of the synthetic biology output makes the threat of environmental contamination or the development of biological weapons so powerful. In this way, the ascription of the term life gives them agency, as though these microbes might seek to destroy us. It shouldn't be surprising then that this framing of the potential of biological engineering taps into the concept of risk and that some of the responses, particularly the regulative strategies outlined earlier that are aimed at identifying 'risky' engineers, are focussed on minimising potential harms whilst enabling scientific progress. However, such concerns are largely utilitarian, 'what might happen if this micro-organism escaped?'

Whilst these arguments are brought to the fore what have been pushed to the edges of the scientific discourse are potentially more fundamental issues about tampering in natural systems and creating 'life itself'. It has been suggested by Edward Machery, a philosopher of science at the University of Pittsburgh, that a stable definition of 'life' is impossible and useless. Machery argues that synthetic biologists (amongst other researchers) are confused over what life is, where it begins and particularly, how complex it must be. This, he suggests, is no surprise and is consistent with a whole programme of 'life definitionism' that fails to confine its object. A similar set of issues have been raised in a recent Nature Editorial, which notes that 'Many a technology has at some time or another been deemed an affront to God, but perhaps none invites the accusation as directly as synthetic biology.' It then goes on to argue that 'It would be a service to more than synthetic biology if we might now be permitted to dismiss the idea that life is a precise scientific concept.'

The final step in Venter's three step process of creating a synthetic organism involves inserting the synthesised genome into a bacterial cell and waiting to see if it springs to life. The publication of this information in January 2008 resulted in quite extensive media coverage with many articles leading with the life aspect: 'Scientist Creates Artificial Life – Almost', 'Synthetic Life: Watch this Space'. The Economist concluded its article on the publication with the lines:

If Dr Venter can take the final step of kicking the new, wholly synthetic genome into reproductive life, he will not only have made a great technological leap forward, he will also have erased one of the last mythic distinctions in science—that between living and non-living matter.

Whilst others were less impressed: But what does doing this really signify? What does it teach us about life that we didn't know before? There was indeed a time when scientists believed there was something fundamentally different about living matter and nonliving matter. It's called the Middle Ages. If Machery is right, that the idea of life is highly complex, but can possibly be defined by science, it would require multiple definitions across multiple fields. What implications might this have for an ethics that sought to trouble synthetic biology at the level of life definition? Put another way, if life is not a stable concept how might one argue that it is fundamentally immoral to create it? In contrast, if Zimmer is right that our definition of life, or at least the scientific definition, hasn't changed since the enlightenment, then perhaps the claim to be creating life is less about heresy and more about hype. He argues that whilst being expertly technical and scientifically significant, the research doesn't reveal the mysteries of existence, in fact he argues that it doesn't even reveal the mysteries of genetics and that creating a new living organism will lead to a whole new set of mysteries. In this sense we are a long way from playing God.

Scientific and Policy Response

This ontology of emerging objects, whether synthetic products are living or not, is being discussed by SynBERC, the NSF funded synthetic biology Engineering Research Centre. SynBERC's 'Human Practices' project, lead by Paul Rabinow (UCB) and Ken Oye (MIT), is also interested in general bioethical issues, security, health, environmental effects, and IP. The 'life' side of the project seeks to do such things as:

- Reflect on the form and essence of the parts, devices, chassis, and systems being created by synthetic biology.
- Analyse the differences between the objects created in older recombinant technologies and those projected in synthetic biology.
- Empirical research tracking how these parts, devices, chassis, systems, and test beds are designed and the ways that evolution and contemporary synthetic approaches differ from and enforce each other.
- Observe and design new institutional arrangements and interventions appropriate to the new objects being brought into the world.
- Eventual standardisation of this new mode of productively assembling scientific, technological, economic, cultural, ethical, and security components. Similarly, researchers from the PACE consortium have acknowledged ethical exploration to be part of its remit, though the development of this work is limited to date.

A number of the scientists involved in the chell programme have argued the case for a modified version of Turing's test for life imitation. Turing developed a test as a response to the perceived uselessness of the question 'can this machine think?' Turing argued that the more pertinent and pragmatic proposal should be to assess to what degree the machine is capable of imitating living beings. He believed, incorrectly, that machine imitations would be sufficiently sophisticated by the year 2000 to be indistinguishable from human communications. Others have found a longer history to the concept of an imitation test, with some tracing it to descartes observations on machines and men in his discourse on method.

The proposal made by the chell scientists is that the imitation test (or game) could be modified to allow for a more universal means of assessing whether something is living or not. Scientist argue that such a method is required so 'researchers from a variety of communities may objectively recognise success' in creating life-like cells. Their version of life is one that requires individual self-replication, self sustaining systems, and a mechanism that allows for spatio-temporally resolved organisation of information within these systems, though they themselves find this somewhat restrictive. The equivalent of the Turing test would be one in which the chell was able to interact with natural cells in an appropriate manner so as to be unrecognisable from those same cells. They foresee an ever increasing level of complexity in both their understanding of the cell in its natural environment and their capacity to imitate those processes such that the test for life becomes ever more stringent.

However, taking into account Machery's observations we may find that even the obfuscation of the more intangible questions, via use of a Turing-like test, there remains a fundamental barrier to translating the concept of life into a scientifically robust concept. Furthermore, it is unclear if these moves to undermine folk or lay concepts of life will ameliorate deeper fears about the blurring of the boundary between the artificial and the natural world.

Thus, synthetic biology should be understood in terms of both well established traditions within molecular biology and as an emerging field in its own right. The idea of biological engineering has a long history and can be seen as a central motif in 20th century biology. However, this promise has only started to be realised as the speed and scale of existing technologies has increased. In this sense, there is nothing completely new about synthetic biology that hasn't already been discussed in relation to the earlier development of molecular biology, recombinant DNA and genetic engineering. Debates about biosafety, bioweapons and the ethics of engineering life all took place in the 1970s and 80s. However, it is also important to recognise that something new and important is happening. In part this represents a growing confidence in the scientific community to undertake the project of engineering life, but it also marks the maturity of a series of powerful technologies, which are converging with other developments in computing, materials science and nanotechnology. Furthermore, synthetic biology can point to some important success, both in terms of creating new technology platforms, and in developing practical applications in the manufacturing of drugs and the synthesis of pathogenic viruses.

Despite its novelty, it is clear that the emergence of synthetic biology is following a now well established path in terms of the debates about the social and ethical issues. Many of the early fears surrounding the growth of recombinant DNA have never come to pass, but this is, in large part, due to the creation of robust governance regimes at local, national and international levels that have controlled the applications of the science and technology. These have included rigorous containment measures and multilateral controls on some aspects of their military use, as well as public debates over sensitive ethical issues. This is not to say that all concerns have been successfully resolved, but it points to a continuing dynamic in relation to synthetic biology, where societal issues will have a major influence on the funding of science, the types of technologies developed, their application in the real world, how they are ethically framed and the extent of regulation. The history of genetic engineering tells us that these debates can sometimes be long and difficult, but that they have been essential to negotiating uncertainty around the risks and benefits of the technology, regulating its socially acceptable use, and addressing concerns over who should control it. In this way, we can think of the science, technology, regulatory frameworks and social implications as coevolving through a process of mutual shaping.

Another important lesson from the development of biotechnology over the last 30 years is that whilst the technology holds great social and economic potential and rapid scientific progress is possible, it is far more problematic to translate this knowledge into real world applications outside the laboratory. High expectations of both the promise and threat of synthetic biology should therefore be tempered by a realistic sense of how difficult it is to create successful new biotechnologies.

Responding to the Challenge

How then should different stakeholders respond to the challenging issues raised by synthetic biology? Firstly, it is vital to recognise the importance of maintaining public legitimacy and support. This is an important principle in its own right, but is also imperative if funding and other forms of institutional support are to be maintained. This was clearly shown by the decline in public funding for the genetic modification of crops following the GM food controversy in Europe in the 1990s. In order to avoid this scientific research must not get too far ahead of public attitudes and potential applications should demonstrate clear social benefits. Furthermore, the potential benefits of the technology must not be overhyped or this risks both creating excessive public anxiety and unrealistic hopes that cannot be fulfilled.

Secondly, the scientific community must take, and be seen to be taking, a lead in debating the implications of their research and engaging with broader society around the issues raised by synthetic biology. It is not sufficient to wait until particular issues arise through the practical application of the technology, as this will be too late. Public debates do not develop in a linear or rational fashion, but are unpredictable and driven by often deeply held cultural attitudes to nature, the environment and the place of science. Anticipatory intervention is therefore essential.

Thirdly, partnership with civil society groups, social scientists and ethicists should be pursued as a highly effective way of understanding critical issues, engaging with publics and winning support for emerging scientific fields. However, at the same time it must be recognised that this is a two-way process and that some ethically problematic scientific projects and potentially controversial technologies may have to be abandoned in order to maintain trust. From this perspective, experiments in upstream engagement and public consultation should be undertaken as they provide a valuable channel for helping negotiate the boundaries of what is socially acceptable science.

Finally, a robust governance framework must be in place before many of the applications of synthetic biology are realised. This will require a thorough review of existing controls and regulations, and the development of new measures in the areas highlighted in this chapter, particularly relating to biosafety, environmental release and biosecurity. Research agencies, such as the BBSRC, therefore have an important role, not just in terms of funding the best science, but also in steering and shaping the field so that research is undertaken in a way that ensures ongoing public support and helps realise the potential social and economic benefits of these powerful technologies, whilst controlling their risks in a way that reassures both the public and the scientific community.

Given the pervasive nature of synthetic biology and its potential for widespread application in what ultimately may be a mundane fashion, its development and application will need to be governed at multiple levels and using a range of policies and practices. These may include the establishment of new professional norms in the scientific community (e.g. codes of conduct concerning dual use technology), local and national research oversight, statutory regulation (e.g. new laws and formal regulatory agencies) and international co-operation and treaties. Such a multi-level governance framework will have to provide a robust overarching framework, whilst respecting different national traditions and empowering local enforcement. It will also have to be fully supported by the scientific community and other professional groups involved, through a process of training and awareness-raising. Finding the right balance between formal statutory regulation and self-regulation of the scientific community remains a contentious issue and will occur only after the risks of synthetic biology are more widely understood and debated.

Implementation of Synthetic Biology

In thinking about how synthetic biology might be governed a number of important questions must be answered:

Biosafety

- Are there new potential threats posed by synthetic biology in terms of risks to health?
- Does synthetic biology require new forms of risk assessment and governance beyond those already used in relation to established practices of genetic engineering?

Environmental release

- Are there new potential threats posed by synthetic biology in terms of the risk of unplanned release and damage to the environment?
- Under what circumstances could synthetic biology based products be safely released into the environment?
- Do existing risk assessment procedures and controls on the release of GMOs adequately cover novel organisms created using synthetic biology?

Bioterrorism

- What problems are posed by synthetic biology in terms of the development of new technologies and capabilities for the development of biological weapons by individuals, states and non-state groups?
- Do established international regimes for the control of bioweapons need to be amended to incorporate the introduction of synthetic biology?
- What measures should be taken to increase awareness within the scientific community of the biosecurity issues surrounding synthetic biology?

Scientific and economic monopolies

- To what extent are broad patents being granted that might lead to monopolies over the exploitation and application of synthetic biology?
- How can policy be developed to balance the claims of inventors and broader public interests to promote scientific research and affordable access to new technology?

Exacerbating global inequalities in trade

- To what extent will synthetic biology create new, or exacerbate existing, inequalities in international trade and development?
- What measures can be taken to promote global equity in areas most affected by new technologies such as synthetic biology?

Creating artificial life

- To what extent does synthetic biology fundamentally challenge established notions of what constitutes life?
- How can constructive public debate on the cultural and philosophical implications of advances in synthetic biology be fostered?

Addressing the important questions raised by synthetic biology should be a policy priority for government, research funders, and the scientific community in order to ensure that it realises its potential in a way that is ethically acceptable and commands broad public support.

References

Adams, J.L., and Roberts, K.J., *Molecular Biology of the Cell*, Garland Science, Taylor & Francis Group, London.

Brown, M.E., *Molecular Biology of Cell*, Marcel Dekker, New York.

Collin, R.K., *Cell Biology*, Cambridge University Press, Cambridge.

Didier, M.B., *Lichen Physiology and Cell Biology*, Kluwer Academic/Plenum Publishers, New York.

David, K.N., *Fundamental of Cell Biology*, Peragam, Oxford.

Eklun, R.W, *Plant Cell and Its Growth*, Academic Press, London.

Frische, B., *DNA Molecular Gymnastics*, Marcel Dekker Inc., New York.

George Plopper, *Principles of Cell Biology*, Jones and Bartlett Publishers, Inc, United States.

Hall, D.R., *Molecular Neurobiology*, Humana Press Inc., New Jersey.

Harvey Lodish, *Molecular Cell Biology*, W. H. Freeman and Company, New York.

Jetten, N.S., *Gene regulation by MicroRNAs*, McGraw Hill, Columbus, Ohio, USA.

Karp, G.C., *Cell and Molecular Biology*, John Wiley & Sons Inc., New York.

Keith, V.G, *Nucleus and Gene Expression*, Pergamon Press, Oxford, New York.

Lewis, D.A, *Ten Commandments of Enzymology*, Science Publishers, New York.

Liebier, F.T, *Biology of Cancer*, Tata McGraw Hill, New York.

Machacon, L.M, *Cell and Molecular Immunology*, Oxford University Press, Oxford.

Martin Raff,, *Molecular Cell Biology*, McGraw-Hills, New York.

Nelson, D.L., *Lehninger, Principles of Biochemistry*, W. H. Freeman and Company, New York.

Pinto, B.C., *The Cell*, Science Publishers, New York.

Peter Walter, *Molecular Biology*, Applied Science Publishers, London.

Phat Dinh, *DNA and Cell Biology*, Mary Ann Liebert, Inc., Publishers, New York.

Reeve, O.M., *Membranes and Their Applications*, Prentice-Hall of India Pvt. Ltd., New Delhi.

Sadava, D.E., *Cell Biology: Organelle Structure and Function*, Jones and Bartlett Publishers, Boston.

Shoshkes, C.R., *DNA and Cell Biology*, Mary Ann Liebert, Inc., Publishers, New York.

Smith, W.D., *Microbial Biotechnology*, John Wiley & Sons, New York.

Tellez, P.E., *Gene Expression*, Affiliated East-West Press, Pvt. Ltd. Moscow

Umetsu, P.N, *Biology and Biotechnology*, Plenum Publishing Corporation, London.

Voet, D., *Biochemistry*, Tata McGraw Hill, New York.

Watson, K.C., *Replication and Repair of DNA*, Routledge, New York.

Wrobel, A.P, *Energy and Metabolism*, Ellis Harwood, New York.

Zeikus, J.G., *Mitochondrion and Bioenergetics*, Marcel Dekker Inc., New York.

Index

Volume II

The Cell

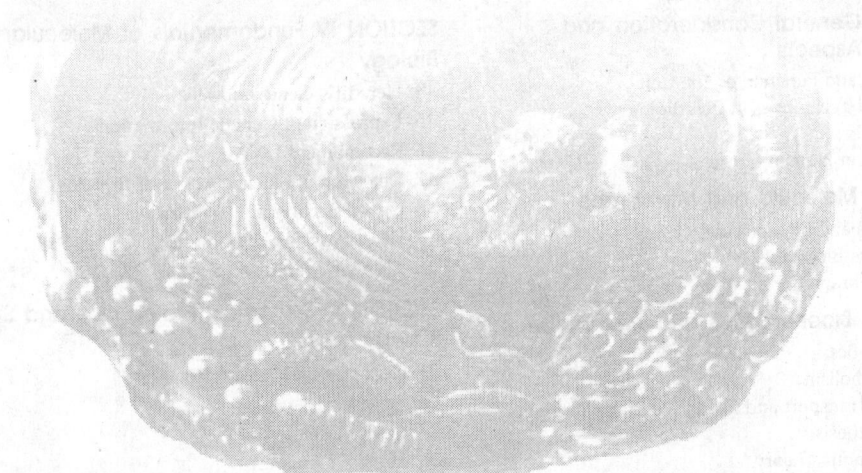

Contents at a Glance

Volume II

Volume I

Volume II

The Cell

S Kemper

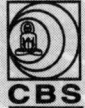

CBS Publishers & Distributors Pvt Ltd

New Delhi • Bengaluru • Chennai • Kochi • Kolkata • Mumbai

Bhopal • Bhubaneswar • Hyderabad • Jharkhand • Nagpur • Patna • Pune • Uttarakhand • Dhaka (Bangladesh)

The Cell
Volume II

ISBN: 978-93-89261-68-4

First Edition: 2020

Published by Satish Kumar Jain and produced by Varun Jain for

CBS Publishers & Distributors Pvt Ltd

4819/XI Prahlad Street, 24 Ansari Road, Daryaganj, New Delhi 110 002, India.
Ph: 23289259, 23266861, 23266867   Fax: 011-23243014   Website: www.cbspd.com
e-mail: delhi@cbspd.com; cbspubs@airtelmail.in

Corporate Office: 204 FIE, Industrial Area, Patparganj, Delhi 110 092
Ph: 4934 4934   Fax: 4934 4935   e-mail: publishing@cbspd.com; publicity@cbspd.com

Branches

- **Bengaluru:** Seema House, 2975, 17th Cross, K.R. Road,
  Banasankari 2nd Stage, Bengaluru 560 070, Karnataka
  Ph: +91-80-26771678/79   Fax: +91-80-26771680   e-mail: bangalore@cbspd.com
- **Chennai:** 7, Subbaraya Street, Shenoy Nagar, Chennai 600 030, Tamil Nadu
  Ph: +91-44-26680620, 26681266   Fax: +91-44-42032115   e-mail: chennai@cbspd.com
- **Kochi:** 42/1325, 1326, Power House Road, Opposite KSEB Power House,
  Ernakulam 682 018, Kochi, Kerala
  Ph: +91-484-4059061-65   Fax: +91-484-4059065   e-mail: kochi@cbspd.com
- **Kolkata:** 6/B, Ground Floor, Rameswar Shaw Road, Kolkata-700 014, West Bengal
  Ph: +91-33-22891126, 22891127, 22891128   e-mail: kolkata@cbspd.com
- **Mumbai:** 83-C, Dr E Moses Road, Worli, Mumbai-400018, Maharashtra
  Ph: +91-22-24902340/41   Fax: +91-22-24902342   e-mail: mumbai@cbspd.com

Representatives

- **Bhopal**   0-8319310552
- **Jharkhand**   0-9811541605
- **Pune**   0-9623451994
- **Bhubaneswar**   0-9911037372
- **Nagpur**   0-9421945513
- **Uttarakhand**   0-9716462459
- **Hyderabad**   0-9885175004
- **Patna**   0-9334159340
- **Dhaka (Bangladesh)** 01912-003485

Printed at: Mudrak, Noida, UP, India

Preface

Cells are the basic unit of life. In the modern world, they are the smallest known world that performs all of life's functions. All living organisms are either single cells, or are multicellular organisms composed of many cells working together. Cells are the smallest known unit that can accomplish all of these functions. Defining characteristics that allow a cell to perform these functions include: A cell membrane that keeps the chemical reactions of life together, at least one chromosome, composed of genetic material that contain the cell's *blueprints* and *software*, cytoplasm—the fluid inside the cell, in which the chemical processes of life occur. Thus, cells are the basic building blocks of living things. The human body is composed of trillions of cells, all with their own specialised function. Cells are the basic structures of all living organisms. Cells provide structure for the body, take in nutrients from food and carry out important functions. Cells group together to form tissues, which in turn group together to form organs, such as the heart and brain. Our cells contain a number of functional structures called organelles. These organelles carry out tasks such as making proteins, processing chemicals and generating energy for the cell. The nucleus is based at the centre of the cell and is the 'control room' for the cell. The genome is found within the nucleus.

This reference textbook *The Cell* is divided in two volumes. Second volume contains 12 sections and 1 to 34 chapters.

Section I discusses *genes and genomes*. Chapter 1 is devoted to structure of eukaryotic genes. Eukaryotic cells are cells that contain a nucleus and organelles, and are enclosed by a plasma membrane. Chapter 2 deals with non-coding sequences. The non-coding regions are segments of DNA that do not comprise a gene and do not code for a protein. These regions sometimes referred to as 'junk DNA' are interspersed throughout the genome. Chapter 3 concentrates on chromosomes and chromatin. A chromosome is a deoxyribonucleic acid (DNA) molecule with part or all of the genetic material (genome) of an organism. Most eukaryotic chromosomes include packaging proteins which, aided by chaperone proteins, bind to and condense the DNA molecule to prevent it from becoming an unmanageable tangle. Chromatin is a complex of DNA, RNA, and protein found in eukaryotic cells. Its primary function is packaging very long DNA molecules into a more compact, denser shape, which prevents the strands from becoming tangled and plays important roles in reinforcing the DNA during cell division, preventing DNA damage, and regulating gene expression and DNA replication.

Chapter 4 focuses on discovery of introns. Spliceosomal introns are one of the eukaryotic defining characters. Intron density ranges from a handful in the entire genome of some protists, to about eight per gene in human. Chapter 5 explains ENCODE project. The major goal of ENCODE is to provide the scientific community with high-quality, comprehensive annotations of candidate functional elements in the human genome.

Section II discusses *replication, maintenance, and rearrangements of genomic DNA*. Chapter 6 is devoted to DNA replication. DNA replication is the biological process of producing two identical replicas of DNA from one original DNA molecule. Chapter 7 deals with DNA repair. DNA repair is a collection of processes by which a cell identifies and corrects damage to the DNA molecules that encode its genome. Chapter 8 focuses on DNA rearrangements. Chapter 9 concentrates on colon cancer and DNA repair. Colon cancer is cancer of the large intestine (colon), which is the final part of your digestive tract. Most cases of colon cancer begin as small, noncancerous (benign) clumps of cells called adenomatous polyps. Chapter 10 explains rearrangement of immunoglobulin genes.

Section III discusses *RNA synthesis and processing.* Chapter 11 is devoted to RNA synthesis and processing: An overview. Gene expression can be regulated at multiple levels, including transcription, RNA processing, messenger RNA (mRNA) stability, translation and post-translation. Chapter 12 deals with transcription in bacteria. Chapter 13 focuses on chromatin and epigenetics. Chapter 14 concentrates on role of small nuclear RNAs in eukaryotic gene expression.

Section IV discusses *protein synthesis, processing and regulation.* Chapter 15 is devoted to protein synthesis and degradation. The regulation of protein synthesis is an important part of the regulation of gene expression. Chapter 16 deals with translation of mRNA. The control of mRNA translation plays a key role in regulating gene expression under a wide range of circumstances in eukaryotic cells, and to a lesser extent in bacteria.

Section V discusses *importance of cell structure and function.* Chapter 17 is devoted to nucleus and nuclear bodies. The nucleus is the most obvious organelle in any eukaryotic cell. It is a membrane-bound organelle and is surrounded by a double membrane. Chapter 18 explains nuclear lamina diseases. The nuclear lamina is a proteinaceous structure located underneath the inner nuclear membrane (INM), where it associates with the peripheral chromatin.

Section VI discusses *protein sorting and transport: Golgi apparatus and lysosomes.* Chapter 19 is devoted to protein sorting and transport. The protein sorting and translocation is a complex task involving multiple decision makings at multiple stages. Chapter 20 deals with endoplasmic reticulum. The endoplasmic reticulum (ER) is a continuous membrane system but consists of various domains that perform different functions. Chapter 21 concentrates on Golgi apparatus. Golgi apparatus is a complex network of smooth membrane enclosed organelle which helps in collection, packaging, distribution and secretion of biomolecules. Chapter 22 focuses on lysosomes. Lysosomes are large, spherical organelles that contain enzymes (acid hydrolases). They break up food so it is easier to digest.

Section VII discusses *mitochondria, chloroplasts and peroxisomes.* Chapter 23 is devoted to mitochondria. Mitochondria are now known to be more than the hub of energy metabolism. They are the central executioner of cells, and control cellular homeostasis through involvement in nearly all aspects of metabolism. Chapter 24 deals with chloroplasts and others plastids. Chloroplasts are members of a class of organelles known as plastids. Chloroplasts are organelles found in plant cells and other eukaryotic organisms that conduct photosynthesis.

Section VIII discusses *cytoskeleton and cell movement.* Chapter 25 concentrates on cytoskelton. A cytoskeleton is present in the cytoplasm of all cells, including bacteria, and archaea. It is a complex, dynamic network of interlinking protein filaments that extends from the cell nucleus to the cell membrane. Chapter 26 focuses on motor protein kinesin.

Section IX discusses *cell walls, the extracellular matrix and cell interactions.* Chapter 27 is devoted to cell walls. The cell wall is the tough, usually flexible but sometimes fairly rigid layer that surrounds some types of cells. It is located outside the cell membrane and provides these cells with structural support and protection, in addition to acting as a filtering mechanism. Chapter 28 deals with extracellular matrix. In cell biology, molecular biology and related fields, the word extracellular (or sometimes extracellular space) means 'outside the cell'. This space is usually taken to be outside the plasma membranes, and occupied by fluid. The term is used in contrast to intracellular (inside the cell).

Section X discusses *cell signalling and cancer: signal transduction and oncogenes*. Chapter 29 focuses on cell signalling. Cell signalling is part of any communication process that governs basic activities of cells and co-ordinates all cell actions. The ability of cells to perceive and correctly respond to their micro environment is the basis of development, tissue repair, and immunity, as well as normal tissue homeostasis. Chapter 30 concentrates on cancer: signal transduction and oncogenes.

Section XI discusses *cell death and cell renewal*. Chapter 31 is devoted to cell death. Cell death is the event of a biological cell ceasing to carry out its functions. Chapter 32 deals with stem cells. Stem cells have the remarkable potential to develop into many different cell types in the body during early life and growth. In addition, in many tissues they serve as a sort of internal repair system, dividing essentially without limit to replenish other cells as long as the person or animal is still alive.

Section XII discusses *cancer its causes and cure*. Chapter 33 concentrates on cancer. Cancer can be defined as a disease in which a group of abnormal cells grow uncontrollably by disregarding the normal rules of cell division. Chapter 34 focuses on molecular approaches to cancer treatment.

Diagrams, figures, tables and index supplement the text. All topics have been covered in a cogent and lucid style to help the reader grasp the information quickly and easily.

It may not be wrong to hold that the present reference textbook *The Cell* is a complete treatise on this subject. It is an essential reading for BTech (environmental biotechnology/microbiology/food microbiology/biomedical and biochemical engineering) and students pursuing BSc/MSc course in biotechnology and microbiology. Besides students, this book will prove useful to industrialists and consultants in their respective fields.

This reference textbook also caters to the requirement of the syllabus prescribed by various universities for undergraduate and postgraduate courses in the above subjects. It has been prepared with meticulous care, aiming at making the book error-free. Constructive suggestions are always welcome from the readers of this book.

S Kemper

Contents

Section II
REPLICATION, MAINTENANCE, AND REARRANGEMENT OF GENOMIC DNA

Section III
RNA SYNTHESIS AND PROCESSING

Section VII
MITOCHONDRIA, CHLOROPLASTS AND PEROXISOMES

Section VIII
CYTOSKELETON AND CELL MOVEMENT

SECTION I

Genes and Genomes

Chapter 1

Structure of Eukaryotic Genes

INTRODUCTION

Eukaryotic cells are cells that contain a nucleus and organelles, and are enclosed by a plasma membrane. Organisms that have eukaryotic cells include protozoa, fungi, plants and animals. These organisms are grouped into the biological domain Eukaryota. Eukaryotic cells are larger and more complex than prokaryotic cells, which are found in *Archaea* and Bacteria, the other two domains of life. Eukaryotic cell are the developed, advanced and complex forms of cells.

They are the building block or smallest unit of life of organisms as simple as amoeba and protozoa to the most complicated plants and animals. Significantly bigger than the prokaryotic cells, eukaryotic cells have diameter ranging from 10–100 μm. Inside it are various cell organelles which performs individual functions and support cell life.

CHARACTERISTICS OF EUKARYOTIC CELLS

Eukaryotic cells contain a variety of structures called organelles, which perform various functions within the cell. Examples of organelles are ribosomes, which make proteins, the endoplasmic reticulum, which sorts and packages the proteins, and mitochondria, which produce the energy molecule adenosine triphosphate (ATP). They also have a true nucleus, which contains the genetic material DNA and is surrounded by a nuclear envelope.

All of the organelles are stabilised and given physical support through the cytoskeleton, which is also involved in sending signals from one part of the cell to the other. In eukaryotic cells, the cytoskeleton is composed mainly of three types of filaments: microtubules, microfilaments, and intermediate filaments. The gel-like substance that surrounds all the organelles in the cell is called cytosol. The cytosol is the blue substance surrounding all of the organelles. Together, the cytosol with all organelles besides the nucleus are grouped as cytoplasm.

Eukaryotic cells (Fig. 1.1) have defined nucleus along with other membrane bound cell organelles such as mitochondria, ribosome, lysosome, Golgi bodies, endoplasmic reticulum, etc. All these cell organelles are held in their position by cytoplasm which is protected by plasma membrane. And the plasma membrane is further protected by the cell wall.

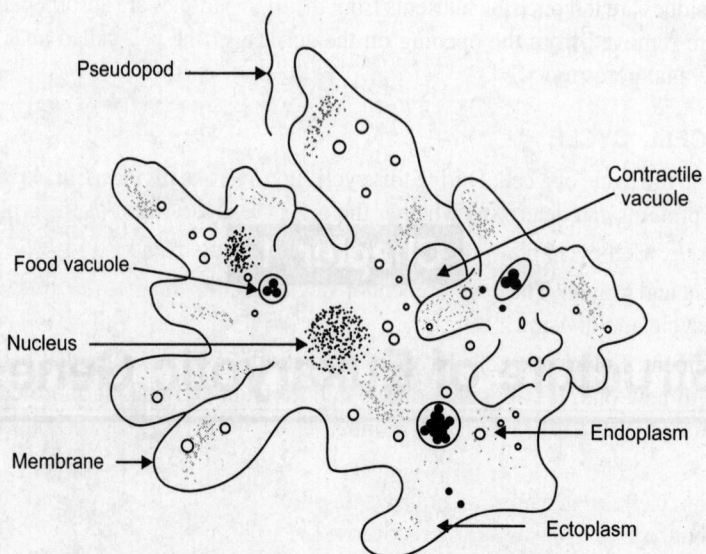

Fig. 1.1: Eukaryotic cells.

Unicellular Cell

There are several organisms made up of a single eukaryotic cell. For example, amoeba, protozoa, slime mold, and some forms of algae are single celled eukaryotes. Sperms, on the other hand, are singular cells found in animals (multicellular).

Eukaryotic unicellular cell consists of several organelles which carry out functions such as respiration, digestion, excretion, reproduction, locomotion, circulation and all others.

Cell membrane: It is the outermost covering of the cell which protects the cell from external environment.

Cytoplasm: The jelly-like substance that fills the cell is known as cytoplasm. In some organisms, it is divided into two types – ectoplasm and endoplasm.

Ectoplasm: Ectoplasm is the outer lining of cytoplasm, just below the cell membrane, which is much denser and clearer. It contains no organelles. It is thinner than the endoplasm.

Endoplasm: Endoplasm is the cytoplasm that lies towards the center of the cell. It is granulated with various cell organelles embedded into it.

Pseudopodium: It is a temporary protrusion on the surface of amoeboid body. It helps in locomotion and in catching preys.

Cilia: Cilia are thin thread like structures which help the cell to swim or move in liquid.

Oral groove: It is an opening on the surface on the cell which leads to cell mouth and to the gullet. Foods that are swept into the oral groove are stored and digested inside the food vacuole.

Food vacuole: It is membrane-bound space in the cytoplasm with digestive enzymes which helps in degrading the food particles engulfed by the cell.

Contractile vacuole: It is a sub-cellular organelle which conducts osmoregulation, the process of removing excessive water along with waste products like ammonia and other salts from the cell in order to prevent the cell from bursting.

Anal pore: Residues are left once the nutrients from the food particles are absorbed into the cytoplasm. These residues are removed from the opening on the surface of the cell called anal pore. Some cells have two or more anal pores too.

EUKARYOTIC CELL CYCLE

The cell cycle is the life cycle of a cell. During this cycle, it grows and divides. Checkpoints exist between all stages so that proteins can determine whether the cell is ready to begin the next phase of the cycle.

Role of cell-cycle: Cell cycle plays important role in following events:

1. Development and growth: The development of single cell into the multi-cellular system is possible due to cell cycle and division.
2. Cell replacement: Eukaryotic cells have pre-defined life span and after that period it needs to be replaced with new one. It is possible due to cell division and making more cellular copies. For example, human RBC has life span of 3 months, new RBCs are formed from bone marrow by cell division.
3. Regeneration: Cellular damage and injury is the integral part of living system. Cell division is the primary event required for the synthesis of lost or damaged organ.
4. Asexual reproduction: Asexual reproduction is common in lower invertebrate. In these organisms cell divide to form new cells and these newly formed ceklls give rise to new organism. For example hydra.

Control of cell-cycle: Cell cycle at different step is tightly controlled by cell-cycle check points. These cell cycle check points are used to ensure the completion of different steps and repair of DNA damage. The main check points are present at G1/S, G2/M and M. Each check point is controlled by the mutual interaction between cyclin and cyclin dependent protein kinase. p53 gene products are known to control many events through G1/S and G2/M checkpoints.

Quiescence (G$_0$)

Quiescence, also known as senescence or resting, is a phase in which the cell is not actively dividing. It is also known as Gap 0, or G$_0$. This stage is considered the start of the cell cycle, although it is one that cells can reach and then stop dividing indefinitely, which ends the cell cycle. Liver, stomach, kidney cells, and neuron are all examples of cells that can reach this stage and remain in it for long periods of time. It can also occur when a cell's DNA is damaged. However, most cells do not go into the G$_0$ stage at all, and can divide indefinitely throughout the life of an organism.

Interphase

In interphase, the cell grows and takes in nutrients in preparation for division. Interphase takes up about 90 per cent of the cell cycle. It consists of three parts: Gap 1, Synthesis, and Gap 2.

- Gap 1 (G$_1$) is also known as a growth phase. The cell gets larger and increases its stock of proteins, along with organelles such as the energy-producing mitochondria.
- Synthesis (S) is the phase in which DNA replicates. During synthesis, the chromosomes replicate so that each chromosome is made up of two sister chromatids. At the end of this phase, there is double the amount of DNA in the cell.
- Gap 2 (G$_2$) is another growth phase. The cell becomes even larger in order to prepare for mitotic division.

Mitosis (M)

Mitosis, or M phase, is when the cell begins to organise its duplicated DNA for separation into two daughter cells. The chromosomes separate so that one of each chromosome goes into each daughter cell. This results in the daughter cells having identical chromosomes to the parent cell. Mitosis itself is divided into prophase, metaphase, anaphase, and telophase, which mark various points in the DNA separation process. Mitosis is then followed by a process called cytokinesis, during which the cell separates its nuclei and other organelles in preparation for division and then physically divides into two cells.

TYPES OF EUKARYOTIC CELLS

Eukaryotic Plant Cell

Plant cells are unique among eukaryotic cells for several reasons. They have reinforced, relatively thick cell walls that are made mostly of cellulose and help maintain structural support in the plant. Each plant cell has a large vacuole in the center that allows it to maintain turgor pressure, which is pressure from having a lot of water in the cell and helps keep the plant upright. Plant cells also contain organelles called chloroplasts which contain the molecule chlorophyll.

This important molecule is used in the process of photosynthesis, which is when a plant makes its own energy from sunlight, carbon dioxide, and water. Eukaryotic plant cell (Fig. 1.2) are developed and advanced form or cell which is similar to animal cell in several ways. However, these cells are bigger than the animal cells and have some added cell organelles.

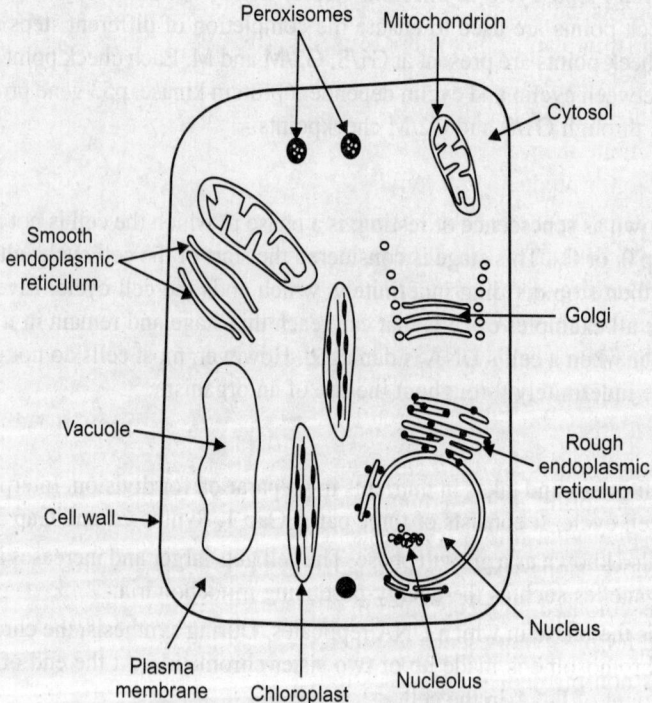

Fig. 1.2: Eukaryotic plant cell.

Cell wall: It is the outermost layer which is present only in plant cell. It is slightly rigid and provides specific shape to the cell.

Plasma membrane: It lies below the cell wall and surrounds the entire cell. The thin layer acts as a protection layer.

Cytoplasm: It is the semi-fluid or jelly like structure which hold all cell organelles in place. It also prevents cells from being flaccid.

Ribosome: It is a complex molecule of RNA-protein which synthesises protein in the cell.

Rough endoplasmic reticulum: Endoplasmic reticulum (ER) which has ribosomes attached to its surface is known as rough ER. Its major function is to carry out the protein synthesising process called translation.

Smooth endoplasmic reticulum: Endoplasmic reticulum (ER) which lacks ribosome is called smooth endoplasmic reticulum. Basically, smooth ER's function is to produce molecules according to the need of specific cell. In plant cell, smooth ER manufactures lipids or fatty acids.

Centrosome: It is round organelle present near to the nucleus. During mitosis, when the nuclear membrane breaks down, microtubules associated with centrosome interact with the chromosome and builds mitotic spindle.

Nuclear membrane: Nuclear membrane which is also called nucleolemma, nuclear envelope or karyotheca, is the covering membrane of nucleus. It is a bilayer of lipid which encases the genetic material.

Nucleus: Regarded as the brain of the cell, nucleus is the controlling unit. It controls every activity of the cell. Particularly, in plant cell, it is not located in the center, also it's not towards the edge of the cell.

Nucleolus: It is the spherical body inside the nucleus. Its major function is to produce ribosomal subunits and to distribute them throughout the cell. These units combine together to form ribosomes which are responsible for producing protein.

Vacuole: It is an empty space or bubble found in the cytoplasm. It is much larger and is located more to the center in a eukaryotic plant cell. It helps in storing foods and other nutritional substances which support cell survival. It also stores waste products in order to prevent contamination of the entire cell. Usually, a single plant cell has single vacuole.

Mitochondria: Often referred to as the powerhouse of the cell, mitochondria are the cell organelles where biochemical respiration occurs. They have double layer of which the inner layer is folded inwards creating layers called cristae.

Golgi bodies: Golgi bodies are the composite of vestibules and folded membranes. It carries out various functions such storing and absorbing lipids, protein, and certain enzymes. Specifically in plant cells, Golgi bodies play vital role in synthesising polysaccharides such as pectin, microfibrils of a cellulose, hemicellulose, along with various mucilaginous products essential to form cell wall.

Chloroplast: It is coloured pigment found in all plant cells and in algae too, which photosynthesis (the process of food for plant in presence of water, carbon dioxide gas and sunlight).

Amyloplast: It is non-pigmented organelles found only in certain plant cells. It synthesises starch granules from polymerisation of glucose and stores them. It can also revert the process to form glucose from starch granules in cases when plant is in need of energy.

Eukaryotic Animal Cell

Animal cells do not have cell walls. Instead, they have only a plasma membrane. The lack of a cell wall allows animal cells to form many different shapes, and allows for the processes of phagocytosis 'cell eating' and pinocytosis 'cell drinking' to occur. Animal cells differ from plant cells in that they do not have chloroplasts and have smaller vacuoles instead of a large central vacuole (Fig. 1.3).

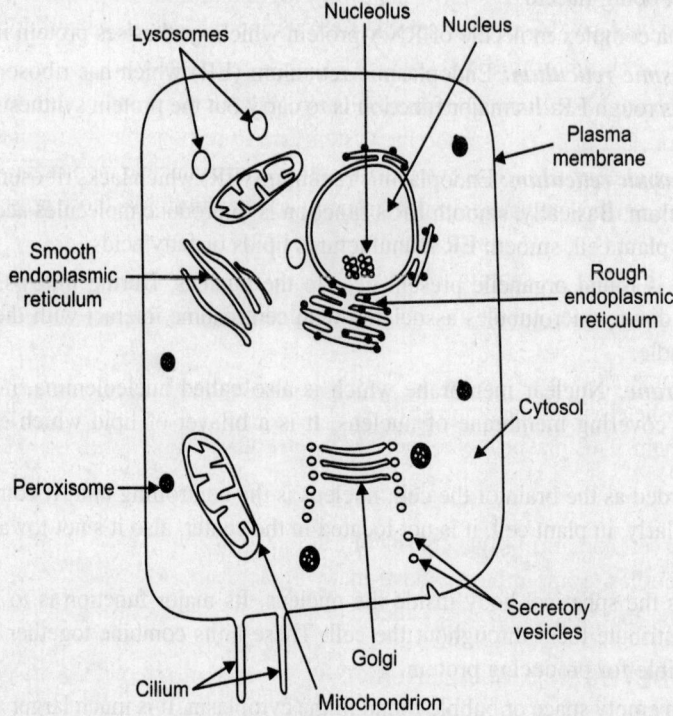

Fig. 1.3: Eukaryotic animal cell.

Slightly smaller than the plant cell, animal cells are also advanced form of cell containing various cell organelles of various purposes.

Plasma membrane: Unlike in plant cells, plasma membrane is the outermost covering in eukaryotic animal cells. These cells are capable of adopting various shapes while some phagocytic cells can even consume other cells as they lack cell wall.

Golgi bodies: Golgi bodies in animal cells have more functions to perform than in plant cells. Some functions of this organelle are:

• They absorb various compounds such as bismutose, protargol, etc.

• Removes water from products that are being synthesised while forming secretory granules.

• Produces various enzymes such as follicular fluid in granulosa cells of ovary, zymogen granules, etc.

• Helps in producing hormones, especially of cells in thyroid gland.

• Stores proteins and lipids.

• Produces milk protein droplets in mammary glands.

Lysosome: It is membrane bound organelle in the cell whose major function is to digest or degrade waste and other excessive particles in the cell. It also digests engulfed cells like bacteria and viruses. Many plant cells may lack lysosome as they have larger vacuole which substitutes the role of lysosome.

Centrosome: Its structure and function is similar to that of the centrosome of plant cells. The only difference is that the centrosome in animal cells contains centriole.

Centriole: Present in animal cells only, centrioles a circular body associated with the centrosome which is responsible for development of spindle fibre during the process of cell division. Spindle fibre helps in separation of chromosomes.

Smooth endoplasmic reticulum: In animal cells, smooth ER plays major role in producing calcium ions. Smooth ER present in cells of endocrine system is also responsible for regulating hormones.

Cell organelles or inclusions such as cytoplasm, mitochondria, nuclear membrane, nucleus, nucleolus, rough ER, vacuole and ribosome have similar structure and functions like those present in the eukaryotic plant cells. However, the vacuole is much smaller than it is in plant cells and may be present in multiple numbers. Also, the nucleus is centrally located.

Fungal Cells

Like plant cells, fungal cells also have a cell wall, but their cell wall is made of chitin (the same substance found in insect exoskeletons). Some fungi have septa, which are holes that allow organelles and cytoplasm to pass between them. This makes the boundaries between different cells less clear.

Protozoa

Protozoa are eukaryotic organisms that consist of a single cell. They can move around and eat, and they digest food in vacuoles. Some protozoa have many cilia, which are small 'arms' that allow them to move around. Some also have a thin layer called a pellicle, which provides support to the cell membrane.

DIFFERENCES BETWEEN ANIMAL, PLANT, FUNGAL, AND PROTISTAN CELLS

Differences between animal, plant, fungal, and protistan cells is given below:

All plant cells have the following:

- A cell wall made of cellulose
- A large central vacuole
- Chloroplasts

Some animal and protistan cells have:

- Flagella
- Cilia

But all animal cells have:

- Centrioles (Well that was shorter than we expected.)

All fungal cells have:

- A cell wall made of chitin.

Table 1.1 shows difference between prokaryotic and eukryotic cells and Table 1.2 shows difference between plants and animal cells.

Table 1.1: Difference between prokaryotic and eukaryotic cells.

Feature	Prokaryote	Eukaryote
Size	Small, in μm range	Variable size, upto 40 μm in diameter
Genetic material	Circular DNA present in cytosol as free material	DNA in the form of linear chromosome present in well defined double membrane nucleus, no direct connection with cytosol
Replication	Single origin of replication	Multiple origin of replication
Genes	No intron	Presence of intron
Organelles	No membrane bound organelles	Membrane bound orgelles with well defined function.
Cell walls	Very complex cell wall	Except Fungi and plant, eukaryotic cells are devoid of a thick cell wall
Ribosome	70S	80S
Trancription and translation	Occurs together	Transcription in nucleus and translation in cytosol

Table 1.2: Difference between plants and animal cells.

Feature	Plant cell	Animal cells
Cell wall	Present	Mostly absent
Size	Large	Comparatively small
Chlorophyll	Present	Absent
Vacuole	Large central	Small and many in number
Mitochondria	Few	More
Lysosome	Almost absent	Present
Glyoxysomes	Present	Absent
Cytokinesis	By plate method	By constriction

Chapter 2

Non-coding Sequences

INTRODUCTION

In the 70s a number of laboratories converged in revealing coding and non-coding regions in nuclear DNAs. Today one goal of genetic projects is to systematically localise all these regions, characterise their function and get a comprehensive understanding of how they act together. But the estimated number of genes continues to fluctuate, the reason being the genes are either not well – clear or easily identifiable. The current available data depends on three techniques such as cDNA cloning and EST (Expressed Sequence Tag) sequencing of polyadenylated messenger RNAs. Conserved coding exon identification by comparative analysis of genome Prediction of genes by computationally. These techniques are most excellent for highly expressed, phylogenetically conserved protein coding regions and large data sets, except for one class of genes – the non-coding regions of the genome.

The non-coding regions are segments of DNA that do not comprise a gene and do not code for a protein. These regions sometimes referred to as 'junk DNA' are interspersed throughout the genome. The non-coding regions get transcribed but are neither translated nor directly involved with the process of translation and hence no functional protein is produced. However, some of these regions are thought to have known biological function. Certain regions also produce transcripts that are involved directly in RNA processing and translation, rather than being expressed into messenger RNAs that encode proteins. It includes transfer RNAs (tRNA), ribosomal RNAs (rRNA), small nuclear RNAs (snRNA), small nucleolar RNAs (snoRNA), etc. The number and diversity of these non-coding regions remain essentially unknown, even after the completion of many genome sequences. Some questions like the number of non-coding genes in a genome, their importance, their function inside a cell and whether these large set of genes have gone undetected because of their inability to be translated into proteins have always remained a mystery. To address such questions, development of new systematic gene discovery approaches specifically aimed at non-coding regions is of utmost necessity. The idea that these classes of genes have remained undetected is stimulating, if not skeptical. Non-coding regions are almost absent in bacterial genomes but makes up as much as 90% or more of the genome in higher organisms. Modern comparative genomics studies suggest that genetic variations between any two allied species are more because of the modifications in the non-coding regions slightly than in the protein–coding genes.

11

Transcription – the process which results in the formation of RNA molecules is the primary way in which genetic information affects a cell's function. Studies that employ metabolic labelling of newly synthesised RNA indicated that a vast proportion of nuclear DNA was actually transcribed and bulk of this heterogeneous RNA (hnRNA) never access the cytoplasm and hence did not get decoded into proteins. Novel genomics and RNomic research have cross verified these findings.

Understanding the phenomena of RNAi and the discovery of post – transcriptional gene silencing has brought the functional significance of non-coding DNA sequences, especially the non-coding RNA's into light. Recently, researchers have elucidated the roles of non-coding regions in causing diseases in humans. Alteration in these region are coupled with disease propensity, but accurately how these functional changes is ambiguous. There are several segments of non-coding regions including: *Cis-* and *Trans-*regulatory elements, Introns, Non-coding functional RNA, Pseudo genes, Repeat sequences, Telomeres, transposons and viral elements. These regions assumed to be 'junk' seem to be responsible for a varied number of disorders in humans. Understanding what these segments are composed of and annotating them would help in understanding their specific roles in the genome.

NON-CODING DNA

Non-coding DNA sequences are components of an organisms DNA that do not encode protein sequences. Some non-coding DNA is transcribed into functional non-coding RNA molecules (e.g. transfer RNA, ribosomal RNA, and regulatory RNAs). Other functions of non-coding DNA include the transcriptional and translational regulation of protein-coding sequences, scaffold attachment regions, origins of DNA replication, centromeres and telomeres. The amount of non-coding DNA varies greatly among species. Often, only a small percentage of the genome is responsible for coding proteins, but a rising percentage is being shown to have regulatory functions. When there is much non-coding DNA, a large proportion appears to have no biological function, as predicted in the 1960s. Since that time, this non-functional portion has controversially been called 'junk DNA'.

The international Encyclopedia of DNA Elements (ENCODE) project uncovered, by direct biochemical approaches, that at least 80% of human genomic DNA has biochemical activity. Though this was not necessarily unexpected due to previous decades of research discovering many functional non-coding regions, some scientists criticised the conclusion for conflating biochemical activity with biological function. Estimates for the biologically functional fraction of our genome based on comparative genomics range between 8 and 15%. However, others have argued against relying solely on estimates from comparative genomics due to its limited scope. Non-coding DNA has been found to be involved in epigenetic activity and complex networks of genetic interactions, and is being explored in evolutionary developmental biology.

Fraction of Non-coding Genomic DNA

The amount of total genomic DNA varies widely between organisms, and the proportion of coding and non-coding DNA within these genomes varies greatly as well. For example, it was originally suggested that over 98% of the human genome does not encode protein sequences, including most sequences within introns and most intergenic DNA, whilst 20% of a typical prokaryote genome is non-coding.

In eukaryotes, genome size, and by extension the amount of non-coding DNA, is not correlated to organism complexity, an observation known as the C-value paradox. For example, the genome of the unicellular Polychaos dubium (formerly known as Amoeba dubia) has been reported to contain more than 200 times the amount of DNA in humans. The pufferfish Takifugu rubripes genome is only about one eighth the size of the human genome, yet seems to have a comparable number of genes, approximately 90% of the Takifugu genome is non-coding DNA. Therefore, most of the difference in genome size is not due to variation in amount of coding DNA, rather, it is due to a difference in the amount of non-coding DNA. In 2013, a new 'record' for the most efficient eukaryotic genome was discovered with Utricularia gibba, a bladderwort plant that has only 3% non-coding DNA and 97% of coding DNA. Parts of the non-coding DNA were being deleted by the plant and this suggested that non-coding DNA may not be as critical for plants, even though non-coding DNA is useful for humans. Other studies on plants have discovered crucial functions in portions of non-coding DNA that were previously thought to be negligible and have added a new layer to the understanding of gene regulation.

Types of Non-coding DNA Sequences

Non-coding functional RNA

Non-coding RNAs are functional RNA molecules that are not translated into protein. Examples of non-coding RNA include ribosomal RNA, transfer RNA, Piwi-interacting RNA and microRNA.

MicroRNAs are predicted to control the translational activity of approximately 30% of all protein-coding genes in mammals and may be vital components in the progression or treatment of various diseases including cancer, cardiovascular disease, and the immune system response to infection. Transfer RNA and ribosomal RNA are not translated into protein, but they are functional, synthesising proteins by translating the coding messenger RNA are shown in Fig. 2.1.

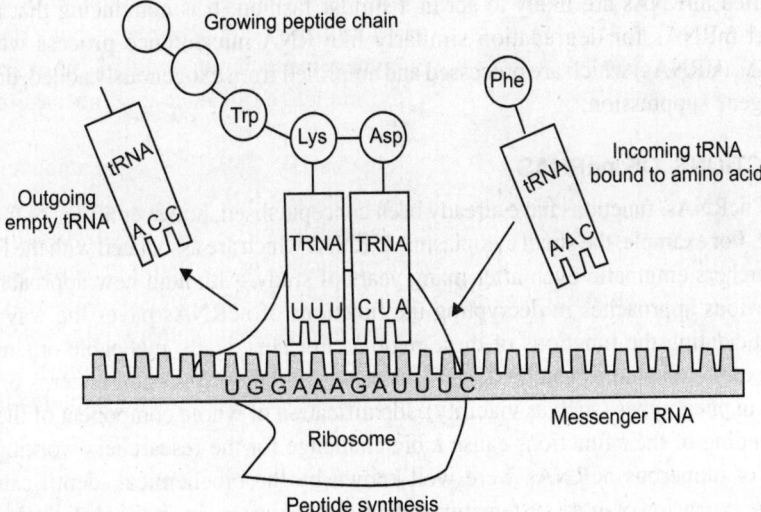

Fig. 2.1: Transfer RNA and ribosomal RNA are not translated into protein, but they are functional, synthesising proteins by translating the coding messenger RNA.

NON-CODING RNA

Non-coding RNA's are functional RNA molecules that do not get translated into a protein. These regions are thought to be involved in many cellular processes as in gene regulation and disease states. These RNA's that does not act as messenger RNAs (mRNAs), ribosomal RNAs (rRNAs) or transfer RNAs (tRNAs) has been given by various names where the term small RNAs (sRNAs) has been dominant in bacteria, whereas the term non-coding RNAs (ncRNAs) has been predominant in eukaryotes. These ncRNA's vary in size greatly. For example, regions of 21–25 nucleotides length form the large family of microRNAs (miRNAs). Those miRNAs are involved in regulation of development in Caenorhabditis elegans, *Drosophila*, and mammals those that are 100–200 nucleotides in length are sRNAs commonly found as translational regulators in bacterial cells and those that are >10,000 nucleotides in length are involved in gene silencing in higher eukaryotes. Thus, ncRNAs vary greatly in function and some RNAs is below.

RNA PROCESSING AND MODIFICATION

Processing of the 5′ end of precursor tRNA and some rRNA's is done by the catalytic ribonuclease P (RNase P) RNA, which is found in all organisms. For splicing of pre-mRNAs in eukaryotes, small nuclear RNAs (snRNAs) are important. Small nucleolar RNAs (snoRNAs) direct the metylation of 29-O-ribose sugar (C/D-box type) and pseudouridylation (H/ACA-box type) of rRNA, tRNA, and ncRNAs by base-pairing with sequences close to the sites has to be altered. The lead RNAs (gRNAs) are available in kinetoplasts to regulate insertions or deletions of uridine residues into mRNA as described by base-paring methods.

REGULATION OF mRNA STABILITY AND TRANSLATION

The process of translation is repressed by *C. elegans* lin-4 and let-7, the first discovered miRNAs. This suppression is because of the formation of base pairs with the 3′ end of target mRNAs. Numerous recently identified miRNAs are likely to act in a similar fashion. It is convincing that a few of these miRNAs target mRNAs for degradation similarly like RNA interference process where the small interfering RNAs (siRNAs) which are processed and amplified from exogenously added, double-stranded RNA leads to gene suppression.

OTHER FUNCTIONS OF ncRNAS

For a variety of ncRNAs, functions have already been conceptualised, however scores of the cellular roles remains elusive. For example, the small cytoplasmic Y RNAs which are associated with the Ro autoantigen leave the researchers enigmatic even after many years of study. Although new approaches need to be developed, previous approaches in decrypting the functions of ncRNAs paves the way to answer the question for elucidating the functions of these regions. For genetically malleable organisms, knock – out or over – expression studies can be done for whole – genome expression patterns or for screening the differences in phenotypes (such as viability). Identification of whole component of these regions for better understanding of their functions cause a big challenge for the researchers working on ncRNAs. The functions of numerous ncRNAs were well-known by the biochemical identification of related proteins, and the expansion of more systematic methods for characterising ncRNA-linked proteins should be fruitful. As computational biology tools expand and improve, comparative genomics approaches should serve as the central avenue for determining the functions of ncRNAs.

CIS- REGULATORY ELEMENTS

These are non-coding DNA sequences that are present in or near a gene and required for the proper expression of genes, usually containing binding sites for transcription factors. A classic example of a *cis* – acting element is the SECIS (SElenoCysteine Insertion Sequence) element, which is an RNA element having a stem – loop structure of 60 nucleotides in length, channelises the cell to translate the 'UGA' codon as 'Selenocysteine' rather than translating into a stop codon. The *cis*-acting elements may be classified into four types:

1. Promoter: This is the DNA element where transcription initiation begins.
2. Enhancer: This element can enhance the transcription process upon binding with the transcription factors (TFs). The TFs that bind to enhancers are known as transcription activators.
3. Silencer: This element can repress the transcription process upon binding with the transcription factors (TFs). The TFs binding silencers are referred to as repressors.
4. Response element: These are the identification sites for certain transcription factors. They are mostly positioned within 1 kb from the upstream of the transcriptional start site.

For the transcriptional regulation of gene expression, binding of transcription factors to *cis*-regulatory elements or transcription factor binding sites (TFBSs) is mandatory. Hence, discovering the *cis*- regulatory elements has brought into vital research challenge for few years. The conventional wet – lab experiments for the investigation of these elements is expensive and impractical on large number of genes. As more genome sequences become accessible, computational approaches provide an alternate low – cost efficient method to deal with large data sets. Many approaches have been projected to spot the putative *cis* – regulatory elements through varied algorithms. For predicting precision of the algorithms, *cis*-regulatory elements derived computationally are compared with known TFBSs from databases and/or literature. This along with Gene Ontology (GO) annotations helps in validating or associating the purported elements with biological functions.

TRANS- REGULATORY ELEMENTS

These are diffusible proteins, which modify gene expression by binding to the *cis*-acting sequences. Some of the general properties of different *trans*-acting factors are:

1. Considered to be the subunits of RNA polymerase.
2. Helps in stabilisation of initiation complex by binding to RNA polymerase.
3. Binds at specific sequences to few promoters and required for initiation of transcription and considered as the 'positive regulators' of gene expression.

Introns

After transcription, the introns are detached by the process of 'splicing' leaving only the 'exons' which further get translated into proteins. Introns consist of large stretches of DNA whose biological functions are in the process of being elucidated. All higher organisms have introns, and the more complex organisms own a higher part of introns. These indicate that they play functions ranging from minor to major. Recent research elucidates a high level of conservation in some introns, indicating that they have some useful function. Many studies show the involvement of introns in cancer causation either directly or indirectly. For example, introns are may be involved in the transcriptional regulation of apoprotein B, E, and A-11 and few introns in regulating neoplasm developments. Conclusions relating introns and cancer are not plausible for varied reasons including studies on determining if intronic mutations responsible for tumour progression or due to collateral or unrelated damage.

Pseudogenes

Pseudogenes are non – functional DNA sequences resembling functional genes. The first pseudogene was reported in 1977 and since then a large number of these genes have been reported and described in humans and many other species. There are two accepted processes during which pseudogenes may arise:

1. Duplication: These genes also known as 'unprocessed pseudogenes' get modified due to mutations, insertions and deletions which usually results in the loss of gene function at the transcription or translation level (or both).

2. Retrotransposition: These genes also termed as 'processed pseudogenes' are located on different chromosomes from their functional counterparts. These segments lack introns and regulator genes and are flanked by direct repeats. This occurs due to the activity of long interspersed nuclear element (LINE), which mimics a genomic virus. LINEs follow their own way of making DNA copies of themselves to get integrated into the genome.

Telomeres

Telomeres are complex, essential, protective nucleoprotein structures located at the ends of eukaryotic chromosomes required for genome stability maintained by the special reverse transcriptase, telomerase. In most eukaryotic cells, telomeres has repetitive GT-rich sequences, which mostly made up of double-stranded DNA (dsDNA) which terminate with 32 single-stranded tails, called as G-tails. Until recently, these regions were considered as transcriptionally 'silent, but now are recognised to be transcribed into non-coding RNA molecules called TERRA. The function(s) of TERRA in telomere metabolism is now the subject of extreme study given the implications these may have on fundamental biological processes such as aging and cancer. In human cells, telomeres are bound and protected by a 'shelterin' complex- a six- subunit protein complex consisting of TRF1, TRF2, RAP1, POT1, TPP1 and TIN2. This complex binds specifically to telomeric DNA and regulates telomere function. TRF1 and TRF2 bind specifically to dsDNA telomeric repeats wherein TRF2 is important for repressing ATM activation at telomeres and have been shown to interact with both ATM and Chk2 kinases and thus might play a role in the inhibition of ATM – dependent check point establishment by interfering with the contact between ATM and Chk2. The DNA repair proteins like Apollo and MRN complex associate with TRF2 hypothesising that their activities may be regulated by TRF2 at the telomeric region. POT1 binds to G- tails and is important for repressing ATR activation at telomeres. This complex also promotes insertion of 32 telomeric G-tails into the dsDNA thereby generating a 't-loop' structure. This hides the telomeric 32 ends from checkpoint proteins and DNA repair. The mammalian shelterin complex is also thought to promote insertion of 32 telomeric G-tails into the dsDNA portion of telomeres to generate a 't-loop' structure, in that way hiding telomeric 32 ends from DNA repair and check point proteins.

Transposons

Transposons also identified as transposable elements (TEs) are DNA sequences that translocate from one genomic locus to another. First identified by Barbara McClintock, these elements are found in almost all organisms in great numbers. For example, TEs make up roughly 50% of the human genome and up to 90% of the maize genome. These elements were once considered as 'selfish' DNA but recent studies show their vitality in host genomes as epitomised by immunoglobulin V (D) J rearrangement, telomere maintenance, horizontal gene transfer, and intron origination. Besides jumping, the behaviour of these transposons depends on where it lands in the genome. Landing inside a gene may result in a mutation, for example, insertions of L1 into the factor VIII gene caused hemophilia.

Studies later on suggested that L1 was present in the APC genes in colon cancer cells but not in the APC genes in healthy cells in the identical individuals. It strongly confirms that L1 transposes in somatic cells in mammals, and this element might play a causal function in disease development. Most TE's appear silent, i.e. no phenotypic effect is seen nor they translocate themselves around the genome. Some are inactive and are unable to move from chromosomal location to another because they have deleterious mutations in them. In spite of being intact and able to move, a few transposons are kept inactive by epigenetic defence mechanisms such as DNA methylation, chromatin remodelling, and miRNAs. Transposon silencing also occurs in the plant genus Arabidopsis. Studies reveal that these plants contain more than twenty different mutator transposon sequences, wherein these sequences are silenced or methylated in wild-type plants. If one of the methylating enzymes becomes defective, then these transposons are transcribed. All of these transposable elements are not detrimental. Transposons have the ability to understand the evolution of genomes by expediting translocation of genomic sequences, shuffling of exons and repair of double stranded breaks.

The ability of transposons to enhance genetic diversity, together with the capacity of the genome to reduce most TE activity, results in a balance that makes transposable elements an crucial part of evolution and genome regulation in all organisms that carrying these sequences.

Repeat sequences, transposons and viral elements

Transposons and retrotransposons are mobile genetic elements. Retrotransposon repeated sequences, which include long interspersed nuclear elements (LINEs) and short interspersed nuclear elements (SINEs), account for a large proportion of the genomic sequences in many species. Alu sequences, classified as a short interspersed nuclear element, are the most abundant mobile elements in the human genome. Some examples have been found of SINEs exerting transcriptional control of some protein-encoding genes. Endogenous retrovirus sequences are the product of reverse transcription of retrovirus genomes into the genomes of germ cells. Mutation within these retro-transcribed sequences can inactivate the viral genome.

Over 8% of the human genome is made up of (mostly decayed) endogenous retrovirus sequences, as part of the over 42% fraction that is recognisably derived of retrotransposons, while another 3% can be identified to be the remains of DNA transposons. Much of the remaining half of the genome that is currently without an explained origin is expected to have found its origin in transposable elements that were active so long ago (>200 million years) that random mutations have rendered them unrecognisable. Genome size variation in at least two kinds of plants is mostly the result of retrotransposon sequences.

Junk DNA

The term 'junk DNA' became popular in the 1960s. According to T. Ryan Gregory, the nature of junk DNA was first discussed explicitly in 1972 by a genomic biologist, David Comings, who applied the term to all non-coding DNA. The term was formalised that same year by Susumu Ohno, who noted that the mutational load from deleterious mutations placed an upper limit on the number of functional loci that could be expected given a typical mutation rate. Ohno hypothesised that mammal genomes could not have more than 30000 loci under selection before the 'cost' from the mutational load would cause an inescapable decline in fitness, and eventually extinction. This prediction remains robust, with the human genome containing approximately 20000 genes. Another source for Ohno's theory was the observation that even closely related species can have widely (orders-of-magnitude) different genome sizes, which had been dubbed the C-value paradox in 1971.

Though the fruitfulness of the term 'junk DNA' has been questioned on the grounds that it provokes a strong a priori assumption of total non-functionality and though some have recommended using more neutral terminology such as 'non-coding DNA' instead, 'junk DNA' remains a label for the portions of a genome sequence for which no discernible function has been identified and that through comparative genomics analysis appear under no functional constraint suggesting that the sequence itself has provided no adaptive advantage. Since the late 70s it has become apparent that the majority of non-coding DNA in large genomes finds its origin in the selfish amplification of transposable elements, of which W. Ford Doolittle and Carmen Sapienza in 1980 wrote in the journal Nature: 'When a given DNA, or class of DNAs, of unproven phenotypic function can be shown to have evolved a strategy (such as transposition) which ensures its genomic survival, then no other explanation for its existence is necessary.' The amount of junk DNA can be expected to depend on the rate of amplification of these elements and the rate at which non-functional DNA is lost. In the same issue of Nature, Leslie Orgel and Francis Crick wrote that junk DNA has 'little specificity and conveys little or no selective advantage to the organism'. The term occurs mainly in popular science and in a colloquial way in scientific publications, and it has been suggested that its connotations may have delayed interest in the biological functions of non-coding DNA. Several lines of evidence indicate that some 'junk DNA' sequences are likely to have unidentified functional activity and that the process of exaptation of fragments of originally selfish or non-functional DNA has been commonplace throughout evolution.

Evidence of Functionality

Many non-coding DNA sequences must have some important biological function. This is indicated by comparative genomics studies that report highly conserved regions of non-coding DNA, sometimes on time-scales of hundreds of millions of years. This implies that these non-coding regions are under strong evolutionary pressure and positive selection. For example, in the genomes of humans and mice, which diverged from a common ancestor 65–75 million years ago, protein-coding DNA sequences account for only about 20% of conserved DNA, with the remaining 80% of conserved DNA represented in non-coding regions. Linkage mapping often identifies chromosomal regions associated with a disease with no evidence of functional coding variants of genes within the region, suggesting that disease-causing genetic variants lie in the non-coding DNA. The significance of non-coding DNA mutations in cancer was explored in April 2013. Non-coding genetic polymorphisms play a role in infectious disease susceptibility, such as hepatitis C. Moreover, non-coding genetic polymorphisms contribute to susceptibility to Ewing sarcoma, an aggressive pediatric bone cancer.

Some specific sequences of non-coding DNA may be features essential to chromosome structure, centromere function and recognition of homologous chromosomes during meiosis.

According to a comparative study of over 300 prokaryotic and over 30 eukaryotic genomes, eukaryotes appear to require a minimum amount of non-coding DNA. The amount can be predicted using a growth model for regulatory genetic networks, implying that it is required for regulatory purposes. In humans the predicted minimum is about 5% of the total genome.

Over 10% of 32 mammalian genomes may function through the formation of specific RNA secondary structures. The study used comparative genomics to identify compensatory DNA mutations that maintain RNA base-pairings, a distinctive feature of RNA molecules. Over 80% of the genomic regions presenting evolutionary evidence of RNA structure conservation do not present strong DNA sequence conservation.

Non-coding DNA separates genes from each other with long gaps, so mutation in one gene or part of a chromosome, for example deletion or insertion, does not have a frameshift effect on the whole chromosome. When genome complexity is relatively high, like in the case of human genome, not only between different genes, but also inside many genes, there are gaps of introns to protect the entire coding segment and minimise the changes caused by mutation. Non-coding DNA may perhaps serve to decrease the probability of gene disruption during chromosomal crossover.

Regulating Gene Expression

Some non-coding DNA sequences determine the expression levels of various genes, both those that are transcribed to proteins and those that themselves are involved in gene regulation.

Transcription factors

Some non-coding DNA sequences determine where transcription factors attach. A transcription factor is a protein that binds to specific non-coding DNA sequences, thereby controlling the flow (or transcription) of genetic information from DNA to mRNA.

Operators

An operator is a segment of DNA to which a repressor binds. A repressor is a DNA-binding protein that regulates the expression of one or more genes by binding to the operator and blocking the attachment of RNA polymerase to the promoter, thus preventing transcription of the genes. This blocking of expression is called repression.

Enhancers

An enhancer is a short region of DNA that can be bound with proteins (trans-acting factors), much like a set of transcription factors, to enhance transcription levels of genes in a gene cluster.

Silencers

A silencer is a region of DNA that inactivates gene expression when bound by a regulatory protein. It functions in a very similar way as enhancers, only differing in the inactivation of genes.

Promoters

A promoter is a region of DNA that facilitates transcription of a particular gene when a transcription factor binds to it. Promoters are typically located near the genes they regulate and upstream of them.

Insulators

A genetic insulator is a boundary element that plays two distinct roles in gene expression, either as an enhancer-blocking code, or rarely as a barrier against condensed chromatin. An insulator in a DNA sequence is comparable to a linguistic word divider such as a comma in a sentence, because the insulator indicates where an enhanced or repressed sequence ends.

STRUCTURAL VARIANTS

Structural variants are modifications in an organisms chromosome due to insertions, deletions, inversions, translocations and duplications commonly referred to as copy – number variants (CNV's) which are usually >1 Kb in length. If present at >1% in a population a CNV may be referred to as copy number polymorphism (CNP). Most of these variants lead to genetic disorders. For example, the Charcot-Marie Tooth (CMT) disease, a autosomal dominant disease associated with a gene dosage effect due to an inherited DNA rearrangement was the first to be elucidated in 1991.

In most cases, this disease was associated with a tandem duplication of length 1.5Mb in 17p11.2-p12 propitiated by flanking segmental duplications which surrounds the PMP22 gene. The disease phenotype results from having three copies of the normal gene. The mutual product of the recombination, a single copy of the PMP22 gene and results in the clinically distinct hereditary neuropathy with liability to pressure palsies.

SIMPLE AND TANDEM REPEATS

Tandem repeats are pervasive repetitive patterns of nucleotides that occur adjacent to each other varying in length from 2–50 base pairs in length. By identification of these patterns, an individual's genetic profile can be created. This method is widely used in forensic analysis by using the fingerprints of the culprit. Estimates from the human genome Sequencing project indicate that such repeats make up ~3% of the sequenced human genome. For example, most of the humans have nearly 30 CGG•CGG repeats in the 52 UTR of their FMR1 gene. However, population studies in Caucasians, the only population for which significant data exist, indicate that 246 to 468 females has 55–200 repeats and 3717 to 8918 males has 200 to >1000 repeats at this locus.

Segmental Duplications

Segmental duplications are repetitive segments of the genome that are 1 to >400 kb in length and 90–100% sequence identity. The evidences show that paralogous segmental duplications, also called as low-copy repeats (LCRs), may be significant determinants of genomic plasticity in all eukaryotes. Computational analysis revealed that these duplications occur frequently in the genome wide analysis of nine model eukaryotes even after concealing of the repetitive elements. Inverted repeats have the ability to form secondary structural elements like palindromes or stem-loops which can recombine and lead to chromosomal rearrangements. This contrivance predisposes many genetic disorders in humans bestowing to tumorigenesis and a vital role in primate karyotype evolution.

   As researchers sift through the long-neglected introns and intergenic stretches of DNA, comparative genomics tools will only help in functional annotation but also in identifying the genetic source of diseases but also in identification of appropriate drugs and understanding of the pharmacological effects of these segments. In cases where organisms vary distantly, the most conserved genes are used, such as rRNA genes (16s rRNA) are found to play vital roles. These segments have been conserved for over millions of years such that they do not seem diverse that they all seems equally unrelated, but cannot give sufficient 'resolution' to determine the relationship between closely related species as they may be almost or completely identical. Thus, using comparative and functional genomics, studies on non-coding segments seems plausible in the near future.

SCALING FEATURES OF NON-CODING DNA

Scaling concepts have played a key role in our understanding of phenomena occurring near critical points. A scale invariant function $f(x)$ has the remarkable property that each time x is doubled, the function $f(x)$ changes by the same factor. There is thus no way to set a characteristic scale for such a function. Stated mathematically, if the variable x is increased by an arbitrary factor λ^p, then the function is changed by a factor p which is independent of the value of x,

$$f(\lambda x) = \lambda^p f(x) \qquad \ldots(2.1)$$

for all λ. A functional equation, such as (Eq 2.1), constrains the set of possible functional forms of $f(x)$: any function $f(x)$ satisfying (Eq 2.1) must be a power-law, as may be seen by substituting the choice $\lambda = 1/x$ in (Eq 2.1):

$$f(x) = Ax^p \qquad \qquad \dots(2.2)$$

We say that scale invariance (Eq 2.1) implies power-law behaviour (Eq 2.2). Conversely, power-law behaviour implies scale invariance, since any function $f(x)$ obeying (Eq 2.2) also obeys (Eq 2.1) one can verify this by substitution. Thus, scale invariance is mathematically equivalent to power-law behaviour.

Power laws are found to describe various functions in the vicinity of critical points. These include not only systems with Hamiltonians (such as the Ising and Heisenberg models) but also purely geometric systems, such as percolation. Scaling is also found to hold for polymeric systems, including both linear and branched polymers. Here power-law correlations develop in the asymptotic limit in which the number of monomers approaches infinity.

The list of systems in which power-law correlations appear has grown rapidly in recent years, including models of rough surfaces, turbulence, and earthquakes. Recent work suggest that—under suitable conditions—the sequence of base pairs or 'nucleotides' in non-coding DNA also displays power-law correlations. The underlying basis of such power-law correlations is not understood at present, but it is at least possible that this reason is of as fundamental importance as it is in other systems in nature that have been found to display power-law correlations.

INFORMATION CODING IN DNA

Genomic sequences contain numerous 'layers' of information. These include specifications for mRNA sequences responsible for protein structure, identification of coding and non-coding parts of the sequence, information necessary for specification of regulatory (promoter, enhancer) sequences, information directing protein–DNA interactions, directions for DNA packaging and unwinding. The genomic sequence is likely the most sophisticated and efficient information database created by nature through the dynamic process of evolution. Equally remarkable is the precise transformation of different layers of information (replication, decoding, etc.) that occurs in a short time interval. While means of encoding some of this information is understood (for example, the genetic code directing amino acid assembly, sequences directing intron/exon splicing, etc.) relatively little is known about other layers of information encrypted in a DNA molecule. In the genomes of high eukaryotic organisms, only a small portion of the total genome length is used for protein coding. The role of introns and intergenomic sequences constituting a large portion of the genome remains unknown. Furthermore, only a few quantitative methods are currently available for analysing such information.

CONVENTIONAL STATISTICAL ANALYSIS OF DNA SEQUENCES

DNA sequences have been analysed using a variety of models that can basically be considered in two categories. The first types are 'local' analyses, they take into account the fact that DNA sequences are produced in sequential order, so the neighbouring base pairs will affect the next attaching base pair. This type of analysis, such as n-step Markov models, can indeed describe some observed short-range correlations in DNA sequences. The second category of analyses is more 'global' in nature, concentrating on the presence of repeated patterns (such as periodic repeats and interspersed base sequence repeats) that can be found mostly in eukaryotic genomic sequences. A typical example of analysis in this category is the Fourier transform analysis which can identify repeats of certain segments of the same length in base pair sequences. However, DNA sequences are more complicated than these two standard types of analysis can describe. Therefore, it is crucial to develop new tools for analysis with a view toward uncovering the mechanisms used to code other types of information in DNA sequences.

SCALE-INVARIANT (FRACTAL) ANALYSIS OF DNA SEQUENCES

In the last decade, scaling analysis (fractal) techniques have been developed for detecting scale-invariant statistical patterns and study physical properties in complex fluids and other random systems. These methods have been successfully applied in a number of disciplines and to a number of problems including stochastic growth processes in physics and chemistry, polymer physics, as well as other problems. Since DNA sequences are long polymer chains, some general scale-invariant properties found in polymer physics may appear in DNA, and alterations of those general properties may serve for characterisation of DNA sequences. A useful approach to studying stochastic properties of DNA involves the construction of a 1 : 1 map of the base pair sequence projected onto a walk–which we term a 'DNA walk'. The mapping is then used to obtain a quantitative measure of the correlation between base pairs over long distances along the DNA chain. In addition, the technique provides a novel graphical 'fingerprint' representation of DNA structures.

In this fashion we uncovered in the base pair sequence a remarkably long-range power-law correlation that is significant because it implies a new scale invariant (fractal) property of DNA. Such long-range correlations are limited to non-coding sequences (introns, regulatory untranscribed gene elements and intergenomic sequences) and occur in organisms as diverse as hepatitis delta agent, cytomegalovirus, yeast chromosome and a large number of eukaryotic genes encoding a variety of proteins.

The power-law decay correlations are of interest because they cannot be accounted for by the standard Markov chain model or other short-range correlations models (which will only give rise to an exponential decay in correlation). On the other hand, unlike the standard Fourier transform analysis that detects the periodical repeats described by a few characteristic length scales, the analysis shows that there exist statistically self-similar patterns on all length scales.

DNA walk or fractal landscape representation: The DNA walk provides a graphical representation for each gene and permits the degree of correlation in the base pair sequence to be directly visualised. This naturally motivates a quantification of this correlation by calculating the 'net displacement' of the walker.

Coding Sequence Finder (CSF) Algorithm

To provide an 'unbiased' test of the thesis that non-coding regions possess but coding regions lack long-range correlations, Ossadnik and others analysed several artificial uncorrelated and correlated 'control sequences' of size 105 nucleotides using the GRAIL neural net algorithm. The GRAIL algorithm identified about 60 putative exons in the uncorrelated sequences, but only about 5 putative exons in the correlated sequences. Using the DFA method, we can measure the local value of the correlation exponent along the sequence and find that the local minima of as a function of a nucleotide position usually correspond to coding regions, while the local maxima correspond to non-coding regions. Statistical analysis using the DFA technique of the nucleotide sequence data for yeast chromosome III (315, 338 nucleotides) shows the probability that the observed correspondence between the positions of minima and coding regions is due to random coincidence is less than 0.0014. Thus, this method—which we called the 'coding sequence finder' (CSF) algorithm–can be used for finding coding regions in the newly sequenced DNA, a potentially important application of DNA walk analysis.

Chapter 3

Chromosomes and Chromatin

INTRODUCTION

All cellular genetic material exists as a compact mass in a relatively confined volume. In bacteria, the genetic material is seen in the form of a nucleoid that forms a discrete clump within the cell. In eukaryotic cells, it is seen as the mass of chromatin within the nucleus at interphase. The packaging of chromatin is flexible and changes during the eukaryotic cell cycle. Interphase chromatin becomes even more tightly packaged at the time of division (mitosis or meiosis), when individual chromosomes become visible as discrete entities.

A chromosome is a device for segregating genetic material at cell division. The crucial structural feature by which this is accomplished is the centromere, often visible as a constriction in the length of the chromosome under the light microscope. At a greater level of detail, the centromere can be seen to include the kinetochore, a structure by which it is attached to microtubules. A eukaryotic chromosome usually consists of a very long linear segment of DNA, and another crucial feature is the telomere, which stabilises the ends and is extended by special mechanisms that bypass the difficulties of replicating the ends of linear DNA. The density of DNA is high. In a bacterial nucleoid it is ~10 mg/mL, in a eukaryotic nucleus it is ~100 mg/mL, and in the head of the phage T4 virus it is >500 mg/mL. Such a concentration in solution is equivalent to a gel of great viscosity and has implications (not fully understood) for the ability of proteins to find their binding sites on DNA. The various activities of DNA, such as replication and transcription, must be accomplished within this confined space. The organisation of the material must accommodate transitions between inactive and active states.

Table 3.1 shows the range of genome sizes and makes the point that they are divided into chromosomes varying greatly in DNA content. The length of the DNA as an extended molecule would vastly exceed the dimensions of the region that contains it. Its condensed state results from its binding to basic proteins. The positive charges of these proteins neutralise the negative charges of the nucleic acid. The structure of the nucleoprotein complex is determined by the interactions of proteins that condense the DNA into a tightly coiled structure. Therefore, in contrast with the customary picture of DNA as an extended double helix, structural deformation of DNA to bend or fold into a more compact form is the rule rather than exception.

23

Table 3.1: The number of chromosomes in the haploid genome and the chromosome size vary extensively.

Organism	Genome (Mb)	Haploid chromosomes	Range of chromosome length (Mb DNA)	Total genes
E. coli	4.6	1	4.6	4401
S. cerevisiae	12.1	16	(0.2)–1.5	6702
D. melanogaster	165	4	(1.3)–28	14399
Rice	389	12	24–45	37544
Mouse	2500	20	60–195	26996
Man	2900	23	49–245	24194

Most chromatin has a relatively dispersed appearance, this material is called euchromatin, and it contains the majority of active genes. Some regions of chromatin are more densely packed, this material is called heterochromatin and is usually not transcriptionally active.

What is the general structure of chromatin, and what is the difference between active and inactive sequences? The high overall packing ratio of the genetic material immediately suggests that DNA cannot be directly packaged into the final structure of chromatin. There must be hierarchies of organisation. A major question concerns the specificity of packaging. Is the DNA folded into a particular pattern, or is it different in each individual copy of the genome? How does the pattern of packaging change when a segment of DNA is replicated or transcribed?

The building block of chromatin is the nucleosome, and it has the same fundamental structure in all eukaryotes. The nucleosome contains ~200 base pair (bp) of DNA, organised by an octamer of small, basic proteins into a beadlike structure. The protein components are the histones. They form an interior core, the DNA lies on the surface of the particle. Nucleosomes are an invariant component of euchromatin and heterochromatin in the interphase nucleus and of mitotic chromosomes. The nucleosome provides the first level of organisation. It packages 67 nm of DNA into a body of diameter 11 nm. Its components and structure are well characterised. A linear string of nucleosomes forms a structure referred to as the '10-nm fibre.' The second level of organisation is the coiling of the series of nucleosomes into a helical array to constitute the fibre of diameter ~30 nm that is found in interphase chromatin as well as in mitotic chromosomes. This condenses the nucleosomes by a factor of 6 to 73 per unit length.

The final packing ratio is determined by the third level of organisation, the packaging of the 30-nm fibre itself. Euchromatin is about 50 times more condensed relative to the 30-nm fibre. Euchromatin is cyclically interchangeable with packing into mitotic chromosomes, which are about 5–10 times more compact. Heterochromatin generally has the same packing density as mitotic chromosomes.

The mass of chromatin contains up to twice as much protein as DNA. Approximately half of the protein mass is accounted for by the nucleosomes. The mass of RNA is <10% of the mass of DNA. Much of the RNA consists of nascent transcripts still associated with the template DNA.

Changes in chromatin structure are accomplished by association with additional proteins or by modifications of existing chromosomal proteins. Both replication and transcription require unwinding of DNA and, thus, must involve an unfolding of the structure that allows the relevant enzymes to manipulate the DNA. This is likely to involve changes in all levels of organisation.

The nonhistones include all the proteins of chromatin except the histones. Non-histones are more variable between tissues and species and comprise a smaller proportion of the mass than the histones. They also comprise a much larger number of proteins, so that any individual protein is present in amounts much smaller than any histone.

CHROMATIN IS DIVIDED INTO EUCHROMATIN AND HETEROCHROMATIN

Each chromosome contains a single, very long duplex of DNA that is folded into a fibre that runs continuously throughout the chromosome. In accounting for interphase chromatin and mitotic chromosome structure, we have to explain the packaging of a single, exceedingly long molecule of DNA into a form in which it can be transcribed and replicated and can become cyclically more or less compressed.

Individual eukaryotic chromosomes are visible as such only during the act of cell division, when each can be seen as a compact unit. (The sister chromatids are daughter chromosomes produced by the previous replication event, still joined together at this stage of mitosis.) Each consists of a fibre with a diameter of ~30 nm and a nubbly appearance. The DNA is 5–10 times more condensed in chromosomes than in interphase chromatin. During most of the life cycle of the eukaryotic cell, however, its genetic material occupies an area of the nucleus in which individual chromosomes cannot be distinguished. The 30-nm fibre from which chromatin is constructed is similar or identical to that of the mitotic chromosomes.

Chromatin can be divided into two types of material, which can be visualised by staining with DNA-specific dyes and are given below:

1. In most regions, the fibres are much less densely packed than in the mitotic chromosome. This material is called euchromatin. It has a relatively dispersed appearance in the nucleus and occupies most of the nuclear region.

2. Some regions of chromatin are very densely packed with fibres, displaying a condition comparable with that of the chromosome at mitosis. This material is called heterochromatin. It is typically found at centromeres but also occurs at other locations, such as telomeres and highly repetitive sequences. It passes through the cell cycle with relatively little change in its degree of condensation. It forms a series of discrete clumps, but often the various heterochromatic regions aggregate into a densely staining chromocenter. (This description applies to regions that are always heterochromatic, called constitutive heterochromatin, in addition, there is another class of heterochromatin, called facultative heterochromatin, in which regions of euchromatin are converted to a heterochromatic state.)

The same fibres run continuously between euchromatin and heterochromatin, because these states represent different degrees of condensation of the genetic material. In the same way, euchromatic regions exist in different states of condensation during interphase and during mitosis. Therefore, the genetic material is organised in a manner that permits alternative states to be maintained side by side in chromatin and allows cyclic changes to occur in the packaging of euchromatin between interphase and division.

The structural condition of the genetic material is correlated with its activity. The common features of constitutive heterochromatin are as follows:

• It is permanently condensed.

• It often consists of multiple repeats of a few sequences of DNA that are not transcribed or are transcribed at very low levels.

• Probably resulting from the condensed state, it replicates later than euchromatin and has a reduced frequency of genetic recombination relative to euchromatic gene-rich areas of the genome.

• The density of genes in this region is very much reduced compared with euchromatin, and genes that are translocated into or near it are often inactivated. The one dramatic exception to this is the ribosomal DNA (rDNA) in the nucleolus, which has the general compacted appearance and behaviour of heterochromatin (such as late replication) yet is engaged in very active transcription.

Numerous molecular markers exist for changes in the properties of the DNA and protein components in heterochromatic regions. They include reduced acetylation of histone proteins, increased methylation at particular sites on histone proteins, and methylation of cytosine bases in specific regions of DNA. These molecular changes cause the condensation of the chromatin, which is responsible for its inactivity.

Although active genes are contained within euchromatin, only a subset of the sequences in euchromatin are transcribed at any time. Therefore, although location in euchromatin is necessary for expression of many genes, it is not sufficient for it. In addition to the general distributions observed for heterochromatin and euchromatin, studies have addressed whether there is an overall chromosome organisation within the nucleus. The answer in many cases is yes, chromosomes appear to occupy distinct three-dimensional spaces known as chromosome territories. The chromosomes occupying these territories are not entangled with each other but do share areas of interaction and some common functional organisation. For example, heterochromatic and other silent regions are found primarily at the nuclear periphery, whereas gene-dense regions are internally located. Active genes are often found at the borders of territories, sometimes clustered together in interchromosomal spaces that are enriched in transcriptional machinery, known as 'transcription factories.' How chromosome territories are established and how they vary by cell cycle and cell type are not yet understood.

CELL CYCLE AND REPLICATION OF GENOME

The period in the cell cycle when the genome is replicated (S phase) is crucially important for the establishment and maintenance of programmes of differential gene activity. Not only must DNA be replicated, but the chromosome itself must be duplicated. The majority of genes in the proliferating cell of a defined type retain the same states of transcriptional activity through cell division. This requires the duplication of the precise nucleoprotein complexes directing gene transcription or repression on the nascent DNA templates. The maintenance of these specific regulatory complexes through replication reflects the commitment of a defined cell type or line to a particular state of determination. Pre-existing chromosomal structures are transiently disrupted by transit through the replication elongation complex. Most of these structures are faithfully reassembled following replication through mechanisms discussed in this chapter. However, the transient disruption of these structures also offers a window of opportunity for modifying regulatory nucleoprotein complexes. These alterations can either activate genes through the disruption of repressed states, or direct the repression of previously active genes. Thus, cell division offers a molecular mechanism to redirect the commitment of a cell towards a particular determined state. A consideration of the processes occurring at the eukaryotic replication fork suggests how this important development process might be accomplished.

IMPLICATIONS OF DNA REPLICATION FOR STABLE STATES OF TRANSCRIPTIONAL ACTIVITY

Active and Repressed States of Eukaryotic Genes

The local nucleoprotein complexes required to maintain a eukaryotic gene in an active or repressed state have been defined in some detail. Transcriptional activity for a given gene depends on a number of sequence-specific transcription factors (e.g. SPI), structural proteins (e.g. HMGIE), and non-DNA binding proteins associated with the promoter interacting to recruit general transcription factors (e.g. TFIIA, TFIIB) together with the TFIID complex [containing TBP (TATA binding protein) and the TAFs (TATA associated factors)]. The assembly of this large nucleoprotein complex is initiated through the association of DNA-binding proteins and requires many intermediate steps leading to the recruitment of RNA polymerase II and, eventually, to transcription itself. Conversely, several features may determine a gene to be transcriptionally inactive. A common mechanism appears to be a deficiency in an essential component required for the assembly of the active complex. If this component is a DNA-binding protein, the cognate DNA sequence might become associated with the histone proteins. Specific nucleosomal structures assembled by the core histones (H2A, H2B, H3, and H4) might restrict the subsequent association of either sequence-specific DNA-binding proteins or the basal transcriptional machinery. Other proteins may stabilise repressive higher-order chromatin structures dependent on prior association of the core histones, these include linker histone variants or the chromodomain (chromatin modification organiser) proteins such as HPl and Polycomb. Generally, the assemblies of nucleosomes or transcription complexes on the promoter of a eukaryotic gene are mutually exclusive.

The prior assembly of nucleosomes can prevent transcription factors from binding to DNA and, conversely, the prior assembly of a transcription complex prevents nucleosome formation from repressing transcription (Fig. 3.1). Although these results provide an excellent molecular basis for the maintenance of stable states of gene expression in a terminally differentiated nondividing cell, they do not explain why either transcriptionally active or inactive states are assembled onto DNA in the first place, nor do they explain how such states can be propagated through cell division. Clearly, because both nucleoprotein structures can incorporate the same DNA molecule, the possibility exists of a competition occurring between the assembly of the two structures. This competition, in fact, occurs during the staged assembly of either active or repressed states following replication. Molecular mechanisms that influence the outcome of this competition direct the commitment of a cell to a particular state of determination or facilitate developmentally regulated switches in cell fate. However, to appreciate how this competition occurs, we must first discuss the consequences of DNA replication for pre-existing chromatin structures.

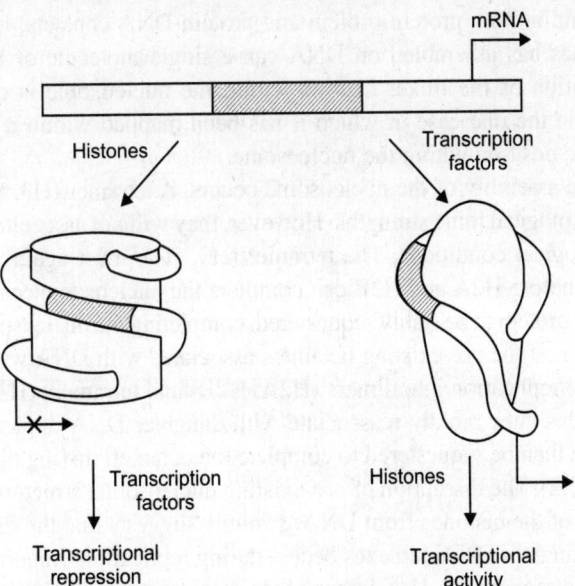

Fig. 3.1: Nucleosome assembly and transcription complex assembly are often mutually exclusive. Two alternate pathways are shown for the association of DNA-binding proteins with a promoter containing a TATA homology. The start site of transcription of mRNA is indicated by the bent arrow.

Impact of DNA replication on pre-existing chromatin structures

Chromatin consists of long arrays of nucleosomal DNA interspersed with specific regulatory nucleoprotein complexes. The replication fork moves through chromatin without apparent impediment. Replication fork progression disrupts pre-existing nucleosomes, however, the fate of regulatory nucleoprotein complexes depends on the particular structure examined.

Nucleosomes: Major considerations for pre-existing nucleosomes during the replication process are whether the histones present in the nucleosome stay together on nascent DNA, and whether nucleosomes are randomly or conservatively segregated to daughter DNA strands. DNA replication requires the transient unwinding of duplex parental DNA into two single-stranded regions. Although histones associate with single-stranded DNA, they do not assemble nucleosomes. This property, coupled with the competing protein-DNA interactions involved in DNA synthesis at the replication fork, probably accounts for nucleosome disruption. Histones released from the parental chromatin during replication *in vitro* can be easily sequestered onto competitor DNA. However, *in vivo* these histones are sequestered onto daughter DNA molecules close to the replication fork (Fig. 3.2). A nucleosome contains an octamer consisting of two molecules each of the four core histones (H2A, H2B, H3, and H4) and a single molecule of a fifth linker histone (Hl). The four core histones and the linker histone have very selective interactions with each other. Our most detailed understanding of nucleosomal architecture and construction has relied on *in vitro* experiments that have attempted to reconstruct nucleosomes with purified histones. These experiments have been informative, although they involve dialysis from high salt to low salt concentrations and do not employ the molecular chaperones used *in vivo*.

The central 'kernel' of the nucleosome is made up of two heterodimers of histones H3 and H4. Only when this 'tetramer' is bound to DNA can two heterodimers of H2A and H2B bind to complete assembly of the histone octamer. One heterodimer of H2A and H2B binds to either side of the histone tetramer in an interaction dependent on both protein-protein and protein-DNA contacts. Only when the complete octamer of core histones has assembled on DNA can a single molecule of linker histone be stably bound. The exact position of the linker histone within the nucleosome is currently the subject of controversy, however, in the one case in which it has been mapped within a specific nucleosome, it occupies an asymmetric position within the nucleosome.

In vivo a comparable assembly of the nucleosome occurs. A tetramer (H3, H4), and a dimer (H2A, H2B) are stable at physiological ionic strengths. However, they will not associate together in the absence of DNA under physiological conditions. The tetramer (H3, H4), must again associate with DNA on newly replicated DNA before H2A and H2B can complete the nucleosome core.

Histone H1 is the last protein to be stably sequestered, completing the nucleosome. Jackson determined that a substantial fraction of the pre-existing octamers associated with DNA within the chromosome *in vivo* fell apart following replication into dimers (H2A, H2B) and tetramers (H3, H4)2. Tetramers from these pre-existing nucleosomes rapidly reassociate with daughter DNA duplexes. Newly synthesised dimers (H2A, H2B) can then be sequestered to complete the octamer, mixing old and new histones into a single structure (Fig. 3.2). The disruption of pre-existing nucleosomal structure at the replication fork, coupled to dissociation of the histones from DNA, strongly suggests that the dispersive segregation of these histones to both daughter DNA duplexes occurs during replication. Importantly, the incorporation of pre-existing histone tetramers (H3, H4), into nascent chromatin provides a means of maintaining and propagating a stable state of gene activity. The old H3 and H4 present in the nascent chromatin retain their pre-existing posttranslational modification state. This differs from that of newly synthesised H3 and H4 and can potentially influence subsequent transcription of the associated DNA. The dispersive

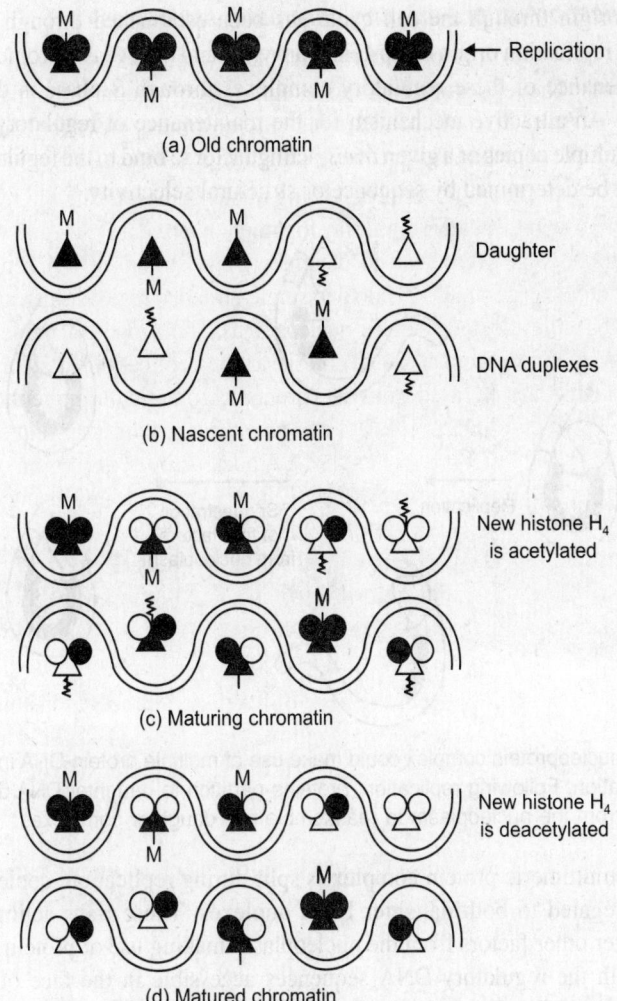

(a) Old chromatin

Daughter

(b) Nascent chromatin

DNA duplexes

New histone H$_4$
is acetylated

(c) Maturing chromatin

New histone H$_4$
is deacetylated

(d) Matured chromatin

Fig. 3.2: Nucleosome disruption during replication and reassembly following replication. (a) Old chromatin consisting of preexisting nucleosomes (histone octamer plus DNA) containing a tetramer (H3, H4), (filled triangle) and two dimers (H2A, H2B) (filled circles). The histones in the tetramer are modified (M). Replication displaces these histones from DNA; the octamer can fall apart into tetramers and dimers, (b) Nascent chromatin. Old tetramers associate with both daughter DNA duplexes. Newly synthesized tetramers (open triangles) containing diacetylated histone H4 (zigzag line) also associate with daughter DNA in a process facilitated by CAF-I, (c) Maturing chromatin. Old and new dimers (open circles) bind to the tetramers and (d) Matured chromatin. New tetramers are deacetylated.

segregation of 'old' histones coupled to maintenance of their pre-existing states of modification provides a molecular mechanism whereby an epigenetic imprint might be propagated through replication.

Regulatory complexes

A special case for a regulatory nucleoprotein complex maintaining association with DNA throughout the cell cycle is the protein assembly that regulates use of an origin of replication itself. Stable association of proteins with an origin through the cell cycle has been established through *in vivo* footprinting methodologies on the replication origin of Epstein-Barr virus and on a yeast chromosomal ARS element. Implicit in the maintenance of these regulatory complexes through S phase is the concept that they duplicate themselves. An attractive mechanism for the maintenance of regulatory complexes through replication requires multiple copies of a given *trans*-acting factor to bind to the regulatory DNA sequences (Fig. 3.3). This could be determined by sequence or structural selectivity.

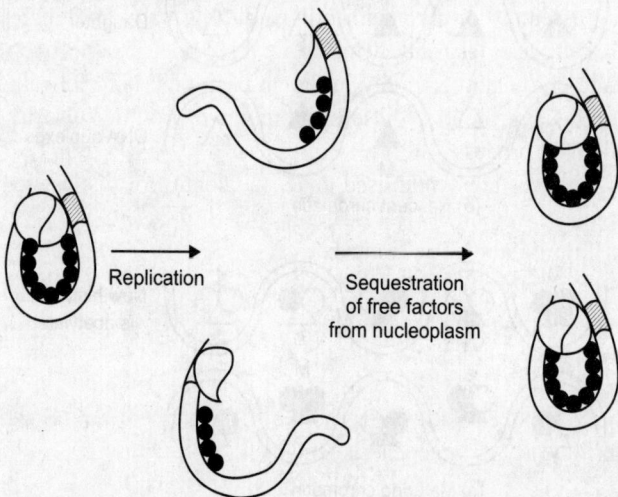

Fig. 3.3: A regulatory nucleoprotein complex could make use of multiple protein-DNA interactions to maintain integrity through replication. Following replication, proteins partition to daughter DNA duplexes. Free factors are then sequestered from the nucleoplasm to reassemble two daughter complexes.

If the pre-existing multimeric protein complex is split during replication, copies of the trans-acting factors could be segregated to both daughter DNA duplexes. These trans-acting factors could then either directly *sequester* other factors from the nucleoplasm making use of protein-protein interactions, or they could maintain the regulatory DNA sequences accessible in the face of ongoing chromatin assembly, such that when other factors became available they could bind to DNA. Structurally driven protein association is consistent with the maintenance of DNA distortion throughout the cell cycle at the Epstein-Barr viral origin.

In contrast to origin complexes, the basal transcriptional machinery appears to be removed from promoter elements by the passage of a replication fork. Replication is found to be dominant to the transcription process, and a direct consequence of replication fork progression through an active 5s rRNA gene is the displacement of transcription factors. Several correlations from *in vivo* work support the generality of this observation. There is a clear antagonism between transcription and replication on efficiently replicating SV40 DNA molecules. Replication forks invade the transcriptionally active ribosomal, RNA genes in yeast.

Thus, replication apparently resets the transcriptional status of a chromosome to 'ground zero.' The component protein molecules that determine transcriptional activity have to reassemble regulatory complexes *de novo* on the daughter DNA duplexes. This reassembly occurs not on naked DNA, but on a nascent chromatin template.

Chromatin Assembly has Replication-dependent and Independent Pathways

Replication-independent pathways

Early work on physiological chromatin assembly pathways made use of cell-free preparations from *Xenopus* oocytes and eggs. More recently, extracts of *Drosophila* embryos have been used with similar results. For both systems, chromatin assembly on non replicating DNA is relatively slow, taking several hours to assemble nucleosomes to a physiological density (one nucleosome per 180–200 bp). This contrasts with the rapid assembly of chromatin *in vivo* during early embryogenesis in *Xenopus* and *Drosophifa,* where entire cell cycles take only 30 minutes and 10 minutes, respectively. Thus, the molecular mechanisms that mediate chromatin assembly in the absence of DNA replication have questionable physiological relevance. Nevertheless, these systems have provided useful information on the biochemistry of the assembly process.

In *Xenopus* oocytes, histones are synthesised under the control of distinct regulatory mechanisms that operate outside of S phase. Tetramers (H3, H4), are stored in a complex with the molecular chaperone NUN2. Dimers (H2A, H2B) are stored in a complex with the chaperone nucleoplasmin. Both chaperones exchange histones onto DNA at physiological ionic strength. NUN2 must function before nucleoplasmin to assemble a nucleosome. During normal development, nucleoplasmin has a specialised role in the remodelling of *Xenopus* sperm chromatin, where it facilitates the exchange of sperm-specific basic proteins for histones H2A and H2B. Nucleoplasmin and NUN2 allow large amounts of histones to be stably sequestered in the Xenopus oocyte and egg, however, a role for these proteins in directly mediating chromatin assembly during early embryogenesis remains to be established.

Replication-dependent pathways

In vivo in normal somatic cells, the vast bulk of the histone proteins are synthesised during S phase. These histones are immediately assembled onto nascent DNA at the replication fork. Stillman discovered that the chromatin assembly process is coupled to replication. The molecular chaperone mediating the process is chromatin assembly factor 1 (CAF-l), which requires ongoing DNA replication to function. CAF-1 directs the association of the tetramer (H3, H4), with replicating DNA. Dimers (H2A/H2B) then bind in a CAF-l-independent process to complete the histone octamer. CAF-1 requires a modified tetramer (H3, H4), from the cytosol of human cells in order to function. This is potentially a key regulatory event in distinguishing the biochemistry of replication-dependent and independent chromatin assembly pathways. It is possible that the phosphorylation and diacetylation of histone H4 coupled to its synthesis may be necessary for chromatin assembly. Whether CAF-1 has specific interactions either with highly modified H4 and/or with the replication machinery itself are important questions yet to be resolved.

Almouzni and colleagues established that replication-coupled pathways of chromatin assembly also exist in Xenopus. However, the molecular chaperones that couple replication to chromatin assembly, such as the CAF-1 found in somatic cells, remain to be defined. These replication dependent pathways direct the efficient assembly of nucleosomes both *in vitro* and *in vivo* with kinetics that could easily accommodate a cell cycle duration of 30 minutes. The mechanism of enhanced assembly involves both the rapid deposition of the histone tetramer (H3, H4), and facilitation of the subsequent deposition of dimers (H2A, H2B). Similar results consistent with a facilitated two step assembly of chromatin have been obtained in mammalian systems. The *de novo* assembly of chromatin on replicating templates *in vitro* provides a useful independent confirmation of earlier work on the staged assembly of chromatin during S phase *in vivo*. As discussed earlier, DNA replication disrupts pre-existing nucleoprotein structures within the chromosome. Histones that are displaced during replication reassociate with newly synthesised DNA, but do so randomly on both daughter.

DNA duplexes: A consequence of this segregation is that nascent chromatin has a 50% enrichment of pre-existing histones. The remainder of the histones incorporated into chromatin are newly synthesised. Radio labelling of these newly synthesised histones has allowed the kinetics of their incorporation into chromatin and subsequent modification to be determined.

Newly synthesised and pre-existing histone tetramers (H3, H4), associate with nascent DNA, this is followed over the space of several minutes by the sequestration of both pre-existing and newly synthesised histone dimers (H2A, H2B). Thus, the majority of nucleosomes behind a replication fork are hybrids of both old and new core histones. Finally, a mixture of newly synthesised and pre-existing histone H1 stably associates with the nascent chromatin. The overall process of chromatin maturation as assayed by nuclease sensitivity requires as long as 10–20 minutes in a rapidly proliferating mammalian cell. Assuming a rate of replication fork movement of 0.5–1 kb of DNA per minute, this implies that 25–100 nucleosomes are present on both of the nascent DNA duplexes as 'immature' chromatin during S phase. The initial rapid deposition of old and new histones H3 and H4 on newly synthesised DNA reflects the nuclease-sensitive stage, whereas the subsequent deposition of histone dimers (H2A, H2B) and histone H1 correlates with the appearance of regular nucleosomal arrays and nuclease resistance. The sequential sequestration of histones is clearly once again related to the structure of the nucleosome, since the tetramer (H3, H4), forms the core of the structure, whereas histones H2A and H2B bind at the periphery of the nucleosome, and histone H1 can only associate in its proper place after two turns of DNA are wrapped around the core histones.

Newly synthesised histone H4 is phosphorylated and acetylated in the amino-terminal tail domain. Approximately 30 minutes after deposition during chromatin assembly, the diacetylated H4 is deacetylated to its mature form. If H4 deacetylation is inhibited, chromatin never achieves the nuclease resistance of bulk chromatin, indicative of the formation of stable higher order structures. Histone H1 may be less efficiently incorporated into chromatin containing acetylated H4.

Thus, histone diacetylation is likely to maintain nascent chromatin in a structure that is more accessible to other DNA-binding proteins. In summary, chromatin assembly *in vivo* is coupled to replication, most probably through the activity of specific molecular chaperones such as CAF-1. Nucleosome assembly occurs in stages and involves transient posttranslational modifications of core histones synthesised during *S* phase already shown in Fig. 3.2.

Epigenetic Mechanisms: The Assembly of Active and Repressed Transcriptional States

In vivo experiments using *Saccharomyces* cerevisiae suggest that replication disassembles repressed chromatin states and facilitates the access of trans-acting factors to DNA. Other experiments using yeast suggest that replication has an essential role in facilitating the repression of specific genes. We have discussed how biochemical experiments indicate that replication introduces a dynamic aspect to chromosomal structure, both directing the disassembly of pre-existing structures and facilitating the assembly of nucleosomes. A central issue in gene regulation is how the assembly of nucleoprotein structures following replication can maintain or alter states of potential transcriptional activity.

Repression

Replication and transcription are most clearly seen to be linked in yeast. Components of the yeast origin recognition complex (ORC) regulate both the initiation of replication within the chromosome and the repression of transcription within the same chromosomal domain. The molecular mechanisms responsible for the repression of transcription directed by ORC are unknown. Two possible explanations are: (i) that the ORC compartmentalises adjacent chromatin into a transcriptionally incompetent environment within the nucleus and (ii) that the ORC influences the type of chromatin assembled adjacent to it. The ORC complex may be a greatly streamlined version of the replication factories of larger eukaryotes. These replication factories represent special nuclear compartments at which proteins involved in the replication process are sequestered. It is possible that a gene adjacent to the origin is directed by the ORC to reside in a replication-competent but transcriptionally incompetent environment. Alternatively, if replication itself is essential for transcriptional repression, then the coupling of chromatin assembly to the replication process could contribute to repression. Pre-existing transcriptionally active complexes would be displaced by the replication fork. trans-Acting factors would then have to compete for assembly against the deposition of histones. In vivo and in vitro experiments in Xenopus demonstrate that the coupling of nucleosome assembly to replication can very effectively repress basal transcription. As discussed earlier, the ORC complex provides one biological example of the maintenance of sequence specific or structure-dependent protein-DNA interactions through the replication process.

However, since the ORC also serves to initiate the replication process, maintenance of the ORC may occur under circumstances distinct from the transcription complexes or chromatin structures that are exposed to the fully assembled replication-elongation complex. We have discussed how the histones already on the template during replication are segregated randomly to the daughter DNA duplexes, but within the context of small groups of nucleosomes. This maintenance of histone modification states potentially influences transacting factor access to DNA. Moreover, if proteins that modify the subsequent folding of nucleosomal arrays or that modify histones themselves, for example, by acetylation or deacetylation, are also partitioned in this way, the properties of a chromatin domain might be stably propagated. For example, histone H4 acetylation may interfere with the association of histone H1 with chromatin. Histone H1 is known to repress specific genes in vivo. Other proteins that might recognise properties of the 'old' histones within nascent chromatin include the chromodomain proteins that initiate the formation of heterochromatin. These are also good candidates for propagating pre-existing states of chromatin-mediated transcriptional repression (Fig. 3.4).

Activation

In vitro experiments using cell-free preparations of Xenopus eggs indicate that stable states of gene activity can be propagated in a nuclear environment. How might this occur? The simplest situation leading to continued gene activity would be the case in which a superabundance of transcription factors specific for a given gene was available within the nucleus throughout the cell cycle, including S phase. The factors would always be able to bind to their regulatory elements should they become accessible, recruiting the basal transcriptional machinery to the nascent promoter DNA, and thereby preventing histones or other proteins from binding to the TATA homology. Several features of nascent chromatin facilitate the association of transcription factors. For example, the complex of the 5s rRNA gene with the tetramer (H3, H4), is not repressive to transcription, whereas the complete octamer of core histones (H2A, H2B, H3, H4), is repressive at high densities of octamers bound to DNA. Moreover, acetylation of the core histones facilitates transcription factor access to DNA even when the complete octamer is bound. The histone tetramer (H3, H4), recognises the DNA sequences that position the nucleosome containing the 5s rRNA gene, hence it is probable that the formation of a specific chromatin structure also has a role in allowing transcription factors access to the template. Thus, following replication, it is

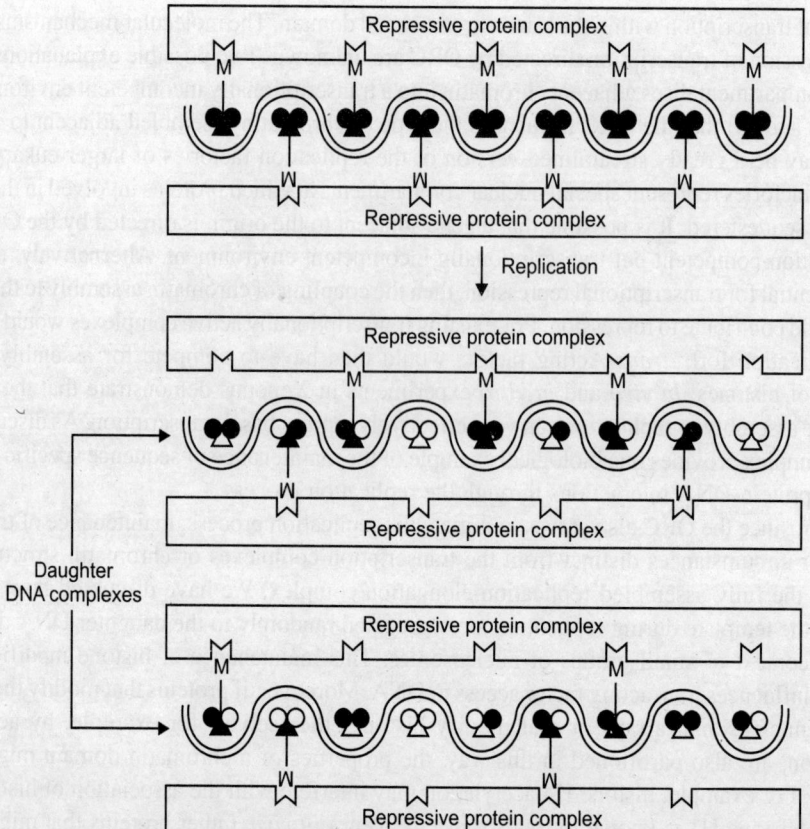

Fig. 3.4: Preexisting histone modifications could provide an epigenetic imprint. A repressive protein complex (e.g. containing chromodomain proteins) recognizes a histone modification (M). Following replication, modified histones are segregated to both daughter DNA duplexes sufficient to sustain interaction with the repressive protein complex.

probable that sequence-specific DNA-binding proteins have an opportunity to reassociate with daughter DNA molecules (Fig. 3.5). Replication might under certain circumstances facilitate gene activation. The regulated activity of a transcription factor, such that it becomes able to bind to DNA or to function during S phase, could lead to transcription activation in a way that is replication-dependent. In a developmental context, this event might be coupled to a particular embryonic cleavage cycle or to a regulated period of cell division. For example, in *Caenorhabditis elegans* and the sea urchin, replication events are correlated with changes in the commitment of cells to a particular developmental fate. Similar changes can occur in differentiated cells that express one set of specialised genes and that can switch to another programme of gene expression only after one or more cell divisions. However, replication events are not necessarily essential for changing gene expression within a particular cell. This is not surprising, since chromatin structure is not completely inert *in vivo*. Histones H2A, H2B, and H1 are known to exchange with a pool of free histones in a cell. Complexes of DNA with only histones H3 and H4 therefore exist for a limited amount of time. However, a comparison of the rate and efficiency of gene activation in the presence or absence of cell proliferation has not yet been made.

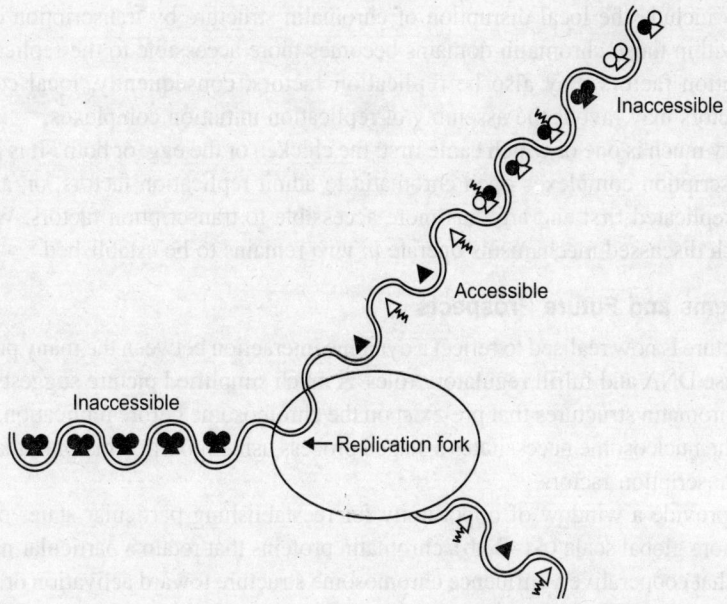

Fig. 3.5: Replicative disruption of preexisting chromatin structures provides a window of opportunity for transcription factors to program genes. The accessibility of nascent, maturing, and mature chromatin to *trans*-acting factors is indicated.

The maintenance of specific transcription factor-DNA interactions through replication, as discussed earlier for the ORC, might be facilitated by considering the promoter, the enhancer, and locus control regions not as separate entities, but as contributory components to a single structure. This could be achieved through protein-protein interactions between the distinct nucleoprotein complexes assembled at each regulatory element. One reason for the separation of these regulatory elements over extensive distances may be that any single structure might be independently disrupted by DNA replication, while the other would remain intact. If protein binding to one sequence element influences the binding of proteins to the other, then the intact nucleoprotein complex might facilitate the re-formation of the disrupted one.

Replication timing

Chromatin organisation outside the ORC may also have significance for the initiation of replication and the timing of this initiation in S phase. If replication disrupts both active and repressed chromatin structures, then the entire nucleus has to be remodelled after each replication event. If there are limiting transcription factors available in a cell, then a gene that is replicated early in S phase has more opportunity for the assembly of an active transcription complex than a gene that replicates late. This is simply because the gene that replicates early is available for transcription factors to bind before all of the early-replicating portion of the genome has sequestered these factors. A late-replicating gene therefore experiences a relative deficiency in factor availability. Conversely, it is also possible that the type of chromatin assembled early in S phase is more accessible to transcription factors than chromatin assembled late in S phase. For example, earlyreplicating chromatin may sequester histones that are more highly acetylated and, consequently, more accessible to the transcription factors that maintain continued transcription activity. Transcriptionally active genes replicate early in S phase. The reason for this early replication is unknown, but possibilities include the local disruption of chromatin structure by transcription complexes, such that the DNA within those chromatin domains becomes more accessible to the replication machinery. Many transcription factors may also be replication factors, consequently, local concentrations of transcription factors may favour the assembly of replication initiation complexes.

The issue very much is one of which came first: the chicken or the egg, or both? It is possible to argue that active transcription complexes open chromatin to admit replication factors, or, alternatively, that these sites are replicated first and are thus more accessible to transcription factors. Whether either or both of the much discussed mechanisms operate *in vivo* remains to be established.

Current Problems and Future Prospects

Chromatin structure is now realised to reflect a dynamic interaction between the many protein complexes that both organise DNA and fulfill regulatory roles. A much simplified picture suggests that replication disrupts local chromatin structures that pre-exist on the chromosome before replication. The subsequent reassembly of the nucleosome necessitates a staged process using modified histones that might be more accessible to transcription factors.

This would provide a window of opportunity for reestablishing particular states of transcriptional activity. On a more global scale (>1–2 kb), chromatin proteins that retain a particular modification (e.g. acetylation) or that cooperatively influence chromosome structure toward activation or repression could provide an imprint on chromatin activity through DNA replication and chromosome duplication. Replication is established as having a major impact on pre-existing nucleoprotein structures and a major role in their reassembly. Although significant attention has been given to the enzymology of the duplication of DNA, relatively little progress has been made concerning the enzymology of chromosomal duplication. The molecular mechanisms of chromatin assembly are not defined in any detail. The definition of molecular chaperones such as CAF-1 is a major advance, however, how CAF-1 functions is unknown. Does CAF-1 have a catalytic or structural role? Does it interact with the elongation complex? What are the special features of the histones that allow CAF-1 to utilise them for nucleosome assembly? On a more mundane level, we do not know the precise sequences or structures of the histone proteins necessary for chromatin assembly. The enzymes that transform nascent chromatin into a mature structure are yet to be defined at the molecular level. How mature chromatin is recognised by other proteins that influence states of gene repression, such as the chromodomain proteins, is unknown.

The impact of DNA replication on gene expression is readily analysed through yeast genetics, however, homologous biochemical systems are currently lacking to test the many hypotheses proposed to explain the phenomena observed. Much progress in the biochemistry of yeast replication can be anticipated. The further reconstruction of determinative events in development will require continued consideration of the fate of regulatory nucleoprotein complexes during replication. This is an important focus for future research. At a biochemical level, *in vitro* systems capable of maintaining states of gene expression through replication offer considerable promise. The future clearly has the exciting prospect of understanding and thus reconstructing chromosomal duplication in all its complexity at a molecular level.

Chapter 4

Discovery of Introns

INTRODUCTION

Spliceosomal introns are one of the eukaryotic defining characters. With the exception of the highly reduced nucleomorph genome of *Hemiselmis andersenii*, introns are found in all fully sequenced eukaryotic genomes, including other nucleo-morphs. Intron density ranges from a handful in the entire genome of some protists, to about eight per gene in human.

The presence of introns in a genome is believed to impose substantial burden on the host. First, unlike self-splicing introns, the excision of spliceosomal introns requires a spliceosome, which is among the largest molecular complexes in the cell, comprising 5 snRNAs and more than 150 proteins. Intron-bearing genomes must, of course, code for all these proteins and snRNAs. Many eukaryotes even harbour a second class of spliceosomal introns, called U12 introns, that are removed by another spliceosome (the minor spliceosome) whose protein content only partially overlaps with that of the major spliceosome. Second, intron transcription is costly in terms of time and energy. The energetic burden is probably tolerable, but an average RNA polymerase II (RNAP II) elongation rate of 60 bases per second means that the transcription of some long introns lasts many hours. Third, recognition of splicing junctions by the spliceosome is directed by a host of *cis* regulatory elements. This makes an organism vulnerable to synonymous (or even non-coding) mutations that otherwise would not have a noticeable effect. Indeed, it is estimated that more than 50% of human genetic disorders are caused by disruption of the normal splicing pattern. Finally, malfunction of any of the snRNAs and proteins that are necessary for proper splicing will have a general detrimental effect on the cell.

The recognition of the potentially hazardous nature of introns had initiated a quest for function that would counter these deleterious effects. This had triggered Walter Gilbert to suggest, shortly after the discovery of the introns, what is now known as the intron-early theory. According to this theory, introns were pivotal in the formation of modern, complex, genes, by allowing for constant shuffling of small, primordial, mini-exons. Hence, introns must have existed in prokaryotes, only to be later eliminated completely from their genomes due to genome streamlining. The accumulation of fully sequenced eukaryotic genomes allowed for high resolution reconstruction of the evolutionary history of introns. Consequently, the intron-early theory gave way to the view that spliceosomal introns first appeared during the early stages of eukaryogenesis, possibly from self-splicing intron forebears, and that their debut was shortly followed by massive invasion into the eukaryotic nuclear genome. It is currently estimated that the last eukaryotic common ancestor was intron-rich, populated with introns whose density was perhaps as high as 50–75% of the intron density in contemporary intron-rich mammals. According to this view, the first introns were, indeed, deleterious elements, and their spreading in eukaryotic genomes was possible due to severe population bottlenecks. At later times, episodes of massive intron gains seem to have been rare, generally limited to lineages that experienced significant evolutionary innovations, such as the emergence of opisthokonts (common ancestor of metazoan and fungi), metazoans, and plants. Many other lineages seem to have gone through phases of massive intron losses, leading to all those present-day intron-poor species.

This evolutionary scenario is compatible with the view that early introns lacked function. However, the mere existence of transcribed gene parts, that are free from selective constraints triggered an increase in genetic diversity that eventually led to the gain of many intron-related functions, up to the point that today they are absolutely essential in intron-rich species, as well as in many intron-poor ones.

One of the best examples to a crucial intronic function in contemporary eukaryotes is the increase in protein abundance of intron-bearing genes. This effect was initially observed in simian vacuolating virus 40 constructs whose protein product was rendered undetachable upon the elimination of their introns. Using similar viral constructs, it was shown that intron removal already affects the mRNA level. In some cases intron-bearing constructs were expressed up to 400 times more than their intron less counterparts. Subsequent works reported the same phenomenon to be associated with numerous other introns in many eukaryotic species, suggesting that this intronic function is wide-ranging. In plants, for example, this intronic effect had been widely described, and was even privileged in getting a unique name – intron-mediated enhancement. In fact, some introns are so efficient in boosting expression levels, that they are regularly included in constructs in order to guarantee high expression. Some introns were even engineered to this purpose. It was shown, for example, that a hybrid intron made of an adenovirus 5′ splice site and an immunoglobulin G 3′ splice site, is boosting the expression level of various genes in transgenic mice up to 300-fold.

Large-scale analyses further corroborated these observations. Intron-bearing genes in yeast were shown to produce more mRNA and more protein than intronless genes. Similarly, intron-bearing genes in mammals were shown to have higher and broader expression than intronless genes. Reconstruction of the intron–exon evolutionary history in 19 eukaryotes revealed that highly expressed genes tend to have higher intron gain rates. As we shall see, there is no single mechanism by which introns enhance expression. In many cases, the mechanism is not yet known, but in those cases in which it had been revealed, introns seem to affect virtually any step of mRNA maturation, including transcription initiation, transcription elongation, transcription termination, polyadenylation, nuclear export, and mRNA stability. We view this functional diversity as a reflection of the fact that introns gained this function on many independent occasions in a rather 'opportunistic' manner. This chapter discusses examples to the great variety of functions carried out by introns. Scientist found it illuminating to divide the life span of an intron to five phases, and to separately refer to the functions that are associated with each phase (Fig. 4.1). The first phase is the genomic intron, which is the DNA sequence of the intron. The second phase is the transcribed intron, which is the phase in which the intron is under active transcription. The third phase is the spliced intron, in which the spliceosome is assembled on the intron and is actively excising it. The fourth phase is the excised intron, which is the intronic RNA sequence released upon the completion of the splicing reaction. The final phase is the exon-junction complex (EJC)-harbouring

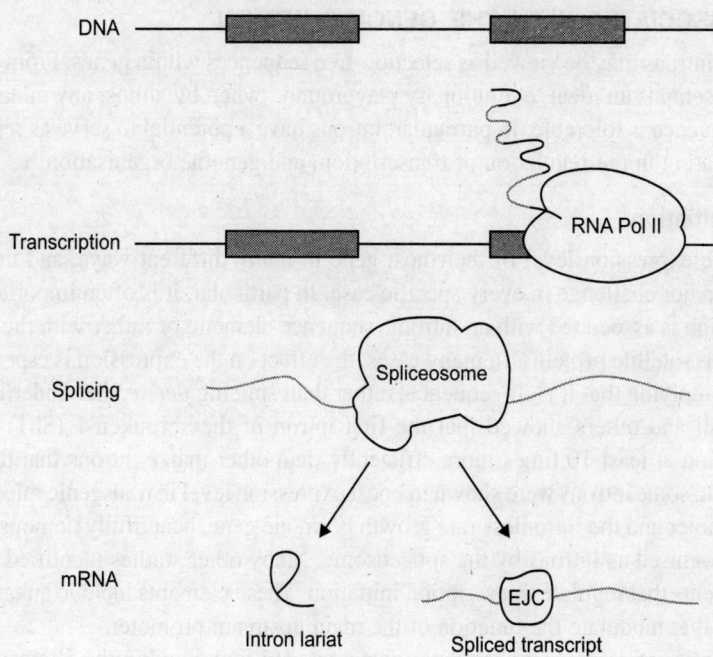

DNA

Transcription

RNA Pol II

Splicing

Spliceosome

mRNA

Intron lariat

EJC

Spliced transcript

Fig. 4.1: Schematic description of the five phases of an intron life span.

transcript, which is the mature mRNA in which the location of the exon–exon junctions is marked by the EJC. Another distinction found useful is between the various intronic properties that mediate the function (Table 4.1). Sequence-dependent functions are mediated by sequence elements within the intron, length-dependent functions are mediated by the length of the intron, regardless of its nucleotide content, position-dependent functions are mediated by the position of the intron with respect to the exons, and splicing-dependent functions are mediated by the mere fact that splicing had occurred during the maturation of the mRNA.

Table 4.1: Summary of the intronic functions covered in this review.

Phase	*Function*	*Intronic property*
Genomic intron	Transcription initiation	Sequence, position
	Transcription termination	Sequence, position
	Genome organisation	Sequence, position, length
Transcribed intron	Time delays	Length
Spliced intron	Transcription regulation	Splicing
	Alternative splicing	Splicing, sequence
Excised intron	Expressing noncoding RNAs	Splicing, sequence
EJC-harboring transcript	Nonsense-mediated decay	Splicing
	Nuclear export	Splicing
	Cytoplasmic localisation	Splicing, sequence
	translation yield	Splicing

Note: The functions are grouped according to the intron life span phase to which they are associated. The intronic properties that enable each function are listed on the rightmost column.

FUNCTIONS ASSOCIATED WITH THE GENOMIC INTRON

At the DNA level introns may be viewed as selection-free sequences within genes. From an evolutionary perspective, such setup is an ideal 'evolutionary playground,' whereby almost any mutational tinkering of the intronic sequence is tolerable. In particular, introns have a potential to serve as repositories of *cis* elements, participating in the regulation of transcription, and genome organisation.

Transcription Initiation

Introns modify the expression level of their host gene in many different ways, and underpinning the mechanism is of major challenge in every specific case. In particular, it is often important to determine whether the function is associated with an intronic sequence element, or rather with the spliceosome or any of its numerous satellite proteins. In many cases, the effect on the expression is especially strong for a specific intron, implying that it is its sequence, rather than splicing *per se*, that underlies the function. For example, Vasil and others showed that the first intron of the shrunken-1 (Sh1) locus in maize increased expression at least 10 times more efficiently than other maize introns that they checked. In another experiment, some introns were shown to boost expression level in transgenic mice, when inserted in between a promoter and the intronless rate growth hormone gene, beautifully demonstrating function without being recognised as introns by the spliceosome. Many other studies identified specific intron-hosted DNA elements that regulate transcription initiation. These elements include enhancers, silencers, or other elements that modulate the function of the main upstream promoter.

In the vast majority of cases, these regulatory elements are found within the 5'-most introns. Large-scale studies provide further credence to the special regulatory role of first introns, showing that 5'-proximal introns, and especially those in the 5' UTR, are significantly longer than more distal introns. The accepted interpretation of this finding is that these introns are longer because they harbour more *cis* regulatory sequences, likely related to transcription initiation. This is not the only case that multitude of regulatory elements is suggested as an explanation to long introns. Another example discuss later on, when similar arguments were recruited to explain why alternative exons tend to be flanked by long introns. And yet, the validity of this surmise is questionable. For example, contrary to the expectations, a clear association between intron length and expression breadth in human was not found.

Genome-wide analysis in *A. thaliana* found that promoter-proximal introns that cause expression enhancement are characterised by unique sequence profile, enriched with certain motifs. Later, such motifs were claimed to have been identified in other plant species, although a comprehensive survey in rice could not find a correlation between the presence of these motifs and expression boost.

Some introns do not harbour elements that modify the efficiency of the main promoter, but rather host an alternative promoter that gives rise, when activated, to an isoform with a different transcription start site. For example, Scohy and others found an alternative promoter within the first intron of the α-fetoprotein (AFT) gene, bringing about an isoform whose transcription start site is 295 bases downstream of the original transcription start site, and is expressed in the yolk sac and fetal liver. Similarly, Petit and others found an SRF-dependent alternative promoter in the second intron of the lipoma preferred partner (LPP) gene, yielding an isoform specific to certain tissues.

Transcription Termination

As will be shown later, splicing is strongly coupled with 3'-end formation. But intronic sequence elements that regulate 3'-end processing in a splicing-independent manner also exist. A well-known example is the second intron of the human β-globin gene. A removal of this intron or its replacement by other introns substantially reduces the efficiency of the 3′-end formation. More-over, mutants that have defective splicing do have intact 3′-end formation, indicating that there is no coupling between 3′-end processing and the splicing itself. Further experiments with hybrid introns showed that it is a 60-bp-long segment toward the 3′-end of the second intron that enhances the 3′-end processing.

Genome Organisation

In an attempt to explain the negative correlation between intron length and expression breadth in multicellular eukaryotes, Vinogradov suggested the 'genomic design' hypothesis, stating that introns are longer in tissue-specific genes because they host regulatory elements, and, importantly, because they serve as scaffold elements to assure correct assembly of nucleosomes. Recently, when genome-wide mapping of nucleosome positions became available, several large-scale studies have found that nucleosomes preferentially occupy exons, and are depleted in introns. This preferential nucleosome coverage of exons was shown to be independent of whether the exon is constitutive or alternative, of its expression level, and of its GC content. It is currently unknown what drives this nucleosome marking of exons, but it had been suggested that sequence elements near the intron ends function as nucleosome disfavouring elements, pushing the nucleosomes away toward the exons.

This exon marking by nucleosomes seems to be interconnected to their marking by specific histone modifications, like H3K36me3, but the full extent of the association between gene architecture, chromatin structure, nucleosome positioning, and histone modifications still has to be clarified. These conclusions from large-scale analyses are supported by a few experiments showing that the ability of nucleosomes to form in some genes is severely perturbed when their introns are deleted.

Nested Genes

Some genes, called nested genes, appear within introns of other genes. The number of nested genes ranges from 158 in human to almost 800 in *Drosophila*. However, in the vast majority of cases nested genes have their own promoters, and their pattern of expression is different from that of their host. Therefore, the presence of nested genes within introns seems a result of stochastic process, only weakly related to the fact that they reside within introns.

FUNCTIONS ASSOCIATED WITH TRANSCRIBED INTRONS

Introns go through transcription just like exons, to form the pre-mRNA. Large-scale transcription studies found that sense transcription is typically accompanied by substantial antisense transcription. Many seemingly functional anti-sense elements come from intronic regions, and may therefore be regarded as intron-hosted RNA genes that are activated during transcription rather than following intron excision. This section focuses on a different, very unique function of introns, associated only with the fact that they are transcribed, regardless of their sequence content, or their position, or of the fact that they are later excised from the pre-mRNA. RNA polymerase II elongation rate had been estimated using various techniques. Recent measurement on different regions of nine long human genes found a rather homogeneous rate of 3.8 kb min^{-1}, although rates higher than 50 kb min^{-1} had also been reported. Many introns, therefore, require minutes, hours, and even days to transcribe. This raises the intriguing possibility that introns may serve as tools to orchestrate time delays between activation of a gene, and the appearance of its protein product. Indeed, such a role was nicely demonstrated in the E74 gene that switches on at the beginning of the metamorphosis of *Drosophila melanogaster* (Fig. 4.2). This complex gene consists of three transcripts, of which the primary one is the 60-kb long E74A gene that matures, after splicing,

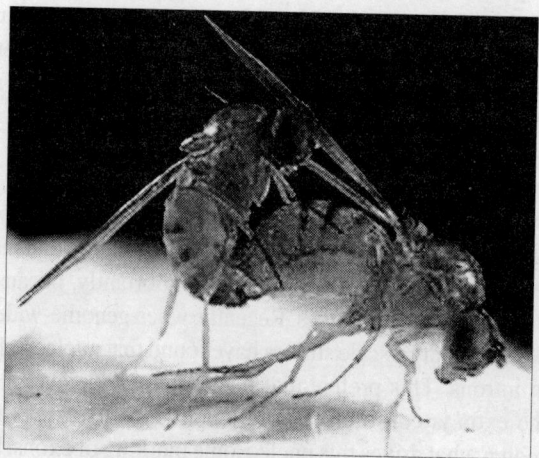

Fig. 4.2: *Drosophila melanogaster.*

to a 6-kb mRNA. The gene is induced by the steroid hormone Ecdysone, and appears in the cytoplasm after about an hour from the time of induction. Thummel and others measured an elongation rate of RNAP II along this gene of about 1.1 kb min^{-1}, suggesting that it is the introns transcription time alone that underlies this delay.

It is a known theoretical result that negative feedback loops with a time delay may end up in oscillatory behaviour. This was demonstrated in an artificial setup by engineering gene networks with time delays, and obtaining expression pulses whose cycle depended on the intron length. But it was also shown in physiological transcripts. The gene Hes7 is cyclically expressed in the presomitic mesoderm and regulates the somite segmentation. It had been recently shown that introns within the mouse Hes7 cause a 19-min delay in transcription, and that without this delay (i.e. if the introns are removed) the oscillations disappear and Hes7 is expressed steadily, leading to severe segmentation defects. As expected from a length-dependent intronic function, the total length of all introns in Hes7 was found to be highly conserved across the eukaryotic domain. Large-scale analysis of additional 1875 genes identified at least 10 more genes whose total intron length is conserved much more than expected, suggesting a similar role in time delays. Interestingly, many of these genes are related to developmental processes, in which negative feedback time delay loops are expected to play an important role.

FUNCTIONS ASSOCIATED WITH SPLICED INTRONS

Pre-mRNA splicing is carried out by the spliceosome, that is built from five core snRNAs (U1, U2, U4, U5, and U6), many core proteins, and numerous other satellite proteins. The spliceosome is increasingly recognised as a huge cellular machine that carries with it proteins that participate in a host of RNA maturation processes, other than splicing. Here, we will discussed the functions that come about by the fact that the spliceosome was recruited to the pre-mRNA.

Transcription Regulation

Many studies show that splicing of most of the introns occurs concomitantly with transcription, and that these two cellular processes are strongly coupled, mainly through the carboxyl-terminal domain (CTD) of RNAP II. In general, RNAP II was shown to be preferentially associated with all of the U1 snRNP core proteins, as well as with some SR-proteins splicing factors. The original interpretation of this finding was that RNAP II brings along factors that facilitate fast spliceosome assembly on the nascent pre-mRNA. Now-a-days, however, despite some works that suggest otherwise, this coupling is generally believed to be bidirectional, in the sense that transcription modulates splicing (see next section), and splicing modulates transcription. It is this latter effect of splicing on transcription that would be the focus of this section. We will show how splicing modulates all phases of transcription, including initiation, elongation, and termination.

Transcription initiation, or re-initiation, is thought to be affected by U1 snRNA. U1 snRNA was shown to associate with TFIIH, a general transcription initiation factor, and to stimulate the rate of formation of the first phosphodiester bond by RNAP II. Further research showed that besides TFIIH, two other transcription initiation factors, TFIID and TFIIB, are preferentially associated with donor splice junctions, leading to the hypothesis that 5′-most introns stimulate transcription initiation at the upstream promoter through U1 snRNA-mediated pre-initiation complex assembly at the donor splice site. However, it is not known whether this role of U1 snRNA is related to the role it plays at the spliceosome, or is it a splicing-independent function of U1 snRNA.

Splicing was also found to directly promote transcription elongation, through interactions between splicing factors or spliceo-somal components and transcription elongation factors. Some experiments suggest that U2 snRNP, apart from its role in the spliceosome, also promotes transcription elongation by interacting with the transcription elongation factors TAT-SF1 and P-TEFb. The generality of this mechanism is questionable, though, as it could not be reproduced in yeast. The splicing factor SC35 was also shown to enhance RNAP II elongation of some mammalian genes via interaction with P-TEFb. Actually, it had been shown that SC35 depletion attenuates transcription, and that this defective phenotype can be rescued by adding recombinant SC35. The splicing-associated c-Ski-interacting protein (SKIP) was similarly shown to promote RNAP II elongation by associating, yet again, with P-TEFb. In this case, however, SKIP seems to have a function that is independent of its role in splicing.

At the final stage of transcription, mRNAs undergo 3′-end processing, involving endonucleolytic cleavage and the addition of a poly(A) tail. Splicing was found to modify the efficiency of this mRNA processing stage as well. In general, functional coupling between splicing, and in particular of the 3′-most intron, and 3′-end formation had been demonstrated. In search for mechanism, at least two snRNPs (U1 and U2) were found to modulate 3′-end processing, in addition to several splicing factors. U2 snRNP was shown to physically interact with the cleavage/polyadenylation specificity factor (CPSF), and that its presence is required for efficient cleavage. In fact, mutations to the U2 snRNP binding site of the pre-mRNA resulted not only in aberrant splicing, but also in reduced cleavage efficiency. However, it is unknown whether this role of U2 snRNP is linked to its splicing role, because it was later shown that U2 snRNP contributes to 3′-end formation of the intronless non-polyadenylated histone genes.

While U2 snRNP seems to enhance 3′-end processing, it was found that binding of U1 snRNA upstream of a polyadenylation signal represses 3′-end formation. For example, bovine papillo-mavirus type 1 genes are expressed only in late stages of the infection. In early stages, expression is repressed by 3′-end formation inhibition caused by U1 snRNA-bound 5′ splice site-like elements upstream of the polyadenylation signal. It was shown that bases at the 5′-end of the U1 snRNA are critical for this inhibition, and that mutations in this part of the U1 snRNA repress expression of many endogenous mammalian genes by binding to their terminal exon. Recently, using morpholinos to knockdown U1 snRNA in human HeLa cells, it was demonstrated that except for the expected accumulation of unspliced pre-mRNA, premature cleavage, and polyadenylation was observed in numerous pre-mRNAs at cryptic polyadenylation sites, mostly within introns. Interestingly, knockdown of U2 snRNA did not show this effect, suggesting that it may be a splicing-independent function of U1 snRNA, which explains the overabundance of U1 snRNA with respect to the other snRNAs. The role of U1 snRNA in repressing 3'-end processing is probably because it brings with it the U1 snRNP proteins that actually mediate the suppression. For example, the inhibition of the 3'-end formation in the bovine papillomavirus type 1 mentioned above was found to be caused by a direct interaction between the U1 snRNP protein U1 70K and the poly(A) polymerase. The U1 snRNP protein U1A was also found to have similar inhibitory roles by interacting with PAP, although, interestingly, it was also suggested to have stimulating effect on 3'-end processing via interaction with the 160-kDa subunit of CPSF.

Further splicing factors have been shown to have an impact on the cleavage/polyadenylation process, such as hnRNP F and SRP75 that have inhibitory roles, Srm160 with a stimulating role, and U2AF65 that probably has a stimulating effect, although it had also been claimed to have an inhibitory role.

Alternative Splicing

Some splice sites are recognised as such by the spliceosome in every tissue, time, and condition. Other splice sites have, at least in certain tissues, times, or conditions, some probability to be missed by the spliceosome, giving rise to alternative splicing. Alternative splicing allows for proteome diversity that much exceeds the number of genes in the genome. One remarkable example is the Dscam gene of *D. melanogaster*, which potentially generates more than 38,000 isoforms. This means that Dscam's protein repertoire is larger than the number of genes in the fruit fly! Recent genome-wide analyses based on RNA-seq data found that in human, nearly 95% of the multiexon genes undergo alternative splicing, mostly in a very tissue-specific way. While alternative splicing is probably widespread in human and in many other eukaryotes, it is still undetermined what fraction of it is functional, and what fraction is simply splicing noise.

Proving function of alternative splicing at the systems level is challenging, but specific examples are accumulating. Here, we shall mention just a few. The fibronectin (FN) gene in human is an extracellular matrix protein. It has several different isoforms, some of which have different patterns of localisation and slightly different functions in human cells, The Slo avian gene coding for a K+ channel protein has 576 possible isoforms, of which several are expressed in a specific gradient along the sensory receptor cells of the inner ear, contributing to the highly accurate perception of different sound frequencies in birds, A beautiful autoregulation based on alternative splicing is demonstrated by the ADAR2 gene, which is a key factor in A-to-I RNA editing. Strikingly, one of the acceptor splice sites in this gene, which has the typical AG dinucleotide at the end of the intron, is preceded by an AA dinucleotide 47 bases upstream. Normally, AA is not recognised as an acceptor splice site, but high levels of ADAR2 edit it to AI, which is recognised as AG, and thus as an acceptor splice site, by the spliceosome. Preference of this new splice site over the original one leads to the production of non-active isoforms of ADAR2, following a decrease in its levels.

Conserved alternative exons are orthologous exons that are alternative in several organisms. Likewise, conserved constitutive exons are orthologous exons that are constitutive in several organisms. Human–mouse comparative study showed that 77% of the introns flanking conserved alternative exons are made of long conserved sequences, while the same held for only 17% of the introns flanking conserved constitutive exons. This observation puts forward the notion that introns host *cis* regulatory elements that facilitate alternative splicing. Indeed, introns not only passively allow for alternative splicing because of their mere existence, but also actively regulate splicing by hosting splicing regulatory elements.

These are short *cis* motifs that generally bind to splicing factors that enhance or repress the spliceosome assembly on a nearby potential splice site. Some SREs are found within exons, and some are harboured within introns and are divided into intronic splicing silencers (ISSs) and intronic splicing enhancers. For example, Nova-1isa neuron-specific RNA binding protein that functions mainly in the brain, and regulates alternative splicing by binding to intronic motifs – such asYCAY – and enhancing splicing of the downstream splice site. Fox-1 is another splicing factor that induces exon skipping in heart and skeletal muscles by binding to the intronic motif GCAUG. In general, ISSs and ISEs are short, degenerate, and of variable distance for the splice site, and are therefore hard to detect and identify, and many putative elements await experimental validation.

FUNCTIONS ASSOCIATED WITH EXCISED INTRONS

Once an intron had been excised, it typically becomes part of post-splicing complexes that lead to efficient debranching and degradation. But when an RNA gene is embedded within the intron, it is expressed upon intron removal, and outlives its intronic host. Many families of non-coding RNAs (ncRNAs) have been characterised, such as microRNAs (miRNAs), small nucleolar RNAs (snoRNAs), piwi-interacting RNAs (piR-NAs), small-interfering RNAs (siRNAs), and various long non-coding RNAs (lncRNAs). Except for piRNAs, Rearick and others found that members of these families are preferentially associated with introns in human, leading to the hypothesis that genes may autoregulate their expression by hosting relevant ncRNAs within their introns.

MicroRNA are small ncRNAs of about 22–23 nucleotides that bind to target sites along mRNAs, usually within their 3' UTRs, and direct them for degradation or translation repression. It is thought that – at least in vertebrates – miRNAs affect thousands of genes, and that in general they form an important layer of regulation. Roughly half of the human miRNAs lie in intergenic regions and are associated with their own transcriptional promoter. The other half reside within introns, usually lack independent promoter, and are co-expressed with their host gene, potentially regulating its expression by feedback loops. It is generally believed that miRNAs are processed from the excised intron, although some evidence points to the possibility that they are processed already on the pre-mRNA. Usually, miRNAs lie within a long transcriptional unit, called pri-miRNA, that is cleaved by *Drosha* to a shorter hairpin structure known as pre-miRNA. The pre-miRNA is then exported to the cytoplasm, where it is cleaved again, this time by Dicer, to form a double-stranded RNA. One of the strands is then associated with the RISC complex to form functional miRNA. Ruby and others reported an alternative miRNA biogenesis pathway. They found that certain debranched introns have the structural features of pre-miRNAs, and that they are generated following splicing without the need to cleave a precursor transcriptional unit by *Drosha*. These miR-NAs that require splicing but not *Drosha* for their maturation are termed mirtrons. They were first identified in *D. melanogaster* and *C. elegans*, but later discovered in mammals, birds, and even plants.

Small nucleolar RNAs comprise a rather large family of small RNAs, mainly known for their role in post-transcriptional methylation and pseudouridylation of various RNA genes like rRNAs, tRNAs, and snRNAs. Similarly to miRNAs, members of this family can reside in intergenic regions and have their own transcriptional promoter, or dwell in introns and rely on splicing for their maturation. In fact, snoRNAs are rather abundant in introns of both vertebrates and insects, where they are processed by the exonucleolytic digestion of debranched introns after their excision from the pre-mRNA. The introns of some ribosome-associated genes were found to host snoRNAs that guide rRNA modifications, but it is generally not the rule that snoRNAs are related to the regulation of their host genes. Strikingly, the sole function of some genes seems to be harbouring snoRNAs in their introns, and their mRNA does not look as if it has a protein-coding potential. Endogenous siRNAs form yet another family of small RNAs that is involved in the RNA interference pathway and in many other cellular processes such as post-transcriptional gene silencing. These are double stranded, 20–25 nucleotides long RNA molecules, whose identification is hindered by the abundance of hairpin structures in eukaryotic genomes. The number of verified intronic siR-NAs is small, but recent large-scale studies found a large number of potential hairpin endogenous siRNAs within introns in human and rice. Introns were also found to host lncRNAs. These are RNA genes longer than 200 bases, that have diverse regulatory functions, presumably affecting the expression of protein-coding genes in *cis* or in *trans*.

FUNCTIONS ASSOCIATED WITH EJC-HARBOURING TRANSCRIPTS

In metazoans, the splicing reaction leaves traces in the form of a protein complex deposited 20–24 nucleotides upstream of the exon–exon junction, known as the EJC. It contains four core proteins, MAGO, Y14, eIF4AIII, and MLN51, and many others that are transiently associated with it. Subject to changes in its composition, the EJC survives from the splicing in the nucleus to the pioneer round of translation in the cytoplasm. During all this time, it serves as a memory device, marking the position of excised introns. It had been gradually appreciated that by interacting with many other factors, EJC participates in a range of mRNA-related cellular processes (Fig. 4.3).

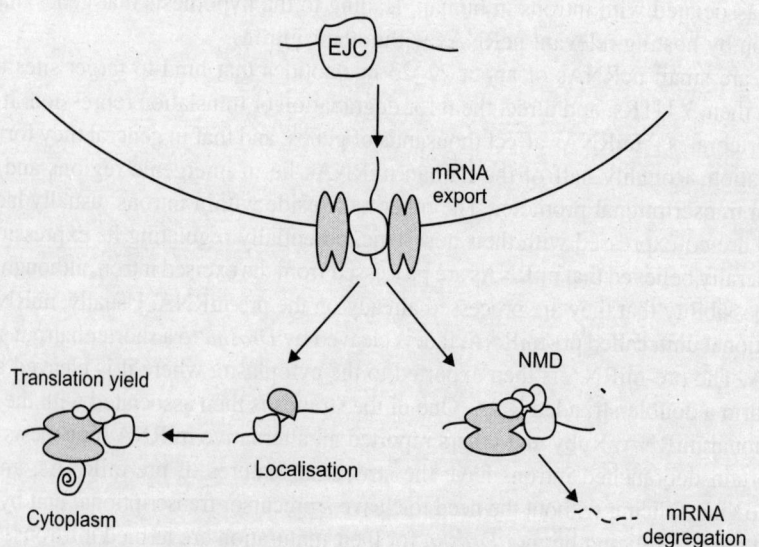

Fig. 4.3: Schematic description of the different roles played by the exon-junction complex (EJC).

Nonsense-Mediated Decay

Nonsense-mediated decay (NMD) is a eukaryotic surveillance mechanism that selectively degrades mRNAs harbouring premature termination codons (PTCs). PTCs arise frequently, mostly as a result of mutations in the DNA level, alternative splicing in the RNA level, and errors in transcription. NMD prevents such transcripts from being translated, as otherwise they can give rise to truncated proteins with dominant-negative or deleterious gain-of-function activities. A major puzzle in the field is what makes a termination codon recognised as premature by NMD. Several properties of the 3′ UTR had been suggested as possible NMD triggers, including sequence motifs, protein context, and the 3′ UTR length.

In mammals, and possibly in other vertebrates as well, the dominant form of NMD is splicing-dependent, in which EJCs that are more than 50–55 nucleotides downstream of a termination codon mark it as premature. Mechanistically, it is believed that NMD is triggered by a phosphorylation–unphosphorylation cycle of the UPF1 protein. The UPF3 protein (which has two par-alogs in vertebrates and one copy in invertebrates) is associated with the EJC, to which it recruits the UPF2 protein. Upon transcription termination, the ribosome deposits a complex named SURF on the mRNA, containing the release factors eRF1 and eRF3. These factors recruit unphosphorylated UPF1. In the presence of nearby EJC, and in particular of UPF2 and UPF3, the UPF1 is phosphorylated by SMG-1.

Interestingly, NMD may sometimes be linked to alternative splicing. A nice demonstration of such coupling is the autoregulation of the PTB protein. This protein has many functions related to mRNA processing, and is also an hnRNP splicing repressor. It was found that is has two isoforms – one is functional and contains all the exons, and the other lacks exon 11 and as a result has a PTC and is degraded by NMD. Wollerton and others found that PTB promotes exon 11 skipping, thereby controlling its own expression level in a negative feedback loop. A few other similar examples have been described, in particular in genes that are regulators of alternative splicing. In a more general context, however, the extent to which the coupling between NMD and alternative splicing is widespread is debated. In an attempt to explain the high percentage of human alternative transcripts that are NMD targets, Hillman and others carefully analysed existing data of mRNA and protein expression in human, and concluded that NMD participates in the regulation of many genes. Using a splicing-sensitive custom microarray Hansen and others identified at least 45 genes in *Drosophila* with an isoform that is NMD-sensitive, leading an NMD-dependent regulation of their expression level. On the other hand, Pan and others used both mouse and human exon arrays to show that PTC-containing iso-forms are expressed at low levels, and thus have no measurable effect on the total abundance of the gene. They supported this finding by knocking down Upf1 in human, and showing that only a minority (6%) of the genes is affected, and that 80% of the PTC-generating alternative splicing events (one third of all alternative splicing events) result in transcripts with low abundance, independent of whether NMD is active or not.

Nuclear Export

In eukaryotes, mature mRNAs must be exported from the nucleus to the cytoplasm before they can start being translated. Mature nuclear mRNAs bind to mRNA-specific transport factors, and are shuttled through pores in the nucleus membrane, formed by the nuclear pore complexes. A link between splicing and export was sought by comparing export rates of spliced transcripts to that of their unspliced counterparts. The first studies pointed at significantly more efficient export of spliced mRNA in mammals and amphibians, but this was called into question by subsequent works. Recently, however, Valencia and others introduced intron-bearing and the corresponding intronless constructs into human and mouse cell nuclei, and then used FISH to study the distribution of transcripts across the nuclear and cytoplasmic compartments. They found that spliced transcripts were mostly cytoplasmic, whereas unspliced transcripts were mostly nuclear. Overall, they reported that the kinetics and efficiency of mRNA export of mammalian cells were enhanced 6- to 10-fold by splicing. The link between splicing and export is presumably caused by the fact that the spliceosome assembly on the pre-mRNA facilitates the recruitment of export factors. This can be done directly by the spliceosome, or by the EJC that is deposited near the exon–exon junction. For example, it was found that the ALY/REF export factor binds mRNAs that have gone through splicing, but is absent from identical mRNAs that were generated from intronless pre-mRNAs. In fact, the EJC seems to provide strong binding sites for this export factor. Further work revealed that

ALY/REF binds to intronless transcripts too, via a different, splicing-independent, mechanism. Other examples include the export-associated THO complex which associates with spliced mRNAs but not with unspliced ones, and the UAP56 splicing factor which also has a key role in export.

Cytoplasmic Localisation

Some eukaryotic cellular processes require certain mRNAs to be translated only within a demarcated region of the cell. mRNA localisation is achieved with the help of a diverse family of shuttling proteins. Some bind the mRNA cotranscriptionally in the nucleus, while others are recruited in the cytoplasm, right after the nuclear export. It is believed that the EJC plays an important role in recruiting shuttle proteins to the mRNA. One well-known example is the localisation of the oskar mRNA in the cytoplasm of *D. melanogasters* oocytes, which affects germline and abdomen development. Although it has not yet been formally proven that splicing deposits EJCs on *Drosophila* mRNAs, fly homologs of the EJC proteins Y14 and MAGO were found to be essential for proper localisation of oskar during oogenesis. Moreover, Hachet and Ephrussi demonstrated that this localisation depends on the splicing of the 5′-most intron. They generated constructs of oskar with all possible combinations of its introns, and showed that transcripts that included the first intron were correctly localised, whereas it was not the case in other versions of the gene. It is worth noting that the intron removal did not affect export, as the same amounts of mRNA were obtained as in the wild type. Interestingly, using intronless constructs in eggs led to over two thirds of the embryos to fail to hatch. As expected from an EJC-dependent function, substituting the third intron in place of the first one did not disrupt the proper localisation. Although not an EJC-dependent function, we shall mention here that splicing can affect mRNA localisation by inclusion/exclusion of sequence localisation signals via alternative splicing and/or alternative polyadenylation. Such sequence signals are thought to drive localisation by serving as targets for shuttle proteins. Such sequence elements appear everywhere, but they are particularly abundant within 3′ UTRs. For example, Horne-Badovinac and Bilder have shown in *Drosophila*, that the mRNA of the Stardust protein (sdt), which forms a vital complex for epithelial polarity, is apically localised in the membrane. This localisation is a result of an inclusion of the alternative third exon that contains a localisation motif. In the absence of this exon, sdt mRNA is uniformly distributed. Regulation of this exon inclusion and exclusion generates a switch, producing the Stardust complex when it is needed during the early stages of epithelial development. Another illuminating example was found in the mouse's brain. Brain cells generate two isoforms of the brain-derived neurotrophic factor (BDNF), one with short 3′ UTR and another with long 3′ UTR. Smith and others compared BDNF mRNA quantities in different brain regions and found great differences in the relative abundance of the long and the short versions. The long isoform was found to be mainly positioned in the dendrites, while the short isoform was shown to be in the soma. More generally, alternative polyadenylation is considered as an important regulator of mRNA localisation.

Translation Yield

Greater amounts of protein are produced per molecule of spliced mRNA than from otherwise identical mRNA molecules not produced by splicing. In some cases, it was possible to show that this is due to direct effect of splicing on the translation yield. For example, having an EJC appears to promote mRNA polysome association, which can also be obtained by tethering the EJC proteins Y14, MAGO, and RNPS1 on intronless transcripts. The mechanism by which EJC promotes translational yield is still unclear. It had been suggested that the EJC proteins Y14 and MAGO, when associated with the cytoplasmic transcript, bind to the PYM protein, which, in turn, binds to the ribosome and therefore serves as a bridge between the EJC and the translation mechanism. Indeed, it had been shown that PYM knockdown reduces translation efficiency of intron-bearing transcripts, but does not affect intronless transcripts. Another work showed that the EJC recruits the SKAR protein, which, in turn, recruits S6K1 and that together, SKAR and S6K1 increase the translational efficiency of spliced mRNA. Greater protein levels can also be a result of splicing conferring enhanced stability to the protein product, or to its mRNA forebear. For example, the Dihydrofolate reductase protein expressed from stably transfected minigenes was found to have a 2.7-fold longer half-life when expressed from an intron-containing construct than from an identical cDNA construct. Another example is the mouse's chemokine gene CXCL1. It has been demonstrated that mRNA derived from a transcript that contains introns is significantly more stable than that derived from an intron-free transcript. Only a single intron is required to produce this effect, and the intron position and sequence do not appear to be important. Although the presence of at least one intron modulates the rate of mRNA decay, it does not modulate the nuclear/cytoplasmic distribution, the rate of translation, or the ability of extracellular stimulus to stabilise the mRNA.

INTRON POSITIONAL CONSERVATION

A fundamental supposition in comparative genomics is that evolutionary conservation is indicative of biological function. This makes the identification of highly conserved genomic regions a chief strategy in looking for function. Evolutionary conservation is mainly identified with sequence conservation, but also with conservation of secondary and tertiary structure of DNA, RNA, and proteins, and with conservation of genome-wide organisation. The success of this strategy notwithstanding, it is increasingly recognised that many functional elements – mostly non-coding – still evade detection. Thus, this section has developed the idea that introns invaded in great numbers to early eukaryotic genomes as slightly deleterious selfish elements, but later gained many functions up to the point that today higher eukaryotes cannot survive without them. This fact implies that the level of conservation of intron position may be correlated with the functional importance of this intron.

Analysing the intron–exon structure – the gene architecture – of orthologous genes makes the comparison of their respective intron positions straightforward (Fig. 4.4). Using such alignments of orthologous genes, it had been noticed that intron positions are sometimes conserved throughout long evolutionary times, in a frequency that is significantly above random expectation. Current intron populations are regarded as a result of intron gain and loss processes. If an intron becomes associated with a function, of whatever type, its chances to be lost will decrease. Therefore, conservation of intron position should be indicative of function of any type, even if the function is not directly related to the intron position.

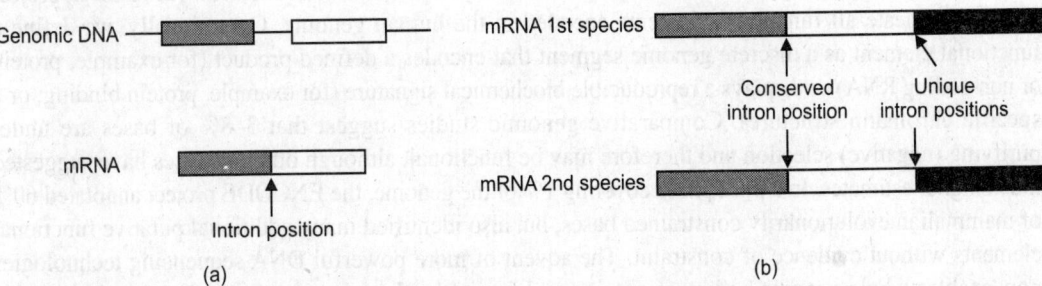

Fig. 4.4: (a) Intron position is defined as the point of intron insertion along the mRNA, and (b) comparison of intron positions between orthologous genes.

Chapter 5

ENCODE Project

INTRODUCTION

The human genome encodes the blueprint of life, but the function of the vast majority of its nearly three billion bases is unknown. The Encyclopedia of DNA Elements (ENCODE) project has systematically mapped regions of transcription, transcription factor association, chromatin structure and histone modification. These data enabled us to assign biochemical functions for 80% of the genome, in particular outside of the well-studied protein-coding regions. Many discovered candidate regulatory elements are physically associated with one another and with expressed genes, providing new insights into the mechanisms of gene regulation. The newly identified elements also show a statistical correspondence to sequence variants linked to human disease, and can thereby guide interpretation of this variation. Overall, the project provides new insights into the organisation and regulation of our genes and genome, and is an expansive resource of functional annotations for biomedical research. The human genome sequence provides the underlying code for human biology. Despite intensive study, especially in identifying protein-coding genes, our understanding of the genome is far from complete, particularly with regard to non-coding RNAs, alternatively spliced transcripts and regulatory sequences. Systematic analyses of transcripts and regulatory information are essential for the identification of genes and regulatory regions, and are an important resource for the study of human biology and disease. Such analyses can also provide comprehensive views of the organisation and variability of genes and regulatory information across cellular contexts, species and individuals. The Encyclopedia of DNA Elements (ENCODE) project aims to delineate all functional elements encoded in the human genome. Operationally, we define a functional element as a discrete genome segment that encodes a defined product (for example, protein or non-coding RNA) or displays a reproducible biochemical signature (for example, protein binding, or a specific chromatin structure). Comparative genomic studies suggest that 3–8% of bases are under purifying (negative) selection and therefore may be functional, although other analyses have suggested much higher estimates. In a pilot phase covering 1% of the genome, the ENCODE project annotated 60% of mammalian evolutionarily constrained bases, but also identified many additional putative functional elements without evidence of constraint. The advent of more powerful DNA sequencing technologies now enables whole-genome and more precise analyses with a broad repertoire of functional assays.

The major goal of ENCODE is to provide the scientific community with high-quality, comprehensive annotations of candidate functional elements in the human genome. For the purposes of this chapter, the term 'functional element' is used to denote a discrete region of the genome that encodes a defined product (e.g. protein) or a reproducible biochemical signature, such as transcription or a specific chromatin structure. It is now widely appreciated that such signatures, either alone or in combinations, mark genomic sequences with important functions, including exons, sites of RNA processing, and transcriptional regulatory elements such as promoters, enhancers, silencers, and insulators. However, it is also important to recognise that while certain biochemical signatures may be associated with specific functions, our present state of knowledge may not yet permit definitive declaration of the ultimate biological role(s), function(s), or mechanism(s) of action of any given genomic element. At present, the proportion of the human genome that encodes functional elements is unknown. Estimates based on comparative genomic analyses suggest that 3%–8% of the base pairs in the human genome are under purifying (or negative) selection. However, this likely underestimates the prevalence of functional features, as current comparative methods may not account for lineage-specific evolutionary innovations, functional elements that are very small or fragmented, elements that are rapidly evolving or subject to nearly neutral evolutionary processes, or elements that lie in repetitive regions of the genome.

The current phase of the ENCODE Project has focused on completing two major classes of annotations: genes (both protein-coding and non-coding) and their RNA transcripts, and transcriptional regulatory regions. To accomplish these goals, seven ENCODE Data Production Centers encompassing 27 institutions have been organised to focus on generating multiple complementary types of genome-wide data. These data include identification and quantification of RNA species in whole cells and in sub-cellular compartments, mapping of protein-coding regions, delineation of chromatin and DNA accessibility and structure with nucleases and chemical probes, mapping of histone modifications and transcription factor (TF) binding sites by chromatin immuno precipitation (ChIP), and measurement of DNA methylation. In parallel with the major production efforts, several smaller-scale efforts are examining long-range chromatin interactions, localising binding proteins on RNA, identifying transcriptional silencer elements, and understanding detailed promoter sequence architecture in a subset of the genome.

HISTORY OF ENCODE

Encode was launched by the US National Human Genome Research Institute (NHGRI) in September 2003. Intended as a follow-up to the Human Genome Project, the ENCODE project aims to identify all functional elements in the human genome. The project involves a worldwide consortium of research groups, and data generated from this project can be accessed through public databases. The project began its fourth phase as of February 2017.

Motivation and Significance

Humans are estimated to have approximately 20,000 protein-coding genes, which account for about 1.5% of DNA in the human genome. The primary goal of the ENCODE project is to determine the role of the remaining component of the genome, much of which was traditionally regarded as 'junk.' The activity and expression of protein-coding genes can be modulated by the regulome - a variety of DNA elements, such as the promoter, transcriptional regulatory sequences, and regions of chromatin structure and histone modification. It is thought that changes in the regulation of gene activity can disrupt protein production and cell processes and result in disease. Determining the location of these regulatory elements and how they influence gene transcription could reveal links between variations in the expression of certain genes and the development of disease. ENCODE is also intended as a comprehensive resource to allow the scientific community to better understand how the genome can affect human health, and to 'stimulate the development of new therapies to prevent and treat these diseases'.

ENCODE Consortium

The ENCODE Consortium is composed primarily of scientists who were funded by US National Human Genome Research Institute (NHGRI). Other participants contributing to the project are brought up into the Consortium or Analysis Working Group. The pilot phase consisted of eight research groups and twelve groups participating in the ENCODE Technology Development Phase. After 2007, the number of participants grew up to 440 scientists from 32 laboratories worldwide as the pilot phase was officially over. At the moment the consortium consists of different centers which perform different tasks. ENCODE is a member of the International Human Epigenome Consortium (IHEC).

ENCODE PROJECT

ENCODE is currently implemented in four phases: the pilot phase and the technology development phase, which were initiated simultaneously, and the production phase. The fourth phase is a continuation of the third, and includes functional characterisation and further integrative analysis for the encyclopedia.

The goal of the pilot phase was to identify a set of procedures that, in combination, could be applied cost-effectively and at high-throughput to accurately and comprehensively characterise large regions of the human genome. The pilot phase had to reveal gaps in the current set of tools for detecting functional sequences, and was also thought to reveal whether some methods used by that time were inefficient or unsuitable for large-scale utilisation.

Some of these problems had to be addressed in the ENCODE technology development phase, which aimed to devise new laboratory and computational methods that would improve our ability to identify known functional sequences or to discover new functional genomic elements. The results of the first two phases determined the best path forward for analysing the remaining 99% of the human genome in a cost-effective and comprehensive production phase.

ENCODE Phase I Project: The Pilot Project

The pilot phase tested and compared existing methods to rigorously analyse a defined portion of the human genome sequence. It was organised as an open consortium and brought together investigators with diverse backgrounds and expertise to evaluate the relative merits of each of a diverse set of techniques, technologies and strategies. The concurrent technology development phase of the project aimed to develop new high throughput methods to identify functional elements. The goal of these efforts was to identify a suite of approaches that would allow the comprehensive identification of all the functional elements in the human genome.

Through the ENCODE pilot project, National Human Genome Research Institute (NHGRI) assessed the abilities of different approaches to be scaled up for an effort to analyse the entire human genome and to find gaps in the ability to identify functional elements in genomic sequence. The ENCODE pilot project process involved close interactions between computational and experimental scientists to evaluate a number of methods for annotating the human genome. A set of regions representing approximately 1% (30 Mb) of the human genome was selected as the target for the pilot project and was analysed by all ENCODE pilot project investigators. All data generated by ENCODE participants on these regions was rapidly released into public databases.

Target selection

For use in the ENCODE pilot project, defined regions of the human genome - corresponding to 30Mb, roughly 1% of the total human genome - were selected. These regions served as the foundation on which to test and evaluate the effectiveness and efficiency of a diverse set of methods and technologies for finding various functional elements in human DNA.

Prior to embarking upon the target selection, it was decided that 50% of the 30Mb of sequence would be selected manually while the remaining sequence would be selected randomly. The two main criteria for manually selected regions were: (i) the presence of well-studied genes or other known sequence elements, and (ii) the existence of a substantial amount of comparative sequence data. A total of 14.82Mb of sequence was manually selected using this approach, consisting of 14 targets that range in size from 500kb to 2Mb. The remaining 50% of the 30Mb of sequence were composed of thirty, 500kb regions selected according to a stratified random-sampling strategy based on gene density and level of non-exonic conservation. The decision to use these particular criteria was made in order to ensure a good sampling of genomic regions varying widely in their content of genes and other functional elements.

The human genome was divided into three parts - top 20%, middle 30%, and bottom 50% - along each of two axes: (i) gene density and (ii) level of non-exonic conservation with respect to the orthologous mouse genomic sequence, for a total of nine strata. From each stratum, three random regions were chosen for the pilot project. For those strata under represented by the manual picks, a fourth region was chosen, resulting in a total of 30 regions. For all strata, a 'backup' region was designated for use in the event of unforeseen technical problems. In greater detail, the stratification criteria were as follows:

- Gene density: The gene density score of a region was the percentage of bases covered either by genes in the Ensembl database, or by human mRNA best BLAT (BLAST-like alignment tool) alignments in the UCSC Genome Browser database.
- Non-exonic conservation: The region was divided into non-overlapping subwindows of 125 bases. Subwindows that showed less than 75% base alignment with mouse sequence were discarded. For the remaining subwindows, the percentage with at least 80% base identity to mouse, and which did not correspond to Ensembl genes, GenBank mRNA BLASTZ alignments, Fgenesh++ gene predictions, TwinScan gene predictions, spliced EST alignments, or repeated sequences (DNA), was used as the non-exonic conservation score.

The above scores were computed within non-overlapping 500 kb windows of finished sequence across the genome, and used to assign each window to a stratum.

Pilot phase results

The pilot phase was successfully finished and the results were published in June 2007 in Nature and in a special issue of Genome Research, the results published in the first paper mentioned advanced the collective knowledge about human genome function in several major areas, included in the following highlights:

- The human genome is pervasively transcribed, such that the majority of its bases are associated with at least one primary transcript and many transcripts link distal regions to established protein-coding *loci*.
- Many novel non-protein-coding transcripts have been identified, with many of these overlapping protein-coding loci and others located in regions of the genome previously thought to be transcriptionally silent.

- Regulatory sequences that surround transcription start sites are symmetrically distributed, with no bias towards upstream regions.
- Numerous previously unrecognised transcription start sites have been identified, many of which show chromatin structure and sequence-specific protein-binding properties similar to well-understood promoters.
- Chromatin accessibility and histone modification patterns are highly predictive of both the presence and activity of transcription start sites.
- Distal DNaseI hypersensitive sites have characteristic histone modification patterns that reliably distinguish them from promoters, some of these distal sites show marks consistent with insulator function.
- DNA replication timing is correlated with chromatin structure.
- A total of 5% of the bases in the genome can be confidently identified as being under evolutionary constraint in mammals, for approximately 60% of these constrained bases, there is evidence of function on the basis of the results of the experimental assays performed to date.
- Although there is general overlap between genomic regions identified as functional by experimental assays and those under evolutionary constraint, not all bases within these experimentally defined regions show evidence of constraint.
- Different functional elements vary greatly in their sequence variability across the human population and in their likelihood of residing within a structurally variable region of the genome.
- Surprisingly, many functional elements are seemingly unconstrained across mammalian evolution. This suggests the possibility of a large pool of neutral elements that are biochemically active but provide no specific benefit to the organism. This pool may serve as a 'warehouse' for natural selection, potentially acting as the source of lineage-specific elements and functionally conserved but non-orthologous elements between species.

ENCODE phase II project: The production phase project

In September 2007, National Human Genome Research Institute (NHGRI) began funding the production phase of the ENCODE project. In this phase, the goal was to analyse the entire genome and to conduct 'additional pilot-scale studies'. As in the pilot project, the production effort is organised as an open consortium. In October 2007, NHGRI awarded grants totalling more than $80 million over four years. The production phase also includes a Data Coordination Center, a Data Analysis Center, and a Technology Development Effort. At that time the project evolved into a truly global enterprise, involving 440 scientists from 32 laboratories worldwide. Once the pilot phase was completed, the project 'scaled up' in 2007, profiting immensely from new-generation sequencing machines. And the data was, indeed, big, researchers generated around 15 terabytes of raw data. By 2010, over 1,000 genome-wide data sets had been produced by the ENCODE project. Taken together, these data sets show which regions are transcribed into RNA, which regions are likely to control the genes that are used in a particular type of cell, and which regions are associated with a wide variety of proteins. The primary assays used in ENCODE are ChIP-seq, DNase I Hypersensitivity, RNA-seq, and assays of DNA methylation.

Production phase results

In September 2012, the project released a much more extensive set of results, in 30 papers published simultaneously in several journals, including six in Nature, six in Genome Biology and a special issue with 18 publications of Genome Research. The authors described the production and the initial analysis of 1,640 data sets designed to annotate functional elements in the entire human genome, integrating results from diverse experiments within cell types, related experiments involving 147 different cell types, and all ENCODE data with other resources, such as candidate regions from genome-wide association studies (GWAS) and evolutionary constrained regions. Together, these efforts revealed important features about the organisation and function of the human genome, which were summarised in an overview paper as follows:

1. The vast majority (80.4%) of the human genome participates in at least one biochemical RNA and/or chromatin associated event in at least one cell type. Much of the genome lies close to a regulatory event: 95% of the genome lies within 8kb of a DNA-protein interaction (as assayed by bound ChIP-seq motifs or DNaseI footprints), and 99% is within 1.7kb of at least one of the biochemical events measured by ENCODE.

2. Primate-specific elements as well as elements without detectable mammalian constraint show, in aggregate, evidence of negative selection, thus some of them are expected to be functional.

3. Classifying the genome into seven chromatin states suggests an initial set of 399,124 regions with enhancer-like features and 70,292 regions with promoters-like features, as well hundreds of thousands of quiescent regions. High-resolution analyses further subdivide the genome into thousands of narrow states with distinct functional properties.

4. It is possible to quantitatively correlate RNA sequence production and processing with both chromatin marks and transcription factor (TF) binding at promoters, indicating that promoter functionality can explain the majority of RNA expression variation.

5. Many non-coding variants in individual genome sequences lie in ENCODE- annotated functional regions, this number is at least as large as those that lie in protein coding genes.

6. SNPs associated with disease by GWAS are enriched within non-coding functional elements, with a majority residing in or near ENCODE-defined regions that are outside of protein coding genes. In many cases, the disease phenotypes can be associated with a specific cell type or TF.

The most striking finding was that the fraction of human DNA that is biologically active is considerably higher than even the most optimistic previous estimates. In an overview paper, the ENCODE Consortium reported that its members were able to assign biochemical functions to over 80% of the genome. Much of this was found to be involved in controlling the expression levels of coding DNA, which makes up less than 1% of the genome.

The most important new elements of the 'encyclopedia' include:

- A comprehensive map of DNase 1 hypersensitive sites, which are markers for regulatory DNA that is typically located adjacent to genes and allows chemical factors to influence their expression. The map identified nearly 3 million sites of this type, including nearly all that were previously known and many that are novel.

- A lexicon of short DNA sequences that form recognition motifs for DNA-binding proteins. Approximately 8.4 million such sequences were found, comprising a fraction of the total DNA roughly twice the size of the exome. Thousands of transcription promoters were found to make use of a single stereotyped 50-base-pair footprint.

- A preliminary sketch of the architecture of the network of human transcription factors, that is, factors that bind to DNA in order to promote or inhibit the expression of genes. The network was found to be quite complex, with factors that operate at different levels as well as numerous feedback loops of various types.

- A measurement of the fraction of the human genome that is capable of being transcribed into RNA. This fraction was estimated to add up to more than 75% of the total DNA, a much higher value than previous estimates. The project also began to characterise the types of RNA transcripts that are generated at various locations.

Data management and analysis

Capturing, storing, integrating, and displaying the diverse data generated is challenging. The ENCODE Data Coordination Center (DCC) organises and displays the data generated by the labs in the consortium, and ensures that the data meets specific quality standards when it is released to the public. Before a lab submits any data, the DCC and the lab draft a data agreement that defines the experimental parameters and associated metadata. The DCC validates incoming data to ensure consistency with the agreement. It also ensures that all data is annotated using appropriate Ontologies. It then loads the data onto a test server for preliminary inspection, and coordinates with the labs to organise the data into a consistent set of tracks. When the tracks are ready, the DCC Quality Assurance team performs a series of integrity checks, verifies that the data is presented in a manner consistent with other browser data, and perhaps most importantly, verifies that the metadata and accompanying descriptive text are presented in a way that is useful to our users. The data is released on the public UCSC Genome Browser website only after all of these checks have been satisfied. In parallel, data is analysed by the ENCODE Data Analysis Center, a consortium of analysis teams from the various production labs plus other researchers. These teams develop standardised protocols to analyse data from novel assays, determine best practices, and produce a consistent set of analytic methods such as standardised peak callers and signal generation from alignment pile-ups. The National Human Genome Research Institute (NHGRI) has identified ENCODE as a 'community resource project'. This important concept was defined at an international meeting held in Ft. Lauderdale in January 2003 as a research project specifically devised and implemented to create a set of data, reagents, or other material whose primary utility will be as a resource for the broad scientific community. Accordingly, the ENCODE data release policy stipulates that data, once verified, will be deposited into public databases and made available for all to use without restriction.

Other Projects

With the continuation of the third phase, the ENCODE Consortium has become involved with additional projects whose goals run parallel to the ENCODE project. Some of these projects were part of the second phase of ENCODE.

modENCODE project

The MODel organism ENCyclopedia Of DNA Elements (modENCODE) project is a continuation of the original ENCODE project targeting the identification of functional elements in selected model organism genomes, specifically *Drosophila melanogaster* and *Caenorhabditis elegans*. The extension to model organisms permits biological validation of the computational and experimental findings of the ENCODE project, something that is difficult or impossible to do in humans. Funding for the modENCODE project was announced by the National Institutes of Health (NIH) in 2007 and included several different research institutions in the US. The project completed its work in 2012.

In late 2010, the modENCODE consortium unveiled its first set of results with publications on annotation and integrative analysis of the worm and fly genomes in Science. Data from these publications is available from the modENCODE web site.

modENCODE was run as a Research Network and the consortium was formed by 11 primary projects, divided between worm and fly. The projects spanned the following:

- Gene structure.
- mRNA and ncRNA expression profiling.
- Transcription factor binding sites.
- Histone modifications and replacement.
- Chromatin structure.
- DNA replication initiation and timing.
- Copy number variation.

modERN

modERN, short for the model organism encyclopedia of regulatory networks, branched from the modENCODE project. The project has merged the *C. elegans* and *Drosophila* groups and focuses on the identification of additional transcription factor binding sites of the respective organisms. The project began at the same time as Phase III of ENCODE, and plans to end in 2017. To date, the project has released 198 experiments, with around 500 other experiments submitted and currently being processed by the DCC.

Genomics of gene regulation

In early 2015, the NIH launched the Genomics of Gene Regulation (GGR) programme. The goal of the programme, which will last for three years, is to study gene networks and pathways in different systems of the body, with the hopes to further understand the mechanisms controlling gene expressions. Although the ENCODE project is separate from GGR, the ENCODE DCC has been hosting GGR data in the ENCODE portal.

Roadmap

In 2008, NIH began the Roadmap Epigenomics Mapping Consortium, whose goal was to produce 'a public resource of human epigenomic data to catalyse basic biology and disease-oriented research'. On February 2015, the consortium released an article titled 'Integrative analysis of 111 reference human epigenomes' that fulfilled the consortium's goal.

The consortium integrated information and annotated regulatory elements across 127 reference epigenomes, 16 of which were part of the ENCODE project. Data for the Roadmap project can either be found in the Roadmap portal or ENCODE portal.

fruitENCODE project

The fruitENCODE: An encyclopedia of DNA elements for fruit ripening is a plant ENCODE project that aims to generate DNA methylation, histone modifications, DHS, gene expression, transcription factor binding datasets for all fleshy fruit species at different developmental stages. Prerelease data can be found in the fruitENCODE portal.

Criticism of the Project

Although the consortium claims they are far from finished with the ENCODE project, many reactions to the published papers and the news coverage that accompanied the release were favourable. The Nature editors and ENCODE authors 'collaborated over many months to make the biggest splash possible and capture the attention of not only the research community but also of the public at large'. The ENCODE project's claim that 80% of the human genome has biochemical function was rapidly picked up by the popular press who described the results of the project as leading to the death of junk DNA.

However the conclusion that most of the genome is 'functional' has been criticised on the grounds that ENCODE project used a liberal definition of 'functional', namely anything that is transcribed must be functional. This conclusion was arrived at despite the widely accepted view, based on genomic conservation estimates from comparative genomics, that many DNA elements such as pseudogenes that are transcribed are nevertheless non-functional. Furthermore, the ENCODE project has emphasised sensitivity over specificity leading possibly to the detection of many false positives. Somewhat arbitrary choice of cell lines and transcription factors as well as lack of appropriate control experiments were additional major criticisms of ENCODE as random DNA mimics ENCODE-like 'functional' behaviour.

In response to some of the criticisms, other scientists argued that the wide spread transcription and splicing that is observed in the human genome directly by biochemical testing is a more accurate indicator of genetic function than genomic conservation estimates because conservation estimates are all relative and difficult to align due to incredible variations in genome sizes of even closely related species, it is partially tautological, and these estimates are not based on direct testing for functionality on the genome. Conservation estimates may be used to provide clues to identify possible functional elements in the genome, but it does not limit or cap the total amount of functional elements that could possibly exist in the genome.

Furthermore, much of the genome that is being disputed by critics seems to be involved in epigenetic regulation such as gene expression and appears to be necessary for the development of complex organisms. The ENCODE results were not necessarily unexpected since increases in attributions of functionality were foreshadowed by previous decades of research. Additionally, others have noted that the ENCODE project from the very beginning had a scope that was based on seeking biomedically relevant functional elements in the genome not evolutionary functional elements, which are not necessarily the same thing since evolutionary selection is neither sufficient nor necessary to establish a function. It is a very useful proxy to relevant functions, but an imperfect one and not the only one.

In response to the complaints about the definition of the word 'function' some have noted that ENCODE did define what it meant and since the scope of ENCODE was seeking biomedically relevant functional elements in the genome, then the conclusion of the project should be interpreted 'as saying that 80 % of the genome is engaging in relevant biochemical activities that are very likely to have causal roles in phenomena deemed relevant to biomedical research.' The issue of function is more about definitional differences than about the strength of the project, which was in providing data for further research on biochemical activity of non-protein coding parts of DNA. Though definitions are important and science is bounded by the limits of language, it seems that ENCODE has been well received for its purpose since there are now more research papers using ENCODE data than there are papers arguing over the definition of function, as of March 2013. Ewan Birney, one of the ENCODE researchers, commented that 'function' was used pragmatically to mean 'specific biochemical activity' which included different classes of assays: RNA, 'broad' histone modifications, 'narrow' histone modifications, DNaseI hypersensitive sites, Transcription Factor ChIP-seq peaks, DNaseI Footprints, Transcription Factor bound motifs, and Exons.

In 2014, ENCODE researchers noted that in the literature, functional parts of the genome have been identified differently in previous studies depending on the approaches used. There have been three general approaches used to identify functional parts of the human genome: genetic approaches (which rely on changes in phenotype), evolutionary approaches (which rely on conservation) and biochemical approaches (which rely on biochemical testing and was used by ENCODE). All three have limitations: genetic approaches may miss functional elements that do not manifest physically on the organism, evolutionary approaches have difficulties using accurate multispecies sequence alignments since genomes of even closely related species vary considerably, and with biochemical approaches, though having high reproducibility, the biochemical signatures do not always automatically signify a function. They concluded that in contrast to evolutionary and genetic evidence, biochemical data offer clues about both the molecular function served by underlying DNA elements and the cell types in which they act and ultimately all three approaches can be used in a complementary way to identify regions that may be functional in human biology and disease. Furthermore, they noted that the biochemical maps provided by ENCODE were the most valuable things from the project since they provide a starting point for testing how these signatures relate to molecular, cellular, and organismal function.

The project has also been criticised for its high cost (~$400 million in total) and favouring big science which takes money away from highly productive investigator-initiated research. The pilot ENCODE project cost an estimated $55 million, the scale-up was about $130 million and the US National Human Genome Research Institute NHGRI could award up to $123 million for the next phase. Some researchers argue that a solid return on that investment has yet to be seen. There have been attempts to scour the literature for the papers in which ENCODE plays a significant part and since 2012 there have been 300 papers, 110 of which come from labs without ENCODE funding. An additional problem is that ENCODE is not a unique name dedicated to the ENCODE project exclusively, so the word 'encode' comes up in many genetics and genomics literature. Another major critique is that the results do not justify the amount of time spent on the project and that the project itself is essentially unfinishable. Although often compared to Human Genome Project (HGP) and even termed as the HGP next step, the HGP had a clear endpoint which ENCODE currently lacks. The authors seem to sympathise with the scientific concerns and at the same time try to justify their efforts by giving interviews and explaining ENCODE details not just to the scientific public, but also to mass media. They also claim that it took more than half a century from the realisation that DNA is the hereditary material of life to the human genome sequence, so that their plan for the next century would be to really understand the sequence itself.

ENCODE Data Integration with known Genomic Features

Promoter-anchored integration

Many of the ENCODE assays directly or indirectly provide information about the action of promoters. Focusing on the TSSs of protein coding transcripts, we investigated the relationships between different ENCODE assays, in particular testing the hypothesis that RNA expression (output) can be effectively predicted from patterns of Consistent with previous reports, we observe two relatively distinct types of promoter: (i) broad, mainly (C1G)-rich, TATA-less promoters, and (ii) narrow, TATA-box-containing promoters. These promoters have distinct patterns of histone modifications, and transcription-factor-binding sites are selectively enriched in each class. Predictive models have been develop to explore the interaction between histone modifications and measures of transcription at promoters, distinguishing between modifications known to be added as a consequence of transcription. In analyses, the best models had two components: an initial classification component (on/off) and a second quantitative model component. The models showed that activating acetylation marks are roughly as informative as activating methylation marks.

Limitations of ENCODE Annotations

All ENCODE datasets to date are from populations of cells. Therefore, the resulting data integrate over the entire cell population, which may be physiologically and genetically inhomogeneous. Thus, the source cell cultures in the ENCODE experiments are not typically synchronised with respect to the cell cycle and, as with all such samples, local micro-environments in culture may also vary, leading to physiological differences in cell state within each culture. In addition, one Tier 1 cell line (K562) and two Tier 2 cell lines (HepG2 and HeLa) are known to have abnormal genomes and karyotypes, with genome instability. Finally, some future Tier 3 tissue samples or primary cultures may be inherently heterogeneous in cell type composition. Averaging over heterogeneity in physiology and/or genotype produces an amalgamation of the contributing patterns of gene expression, factor occupancy, and chromatin status that must be considered when using the data. Future improvements in genome-wide methodology that allow the use of much smaller amounts of primary samples, or follow-up experiments in single cells when possible, may allow us to overcome many of these caveats.

The use of DNA sequencing to annotate functional genomic features is constrained by the ability to place short sequence reads accurately within the human genome sequence. Most ENCODE data types currently represented in the UCSC browser use only those sequence reads that map uniquely to the genome. Thus, centromeric and telomeric segments (collectively ,15% of the genome and enriched in recent transposon insertions and segmental duplications) as well as sequences not present in the current genome sequence build are not subject to reliable annotation by our current techniques. However, such information can be gleaned through mining of the publicly available raw sequence read datasets generated by ENCODE.

It is useful to recognise that the confidence with which different classes of ENCODE elements can be related to a candidate function varies. For example, ENCODE can identify with high confidence new internal exons of protein-coding genes, based on RNA-seq data for long polyA+ RNA. Other features, such as candidate promoters, can be identified with less, yet still good, confidence by combining data from RNA-seq, CAGE-tags, and RNA polymerase 2 (RNA Pol2) and TAF1 occupancy. Still other ENCODE biochemical signatures come with much lower confidence about function, such as a candidate transcriptional enhancer supported by ChIP-seq evidence for binding of a single transcription factor.

Identification of genomic regions enriched by ENCODE biochemical assays relies on the application of statistical analyses and the selection of threshold significance levels, which may vary between the algorithms used for particular data types. Accordingly, discrete annotations, such as TF occupancy or DNaseI hypersensitive sites, should be considered in the context of reported p values, q values, or false discovery rates, which are conservative in many cases. For data types that lack focal enrichment, such as certain histone modifications and many RNA Pol2-bound regions, broad segments of significant enrichment have been delineated that encompass considerable quantitative variation in the signal strength along the genome.

Future Plans and Challenges

Data production plans

The challenge of achieving complete coverage of all functional elements in the human genome is substantial. The adult human body contains several hundred distinct cell types, each of which expresses a unique subset of the ~1,500 TFs encoded in the human genome. Furthermore, the brain alone contains thousands of types of neurons that are likely to express not only different sets of TFs but also a larger variety of non-coding RNAs. In addition, each cell type may exhibit a diverse array of responses to exogenous stimuli such as environmental conditions or chemical agents. Broad areas of fundamental chromosome function, such as meiosis and recombination, remain unexplored. Furthermore, ENCODE has focused chiefly on definitive cells and cell lines, by passing the substantial complexity of development and differentiation. A truly comprehensive atlas of human functional elements is not practical with current technologies, motivating our focus on performing the available assays in a range of cell types that will provide substantial near-term utility. ENCODE is currently developing a strategy for addressing this cellular space in a timely manner that maximises the value to the scientific community. Feedback from the user community will be a critical component of this process.

Integrating ENCODE with other projects and the scientific community

To understand better and functionally annotate the human genome, ENCODE is making efforts to analyse and integrate data within the project and with other large-scale projects. These efforts include (i) defining promoter and enhancer regions by combining transcript mapping and biochemical marks, (ii) delineating distinct classes of regions within the genomic landscape by their specific combinations of biochemical and functional characteristics, and (iii) defining transcription factor co-associations and regulatory networks. These efforts aim to extend our understanding of the functions of the different biochemical elements in gene regulation and gene expression.

One of the major motivations for the ENCODE Project has been to aid in the interpretation of human genome variation that is associated with disease or quantitative phenotypes. The Consortium is therefore working to combine ENCODE data with those from other large-scale studies, including the 1,000 Genomes Project, to study, for example, how SNPs and structural variation may affect transcript, regulatory, and DNA methylation data. We foresee a time in the near future when the biochemical features defined by ENCODE are routinely combined with GWAS and other sequence variation–driven studies of human phenotypes. Analogously, the systematic profiling of epigenomic features across *ex vivo* tissues and stem cells currently being undertaken by the NIH Roadmap Epigenomics programme will provide synergistic data and the opportunity to observe the state and behaviour of ENCODE-identified elements in human tissues representing healthy and disease states.

These are but a few of many applications of the ENCODE data. Investigators focused on one or a few genes should find many new insights within the ENCODE data. Indeed, these investigators are in the best position to infer potential functions and mechanisms from the ENCODE data—ones that will also lead to testable hypotheses. Thus, we expect that the work of many investigators will be enhanced by these data and that their results will in turn inform the development of the project going forward. Finally, we also expect that comprehensive paradigms for gene regulation will begin to emerge from our work and similar work from many laboratories. Deciphering the 'regulatory code' within the genome and its associated epigenetic signals is a grand and complex challenge. The data contributed by ENCODE in conjunction with complementary efforts will be foundational to this effort, but equally important will be novel methods for genome-wide analysis, model building, and hypothesis testing. We therefore expect the ENCODE Project to be a major contributor not only of data but also novel technologies for deciphering the human genome and those of other organisms.

To sum up, the project yielded invaluable information on the human transcriptional regulatory network with systematic analyses of transcription factors, chromatin structure and regulatory modifications. All these findings shine new light on our concept of the gene. This impressive undertaking brings new understanding to the functional aspects of the genome and can probably be considered the most significant genomic discovery step since the sequencing of the whole human genome in 2000. The ENCODE project assigned biochemical function to about 80% of the genome, and in particular to elements outside of the well-studied protein-coding regions. The mapping provides new insights into gene organisation and most of all, mechanisms of regulation. A central goal in biology - understanding the enormous diversity of gene expression in different cell types under various physiological conditions - can be considered partly achieved. It would be a shame that the phenomenal effort that brought forth ENCODE might be misused to attempt to breach the foundations of forensic DNA typing. ENCODE's value is in laying a foundation of the intricate functionality of the human genome that someday may help improve the human condition. Certainly, claims of privacy violations via human identification by STR typing are unfounded and criticizing this powerful forensic tool, based on ENCODE data, does not improve the human condition.

Some of the newly identified elements correspond to sequence variants linked to human disease, and can therefore guide interpretation of these variations. Genome-wide association studies have previously identified many noncoding variants associated with common diseases and traits. Such variants systematically perturb transcription, alter chromatin states, and form regulatory networks. ENCODE's results point to the involvement of regulatory DNA variation in common human disease and provide pathogenic insights into diverse disorders. The publication of such a detailed analysis of the functionalities of the human genome has understandably generated much enthusiasm among scientists and general public alike. Confirmation that a far larger chunk of our genome is biologically active than previously thought has been an exciting discovery and researchers hope the findings will lead to a deeper understanding of numerous diseases. It is however important to remember, and for the scientific community to clearly acknowledge, that despite these fantastic results it may be many years before patients see any benefits from the project. Better understanding of the functional complexity of the human genome will undeniably lead to improved control of disease and to better treatments, but the road to clinical implications and applications is still long and difficult.

SECTION II

Replication, Maintenance, and Rearrangements of Genomic DNA

Chapter 6

DNA Replication

INTRODUCTION

DNA replication is the biological process of producing two identical replicas of DNA from one original DNA molecule. DNA replication occurs in all living organisms acting as the basis for biological inheritance. The cell possesses the distinctive property of division, which makes replication of DNA essential. Before a cell divides, its DNA is replicated (duplicated.) Because the two strands of a DNA molecule have complementary base pairs, the nucleotide sequence of each strand automatically supplies the information needed to produce its partner. If the two strands of a DNA molecule are separated, each can be used as a pattern or template to produce a complementary strand. Each template and its new complement together then form a new DNA double helix, identical to the original. Before replication can occur, the length of the DNA double helix about to be copied must be unwound. In addition, the two strands must be separated, much like the two sides of a zipper, by breaking the weak hydrogen bonds that link the paired bases. Once the DNA strands have been unwound, they must be held apart to expose the bases so that new nucleotide partners can hydrogen-bond to them.

COMMON STEPS IN DNA REPLICATION

In the most fundamental sense, the general mechanism of DNA replication was first suggested by Watson and Crick as an immediate and obvious consequence of the complementarity of the two strands of the DNA structure. Thus, all replication processes simply involve the melting apart of the two strands followed by the polymerisation of each complementary strand on the resulting single-stranded templates. However, when one looks a bit closer at the details of the process of genome duplication, one finds that cells, plasmids, and viruses have evolved a bewildering variety of particular solutions to the problem. In many cases, the level of complexity of the enzymatic machinery for DNA replication is considerably greater than might have been expected, given that the information required to generate two daughter genomes is encoded in the structure of the parental genome in such a simple way. Such complexity presumably evolved to increase the efficiency and fidelity of DNA replication and to ensure that the duplication of the genome is coordinated with other events in the life of a cell. Below we attempt to distill the observed complexity down to the few basic processes that are common to most DNA replication pathways.

Initial Opening of the Duplex at Origins of Replication

DNA replication usually begins at one or more specific sites within the genome, referred to as origins of DNA replication. The first essential event in the initiation of DNA synthesis is the local opening of the duplex to provide access to the template strands. Origins of replication serve to increase the efficiency of initiation of DNA replication by providing loci for the assembly of multiprotein complexes that mediate DNA synthesis. If the individual components required for DNA synthesis were capable of interacting with random sites along the DNA, a sufficient local concentration of all of the essential factors might be achieved infrequently. Thus, the required components are usually brought together in one place by specific protein-DNA and protein-protein interactions. Origins of replication also provide specific points for the control of cellular DNA replication, ensuring that replication occurs at the right point in the cell cycle and that each segment of DNA is replicated precisely once. The initial opening of the DNA duplex at origins is generally mediated by specific initiator proteins and can be facilitated by certain structural features of the DNA [e.g. negative supercoiling, easily unwound sequences) and by certain accessory proteins e.g. singlestranded DNA binding proteins (SSBs)].

Duplex Unwinding at Replication Forks

The initial opening of the duplex allows the establishment of a replication fork(s). The essence of this process is the loading of a DNA helicase on one or both of the exposed single strands. DNA helicases are enzymes that utilise the energy of ATP hydrolysis to translocate unidirectionally along a DNA strand, melting the duplex. At some origins, helicases are loaded onto both DNA strands, resulting in the establishment of two active replication forks (bidirectional DNA replication). In other cases, only a single fork is established (unidirectional DNA replication). An important characteristic of a given helicase activity is its polarity of translocation. Some helicases track along in the 3′ to 5′ direction of the so called 'leading strand' template of the replication fork, and others move in the 5′ to 3′ direction of the 'lagging strand' template.

Priming of DNA Synthesis

In most DNA replication systems, the process of starting new DNA chains is distinct from the process of elongating established chains. Thus, all of the known DNA polymerases are incapable of starting chains *de novo* and require a primer to begin DNA synthesis. In eukaryotic cells, DNA synthesis is generally primed by short RNA chains. The separation of initiation from elongation and the use of RNA, rather than DNA, to initiate DNA synthesis are probably consequences of the requirement for extremely high fidelity in DNA replication. One major mechanism for achieving high fidelity involves proofreading the products of a given polymerisation step before proceeding to the next polymerisation step. A proofreading exonuclease built into most DNA polymerases recognises and efficiently excises mismatched nucleotides at the primer terminus. It is likely that this type of proofreading mechanism would be rather inefficient in detecting errors at or near the beginning of a new DNA chain. This problem is apparently solved by 'marking' sites of initiation with a chemically distinct RNA chain. The replication machinery can later remove the RNA and fill the resulting gap by extension of an upstream DNA chain by DNA polymerase with proofreading function. This is a relatively costly solution, but one that maintains the accuracy of the genome. Although both nuclear and mitochondrial DNA replication make use of RNA priming, the enzymatic mechanism of primer synthesis is different in the two cases. The synthesis of RNA primers for nuclear DNA synthesis is accomplished by a primase enzyme that is a component of DNA polymerase-α (pol-α:primase). This primase appears to be the only enzyme that is capable of priming chromosomal DNA synthesis in eukaryotes and is distinct from the RNA polymerases involved in the transcription of nuclear genes. A few eukaryotic viruses, such as SV40, utilise the cellular priming apparatus for the replication of their genomes. There is no evidence for the presence of pol-α:primase in mitochondria, and it is believed that the synthesis of RNA primers for mitochondrial DNA replication is carried out by uniquely mitochondrial enzymes. Interestingly, initiation of DNA synthesis at the primary origin of DNA replication in the mitochondrial genome is mediated by mitochondrial RNA polymerase, the same enzyme that is responsible for mitochondrial transcription.

Some eukaryotic viruses have evolved mechanisms for priming DNA synthesis that do not involve oligoribonucleotide synthesis. Two examples are discussed below. The parvovirus genomes have selfcomplementary hairpin termini that allow the 3′ termini of the genomic single strands to prime DNA synthesis. This example represents a very simple case, since the primers for DNA replication are incorporated into the viral genome itself. Adenoviruses make use of a protein to prime DNA replication. In this interesting case, the first phosphodiester bond is formed between the terminal nucleotide and a serine residue of a virus encoded protein. The distribution and frequency of priming events on the two parental strands determine the general pattern of DNA replication in a given system (Fig. 6.1). In continuous DNA replication there is only a single priming event per template strand, so each progeny DNA strand is synthesised continuously from one end to the other. Examples include mitochondrial DNA replication and the replication of the parvoviruses and adenoviruses.

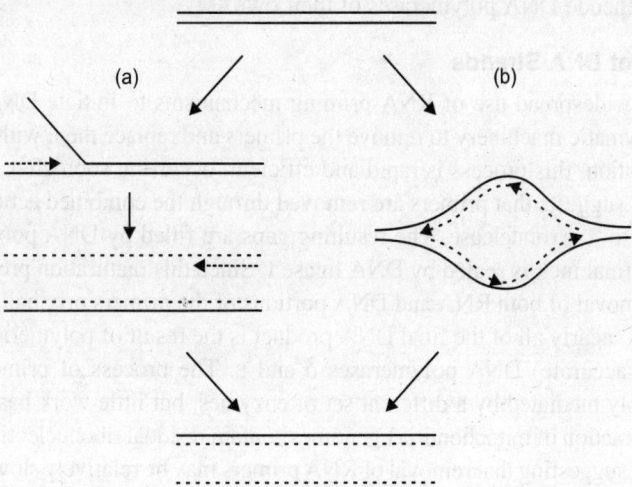

Fig. 6.1: Continuous (A) versus semidiscontinuous (B) DNA replication. The two basic mechanisms for replicating DNA are shown, with nascent DNA (broken lines) synthesised from primers in the direction of the arrows.

In semidiscontinuous DNA replication one progeny strand (leading strand) is elongated continuously from a single primer, whereas the other progeny strand (lagging strand) is constructed from many short DNA chains elongated from multiple primers. Polymerisation of the leading strand occurs in the same direction as replication fork movement, and polymerisation of the lagging strand occurs in the opposite direction. Nuclear DNA replication and the replication of some viruses (e.g. SV40, herpesviruses) proceed by a semidiscontinuous mechanism. In semidiscontinuous DNA synthesis, completion of the lagging strand requires a repair system to remove the primers, fill in the resulting gaps, and join together the short nascent DNA strands.

Elongation of Nascent DNA Strands

Eukaryotic cells contain several DNA polymerase activities. The nuclear pol-α:primase complex mentioned above appears to be largely concerned with the synthesis of primers during semi discontinuous DNA synthesis. The DNA polymerase activity of the enzyme is capable of extending the oligoribonucleotides synthesised by the intrinsic primase activity. However, pol-α:primase is relatively nonprocessive, so that only a short DNA chain is synthesised before the enzyme dissociates from the template. The relatively rapid turnover of the enzyme is consistent with its primary role in the synthesis of multiple primers on the lagging strand as the replication fork advances. The RNA-DNA primers synthesised by pol-α: primase can be extended by the highly processive DNA polymerases δ (pol-δ) and ε (pol-ε). Both of these enzymes can be assembled into complexes with the eukaryotic processivity factor proliferating cell nuclear antigen (PCNA) at primer termini.

PCNA serves as a topological clamp, tethering pol-δ or pol-ε to the template, so that many thousands of nucleotides can be polymerised before the enzyme dissociates. It is likely that the bulk of chromosomal DNA synthesis is mediated by either pol-δ or pol-ε or both. In addition to their high processivity, which contributes to the efficiency of DNA replication, both enzymes have active proofreading exonuclease activities that enhance the fidelity of DNA replication. As described in greater detail below, mitochondria possess a DNA polymerase activity distinct from the enzymes involved in nuclear DNA replication. Although some eukaryotic viruses, like SV40, utilise the resident cellular DNA polymerases, others, like the adenoviruses, encode DNA polymerases of their own.

Maturation of Nascent DNA Strands

A consequence of the widespread use of RNA priming mechanisms to initiate DNA synthesis is the requirement for an enzymatic machinery to remove the primers and replace them with DNA. In the case of nuclear DNA replication, this process is rapid and efficient, occurring soon after Okazaki fragment synthesis. Recent work suggests that primers are removed through the combined action of ribonuclease H (RNase H) and a 5' to 3' exonuclease. The resulting gaps are filled by DNA polymerase, probably pol-δ or pol-ε, and the final nick is sealed by DNA ligase I. Since this maturation process may result in the nearly complete removal of both RNA and DNA portions of the primers originally generated by the pol-α:primase complex, nearly all of the final DNA product is the result of polymerisation by the more processive (and more accurate) DNA polymerases δ and ε. The process of primer replacement in mitochondria is probably mediated by a different set of enzymes, but little work has been done on the problem. A significant fraction of mitochondrial genomes contain residual ribonucleotides at the initiation sites of DNA synthesis, suggesting that removal of RNA primers may be relatively slow and/or inefficient within the organelle.

The DNA-priming mechanism utilised by the parvoviruses requires a maturation mechanism that is quite different from that needed for RNA priming. Since DNA synthesis is primed by a duplex hairpin at the terminus of the genome (see below), there remains the problem of replicating the hairpin primer sequence itself. This is accomplished by a novel and interesting mechanism in which the hairpin sequence first serves as a primer and then is transferred to the newly synthesised DNA strand where it can serve as a template for DNA synthesis. This maturation scheme regenerates the full-length parvovirus genome. Although a similar scheme could, in principle, be used for the maturation of the ends (telomeres) of linear cellular chromosomes, it is now clear that telomeres are synthesised by a special enzyme, telomerase, which polymerises short DNA repeats at chromosome termini using an RNA template that is intrinsic to the enzyme.

CONTINUOUS DNA REPLICATION

As indicated above, mitochondrial DNA and a number of viruses that replicate in eukaryotic cells have evolved replication mechanisms in which both progeny strands are synthesised continuously from one end to the other. To illustrate this general mode of DNA replication, we summarise the replication pathways of two viral systems, the parvoviruses and the adenoviruses, and then discuss mammalian mitochondrial DNA replication. The examples chosen also illustrate the major modes of priming DNA synthesis: DNA self-priming, protein priming, and RNA priming.

Mechanism of Panrovirus (AAV) DNA Replication

The parvoviruses are the simplest of the viruses that infect animal cells. They contain linear single-stranded DNA genomes that are converted to duplex replicating intermediates within infected cells. Progeny single strands are generated from the duplex intermediates by a self-priming, strand-displacement mechanism. Viral DNA replication is largely dependent on host enzymes, probably the factors normally involved in leadingstrand synthesis at chromosomal replication forks. Only one viral gene, *rep,* is required for DNA replication, and its product(s) is mainly concerned with processing of the termini of the genome.

Two general classes of parvoviruses have been identified. Adeno-associated viruses (AAV) generally require coinfection with a helper virus for efficient replication, although the basis for this requirement is not understood. Other parvoviruses are capable of autonomous replication in the absence of any helper virus. All members of the parvovirus group have a similar genetic organisation and follow a roughly similar replication pathway. The replication mechanism of AAV is discussed here as prototypical of the group.

AAV genome

The AAV genome contains two large open reading frames (ORFs). The 5' ORF, referred to as the *rep* gene, encodes four distinct, but overlapping, polypeptide chains generated by alternate promoter utilisation and alternate splicing. The two largest gene products, Rep78 and Rep68, have been implicated in AAV DNA replication by genetic studies. It is not known whether they play different roles in DNA replication *in vivo*, but either protein appears to be capable of supporting AAV DNA replication *in vitro*. The Rep proteins have site-specific endonuclease and helicase activities that mediate the novel processing reaction responsible for regenerating AAV termini.

Replication pathway

Current evidence indicates that AAV DNA replication is completely continuous. The termini of the viral genome contain 145-bp palindromic sequences, referred to as inverted terminal repeats (ITRs). When folded in such a way as to maximise base-pairing, the ITRs are capable of forming T-shaped hairpin structures containing only seven unpaired bases. The 3' end of the genome represents a primer terminus that is used initially to convert the infecting single-stranded genome to a linear duplex form whose strands are covalently linked at one end via the terminal hairpin.

The hairpin terminus is converted to an open duplex through the action of the Rep protein(s) and host enzymes. This processing event, called terminal resolution or hairpin transfer, is initiated by a single endonucleolytic cleavage at a site opposite the original 3' terminus of the genome. Cleavage at the terminal resolution site (TRS) is carried out by the Rep protein, which becomes covalently linked to the 5'-phosphoryl terminus at the TRS cleavage site. The 3'-OH terminus is then extended by a cellular polymerase(s) to replicate the terminal hairpin.

It is likely that the helicase activity of the covalently bound Rep protein facilitates this process by unwinding the hairpin. The result of the terminal resolution reaction is the generation of a linear duplex replication intermediate whose strands are identical to those of the infecting AAV genome except for inversion of the terminal palindromic sequence. The intermediate is then replicated via a selfpriming, strand-displacement mechanism. Priming of this reaction probably involves a rearrangement of the termini reforming the hairpin structures. The resulting structure resembles a replication fork and is presumably a competent substrate for the cellular elongation machinery. It is not clear whether rearrangement of the termini is catalysed by Rep or a cellular protein or whether it occurs spontaneously. The products of the second stage of the AAV replication reaction are a displaced single strand and a linear duplex with covalently joined termini. The latter can be resolved to an open duplex by Rep and the process can be repeated. Since the two termini of AAV are essentially equivalent, equal numbers of the two complementary strands are synthesised. Both strands are packaged into progeny virus particles.

Entymology of AAV DNA replication

Several *in vitro* systems that carry out various aspects of the AAV DNA replication reaction have been developed. When duplex DNA molecules containing functional AAV origins are used as templates, either Rep68 or Rep78 is required for extensive DNA synthesis. It has also been reported that DNA synthesis *in vitro* can be stimulated significantly when the extracts are prepared from adenovirus-infected cells, suggesting that a protein(s) encoded or induced by the helper may play some role in AAV DNA replication. However, it seems likely that most of the proteins involved in viral DNA replication are derived from the host cell. Recent work indicates involvement of the cellular replication proteins PCNA, replication factor C (RF-C), and replication protein A (RP-A) (N. Muzyczka, pers. comm.). The DNA polymerase responsible for AAV DNA chain elongation has not yet been identified with certainty, but, given the involvement of the processivity factor PCNA, pol-δ and pol-ε are likely candidates. Thus, AAV is probably replicated mainly by the apparatus responsible for leading-strand synthesis at cellular replication forks (see below). It is not known whether movement of the AAV replication fork is catalysed by the helicase activity of Rep68/78 or whether a cellular helicase mediates this function. Since the AAV genome is linear and rather short, there is no apparent need for a DNA topoisomerase, consistent with the observation that antibodies against mammalian topoisomerase I and II do not inhibit DNA replication *in vitro*.

Mechanism of Adenovirus DNA Replication

Adenovirus genome

The mechanism of adenovirus DNA replication has been well characterised because of the early development of a cell-free replication system. The most extensively studied viral serotypes are the closely related Ad2 and Ad5. The Ad2/5 genome is a linear doublestranded DNA molecule of 36 kb with two novel structural features: (i) The nucleotide sequences at the ends of the genome are identical for the first 103 nucleotides and (ii) the 5'end of each strand is covalently linked to the virus-encoded, 55-kD terminal protein (TP). Viral DNA replication requires three viral proteins: an 80-kD precursor to the terminal protein (pTP), a 140-kD DNA polymerase (Ad pol), and a singlestranded DNA-binding protein (Ad DBP). The efficiency of DNA replication is increased significantly by several cellular proteins, including the transcription factors nuclear factor I (NFI) and octamer-binding protein 1 (Oct-1) and a DNA topoisomerase (NFII). Initiation of adenovirus DNA replication takes place by a proteinpriming mechanism at the termini of the genome, and each daughter strand is synthesised continuously from one end to the other.

Initiation of adenovirus DNA replication

The adenovirus origin of replication, encompassing roughly the first 50 bp of the viral genome, is the locus of binding of several proteins. NFI and Oct-1 bind to specific recognition sites within the region between nucleotides 19 and 51. A complex of the two viral proteins, pTP and Ad pol (pTP-pol), appears to recognise sequence elements within the first 18 nucleotides that constitute the minimal essential origin. Binding of pTP-pol to the viral origin of replication is the critical first step in the initiation reaction. This step is greatly facilitated by protein-protein interactions between pTP-pol and the bound cellular proteins, NFI and Oct-1. The binding reaction may also be stimulated by the presence of the 55-kD terminal protein at the 5 end of one of the parental strands. Once the pTP-pol is bound at the terminus of the genome, DNA synthesis is initiated by the formation of a phosphodiester bond between the first nucleotide in the new DNA chain, dCMP, and the p-hydroxyl group of a serine residue in the pTP. This novel proteinpriming reaction is presumably catalysed by the adenovirus DNA polymerase, which then functions to extend the nascent chain. An early intermediate in the elongation reaction of Ad5 is a trinucleotide covalently attached to the pTP (pTPCAT). Interestingly, it has recently been demonstrated that the template for synthesis of pTP-CAT is not the first three nucleotides in the parental strand, but nucleotides 4–6. The sequence at the terminus of the template strand (3 GTAGTAGTTA ... 5′) is repetitive, so it is thought that the pTP-CAT, synthesised opposite residues 4–6, translocates to positions 1–3 to start elongation. The function of this rather baroque mechanism is not yet clear, but it has been suggested that it may serve to protect the integrity of the terminal sequences of the viral genome during DNA replication.

Elongation of adenovirus DNA strands

Following initiation at one of the termini, DNA synthesis proceeds by a displacement mechanism, producing a daughter duplex and a free single strand. The latter can cyclise via selfcomplementary termini to form a panhandle structure. Since the duplex panhandle is identical to the termini of the original genome, initiation of DNA synthesis can presumably occur by the same mechanism, leading to the completion of a second daughter duplex. *In vitro* studies have demonstrated that the elongation of nascent adenovirus DNA strands requires only two proteins, Ad pol and Ad DBP. The adenovirus DNA polymerase is a highly processive enzyme that extends DNA primers much more efficiently than RNA primers. Its activity is specifically stimulated by the Ad DBP; prokaryotic or other eukaryotic DBPs cannot replace Ad DBP in the replication reaction. Movement of the displacement fork during adenovirus DNA replication does not appear to require a separate helicase activity.

The Ad DNA pol, acting in concert with the Ad DBP, is sufficient to unwind the parental duplex. The energy required for unidirectional fork movement is derived exclusively from hydrolysis of the deoxyribonucleoside triphosphate precursors for DNA synthesis. Thus, adenovirus appears to have evolved a highly efficient two-protein engine for DNA synthesis that combines the functions of helicase and polymerase. Interestingly, *in vitro* studies have suggested that the replication of the adenovirus genome is facilitated by a cellular DNA topoisomerase (NFII) even though the genome is linear. Replication proceeds efficiently in the presence of Ad DNA pol and Ad DBP until replication is about 25% complete, after which fork movement is slow unless topoisomerase activity is present. The basis for this requirement is not completely clear, but presumably it reflects some hindrance to the free rotation of the unreplicated parental duplex in adenovirus replication intermediates.

Mechanism of Mitochondrial DNA Replication

General features of mitochondria DNA replication

Much of the early work on the mechanism of mitocondria DNA replication was done in mammalian systems, but studies in other organisms, particularly yeast, have been increasingly important for dentifying and characterising required replication proteins. The available evidence suggests that the basic features of mitochondrial DNA replication have been conserved from yeast to man, so the following description focuses primarily on mammalian cells (Fig. 6.2). The mammalian mitochondrial genome is a closed duplex circle of about 16 kb. Cells contain on the order of 10^3–10^4 mitochondrial genomes with an average of 5–10 per organelle. Unlike the nuclear DNA, mitochondrial genomes are replicated throughout the cell cycle, and templates appear to be drawn at random from the pool of genomes. Thus, in a given cell cycle, some mitochondrial genomes are replicated more than once and some are not replicated at all. The regulatory mechanisms that determine the total number of mitochondrial genomes per cell are not understood:

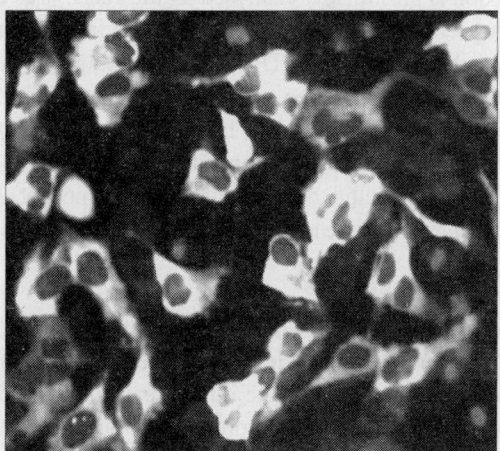

Fig. 6.2: Mammalian cells.

Studies of the structures of replication intermediates have provided strong evidence that the replication of the mitochondrial genome occurs by a completely continuous mechanism (Fig. 6.3). In mammalian cells there are two origins of DNA replication, one for each strand, which are located about 11 kb apart. At each of these origins, DNA synthesis is primed by specific RNA molecules. A single priming event apparently suffices for the complete synthesis of each strand. The origin for heavy (H) strand synthesis (O_H) is activated first, resulting in the establishment of a replication fork that moves unidirectionally. At this fork a new H strand is continuously elongated, and the parental H strand is displaced. The origin for light (L) strand synthesis (O_L) is activated only when it has been rendered single-stranded by the passage of the Hstrand replication fork. It is likely that a specific secondary structure that forms in the displaced strand is recognised by the protein(s) responsible for RNA primer synthesis. The L strand is continuously elongated from the primer in what is essentially a large gap-filling reaction. Since the two origins of DNA replication are separated by approximately two-thirds of the genome, the replication of the two strands of mitochondrial DNA is quite asynchronous. When the synthesis of the H strand is completed, a process that takes about an hour, two products are generated. One product is a duplex circle with a

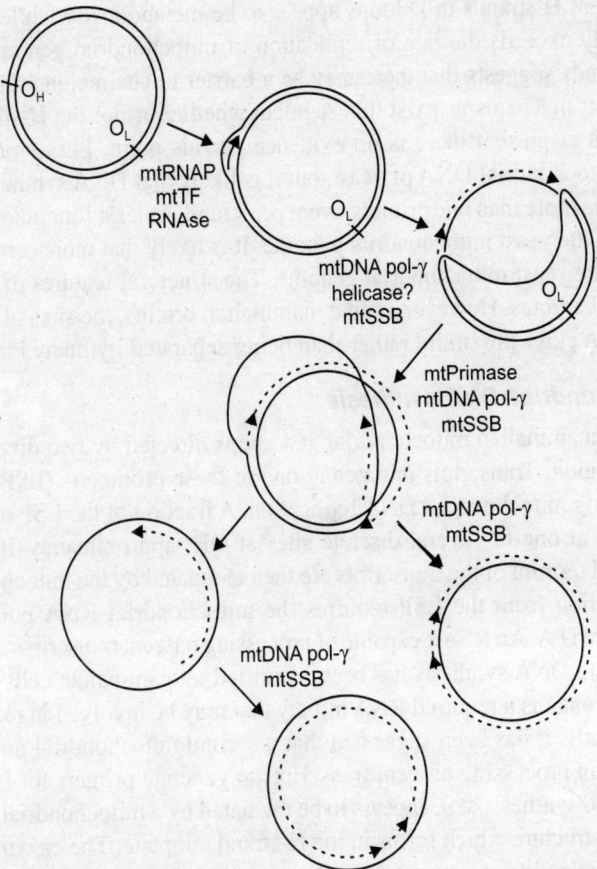

Fig. 6.3: Model for mammalian mitochondrial DNA replication. The two mitochondrial origins 0, and 0, are located about two-thirds of the genome apart. Initiation of DNA replication begins with the synthesis of a transcript by the mitochondrial RNA polymerase (mtRNAP) and an essential transcription factor (mtTF). The transcripts are either processed by an endoribonuclease (RNase) to form a primer for mitochondrial DNA replication or continue to be extended to form mRNA. If cleavage occurs, a nascent H strand (broken line) is synthesised by the mitochondrial DNA polymerase (mtDNA pol-y). Other proteins, including a putative mitochondrial helicase and SSB (mtSSB) probably participate in the chain elongation process. Synthesis of the L strand is initiated by a mitochondrial primase (mtPrimase) after the displacement fork passes 0,. Completion of H-strand synthesis and separation of the two progeny molecules occurs before completion of L-strand synthesis.

full-length progeny H strand, and the other is a gapped circle with an incomplete progeny L strand, which is subsequently extended to full length.

The primary event in mitochondrial DNA replication is the activation of the H-strand origin, since the activation of the L-strand origin is secondary to the establishment of the H-strand replication fork. Thus, one likely point of regulation of mitochondrial DNA synthesis is the generation of the initial RNA primer. There may also be a second control point that operates at the level of elongation of the H strand. A majority of mitochondrial genomes in mammalian cells contain a so-called D loop in the vicinity of O_H. This structure consists of a short nascent H DNA whose 5′ end is located at the origin for H strand synthesis. The nascent H strands in D loops appear to be metabolically labile and are turned over at a rate that significantly exceeds the rate of replication of mitochondrial genomes. The existence of the short nascent H strands suggests that there may be a barrier to chain elongation just downstream from O_H. It is possible that mechanisms exist that regulate whether or not the H-strand replication fork can pass this barrier, but at present there is no evidence on this point. Less work has been done on the replication of the mitochondrial DNA of yeast, but it is likely that DNA synthesis is largely continuous, although there may be more than one priming event per strand. At least four putative origins of replication have been located in the yeast mitochondrial genome. It is likely that more origins are required because of the large size of the yeast mitochondrial genome. The structural features of yeast origins are similar to those of higher eukaryotes. However, unlike mammalian origins, the sites of initiation of synthesis of the two strands are in close proximity rather than being separated by many kilobases.

Priming of mitochondrial DNA synthesis

Transcription of the mammalian mitochondrial genome is directed by two divergent promoters located within the D-loop region. Transcripts initiated at one of these promoters (LSP) also serve to prime H-strand synthesis during mitochondrial DNA replication. A fraction of the LSP transcripts are cleaved by an endoribonuclease at one of several discrete sites at OH, approximately 100 nucleotides from the promoter. The 3'- OH termini of the transcripts are then elongated by the mitochondrial DNA replication apparatus. Transcription from the LSP requires the mitochondrial RNA polymerase and a specific transcription factor, mtTFA. An RNase capable of processing nascent transcripts at sites near the transition from RNA synthesis to DNA synthesis has been identified in mammalian cells and yeast. The enzyme, called RNase MRP, contains a required RNA moiety that may be involved in recognition of the specific cleavage sites. Recently, it has been suggested that a second mitochondrial nuclease, endonuclease G, may also play a role in processing nascent transcripts to generate primers for DNA replication.

Priming of L-strand synthesis at 0, appears to be mediated by a mitochondrial primase that recognises a specific stem-loop structure which forms in the H-strand template. The enzyme initiates the synthesis of a short oligoribonucleotide at a run of T residues in this loop. The transition from RNA synthesis to DNA synthesis occurs immediately adjacent to the base of the stem. The mitochondrial primase appears to require an RNA component for activity, and the most likely candidate is cellular 5.8s RNA. Thus, the priming mechanisms for the synthesis of both strands of the mitochondrial genome require ribonucleoprotein enzymes.

Mechanism of chain elongation

Although some of the required enzymes have been identified, the detailed mechanism of continuous DNA synthesis in mitochondria is not well understood. This is mainly due to the absence of an efficient cellfree replication system. All of the components involved in mitochondrial DNA replication, including both the priming and elongation stages, are encoded by nuclear genes and imported into the organelle. A highly processive mitochondrial DNA polymerase, referred to as DNA polymerase-y, has been purified from several sources. The human enzyme consists of subunits of 140 kD and 54 kD. The larger subunit contains the polymerase active site as well as a potent 3' to 5' exonuclease activity. The latter shows strong preference for unpaired primer termini and presumably plays a proofreading role. The yeast gene encoding the catalytic subunit of DNA polymerase-y (MIPl) has been cloned. The amino acid sequence of the Mipl protein is similar to both eukaryotic nuclear DNA polymerases and reverse transcriptases, but has no discernible resemblance to prokaryotic DNA polymerases.

Mitochondria1 DBPs have also been identifed from several organisms. Interestingly, these proteins are homologous to *Escherichia coli* SSB, and their physicochemical properties are quite similar to the prokaryotic enzyme as well. Yeast mutants lacking the RIM1 gene, which encodes the mitochondrial SSB, are completely devoid of mitochondrial DNA, consistent with an essential role for the protein in mitochondrial DNA replication. Presumably, the mitochondrial SSB facilitates the elongation of nascent DNA chains by the mitochondrial DNA polymerase. However, the functional interactions of the two proteins have not been extensively analysed to date.

Another likely accessory protein for mitochondrial DNA synthesis is a DNA helicase, since H-strand synthesis requires melting of the parental strands at the replication fork. A helicase activity has been identified in highly purified mitochondria from bovine brain. This activity, which translocates in the 3′ to 5′ direction on the single-stranded portion of partially duplex substrates, is a likely candidate for a replicative helicase in mitochondria, but this role has not been verified directly. The Pifl helicase of budding yeast has been implicated in the repair, recombination, and replication of the mitochondrial genome. Genetic interactions have been observed between the *PIFl* gene and the *RIM1* gene, encoding the mitochondrial SSB. Moreover, a yeast strain deficient in the Pifl enzyme loses mitochondrial DNA at elevated temperatures. Mitochondria1 DNA replication remains the best example of a naturally occurring, completely continuous DNA replication system in eukaryotic cells. Although a number of the components required for DNA replication have been identified, and we have a general picture of the overall replication pathway, much remains to be learned about the biochemical mechanisms involved. Future *in vitro* studies of mitochondrial DNA synthesis with purified components will likely fill in many of the gaps in our knowledge.

SEMIDISCONTINUOUS DNA SYNTHESIS

Replication of Chromosomal DNA

In the continuous DNA replication systems that we have discussed so far, the two complementary DNA strands are synthesised relatively independently and asynchronously. In contrast, the replication of eukaryotic chromosomal DNA occurs by a semidiscontinuous mechanism in which the synthesis of the two strands is strongly coupled in space and time. One advantage of semidiscontinuous DNA replication over completely continuous DNA replication is that the generation of single-stranded DNA is much more localised and transient. This may help preserve the integrity of the genome, since breaks and other lesions in single-stranded DNA are difficult to repair.

Semidiscontinuous DNA replication is mediated by a complex protein machine assembled at each replication fork. The proteins comprising this replication machine act in concert to unwind the parental strands and carry out the simultaneous synthesis of the two progeny strands. Both progeny strands are synthesised in the 5′ to 3′ direction, but since the parental DNA strands are antiparallel, two distinct mechanisms of DNA synthesis are required. One of the two progeny strands (leading strand) is synthesised continuously in the direction of fork movement. The other strand (lagging strand) is synthesised discontinuously in the direction opposite to fork movement. Discontinuous DNA synthesis on the laggingstrand template involves the repeated synthesis of oligoribonucleotide primers, which are then elongated into short DNA chains (Okazaki fragments). Following their synthesis, Okazaki fragments are processed to remove the RNA primers and joined together to form an uninterrupted progeny strand.

The semidiscontinuous DNA replication mechanism appears to be quite ancient in origin, as its essential features have been conserved from bacteria to man. Although the basic biochemical processes that occur at eukaryotic and prokaryotic replication forks are similar, there are many differences in detail. For example, in *E. coli,* a single DNA polymerase is thought to form a dimeric complex that mediates DNA synthesis on both the leading and lagging strands, whereas eukaryotes contain at least three distinct DNA polymerase activities, all of which participate in DNA replication. The critical proteinprotein interactions that are required for formation of an efficient replica tion machine also appear to differ between prokaryotes and eukaryotes. In *E. coli,* the primase activity responsible for initiating new DNA chains forms a specific complex with the helicase activity responsible for unwinding the parental strands as the fork moves whereas in eukaryotes, the primase is a subunit of one of the DNA polymerase molecules. Some of the accessory proteins involved in DNA synthesis have more complex structures in eukaryotes than in prokaryotes. One example is the singlestranded DNA-binding protein, which is a single polypeptide chain in *E. coli* but a large heterotrimeric protein in eukaryotes. The greater complexity may be related to the more complex mechanisms required to regulate DNA replication in eukaryotes. Despite these apparent differences, there are many similarities between prokaryotic and eukaryotic DNA replication that reflect a common evolutionary origin. One particularly striking example is the remarkable structural similarity of the *p*-subunit of *E. coli* DNA polymerase III and the eukaryotic protein PCNA, both of which function as 'sliding clamps' to increase the processivity of DNA synthesis. A novel feature of eukaryotic chromosomes is the packaging of DNA into chromatin. This fact may account for the surprising disparity in the rate of fork movement in prokaryotes and eukaryotes. Whereas the *E. coli* replication machinery moves at the prodigious rate of 100 kb/minute, unwinding DNA at some 10,000 rpm, eukaryotic fork movement is much slower (0.5–5 kb/min). The presence of histones may limit the maximal rate at which DNA polymerisation can occur. Such a constraint might have contributed to the evolution of intrinsically slower polymerases in eukaryotes. In addition, special mechanisms may have evolved to allow fork movement without disruption of either the replication complex or the nucleosomes. In this manner, the DNA remains packaged even while DNA synthesis is taking place. However, the ability of large protein assemblies to negotiate one another is not unique to eukaryotes, as *in vitro* experiments have shown that the phage T4 replication apparatus can bypass an RNA polymerase complex moving in either direction without complete dissociation of either set of proteins.

Viral Model Systems

Direct biochemical investigation into the mechanisms underlying cellular DNA replication has proven difficult. With the exception of special cases such as *Xenopus* eggs (Fig. 6.4), it has not yet been possible to develop an *in vitro* cellular DNA replication system. In the absence of such a system, investigators have turned to viral models to study the mechanism of cellular DNA replication. Viruses present several advantages, including small genomes and well-defined origins of replication. The Papovaviridae, which include the SV40, polyoma, and papilloma viruses, have been particularly important to the study of chromosomal replication. Upon infection of suitable host cells, the genomes of these viruses are transported to the nucleus, where the double-stranded viral minichromosomes are replicated by mechanisms that closely resemble the cellular process. Initiation occurs at a single origin within the viral genome and proceeds bidirectionally in a semidiscontinuous manner. The great advantage of SV40 and other papovaviruses is that many of the important steps in DNA replication are performed by host proteins. A significant advance in the study of eukaryotic DNA replication came with the development of a cell-free SV40 system in 1984. Primate cytoplasmic extract and a single viral protein, the large T antigen, carry out all the functions required for complete replication of SV40-origin-containing plasmid DNA. T antigen recognises the origin and unwinds the duplex, providing access for the numerous host replication proteins

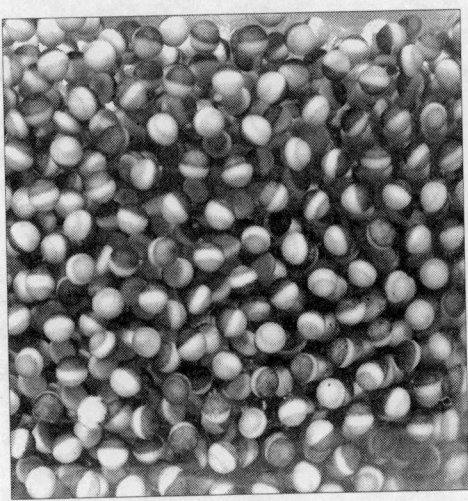

Fig. 6.4: Xenopus eggs.

that function coordinately to synthesise the daughter DNA strands. Fractionation of human extract and reconstitution of replication activity using an *in vitro* complementation assay have led to the identification of those cellular proteins necessary and sufficient for viral DNA replication. Given that the mechanisms of SV40 and cellular DNA replication appear to be very similar, there is considerable confidence that the same proteins have identical functions in the replication of the chromosomes. It should be noted that analysis of the viral system has not identified all of the proteins involved in eukaryotic DNA replication. For example, genetic studies in yeast strongly suggest that pol-ε is necessary for DNA replication *in vivo*, but this enzyme was not originally identified as necessary for SV40 DNA replication. As discussed previously, the natural template for eukaryotic DNA replication is chromatin. Whereas the cell-free system was originally developed with naked DNA templates, a number of studies have attempted to more accurately reflect the *in vivo* replicative process by employing chromatin templates. Although *in vitro* replication of such minichromosomes is very inefficient relative to that of naked DNA, the repression of initiation due to tightly bound histones can be relieved by the presence of transcription factors bound near the origin. A similar stimulatory effect of transcription factors on replication efficiency has been observed *in vivo*. Several possible mechanisms could account for this derepression, including increased accessibility of the origin to the initiator protein or activation of the replication apparatus by contact with factors bound near the origin. Further studies have focused on the fate of parental nucleosomes during DNA replication and indicate that nucleosomes remain associated with the replicating DNA during DNA synthesis. In addition, the assembly of new chromatin appears to be coupled to SV40 DNA replication *in vitro*. Experiments such as these have added to our understanding of the mechanism by which the replication machinery negotiates other DNA-bound structures, a process that must occur continuously in the nucleus.

Enzymology of the Replication Fork

Replication proteins

Studies employing the SV40 model system have resulted in the identification of many cellular replication proteins. Recent work employing both genetic and biochemical techniques has added to this list. A summary of known replication proteins is presented in Table 6.1.

Table 6.1: Cellular replication proteins.

Protein	Subunit (kD)^a	Replicative function
DNA polymerases		
pol-α:primase	180, 70, 58,48	DNA polymerase, primase
pol-δ	125,48	DNA polymerase, 3′ to 5′ exonuclease
pol-ε	258,55	DNA polymerase, 3′ to 5′ exonuclease
Accessory proteins		
RP-A	70, 32, 14 S	ingle-stranded DNA binding
PCNA	36	Pol-δ/processivity factor
RF-C	145, 40, 38, 37, 36.5	Loads PCNA onto template
Nucleases		
Ribonuclease H1	89	Okazaki fragment maturation
FEN-1 (MF-I)	44	Okazaki fragment maturation
Others		
DNA ligase I	102	Joins Okazaki fragments
Topoisomerase I	100	Unlinks parental strands
Topoisomerase I1	172	Unlinks parental strands and progeny duplexes

Helicases

The focal point of all replication forks is the helicase, which catalyses the transition from double- to single-stranded DNA. In *E. coli*, the DNAB helicase translocates in a 5' to 3' direction while unwinding DNA and therefore is bound to the laggingstrand template during DNA replication. The same mechanism is employed by the phages T4 and T7, which induce their own helicases to engage in semidiscontinuous replication. In direct contrast, SV40 T antigen is bound to the leading-strand template and moves in the 3' to 5' direction advancing the fork. Although the polarity of translocation is not conserved, the replicative helicases of *E. coli*, T4, T7, and SV40 are all hexamers, suggesting a common quaternary structure for enzymes with this function. To date, several eukaryotic helicases have been identified, but conclusive identification of the enzyme that acts at chromosomal replication forks must await further biochemical and genetic investigation.

Single-stranded DNA-binding protein

As the replication fork advances, a helix-destabilising protein is required to maintain the single-stranded DNA structure that serves as a template for RNA priming and DNA synthesis. In eukaryotic cells, replication protein A (RP-A; RF-A; HSSB) performs this function. This phosphoprotein has three subunits with molecular weights of 70,000, 32,000, and 14,000. The large subunit contains the DNA-binding activity but cannot support SV40 DNA replication *in vitro* by itself, therefore, at least one of the two smaller subunits is likely to be required for replication. In support of this hypothesis, all three yeast genes encoding RP-A are essential for viability, and antibodies directed against any of the three subunits inhibit SV40 DNA replication *in vitro*. Although the roles of the two smaller RP-A subunits remain unknown, the middle subunit is phosphorylated during S phase of the cell cycle, suggesting that this subunit may play some role in regulating DNA replication.

The DNA-binding properties of RP-A have been investigated extensively, but there remains some disagreement about fundamental aspects of the protein-DNA interaction. RP-A binds relatively nonspecifically to single-stranded DNA but exhibits a modest preference for DNA sequences rich in pyrimidines. Several different binding site sizes have been reported, ranging from 8 to 30 nucleotides for human RP-A and up to 100 nucleotides for the yeast protein. Some evidence has been presented that RP-A forms two different types of complexes with DNA, which may account for the variability in site size estimates. Further disagreement centers on the degree of cooperativity of the DNAbinding reaction. Most prokaryotic single-stranded DNA-binding proteins display a high level of cooperativity, allowing the rapid and complete binding of any exposed single-stranded regions in the genome. Steady-state fluorescence experiments indicate that this is also the case with yeast RP-A. However, a series of studies employing electrophoretic mobility shift of oligonucleotides in the presence of human RP-A have demonstrated little cooperativity. Other studies employing a similar technique suggest that only one of two proposed binding modes is highly cooperative. The lack of consensus with regard to the DNA-binding properties may result from differences in experimental technique, or possibly differences in the state of the protein itself, such as the extent of phosphorylation.

DNA Pol-α:primase complex

DNA synthesis is initiated by the bifunctional pol-α:primase complex, a heterotetrameric phosphoprotein. The primase activity resides in the 48-kD D subunit and is tightly associated with the 58-kD C subunit, which is thought to tether the primase to the 180-kD polymerase A subunit. With the exception of the *Drosophila* enzyme, there is no proofreading exonuclease activity associated with the A subunit. The remaining 70-kD B subunit has no known catalytic function, but it may contribute to recruitment of pol-α:primase to the replication fork.

The main function of pol-α:primase is to serve as a priming enzyme. The primase catalyses the synthesis of complementary oligoribonucleotides, which are then extended a short distance by the A subunit DNA polymerase activity. Although high concentrations of pol-α:primase can support the complete replication of SV40 origin-containing plasmid DNA *in vitro*, it is unlikely that cellular replication relies heavily on this polymerase during elongation. The low processivity of the enzyme and the lack of an associated proofreading exonuclease suggest that pol-α:primase serves exclusively to initiate DNA synthesis on the lagging strand. Dissociation of pol-α:primase from the DNA provides a primer terminus for the assembly of the PCNNpol-δ or /pol-ε complexes, highly processive polymerases that can efficiently extend the RNNDNA primers originally synthesised by pol-α:primase.

DNA polymerases δ and ε

The heterodimeric DNA polymerases δ and ε are involved in the elongation stage of DNA replication. Unlike pol-α:primase, polymerases α and ε do not act alone but require the action of two auxiliary factors. The multisubunit replication factor C (RF-C) binds to the primer terminus immediately after RNADNA primer synthesis has been completed by pol-α:primase, allowing the subsequent assembly of a functional pol-δ or pol-ε complex. Once bound to the primer-template junction, RF-C loads PCNA onto the DNA in an energy-dependent reaction. PCNA then functions as a processivity factor, binding to pol-δ or pol-ε and maintaining a stable interaction between polymerase and template. Ultimately, one or both of these processive polymerases, with their intrinsic proofreading activities, probably synthesise all of the cellular DNA, thereby ensuring faithful duplication of the genome.

DNA polymerases δ and ε have some similarities in catalytic function and are both essential for viability in yeast. However, it is not yet clear whether they have specialised roles in replication. pol-ε does not substitute well for pol-δ in the cell-free SV40 DNA replication system with purified proteins, so it may contribute to DNA synthesis only when certain additional factors are present. It is also possible that these enzymes have important roles that are not limited to DNA replication. For example, recent experiments indicate that pol-ε is one member of the S-phase checkpoint pathway , a biochemical feedback mechanism that delays cell-cycle progression upon damage to the DNA or inhibition of DNA synthesis during the replicative phase. Thus, in addition to synthesising DNA, pol-ε may be involved in monitoring the status of DNA replication.

Nucleases

Synthesis of the lagging strand results in the generation of DNA fragments with RNA primers at the 5' ends. For lagging-strand synthesis to be completed, these primers must be removed and the resulting gap must be filled. In *E. coli*, DNA polymerase I, with its intrinsic 5' to 3' exonuclease activity, mediates both functions. None of the replicative eukaryotic polymerases contains a 5' to 3' exonuclease, indicating that other factors are involved in the initial processing of Okazaki fragments. A 44-kD 5' to 3' exonuclease (FEN-1, MF-1) that is required for the formation of covalently closed circular DNA during *in vitro* SV40 DNA replication has been identified in human cells. Recently, studies employing purified calf proteins and a model laggingstrand template have shown that FEN-1 and RNase H1 act together to process Okazaki fragments. RNase H1 nicks the primer on the 5' side of the 3' ribonucleotide, providing a suitable substrate for FEN-1, which removes the 3'-terminal ribonucleotide of the RNA primer. The oligoribonucleotide is displaced and the gap is filled by DNA polymerase, resulting in nicked double-stranded DNA.

DNA ligase

After removal of the RNA primers and extension of the DNA chains through the resulting gaps, the nascent DNA fragments must be joined to complete the synthesis of the lagging strand. Of the three DNA ligases that have been identified in mammalian cells, DNA ligase I is the most likely candidate to carry out this function *in vivo*. In a cell-free SV40 system containing highly purified proteins, DNA ligase I, but not DNA ligase III, catalyses the formation of covalently closed daughter molecules. Although DNA ligase II has not been tested, this enzyme is present at low abundance and is likely to be involved in DNA repair. Genetic studies support the conclusion that DNA ligase I is involved in cellular replication *in vivo*. It has been shown that the human DNA ligase I gene can complement a *Saccharomyces cerevisiae* cdc9 mutant, which is defective in DNA replication due to DNA ligase deficiency.

Topoisomerases

As replication proceeds and the parental strands are unwound, positive supercoils are potentially introduced ahead of the replication fork. The resulting accumulation of torsional strain could lead to inhibition of fork movement if not relieved by a DNA topoisomerase. In eukaryotic cells, two types of topoisomerases have been discovered. The type I enzyme introduces a transient single-strand break in the DNA, thereby relaxing either negatively or positively supercoiled DNA. Type II topoisomerase introduces a transient double-strand DNA break through which duplex DNA is passed. In addition to relaxing DNA, this enzyme can decatenate intertwined molecules. Studies with the SV40 model system employing naked DNA have revealed that either type of topoisomerase is capable of removing the positive supercoils ahead of the fork, allowing rapid and efficient DNA synthesis. However, the progeny DNA molecules that are formed remain multiply intertwined because of failure to remove all of the links between the parental strands during DNA synthesis. Topoisomerase II is required to resolve this tangled structure into two separate progeny genomes, allowing subsequent segregation.

The topological problems accompanying SV40 DNA replication *in vitro* are likely to arise during cellular replication as well. The length of chromosomal DNA and its association with nuclear proteins to form chromatin probably precludes free rotation of the DNA during replication. Therefore, the two eukaryotic topoisomerases are likely to function *in vivo* as they do in the SV40 system. It has been suggested that topoisomerase II may have a special role in the completion of DNA synthesis where two adjacent forks converge. However, this conclusion is based on studies of a cell-free SV40 system containing only one DNA polymerase (pol-α:primase) and may not accurately reflect the normal cellular process.

Organisation of the Replication Fork

Most of the studies aimed at defining the organisation of the cellular replication fork have revolved around the SV40 system. Although the identity and mechanism of the cellular helicase remain unknown, it is likely that the known cellular proteins play similar roles in chromosomal replication as in the viral model. Leading-strand synthesis is performed by a processive polymerase complex (PCNA/pol-α or PCNA/ pol-ε) and a single auxiliary protein (RP-A). Lagging-strand synthesis requires additional proteins. pol-α:primase synthesises RNA/DNA primers that are extended by complexes similar to those operating on the leading strand. Primer removal and completion of DNA synthesis require FEN-1 nuclease, RNase H1, and DNA ligase I as described above. Studies with both crude and purified systems have demonstrated that assembly of replication proteins at the replication fork is mediated by specific protein-protein contacts. These interactions are critical for the coordinated synthesis of both leading and lagging strands, and are likely to be important at all stages of the replicative process. Specific mechanisms involving multiple proteins at the replication fork are discussed below.

Protein-protein interactions

In the SV40 system, the viral T antigen and the cellular proteins pol-α: primase and RP-A are required for initiation of DNA replication, and a variety of studies have provided evidence for significant molecular interactions among the three proteins. For example, biochemical analysis of model reactions has uncovered a number of instances in which one protein affects the activity of another. These biochemical data are supported by physical studies demonstrating direct association of each combination of two proteins. In particular, much information has been gathered on the polam-antigen interaction. This association appears complex, possibly involving three of the four pol-α subunits (A, B, and D).

It is very likely that the molecular interactions among initiation proteins are important determinants of efficiency and specificity in the initiation reaction. Unwinding of the SV40 origin requires T antigen and RP-A, and contact between these two proteins is likely to be important at this early stage of replication. Although the isolated large subunit of RPA does not interact with T antigen, intact RP-A does, suggesting that one or both of the smaller subunits could play a role in this interaction. Once the duplex is unwound, interaction between T antigen and pol-α may contribute to efficient priming on the RP-Acoated, single-stranded DNA template. It is possible that the different in teraction domains on pol-α have different functional roles during replication. For example, the D subunit may help to coordinate initiation at the origin, and the A and B subunits may be important for tethering pol-α:primase to the advancing helicase. Priming is also likely to be influenced by an RP-A/primase interaction, which has been demonstrated to occur *in vitro* through the large subunit of RP-A. The close association of the three proteins involved in initiation of SV40 DNA replication is quite striking and suggests that similar interactions may occur at cellular origins of replication. Confirmation of this possibility awaits identification of the cellular counterpart(s) of T antigen.

Protein-protein interactions are also critically important during elongation of the nascent DNA chains. As discussed above, efficient elongation requires a highly processive polymerase, and it is likely that pol-δ (or pol-ε), with its auxiliary factors RF-C and PCNA, carries out this function on both leading and lagging strands. The processivity of pol-δ is absolutely dependent on interaction with PCNA, which is topologically linked to the template DNA. There is no evidence for interaction between the processive polymerases and other replication proteins, although RP-A does stimulate pol-δ activity to some extent.

Recent data suggest the possibility that protein-protein interactions may even be important during the final stage of DNA replication, when the Okazaki fragments are joined to form a continuous DNA chain. Studies with purified proteins have shown that DNA ligase I, but not DNA ligase 111, can catalyse the formation of covalently closed daughter DNA molecules in the SV40 model system. Since both ligases are capable of sealing nicks in double-stranded DNA, the strict requirement for DNA ligase I may reflect specific contacts between the enzyme and other proteins involved in the maturation of nascent strands.

A number of interesting interactions between replication proteins and other cellular factors have been uncovered. Although the functions of these interactions are not entirely clear, some of these may be involved in regulating replication. RP-A interacts with several proteins, including the transcription factors p53, GAL4, and VP16 and the repair proteins XPA and XPG. Another example, discovered with the SV40 model system, is the coupling of chromatin assembly to DNA replication. This coupling is strongly suggestive of a direct interaction between the chromatin assembly apparatus and the replication machinery and probably evolved to ensure rapid and efficient packaging of the progeny DNA following synthesis.

Synthesis of Okazaki fragments and cycling of pol-α:primase

Because synthesis of the lagging strand proceeds in the direction opposite to fork movement, repeated priming events by the pol-α:primase are required. There are two general mechanisms by which this priming could occur. One possibility is that pol-α:primase completely dissociates from the template following completion of each RNA/DNA primer (distributive mechanism). In this scenario, synthesis of each RNA/DNA primer would involve association of a different molecule of pol-α:primase with the template. Alternatively, pol-α:primase might be tethered to the replication complex at the fork via specific protein-protein interactions. In this case, the enzyme would not leave the domain of the template following the completion of an RNA/DNA primer but would immediately reassociate with the template at a new site to initiate primer synthesis (processive mechanism).

At this point, the available data are not sufficient to choose between the two mechanisms. Evidence supporting a distributive model has come from dilution experiments in the cell-free SV40 DNA replication system. When the pol-α:primase concentration is decreased by dilution, the rate of DNA replication decreases proportionately. Although these data clearly indicate that pol-α:primase dissociates from the template at a measurable rate during DNA synthesis, it has not yet been possible to directly measure the number of priming events mediated by a given pol-α:primase prior to dissociation. Evidence for processive priming has been provided by the strong physical interaction between pol-α and T antigen. It is known that T antigen is capable of unwinding long segments of DNA without dissociation. Binding of pol-α:primase to T antigen could significantly increase the lifetime of pol-α:primase at the fork. Thus, a single pol-α:primase molecule could proceed through several priming cycles, allowing efficient synthesis of the lagging strand. In agreement with this model, the presence of T antigen increases the apparent processivity of pol-α: primase on model templates. In addition to possibly increasing processivity of priming, interaction between pol-α:primase and T antigen may facilitate access of pol-α:primase to the template during replication. Experiments with model templates have shown that RP-A-coated single-stranded DNA is resistant to priming. In the presence of T antigen, this inhibition is relieved. Therefore, interaction of pol-α:primase with T antigen may be required for primase to productively interact with the template DNA. During cellular DNA replication, a similar mechanism must be employed to allow efficient priming of the RP-A-coated DNA. It is possible that the cellular process is also mediated by a direct physical interaction between pol-α:primase and the replicative helicase.

Proofreading mechanisms

The catalytic subunits of polymerases δ and ε contain 3' to 5' exonuclease activities, allowing high-fidelity DNA synthesis. Therefore, the majority of nuclear DNA synthesis employs the conventional proofreading mechanism first outlined in prokaryotic systems. However, pol-α:primase contains no obvious proofreading activity. It has been reported that a cryptic 3' to 5' exonuclease is uncovered when the *Drosophila* pol-α:primase complex is dissociated, but this phenomenon has not been observed with pol-α:primase complexes from other species. It is not clear how errors are corrected in DNA synthesised by pol-α:primase. One possibility is that a separate exonuclease proofreading activity exists. However, it is more likely that maturation of lagging-strand DNA fragments leads to removal of mismatches downstream from the RNA primer in pol-α-catalysed regions. Prior to ligation of the nicked strand, FEN-1 nuclease and a proofreading polymerase could act in conjunction to accurately replace the DNA originally polymerised by pol-α. Since FEN-1 does not function on a gapped template but requires a nick, removal of DNA and resynthesis would have to occur concurrently. Alternating nucleolytic and synthetic steps by these two enzymes would closely resemble the 'nick translation' reaction of *E. coli* DNA polymerase I.

Replication centers

An interesting recent development has been the discovery that DNA replication may occur in relatively discrete foci in the nuclei of mammalian cells. When nascent DNA is labeled by exposure of cells to a short pulse of BrdU, the label is localised to a relatively small number of intranuclear sites. Enumeration of these sites or 'replication centers' suggests that each may contain as many as 100 replication forks. Thus, DNA replication may be highly compartmentalised in eukaryotic cells. Both PCNA and RP-A have been detected at these replication centers by immunofluorescence. Interestingly, the large subunit of RP-A has been detected at foci prior to the onset of replication and is a possible component of a prereplication complex at the origin. The organisation of replication centers is not well understood. One hypothesis invokes the nuclear matrix as an insoluble support that serves as a foundation for DNA replication and organises the replication centers. However, a clear understanding of the structure and function of foci will have to await further biochemical investigation.

Control of Eukaryotic DNA Replication-Unanswered Questions

The basic enzymology of the eukaryotic replication fork has been uncovered through the identification and characterisation of the replication proteins required for DNA synthesis *in vitro*. However, many fundamental questions remain regarding the control of replication *in vivo*. These problems focus on the coordination of DNA replication with other events in the cell cycle, including the timing of initiation, the prevention of multiple rounds of replication during a single replicative phase of the cell cycle, and the response to insults that may compromise the faithful duplication of the genetic material. Much of the current research on eukaryotic DNA replication is directed at characterising these mechanisms. Initiator proteins, which recognise origins of replication and unwind the double-stranded DNA, are likely to be central to the regulation of cellular DNA replication. The presence or the activation of these proteins may be responsible for controlling the timing of initiation during the cell cycle, and their subsequent removal or inactivation may be necessary to prevent re-replication during a single S phase. Identification of eukaryotic initiator proteins has proven to be quite difficult. However, a complex of six polypeptides that specifically recognises yeast origin sequences has been purified recently. This origin recognition complex (ORC) is likely to function as an initiator, and thorough characterisation of the protein should provide insight into the mechanisms that operate to regulate initiation. Studies have already shown that ORC protein level is constant through the cell cycle. This observation suggests that the initiator protein is activated at the G_1/S transition, possibly by protein phosphorylation or by specific interactions with other cellular proteins.

Studies with the cell-free SV40 system have provided some evidence that protein phosphorylation may be involved in replication control. SV40 DNA replication does not occur until the G_1/S transition has been reached in the host cell. Interestingly, extracts prepared from cells in GI are incompetent for *in vitro* SV40 DNA replication unless supplemented with protein phosphatase 2Ac (PP2Ac) or cdc2 kinase. Although the key target of these GI-activating enzymes is not yet clear, T antigen is one possible candidate. Both PP2Ac and cdc2 kinase can directly modify the phosphorylation state of T antigen *in vitro*, thereby regulating its ability to unwind the SV40 origin. It is possible that cellular initiator proteins may be activated at the G_1/S boundary by similar phosphorylation and/or dephosphorylation events.

Two cellular proteins involved in the initiation of SV40 DNA replication *in vitro*, pol-α:primase and RP-A, are phosphorylated in cell-cycledependent manners. There has been no clear demonstration that phosphorylation affects the replicative function of either protein, but this remains a reasonable possibility. It has also been suggested that RP-A phosphorylation might be involved in a signaling pathway that coordinates DNA replication with the cell cycle. In this case, RP-A would have both a replicative and a regulatory role. Such bifunctionality has recently been demonstrated with pol-ε, which appears to act as a replicative polymerase and as a member of the S-phase checkpoint pathway. This finding may help to explain the need for two rather redundant DNA polymerase activities in eukaryotic cells. Observations such as those described above have provided some clues into the mechanism of DNA replication control, but it is clear that the majority of the process is not well understood. The characterisation of the pathways and their components that allow communication between the replication machine and other cellular apparati will rely on both the biochemistry of the viral model systems and the genetics afforded by yeast. Since the basic mechanism of DNA replication has been conserved from yeast to humans, many of the regulatory mechanisms are likely to be conserved as well. As a result, these systems will continue to be used interchangeably to provide us with an understanding of how the cell efficiently and faithfully replicates its DNA in preparation for cell division.

ENZYMES INVOLVED IN DNA REPLICATION

The enzymes involved in DNA replication are: (i) DNA polymerase, (ii) DNA gyrase, (iii) DNA ligase, (iv) helicase, and (v) primase.

DNA Polymerase

The primary enzyme which carries out the condensation of the nucleotides to form a polynucleotide chain is the DNA polymerase. It is a single polypeptide with a molecular weight of 109 KD. It catalyses the synthesis of the DNA from 5 to 3 direction, i.e. starts copying the template DNA from its 3 end. It can not act in opposite direction. DNA polymerase has three distinct properties.

1. One of the important functions of DNA polymerase is 5→3 polymerase activity, which is the predominant function of the enzyme and is responsible for the nucleotides to form the DNA chain. A new nucleotide is added to an existing oligonucleotide at the 3-OH group. For the formation of a new strand, a single-stranded DNA is required which is to be copied and is known as template. The enzyme thus depends on a template DNA and is referred to as the DNA dependent DNA polymerase.

2. Another function of DNA polymerase is 5→3 exonuclease activity, which helps in the removal of nucleotides from the DNA chain. RNA primer is removed from the newly synthesised chain by 5→3 exonuclease activity.

3. DNA polymerase shows another function of 3→5 exonuclease activity, which catalyses the removal of nucleotides from the 3 end of the DNA chain.

Arthur Kornberg was the first scientist who discovered the DNA polymerase and thought that it is the only DNA polymerase found in the cells, which has the polymerisation activity. After that, various enzymes have been discovered with the similar activity as that of the Kornberg's enzyme. Kornberg's enzyme was designated as polymerase I (Pol I). Later on, it was proved that Pol I is not involved in DNA synthesis. The basic function of Pol I was proofreading and DNA repair. Another enzyme designated as Pol II is involved in DNA repair. The third enzyme Pol III is the main enzyme responsible for the DNA replication.

DNA Polymerase I

DNA Polymerase I was the first enzyme suggested to be involved in DNA replication. The enzyme is now considered to be a DNA repair enzyme and has five active sites. The enzyme is mainly involved in removing RNA primers from okazaki fragments and fills up the gap due to its 5→3 polymerising activity. The important function of this enzyme is proofreading which includes polymerising activity and exonuclease activity (exonuclease activity means cleavage of nucleotides only at the end). DNA polymerase I consists of two fragments: (i) a larger fragment, called Klenow fragment, which contains 3′–5′ exonuclease activity with 5′–3′ polymerising activity and (ii) a smaller fragment which contains 5′–3′ exonuclease activity.

DNA Polymerase II

DNA Polymerase II resembles DNA polymerase I in its activity to bring about the growth in 5′–3′ direction, using free 3′-OH groups, but mainly uses duplexes with short gaps only. It can not use nicked duplexes. Although it has 3′–5′ exonuclease activity, It lacks 5′–3′ exonuclease activity. DNA polymerase II is not the replication enzyme, and is involved in DNA repair.

DNA Polymerase III

DNA Polymerase III (Pol III) is a hetero-multemeric enzyme with a molecular mass of about 900 KD in its complex or holoenzyme form. The core polymerase that has catalytic activity consists of three subunits: α-subunit (coded by *dnaE* gene) has 5′–3′ synthetic activity; ε (coded by *dnaQ* gene) has 3′–5′ exonuclease activity; and θ (coded by *holE* gene) is stimulator of the 3′–5′ exonuclease activity. The core enzyme which has the ability to synthesise DNA, consists of subunits α, β and θ. The τ subunit (coded by *dnaX* gene) is responsible for dimerisation of catalytic core and increased activity. The catalytic core synthesises rather short DNA strands because of its tendency to fall off the DNA template. In order to synthesise the long DNA molecules present in chromosomes, this frequent dissociation of the polymerase from the template must be eliminated. For this purpose two homodimers of the β subunit (coded by *dnaN* gene), provides the ring structure that encircles the replicating DNA molecule and allows DNA polymerase III to slide along the DNA while remaining tethered to it. The DNA polymerase III holoenzyme, which is responsible for the synthesis of both nascent DNA strands at a replication fork, contains at least 20 polypeptides. The structural complexity of the DNA polymerase III holoenzyme shows 16 of the best characterised polypeptides encoded by seven different genes.

DNA Gyrase/Topoisomerases

Two strands of a ds DNA are wound with each other in a spiral manner. Further, the DNA molecule is supercoiled under normal cellular conditions. It is, therefore, necessary to unwind the DNA, so that the two strands can be opened and form ss regions during the DNA replication. In order to get the DNA strands unwound, it will require to rotate at a speed of about 4500 rpm. The rotation will require a large amount of energy. The rotation of long strands of DNA at such a high speed can also cause mechanical shearing of the DNA. Thus the entire process will create an undesirable condition for the cell. This problem is overcome by the enzyme topoisomerase which opens the coiled turns by creating a small nick in one strand, letting the molecule uncoiled by one turn and closing the gap. The topoisomerases are of two types: (i) DNA topoisomerase I enzyme produce temporary single stranded break or nick in DNA and (ii) DNA topoisomerase II enzyme produce transient double stranded break in DNA. Type I topoisomerase are remarkable in that they don't require ATP to work, they bind covalently to the cut DNA strand storing the chemical energy of the phosphodiester bridge, which they then use to reseal the strand after the tension has been removed from the DNA. An important result of this difference is that topoisomerase I activities remove supercoils from DNA one at a time, whereas, topoisomerase II enzyme remove and introduce supercoils two at a time. The best characterised type II topoisomerase is an enzyme named DNA gyrase in *E. coli*. Gyrases or topoisomerases II is a tetramer with 2 α-subunits encoded by the gene *gyrA* and 2 β-subunits encoded by gene *gyrB*.

DNA Ligase

It can join two pieces of DNA by the formation of a phosphodiester bond between these molecules. For this, the two DNAs should have a free 3-OH and a 5-PO$_4$ groups respectively. It should be noted that the DNA ligase can only close a nick but cannot incorporate any new nucleotide to fill the gap. The enzyme is used to join the polypeptide fragments in the lagging strand during the DNA replication. DNA ligase catalyses the covalent closure of nicks in DNA molecules by using energy from NAD (Nicotiamide adenine dinucleotide) or ATP (Adenosine triphosphate).

Helicase

The enzyme also referred as unwinding protein. It is responsible for the melting of DNA and formation of ss DNA at the beginning of the replication fork. The major DNA replicative helicase in *E. coli* is the product of *dnaB* gene. DNA helicases unwind DNA molecules using energy derived from ATP. The active form of helicase is the homo-hexamer of a 330 KD protein.

Primase

It is a specific RNA polymerase which is responsible for the synthesis of a sequence specific RNA molecule which serves as the primer to initiate the DNA synthesis. This is a monomer of 66 KD and is the product of the gene DnaG. This enzyme is simpler and much smaller than the RNA polymerase involved in the transcription and is distinct from it.

Chapter 7

DNA Repair

INTRODUCTION

DNA repair is a collection of processes by which a cell identifies and corrects damage to the DNA molecules that encode its genome. In human cells, both normal metabolic activities and environmental factors such as radiation can cause DNA damage, resulting in as many as 1 million individual molecular lesions per cell per day. Many of these lesions cause structural damage to the DNA molecule and can alter or eliminate the cells ability to transcribe the gene that the affected DNA encodes. Other lesions induce potentially harmful mutations in the cells genome, which affect the survival of its daughter cells after it undergoes mitosis.

TYPES OF DAMAGE

A variety of defects can be present in DNA. These defects can be introduced by spontaneous *in situ* reactions, insults from external physical and chemical agents, and reaction with intermediates present during normal metabolism. In this chapter, we consider some representative examples of different types of damage, but a comprehensive list of all known varieties of damage is beyond the scope of this chapter.

Mismatches

Mismatches involve an incorrect base in one strand that does not pair correctly with a base in the other strand. Replication errors can result in the incorporation of an incorrect base into the new daughter strand. The replicating fork contains many accessory proteins in addition to the main polymerase that result in a great increase in the fidelity of replication. However, a few replication errors are still made and are left behind after replication. Spontaneous deamination of bases in DNA occurs at a low but significant rate. Two of the most frequent events are the deamination of cytosine to form uracil (which then codes like thymine) and the deamination of adenine to form hypoxanthine (which codes like guanine).

Missing Bases (AP Sites)

Missing bases in DNA, also called a basic or AP sites (AP is an abbreviation for both apurinic and apyrimidinic), are the result of cleavage of the bond linking the base to the deoxyribose in the sugar phosphate backbone of DNA. Such cleavage can occur spontaneously, most often in the case of purines, or after alkylation of the base which causes the bond linking the base to the sugar-phosphate backbone to become more labile. AP sites can also be formed in DNA as intermediates in the repair process when a DNA glycosylase removes a particular base from the backbone.

Altered Bases

Altered bases in DNA can be formed after irradiation with UV or ionising radiation and also as a consequence of exposure to certain chemicals. The effects of radiation can be direct, that is, a consequence of the interaction of the radiation directly with DNA, such as the formation of cyclobutane pyrimidine dimers after exposure of the DNA to UV light. Ionising radiation can cause alterations either directly by the direct deposition of energy in the DNA or indirectly by the action of reactive solvent species such as radiation-produced radicals and ions. DNA can also become damaged after reaction with a variety of chemicals. Some chemicals interact directly to damage DNA, while others may need to be converted to a more reactive species. In some cases, the cell is responsible for converting a chemical to an active form, while in other cases (such as psoralen and its relatives), the chemical is activated by light only after it has bound noncovalently to DNA. Other possible chemical sources for DNA damage come from the metabolic intermediates of the cell itself. For example, S-adenosylmethionine, the metabolic methyl donor, is able to transfer methyl groups to DNA. Intermediates in oxidative processes are capable of oxidising DNA bases to make them non-instructive or mutagenic, while some enzymes, such as DNA methylases, can cause deamination of cytosine to uracil under certain conditions.

Single-Strand Breaks

Single-strand breaks (and sugar damage that leads to breaks) can be introduced by several means, including ionising radiation, various chemicals, and attack by nucleases.

Double-Strand Breaks

Double-strand breaks can result from the chance occurrence of two single-strand breaks that occur close to each other in the complementary strands or can result from a single event, as in deposition by ionising radiation of a large amount of energy that is sufficient to break both strands.

Cross-links

Cross-linking of complementary strands occurs with some chemicals, particularly with bifunctional alkylating agents but also with some chemicals such as psoralen derivatives, which intercalate into the DNA backbone and have two reactive sites that react with pyrimidines in the complementary strands with high efficiency when the chemical is photoactivated. With the psoralens, the activating wavelength is longer than that absorbed by the DNA itself, so psoralen can be added to form monoadducts and cross-links with minimal other photodamage to the DNA when appropriate care is taken with the experimental protocol.

POSSIBLE STRATEGIES FOR DNA REPAIR

In principle, there are several strategies that cells could use to repair the effects of damage to DNA, and in fact, during evolution, *Escherichia coli* has accumulated a battery of responses that includes a variety of these possibilities. The simplest and most direct mechanism is reversal of the effects of the damage directly without otherwise altering the DNA structure. Two protein reactions that use this strategy are the methyltransferase activity on O^6-methylguanine (O^6-MeG), which removes the methyl to regenerate G in the DNA, and the photolyase reaction, which reverses cyclobutane pyrimidine dimers to regenerate the two original pyrimidines. Other repair or recovery processes use several different specific mechanisms to remove damaged segments from one strand and then utilise the redundancy of information in the two strands of DNA to reconstruct the original sequence by copying the undamaged strand. In other cases, the actual damaged portion may not need to be removed from the DNA molecule, recombinational exchanges can restore information to at least one strand of the DNA even though the correct information was previously absent from both strands.

DIRECT REVERSAL OF DAMAGE

Direct reversal of damage by repair proteins without any breakage of the sugar-phosphate backbone occurs in several cases.

DNA Repair Methyltransferase

DNA repair activity removes methyl groups from several specific sites in DNA, including O^6-MeG, O^4-MeT, and the methyl phosphotriesters that result from methylation of the phosphate in the sugar-phosphate backbone. This activity was first identified when the phenomenon of adaptation was studied in detail. During adaptation, exposure of cells to low concentrations of methylating agents (and other alkylating agents) causes the cells to develop resistance to the lethal and mutagenic effects of subsequent exposure to much higher amounts of the adapting agents. Biochemical studies revealed that the disappearance of O^6-MeG from the DNA accompanied this phenomenon. More extensive biochemical and genetic studies showed that during this process, a methyl group is actually transferred from the O^6-MeG in DNA to a specific 39-kDa protein, leaving behind a normal G in the DNA. Furthermore, this protein is also involved in the regulation of the adaptation response. The 39-kDa protein is the gene product of the *ada* gene and is designated *ada*. The role of *ada* in regulation is discussed in a later section. The *ada* protein has two domains that act as acceptors in methyltransferase reactions from methylated sites in DNA. The site to which a methyl is transferred from O^6-MeG in DNA is a cysteine (Cys-321) near the carboxyl terminus. In addition to this active site on the *ada* protein, the methyl group from methyl phosphotriesters in DNA can be transferred to a different site (Cys-69) in the *ada* protein near its amino terminus, and methylation of this amino-terminal site correlates with the function of *ada* as a transcriptional activator. An interesting property of the *ada* protein is that when a site on *ada* is methylated, the methyl group remains indefinitely. This means that the protein is used once for each site and does not recycle in the catalytic way that is typical for enzymes. Thus, to remove many methyl groups from DNA, a separate protein must be used for each methyl that is removed. (More precisely, each polypeptide can remove one methyl from an alkylated base and one methyl from a methyl phosphotriester, since the two methyl-accepting sites are separate and distinct in their locations and functions.) Because the transfer of the methyl group from DNA to *ada* is a one-way process in which the methyl remains permanently attached to *ada*, *ada* has been called a suicide DNA repair protein.

Recent studies have demonstrated the presence of a second DNA repair methyltransferase that removes methyl groups from O^6-MeG of the DNA of cells in which the *ada* gene has been inactivated by mutation. This protein is now known to be the gene product of the *ogt* gene (shorthand for DNA O^6-MeG transferase), which has been identified and mapped at min 30.1 on the *E. coli* chromosome. In contrast to the regulation of *ada*, the expression of *ogt* is constitutive, with no apparent activators or repressors known to be involved in its transcription.

Cyclobutane Dimer Photolyase (Photoreactivating Enzyme)

Another reaction in *E. coli* that operates by the direct reversal of damage in the DNA is that of the DNA photolyase. The substrates for DNA photolyase are *cis-syn* cyclobutane pyrimidine dimers (Pyr<>Pyr) that are formed in UV-irradiated DNA in which two pyrimidines are adjacent in the same strand. A large number of careful, detailed studies have shown quite clearly how this enzyme works. The *E. coli* DNA photolyase is a monomeric polypeptide of 471 amino acids (54 kDa). Two essential non-covalent cofactors that are also chromophores (flavin adenine dinucleotide and methenyltetrahydrofolate) play key roles in its action. Photolyase attaches to the DNA substrate in the dark. Upon exposure to light of the appropriate activating wavelength (350 to 500 nm), methylenetetrahydrofolate absorbs energy from the light and transfers energy to the reduced flavin adenine dinucleotide by dipole-dipole interaction. This activated intermediate then transfers an electron to the Pyr<>Pyr to split it. Further electron transfers then restore the original pyrimidines and regenerate the original form of the DNA photolyase enzyme. This polypeptide, in contrast to the DNA methyltransferase, recycles many times and operates in the typical catalytic mode that is familiar for most enzymes.

BASE EXCISION REPAIR

Base excision repair is a repair process that begins when a damaged base is removed through the action of a DNA *N*-glycosylase that cuts the bond linking the base to the sugar-phosphate backbone of DNA (Fig. 7.1). This a basic (AP) site is then further processed by an AP endonuclease to cut the sugar-phosphate backbone. Some DNA *N*-glycosylases (uracil DNA *N*-glycosylase) have only glycosylase activity, while others, such as endonuclease III and MutM (formamidopyrimidine [Fapy]) glycosylase, have an associated AP endonuclease activity that is an integral part of the same polypeptide chain. After nuclease activity has cleaned up the ends, the small gap that remains is filled by a DNA polymerase, ligation of the ends then completes the base excision repair cycle. The specificity in this repair pathway is determined by the properties of the particular DNA *N*-glycosylase that initiates the process. A battery of different glycosylases provides the cell with the ability to recognise and repair many of the most common alterations in DNA. Some of these DNA *N*-glycosylases (particularly uracil DNA *N*-glycosylase) are highly specific for a particular substrate, while others (Fapy glycosylase and endonuclease III) have a wider range of substrates that includes several different damaged bases. Several years ago, researchers anticipated finding many different glycosylases with high specificities for their substrates, but it is now recognised that some of the enzymes act on multiple substrates, so these various activities are actually performed by a relatively small number of separate DNA *N*-glycosylases.

Glycosylases

Uracil DNA N-Glycosylase: Uracil is produced in DNA by deamination of cytosine and is removed by uracil DNA *N*-glycosylase (Fig. 7.1), the product of the *ung* gene. This enzyme is very specific for U as a substrate. As mentioned above, this enzyme is a simple glycosylase and does not have associated AP endonuclease or lyase activity.

Tag (3-MeA DNA Glycosylase I) and alkA (3-MeA DNA Glycosylase II): Alkylation products in DNA are substrates for at least two different 3-MeA DNA glycosylases that are products of the *tag* and *alkA* genes. Tag has greater selectivity than *alkA*, removing 3-MeA much better than 3-MeG, while *alkA* has a broader specificity and removes them both quite efficiently. *alkA* is also known to remove hypoxanthine from DNA. (Hypoxanthine is a mutagenic product formed by deamination of A.) The expression of the *tag* gene is constitutive, while the *alkA* gene product is under the control of *ada*. This

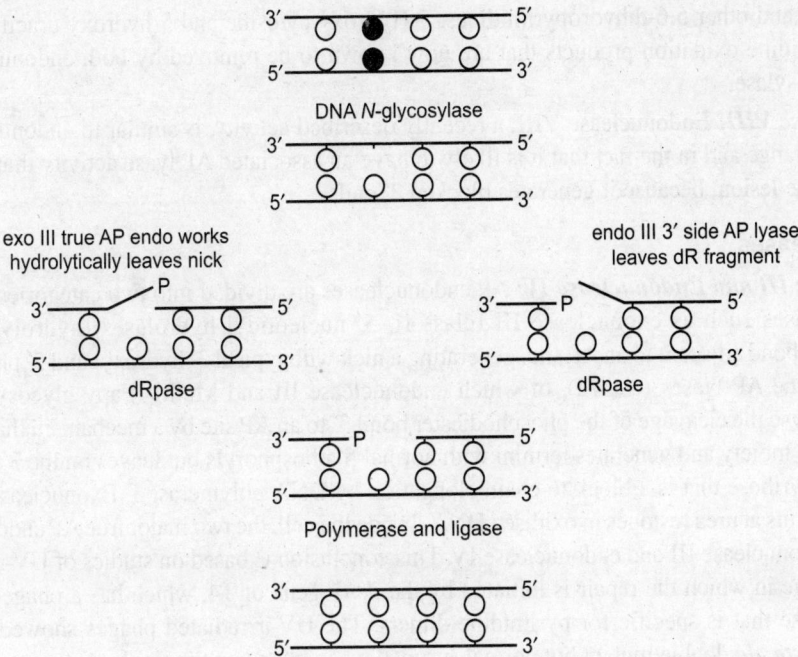

Fig. 7.1: Base excision repair. A DNA N-glycosylase starts the process by removing a base. Some glycosylases have associated AP endonuclease (lyase) activities, while others do not and require the action of a separate true AP endonuclease such as exonuclease III or endonuclease IV. dR, deoxyribose, dRpase, deoxyribophosphodiesterase

coordinated expression of *alkA* and *ada* is noteworthy in that the two gene products repair different types of alkylation damage by different mechanisms. The linked regulation of these two proteins thus optimises the repair of several diverse lesions that are likely to be formed in DNA by a single alkylating agent.

Glycosylases with Associated AP Endonuclease (Lyase) Activities

MutM (Fapy) Glycosylase: Oxidative damage to purines and pyrimidines is a consequence of exposure to metabolic intermediates and certain other chemicals as well as exposure to radicals produced by ionising radiation. Two proteins, Fapy glycosylase and endonuclease III, are glycosylases with associated AP endonuclease activities that remove many of the most significant oxidative lesions. Although there is some overlap in the substrates of the two proteins, endonuclease III acts primarily on pyrimidine products, while Fapy glycosylase acts primarily on damaged purines. Fapy is formed when the imidazole ring of a damaged purine is opened. Fapy DNA glycosylase is known by various names, including 8-oxoguanine (8-oxoG) DNA glycosylase, Fapy glycosylase, FPG protein, and MutM protein. It has *N*-glycosylase activity that releases 8-oxoG and Fapy from oxidatively damaged DNA. (Fapy is a purine oxidation product in which the five-member ring has been opened.) This enzyme also releases 5-hydroxy cytosine and 5-hydroxy uracil, common pyrimidine oxidation products that are now known to be removed by endonuclease III as well as by Fapy glycosylase.

Endonuclease III: Endonuclease III was originally identified as an enzyme that cut DNA irradiated with high fluences of UV light. It is now known that endonuclease III acts as a DNA glycosylase on pyrimidine derivatives with rings that are saturated, contracted, and rearranged. These derivatives include thymine glycol and other 5,6-dihydropyrimidines. 5-Hydroxy cytosine and 5-hydroxy uracil are other common pyrimidine oxidation products that are now known to be removed by both endonuclease III and Fapy glycosylase.

Endonuclease VIII: Endonuclease VIII, a recently described activity, is similar to endonuclease III in its substrate range and in the fact that it is likely to have an associated AP lyase activity that nicks on the 3′ side of the lesion, because it generates blocked 3′ ends.

AP Endonucleases

Exonuclease III and Endonuclease IV: AP endonucleases are divided into two categories: the true AP endonucleases such as exonuclease III (class II, 5′ nucleotidyl hydrolases) hydrolyse the 5′ phosphodiester bond adjacent to an AP site, generating a nick with typical 3′ hydroxyl and 5′ phosphoryl termini, while the AP lyases (class I), of which endonuclease III and MutM (Fapy glycosylase) are examples, catalyse the cleavage of the phosphodiester bond 3′ to an AP site by a mechanism that cleaves the deoxyribose moiety and generates termini with normal 5′ phosphoryls but leaves on the 3′ end only an altered deoxyribose that is a block to chain elongation by DNA polymerase I. Exonuclease III also recognises and cuts at urea residues in oxidised DNA. Inside the cell, the two major true AP endonuclease activities are exonuclease III and endonuclease IV. This conclusion is based on studies of UV-irradiated T4 bacteriophage in which the repair is initiated by the *denV* gene of T4, which has a phage-encoded DNA glycosylase that is specific for pyrimidine dimers. The UV-irrradiated phages showed reduced survival on the *xth nfo* double mutant but normal survival when plated on the single mutants, indicating that either protein provided enough activity for optimal survival.

The deoxyribose fragment left at the end of a strand by the action of an AP endonuclease or AP lyase needs processing, because it is a block for gap filling by a DNA polymerase. An activity that removes this a basic residue was described by Franklin and Lindahl and named DNA deoxyribophosphodiesterase. In subsequent studies, the two groups attempting to assign this activity to a specific enzyme came to different conclusions. Sandigursky and Franklin assigned this activity to exonuclease I, while Dianov and others reported that the deoxyribophosphodiesterase is associated with the RecJ protein.

SoxRS control of endonuclease IV: A number of functions that are responsive to oxidative stress are under *SoxRS* control. Of these, *nfo,* the structural gene for endonuclease IV, is the only one that is directly concerned with DNA repair. The regulatory control is complex in that *SoxR* is produced constitutively and senses the redox state of the cell by a mechanism that is only vaguely understood. Under conditions of oxidative stress, *SoxR* becomes a transcriptional activator of *soxS,* whose gene product in turn activates the *nfo* gene to increase the synthesis of endonuclease IV.

GO (OXIDISED GUANINE) REPAIR

Oxidised guanines must be a significant problem for the cell, as evidenced by the fact that *E. coli* has devised a multifaceted approach for dealing with the products of guanine oxidation (Fig. 7.2). This approach has been called the GO system and includes two different glycosylases (MutY adenine glycosylase and MutM Fapy glycosylase) along with MutT, a novel 8-oxoguaninedeoxyribotriphosphatase (8-oxodGTPase) that acts to cleanse the precursor pool. Oxidised guanine precursors of DNA can be misincorporated into DNA opposite A during DNA replication. To decrease this probability, the cells have developed a particular enzyme, the MutT protein, that converts 8-oxodGTP to the monophosphate form before it becomes incorporated into DNA. When a G in DNA is oxidised to 8-oxoG, this altered base is a substrate for the glycosylase that is the product of the *mutM* gene. This protein is known by

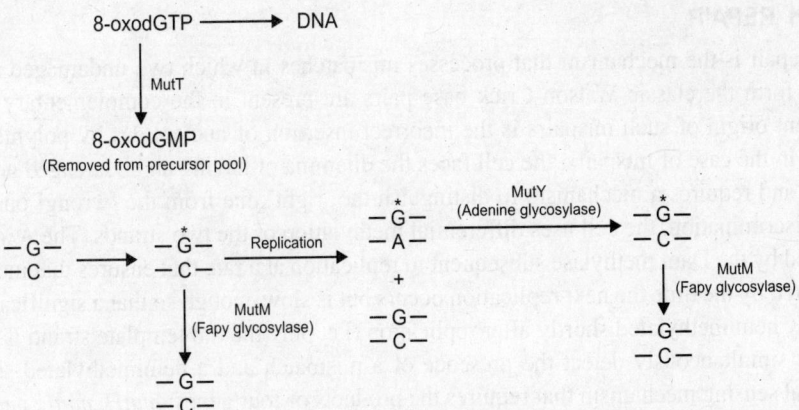

Fig. 7.2: GO system for repair of oxidised G. Several enzyme activities work in concert to over-come the effects of guanine oxidation on different stages, including the precursor pool and double-stranded DNA, before and after replication.

various names, including Fapy glycosylase, Fapy DNA glycosylase, 8-oxoG DNA glycosylase, FPG protein, and MutM protein. It has *N*-glycosylase activity that releases 8-oxoG and Fapy from oxidatively damaged DNA. This protein is one of those glycosylases that also has an associated AP endonuclease activity that cuts the phosphodiester backbone. Exonuclease processing of the gap generated by MutM creates a substrate that can then be restored with DNA polymerase and ligase. Replication of a template with 8-oxoG can result in the significant misincorporation of A opposite the 8-oxoG. In yet another strategy for coping with the consequences of guanine oxidation, *E. coli* has an additional enzyme, the MutY protein, which is an adenine DNA glycosylase with associated AP lyase that acts to remove the A from DNA structures containing mismatches of A with 8-oxoG. Repair of this structure results in the formation of a structure with C paired with 8-oxoG, which is the substrate for the MutM glycosylase. This system is fascinating because it demonstrates the response of the cell to damage in the DNA precursors, in the DNA itself, and in the aberrant products resulting from the replication of DNA with the oxidised guanine lesion.

STRAND BREAK REPAIR

Many of the single-strand breaks introduced by X irradiation are repaired very rapidly with a half-life of a few seconds, as in the joining of newly synthesised Okazaki fragments into longer DNA molecules. Thus, when there is no intrinsic block to joining, repair of single-strand breaks is very rapid and is carried out by DNA polymerase I and DNA ligase. Most breaks made by X rays are more complex and may even be formed indirectly as a consequence of chemical or enzymatic conversion of other radiation products. Several of the most common single-strand breaks inferred to be present after irradiation have been studied in a φX174 replicative-form transfecting DNA model system. Ligatable nicks with 3′ hydroxyl and 5′ phosphate termini were not lethal. Other breaks were made from substrates with thymine glycols, urea residues, or a basic (AP) sites by treatment with endonuclease III to generate a single-strand nick with a 3′ α,β- unsaturated aldehyde (4-hydroxy-2-pentenal). Single-strand breaks with a 5′ deoxyribose or a 5′ deoxyribosylurea were made by treating the AP or urea substrates with endonuclease IV. These enzymegenerated breaks had inactivation efficiencies of 0.12 to 0.14, which is similar to the inactivation of the damaged molecules without the enzyme treatment.

MISMATCH REPAIR

Mismatch repair is the mechanism that processes mismatches in which two undamaged normal bases that cannot form the classic Watson-Crick base pairs are present in the complementary strands. The most frequent origin of such mispairs is the incorrect insertion of nucleotides by polymerases during replication. In the case of mispairs, the cell faces the dilemma of having an undamaged normal base in each strand and requires a mechanism to distinguish the 'right' one from the 'wrong' one. In order to make this discrimination, the cell uses differential methylation of the two strands. The A in GATC sites is methylated by the Dam methylase subsequent to replication at a rate that ensures that most or all sites are methylated by the time the next replication occurs but is slow enough so that a significant number of sites are only hemimethylated shortly after replication (i.e. only the old template strand is methylated).

The cells simultaneously detect the presence of a mismatch and a hemimethylated site through a complex dual sensing mechanism that requires the products of four genes: *mutH, mutL, mutS,* and *uvrD* (alternately named *mutU,* whose gene product UvrD is also known to be helicase II). The first step is the detection of a mismatch through the binding of MutS to the mismatch. MutL then binds and in some way activates MutH endonuclease activity, which interacts with hemimethylated sites to cut the unmethylated strand at the GATC site. Unidirectional exonucleolytic degradation from the cut toward and past the mismatch results in preferential removal of the mismatched nucleotide from the undermethylated (i.e. the newly replicated) strand. The specific enzymes participating in this exonucleolytic degradation depend on the orientation of the cleaved GATC site relative to the mismatch. When the cut at the GATC site is on the 5′ side of the mismatch, exonuclease VII or RecJ provides the exonuclease function, in the other case, when the cut at the GATC site is 3′ to the mismatch, exonuclease I does the digestion. In either case, the degraded strand (which may be as long as several kilobases) is replaced by using DNA polymerase III holoenzyme and single-strand binding protein, with repair being completed by ligation of the resulting nick by DNA ligase. This mechanism ensures that the information retained at the site of a mismatch will be that of the old original strand and that the incorrect nucleotide inserted at replication will be the one removed, thus maintaining the correct DNA sequence (Fig. 7.3).

MutS and MutL proteins also reduce recombination between related DNAs that are not exactly homologous, and they account for much of the barrier to genetic exchange between related organisms such as *E. coli* and *Salmonella* spp. This phenomenon has been studied in a cell-free system with purified components, including MutS, MutL, and RecA, where it was demonstrated that MutS and MutL greatly reduce the strand exchange between molecules with several percent mismatches but do not inhibit the exchange of completely homologous DNAs. Presumably, the binding of MutS and MutL to mismatches effectively blocks the orderly exchange of strands by RecA.

VSP REPAIR

VSP (very short patch) repair (Fig. 7.4) operates on the specific sequences -CC(A/T)GG-, in which the second cytosine is methylated at position 5 by Dcm. When 5-MeCs are deaminated, they are converted to thymine. Consequently, they are not recognised by uracil glycosylase, the enzyme that recognises and removes uracils that are formed during deamination of normal unmethylated cytosine. The VSP system specifically recognises thymine-guanine mismatches in the sequence context that is the substrate for methylation of C by the Dcm methylase and then repairs the thymine-containing strand by a combination of Vsr endonuclease (the *vsr* gene product), repair synthesis, and ligation that results in a replacement patch of only several nucleotides, accounting for the term 'very short patch repair.' The Vsr nuclease provides the specificity in this reaction, causing incision only on the 5′ side of the T in the

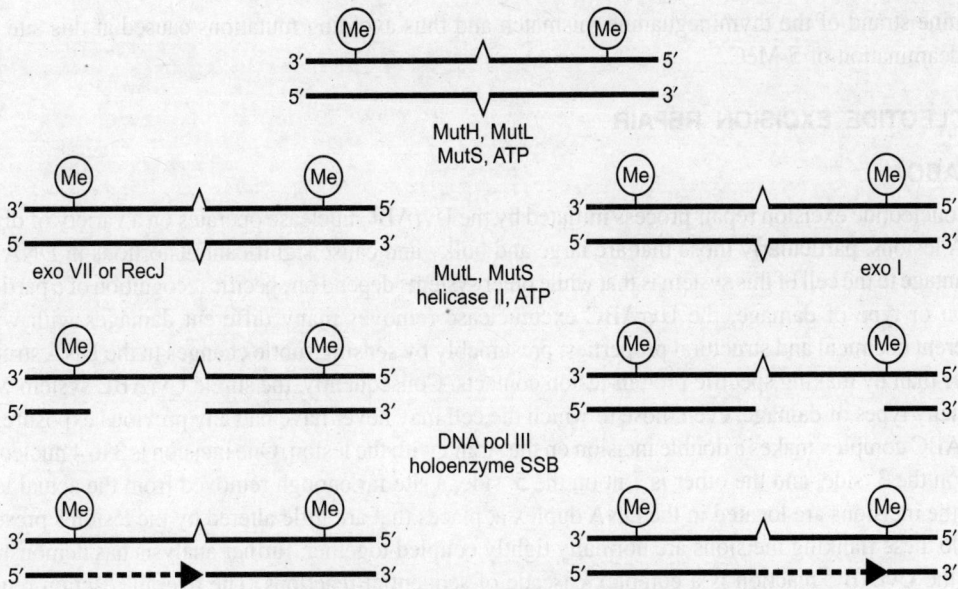

Fig. 7.3: Mechanism of methyl-directed mismatch repair.

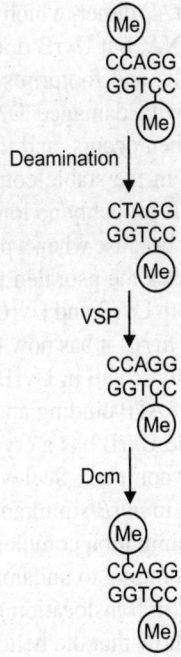

Fig. 7.4: VSP repair of mismatches resulting from the conversion of 5-MeC to T by deamination. This is a specialised repair process that occurs in sequences where cytosine is methylated because of its presence in the Dcm recognition sequence. (Deamination of cytosines in other sequences converts them to U, the substrate for uracil glycosylase.) The specificity is provided by the VSR nuclease, which makes a strand-specific cut immediately 5′ to the T in the TG mismatch.

thymine strand of the thymineguanine mismatch and thus avoiding mutations caused at this site from the deamination of 5-MeC.

NUCLEOTIDE EXCISION REPAIR

UvrABC

The nucleotide excision repair process initiated by the UvrABC nuclease operates on a variety of diverse DNA lesions, particularly those that are large and bulky and cause significant distortions in DNA. The advantage to the cell of this system is that while other systems depend on specific recognition of a particular lesion or type of damage, the UvrABC excinuclease removes many different damages with widely different chemical and structural properties, presumably by sensing subtle changes in the DNA structure rather than by making specific protein-lesion contacts. Consequently, the single UvrABC system works on many types of damage, even those to which the cell may never have had any previous exposure. The UvrABC complex makes a double incision on the strand with the lesion. One incision is 3 to 4 nucleotides (nt) on the 3′ side, and the other is 7 nt on the 5′ side, a site far enough removed from the actual lesion that the incisions are located in the DNA duplex at places that are little altered by the lesion's presence. While these flanking incisions are normally tightly coupled together, further analysis has demonstrated that the UvrABC reaction is a complex cascade of sequential reactions. The overall reaction requires ATP, and much is now known about individual steps that require ATP binding and/or hydrolysis, although interpretation is complicated by the fact that UvrA has multiple nucleotide-binding motifs and UvrB has only one. UvrA dimerises to form a UvrA2 dimer, which then interacts with UvrB to form a UvrA2B complex. UvrA by itself has affinity for DNA, but UvrB does not bind to DNA unless UvrA is present. UvrA has the ability to interact specifically, and footprints at damaged sites are observed with UvrA alone. However, tight, stable complexes with damaged DNA are formed only when both UvrA and UvrB are present. Interaction with UvrC then occurs, and the dual incision takes place.

Studies by Shi and others indicate that in the stable complex formed in the presence of UvrA and UvrB, the DNA is sharply bent, and UvrA is probably no longer present. In this complex, UvrB must be in very close proximity to the damaged site, because when a psoralen monoadduct is used as the substrate, subsequent exposure to near-UV light causes the psoralen monoadduct to be photocross-linked to the UvrB protein. The dual incisions require both UvrB and UvrC and are normally tightly coupled. Through the use of site-specific mutants in *uvrB* and *uvrC,* it has now been concluded that the first incision occurs on the 3′ side of the lesion and uses a catalytic site in UvrB, while the second incision, on the 5′ side, utilises a catalytic site in UvrC. The role of ATP binding and hydrolysis is complex, because UvrA has multiple nucleotide-binding domains, while UvrB has a cryptic ATPase activity that is associated with a limited helicase activity of the UvrA2B complex. Seeley and Grossman observed that site-specific mutagenesis of the nucleotide-binding site in *uvrB* simultaneously inactivates the helicase activity and prevents the formation of tight specific preinitiation complexes with damaged DNA but does not affect formation of the UvrA2B complex and its binding to undamaged DNA. Although it has been suggested that this helicase activity may be involved in translocation of the UvrA2B complex along undamaged DNA searching for lesions, other studies show that the helicase activity is very limited in the length of oligonucleotide that can be released. This activity may thus be a very localised action in which the complex is flexing and probing the DNA to determine whether there is a lesion present and then, if there is, to correctly assemble the components in preparation for incision. The localised bending and unwinding of DNA associated with locating the lesion and precisely loading UvrB may account for the observed separation of positive and negative domains when UvrA and UvrB act on supercoiled DNA.

How Does UvrABC Recognise a Substrate?

Although it is clear that many repair enzymes such as the alkyltransferases, DNA photolyase, and the DNA glycosylases 'recognise' their substrates by interacting with them in highly specific protein-lesion contacts, the variety of lesions recognised by the UvrABC system requires a much different process. Although the UvrABC system is the only system for removing a variety of bulky DNA adducts, other types of damage that are handled by some of the other more specific systems can also be removed by UvrABC, and it has been suggested that UvrABC actually 'repairs everything'. Since a static interaction of protein with substrate seems inadequate to account for the wide variety of substrates utilised by UvrABC, it was suggested that recognition of lesions might require a more active process in which UvrAB flexes and distorts DNA while looking for an atypical response, much as a physician flexes an injured limb while checking on its range of motion. The results showing the extreme bending of DNA in the UvrB complex are consistent with this expectation. Snowden and Van Houten observed that the formation of the stable UvrAB complex at a damaged site is the limiting step for incision. However, with a psoralen DNA cross-link and with cisplatin DNA adducts, other steps later in the reaction sequence can be rate limiting for incision. A model for the overall reaction cascade is presented in Fig. 7.5.

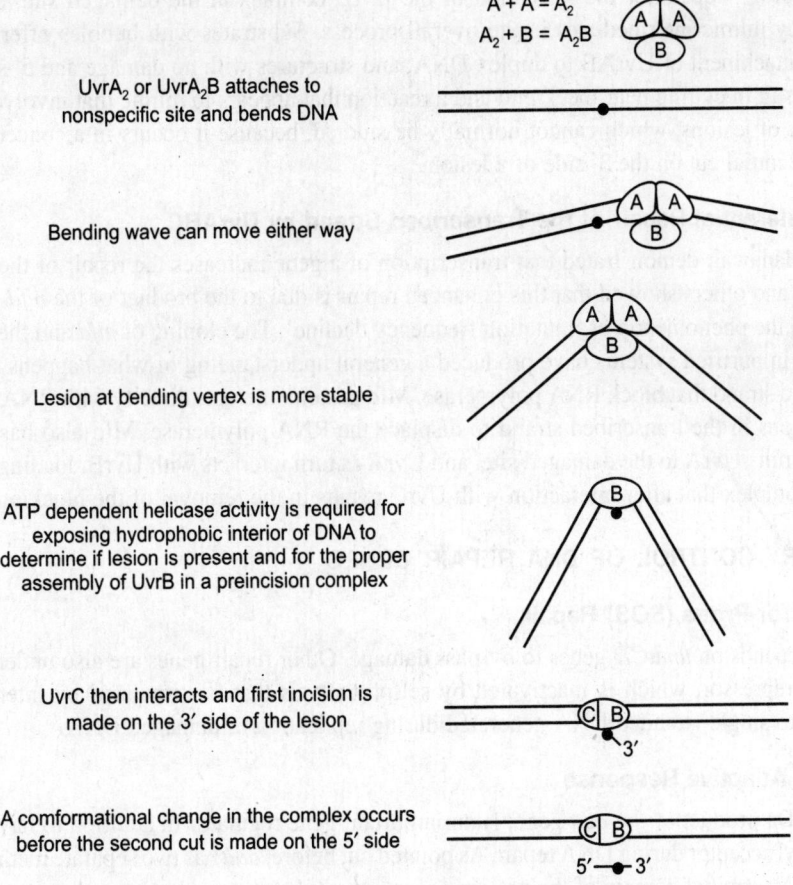

$$A + A = A_2$$
$$A_2 + B = A_2B$$

UvrA$_2$ or UvrA$_2$B attaches to nonspecific site and bends DNA

Bending wave can move either way

Lesion at bending vertex is more stable

ATP dependent helicase activity is required for exposing hydrophobic interior of DNA to determine if lesion is present and for the proper assembly of UvrB in a preincision complex

UvrC then interacts and first incision is made on the 3' side of the lesion

A comformational change in the complex occurs before the second cut is made on the 5' side

Fig. 7.5: Nucleotide excision repair: UvrABC mechanism.

The overall specificity and selection for substrates are determined by the net contribution of all the various individual steps, not by one single highly selective reaction. This can account for the high selectivity of the overall process, which is greater than the selectivity at any one specific step, presumably because different parameters of the structure can be tested at different stages. For example, the parameter being tested at the first step might be the presence of a 'weak' place in the helix that allows the helix to be bent or deformed at a particular site. Subsequent steps involving the UvrAB probing of a limited region might then provide a higher-resolution test to determine whether there actually is at that position a lesion that can be converted into a complex suitable for incision. For example, after comparing results for model substrates containing a bulky lesion (AAF) that is a particularly good substrate for incision with results for a substrate containing a mismatch that is incised very infrequently if at all, Gordienko and Rupp (unpublished data) suggested that while both substrates can initially be recognised by UvrA2B, the reaction cascade with the AAF substrate proceeds well, while the reaction with the mismatch is usually aborted and only rarely proceeds to successful incision. With a psoralen monoadduct, the cascade proceeds through incision, with a psoralen cross-link, a similar stable complex is formed in the presence of UvrA and UvrB, and in the presence of UvrC, incision was inefficient in relaxed DNA but rapid when the DNA was negatively supercoiled. Visse and others also noted with cisplatin adducts that there were rate-limiting steps after the formation of the UvrB complex at the damaged site. Some model substrates may mimic intermediates in the overall process. Substrates with bubbles offer preferential sites for the attachment of UvrAB to duplex DNA, and structures with no damage and 5' single-strand extensions result in cutting near the 3' end and a reaction that appears to mimic that involved in cutting on the 5' side of lesions, which cannot normally be studied, because it occurs in a concerted reaction following the initial cut on the 3' side of a lesion.

Mfd and Preferential Repair of the Transcribed Strand by UvrABC

Mellon and Hanawalt demonstrated that transcription of a gene increases the repair of the transcribed strand. Selby and others showed that this enhanced repair is due to the product of the *mfd* gene, which is involved in the phenomenon of 'mutation frequency decline'. The cloning of *mfd* and the study of its gene product in purified systems have produced a general understanding of what happens at lesions in the transcribed strand that block RNA polymerase. Mfd protein interacts directly with RNA polymerase stalled at lesions in the transcribed strand to displace the RNA polymerase. Mfd also has affinity for UvrA and recruits UvrA to the damaged site, and UvrA in turn interacts with UvrB, loading it to form a preincision complex that after interaction with UvrC results in the removal of the blocking lesion.

REGULATORY CONTROL OF DNA REPAIR GENES

Inducible Error-Prone (SOS) Repair

SOS repair depends on *umuCD* genes to by-pass damage. Other repair genes are also under the control of the LexA repressor, which is inactivated by selfproteolysis that is stimulated by interaction with RecA bound to single-stranded DNA generated during replication of damaged DNA.

ada and the Adaptive Response

ada, the 39-kDa product of the *ada* gene, is an important gene regulator in addition to having a direct role as a methyl acceptor during DNA repair. As pointed out before, *ada* has two separate methylaccepting domains: the *N*-terminal domain of the protein accepts methyls from methyl-phosphotriesters in DNA, while the C-terminal domain contains the site that receives the methyls transferred from the alkylated DNA bases O6-MeG and O4-MeT. The *N*-terminal domain of *ada* is now known to be the part of the protein most important for the regulatory activity in modifying transcription (Fig. 7.6). When the Nterminal domain of *ada* is methylated as a consequence of its methyltransferase activity acting on DNA phosphotriesters, *ada* becomes a transcriptional activator for its own gene *ada* and also for the *alkA* gene, which codes for the synthesis of 3-MeA DNA glycosylase II. The methylated *ada* protein binds to a regulatory sequence, designated the *ada* box, that precedes the regulated genes. (*ada* protein that is not methylated at Cys-69 in its *N*-terminal domain binds much less strongly to the *ada* box.) Interaction of the bound *ada* with RNA polymerase increases transcription of the gene, thus increasing the synthesis of the gene products *ada* and *alkA*.

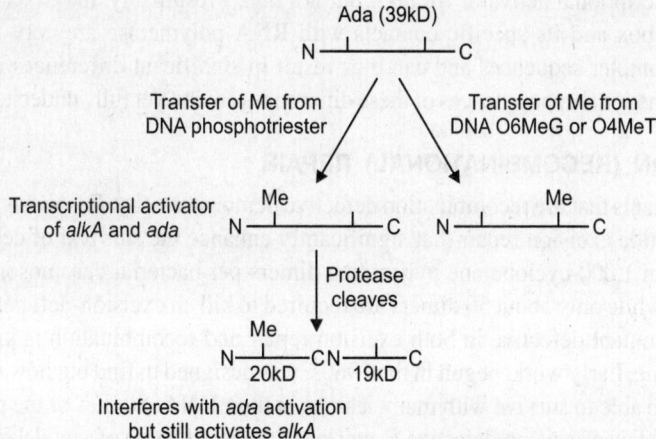

Fig. 7.6: Methylation of Ada and regulation of transcription. Methyl groups from DNA are transferred to either Cys-69 or Cys-321 of the Ada protein. The Omp T protease cleaves Ada, but this reaction is not believed to be physiologically relevant, although it has been useful in studying the mechanism by which methylation of Ada converts Ada to a transcriptional activator.

This mechanism explains the induction of these genes after their exposure to methylating agents. However, there is a conceptual problem in a mechanism for turning off the induction, because the *ada* transmethylase activity is not catalytic but instead is a unidirectional 'suicidal' process in which the protein that receives a methyl group apparently retains that methyl group indefinitely and would thus be expected to continue stimulating expression even when all methyl lesions are removed from the DNA. An observation of a cellular protease activity that cleaves *ada* near the middle seemed to provide a possible solution to this regulatory challenge. The protease cleavage generates two similarly sized fragments of *ada*: a 20-kDa fragment from the *N*-terminal end and a 19-kDa fragment from the C terminus. The methylated *N*-terminal 20-kDa fragment still binds to *ada* boxes, but when the fragment is bound to the regulatory region of the *ada* gene, it does not activate transcription but actually interferes with the activation observed with the intact 39-kDa *ada* methylated in its *N*-terminal domain. Protease cleavage of the methylated *ada* thus might explain how synthesis of *ada* is turned off when repair of methylated DNA is complete and *ada* is no longer needed. However, subsequent studies showed that the cleavage of *ada* is due to OmpT, a protease found in the outer membrane. Since intracellular *ada* is not accessible to OmpT, OmpT does not provide a physiological route for turning off the expression of those genes activated by methylated *ada*. An alternate possibility for a regulatory loop comes from recent studies by Saget and Walker. Their experiments confirm that the methylation of Cys-69 in the *N*-terminal region of *ada* by methyl transfer from a DNA methyl phosphotriester is the critical step in generating the transcription activator for binding to the *ada* box in the *ada* promoter. However, their results indicate that *ada* that is not methylated at Cys-69 does bind weakly to the *ada* box and that at concentrations that are physiologically significant, such *ada* interferes with the transcriptional activation of the *ada* gene. Thus, in this scenario, large quantities of unmethylated *ada* could turn off the continued synthesis of itself, even though methylated *ada* remained in the cell.

The regulation of the *alkA* gene by *ada* differs in some details but resembles the regulation of *ada* in that methylated *ada* is a transcriptional activator. For example, the methylated 20-kDa *N*-terminal product of *ada* acts as a transcriptional activator for *alkA* but not *ada*. Presumably, the exact positioning of the activator at the *ada* box and its specific contacts with RNA polymerase are very sensitive to slight differences in the promoter sequences and can thus result in significant differences in its activation of the two genes. The functional consequences of these differences are not yet fully understood or appreciated.

POST-REPLICATION (RECOMBINATIONAL) REPAIR

The properties of mutants that are recombination defective demonstrate that *E. coli* has other mechanisms in addition to nucleotide excision repair that significantly enhance the survival of cells exposed to UV irradiation. More than 1,000 cyclobutane pyrimidine dimers per bacterial chromosome are required to kill a wild-type cell, while only about 50 dimers are required to kill an excision-deficient cell. In contrast, a *uvrA recA* double mutant defective in both excision repair and recombination is killed by about one lesion per chromosome. Early work, begun in the 1960s, was designed to find out how excision-defective strains of *E. coli* were able to survive with many lesions in their DNA. Studies of the properties of DNA synthesised in UV-irradiated excision-defective *E. coli* led to the formulation of a model for recombinational repair, which was summarised in a review by the Sancars (with the assistance of Paul Howard-Flanders) as follows.

When the polymerase encounters certain nucleotideadducts, such as pyrimidine dimers, it stops replicating and reinitiates about 1000 bp beyond the adduct, thus generating a single-stranded gap that contains a modified nucleotide. This discontinuity or post-replication gap is filled in by the RecA protein, which transfers the complementarystr and from the sister duplex into the gap. This model, which was formulated for *E. coli* two decades agoremains essentially unchanged.

In this section, the focus is on events that occur at a replicating fork when a blocking lesion is present in the template DNA, because those structures initially generated during replication play a key role in repair, mutagenesis, and SOS induction. Many recent studies have led to impressive advances in our understanding of details of the enzymology of DNA replication that could not even have been imagined when the early whole-cell studies were done. Of particular mechanistic interest is the case in which the lesion is on the strand being used as the template for synthesis of the leading strand. Information that may be relevant to this situation has been compiled from a variety of sources, including studies with whole cells and with purified enzyme systems.

Replication Generates Daughter Strand Gaps

From sedimentation of newly synthesised DNA through alkaline sucrose gradients, it was estimated that the lengths of the new strands were similar to the distances between pyrimidine dimers in the template strands. From the amount of radioactivity incorporated, it was calculated that the number of pieces synthesised was much larger than the number of active growing forks. Using the straightforward assumption that these pieces were generated at pre-existing active forks, it followed that replicating forks had proceeded past many lesions in the template strands. The accuracy of the molecular weight estimates obtained from the distribution of radioactivity in alkaline sucrose gradients can legitimately be questioned. (In fact, after the relation between counts, sedimentation velocity, and number- or weight-average molecular weights had been derived, it was a surprise to find that the experimentally determined sizes of the newly replicated DNA agreed as well as they did with the number of lesions in the template strands and with the theoretically calculated curve. This agreement is probably a consequence of the labelling time of 1 to 10 min. Whereas Okazaki fragments are joined with a half-life of a few seconds, these fragments synthesised in UV-irradiated cells are joined with a half-life of about 15 to 20 min.) Although there may be some error in the experimentally determined sizes of these fragments, the error is almost certainly substantially less than a factor of 2. Even more significant, there was no indication of the bimodal distribution that would result from the presence of two discrete molecular weight populations, which would be expected if one strand were synthesised continuously and the other strand were synthesised in small pieces. While this result argues strongly against the continuous synthesis of either strand, it does not rule out the possibility that direct by-pass synthesis might occur at a low frequency (<10%). (Other investigators have sometimes observed various extents of a small, second, faster-sedimenting peak or shoulder in the newly synthesised DNA, but this peak is most likely due to early repair rather than to continuous by-pass. This faster-sedimenting shoulder is not seen in *recA* mutant cells. The experiments of Ganesan clearly demonstrated that the fast-sedimenting shoulder of newly synthesised DNA contains material formed by recombinational exchanges with the parental strand and is therefore not likely to be due to *de novo* synthesis of a continuous new strand.)

Inhibition of DNA Synthesis by UV Irradiation: Inhibition Is Not Equivalent to a Stalled Replication Fork

Although the usual plots, particularly in wild-type repair-proficient cells, can give the impression that DNA synthesis comes to a rapid and complete stop after UV irradiation, closer analysis shows that this is not the case. Inhibition of DNA synthesis is a continuous function of UV exposure. Under conditions in which incorporation continues at low levels for minutes or even hours, it can readily be calculated that every replication fork advancing through duplex DNA at the normal rate of 1,000 bp/s will contact a template strand lesion within a few seconds. These results are not explained satisfactorily by models in which a replication fork is proceeding at a normal rate until it reaches a lesion (either the first lesion or a particular subset of lesions) and then comes to a complete stop, but are more consistent with a model in which replication forks are slowed but not stopped. Although the analysis is complicated by DNA breakdown, DNA synthesis in *uvrA recA* cells also continues past many lesions. It is thus clear that in *uvrA recA* cells, a simple measure of the incorporation of label into DNA significantly underestimates the actual extent of synthesis, because of concurrent breakdown. The interpretation of these results is that the primary problem in *recA* cells is not in getting the replication complex to pass template strand lesions but in the subsequent processing of those structures that are present as a consequence of the replication fork having already passed a significant number of lesions.

Newly Synthesised DNA in UV-Irradiated Cells Is Associated with Single-Stranded Regions

In order to search for and quantitate single-stranded regions associated with newly replicated DNA, a column method that separated DNA molecules as a function of the degree of single strandedness was developed. This method was used to estimate that the DNA synthesised shortly after UV irradiation had single-stranded regions that corresponded roughly to the size of an Okazaki fragment for each lesion in the template strand. In addition, these data also showed that the interruptions in the newly synthesised strands observed previously in alkaline sucrose gradients by Rupp and Howard-Flanders were due to gaps rather than to cryptic lesions that led to alkaline-induced strand breaks.

The data from Iyer and Rupp can also be used to estimate the amount of single-stranded DNA at each replication fork, an interesting calculation that was not done in the original paper. Iyer and Rupp estimated that the DNA synthesised in the first 10 min after UV irradiation was 3.0% single stranded with a UV dose that reduced the DNA synthesis level to 25% of that of the control. The normal *E. coli* replication fork moves at about 1000 bp/s at 37°C. From these numbers, it follows that about 9000 bases of single-stranded DNA are generated at each replicating fork in the first 10 min after irradiation. This should not be considered a precise measurement, because the column method is rather crude, and elution of the experimental sample from the column was more heterogeneous than elution of the standard. However, the experimental design used in this procedure systematically underestimates the amount of single-stranded DNA, because the label is in the newly synthesised strand while the single-stranded bases are expected in the template strand. Intentional shearing to produce a size comparable to that of the standard certainly broke off any long single-stranded tails, which would not then be scored by this method, because the single-stranded fragments would no longer be associated with the label in the newly synthesised strands. Thus, the actual amount of single-stranded DNA might well be considerably greater than the 9000 nt calculated above.

How does this amount of single-stranded DNA relate to the amount of the *E. coli* DNA-binding protein SSB present in a cell? The generally accepted view is that the amount of single-stranded DNA in a cell under normal conditions is quite small and that the amount of SSB exceeds this amount by a considerable margin, so that any single-stranded DNA is rapidly coated by SSB. According to Kornberg and Baker, there are about 270 SSB monomers per replication fork, which are sufficient to cover about 2000 to 4000 nt of single-stranded DNA. In their review, Chase and Williams stated that the SSB in a cell covers an average of about 1,400 nt per replication fork. Since the level of SSB is apparently not increased significantly after UV irradiation, this calculation shows that in a UV-irradiated cell, the amount of single-stranded DNA generated at a replication fork soon exceeds the amount that can be coated by SSB. This exposed single-stranded DNA is highly significant in several respects. It will certainly be a site for binding of RecA protein, leading to strand exchange and activation of SOS responses through cleavage of the LexA repressor. Another highly significant property of single-stranded DNA lacking SSB is that it allows several modes of primer formation by the DnaG primase to occur that are prevented when single stranded DNA is coated with SSB. Such primer formation may play a role in the cycling of polymerase III holoenzyme to new primed sites beyond a blocking lesion on the leading strand template, as discussed in more detail below.

Coupling of DnaB Helicase and Polymerase III Holoenzyme at the Replication Fork

A key element of current DNA replication models is that a replication fork moves in one direction and uses DNA polymerases that have a unique polarity of synthesis (5′ to 3′ for the new strand) to achieve duplication of two DNA strands with differing polarities. Though one strand (the leading strand) can be synthesised continuously in the same direction as fork movement, the other strand (the lagging strand) is synthesised discontinuously in many segments (Okazaki fragments), with the individual pieces being generated in a direction opposite to the direction of overall movement of the fork. Mechanistically, the cell presumably accomplishes this with a replicative polymerase III holoenzyme that acts processively while remaining attached to one side of the fork to synthesise the leading continuous strand, while the discontinuous synthesis of the lagging strand is accomplished by a polymerase III holoenzyme that must repeatedly cycle on and off its template strand. A dimeric polymerase III holoenzyme might be able to accomplish synthesis of both the leading and the lagging strands concurrently.

It is clear that a replication fork is much more complex than just a polymerase copying template strands. The DnaB helicase is a key player in the formation and propagation of replication forks. The insertion of the DnaB helicase in a double-stranded DNA at the replication origin is a keystone event in forming a replication fork to start a round of replication. Once DnaB is inserted into the DNA, it apparently remains at the front of the replication fork until the replication of that replicon is finished. Mok and Marians developed an *in vitro* replication system for rolling-circle molecules and demonstrated a very high rate of fork movement that required polymerase III holoenzyme plus helicase activity from either DnaB or the preprimosomal proteins (a primosome without DnaG primase). In this system, the helicase and polymerase III holoenzyme were extremely processive (>50,000 nt), with a fork moving at a rate similar to the *in vivo* rate. In this coupled system, the fork was moving at a rate faster than the helicase by itself is known to separate strands. (Although this result might suggest specific protein-protein interactions between DnaB and the polymerase III holoenzyme, the fact that the polymerase III holoenzyme's rate of polymerisation on a primed single-stranded DNA template exceeds the rate at which the DnaB helicase can move through duplex DNA to separate the strands could be sufficient to maintain intimate contact between DnaB and the holoenzyme at the replicating fork and perhaps to even 'push' the helicase so that it separates strands faster in the coupled situation than when acting by itself.) Under normal conditions, in which leading-strand elongation is coupled with helicase movement at the fork, the template for leading-strand extension is copied so efficiently that no single-stranded DNA between DnaB and polymerase III interacts with SSB, either because this DNA is too short or because it is protected by proteins in the replication complex or both.

Effect of DNA lesions on activity of DnaB helicase: Oh and Grossman reported that DnaB helicase activity is little affected by UV irradiation of the substrate. As an extension of this observation, a DnaB helicase substrate was constructed to mimic the situation in which a bulky lesion is present in the template for leading-strand synthesis. With this construct, there was no inhibition of the DnaB helicase activity (Fig. 7.7). Extrapolating these results to a replicating fork, it is suggested that the DnaB helicase in a replication complex at a fork will not be blocked by lesions such as pyrimidine dimers in the duplex DNA and can continue to move along and separate the two strands even though they contain lesions that block polymerase III holoenzyme.

Cycling of polymerase III holoenzyme: During replication of *E. coli,* the polymerase III holoenzyme must cycle to the next Okazaki fragment every second or two. In contrast, although the purified enzyme rapidly and processively replicates a primed single-stranded-DNA circle, several minutes are required to cycle to the next primed single-stranded-DNA circle. O'Donnell and his colleagues studied this process and demonstrated that the cycling time can be reduced to 10 s when the primed acceptor single-stranded DNA has an appropriate preinitiation complex that comprises a subassembly of the polymerase III holoenzyme. The preinitiation complex is a 'protein clamp on primed ssDNA formed by the accessory protein β and the five-protein g complex ($\gamma\delta\delta'\chi\psi$),' and it was concluded that the γ complex acts catalytically in forming a β clamp on the primed template. The cycling takes place only when a fragment has been completed, and cycling is thought to proceed through a bimolecular reaction in which part of the holoenzyme is transferred directly from the completed molecule to the subassembly on the acceptor

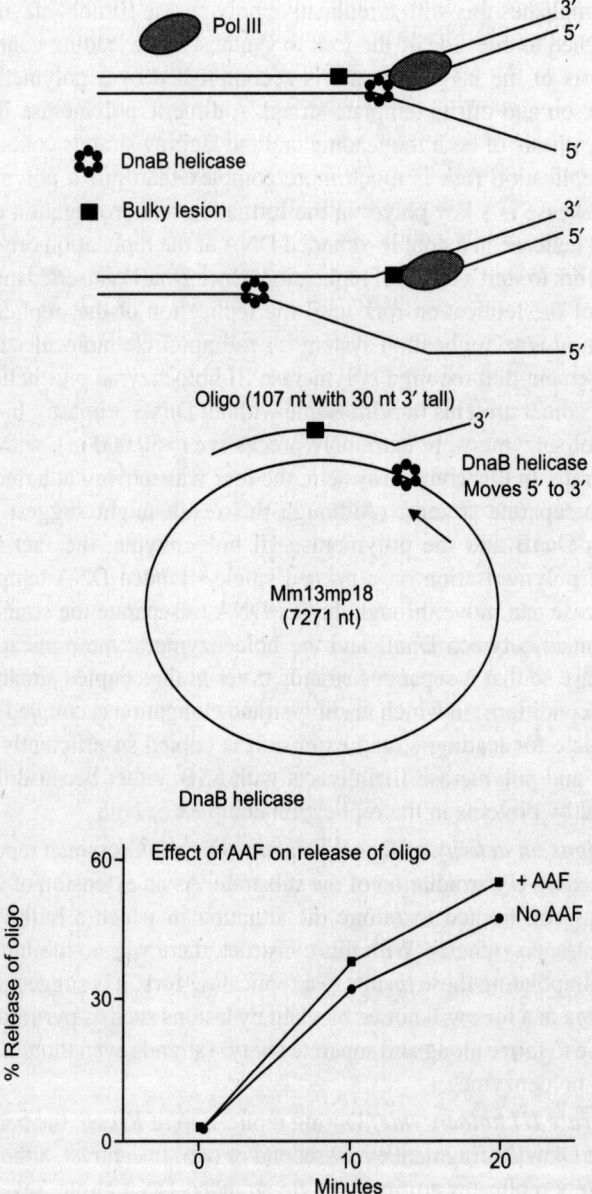

Fig. 7.7: Uncoupling of DnaB helicase and polymerase III at a lesion in the DNA strand coding for synthesis of the continuous strand. (Top) Model for replication fork with polymerase III and DnaB helicase at the replicating fork approaching a bulky lesion. Polymerase III is blocked at the lesion, but the helicase continues past the lesion. (Center) Model substrate for DnaB constructed with the AAF bulky lesion to mimic the structure given about but without polymerase III. (Bottom) The results show that AAF on the oligonucleotide does not prevent release of the oligonucleotide. This finding is consistent with the suggestion that DnaB helicase at the replicating fork might proceed past bulky lesions in the strand that serves as template for synthesis of the continuous strand.

molecule to form an active replication complex on the acceptor. This mode of facilitated transfer without dissociation from the completed fragment is of obvious value for repetitive synthesis of the lagging-strand Okazaki fragments. We expect that these cycling reactions play a central role in the processing of the newly synthesised fragments in UV-damaged cells.

In an earlier study of UV-irradiated DNA, Shavitt and Livneh studied the cycling of polymerase III holoenzyme. Their results showed that cycling from one molecule to another is slowed by UV irradiation but that increasing the amount of the β subunit (known to be part of the preinitiation complex) decreases the cycling time, presumably by facilitating the dissociation of the polymerase III holoenzyme from locations where it was stalled at a photo product. In these experiments, cycling times were in minutes rather than seconds, presumably because these studies did not generate in advance the preformed preinitiation complexes on the acceptor single-stranded DNA molecules that are necessary for the very fast cycling observed by Studwell and others.

Lagging-strand synthesis: During the discontinuous synthesis of the lagging strand on a normal undamaged template, the DnaG primase interacts with DnaB helicase at the fork to synthesise primers for the lagging strand. These primed sites are then used by polymerase III holoenzyme to generate the lagging strand segments that are subsequently joined together to form an intact lagging strand. The polymerase III holoenzyme cycles efficiently from one primed site to another during this process. Although DnaG primase interacts with DnaB helicase at the fork, this interaction seems to be transient, since the reaction of DnaG primase is apparently distributive rather than processive.

Lesion on lagging-strand template at the replication fork: A lesion on the lagging-strand template at the replication fork is similar to that occurring during synthesis of the lagging strand on a normal template. The priming by DnaG can occur normally to generate a primed site for polymerase III holoenzyme. Instead of completing a whole segment, the polymerase III will presumably stop at the lesion, but from here it can be recycled to the next primed site on the lagging-strand template. This gap, which extends from the lesion to the 5′ end of the next fragment, is single stranded and presumably accounts for a significant amount of the single-stranded DNA generated in UV-irradiated cells.

Lesion on leading-strand template at the replication fork: When a replication complex runs into a lesion on the leading-strand template, the resulting structure will be quite different from the normal undamaged case. The DnaB helicase will presumably continue separating strands and will proceed right on past the lesion. However, the situation with the polymerase III holoenzyme will differ, in that the holoenzyme will stall when it reaches the lesion in the template strand, thus uncoupling leading-strand synthesis from the helicase movement at the fork. This abnormal situation with the polymerase III holoenzyme stalled at the lesion while the DnaB helicase at the fork continues separating the two strands will generate a stretch of single-stranded DNA extending from the lesion on the leading-strand template where the polymerase III holoenzyme is stalled to the slowly advancing DnaB helicase at the fork (Fig. 7.7 and 7.8).

Uncoupling of DnaB helicase and polymerase III holoenzyme: Priming and polymerase cycling on leading strand: The continuous synthesis of the leading strand is a generally accepted central tenet of current replication fork models. Thus, the requirement in our interpretation that the leading strand must frequently be restarted seems bizarre. However, in considering known reactions of relevant enzymes, this possibility becomes credible. The first step in the process must be a priming event. The first and most efficient possibility, if it occurs, is a DnaB-DnaG priming event at the fork that is analogous to the priming of the lagging-strand fragments. In the coupled situation, all the priming events are on the

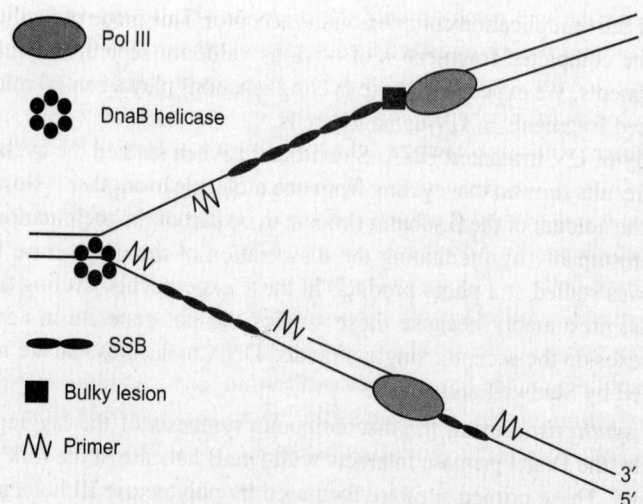

Fig. 7.8: Model for restart of the leading strand when a replication fork reaches a polymerase-blocking lesion.

lagging-strand template. In the uncoupled situation, frequent priming events do occur, but it has not been determined whether these are exclusively on the lagging-strand template or whether they also take place on the leading strand template. In the coupled situation, the exclusive synthesis of primers on the lagging-strand template may be explained simply by differences in the accessibility of the two strands when they are first separated by the advancing DnaB helicase. The leading-strand template is copied efficiently by polymerase III holoenzyme before it is accessible to SSB, so it is not surprising that the DnaG primase could not use it for primer formation. However, when elongation of the leading strand is interrupted by a photo product at which polymerase III is stopped, the separated strands formed by the uncoupled advancing DnaB helicase might well become a substrate for DnaG primase priming on the template for the leading strand as well as for the lagging strand. This is only one of the hypothetical possibilities, and other priming reactions might come into play during uncoupled conditions either instead of or in addition to direct interaction of DnaG with DnaB helicase at the fork. One possibility that is normally considered to be physiologically irrelevant, the general priming reaction, should be mentioned, because as pointed out in the calculation in a previous section, the quantity of single-stranded DNA generated soon after UV irradiation might be greater than can be coated by SSB. Thus, while the general priming reaction may not occur in unirradiated cells, it may become significant after UV irradiation under exactly those conditions in which the leading strand must be restarted.

Primosomes with PriA, PriB, and PriC May Be Involved in Restarts: PriA, PriB, and PriC are not essential for normal replication, since strains with mutants in the single genes are viable, although somewhat sick. However, double mutants with *recA* are not viable. A potential role for these gene products is to facilitate the movement of the replication fork past certain problem areas in the chromosome that might be barriers for replication, such as unexcised bulky lesions. Perhaps bulky lesions are a more serious obstacle for the DnaB helicase in the template for lagging-strand synthesis than in the leading-strand template, since the polarity of DnaB predicts that the lagging-strand template will be tracked. The dual polarity of the primosome with PriABC might provide a backup helicase activity for proceeding beyond such barriers. Once a primer is formed, the polymerase III holoenzyme must bind to and extend the primer to restart the leading strand. When this stage is reached, the extension will be rapid, the polymerase III holoenzyme will catch up with the more slowly moving uncoupled DnaB helicase, a coupled replication complex will be re-established, and this complex will then move at the normal rapid velocity (1 kbp/s) expected for normal replication fork movement. This mechanism requires cycling of the polymerase III holoenzyme on the leading strand at lesions as well as on the lagging strand. In our original study, we estimated that the average delay per dimer was about 10 s. If only the lesions in the leading strand cause a delay, then this rate is equivalent to 20 s per lesion. It was estimated that during normal replication, the lagging strand is primed every 1 to 2 s. In the experiments of Studwell and others, cycling with model substrates was fast and was comparable to the calculated delay at a pyrimidine dimer.

Maintenance of DnaB helicase at a fork may be sufficient to retain a replication fork if polymerase III holoenzyme can recycle past lesions on the leading-strand template, because the polymerase will soon catch up with the slowed helicase when synthesis resumes at a primed site on the leading-strand template. As pointed out before, the limiting factor in forming replication forks is the installation of the DnaB helicase at replication origins, not the availability of the polymerase III holoenzyme.

Translesion synthesis: It is well documented that UV-produced lesions such as pyrimidine dimers are effective blocks to DNA polymerases in purified systems and inside cells. It is also now clear that direct by-pass does occur at low frequencies with purified polymerase I or polymerase III. Results with a thymine-thymine dimer incorporated at a specific site in a vector are particularly clear. When this single-stranded circle was used to transfect an excision-defective host, survival was less than 0.5% of that of the control, demonstrating that by-pass was very rare. However, when the host was UV irradiated to induce SOS functions, survival rose to 25 to 30%, showing that *in vivo* by-pass can occur with a high frequency at a particular lesion. This is a very specialised situation, and the results may have only limited applicability to a lesion in a double-stranded molecule. In the single-stranded circle, the alternatives are limited when a polymerase reaches a blocking lesion, it (or another polymerase) can keep trying to by-pass the lesion until the template molecule is inactivated (for example, by nuclease attack). In a double-stranded molecule, competing reactions such as recombinational exchange or polymerase cycling to another site may decrease the probability of by-pass at a particular site except in cases such as overlapping daughter strand gaps, where recombinational exchanges do not provide feasible alternatives.

What is the contribution of direct translesion synthesis after UV irradiation? UV mutagenesis depends on the *umuC* and *umuD* gene products, presumably as a result of mutagenic translesion synthesis. How frequently does this synthesis actually occur, and what effect does it have on survival of UV-irradiated cells? Experiments were done to determine the effect of constructing a double mutant defective in both *umuC* and *uvrA*. Walker and Dobson did not observe any increased sensitivity due to the *umuC* mutation in either wild-type or *uvrA6* excision-defective strains. Thus, under conditions in which the recombination systems are active, any enhanced survival promoted by translesion synthesis dependent on UmuC is minimal and can represent only a small fraction of those events that occur when a replication fork reaches a blocking lesion. While the UmuCD-dependent by-pass of lesions is quantitatively dominant for UV mutagenesis, these error-producing events arise from a very small fraction of the total repair events.

Inhibition of DNA synthesis by UV irradiation: Induced replisome reactivation and replication restart: Transient inhibition of DNA synthesis in UV-irradiated *E. coli* was studied by Khidir and others and Witkin and others. This phenomenon has been termed Irr (induced replisome reactivation) or replication restart. These studies, which show a requirement for RecA and a second additional factor, are complicated by the fact that most of the experiments were done in an excision-proficient background that allowed rapid removal of lesions after irradiation. However, it is clear from the data in both papers that after irradiation, although DNA synthesis was markedly inhibited, substantial residual synthesis continued even when the Irr or replication restart did not occur. The interpretations of the various authors are that lesions bring the replisome to a complete halt and that the replisome must be 'reactivated' or 'restarted' to allow DNA synthesis to continue. However, if the interpretation offered here is correct, i.e. that blocking lesions cause uncoupling of polymerase III and DnaB activity of the replication complex rather than a complete block, then the interpretation of these data will be rather different.

Thus, if a replisome is not blocked at a lesion, it does not need reactivation or a restart to pass the lesion. Inhibition initially occurs because template strand lesions uncouple the helicase and the polymerase at the replication fork, causing the overall movement of the fork to slow down but not stop. In this model, inhibition might persist if the passage of the replication complex generates structures that might be resistant to the normal modes of repair and thus accumulate to provide a sink that competes with the fork for components that might be limiting, such as the polymerase III holoenzyme. In this situation, translesion synthesis might well be the mechanism to relieve the observed inhibition, but this translesion synthesis would not be required to occur directly at the fork to get it restarted but would occur at structures generated by the previous passing of the DnaB helicase component of the replication complex. The third role of RecA in addition to cleavage of LexA and UmuD, could be a protective effect of its binding to single stranded DNA. This effect might be particularly critical, since the calculations given above indicate that the level of SSB may be insufficient for the amount of single-stranded DNA generated soon after UV irradiation.

In this model, DNA synthesis can be inhibited in at least two ways by uncoupling DnaB helicase activity from polymerase III chain elongation of the leading strand at the replication fork. First, when DnaB helicase is uncoupled, it separates strands much more slowly than when it is coupled with polymerase III in the normal fork configuration. In the second, a somewhat indirect way, unrepaired pieces left in the wake of the advancing uncoupled fork could be competitive sinks for polymerase III holoenzyme, particularly if they retain either the entire polymerase III enzyme or a subassembly of the holoenzyme, as might occur in the facilitated bimolecular transfer of the polymerase III core to a second preprimed location. The accumulation of significant quantities of these unrepaired termini with preinitiation complexes remaining attached could compete with the replication fork for the limited number of polymerase III holoenzyme molecules in the cell. If these locations are at closely spaced lesions or overlapping daughter strand gaps, SOS-mediated translesion synthesis requiring UmuCD' might be required to remove inhibitory unrepaired competitive termini. Sommer and others suggested that the UmuCD' proteins compete with RecA and switch from homologous recombination to SOS mutagenesis and that this switch occurs slowly because the induction of the UmuCD proteins is delayed.

To sum up, although many steps and many polypeptides are required for replication, the single most important element that is required for beginning and maintaining a round of replication is the insertion of the DnaB helicase at the replication origin and its continued ordered processive advance through the replicon. Its entry into the DNA precedes entry of the polymerase III holoenzyme, and its location at the front of the replication fork separates the strands for copying by polymerase III. It is clear from the work of Baker and others that the DnaB helicase can separate strands for long distances on its own and that priming can occur so that the subsequent addition of polymerase III holoenzyme results in rapid copying of the exposed regions, presumably until polymerase III either catches up with the more slowly moving DnaB helicase or comes to another duplex region. For a replication complex in an unirradiated cell, synthesis of the leading strand will be synchronous with advancement of the DnaB helicase, because the rate of chain elongation is greater than the movement of DnaB helicase alone. (It is not clear whether DnaB's higher velocity under coupled conditions is due to specific protein-protein interaction between polymerase III and DnaB or whether the rapid polymerisation on the leading-strand template exposed by DnaB is sufficient to bring the polymerase III holoenzyme into direct contact with DnaB and simply push the DnaB helicase faster without any specific interactions between the proteins.) Coordination with lagging-strand synthesis is accomplished in two ways. First, the lagging-strand primers require the interaction of DnaG primase with DnaB helicase. Second, the polymerase III holoenzyme has a dimeric structure with two core enzyme units, so that polymerisation on the leading and lagging strands can take place simultaneously with the same dimeric polymerase molecule. It has thus been proposed that while one of the core units of the dimeric polymerase III continuously extends the leading strand, the second part of the dimeric molecule continuously recycles to generate the discontinuous Okazaki pieces of the lagging strand.

What effect does DNA damage have on this process? The main points are that the replisome or replication fork may not always behave like a monolithic unit, and that the assumption that the entire replication fork stops at a lesion just because one component of the replication complex, the polymerase III holoenzyme, stops there is probably an inaccurate oversimplification. The continued progress and integrity of a replicating fork may well be determined by what happens to the DnaB helicase rather than by what happens to a particular polymerase III holoenzyme molecule. Although polymerase III can easily start elongating chains from an appropriate primer at any location, the correct insertion of DnaB helicase to create a replication fork is a highly specialised reaction that occurs efficiently only at replication origins.

Chapter 8

DNA Rearrangements

INTRODUCTION

Genetic map is the characteristic of a species. All the members of a species have their genes arranged in the same order. This arrangement of genes remains the same in different tissues of the body and during all stages of development. A plethora of examples exist which astray from these rules, resulting in the rearrangement of genomic DNA. The existence of various kinds of rearrangements hints towards the amount of flexibility that otherwise rigid gene order allows itself. DNA rearrangements are some of the best characterised clonal oncogenic abnormalities, and they frequently involve juxtaposition of cellular protooncogenes with regulatory sequences of other genes. DNA rearrangements can either be programmed or incidental (or unprogrammed). Mutations resulting from errors in DNA replication, repair or recombination could lead to unprogrammed DNA rearrangements. A variety of DNA rearrangements could take place during the formation of tumours. Mobility of transposons, insertion/excision of plasmid or viral DNA, are the other means by which incidental rearrangements may happen. The rearrangements could also result due to the action of certain drugs e.g. amplification in the presence of certain metabolite inhibitors e.g. methotrexate. But, this kind of rearrangements are not a part of normal development. Programmed rearrangements, on the other hand, are part of normal development programme of a species.

The outcome of these rearrangements is largely predictable. The process is usually carried out by specific recombination enzymes, is developmentally regulated, and is heritable. The frequency of switching/rearrangement of genes varies with the system and is generally 10^{-2} per cell cycle or lower. Yeast mating type switch shows exceptionally high frequency of once per cycle. Based on their consequences, the known examples of programmed rearrangements can be categorised as:

1. DNA amplifications and deletions resulting in change in gene copy number.

2. Re-assorting DNA segments to create large and diverse combination of genes.

3. Regulation of gene expression by switching expression from one: Expressing gene to the other gene.

The demarcation between these categories is not always straightforward, but they broadly classify the known examples of DNA rearrangements. A brief description of each category, thus, follows with representative examples.

DNA AMPLIFICATIONS AND DELETIONS

DNA Amplifications

DNA is amplified to different levels and for varied purposes. Polyploidy (e.g. in plants or in fat cells of insects) or Polyteny (e.g. in salivary glands and malpighian tubules of insects) amplifies neatly whole of the genome. The formation of macronuclei in ciliates involves a programmed amplification, again using polyteny as the first step. On the other hand, there are many examples known, where relatively much smaller segments are amplified to varied degrees. A tissue-specific amplification of large ribosomal RNA (18S and 28S rRNAs) genes takes place in the case of amphibian oocytes and of chorion genes in *Drosophila melanogaster* ovaries. Similarly, rDNA amplification in ciliate macronucleus and amplification of DNA in late larval stages of *Rhynchosciara americana* (Fig. 8.1) are other known examples of DNA amplification.

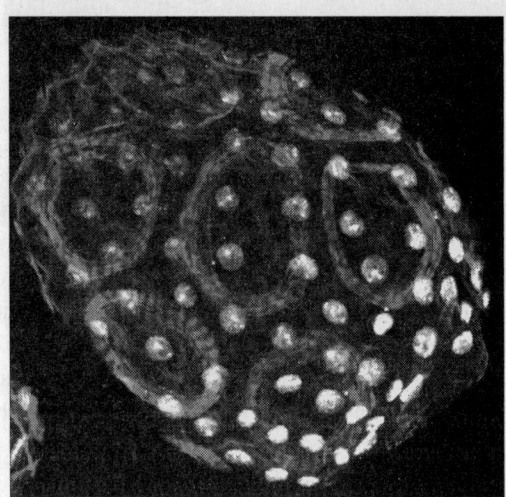

Fig. 8.1: *Rhynchosciara americana.*

Amphibian rRNA genes amplification

The differential amplification of ribosomal RNA genes takes place to meet the demand of huge amounts of rRNA for ribosome synthesis in a short time span during oogenesis. The amplification results in ~2500-fold increase in rDNA even though chromosomal complement contains only 450 copies of each of 28S and 18S rRNA genes. The rRNA genes are 'excised' as circles and amplification takes place by rolling circle method. Thus, eventually, more than 70% of the nuclear DNA in a *xenopus* oocyte (Fig. 8.2) codes for rRNA.

Ribosomal DNA amplification in ciliates

During the formation of macronuclei of holotrichous ciliate, *Tetrahymena,* the total micronuclear DNA undergoes polyploidisation up to ~45°C, before other rearrangements follow. Ribosomal RNA genes, on the other hand, undergo much extensive amplification. One copy of rRNA genes, present in the micronuclear DNA amplifies into ~9000 copies of linear extrachromosomal molecules of 21kb each in macronucleus. Each linear molecule contains two copies of rDNA arranged as palindromic repeats. Thus, rDNA is amplified 200 times in the polyploid macronucleus.

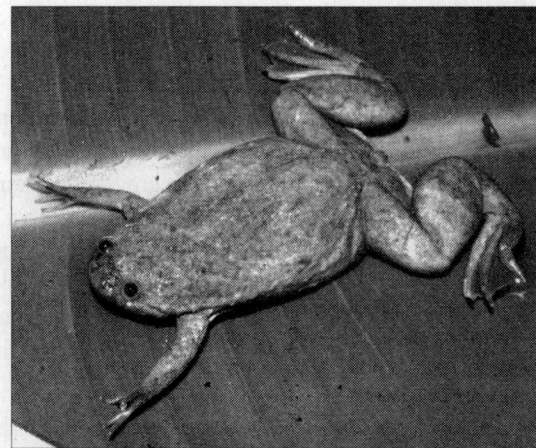

Fig. 8.2: *Xenopus* oocyte.

Chorion gene amplification in Drosophila

During oogenesis in *Drosophila melanogaster,* follicular cells synthesise $1–4 \times 10^{12}$ molecules each of 20 chorion proteins (each encoded by single-copy gene in the haploid genome), and deposit it around each oocyte. The whole process of chorion protein ,synthesis needs completion within 3 hr. Despite the fact that there are nearly 1000 follicle cells with each of them having a ploidy level of 45°C, still the kinetics of chorion protein synthesis exceeds by nearly two orders of magnitudes from the efficiency limits of the protein synthesis by a cell. The deficit is made up by differential amplification of chorion gene clusters in the follicular cells just before and during choriogenesis. The mechanism of amplification seems to involve multiple branched replication forks initiating in or near each cluster of chorion genes and spreading bidirectionally.

Cocoon formation in Sciarids

DNA puffs observed at many sites in the salivary gland polytene chromosomes of the larvae of all species of flies belonging to the family Sciaridae, constitute special cases of developmentally regulated DNA sequence amplification. Just like rDNA and chorion gene amplification, the rationale for DNA amplification seems to be the requirement of high amount of certain gene products in a short period during development. In these flies, DNA puffs are induced to meet the requirement of proteins for communal cocoon formation (for pupation) late in larval stages. Unstable nature of the corresponding mRNAs could be another reason for the 'DNA puff' formation.

DNA deletions

Just like amplifications, the extent of programmed deletions also varies. In the case of formation of macronuclei of a hypotrichous, ciliate, *Oxytricha,* a substantial portion of the genome is deleted. This massive deletion of DNA sequences, which follows polyteny of the entire genome, involves excision and deletion of thousands of transposon-like elements and thousands of other small sequences, cutting of polytene chromosomes band-by-band and finally in some cases, unscrambling the DNA segments and ligating them into a genetically correct order to get multiple copies of roughly gene-sized fragments which are acentromeric but with telomeres at the two ends. Thus, ciliated protozoa actually provide examples of multiple types of programmed DNA rearrangements. It has recently been shown in certain ciliates like *Paramecium* and *Tetrahymena* that the decision about whether a particular sequence is to be amplified or deleted during the formation of macronucleus is inherited epigenetically. It has been proposed that homology and consequent pairing interactions between maternal macronuclear sequences and micronuclear sequences of the sexual progeny induce these epigenetic modifications of homologous germ-line sequences. As compared to massive deletions in ciliates, relatively much smaller and fewer fragments of DNA are deleted from a B-cell in the case of generation of antibody diversity. The rearrangement of immunoglobulin genes involves deletion of intervening DNA placed between distantly located V, D and J segments. Concomitant ligation of the fragments on the two sides of the deletion results in the generation of a continuous immunoglobulin gene.

RE-ASSORTING DNA SEGMENTS

This kind of rearrangement involves piecing together DNA segments, which would be separated by small to large chunks of DNA, or could be present in a scrambled state.

Generation of Antibody Diversity in Mammals

In mammals, the generation of huge repertoire of antibodies with different antigen specificity involves many steps. The joining of just few segments, but in different combinations, is one major mechanism employed to achieve diverse immunoglobulin genes.

Diversity in the antigen-binding region

In the formation of immunoglobulin light chain genes, either κ or λ the joining of different Variable (V) segments to any of the Joining (0) segments makes up the repertoire for IgL chains. For heavy chains, IgH, any Diversity (D) segment is first spliced to any Joining (0) segment. This D-J combination is then joined to any of the different Variable (V) segments. The V-J or V-D-J segment is finally joined to the Constant (C) segment by RNA splicing to form the complete protein in the end. Besides generating diversity, V-J/V-D-J joining brings the promoter of the V segment under the control of transcriptional enhancer located between J and C segments, thereby stimulating transcription.

There are other means by which additional levels of diversity is accrued by immunoglobulin genes. Impreciseness of joining of these different segments, including *de novo* addition or removal of nucleotides increases the diversity by many folds. Finally, somatic diversification process, such as point mutations amplify the number of available functional variable sequences. 'Somatic mutations' are induced specifically in the active B lymphocytes, in all regions of the variable domain of immunoglobulin. The variation is in the range of 1–4% divergence from the germ-line, corresponding upto maximum of 10 amino acid substitutions in the protein. There are certain hotspots for mutations. These 'somatic mutations' generate B cells that have increased affinity for antigen. Most of these, somatically mutated cells are stored as inactive memory cells, which get activated, if there is new exposure to the same antigen. This secondary response is very rapid and involves only clonal expansion, and no further somatic mutation.

Diversity in the effector region

There are five types of Immunoglobulins, IgM, IgD, IgG, IgE and IgA, as determined by the class of the constant region of heavy chain of Immunoglobulin, CH. The genes coding for these five classes are arranged on the mouse chromosome 16 as Cμ, Cδ, (Cγ3, Cγ1, Cγ2b, Cγ2a), Cε and Cα, respectively, in the order of increasing distance from the last segment of heavy chain. V-D-J joining reaction triggers expression of the Cμ gene and the process is accomplished by splicing J segment with Cμ after transcription, as Cμ is the first C_H segment, present at the end of J segments. So, IgM is the first immunoglobulin produced, that too at the stage when B cells are still immature.

Programmed DNA recombinations occurring late in the life of a B-cell can lead to replacement of one C_H segment with another, the process is called 'class switching'. In B-cell ontogeny, variable region formation always precedes class switching. Class switching is accomplished by a recombination to bring a new CH gene into juxtaposition with the expressed V-D-J unit. Cells expressing later C_H genes, delete Cμ and the other genes between Cμ and the expressed C_H gene as circular molecules. Since, Cμ gene is just adjacent to the last J segment, the formation of IgM does not require any DNA rearrangement. The regions of DNA that actually bring about switching between two distantly placed C_H regions are called 'Switch regions' or 'S regions'. S regions lie just upstream of CH genes and contain poorly defined switching sites, the actual sites of recombination. Switching sites may occur preferentially near certain sequence motifs within the G-rich, simple tandem repeat. The lack of homology between S_μ and S_α segments makes homologous recombination an unlikely mechanism for class switching.

It has been postulated that there exists class-specific 'switching' proteins, which recognise their specific S region. These proteins then bind to one another, juxtaposing two S segments, thus facilitating a recombinational event to join them. Consistent with the hypothesis, it has been reported that LR1, a transcription factor binds to one site in Sγ1 and, possibly, to a site in Sγ3. Moreover NF-κB/p50 and SNAP complex/E47 (a helix-loophelix protein), binds to first 30 bp regions (of 49bp repeats) of Sγ3, Sγ1 and Sγ2b. Similarly in the mouse Pax/BSAP, a B-cell lineage specific transcription factor, binds to one or two sites 5′ to or within every S region. Thus the 'class switching' further widens the repertoire of immunoglobulins by allowing one V_H gene to be combinatorially associated with eight different CH genes, allowing distinct effector functions to be employed with each V_H region (antigen-binding specificity) and regulating the expression of the C_H genes.

Generation of T Cell Receptor Diversity

Creation of diversity in the α and β subunits of T-cell receptor (TCR) involves similar mechanisms as are used for immunoglobulins. TCR α and γ have components like IgL chains, and TCR α and γ are like IgH chains. Just like Igs, the diversity of the TCR repertoire is generated through: (i) the joining of distinct V to D to J gene segments, (ii) the imprecise 3′ margins at the joints of the recombined segments, (iii) the use of multiple D segments (in δ chain products), (iv) the insertion of additional non-germline nucleotides at the joint.

Segmental Gene Conversion in Chicken

In chicken there is only one V gene segment, one J segment and only one C segment for the light chain of the immunoglobulin. In the Bursa of Fabricius, an avian lymphoid organ, most of the B-cells produce A light chain by the recombination of same single V region with a single J region and a single C region. But the circulating A light chains exhibit extensive heterogeneity when analysed on isoelectric focusing gels. There are 25 pseudogenes for V segment. The diversification, beginning late in embryonic development, results from the replacement of the V region by these pseudogenes, which serve as donors, in this conversion process. The diversification is detected in the V region only and takes place in bursa alone. The extent of diversification increases with time. Just like mammals, the junctional diversity is achieved by addition or deletion or modification of the nucleotides at the junction between V and J segments. The combinatorial diversity is achieved in a fashion different from mammals. The pseudogenes representing the different parts of the V segment may repeatedly act as donors. Thus, creating a new kind of combinatorial diversity. Additional junctional diversity could arise with the joining of each pseudogene at their border sequences. The rates of conversion is very high- approximately, one event every ten or twenty cell divisions.

Scrambling of Gene Segments order in Ciliates

The comparison of macronuclear and micronuclear gene sequences showed that the gene segments are arranged in a scrambled order in micronucleus. These segments are ligated into a genetically correct order by not only the removal of intervening sequences (called Internal eliminated sequences or IESs) but also by shuffling the order of gene segments as well as by inversion of certain gene segments. Actin gene in *Oxytricha nova* consists of nine segments arranged in scrambled order in its micronucleus. Any two segments to be ligated in the macronucleus have same pair of a repeat sequence at their ends. This repeat acts as the site of recombination and joins the two segments by the removal of IES as well as one of the repeat sequence.

REGULATION OF GENE EXPRESSION

DNA rearrangements leading to regulation at the level of expression, basically control genes involved in similar functions. These rearrangements enable the organism to switch between the different available options e.g. switching between two variant forms of MAT locus involved in the control of mating type of yeast. This kind of switching has been used by many organisms, specially unicellular pathogens to change their surface properties to help evade the immune surveillance as well as to preadapt to sudden~ unforeseen changes in the environment. A huge immune response is mounted by the host against this surface property (e.g. surface antigen) displayed by the majority of the population. A minor population, which has switched its surface antigen, escapes the host's immune response.

Most DNA Rearrangements are Reversible

In most of the cases known the rearrangement causing the change in expression are reversible. The reversibility of the DNA rearrangement has been known to be ensured by different organisms in the following three ways:

1. An invertible DNA segment causes the switch of expression from one gene to another, between the two alternative states.
2. DNA transposition moves a gene from non-expressing to the expression linked site.
3. Addition or deletion of sequences to a protein-coding region to break or restore the reading frame. A control at the translation level.

Expression control by DNA inversion

This kind of rearrangement is adapted by few bacteria and bacteriophages. The frequency of inversion is, generally, very low. One type of inversion control involves switching of DNA segments containing promoter element between two states in such a way that in one orientation it controls one set of gene(s), while the other set is expressed in the flip orientation. The second way of achieving inversion control of expression involves keeping the two genes, to be controlled by a promoter, in the invertible DNA segment, in such a way that flip sides of the invertible DNA segment place either of the two genes, in front of the given promoter, for expression.

Phase inversion in Salmonella: Antigenically different flagellar proteins, flagellin, are encoded by two genes Hl and H2 in *Salmonella.* These bacteria can switch between the two proteins but at a very low frequency of the range of 10^{-5} to 10^{-3} per bacterial division. Thus, as the immune response gets activated to kill all the bacteria, which are displaying on of the two flagellins, it is postulated that few bacteria switch the expression to the other flagellin gene and evade the immune defence.

Genetic and molecular studies revealed that the repressor for H1 protein, rH1, is synthesised by the same operon which synthesises H2 protein. At the time of phase transition, a DNA element called H region containing promoter for H2 rH1 operon is inverted. This kind of promoter switching shuts down the synthesis of both H2 and rH1, resulting in the synthesis/ production of H1 flagellin.

Two imperfect inverted repeats, *hixL* and *hixR,* flanking the H region are recognised by a protein called Hin. The gene coding for Hin protein is contained in the invertible H segment An enhancer element recognised by host (bacterial) DNA binding protein, The gene forFis, is present entirely within the coding sequence for Hin. This enhancer element serves to stimulate the rate of inversion by 150-fold by bringing together Hin and Fis proteins, each bound as a dimer to their respective DNA-bound forms into a complex, called Invertasome. The DNA must be negatively supercoiled for Invertasome formation. Fis binding at the enhancer results in the bending of the DNA. This bending may be necessary for enhancer function.

Host range specificity of Mu phage: By alternating between two operons coding for two different types of tail fibres, bacteriophage Mu can change its host-specificity from *E. coli* K12, a host of G(+)phage to *Citrobacter freundii, E. coli, C. Shigellasonneii,* etc., which are the hosts for G(–) phage. A 3kb invertible segment, called 'Gregion', contains, towards one end, most of an operon consisting of S and U genes, while the other end has most of the second operon consisting of S' and U' genes in opposite orientation. Depending upon which set of genes (S and U or S' and U') are placed in front of the promoter as a result of the inversion, G(+) or G(–) phages are synthesised. Just like *Salmonella,* the invertible G-segment is flanked by 34 bp inverted repeats that are recognised by a specific recombinase called Gin. But unlike *Salmonella,* in Mu phage the promoter element for the expression of the two sets of genes lies outside the invertible G-segment. The frequency of inversion, just as in *Salmonella,* is very low, of the order of 10^{-6}, mainly due to the low level of expression of Gin.

In addition to Hin and Gin recombinases, the products of *cin* and *pin* genes are also known to mediate site-specific inversion. Cin mediates inversion in bacteriophage P1 in much the similar way, as Gin does for Mu phage even though 'C region' is flanked by inverted repeats of 600bp. The inversion of 'P-region' in e14-defective bacteriophage in *E. coli* is carried out by Pin. The amino acid sequences of Pin, Gin, and Hin are more than 60% homologous. Moreover, Hin, Gin and Cin seem to be functionally related, since they can substitute one another in *in vivo* complementation studies. The homology is seen between the recombination sites (inverted repeats) of *gin, pin* and *hin.*

Expression control by DNA transposition

Switching of mating type in Yeast: In the homothallic strains of the budding yeast, *Saccharomyces cerevisiae*, the determination of the mating type, a or α, is controlled by three loci on chromosome ID: a transcriptionally active locus MAT and two silent loci, HMLa and HMRa. According to the 'Casette model', all the three loci carry information ~at codes for the mating type, but only the active cassette at the MAT locus is expressed.

Mating-type switching occurs when the active cassette, is replaced by the information from a silent cassette. The newly installed cassette is then expressed. The Ho endonuclease initiates this unidirectional switch by introducing a double strand break in the MAT locus which then becomes the recipient of the information from donor loci, HML or HMR, by a duplicative gene conversion process.

MATa donor preference is not restricted to a single site. In MATα cells, a big region of 40kb or more on the left arm of chromosome m, including HML, is activated in terms of enhanced recombination/switching potential. Recently, Wu and Haber have narrowed down this 'recombination enhancer' to a nearly 700 bp cis-acting, orientation-independent DNA sequence that is both necessary and sufficient. Surprisingly, there does not seem to be any strong preferential activation of HMR for recombination in MAT α cells, rather a large region (~175 kb) of the left arm of Chromosome III is inactivated.

An interesting aspect of this switch is that only mother cells, defined as cells which have budded in the previous cell cycle and have thus given birth to a daughter cell, typically switch their mating type. Consistent with its role, Ho is expressed only in mother cells as a result of transient transcription late in G1 phase of the cell cycle. The timing of Ho production, just before MAT is replicated, ensures that both the daughter cells have the same mating type, switched from the mother.

SWI genes discovered as mutants unable to switch are involved in mother specific and cell cycle control of transcription of HO gene. SWI5, a transcription factor, is required for HO transcription in the mother cell, but is found in both mother and daughter cells.

Recently a negative regulator of HO expression, encoded by ASH1 (for asymmetric synthesis of Ho), has been identified which is daughter cell specific and prevents daughter cell switching. Ash1p contains a domain with homology to the zinc finger domain of the GATA-like transcription factor family. Genetic data support the view that Ash1p antagonises Swi5p.

Shelp/Myo4p, an unconventional myosin, along with other She proteins: She2p, She3p and She5p, is required for the preferential accumulation of Ash1p in daughter cells, suggesting that actin-based transport may play a role in the generation of HO asymmetry.

Swi4p and Swi6p confine activation of HO transcription by Swi5p to the late Gl phase of the cell cycle. This temporal delay in activation of HO employed by Swi4p and Swi6p might provide a time window in which Ashlp can accumulate in the daughter cell nucleus to levels sufficient to inhibit all Swi5p functions or to prevent binding of transcriptional activators to the HO promoter. This could lead to repression of HO expression in daughter cells.

Coat protein switching in Trypanosomes: African trypanosomes such as *Trypanosoma brucei,* the causative agent of sleeping sickness in humans and 'Nagana' (meaning 'loss of spirits' in Zulu language) disease in cattle, is covered with a dense surface coat of 10 million molecules of a single species, the Variant Surface Glycoprotein (VSG) attached to the plasma membrane. Although the genome of this unicellular protozoan contains more than a thousand VSG genes, a single gene is expressed at any given time. The parasite protects itself from the immune response of the mammalian host on its highly immunogenic protein coat by switching the expression of, VSG from one gene to the other. The rate of switching aries from 1 per 10 million cell divisions to 1 per 100.

The expressed VSG genes, also called Expression Linked Copy (ELC), is always located close to telomere, only 1–3 kb from the start of telomeric repeat (ITAGGG), in a region called Expression Site or, ES. The silent copies, also called the Basic Copies, are present at the telomeres of nearly all the chromosomes as well as at many chromosome-internal sites.

Among the different methods used to switch the', expression of VSG, the most frequently used one involves DNA rearrangement resulting in the change of ELC at the expression site. The silent copy from other 'telomeric and chromosome-internal sites is copied by duplicative transposition or gene conversion. Just as in the case of mating type switch in the yeast, the replacement of a cassette at the active (telomeric) locus takes place by silent cassette. The difference from the yeast lies in the number of silent cassettes, which is a large number in trypanosomes, as compared to two in yeast.

The prototypical gene conversion cassette consists 1.5–1.8 kb VSG, a unique upstream 'cotransposed region' of 1–2 kb and an upstream repetitive region of varying length containing 70 bp repeats. The 5′ boundary of VSG cassette was concluded to lie somewhere within 70bp repeats while 3′ boundary lies within the highly conserved VSG carboxy-terminal coding or 3′ untranslated regions johnson and others. But, according to a recent report by McCulloch and others, deletion of the 70 bp repeats from the ES does not effect the gene transfer by duplicative transposition from the silent copy, thus hinting at the existence of other sequence(s) acting as 5′ boundary of the duplicating sequence. The telomere-transposition differs from the transposition of the chromosome-internal sites in that the segment transposed may start as far 'as 50 kb upstream of the gene and end far down stream of the gene, possibly including the whole telomere. On the other hand, the gene segments transferred from chromosome-internal sites are not complete genes. Chimeric VSG genes of novel type are created if many of these segmental genes act as donors. This often seems to be the case late in chronic infections of the parasite.

Antigenic variation in Borrelia: Just like trypanosomes, *Borrelia hermsii*, a spirochete, which causes relapsing fever in humans and other mammals counters host immunity with multiphasic antigen variation. A single cloned organism can give rise to at least 26 antigenically distinct serotypes. Antigen switching is apparently spontaneous and occurs at the rate of 10^{-4} to 10^{-3} per cell generation. Antigenic variation is the consequence of segmental expression genes for outer membrane lipoproteins called variable major proteins or Vmps. Activation of a different *vmp* gene follows a non-reciprocal recombination event, probably by gene conversion, in which a copy of an untranscribed *vmp* is fused to a common expression site and the formerly active *vmp* is lost. In *B hermsii*, silent and expressed copies of *vmp* genes are located separately on linear plasmids of approximately 30kb. Intraplasmidic deletions and interplasmidic recombinations provide the necessary reportire of *vmp* genes.

Antigenic variation of pili in Neisseria: The pilins are the protein subunits of the pili, which are hair like appendages on the cell surface of *Neisseria gonorrhoeae* (Fig. 8.3), the causative agent of gonorrhoea. The pilins are the immunodominant antigens of these bacteria and the major target of host antibodies. Just like trypanosomes and *Borrelia*, *Neisseria* has an array of silent pilin genes and activation of a gene requires its transposition to an expression site.

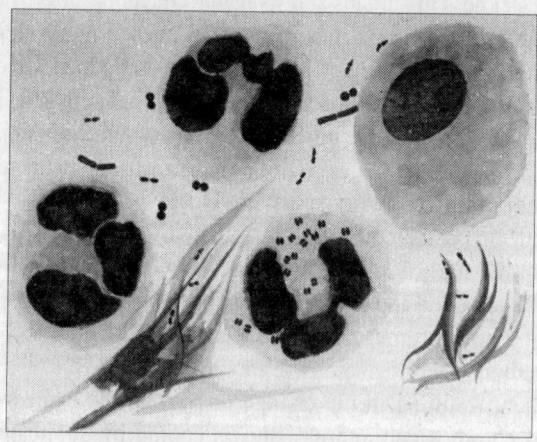

Fig. 8.3: *Neisseria gonorrhoeae.*

The switching occurs at a very low rate. This recA dependent, non-reciprocal exchange of information can be achieved through recombination between 'silent' and 'expression' sites. The more prevalent pathway used by these bacteria involves recombination with extrachromosomal DNA taken up from autolysed neighbours. Unlike *Borrelia* and trypanosomes, the silent genes are incomplete in *Neisseria,* as the amino-terminal invariant domain of pilin is contributed by the expression site, and is absent from silent sites. A feature specific to *Neisseria* is that since pili are not essential for the survival of the' bacterium in the host environment, it can undergo phase variation in addition to antigenic variation. One of the methods of phase variation involves transfer of a non-functional, silent gene copy into the expression site, leading to the loss of pili. While the trypanosomes without surface coat are killed, I hairless *Neisseria* may even be at advantage under some conditions.

Expression control at translation level

Altering the reading frame to truncate the protein very early in its coding region has been used as another means to switch between different genes of a protein. The expression control of opacity *(opa)* proteins, the minor cell surface proteins of *Neisseria,* is the only known example in which this kind of control is exercised at the translation level. In contrast to the silent pilin genes, *opa* genes are not truncated. All *opa* genes are transcribed and code for functional proteins. Addition or removal of one or two pentamer repeats, CTCTI, to the DNA segment coding for the hydrophobic part of the signal sequence of the opacity protein will throw translation out of frame and result in truncated protein. This kind of switching of *opa* genes in and out of frame occurs at a very high rate of nearly 10^{-3} to 10^{-4} per cell per generation. The possible mechanism of variation of the repeat number has been explained by slipped-strand mispairing in the CTCTI repeat region during replication. Why a wasteful process like control at the translation level is adopted is not clear, but it definitely offers a variant theme for gene rearrangements.

Irreversible DNA Rearrangements

Certain DNA rearrangements lead to irreversible alteration in the arrangement of the involved sequences. The resulting cell either cannot revert/switch to other forms or even if it can, the options available for switching get reduced to quite a large extent. This kind of rearrangement occurs while joining V-D-J regions of Immunoglobulins or T-cell receptors, as it involves deletion of the intervening sequences.

Another example of irreversible DNA rearrangement leading to rearranged functional genes is found in the genes involved in N_2 fixation *(nif* genes) in heterocystous cyanobacteria e.g. *Anabaena* (Fig. 8.4). Each of the three operons, (nifHDK), *(nifB, fdxN, nifS, nifU)*, and *(hupSL),* coding for genes related to nitrogen fixation, are interrupted by different sized fragments leading to no expression in vegetative I cells. An 11kb element *nifD* gene in *nifHDK* operon while 55kb sequence is present in *fdxN* gene of *(nifB, fdxN, nifSU)* operon, a 10.5kb element is located in *hupL* gene of *hupSL* operon.

During the formation of heterocysts, the specialised cells capable of fixing free nitrogen from the air, these interrupting elements are excised as circles, by the use of three independent site-specific recombination events. The process of excision is carried out by three different enzymes, *XisA, XisF* and *XisC*, which recognise the different sized direct repeats flanking 11kb element, 55kb element and 10.5kb element, respectively. Interestingly, the gene coding for *Xis* A is present in 11kb element, for *XisF* in 55kb element and for *XisC* in 10.5kb element.

nif gene rearrangement is one of the rare example known which is induced by external stimuli. Other examples, described here, undergo a defined rate of rearrangement which is not affected by the environment.

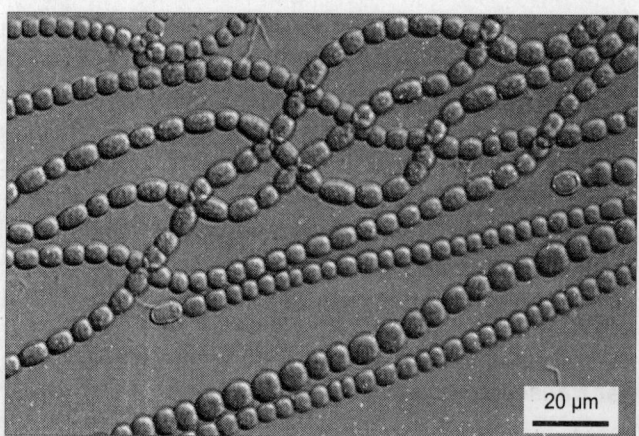

20 µm

Fig. 8.4: *Anabaena*.

To sum up, developmentally programmed deoxyribonucleic acid (DNA) rearrangements are structural reorganisations of the genome that occur reproducibly during the development of a variety of organisms. In the majority of cases, programmed DNA rearrangements function to alter gene expression. V(D)J recombination is a DNA rearrangement that occurs during the development of the human immune system to assemble functional genes encoding antibodies. Some human pathogens use programmed DNA rearrangements to evade the immune system by varying the expression of their antigenic surface proteins. However, in some cases, the function of large-scale developmentally programmed DNA rearrangements remains unknown. In the ciliate protozoan Tetrahymena thermophila, a wide variety of programmed rearrangements occur during the development of the somatic nucleus including chromosome fragmentation and deletion of specific DNA sequences. In a related ciliate Oxytricha trifallax, programmed genome rearrangements are needed to unscramble segments to assemble functional genes.

Chapter 9

Colon Cancer and DNA Repair

INTRODUCTION

Colon cancer is cancer of the large intestine (colon), which is the final part of your digestive tract. Most cases of colon cancer begin as small, noncancerous (benign) clumps of cells called adenomatous polyps. Over time some of these polyps can become colon cancers. DNA damage appears to be a fundamental problem for life. In this chapter we review evidence indicating that DNA damages are a major primary cause of cancer. DNA damages give rise to mutations and epimutations that, by a process of natural selection, can cause progression to cancer. First, we describe the distinguishing characteristics of DNA damage, mutation and epimutation.

DNA damage is a change in the basic structure of DNA that is not itself replicated when the DNA is replicated. A DNA damage can be a chemical addition or disruption to a base of DNA (creating an abnormal nucleotide or nucleotide fragment) or a break in one or both chains of the DNA strands. When DNA carrying a damaged base is replicated, an incorrect base can often be inserted opposite the site of the damaged base in the complementary strand, and this can become a mutation in the next round of replication. Also DNA doublestrand breaks may be repaired by an inaccurate repair process leading to mutations. In addition, a double strand break can cause rearrangements of the chromosome structure (possibly disrupting a gene, or causing a gene to come under abnormal regulatory control), and if such a change can be passed to successive cell generations, it is also a form of mutation. Mutations, however, can be avoided if accurate DNA repair systems recognise DNA damages as abnormal structures, and repair the damages prior to replication. As illustrated in Fig. 9.1, when DNA damages occur, DNA repair is a crucial protective process blocking entry of cells into carcinogenesis.

The DNA damages occurs in both replicating, proliferative cells (e.g. those forming the internal lining of the colon or blood forming 'hematopoietic' cells), and in differentiated, non-dividing cells (e.g. neurons in the brain or myocytes in muscle). Cancers occur primarily in proliferative tissues. If DNA damages in proliferating cells are not repaired due to inadequate expression of a DNA repair gene, this increases the risk of cancer. In contrast, when DNA damages occur in non-proliferating cells and are not repaired due to inadequate expression of a DNA repair gene, the damages can accumulate and cause premature ageing. As examples, deficiencies in DNA repair genes *ERCC1* or *XPF* or in *WRN* cause both increased

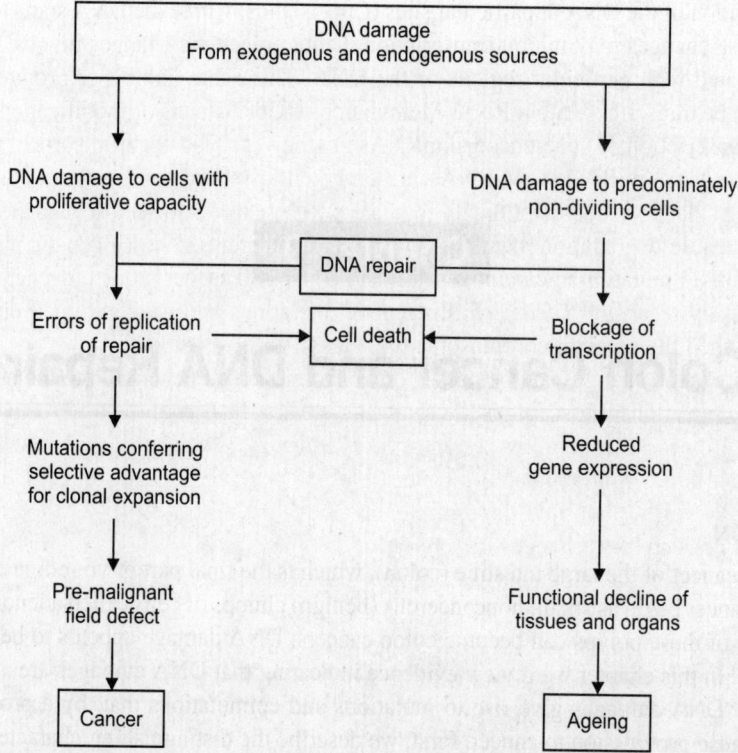

Fig. 9.1: The roles of DNA damage and DNA repair in cancer and ageing.

risk of cancer as well as premature ageing. In Fig. 9.1, DNA repair is indicated as a crucial process impeding both cancer and premature ageing. A mutation is a change in the DNA sequence in which normal base pairs are substituted, added, deleted or rearranged. The DNA containing a mutation still consists of a sequence of standard base pairs, and the altered DNA sequence can be copied when the DNA is replicated. A mutation can prevent a gene from carrying out its function, or it can cause a gene to be translated into a protein that functions abnormally. Mutations can activate oncogenes, inactivate tumour suppressor genes or cause genomic instability in replicating cells, and an assemblage of such mutations, together in the same cell, can lead to cancer. Cancers usually arise from an assemblage of mutations conferring a selective advantage that leads to clonal expansion (Fig. 9.1). Colon cancers, for example, have an average of 15 'driver' mutations (mutations occurring repeatedly in different colon cancers) and about 75 'passenger' mutations (mutations occurring infrequently in colon cancers). Colon cancers also were found to have an average of 9 duplications or deletions of chromosome segments or, more recently, 17 focal amplifications, 28 recurrent deletions and up to 10 translocations. Since mutations have normal DNA structure, they cannot be recognised or removed by DNA repair processes in living cells. Removal of a mutation only occurs if it is sufficiently deleterious to cause the death of the cell.

Another type of inheritable alteration, similar in some ways to a mutation, is an epigenetic change. An epigenetic change refers to a functionally relevant modification of the DNA, or of the histone proteins controlling the relaxation or tightened winding of the DNA within their nucleosome structures. Some epigenetic changes involve specific alterations of the DNA nucleotides. Examples of such changes include methylation of the DNA at particular sites (CpG islands) where the DNA starts to be transcribed into RNA. These changes may inhibit transcription. Other epigenetic changes involve modification of histones associated with particular regions of the DNA. These may inhibit or promote the ability of these regions to be transcribed into mRNA. Methylation of CpG islands or modification of histones can directly alter transcription of gene-encoded mRNAs but they can also occur in parts of the genome that code for microRNAs (miRNAs). MiRNAs are endogenous short non-protein coding RNAs (~22 nucleotides long) that post-transcriptionally regulate mRNA expression in a sequence specific manner. miRNAs either cause degradation of mRNAs or block their translation. Epigenetic modifications can play a role similar to mutation in carcinogenesis, and about 280 cancer prone epigenetic alterations are listed by *Schnekenburger* and *Diederich*. Epigenetic alterations are usually copied onto the daughter chromosomes when the parental chromosome replicates.

Although epigenetic changes can be passed down from one cell generation to the next, they are not regarded as true mutations. Most epigenetic changes appear to be part of the differentiation programme of the cell and are necessary to allow different types of cells to carry out different functions. In most cells of a human body, only about 5% of genes are active at any one time, often due to epigenetic modifications. However, abnormal unprogrammed epigenetic changes may also occur that alter the functioning of a cell and these changes are referred to as 'epimutations.' Programmed epigenetic changes can be reversed. During development, as daughter cells of a stem cell differentiate, some epigenetic changes are programmed for reversal. However, a double strand break in DNA (a type of DNA damage) can initiate unprogrammed epigenetic gene silencing both by causing methylation of a CpG island as well as by promoting silencing types of histone modifications. Another form of epigenetic silencing may occur during DNA repair. The enzyme Parp1 (poly(ADP)-ribose polymerase) and its product poly(ADP)-ribose (PAR) accumulate at sites of DNA damage as part of a repair process. This, in turn, directs recruitment and activation of the chromatin remodelling protein ALC1 that may cause nucleosome remodelling. Nucleosome remodelling has been found to cause, for instance, epigenetic silencing of DNA repair gene *MLH1*. Chemicals previously identified as DNA damaging agents, including benzene, hydroquinone, styrene, carbon tetrachloride and trichloroethylene, were shown to cause considerable hypomethylation of DNA, some through the activation of oxidative stress pathways. Dietary agents also have been shown to affect DNA methylation or histone modification by numerous pathways. Recent evidence indicates that epimutations occur in DNA repair genes that reduce their function. Epimutations in DNA repair genes allow DNA damages to accumulate, and are a cause of progression to cancer.

DNA DAMAGES ARE FREQUENT, AND DNA REPAIR PROCESSES CAN BE OVERWHELMED

Tens of thousands of DNA damages occur per day per cell, on average, in humans, due to reactive molecules produced by metabolism or by hydrolytic reactions in the warm aqueous cellular media. Some types of such endogenous damages, and their rates of occurrence, are shown in Table 9.1. A considerable number of other types of endogenous DNA damages have been identified, many of which are mutagenic. These include propano-, etheno- and malondialdehyde-derived DNA adducts, base propenals, estrogen-DNA adducts, alkylated bases, deamination of each of cytosine, adenine and guanine (to form uracil, hypoxanthine and xanthine, respectively) and adducts formed with DNA by reactive carbonyl species.

While there are repair pathways that act on these DNA damages, the repair processes are not 100% efficient, and further damages occur even as current DNA damages are being repaired. Thus there is a steady state level of many DNA damages, reflecting the efficiencies of repair and the frequencies of occurrence. For instance, Helbock and others estimated the steady state level of oxidative adducts in rat

Table 9.1: DNA damages due to natural endogenous causes in mammalian cells

DNA damages	Reported rate of occurrence
Oxidative	86000 per cell per day in rats
	10000 per cell per day in humans
	100000 per cell per day in rats
	11500 per cell per day for humans
	74000 per cell per day for rats
Specific oxidative damage products 8-hydroxyguanine,	2800 per cell per day in humans
8-hydroxydeoxyguanosine, 5-(hydroxymethyl) uracil	34800 per cell per day in mice
Depurinations	10000 per cell during 20 hr generation period
	13920 per cell per day (580/cell/hr)
	2000 to 10000 per cell per day
	9000 per cell per day
Depyrimidinations	500 pyrimidines per cell during 20 hr generation period
	696 per cell per day (29/cell/hr)
Single-strand breaks	55200 per cell per day (2300/cell/hr)
Double-strand breaks	~10 per cell cycle in humans
	~50 per cell cycle in humans
O^6-methylguanine	3120 per cell per day (130/cell/hr)
Cytosine deamination	192 per cell per day (8/cell/hr)

liver as 24000 adducts per cell in young rats and 66000 adducts per cell in old rats. Nakamura and Swenberg determined the number of AP sites (apurinc and apyrimidinic sites) in normal tissues of the rat (i.e. in lung, kidney, liver, testis, heart, colon and brain). The data indicated that the number of AP sites ranged from about 50000 per cell in liver, kidney and lung to about 200000 per cell in the brain. These steady state numbers of AP sites in genomic DNA were considered to represent the balance between formation and repair of AP sites. DNA repair pathways are usually able to keep up with the endogenous damages in replicating cells, in part by halting DNA replication at the site of damage until repair can occur. In contrast, non-replicating cells have a build-up of DNA damages, causing ageing.

However, some exogenous DNA damaging agents, such as those in tobacco smoke, discussed below, may overload the repair pathways, either with higher levels of the same type of DNA damages as those occurring endogenously or with novel types of damage that are repaired more slowly. In addition, if DNA repair pathways are deficient, due to inherited mutations or sporadic somatic epimutations in DNA repair genes in replicating somatic cells, unrepaired endogenous and exogenous damages will increase due to insufficient repair. Increased DNA damages would likely give rise to increased errors of replication past the damages (by trans-lesion synthesis) or increased error prone repair (e.g. by non-homologous end-joining), causing mutations. Increased mutations that activate oncogenes, inactivate tumour suppressor genes, cause genomic instability or give rise to other driver mutations in replicating cells would increase the risk of cancer.

Cancers are often caused by Exogenous DNA Damaging Agents

Cancer incidence, in different areas of the world, varies considerably. Thus, the incidence of colon cancer among Black Native-Africans is less than 1 person out of 100, 000, while among male Black

African-Americans it is 72.9 per 100, 000, and this difference is likely due to differences in diet. Rates of colon cancer incidence among populations migrating from lower-incidence to higher-incidence countries change rapidly, and within one generation can reach the rate in the higher-incidence country. This is observed, for instance, in migrants from Japan to Hawaii. The most common cancers for men and women and their rates of incidence per 100000, averaged over the more developed areas and less developed areas of the world, are shown in Table 9.2. Overall, worldwide, cancer incidence in all organs combined is 300.1 per 100000 per year in more developed areas and 160.3 per 100000 per year in less developed areas. The differences in cancer incidence between more developed areas of the world and less developed areas are likely due, in large part, to differences in exposure to exogenous carcinogenic factors. The lowest rates of cancers in a given organ (Table 9.2) may be due, at least in part, to endogenous DNA damages (as described in the previous section) that cause errors of replication (trans-lesion synthesis) or error prone repair (e.g. non-homologous end-joining), leading to carcinogenic mutations. The higher rates (Table 9.2) are likely largely attributable to exogenous factors, such as higher rates of tobacco use or diets higher in saturated fats that directly, or indirectly, increase the incidence of DNA damage. It is interesting to note in Table 9.2 that, in cases where cancers occur in the same organs of men and women, men consistently have a higher rate of cancer than women. The basis for this is currently unknown.

Table 9.2: Incidence and mortality rates for the most common cancers in age standardised rates per 100000 (excluding non-melanoma skin cancer).

	More developed areas		Less developed areas	
	Incidence	*Mortality*	*Incidence*	*Mortality*
Breast (women)	66.4	15.3	27.3	10.8
Prostate (men)	62.0	10.6	12.0	5.6
Lung (men)	47.4	39.4	27.8	24.6
Lung (women)	18.6	13.6	11.1	9.7
Colorectum (men)	37.6	15.1	12.1	6.9
Colorectum (women)	24.2	9.7	9.4	5.4
Esophagus (men)	6.5	5.3	11.8	10.1
Esophagus (women)	1.2	1.0	5.7	4.7
Stomach (men)	16.7	10.4	21.1	16.0
Stomach (women)	7.3	4.7	10.0	8.1
Liver (men)	8.1	7.2	18.9	17.4
Liver (women)	2.7	2.5	7.6	7.2
Bladder (men)	16.6	4.6	5.4	2.6
Bladder (women)	3.6	1.0	1.4	0.7
Cervix/Uterine (women)	12.9	2.4	5.9	1.7
Kidney (men)	11.8	4.1	2.5	1.3
Kidney (women)	5.8	1.7	1.4	0.8
Non-Hodgkin lymphoma (men)	10.3	3.6	4.2	3.0
Non-Hodgkin lymphoma (women)	7.0	2.2	2.8	1.9
Melanoma (men)	9.5	1.8	0.7	0.3
Melanoma (women)	8.6	1.1	0.6	0.3
Ovarian (women)	9.4	5.1	5.0	3.1

EXOGENOUS DNA DAMAGING AGENTS IN CARCINOGENESIS

Carcinogenic exogenous factors have been identified as a major cause of many common cancers, including cancers of the lung, colorectum, esophagus, stomach, liver, cervix/uterus and melanoma. Often such exogenous factors have been shown to cause DNA damage, as described below.

EXOGENOUS DNA DAMAGING AGENTS IN LUNG CANCER

In both developed and undeveloped countries, lung cancer is the most frequent cause of cancer mortality (Table 9.2, data for men and women combined). Lung cancer is largely caused by tobacco smoke, since risk estimates for lung cancer indicate that, in the United States, tobacco smoke is responsible for 90% of lung cancers. Also implicated in lung cancer (and somewhat overlapping with smoking) are occupational exposure to carcinogens (approximately 9 to 15%), radon (10%) and outdoor air pollution (perhaps 1 to 2%). Tobacco smoke is a complex mixture of over 5,300 identified chemicals, of which 150 are known to have specific toxicological properties. A 'Margin of Exposure' approach has recently been established to determine the most important exogenous carcinogenic factors in tobacco smoke. This quantitative-type of measurement is based on published dose response data for mutagenicity or carcinogenicity and the concentrations of these components in tobacco smoke (Table 9.3). Using the 'Margin of Exposure' approach, Cunningham and others found the most important tumorigenic compounds in tobacco smoke to be, in order of importance, acrolein, formaldehyde, acrylonitrile, 1,3-butadiene, acetaldehyde, ethylene oxide and isoprene.

Table 9.3: Weight, in µg per cigarette, of several likely carcinogenic DNA damaging agents in tobacco smoke.

Acrolein	122.4
Formaldehyde	60.5
Acrylonitrile	29.3
1,3-butadiene	105.0
Acetaldehyde	1448.0
Ethylene oxide	7.0
Isoprene	952.0
Benzo[α]pyrene	0.014

Acrolein, the first agent in Table 9.3, is the structurally simplest α, β-unsaturated aldehyde (Fig. 9.2). It can rapidly penetrate through the cell membrane and bind to the nucleophilic N^2-amine of deoxyguanine (dG) followed by cyclisation of N^1, to give the exocyclic DNA adduct α-hydroxy-1, N^2-propano-2′-deoxyguanine (γ-HOPdG) (shown in Fig. 9.2) and another product designated α-HOPdG. The adducts formed by acrolein are a major type of DNA damage caused by tobacco smoke, and acrolein has been found to be mutagenic. In tobacco smoke, acrolein has a concentration >8, 000 fold higher than benzo[α]pyrene, with 122.4 µg of acrolein per cigarette. Benzo[α]pyrene has long been thought to be an important carcinogen in tobacco smoke. As reviewed by Alexandrov and others, benzo[α]pyrene damages DNA by forming DNA adducts at the N^2 position of guanine (similar to where acrolein forms adducts). However, by the 'Margin of Exposure' approach, based on published dose response data and its concentration in cigarette smoke of 0.014 µg per cigarette, benzo[α]pyrene is thought to be a much less important mutagen for lung tissue than acrolein and the other six highly likely carcinogens in tobacco smoke listed in Table 9.3.

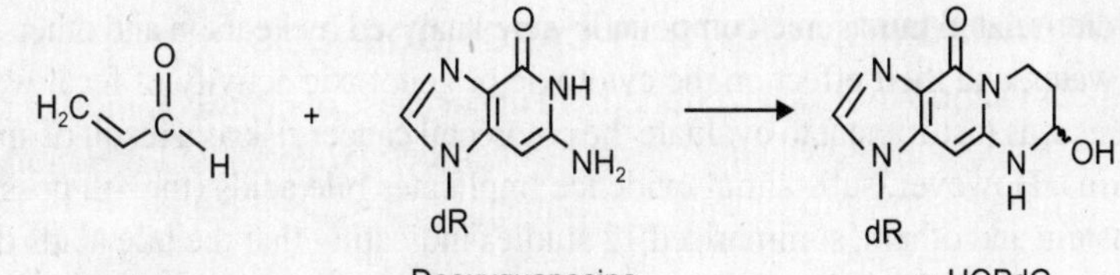

Fig. 9.2. Reaction of acrolein with deoxyguanosine.

The other agents in Table 9.3 cause DNA damages in different ways. Formaldehyde, the second agent in Table 9.3, primarily causes DNA damage by introducing DNA-protein cross-links. These cross-links, in turn, cause mutagenic deletions or other small-scale chromosomal rearrangements and may also cause mutations through single-nucleotide insertions. Acrylonitrile, the third agent in Table 9.3, appears to cause DNA damage indirectly by increasing oxidative stress, leading to increased levels of 8'-hydroxyl-2-deoxyguanosine (8-OHdG) in DNA. Oxidative stress also causes lipid peroxidation that generates malondialdehyde (MDA), and MDA forms DNA adducts with guanine, adenine and cytosine. The fourth agent in Table 9.3, 1,3-butadiene, causes genotoxicity both directly by forming a DNA adduct as well as indirectly by causing global loss of DNA methylation and histone methylation leading to epigenetic alterations. The fifth agent in Table 9.3, acetaldehyde, reacts with 2'-deoxyguanosine in DNA to form DNA adducts. The sixth agent in Table 9.3, ethylene oxide, forms mutagenic hydroxyethyl DNA adducts with adenine and guanine. The seventh agent in Table 9.3, isoprene, is normally produced endogenously by humans, and is the main hydrocarbon of non-smoking human breath. However, smoking one cigarette causes an increase of breath isoprene levels by an average of 70%. Isoprene, after being metabolised to mono-epoxides, causes DNA damage measured as single and double strand breaks in DNA.

A large number of studies have been published in which the levels and characteristics of DNA adducts in the lung and bronchus of smokers and non-smokers have been compared, as reviewed by Phillips. In most of these studies, significantly elevated levels of DNA adducts were detected in the peripheral lung, bronchial epithelium or bronchioalveolar lavage cells of the smokers, especially for total bulky DNA adducts. As further discussed by Phillips, mean levels of DNA adducts in ex-smokers (usually with at least a 1 year interval since smoking cessation) are found generally to be intermediate between the levels of smokers and life-long non-smokers. From these comparisons, the half-life of some DNA adducts in lung tissue are estimated to be ~1–2 years.

EXOGENOUS DNA DAMAGING AGENTS IN COLORECTAL CANCER

Up to 20% of current colorectal cancers in the United States may be due to tobacco smoke. Presumably tobacco smoke causes colon cancer due to the DNA damaging agents described above for lung cancer. These agents may be taken up in the blood and carried to organs of the body. The human colon is exposed to many compounds that are either of direct dietary origin or result from digestive and/or microbial processes. Four different classes of colonic mutagenic compounds were analysed by de Kok and van Maanen and evaluated for fecal mutagenicity. These included (i) pyrolysis compounds from food (heterocyclic aromatic amines and polycyclic aromatic hydrocarbons), (ii) *N*-nitroso-compounds (from high meat diets, from drinking water with high nitrates or produced during ulcerative colitis), (iii) fecapentaenes (produced by the colonic bacteria *Bacteriodes* in the presence of bile acids) and (iv) bile acids (increased in the colon in response to a high fat diet and metabolised to genotoxic form by bacteria in the colon).

Many of these diet-related mutagenic compounds were analysed by Pearson and others in terms of their presence in fecal water, and their effect on the cytotoxic or genotoxic activity of fecal water. Evidence in both of these studies was insufficient to evaluate the colorectal cancer risk as a result of specific exposures in quantitative terms. However, substantial evidence implicates bile acids (the 4th possibility above) in colon caner. Bernstein and others, summarised 12 studies indicating that the bile acids deoxycholic acid (DCA) and/or lithocholic acid (LCA) induce production of DNA damaging reactive oxygen species and/or reactive nitrogen species in colon cells of animal or human origin. They also tabulated 14 studies showing that DCA and LCA induce DNA damage in colon cells. In addition to causing DNA damage, bile acids may also generate genomic instability by causing mitotic perturbations and reduced expression of spindle checkpoint proteins, giving rise to micro-nuclei, chromosome bridges and other structures that are precursors to aneuploidy. Furthermore, at high physiological concentrations, bile acids cause frequent apoptosis, and those cells in the exposed populations with reduced apoptosis capability tend to survive and selectively proliferate. Cells with reduced ability to undergo apoptosis in response to DNA damage would tend to accumulate mutations when replication occurs past those damages, and such cells may give rise to colon cancers. In addition, 7 epidemiological studies between 1971 and 1990, found that fecal bile acid concentrations are increased in populations with a high incidence of colorectal cancer. A similar 2012 epidemiological study showed that concentrations of fecal LCA and DCA, respectively, were 4-fold and 5-fold higher in a population at 65-fold higher risk of colon cancer compared to a population at lower risk of colon cancer. This evidence points to bile acids DCA and LCA as centrally important DNA-damaging carcinogens in colon cancer. Dietary total fat intake and dietary saturated fat intake is significantly related to incidence of colon cancer. Increasing total fat or saturated fat in human diets results in increases in DCA and LCA in the feces, indicating increased contact of the colonic epithelium with DCA and LCA. Bernstein and others added the bile acid DCA to the standard diet of wild-type mice. This supplement raised the level of DCA in the feces of mice from the standard-diet fed mouse level of 0.3 mg DCA/g dry weight to 4.6 mg DCA/g dry weight, a level similar to that for humans on a high fat diet of 6.4 mg DCA/g dry weight. After 8 or 10 months on the DCA-supplemented diet, 56% of the mice developed invasive colon cancer. This directly indicates that DCA, a DNA damaging agent, at levels present in humans after a high fat diet, can cause colorectal cancer.

EXOGENOUS DNA DAMAGING AGENTS IMPLICATED IN OTHER MAJOR CANCERS

It is beyond the scope of this chapter to detail the evidence implicating DNA damaging agents as etiologic agents in all of the significant cancers. Therefore, in Table 9.4 we indicate with a single reference the major DNA damaging agent in five additional prevalent cancers, in order to illustrate the generality of exogenous DNA damaging agents as causes of cancer.

Table 9.4: Selected cancers and relevant implicated exogenous DNA damaging agents.

Cancer	*Exogenous DNA damaging agent*
Esophagus	Bile acids
Stomach	*Helicobacter pylori* infection
Liver	*Aspergillus* metabolite aflatoxin B(1)
Cervix/Uterus	Human papillomavirus plus increased nitric oxide from tobacco smoke or other infection
Melanoma	UV light from solar radiation

In particular, we point out, as reviewed by Handa and others, *Helicobacter pylori* infection increases the production of reactive oxygen and reactive nitrogen species (RNS) in the human stomach, which, in turn, significantly increases DNA damage in the gastric epithelial cells.

Thus, *H. pylori* infection acts as a DNA damaging agent. In the case of human papillomavirus (HPV) infection, Wei and others showed that cervical cells could resist RNS stress when not infected with HPV. However, cervical cells infected by HPV and exposed to RNS had higher levels of DNA double strand breaks as well as a higher mutation rate. This appeared to occur due to the ability of HPV to greatly reduce protein expression of the DNA damage repair/response gene *P53* when infected cells were stressed by RNS. Since reduced *P53* expression leads to greater RNS-induced DNA damage, HPV infection acts as a DNA damaging agent in the presence of RNS stress.

DEFICIENT DNA REPAIR DUE TO A GERM LINE MUTATION ALLOWS DNA DAMAGES LEADING TO INCREASED FREQUENCIES OF MUTATION, EPIMUTATION AND CANCER

Expression of DNA repair genes may be reduced by inherited germ line mutations or genetic polymorphisms, or by epigenetic alterations or mutations in somatic cells, and these reductions may substantially increase the risk of cancer. Overall, about 30% of cancers are considered to be familial (largely due to inherited germ line mutations or genetic polymorphisms) and 70% are considered to be sporadic. In 2 overlapping databases 167 and 169 human genes (depending on the database) are listed that are directly employed in DNA repair or influence DNA repair processes.

The lists were originally devised by Wood and others. The genes are distributed in groups of DNA repair pathways and in related functions that affect DNA repair (Table 9.5). Bernstein and others illustrate many of the steps and order of action of the gene products involved for the first five DNA repair pathways listed in Table 9.5.

Table 9.5: DNA repair pathways and other processes affecting DNA repair.

	Number of genes listed in the two databases
Homologous Recombinational Repair (HRR)	21,21
Non-homologous End Joining (NHEJ)	8,7
Nucleotide Excision Repair (NER)	30,29
Base Excision Repair (including PARP enzymes) (BER)	19,20
Mis-Match Repair (MMR)	11,10
Fanconi Anemia (FANC) [affects HRR (above) and translesion synthesis (TLS)]	10,16
Direct reversal of damage	3,3
DNA polymerases (act in various pathways)	17,15
Editing and processing nucleases (act in various pathways)	6,8
Ubiquitination and modification/Rad6 pathway including TLS	11,5
DNA damage response	12,14
Modulation of nucleotide pools	3,3
Chromatin structure	2,3
Defective in diseases and syndromes	4,5
DNA-topoisomerase cross-links	2,1
Other genes	8,9

Individuals with an inherited impairment in DNA repair capability are often at considerably increased risk of cancer. If an individual has a germ line mutation in a DNA repair gene or a DNA damage response gene (that recognises DNA damage and activates DNA repair), usually one abnormal copy of the gene is inherited from one of the parents and then the other copy is inactivated at some later point in life in a somatic cell. The inactivation may be due, for example, to point mutation, deletion, gene conversion, epigenetic silencing or other mechanisms. The protein encoded by the gene will either not be expressed or be expressed in a mutated form. Consequently the DNA repair or DNA damage response function will be deficient or impaired, and damages will accumulate. Such DNA damages can cause errors during DNA replication or inaccurate repair, leading to mutations that can give rise to cancer. Increased oxidative DNA damages also cause increased gene silencing by CpG island hypermethylation, a form of epimutation. These oxidative DNA damages induce formation and relocalisation of a silencing complex that may result in cancer-specific aberrant DNA methylation and transcriptional silencing. As pointed out above, the enzyme Parp1 (poly(ADP)-ribose polymerase) and its product poly(ADP)-ribose (PAR) accumulate at sites of DNA damage as part of a repair process, recruiting chromatin remodelling protein ALC1, causing nucleosome remodelling that has been shown to direct epigenetic silencing of DNA repair gene *MLH1*. If silencing of genes necessary for DNA repair occurs, the repair of further DNA damages will be deficient and more damages will accumulate. Such additional DNA damages will cause increased errors during DNA synthesis, leading to mutations that can give rise to cancer.

INHERITED MUTATIONS IN GENES EMPLOYED IN DNA REPAIR THAT GIVE RISE TO SYNDROMES CHARACTERISED BY INCREASED RISK OF CANCER

Table 6 lists 36 genes for which an inherited mutation results in an increased risk of cancer. The proteins encoded by 35 of these genes are involved in DNA repair and in some cases also in other aspects of the DNA damage response such as cell cycle arrest and apoptosis. The polymerase coded for by the 36th gene, *XPV (POLH)*, is involved in bypass (rather than repair) of DNA damage, called translesion synthesis. The genes listed in Table 6, when mutated in the germ line, give rise to a considerably increased lifetime risk of cancer, of up to 100%. Thus defects in DNA repair cause progression to cancer. In addition to mutations in genes that may substantially raise lifetime cancer risk, there appear to be many weakly effective genetically inherited polymorphisms [single nucleotide polymophisms (SNPs) and copy number variants (CNVs)]. By the HapMap Project, more than 3 million SNPs have been found, and by Genome Wide Association studies (GWAs), about 30 SNPs were found to increase risk of cancers. However the added risk of cancer by these SNPs is usually small, i.e. less than a factor of 2 increase. A large twin study, involving 44, 788 pairs of twins, evaluated the risk of the same cancer before the age of 75 for monozygotic twins (identical genomes with the same polymorphisms) and dizygotic twins. If one twin had colorectal, breast or prostate cancer, the monozygotic twin had an 11 to 18 per cent chance of developing the same cancer while the dizygotic twin had only a 3 to 9% risk. The differences in monozygotic and dizygotic rates of paired cancer were not significant for the other 24 types of cancer evaluated in this study. Polymorphisms of the DNA repair gene ERCC1 will be discussed below in relation to targeted chemotherapy.

EPIMUTATIONS MAY REPRESS DNA REPAIR GENE EXPRESSION, ALLOWING DNA DAMAGES TO INCREASE, LEADING TO INCREASED FREQUENCY OF FURTHER EPIMUTATION, MUTATION AND CANCER

While germ line (familial) mutations in DNA repair genes cause a high risk of cancer, somatic mutations in DNA repair genes are rarely found in sporadic (non-familial) cancers. Much more often, DNA repair genes are found to have epigenetic alterations in cancers. One example of the epigenetic down-regulation of a DNA repair gene in cancers comes from studies of the MMR protein MLH1. Truninger and others assessed 1048 unselected consecutive colon cancers. Of these, 103 were deficient in protein expression of *MLH1*, with 68 of these cancers being sporadic (the remaining *MLH1* deficient cancers were due to germ line mutations). Of the 68 sporadic MLH1 protein-deficient colon cancers, 65 (96%) were found to be deficient due to epigenetic methylation of the CpG island of the *MLH1* gene. Deficient protein expression of *MLH1* may also have been caused, in the remaining 3 sporadic MLH1 protein-deficient cancers (which did not have germ line mutations), by over expression of the microRNA miR-155. When miR-155 was transfected into cells it caused reduced expression of *MLH1*. Overexpression of miR-155 was found in colon cancers in which protein expression of *MLH1* was deficient and the *MLH1* gene was neither mutated nor hypermethylated in its CpG island. Another example of the epigenetic down-regulation of a DNA repair gene in cancer comes from studies of the direct reversal of methylated guanine bases by methyl guanine methyl transferase (*MGMT*). In the most common form of brain cancer, glioblastoma, the DNA repair gene *MGMT* is epigenetically methylated in 29% to 66% of tumours, thereby reducing protein expression of *MGMT*. However, for 28% of glioblastomas, the *MGMT* protein is deficient but the *MGMT* promoter is not methylated. Zhang and others found, in the glioblastomas without methylated *MGMT* promoters, that the level of microRNA miR-181d is inversely correlated with protein expression of *MGMT* and that the direct target of miR-181d is the *MGMT* mRNA 3′UTR (the three prime untranslated region of *MGMT* mRNA), though they indicated that other miRNAs may also be involved in the reduction of protein expression of *MGMT*.

As summarised above, epimutations can result from oxidative DNA damages. Such damages cause formation and relocalisation of a silencing complex that in turn causes increased gene silencing by CpG island hypermethylation. Epigenetic nucleosome remodelling during DNA repair can also silence gene expression. When CpG island methylation or nucleosome remodelling or other types of epigenetic alterations (e.g. micro RNAs or histone modifications) inhibit DNA repair genes, more damages will accumulate. Accumulated DNA damages cause increased errors during DNA synthesis and repair. Thus epigenetic deficiencies in DNA repair genes can have a cascading effect (a mutator phenotype), leading to genomic instability and accumulation of mutations and epimutations that can give rise to cancer.

Deficiencies in DNA repair genes cause increased mutation rates. Mutations rates increase in MMR defective cells and in HRR defective cells. Chromosomal rearrangements and aneuploidy also increase in HRR defective cells. Thus, deficiency in DNA repair causes genomic instability and genomic instability is the likely main underlying cause of the genetic alterations leading to tumorigenesis. Deficient DNA repair permits the acquisition of a sufficient number of alterations in tumour suppressor genes and oncogenes to fuel carcinogenesis. Deficiencies in DNA repair appear to be central to the genomic and epigenomic instability characteristic of cancer. The chain of consequences of exposure of cells to endogenous and exogenous DNA damaging agents that lead to cancer. The role of germ line defects in DNA repair genes in familial cancer are also indicated. The large role of DNA damage and consequent epigenetic DNA repair defects leading to sporadic cancer are emphasised. The roles of germ line mutation and directly induced somatic mutation in sporadic cancer are indicated as well.

EPIGENETIC ALTERATIONS CAUSED BY MICRO RNAs

MicroRNAs (miRNAs) are endogenous non-coding RNAs, 19–25 nucleotides in length, that can have substantial effects on DNA repair. miRNAs can either directly or indirectly reduce expression of DNA repair or DNA damage response genes. As discussed above, over-expression of miR-155 causes reduced expression of DNA repair protein MLH1, and miR-155 is overexpressed in colon cancers. Similarly, miR-181d is overexpressed in glioblastomas, causing reduced expression of DNA repair protein *MGMT*. Although miRNAs can epigenetically regulate DNA repair gene expression, the expression levels of many miRNAs may themselves be subject to epigenetic regulation. One mechanism of epigenetic regulation of miRNA expression is hypomethylation of the promoter region of the DNA sequence that codes for the miRNA. Schnekenburger and Diederich list miR-155 as one of a long list of mi-RNAs whose expression is increased by hypomythylation in colorectal cancers. In particular, hypomethylated miR-155 (the hypomethylation making it more active) targets genes *MLH1, MSH2* and *MSH6,* causing each of them to have reduced expression.

Wan and others referred to 6 further DNA repair genes that are directly targeted by miRNAs. *ATM, RAD52, RAD23B, MSH2, BRCA1* and *P53*, are each specifically targeted by one or two of the 8 miRNAs miR-21, miR-24, miR-125b, miR-182, miR-210, miR-373, miR-421 and miR-504, with all but miR-210, miR-421 and miR-504 among those identified by Schnekenburger and Diederich as overexpressed through epigenetic hypomethylation. Overexpression of any one of these miRNAs leads to reduced expression of its target DNA repair gene. Wan and others further listed 16 DNA damage response genes targeted by specific miRNAs. Wan and others indicated miR-15a, miR-16, miR-17, miR-20a, miR-21, miR-24, miR-29, miR-34a, miR-106a, miR-93, miR-124a, miR-125b, miR-192, miR-195, miR-215, miR-182, miR-373 as among those targeting DNA damage response genes. Of these, all but miR-124a were identified by Schnekenburger and Diederich, (and Malumbres further identified miR-34a and miR-124a) as being among miRNAs whose expression is subject to epigenetic alteration in tumours. Other miRNAs whose expression is subject to epimutation in colorectal cancers (and their target DNA repair or DNA damage response genes) include miR-17 (*E2F1*), miR-34b/c (*P53*), miR-106a (*E2F1*), miR-200a and miR-200b (*MLH1, MSH2*) and miR-675 (*Rb*).

EPIGENETIC ALTERATIONS CAUSED BY CHROMOSOME REMODELLING AND HISTONE MODIFICATION

Specific miRNAs can also indirectly (and strongly) reduce protein expression of DNA repair genes through their role in repression of proteins designated High Mobility Group A1 (HMGA1) and HMGA2 (the names come from the proteins' high electrophoretic mobility on acrylamide gels). HMGA1 and HMGA2 cause chromatin remodelling at specific sites in DNA and reduce expression at those sites. In particular, these proteins appear to control DNA repair genes *BRCA1* and *ERCC1*. BRCA1 And ERCC1 proteins have key roles in DNA repair, particularly of double-strand breaks and interstrand crosslinks. *HMGA1* and *HMGA2* genes are usually active in embryogenesis, but normally have very low expression levels in adult tissues. Their expression levels in adult tissues are kept low by the actions of specific miRNAs. If expression of these miRNAs is reduced, then the repressive HMGA1 and HMGA2 proteins become highly expressed and, in particular, can reduce expression of *BRCA1* or *ERCC1* respectively.

As reviewed by Resar, all HMG proteins share an acidic carboxyl terminus and associate with chromatin. As an example, HMGA1A, in particular, has three AT-hook domains that allow it to bind to AT-rich regions and recruit an 'enhanceosome' that may displace histones and cause chromosome remodelling and reduce gene expression. Baldassarre and others showed that HMGA1B protein binds to the promoter region of *BRCA1* and inhibits *BRCA1* promoter activity (indicated in Figure 3 as chromatin remodelling causing reduced *BRCA1*). In 12 surgically removed human breast carcinomas, there was an inverse correlation between HGMA1 protein and *BRCA1* mRNA levels. HGMA1 was almost undetectable in normal breast tissue, highly expressed in the tumour samples, and BRCA1 protein was strongly diminished in tumour samples. Baldassarre and others suggested that while only 11% of breast tumours had hypermethylation of the *BRCA1* gene, 82% of aggressive breast cancer specimens have low BRCA1 protein, and most of these could be due to chromatin remodelling by high levels of HMGA1 protein. Similarly, HMGA2 binds to an *ERCC1* promoter site and represses *ERCC1* promoter activity. The miRNAs miR-23a, miR-26a and miR-30a inhibit *HMG2A* protein expression though it has not been reported whether these miRNAs are under epigenetic control.

Resar and Baldassarre and others summarised reports indicating that *HGMA1* is widely overexpressed in aggressive malignancies including cancers of the thyroid, head and neck, colon, lung, breast, pancreas, hematopoetic system, cervix, uterine corpus, prostate and central nervous system. Palmieri and others showed that *HGMA1* and *HMGA2* are targeted (and thus strongly reduced in expression) by miR-15, miR-16, miR-26a, miR-196a2 and Let-7a. The promoter regions associated with miR-16, miR-196a2 and Let-7a miRNAs are epimutated by hypomethylation while Sampath and others showed, in addition, that the coding regions for miR-15 and miR-16 were epigenetically silenced due to histone deacetylase activity. Palmieri and others further showed that these 5 miRNAs are drastically reduced in a panel of 41 pituitary adenomas, accompanied by increases in *HMGA1* and *HMGA2* specific mRNAs. In a more recent study on pituitary adenomas by D'Angelo and others, reduced expression of 18 miRNAs was found, with 5 of them targeting *HMGA1* or *HMGA2*. In this recent study, among the 18 miRNAs with reduced expression, the reduced expression of miR-26b, miR-34b, miR-432 and miR-592 was known to be due to epigenetic alteration. Thus, epigenetic miRNA silencing, causing strong expression of *HMGA1* and *HMGA2,* occurs in many types of cancer and this may be related to reductions found in expression of DNA repair genes *BRCA1, BRCA2* and *ERCC1.*

Suzuki and others, using genome wide profiling, found 174 primary transcription units for miRNAs, called 'pri-miRNAs' (large precursor RNAs which may encode multiple miRNAs), of which they identified 37 as potential targets for epigenetic silencing. Of these 37 pri-miRNAs, 22 were encoded by DNA sequences with CpG islands (all of which were hypermethylated in colorectal cancer cells) while the other pri-miRNAs were subject to regulation by epigenetic 'activating marks' without evidence of deregulated methylation. Activating marks are alterations on histones that cause transcriptional activation of the genes associated with those altered histones. In particular, the nucleosome, the fundamental subunit of chromatin, is composed of 146 bp of DNA wrapped around an octamer of four core histone proteins (H3, H4, H2A, and H2B). Post-translational modifications (i.e. acetylation, methylation, phosphorylation, and ubiquitination) of the *N-* and C-terminal tails of the four core histones play an important role in regulating chromatin biology.

These specific histone modifications, and their combinations, are translated, through protein interactions, into distinct effects on nuclear processes, such as activation or inhibition of transcription. In eukaryotes, methylation of lysine 4 in histone H3 (H3K4), which interacts with the promoter region of genes, is linked to transcriptional activation. There is a strong positive correlation between trimethylation of H3K4, transcription rates, active polymerase II occupancy and histone acetylation. Thus trimethylation of H3K4 is an activating mark.

In addition to pri-miRNAs being regulated by activating marks, some miRNAs appear to be directly regulated by these histone modifications. As summarised by Sampath and others, histone deacetylases catalyse the removal of acetyl groups on specific lysines around gene promoters to trigger demethylation of otherwise methylated lysine 4 on histones (H3K4me2/3) and this causes loss of these activating marks, promoting chromatin compaction, and leading to epigenetic silencing. Sampath and others showed that such histone deacetylase activity mediates the epigenetic silencing of miRNAs miR-15a, miR-16, and miR-29b. As indicated above, miR-15, miR-16 specifically target *HGMA1* and *HMGA2*. If miR-15 and miR-16 lose their activating marks, they have reduced expression, causing *HGMA1* and *HGMA2* to be transcriptionally activated, thus reducing expression of DNA repair genes *BRCA1* and *ERCC1*.

Histone modification and chromatin remodelling are indicated as epigentically altering the expression of many genes in progression to cancer, and specifically causing reduced *BRCA1* and possibly reduced expression of *ERCC1*. In addition, a second dotted line is used to indicate possible repression of *ERCC1* by an miRNA. Klase and others showed that a particular virally coded miRNA down regulates ERCC1 protein expression at the *p*-body level (a *p*-body is a cytoplasmic granule 'processing body' that interacts with miRNAs to repress translation or trigger degradation of target mRNAs).

A survey of human miRNA homology regions to *ERCC1* mRNA indicates at least 21 human coded miRNAs that could act to decrease *ERCC1* mRNA translation (shown in Microcosm Targets). ERCC1 protein expression, assessed by immunohistochemical staining, is deficient due to an epigenetic mechanism in colon cancers, and this could be due to action of one or more miRNAs, acting directly on *ERCC1* mRNA.

DRIVER MUTATIONS AND PATHWAYS TO CANCER PROGRESSION

Recent research indicates a mechanism by which an early driver mutation may cause subsequent epigenetic alterations or mutations in pathways leading to cancer. Wang and others point out that isocitrate dehydrogenase genes *IDH1* and *IDH2* are the most frequently mutated metabolic genes in human cancer. A gene frequently mutated in cancer is considered to be a driver mutation so that mutations in *IDH1* and *IDH2* would be driver mutations. Wang and others further point out that *IDH1* and *IDH2* mutant cells produce an excess metabolic intermediate, 2-hydroxyglutarate, which binds to catalytic sites in key enzymes that are important in altering histone and DNA promoter methylation.

Thus, mutations in *IDH1* and *IDH2* generate a DNA CpG island methylator phenotype that causes promoter hypermethylation and concomitant silencing of tumour suppressor genes such as the DNA repair genes *MLH1*, *MGMT* and *BRCA1*. A study, involving 51 patients with brain gliomas who had two or more biopsies over time, showed that mutation in the *IDH1* gene occurred prior to the occurrence of a *p53* mutation or a 1p/19q loss of heterozygosity, indicating that *IDH1* mutation is an early driver mutation. Work by Turcan and others showed that *IDH1* mutation alone is sufficient to establish the brain glioma CpG island methylator phenotype. Carillo and others showed that when an *IDH1* mutation was present in glioblastoma tumours, 64% of these were hypermethylated in the promoter regions of *MGMT*.

Other initial driver mutations can cause progression to glioblastoma as well. As pointed out above, increased levels of miR-181d also cause reduced expression of *MGMT* protein in glioblastoma. Nelson and others indicate that a single type of miRNA may target hundreds of different mRNAs, causing alterations in multiple pathways. Patients with a glioblastoma that does not harbour an *IDH1* mutation have an overall fairly short survival time, while patients with both mutated *IDH1* and methylated *MGMT* have a subtype of glioblastoma with a much longer survival time (implying a different pathway of cancer progression).

An *IDH1* mutation that gives rise to a CpG island methylator phenotype that causes promoter hypermethylation and concomitant silencing of *MGMT* also causes promoter silencing of other genes as well. In addition to silencing of genes, the CpG island methylator phenotype can cause methylation of the promoter regions of long interspersed nuclear element-1 (LINE-1) DNA sequences. Ohka and others point out that LINE-1 is a class of retroposons that are the most successful integrated mobile elements in the human genome, and account for about 18% of human DNA. Ohka and others found that LINE-1 methylation is directly proportional to *MGMT* promoter methylation in gliomas and suggested that LINE-1 methylation could be used as a proxy to indicate the CpG island methylator phenotype status in glioblastomas. This phenotype, likely associated with methylation of the *MGMT* promoter, in turn, indicates whether treatment with the DNA alkylating agent temozolomide will be beneficial in treatment of a patient with a glioblastoma, since *MGMT* removes the alkyl groups added to guanine by temozolomide.

FIELD DEFECTS

Field defects have been described in many types of gastrointestinal cancers. A field defect arises when an epimutation or mutation occurs in a stem cell that causes that stem cell to give rise to a number of daughter stem cells that can out-compete neighbouring stem cells. These initial mutated cells form a patch of somewhat more rapidly growing cells (an initial field defect). That patch then enlarges at the expense of neighbouring cells, followed by, at some point, an additional mutation or epimutation arising in one of the field defect stem cells so that this new stem cell with two advantageous mutations can generate daughter stem cells that can out-compete the surrounding field defect of cells that have just one advantageous mutation. As illustrated in Fig. 9.3, this process of expanding sub-patches within earlier patches will occur multiple times until a particular constellation of mutations results in a cancer (represented by the small dark patch in Fig. 9.3. It should also be noted that a cancer, once formed, continues to evolve and continues to produce sub clones. A renal cancer, sampled in 9 areas, had 40 ubiquitous mutations, 59 mutations shared by some, but not all regions, and 29 'private' mutations only present in one region.

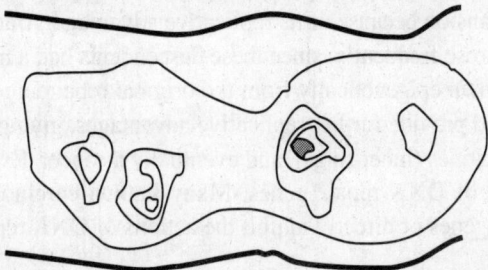

Fig. 9.3: Schematic of a field defect in progression to cancer.

Figure 9.4 shows an opened resected segment of a human colon that has a colon cancer. As illustrated by Bernstein and others, there are about 100 colonic microscopic epithelial crypts per sq mm in the colonic epithelium. The resection shown in Fig. 9.4 has an area of about 6.5 cm by 23 cm, or 150 sq cm, or 15000 sq mm. Thus this area has about 1.5 million crypts. There are 10–20 stem cells at the base of each colonic crypt. Therefore there are likely about 15 million stem cells in the grossly unremarkable colonic mucosal epithelium shown in Fig. 9.4. Evidence reported by Facista and others, indicates that in many such resections, most of the stem cells in such an area up to 10 cm distant (in each direction) from a colon cancer (such as in the grossly unremarkable area shown in Fig. 9.4), and the majority of their differentiated daughter cells, are epigenetically deficient for protein expression of the DNA repair genes *ERCC1, PMS2* and/or *XPF*, although the epithelium is histologically normal.

The stem cells most distant from the cancer, deficient for *ERCC1, PMS2* and/or *XPF,* can be considered to constitute an outer ring, and be deficient as well in the inner rings, of a field defect schematically illustrated in Fig. 9.4. The outer ring in Fig. 9.4 includes, within its circumscribed area, on the order of 15 million stem cells, presumably arising from an initial progenitor stem cell deficient in DNA repair (due to epigenetic silencing). As a result of this repair deficit, the initial stem cell was genetically

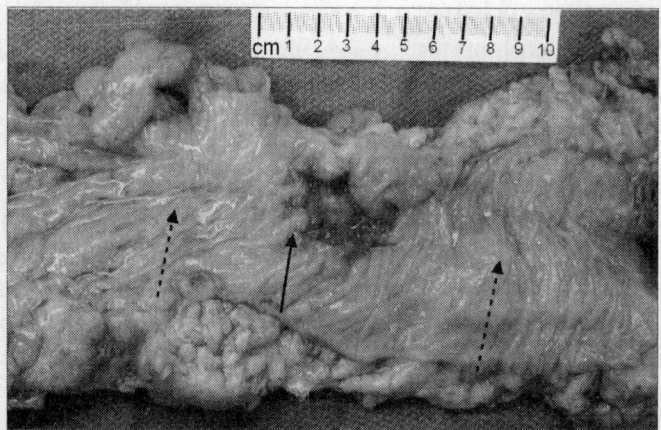

Fig. 9.4: Colon resection including a colon cancer. Dashed arrows indicate grossly unremarkable colonic mucosa. Ulcerated hemorrhagic mass represents a moderately differentiated invasive adenocarcinoma. Solid arrow indicates the heaped up edge of the malignant ulcer.

unstable, giving rise to an increased frequency of mutations in its decendents. One daughter stem cell among its decendents had a mutation that, by chance, provided a replicative advantage. This descendent then underwent clonal expansion because of its replicative advantage. Among the further decendents of the clone, new mutations arose frequently, since these descendents had a mutator phenotype, due to the repair deficiency passed down epigenetically from the original repairdefective stem cell. Among these new mutations, some would provide further replicative advantages, giving rise to a succession of more aggressively growing sub clones (inner rings), and eventually a cancer. Exogenous carcinogenic agents cause reduced expression of DNA repair genes. Many known carcinogenic agents cause reduced expression of DNA repair genes or directly inhibit the actions of DNA repair proteins.

POLYPHENOLS CAN EPIGENETICALLY INCREASE EXPRESSION OF DNA REPAIR GENES

Some polyphenols affect expression of many genes, including DNA repair genes, through epigenetic alterations, are reviewed by Link and others. Examples of DNA repair genes expression increased by epigenetic alteration are listed in Table 9.6.

Table 9.6: Examples of phytochemicals that increase expression of DNA repair genes by an epigenetic mechanism.

Phytochemical	Plant source	Mechanism	Targeted DNA repair genes
Epigalocatechin-3-gallate	Green tea	Reversal of CpG island methylation	MGMT, MLH1
Dihydrocoumarin	Yellow sweet clover	p53 acetylation	P53
Genistein	Soya	Reversal of CpG island methylation	MGMT
Genistein	Soya	Histone acetylation	P53

POSSIBLE PROTECTION AGAINST CANCER BY PHYTOCHEMICALS THAT INCREASE DNA REPAIR BY UNKNOWN MECHANISMS

A recent review article by Collins and others summarises some examples of micronutrients that affect DNA repair gene expression, though by unknown mechanisms. Table 9.7 lists such phytochemicals, without defined mechanisms, that increase DNA repair gene expression, along with commonly known foods that are high in those phytochemicals.

Table 9.7: Examples of phytochemicals that increase expression of DNA repair genes by unknown mechanisms.

Phytochemical (test system)	Examples of foods high in nutrient	Increased DNA repair gene expression
Ellagic acid (mice)	Raspberries, pomeganate	XPA, ERCC5, DNA Ligase 3
Silymarin (cells *in vitro*)	Artichoke, milk thistle	MGMT
Curcumin (cells *in vitro*)	Turmeric	MGMT
Chlorogenic acid (cells *in vitro*)	Blueberries, coffee, sunflower seeds, artichoke	PARP
Caffeic acid (cells *in vitro*)	Coffee, cranberry, carrot	PMS2
m-coumaric acid (cells *in vitro*)	Olives (and metabolite of caffeic acid)	PARP, PMS2
3-(*m*-hydroxyphenyl) propionic	(Major metabolite of caffeic acid and degradation product of proanthocyanidins in chocholate)	PARP, PMS2

Bernstein and others evaluated antioxidants based on their ability to increase DNA repair proteins PARP-1 and Pms2 *in vitro*. They tested 19 anti-oxidant compounds and of these 19 compounds only chlorogenic acid and its metabolic products: chlorogenic acid, caffeic acid, *m*-coumaric acid and 3-(*m*-hydroxy-phenyl) propionic acid, increased expression of the two tested DNA repair genes in HCT-116 cells (Table 9.7).

Chlorogenic acid (CGA) (high in blueberries, coffee, sunflower seeds, artichoke) was then tested as a preventive agent in the recently devised diet-related mouse model of colon cancer. As described above in the section Exogenous DNA damaging agents in colorectal cancer, deoxycholic acid (DCA), a DNA damaging agent, at levels present after a high fat diet, can cause colorectal cancer. When DCA is added to the diet of wild-type mice to raise the level of DCA in the mouse feces to the level in feces of humans on a high fat diet, by 10 months of feeding 94% of the mice develop tumours in their colons with 56% developing colonic adenocarcinomas. This mouse model develops tumours solely in the colon, phenotypically similar to development of colon cancer in humans. When CGA, equivalent to 3 cups of coffee a day for humans, was added to the DCA supplemented diet it was dramatically protective against development of colon cancer, reducing incidence of colon cancer significantly from 56% to 18%.

TARGETING OF CHEMOTHERAPEUTIC AGENTS TO CANCERS DEFICIENT IN DNA REPAIR

As discussed above, DNA repair deficiency often arises early in progression to cancer and can give rise to genomic instability, a general feature of cancers. If cancer cells are deficient in DNA repair they are likely to be more vulnerable than normal cells to inactivation by DNA damaging agents. This vulnerability of cancer cells can be exploited to the benefit of the patient.

Some of the most clinically effective chemotherapeutic agents currently used in cancer treatment are DNA damaging agents, and their therapeutic effectiveness appears to often depend on deficient DNA repair in cancer cells.

In the next four sections we discuss repair deficiencies in cancer cells that can be effectively targeted by DNA damaging chemotherapeutic agents. In addition, deficiency in a DNA repair pathway that arises during tumour development may make cancer cells more reliant on a remaining reduced set of DNA repair pathways for survival. Recent studies indicate that drugs that inhibit one of these alternative pathways in such cancers cells can be useful in cancer therapy.

Targeting cancer cells having a repair deficiency with specific DNA damaging agents, or with agents that inhibit alternative repair pathways, offers a new promising approach for treating a variety of cancers.

TARGETING CANCERS DEFICIENT IN BRCA1

The BRCA1 (breast cancer 1 early onset) protein is employed in an important DNA repair pathway, homologous recombinational repair (HRR). This pathway removes a variety of types of DNA damages, and is the only pathway that can accurately remove double-strand damages such as double-strand breaks and inter-strand cross-links. BRCA1 also has other functions related to preservation of genome integrity. Individuals with a germ-line inherited defect in the *BRCA1* gene are at increased risk of breast, ovarian and other cancers. In addition to inherited germ-line defects in *BRCA1*, deficiencies in expression of this gene may arise in somatic cells either by mutation or by epimutation during progression to sporadic (non-germline) cancer. Patients with a variety of types of cancer are treated effectively with chemotherapeutic agents that cause double-strand breaks (e.g. the topoisomerase inhibitor etoposide), or cause inter-strand cross-links (e.g. the platinum compound cisplatin). These damages can cause cancer cells to undergo apoptosis (a form of cell death). However, patients treated with these agents often prove to be intrinsically resistant, or develop resistance during treatment. Quinn and others demonstrated that BRCA1 expression is necessary for such resistance. This finding suggests that BRCA1-mediated DNA repair can protect cancer cells from therapeutic DNA damaging drugs.

Thus, although high expression of BRCA1 may be initially beneficial to the individual by reducing the risk of developing cancer, it also may be detrimental once cancer has developed by counteracting the therapeutic effect of DNA-damaging agents targeted to the cancer cells. Patients with non-small cell lung cancer (NSLC) are often treated with DNA cross-linking platinum therapeutic compounds such as cisplatin, carboplatin or oxaliplatin. NSCLC is the leading cause of cancer deaths worldwide, and almost 70% of patients with NSCLC have locally advanced or metastatic disease at diagnosis. Improved survival after platinum-containing chemotherapy in metastatic NSCLC correlates with low BRCA1 expression in the primary tumour. This finding indicates that low BRCA1-mediated DNA repair is detrimental to the cancer upon treatment, and thus beneficial to the patient. BRCA1 likely protects cancer cells by participating in a pathway that removes the potentially lethal DNA cross-links introduced by the platinum drugs. Since low BRCA1 expression in the tumour appears to be beneficial to the patient, Taron and Papadek concluded that BRCA1 expression is potentially an important tool for use in cancer management and should be assessed for predicting chemosensitivity and tailoring chemotherapy in lung cancer. Over 90% of ovarian cancers appear to arise sporadically in somatic cells and are associated with BRCA1 dysfunction. Weberpals and others showed for patients having sporadic ovarian cancer treated with platinum drugs, the median survival was longer for patients with lower expression of BRCA1 vs. higher BRCA1 expression (46 vs. 33 months).

TARGETING CANCERS DEFICIENT IN ERCC1

ERCC1 (Excision Repair Cross-Complementaion group 1) is a key protein needed to remove platinum adducts and repair inter- and intra-strand cross-links. ERCC1 dimerizes with XPF (xeroderma pigmentosum complementation group F) protein to form a complex that can excise damaged DNA. Over-expression of ERCC1 is associated with cellular resistance to platinum compounds, whereas ERCC1 down-regulation sensitises cells to cisplatin. Cisplatin has made a major impact in the chemotherapeutic treatment of testicular cancer. Over 90% of patients with newly diagnosed testicular germ cell cancer, and 70 to 80%

of patients with metastatic testicular cancer, can be cured using cisplatin based combination chemotherapy. Hypersensitivity of testicular cancer to cisplatin appears to be due to low levels of the three NER proteins ERCC1, XPF and XPA.

Simon and others evaluated ERCC1 mRNA expression in lung tumours as a predictor of survival of NSCLC patients. They found that patients with relatively low ERCC1 mRNA expression had poor overall survival. This finding suggests that low ERCC1-mediated DNA repair allows DNA damages to persist and give rise to carcinogenic mutations. However, they also noted that those NSCLC tumours with relatively low ERCC1 expression responded better to platinum based therapy. Lord and others found that low *ERCC1* mRNA expression in the primary tumour correlates with prolonged survival after cisplatin plus gemitabine chemotherapy in NSCLC. Median overall survival with low ERCC1 expression tumours was 61.6 weeks compared to 20.4 weeks for patients with high expression tumours.

Zhou and others reported that a particular genetic polymorphism that alters ERCC1 mRNA level predicts overall survival in advanced NSCLC patients treated with platinum based chemotherapy. Olaussen and others found that patients with completely resected NSCLC tumours that were ERCC1-negative benefited from adjuvant cisplatin-based chemotherapy, whereas patients with ERCC1-positive tumours did not benefit. They suggested that determination of ERCC1 expression in NSCLC cells before chemotherapy can make a contribution as an independent predictor of the effect of adjuvant chemotherapy. Papadaki and others found that *ERCC1* mRNA level in the primary tumour of patients with metastatic NSCLC could predict the effectiveness of cisplatin based chemotherapy. Low *ERCC1* mRNA level was significantly associated with higher response rate, longer median progression-free survival and median overall survival. Leng and others found that patients with ERCC1 negative expression had a longer progression free survival and overall survival than ERCC1 positive patients after receiving platinum based adjuvant therapy. Thus *ERCC1* mRNA level, like *BRCA1* mRNA level (discussed above), in the primary tumour at the time of diagnosis could be used to predict platinum sensitivity of NSCLC.

ERCC1 expression also appears to have predictive significance for ovarian cancer. Dabholkar and others found in ovarian tumour tissues that *ERCC1* mRNA expression levels were higher in patients who were resistant to platinum based therapy than in those patients who responded to such therapy. Kang and others observed that a particular polymorphism of the ERCC1 gene sequence was associated with clinical outcome of platinum based chemotherapy in patients with ovarian cancer. Weberpals and others also showed for ovarian cancer patients that higher ERCC1 mRNA level, alone, or especially in combination with higher *BRCA1* mRNA level in the tumour, predicted shorter overall patient survival after platinum therapy.

ERCC1 protein expression is often reduced within colon cancers and in a field defect surrounding these cancers. For metastatic colorectal cancer patients receiving combination oxaliplatin and fluorouracil chemotherapy, lower *ERCC1* mRNA expression in the tumour predicts longer survival. Viguier and others found that a particular ERCC1 genetic polymorphism predicts a better tumour response to oxaliplatin/5-fluorouracil combination chemotherapy in patients with metastatic colorectal cancer.

Low *ERCC1* mRNA levels also predict better response and survival for gastric cancer patients and bladder cancer patients receiving cisplatin-based chemotherapy. Thus numerous studies involving cancer of the testis, lung, ovary, colon, stomach and bladder indicated that platinum based chemotherapy can enhance patient outcome when targeted specifically to tumours with low ERCC1 expression. Such tumours have diminished ability to repair the DNA damages, particularly the cross-links, induced in the tumours by the platinum compound.

TARGETING CANCERS DEFICIENT IN *MGMT*

Alkylating agents, including chloroethylnitrosoureas, procarbazine and temozolomide, are commonly used to treat malignant brain tumours. These agents cause DNA damage by adding alkyl groups to DNA. Such damages may then be repaired or, if unrepaired, trigger cell death. As an example, temozolomide methylates DNA at several sites generating mainly N^7-methylguanine and N^3-methyladenine adducts, which constitute nearly 90% of the total methylation events. However these adducts are efficiently removed and accurately replaced by the base excision repair pathway, and thus have low cytotoxic potential. About 5 to 10% of the methylation events caused by temozolomide produce O^6-methylguanine which is cytotoxic, and this adduct accounts for the beneficial therapeutic effect of temozolomide and other alkylating agents on malignant brain tumours. O^6-methylguanine methyltransferase (*MGMT*) is a DNA repair enzyme that rapidly reverses alkylation (including methylation) at the O^6 position of guanine, thus neutralising the cytotoxic effects of chemotherapeutic alkylating agents such as temozolomide. High *MGMT* activity in tumour tissue is associated with resistance to alkylating agents. *MGMT* activity is controlled by a promoter sequence, and methylation of the CpG island in the promoter silences the gene in cancer cells, so that these cells no longer produce *MGMT*. In addition, as described above, an increased level of miR-181d can also decrease *MGMT* expression and help the ability of temozolomide to give a beneficial therapeutic effect.

Esteller and others showed that methylation of the *MGMT* promoter increases the responsiveness of the gliomas (brain tumours) to chemotherapeutic alkylating agents, leading to regression of the tumours and prolonged overall and disease free survival. Paz and others showed that hypermethylation of CpG islands within the promoter sequence of the *MGMT* gene predicts a better clinical response to temozolomide in primary gliomas. They considered that their results might open up possibilities for more customised treatments of human brain tumours. Hegi and others demonstrated a significantly improved clinical outcome in patients with malignant glioma who had a methylated *MGMT* promoter and were treated with temozolomide. The 18-month survival rate was 62% among patients with a methylated *MGMT* promoter compared with only 8% in the absence of promoter methylation. Hegi and others reviewed further evidence that *MGMT* promoter methylation is associated with improved progression-free and overall survival in malignant glioma patients treated with alkylating agents. They also discussed strategies to overcome *MGMT*-mediated chemoresistance that are currently under investigation. Upon reviewing the relevant evidence, Weller and others concluded that *MGMT* promoter methylation is the key mechanism of *MGMT* gene silencing, and could be used as a biomarker for predicting a favourable outcome in patients with malignant glioma who are exposed to alkylating chemotherapy. They considered that this biomarker is on the verge of entering clinical decision-making.

TARGETING CANCERS WITH A REPAIR DEFICIENCY USING A PARP INHIBITOR, SYNTHETIC LETHALITY

If a tumor is deficient in an essential protein component of a DNA repair pathway, the cancer cells would likely be more reliant on remaining DNA repair pathways for survival. Drugs that inhibit one of these alternative pathways, in principle, might prove to be useful in cancer therapy by selectively killing the cancer cells. An example of such an approach is the use of poly(ADP-ribose) polymerase [PARP] inhibitors against tumours that are deficient in BRCA1 or BRCA2. This approach has provided proof-of-concept for an anticancer strategy termed 'synthetic lethality.' By this strategy the inhibition of a particular repair pathway in cancer cells that are already deficient in another repair pathway preferentially induces greater toxicity in repair deficient cancer cells than in normal non-cancer cells. Current research guided by this strategy is directed at finding new agents that inactivate protein components of major repair pathways, and thus could be targeted against cancers that are already deficient in another repair pathway. A germ-line mutation in one *BRCA1* or *BRCA2* allele substantially increases the risk of developing several cancers, including breast, ovarian, and prostate cancer. Diploid cells heterozygous for either a *BRCA1* or a *BRCA2* mutant allele may lose expression of the remaining wild-type allele, resulting in deficient homologous recombinational repair. This loss causes an increase in unrepaired DSBs that can lead to mutations (through compensatory inaccurate repair) and chromosomal aberrations that drive carcinogenesis. Inactivation of the wild-type allele in the cell lineage leading to the tumor is thought to be an obligate step in this carcinogenesis pathway, a step that does not occur in the normal non-cancer tissues of the patient.

The deficiency in homologous recombinational repair is thus specific to the tumor, and can be exploited by employing PARP inhibitors. Ordinarily, single-strand breaks (SSBs), as distinct from DSBs, are repaired by the base excision repair pathway, in which the enzyme PARP1 plays a key role. The inhibition of PARP1 leads to the accumulation of DNA SSBs. Unrepaired SSBs can give rise to DSBs at replication forks during DNA replication. Thus PARP inhibition in tumor cells with deficient homologous recombinational repair (because of the absence of BRCA1 or BRCA2) generates unrepaired SSBs that are likely to cause an overwhelming accumulation of DSBs leading to tumor cell death. In contrast, the normal tissues of a patient consists of cells that are heterozygous for a *BRCA1* or *BRCA2* mutant allele and therefore retain homologous recombinational repair function, and have a sensitivity to PARP inhibitors similar to that of wild-type cells. Thus PARP inhibition induces selective tumor cell killing while sparing normal cells. Fong and others conducted a preliminary clinical evaluation of the oral PARP inhibitor olaparib. They observed that 63% of patients carrying *BRCA1* or *BRCA2* mutations who had ovarian, breast or prostate cancer had a clinical benefit from treatment with olaparib with few adverse side effects. This is an example of the concept of 'synthetic lethality' which occurs when there is a potent lethal synergy between two otherwise non-lethal events. The two events in this case are: (i) a specific PARP inhibitor blocks repair of SSBs causing an increase in SSBs leading to an increase in DSBs, and (ii) a tumor restricted genetic loss of function or homologous recombinational repair that is ordinarily needed to accurately repair these DSBs.

A subsequent trial of olaparib in BRCA mutation-associated breast cancer demonstrated objective positive response rates of 41%, again with limited toxicity. About 10% of women with ovarian cancer carry a *BRCA1* or *BRCA2* mutant allele. Audeh and others showed that the oral PARP inhibitor olaparib has antitumor activity in women carriers of *BRCA1* or *BRCA2* alleles who have ovarian cancer. The objective positive response rate was 33%.

OVERVIEW OF THE ROLE OF DNA DAMAGE AND REPAIR IN CARCINOGENESIS

In this section we present a brief overview of the relationship of DNA damage and repair to carcinogenesis, and the implications of this relationship for strategies of prevention and therapy, emphasising the evidence reviewed above. Carcinogenesis is generally viewed as a Darwinian process that occurs in a somatic cell lineage by mutation or epimutation and natural selection. Natural selection operates on the basis of the adaptive benefit to individual cells in the lineage of more rapid cell division or higher resistance to cell death (apoptosis) than occurs in neighbouring cells. Most of the random mutations and epimutations that arise during progression to cancer are likely to be disadvantageous or neutral from the prospective of the emerging cancerous cells, and only those that promote more rapid overall growth are advantageous. The cell lineage that ultimately becomes a cancer probably passes through a series of evolutionary pre-cancerous stages involving sequential rounds of mutation/epimutation and selection. The initial stage is probably a lineage of cells with a small selective advantage that forms an early field within a tissue. Within this defective field successive mutation and selection events occur which finally give rise to an invasive and then metastatic cell lineage. During this process the cell lineage acquires the hallmarks of cancer. These include: sustaining proliferative signalling, evading growth suppressors, resisting cell death, enabling replicative immortality, inducing angiogenesis, reprogramming energy metabolism, and evading immune destruction. Mutations arise from unrepaired DNA damages, either by translesion synthesis during DNA replication or by inaccurate repair of DNA damages, as in the inaccurate process of non-homologous end joining of double-strand breaks.

Mutations may also arise by spontaneous replication errors without the intervention of DNA damage, but this source of mutation is likely less frequent than mutations caused by DNA damage. The primary cause(s) of epimutations (such as CpG island methylations) are not well understood, but evidence suggests that epimutations arise during the repair processes that remove DNA damages. The sources of DNA damage underlying carcinogenesis can be extrinsic or intrinsic. Epidemiologic evidence suggests that a large proportion of the DNA damages contributing to cancer arise from extrinsic stressful conditions, including such factors as smoking, high fat diet, certain infections and UV light exposure. The possible contribution from intrinsic causes, such as free radical production during normal metabolism, have not been assessed. A pervasive characteristic of human tumours is genomic instability. A likely major source of this instability is loss of DNA repair capability. Germ line mutations in DNA repair genes generally lead to syndromes characterised by a greatly increased risk of cancer. The majority of cancers arise sporadically, i.e. are not primarily due to germ line mutations. A frequent characteristic of sporadic cancers is loss of expression of one or more DNA repair proteins through epigenetic silencing. The several different DNA repair pathways that occur in mammalian cells each specialise in removing different types of damage, but they are also partially overlapping. Thus reduction of a particular repair pathway may have different carcinogenic consequences from loss of another repair pathway. However, the deleterious effect of loss of one pathway may be partially ameliorated by another functioning pathway.

This general view of the role of DNA damage and repair in carcinogenesis has implications for the prevention and treatment of cancer. Cancer incidence could be substantially reduced by a general avoidance of the known sources of DNA damage such as smoking. In addition to avoiding DNA damage, it should also be beneficial to increase DNA repair, or at least to avoid extrinsic factors that decrease repair. The factors affecting repair capability are less well studied than those causing DNA damage, but several are known, and a significant benefit may be derived from considering such factors as well.

The finding that DNA repair deficiency is a common feature of cancers, and is perhaps the underlying cause of the genetic instability of cancers, has implications for therapy. If a cancer is composed of cells deficient in DNA repair, it is, in principle, vulnerable to agents that cause DNA damage. Thus a chemotherapeutic DNA damaging agent can be targeted to cancers that lack the capability to repair the particular type of DNA damage caused by the agent. This can lead to a level of DNA damages that overwhelms the defenses of the cancer cells and causes their death. Non-cancerous cells with normal repair would not be targeted. Thus the toxicity of such DNA damaging agents to the treated patient would be limited. A dramatic example of such targeted therapy is the high cure rate of testicular cancer due to a defect in the ability of the cancer cells to repair DNA inter-strand cross-links, and the use of cross-linking platinum compounds to kill such cells.

Another strategy, which is currently the basis for numerous ongoing clinical trials, involves synthetic lethality. By this strategy cancers that are deficient in one DNA repair pathway can be made more vulnerable to DNA damage by treatment with agents that inhibit an additional repair pathway. Promising clinical results, so far, have been obtained in the treatment of patients with breast and ovarian cancer due to an inherited genetic defect in the homologous recombinational repair pathway. Such cancers are deficient in the ability to repair double-strand breaks. Treatment of these cancers with an agent that interferes with another pathway that ordinarily repairs single-strand breaks allows such breaks to accumulate and to be converted to double-strand breaks during DNA replication. The increase in doublestrand breaks appears to overwhelm the cancer cells, while sparing normal cells, thus providing positive clinical benefit to the patient without much toxicity.

Chapter 10

Rearrangement of Immunoglobulin Genes

INTRODUCTION

Antibody (or immunoglobulin) structure is made up of two heavy-chains and two light-chains. These chains are held together by disulphide bonds. The arrangement or processes that put together different parts of this antibody molecule play important role in antibody diversity and production of different subclasses or classes of antibodies. The organisation and processes take place during the development and differentiation of B cells. That is, the controlled gene expression during transcription and translation coupled with the rearrangements of immunoglobulin gene segments result in the generation of antibody repertoire during development and maturation of B cells. The immune system protects us from being harmed by a variety of infectious microbial agents in our environment. One key component in the immune response against foreign particles is the antibody (Ab) molecule.

Two functions are characteristic of every Ab molecule: (i) specific binding to an antigenic determinant, and (ii) mediator of effector functions. The latter involves binding and activation of complement, stimulation of phagocytosis by macrophages and triggering of granule release by mast cells. Abs are expressed exclusively by cells of the developmental line of B lymphocytes. Terminally differentiated B cells, so called plasma cells, produce enormous amounts of Abs, which requires the corresponding genes to be very active in these cells. The expression of genes encoding the light and heavy-chain immunoglobulin (Ig) polypeptides is stringently regulated by a variety of different regulatory proteins.

IMMUNOGLOBULIN STRUCTURE

An antibody molecule consists of two identical light (L) polypeptide chains and two identical heavy (H) chains held together by a combination of noncovalent bonds and covalent disulphide bonds (Fig. 10.1). Each polypeptide chain can be divided into one variable (V) and one to four constant (C) domains. The antigen binding site is combined by the VL and VH domains. The variable region can be further divided into more conserved regions, the framework regions (FR), and hypervariable regions, often called the complementarity determining regions (CDR). The effector functions are determined by the structure of the constant region of the heavy chain. Abs are glycoproteins and the presence of carbohydrates on the Ab molecule is essential for some of the effector functions. Cleavage with the enzyme papain splits the

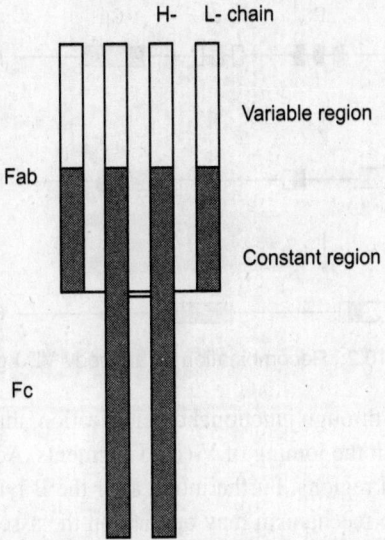

Fig. 10.1: The immunoglobulin molecule.

Ab molecule into a Fab region, the antigen binding site and an Fc region, mediating effector functions. In humans, there are five classes of antibodies, IgM, IgD, IgG, IgA and IgE, each with its own isotype of H chain- μ, δ, γ, α and ε, respectively. The two isotypes of light chain, κ and λ are shared between the different classes. IgM is the first class of antibody secreted in a primary immune response and it is preferentially produced as a pentamer. The low affinity of the molecule is compensated for by the high avidity mediated by its pentameric form. IgD is expressed on the surface of naive mature B cells together with IgM. They are rarely secreted by an activated B cell and their function is unknown. IgG is the major class of Ab in blood and is produced during secondary immune responses. There are four different subclasses IgG1-IgG4 which differ in their ability to activate effector functions. In general, protein antigens mainly induce IgG1 responses, and to a lesser degree IgG3 and IgG4, while polysaccharides induce IgG2 response.

IgA can be expressed either as a monomer or as a dimer. The dimeric form is the dominant class in secretions (milk, respiratory and intestinal secretions). IgA constitutes the first line of defense against pathogen invading the organism via the mucosa.

IgE is involved in some types of allergic responses through its high affinity binding to receptors on mast cells and basophils.

Generation of Antibody Diversity

The immune system is capable of producing a tremendous diversity of antibody specificities. Immunoglobulin genes are assembled during B cell differentiation from different gene segments that are combined through sitespecific recombination. The variable regions are encoded by variable (V), diversity (D) and joining (J) segments. The human immunoglobulin heavy chain (IgH) locus contains approximately 50 VH, 20 DH and 6 JH gene segments. The Igλ locus contains 100 Vκ and 5 Jκ, whereas the Igλ contains 30 Vλ and 8 Jλ. These different segments, in the H chain locus, are joined by recombination as outlined in Fig. 10.2. The L chain locus undergoes a similar recombination process, with the exception that it lacks the D region genes.

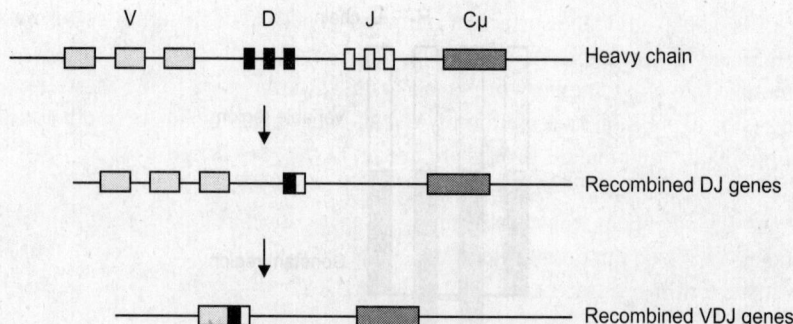

Fig. 10.2: Recombination of antibody VDJ genes.

Further diversity is generated through junctional diversification, that is nucleotides can either be lost or added (P and N nucleotides) in the joining of V-(D)-J segments. Additional diversity can be derived from pairing of different VL/VH regions. Furthermore, after the B lymphocyte has been stimulated by antigen a somatic hypermutation mechanism may operate on the assembled variable regions.

B Cell Development

During the development of B cells, the immunoglobulin gene undergoes sequences of rearrangements that lead to formation of the antibody repertoire. For example, in the lymphoid cell, a partial rearrangement of the heavy-chain gene occurs which is followed by complete rearrangement of heavy-chain gene.

The cells of the immune system which are specialised to make antibodies are called B lymphocytes. They originate in the bone marrow and are derived from a multipotent stem cell. The different stages during differentiation of B lymphocytes, from precursor cells to antibody secreting cells, are outlined in Fig. 10.3. The different steps are defined by changes in the specific gene expression pattern.

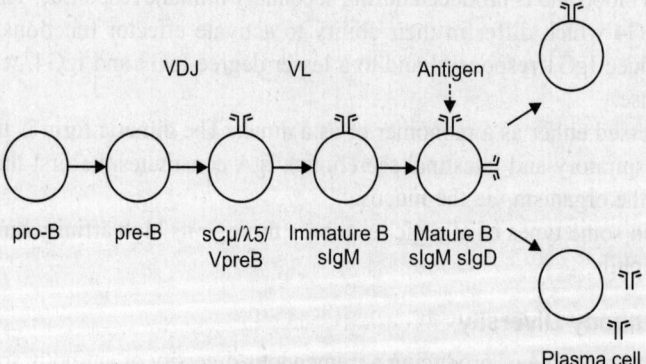

Fig. 10.3: B cell differentiation.

At the pro-B cell stage, the Ig genes are in germline configuration but a sterile transcript is produced. In pre-B cells, VDJ recombination of the IgH variable chain generates μ-chains which can associate with either the surrogate λ5 and VpreB light chains or the κ protein encoded by a germline JCκ transcript. This immature B cell receptor is expressed on the surface of the pre-B cell and can function as a signal-transducing surface receptor. Following the rearrangement of genes encoding Igλκ or Igλ light chain, the IgM receptor is displayed on the surface of immature B cells. The mature B cell is antigen reactive and expresses IgM and IgD receptors. After encountering the correct antigen the mature B cell is activated and can differentiate into either memory or plasma cells. Differentiation to plasma cells include switch from surface Ig (sIg) expression to secretion of Abs and may include somatic mutation of Ig variable regions. SIg on immature and mature B cells are noncovalently associated with the mb-1 gene product Igα and the B29 gene product Igβ. These molecules together form the B cell antigen receptor (BCR) complex. Igα and Igβ facilitates transport of the Ig molecule from the endoplasmatic reticulum to the cell surface and also have an important role in the signal transduction event. Igα and Igβ are expressed at all stages prior to terminal differentiation into plasma cells.

Multigene organisation of immunoglobulin genes

From studies and predictions such as Dreyer and Bennett's, it shows that the light chains and heavy chains are encoded by separate multigene families on different chromosomes. They are referred to as gene segments and are separated by non-coding regions. The rearrangement and organisation of these gene segments during the maturation of B cells produce functional proteins. The entire process of rearrangement and organisation of these gene segments is the vital source where our body immune system gets its capabilities to recognise and respond to variety of antigens.

Light chain multigene family: The light chain gene has three gene segments. These include the light chain variable region (V), joining region (J), and constant region (C) gene segments. The variable region of light is therefore encoded by the rearrangement of VJ segments. The light chain can be either kappa, κ or lambda, λ. This process takes place at the level of mRNAs processing. Random rearrangements and recombinations of the gene segments at DNA level to form one kappa or lambda light chain occurs in an orderly fashion. As a result, 'a functional variable region gene of a light chain contains two coding segments that are separated by a non-coding DNA sequence in unrearranged germ-line DNA'.

Heavy-chain multigene family: Heavy chain contains similar gene segments such as VH, JH and CH, but also has another gene segment called D (diversity). Unlike the light chain multigene family, VDJ gene segments code for the variable region of the heavy chain. The rearrangement and reorganisation of gene segments in this multigene family is more complex . The rearranging and joining of segments produced different end products because these are carried out by different RNA processes. The same reason is why the IgM and IgG are generates at the time.

B Cell Activation

B cell activation initially involves antigen binding to sIg. There are two kinds of antigen, T cell-dependent and T cell-independent. The T cell-independent pathway is triggered by two kinds of antigen, polysaccharides or potent polyclonal activators like lipopolysaccharide, (LPS). These antigen cross-link the sIg and thereby activate the B cells. However, the activation still requires T cell derived cytokines to stimulate Ig secretion. The T cell dependent pathway is triggered by soluble proteins and relies on the possibility of the B cell to act as an antigen-specific presenting cell (APC). The B cell binds the antigen with its sIg. The antigen is internalised, processed into peptides and there after presented on the cell surface bound to the MHC class II molecule. Finally the T cell recognises the processed antigen on the B cell surface and the activation of the B cell starts. This presentation leads to cognate interactions, involving the release of T cell derived cytokines and increased expression of accessory molecules, which results in both T and B cell activation. A key feature of this cognate interaction is the induction on the T cell membrane of a ligand for CD40 (CD40L), which delivers an activational signal to the B cell.

Other important accessory molecules are the CD80, CD86 on the B cell and CD28 and CTLA-4 on the T cell (Fig. 10.4). Cross-linking CD40 promotes B cell proliferation and immunoglobulin class switch. If the CD40-CD40L interaction is blocked *in vitro* with soluble CD40 or CD40L specific Ab, the B cell can not proliferate indicating that this interaction is required for signalling. The interaction of CD28-CD80/CD86 preferentially activates the T cells to produce cytokines and to proliferate. CTLA-4 deficient mice show massive expansion of activated T cells and an increase in serum Ig levels. This data suggest that CTLA-4 may act as a negative regulator of T cell activation, and indirectly, B cell stimulation.

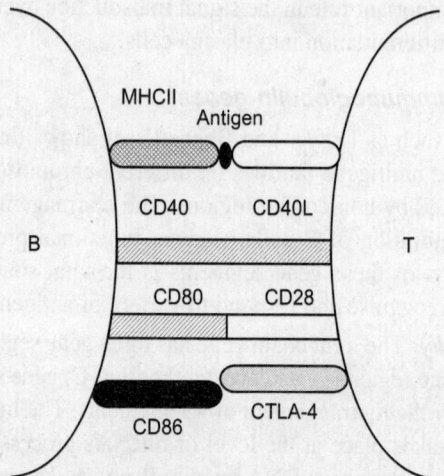

Fig. 10.4: Interaction between B and T cell.

PRODUCTION OF HUMAN ANTIBODIES

Monoclonal Ab became available when Köhler and Milstein demonstrated that cultured mouse myeloma cells could be fused to spleen cells from immunised mice. The hybrid cells (hybridoma) grew continuously in culture (a property acquired from the myeloma cells) and continued to produce large quantities of Ab (a property obtained from the spleen cells). The mAbs have an enormous potential as therapeutic and diagnostic agents because of their remarkable specificity and affinity for their target. Rodent mAb unfortunately has several disadvantages, such as a short half-life in serum, only some of the different classes can trigger human effector functions and the Abs elicit an unwanted immune response in patients (human anti-mouse antibodies or HAMA). HAMA can result in enhanced clearance of the Ab from the serum, blocking of its therapeutic effect. Only a fraction of the anti-mouse immune response is directed to the variable region of the rodent Abs. To reduce the HAMA response it is therefore necessary to express potentially therapeutic Ab either as chimeric, humanised (engraftments of mouse CDR into the human framework region) or human monoclonal Abs. Recent development in both monoclonal Ab strategy and the use of recombinant DNA technology have now made it feasible to produce human mAb with the desired specificity. Below, the different steps, outlined in Fig. 10.5, leading to antigen-specific human Ab will be discussed.

In vitro Generation of Antigen-specific Abs

Due to ethical problems associated with immunisation of humans much interest has been focused on techniques to generate antigen-specific Ab, using *in vitro* systems. Human B cells may be obtained

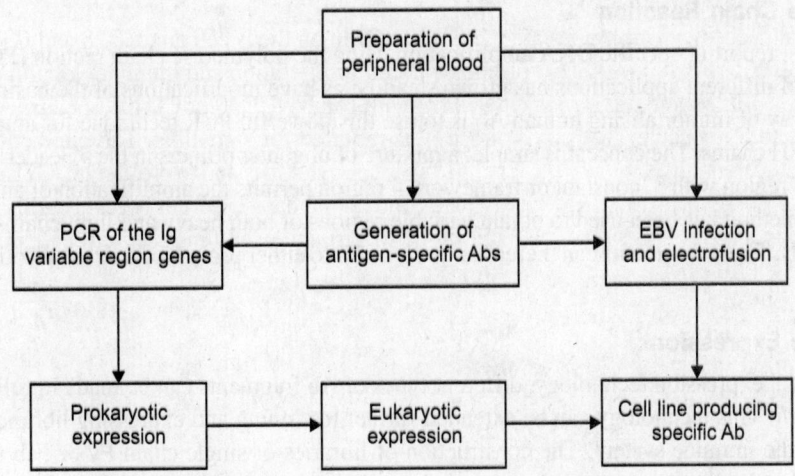

Fig. 10.5: Establishment of human monoclonal Ab-producing cell lines.

from spleen, tonsils, lymph nodes, bone marrow or peripheral blood, the latter being the most accessible source. An approach to generate antigen-specific Abs is to use *in vitro* immunisation techniques. However, *in vitro* immunisation of human lymphocytes was initially more difficult to achieve than that of the murine counterpart. The reason for this might be that peripheral blood cells contain cytotoxic T cells, monocytes, granulocytes and NK cells, which abrogate the antigen-specific activation of B cells. These cells must therefore be removed from the peripheral blood cells by L-leucyl-L-leucine methyl ester (LeuLeuOMe) treatment before an *in vitro* immunisation of the B cells can take place. Briefly, the cells are cultivated with antigen in medium containing supernatant from irradiated pokeweed mitogen (PWM) stimulated T cells and recombinant IL-2. Immunisation of naive B cells using this protocol only generates primary immune responses.

B cells can be activated antigen-specifically and simultaneously be costimulated *in vitro* via their CD40 surface molecules. The stimulation can be delivered using either soluble recombinant CD40L or CD40 specific Ab in combination with cytokines. Using this CD40-system it is possible to maintain a long term B cell culture and polyclonal isotype switch has also been reported.

Antigen-specific activation of B cells *in vitro* could be achieved after stimulating the B cells with anti-sIg Abs in the presence of T helper cells and Staphylococcal Enterotoxin A (SEA). Increased Cross-linking of the sIg enhanced Ig production. In this manner specific Ab was obtained against both primary and secondary antigens. Chin and others have been able to activate B cells antigen-specifically and induce isotype switch to achieve antigen-specific IgG production, using their primary and secondary antigen driven cultures. The secondary immunisation is supported by antigen activated T helper cells and stimulation via the CD40 pathway.

Immortalisation

One of the most important technologies in the production of monoclonal Ab is the establishment of immortal cell lines. The most frequently applied technique uses Epstein-Barr virus (EBV) to infect and activate human B cells. To rescue the transformed B cells they can be further fused to myeloma cells which stabilises the Ab production. Another alternative to immortalising monoclonal Abs is to use DNA recombinant technology, which will be discussed below.

Polymerase Chain Reaction

Since the first report of specific DNA amplification using the polymerase chain rection (PCR) in 1985, the number of different applications has grown steadily, as have modifications of the basic method. An alternative way of immortalising human Ab is to use this powerful PCR technique for amplification of the VL and VH chains. The concept is simple: a mixture of oligomer primers in the 5′ leader sequences or framework 1 region with 3′ constant or framework 4 region permits the amplification of any Ig variable region. The method has been used to obtain variable regions of both heavy and light chains from single human B cells. These fragments can thereafter be cloned into either prokaryotic or eukaryotic expression vectors.

Prokaryotic Expression

Using bacterial expression technology, different types of Ab fragments can be made in fully functional form in *E. coli*. This technology can be extended further to cloning and expressing libraries of VL/VH chains from the immune system. The construction of libraries of single chain Fv or Fab fragments of antibody molecules that are expressed on the surface of filamentous phages and the selection of specific recombinant Ab offers a new and powerful mean for generating monoclonal Ab. A major goal of recombinant Ab technology is to develop Ab libraries of large size and diversity to facilitate the isolation of Abs of every conceivable specificity, among them Abs with high affinity. The rearranged V-genes can be derived from immunised or unimmunised B cells. The naive libraries are easier to obtain but mostly low affinity binders have been isolated. An alternative approach to creating diverse libraries is to use a collection of germline VH segments fused to synthetic CDR3 regions *in vitro* (varying in length between 6 and 15 amino acids) and combined with one or multiple light chains. Fully synthetic libraries have also been described. Several methods for antigen-specific selection of high affinity Abs have been described. These include selection of phage Abs binding to antigen-coated tubes or binding to antigen on a column matrix. One alternative is to use flow cytometry based selection for finding Ab against cell surface antigens. To mimick *in vivo* antigen selection, Duenas and Borrebaeck used a fusion protein consisting of antigen fused to the pIII protein. Using an engineered helper-phage with deleted functional gIII made it possible to select high affinity Abs.

Since most libraries are obtained from naive repertoires, methods for affinity maturation *in vitro* have been developed. These include *in vitro* maturation of Ab using codon based mutagenesis, error prone PCR or spiked oligonucleotide based mutagenesis. One alternative is to use the chain-suffling technique. After selecting a high affinity Ab to a desired antigen, it could be either expressed in *E. coli* and purified, or cloned in an eukaryotic expression vector to produce the entire Ab molecule. The use of Ab fragments may be advantageous in some therapeutical applications, as they penetrate tissue more readily and are cleared more rapidly from serum. This may help in neutralising and clearing drugs from the serum. Engineering of recombinant Ab has also resulted in the construction of a new generation of molecules. Monovalent sFv Abs have been converted into bivalent monospecific or bispecific reagents using e.g. dimerisation domains or direct coupling. In addition, Fv can be fused or coupled to a variety of cytokines, enzymes or radioactive entities.

Eukaryotic Expression

Gene transfection provides a method for making novel Ig molecules. The tranfected cells (transfectomas) grow continuously in culture and produce the Ig specified by the transfected gene. To create a transfectoma cell line synthesising a novel Ab, both Ig heavy and light chains must be transfected into the same recipient cell line. Although both chains can be contained in a single vector, it is usually more convenient to construct separate light and heavy chain vectors, which are simultaneously transferred and expressed. A vector should contain regulatory elements, VL/VH region genes, a genomic constant region including polyA signal and splice signals and a selectable marker.

The variable region genes can be obtained either as genomic DNA from a bacteriophage lambda (Fig. 10.6) library or as cDNA from any B cell, hybridoma or phagedisplay-selected Ab fragment. There are several methods for stably introducing DNA into eukaryotic recipient cells, such as protoplast fusion or electroporation. Stable transfectomas are produced with frequencies of 10^{-3} to 10^{-7} depending on the recipient cell line. The vector must therefore contain a biochemically selectable marker, which permits the selection of the rare, stably transfected cell line. Two frequently used selectable markers are the gpt-gene (bacterial xanthine-guanine phosphoribosyltransferase gene) or the neo-gene (aminoglycoside phosphotransferase gene). Both enzymes, when expressed, endow a dominant biochemically selectable phenotype to mammalian cells so that they can be used for selection in non drug-marked recipient cells.

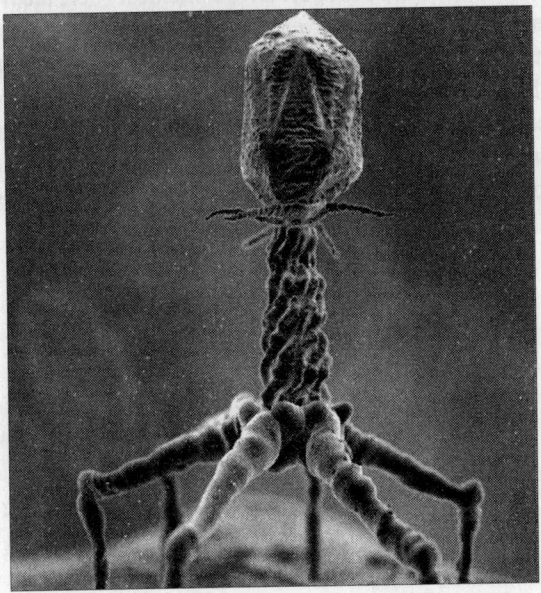

Fig. 10.6: Bacteriophage lambda.

There are two possible ways of creating an eukaryotic expression vector, to use either viral or endogenous regulatory elements. Viral promoter/enhancer pairs from cytomegalovirus (CMV) and SV40 have been used successfully to achieve high levels of Ab expression. Viral based vectors can be transfected into either myeloma cell lines or Chinese hamster ovary cells (CHO). The Ig gene expression was for a long time thought to be regulated by the V promoter and the intron enhancer. Therefore most vectors based on endogenous control elements use this promoter/enhancer combination. The rate of Ab secretion attainable using these vectors is generally considerably lower than those of comparable parent hybridomas. Recent observations indicate that other enhancer elements are important for Ig gene expression. Including the 3'E to the IgH vector increased the IgH expression five fold. Vectors based on endogenous control elements are also transfected in myeloma cells.

Gene amplification can be used to increase the level of Ig expression. Two alternative selectable markers have been described in Ig expression vectors, the glutamine synthetase (GS), and the dihydrofolate reductase (DHFR). Cointroduction of heavy and light chain constructs with subsequent amplification using the DHFR-marker resulted in as much as 25-fold increase in secretion of intact Ab relative to unamplified cells. The GS-marker in combination with a vector, based on viral control elements, containing both heavy and light chain, also resulted in higher secretion levels of Ab.

Using eukaryotic Ig expression vectors it is also possible to introduce novel functions not normally found in the Ig molecule. To achieve optimal effector functions either the constant region can be changed into an other region or the IgG1 can be converted into a pentamer IgG1. It is also possible to produce fusion proteins with e.g. cytokines. One alternative way of producing chimeric Abs is to, through homologous recombination, introduce the desired human constant gene segment into the Ig loci of any hybridoma cell line of interest. The advantages of using this system is that all regulatory elements needed are already in the loci and the variable gene does not have to be isolated from the hybridoma and finally that one recombination vector can be used for all specificities. There are two kinds of recombination vectors available, replacement or integration vectors. The replacement vector contains a two-sided homology flank neighbouring the heterologous region, whereas the integration vector contains one homology flank within which the construct is linearised, thus giving rise to a duplication of the target sequence. Using these vectors, the Ig expression levels are comparable with the original hybridoma levels. The disadvantage in using these vectors is a frequent occurrence of clones that coexpress Ig from two species. So far this approach to produce Abs has only been done using murine hybridomas.

SECTION III

RNA Synthesis and Processing

Chapter 11

RNA Synthesis and Processing: An Overview

INTRODUCTION

Gene expression can be regulated at multiple levels, including transcription, RNA processing, messenger RNA (mRNA) stability, translation and post-translation. In this processional hierarchy, transcription provides the first opportunity for regulation. In fact, the initial step in regulating gene expression is deciding whether or not to transcribe a gene. Transcription is the process of RNA synthesis in which the genetic information that is stored in the nucleus in the form of double-stranded DNA is converted into a single-stranded RNA chain by an enzyme called RNA polymerase (RNAP). The RNA chain is identical to one strand of the DNA, called the coding strand, and complementary to the other strand which provides the template for its synthesis. In prokaryotes, a single form of RNAP shoulders the responsibility of transcribing the genomic DNA. Eukaryotic cells have evolved to accommodate their increased genetic complexity by delegating this function to three nuclear DNA dependent RNAPs, each responsible for the synthesis of different classes of RNA. Despite the partitioning of the transcription workload in eukaryotic cells, the fundamental mechanics of transcription are conserved from bacteria to mammals.

RNA POLYMERASE

Most RNA polymerases (RNAPs), with the exception of those encoded by bacteriophages, are multisubunit enzymes. Analysis of subunit composition reveals a trend that mirrors the evolutionary divergence of prokaryotes and eukaryotes. The prokaryotes are composed of two distinct groups: Bacteria and *Archaea*. Consistent with the fact that Bacteria diverged before *Archaea* and *Eukarya* split, the subunit composition of *archaeal* RNAP is more reminiscent of eukaryotic RNAP than of bacterial RNAP. The core bacterial RNAP consists of five proteins (two α subunits, one β', one β, and one ω subunit). *In vitro*, this five-subunit enzyme is capable of RNA synthesis from nonpromoter DNA in the absence of additional factors. *In vivo*, the nonspecific activity of core RNAP is modulated by sigma (σ) factors, which are essential for the enzymes function. Sigma factors are integral components of the complete bacterial RNAP or holoenzyme and function to recognise specific DNA sequences, called promoter elements, located immediately upstream of the transcription start site. In the context of sigma factor, the a subunit is capable of recognising promoter elements and responding to various regulatory factors. The β and β′ subunits together make up the catalytic centre of RNAP.

The pioneering work of R.G. Roeder and P. Chambon identified three mammalian RNAPs (RNAP I, II and III) by their elution profiles on ion-exchange chromatography (DEAE-Sephadex) and later by their differential sensitivity to the bicyclic octapeptide α-amanitin. In all systems studied, RNAP II is rapidly inhibited by low concentrations of α-amanitin, RNAP I is the most resistant; and RNAP III is inhibited at intermediate concentrations. Since these landmark studies, researchers have been able to define further the precise role of each mammalian RNAP. RNAP I transcribes the multicopy genes encoding large ribosomal RNAs (28S, 18S and 5.8S), RNAP II transcribes all protein-coding genes, as well as some small nuclear

RNAs (snRNA), and RNAP III transcribes the genes for transfer RNAs, 5S ribosomal RNAs and some snRNAs. The *archaeal* RNAP and the three eukaryotic RNAPs are complex enzymes, consisting of 8–14 different subunits. Although the three eukaryotic RNAPs recognise different promoters and transcribe different classes of genes, they share several common features. The two largest subunits of all three eukaryotic RNAPs are related to the B and A′ subunits of *archaeal* RNAP and to the β and β′ subunits of bacterial RNAP. Interestingly, the ω subunit of bacterial RNAP was recently shown to be the homologue of Rbp6, an essential subunit shared by eukaryotic RNAP I, II and III. Rbp6 and o appear to promote RNAP assembly and stability. In addition, five subunits of the eukaryotic RNAPs are common to all three eukaryotic RNAP enzymes. Like the core bacterial RNAP, the purified eukaryotic RNAPs can undertake template dependent transcription of RNA, but are not able to initiate selectively at promoters. However, unlike the bacterial holoenzyme, eukaryotic RNAPs require additional factors to accurately initiate transcription from promoter start sites. This is also true in *archaeal* RNA synthesis. Though the specifics for each RNAP may differ, the general function of the accessory protein factors is to deliver RNAP to the promoter region and position it over the transcription start site.

TRANSCRIPTION CYCLE

The transcription reaction is highly conserved between prokaryotes and eukaryotes. It begins with the binding of RNAP to specific promoter elements. Although RNAP can interact with DNA, it cannot recognise specific promoter DNA elements on its own. The delivery of RNAP to promoter elements is facilitated by auxiliary factors unique to each RNAP. Once at the promoter, RNAP forms a tight stable complex with the DNA. In the presence of nucleotides, this stable complex can initiate RNA synthesis. RNA synthesis occurs within a 'transcription bubble' in which the DNA duplex is temporarily separated into single strands, and one strand serves as the template for synthesis of RNA. As RNAP moves along the DNA, it unwinds the DNA in front of it and rewinds the DNA behind it. In this way, the size of the 'transcription bubble' remains relatively constant while RNAP elongates the RNA chain. As a consequence, the RNA : DNA hybrid within the 'transcription bubble' is short.

The length of the RNA: DNA hybrid has been a topic of intense debate. Most studies are consistent with a hybrid that is approximately 9–12 nucleotides in length. This short RNA: DNA hybrid is important when one considers the processivity of RNAP. The processivity of an enzyme is defined as the ability of the enzyme to continue to act on the substrate and not dissociate between repetitions of the catalytic event. If RNAP dissociates from the template during transcription, the short hybrid would be too unstable and the RNA would be released. Under these circumstances, there is no mechanism for the polymerase to reassociate and continue transcribing where it left off. This is in contrast to DNA synthesis where the newly synthesised DNA is base paired to the template. In principle, if DNA polymerase dissociated from the template, it could conceivably reassociate and resume synthesis where it left off. Therefore, processivity is extremely important during RNA synthesis. As RNAP translocates along DNA, the RNA chain is extended until the polymerase reaches a terminator sequence. The terminator sequence signifies the end of the gene and defines a transcription unit as the RNA chain that is synthesised from DNA sequences that begin at the promoter start site and end at the terminator. At this point, the ternary complex of RNAP, RNA, and DNA dissociates and RNAP is able to recycle for another round of transcription.

The details of the RNA synthesis reaction can be divided into six discrete steps: (i) promoter engagement, (ii) transition from a closed to opened RNAP: promoter complex, (iii) synthesis of initial phospho diester bond and abortive initiation, (iv) promoter clearance, (v) elongation and (vi) termination and RNAP recycling. Except where noted, these steps are common to all RNAPs.

Promoter Engagement

In bacteria, transcription is a process that is largely unregulated. Nevertheless, there are a number of bacterial genes whose expression is governed by regulatory proteins. One of the simplest and most well-studied bacterial regulators is the *Escherichia coli* catabolite activator protein (CAP). In the presence of the allosteric effector cyclic adenosine monophosphate (cAMP), CAP functions by binding to specific DNA sites near target promoters and enhancing the ability of RNAP holoenzyme to bind and initiate transcription. CAP-dependent promoters can be grouped into three classes. Class I promoters require only CAP for transcription activation. In these promoters, the DNA-binding site for CAP is upstream of the binding site for RNAP. Class II promoters also only need CAP for transcription activation but in these promoters the CAP binding site overlaps with the binding site for RNAP. Class III promoters require multiple regulatory proteins including two or more CAP molecules. In all cases, the mechanism is conserved. CAP binds its cognate DNA element and makes specific protein–protein contacts with the C-terminus of the α subunit of RNAP. This interaction enables the α subunit to make specific contacts with the promoter DNA and position the catalytic subunits of RNAP over the transcription start site.

In eukaryotic systems, the mechanism is conserved but the specifics are different. Since eukaryotic RNAPs cannot initiate RNA synthesis at promoter DNA elements on their own, they need the assistance of accessory factors. These factors are called general transcription factors (GTFs). Their function is to make specific protein–DNA and protein–protein contacts to escort RNAP to the promoter. In many ways, these factors serve a similar function to the sigma factors of the bacterial holoenzyme. RNAP II requires five GTFs to accurately initiate RNA synthesis from most promoters of protein coding genes: TFIIB, TFIID, TFIIE, TFIIF and TFIIH. TFIID is a multisubunit complex composed of the TATA-binding protein (TBP) and TBP-associated factors (TAFs). TBP is required for transcription of all genes, including RNAP I and RNAP III genes.

TAFs are required at two levels: (i) for general basal levels of transcription and (ii) to mediate activated transcription. In a manner analogous to the recruitment of bacterial RNAP to the promoter by CAP, transcriptional regulators can target GTFs to facilitate or hinder the delivery of RNAP II to the promoter. Specific interactions have been reported between various regulators and TBP, TAFs, TFIIB, and TFIIH. The importance of these GTF–activator interactions is emphasised by *in vivo* studies showing that artificially tethering TBP to a promoter overcomes the requirement for an activator to achieve stimulated levels of transcription. The essence of these findings is that the delivery of RNAP to the promoter is an important and regulated step in the transcription cycle.

Transition from a Closed to Open RNAP–Promoter Complex

The delivery of RNAP to the promoter results in the binding of RNAP to DNA sequences upstream and around the transcription start site. This complex is referred to as the RNAP–promoter closed (RPc) complex. The RPc complex is very stable as measured by *in vitro* criteria. Specifically, it is stable under nondenaturing gel electrophoresis and is resistant to challenge by nonspecific competitor DNA. Subsequent to the formation of this closed complex, RNAP wraps promoter DNA around its circumference, capturing and interacting with DNA sequences downstream of the transcription start site. As this occurs, there is a conformational change within RNAP that enables it to clamp tightly on to DNA, resulting in an RNAP–promoter intermediate (RPi) complex. RNAP then 'melts' the promoter DNA surrounding the transcription start site to form the 'transcription bubble'. The formation of the bubble renders accessible the genetic information in the template DNA strand to yield an RNAP–promoter open (RPo) complex.

All RNAPs are inherently capable of melting the DNA around the transcription start site with one exception: eukaryotic RNAP II. In the prokaryotic as well as the eukaryotic RNAP I and RNAP III systems, the delivery of RNAP to the promoter signals the completion of promoter engagement. The presence of nucleotide triphosphates (NTPs) triggers the onset of transcription. RNAP II diverges from this paradigm in two ways. First, after the association of the polymerase with the promoter, the complex is not competent to initiate transcription. This system requires the association of two GTFs called TFIIE and TFIIH. The second distinction is that RNAP II requires the input of energy in the form of adenosine triphosphate (ATP) hydrolysis for initiation. Why this particular RNAP requires energy is unclear. What is clear is that the energy derived from ATP is not required for elongation but rather for the formation of a stable RPo complex and for a step subsequent to initiation called promoter clearance. How is this energy utilised? The RNAPII-specific GTFTFIIH is a multisubunit factor that contains as its largest component a protein called XPB/ERCC3. XPB/ERCC3 is an ATP-dependent DNA helicase that appears to function as a 'molecular wrench'. It utilises the energy stored in the β–γ bond of ATP to rotate downstream DNA relative to fixed upstream protein–DNA interactions. This torsion on the DNA helix presumably results in strand separation around the start site of transcription and the establishment of an RPo complex.

Synthesis of Initial Phosphodiester Bond and Abortive Initiation

Once formed, the RPo complex is stabilised by interaction between single-stranded DNA and RNAP. The binding of the initiating NTP confers further stability to the open complex without requiring its hydrolysis or formation of a phosphodiester bond. In the RPo complex, the template strand is accessible and directs base pairing with NTPs to initiate phosphodiester bond formation and RNA synthesis. This generates a ternary complex that contains RNA as well as DNA and RNAP. However, the formation of a ternary complex does not predict productive RNA synthesis. In fact, a significant fraction of complexes engage in abortive RNA synthesis in which short (2–8 nucleotides) RNA transcripts are made and released in a repetitive manner. Escape from this nonproductive cycle occurs when the RNA transcript reaches a critical length (about 10 nucleotides). In the bacterial system, when an RNA chain of this length is synthesised, sigma factor is released. At this point, RNAP leaves the promoter and becomes committed to productive chain elongation. The physical movement of RNAP away from the promoter is referred to as 'promoter clearance' and signals a vacancy at the promoter that can be filled by another RNAP.

Promoter Clearance and Elongation

During promoter clearance, RNAP breaks contact with DNA and with protein components at the promoter and becomes stably associated with the RNA and DNA chains. How does this happen? One possible explanation stems from electron crystallographic, electron microscopic and photo cross-linking data that have been used to deduce low resolution models of RNAP open complexes and RNAP II elongating complexes. These models reveal common features likely shared by all RNAPs. In an RNAP complex that has initiated RNA synthesis, the 8–10 most recently synthesised nucleotides of the nascent RNA are engaged in Watson–Crick hydrogen bonding with the DNA template strand as an RNA–DNA hybrid. Importantly, the 5–8 next most recently synthesised nucleotides of the nascent RNA are engaged in interactions with regions of RNAP that resemble a tunnel or channel.

RNA within this tunnel is protected from enzymatic manipulations. The entry of nascent RNA into an exit tunnel appears to confer stability to the elongating RNAP complex. The formation of a stable and productive RNAP ternary complex correlates with the departure of sigma factor. Perhaps it is the entry of RNA transcripts into the exit tunnel that confers stability to the RNAP ternary complex resulting in the release of sigma factor. Although this model is supported by data from all RNAP systems, the situation for RNAP II is more intricate.

CTD OF RNAP II

For RNAP II, the transition from initiation to elongation is accompanied by covalent modifications of an unusual structure at the C-terminal domain (CTD) of its largest subunit. This structure consists of multiple tandem repeats of a heptapeptide (Tyr-Ser-Pro-Thr-Ser-Pro-Ser) that is conserved between fungi and vertebrates. Although the largest subunits of bacterial, *archaeal*, and eukaryotic RNAPs are members of the same family, the CTD is unique to eukaryotic RNAP II. The length of the heptapeptide repeats seems to correlate with increased genomic complexity; *Saccharomyces cerevisiae* has 26–27 repeats, *Caenorhabditis elegans* 34 repeats, *Drosophila* 43 repeats, and mouse and human 52 repeats. The importance of the CTD is well established, as deletion of the mouse, *Drosophila* or *S. cerevisiae* CTD is lethal.

Owing to the high content of serine and threonine residues in the heptapeptide, the CTD can be found in two states *in vivo*, highly phosphorylated and unphosphorylated. A number of studies have shown that the phosphorylation state of the CTD dictates the activity of RNAP II during the transcription cycle. Specifically, it has been shown that while the nonphosphorylated form of the CTD associates with promoter-bound components prior to initiation of RNA synthesis, it is the hyperphosphorylated form that catalyses RNA chain elongation.

These observations point to a critical role for CTD phosphorylation in the disengagement of RNAP from the promoter during the transition from initiation of RNA synthesis to elongation. Phosphorylation of the CTD presumably induces conformational changes within the initiation complex that disrupt certain protein–protein interactions. This disruption may concomitantly stabilise the nascent RNA chain within the RNAP exit tunnel, thereby triggering clearance of the polymerase from the promoter. The above model implies a cycling of the CTD from an unphosphorylated form to a hyperphosphorylated form during rounds of RNA synthesis, and predicts that one of the RNAP II-specific GTFs would be capable of phosphorylating the CTD. This prediction was validated by the identification of a CTD-specific kinase activity in TFIIH. The TFIIH kinase phosphorylates the CTD after the formation of the first phosphodiester bond and is probably important for promoter clearance.

The function of the RNAP II CTD does not end with promoter engagement and promoter clearance. In the RNAP II system, nascent RNA molecules undergo a number of modifications prior to being exported to the cytoplasm for translation. The transcripts are capped, spliced, cleaved and polyadenylated. These reactions do not proceed independently of one another. *In vivo*, these reactions occur cotranscriptionally; meaning that as the nascent RNA chain protrudes out of the RNAP exit tunnel it becomes a substrate for modification. RNA 'capping' involves three reactions in which the 5'-triphosphate terminus of the RNA is cleaved to a diphosphate by RNA triphosphatase, then 'capped' with guanosine monophosphate (GMP) by RNA guanylyltransferase, and methylated at the N7 position of guanine by RNA methyltransferase.

How is capping enzyme targeted to elongating RNA transcripts? Recently it was shown that components of capping enzyme directly interact with the phosphorylated form of the RNAP II CTD. Specifically, the guanylyltransferase component of the capping apparatus binds the CTD containing phosphoserine at either position 2 or 5 of the heptad repeat. Phosphoserine at position 5 stimulates the guanylyltransferase activity of capping enzyme. *In vivo* only the TFIIH associated CTD kinase is necessary for proper capping enzyme recruitment.

Interestingly, shortly after promoter clearance, TFIIH dissociates from the elongating RNAP II complex. The departure of TFIIH is followed by the departure of capping enzyme. What triggers the release of capping enzyme? Phosphorylation of serine 5 in the heptad by TFIIH promotes the interaction of capping enzyme with the CTD. The release of capping enzyme shortly after promoter clearance invokes a change in the phosphorylation state of the CTD. Current evidence suggests that there is a wave of phosphorylation on serine 2 after promoter clearance. This change in phosphorylation may trigger the release of capping enzyme and recruit factors that are involved in splicing and polyadenylation of RNA. The recruitment of RNA-processing machinery to the CTD of RNAP II provides a mechanism of targeting capping, splicing, and cleavage and polyadenylation of the proper RNA substrate. In this system, the CTD serves as a unique platform from which to coordinate these activities.

The elongation phase of RNAP II is also subject to extrinsic influences. Specifically, RNAP II elongation can respond to *cis* (DNA) and trans (protein)-acting factors. *Cis*-acting factors constitute natural DNA sequences that cause RNAP II to pause during transcription. The paused RNAP II is acted upon by factors that promote transit beyond these sites. One example is TFIIS. This factor caused the paused RNAP II to back up and then proceed forward past the pause site. Another class of factors, including TFIIF and the elongins, influence the rate of RNAP II elongation. Together, these two classes of factors govern the kinetics of RNAP II elongation.

Termination

Once RNAP has cleared the promoter, it synthesises RNA until it encounters a terminator sequence. At this point, RNA synthesis stops, RNAP releases the completed RNA product and dissociates from the DNA template. How does this happen? Many terminators require a hairpin to form in the secondary structure of the RNA being transcribed. This suggests that termination depends on the structure of the RNA product and is not simply determined by specific DNA sequences encountered during transcription.

Termination is best understood in the prokaryotic system. *E. coli* RNAP can terminate RNA synthesis at two types of terminators. One class is called intrinsic terminators because RNAP can terminate at these sequences without the assistance of other factors. The other class of terminators is called Rho-dependent terminators; termination at these sites requires the assistance of rho factor.

Two structural features characterise intrinsic terminators: a hairpin in the secondary structure and a stretch of 7–9 uracil residues at the end of the RNA chain. The uracil residues produce a particularly unstable RNA–DNA hybrid. Typically, when RNAP encounters a weak hybrid it pauses and backtracks to form a more stable hybrid. However, when RNAP encounters a terminator sequence, the resulting hairpin in the RNA prevents RNAP from backtracking and also disrupts critical RNA contacts in the exit channel of RNAP. Rho-dependent termination requires a stretch of 50–90 nucleotides preceding the site of termination that is rich in C and poor in G residues. Rho has an ATPase activity that is dependent on RNA. As RNAP translocates along the DNA template, rho translocates along the RNA transcript. When RNAP pauses at a termination sequence, the secondary structure in the transcript enables rho to disrupt the RNA–DNA hybrid and release the RNA. In the highly regulated RNAP II system, termination of RNA synthesis is coupled to RNA polyadenylation. Once again, the CTD is invoked to execute this final step inRNA synthesis. Once RNAP II has transcribed through the polyadenylation site (poly(A), the resulting RNA chain is acted upon by factors that cleave the RNA chain from the moving RNAP II and catalyse the poly(A) addition to the end of the RNA molecule. This modification completes the synthesis and processing of messenger RNA.

Studies on the mouse β-globin gene have shown that transcription terminates within a region 1400 nucleotides downstream of the poly(A) site. What is the nature of the signal that finally releases RNAP II from the template? Two general models can be proposed to address this question. The first suggests that upon the release of the nascent RNA chain, RNAP II continues to synthesise RNA lacking a proper cap at the new 5′ end.

The absence of a 5′ cap makes this RNA chain susceptible to degradation. The model invokes the recognition of the unprotected 5′ end of the RNA by an exonuclease that degrades the RNA at a faster rate than RNA synthesis by RNAP II. Eventually, the exonuclease catches up with RNAP II, disrupts the ternary complex, and releases RNAP II from the template. The other model suggests that once RNAP II transits past the poly(A) site, a signal is sent to RNAP II, perhaps by processivity factors, causing it to dissociate from the template.

One example that illustrates the latter mechanism is transcription termination factor 2 (HuF2). HuF2 is identical to the *Drosophila* lodestar protein. HuF2/lodestar possesses DNA-dependent ATPase activity and can efficiently dissociate RNAP II from the template. Earlier observations showed that lodestar is cytoplasmic during interphase but translocates to the nucleus during mitosis. Perhaps HuF2/lodestar functions to ensure transcriptional silencing during mitosis. Support for this notion comes from analysis of the lodestar mutant in *Drosophila*. Specifically, mutations in lodestar result in chromatin bridges, chromosome tangling and breakage during anaphase.

This observation suggests that proper chromosome segregation is hindered by the presence of active transcription complexes during mitosis and that HuF2/lodestar preserves the integrity of the chromosomes by displacing active RNAP II complexes from the template.

RNAP Recycling

Once RNAP dissociates from the DNA template, it is free to reassociate with promoter elements and initiate another round of RNA synthesis. Once again, the RNAP II system affords a higher level of regulation. After cleavage of the nascent RNA chain, most of the factors associated with the RNAP II CTD platform have executed their function. As a result, the CTD does not need to remain phosphorylated. Moreover, in order for RNAP II to re-engage the promoter it must be in the dephosphorylated form. This requisite dephosphorylation event is facilitated by a specific phosphatase called FCP1. FCP1 associates with the elongation RNAP II complex and is required for the dissociation of capping enzyme from the complex, presumably by altering the phosphorylation state of the CTD from predominantly serine 5 phosphorylation to mostly serine 2 phosphorylation. When RNAP II encounters certain DNA sequences FCP1 can catalyse the dephosphorylation of the CTD. Importantly, the conversion of the elongating RNAP II to the dephosphorylated form does not promote the release of RNAP II from the template DNA. The ability of FCP1 to dephosphorylate the CTD in the elongation complex suggests that RNAP II is converted to the nonphosphorylated form prior to, or concomitant with, its release from the DNA template. The catalytic activity of FCP1 enables RNAP II to recycle and engage in multiple rounds of productive RNA synthesis.

Chromatin Challenge

In eukaryotic cells, the genetic blueprint, which extends over a meter if unravelled, is stored in a nucleus that is less than 10^{-5} m in diameter. Chromosomes represent the largest and most visible structures of genetic information. This degree of compaction has severe consequences for processes that require access to DNA. The cell has developed compensatory mechanisms that facilitate access to the DNA during the processes of RNA synthesis, DNA synthesis and DNA repair. The interplay of chromatin remodelling activities with the basal transcription machinery undoubtedly has a profound impact on the overall level and regulation of gene expression.

Chapter 12

Transcription in Bacteria

INTRODUCTION

Eukaryotic transcription uses three distinct RNA polymerases, which are specialised for different RNAs. RNA polymerase I makes Ribosomal RNAs, RNA polymerase II makes messenger RNAs, and RNA polymerase III makes small, stable RNAs such as transfer RNAs and 5S ribosomal RNA. Eukaryotic RNA polymerases are differentiated by their sensitivity to the toxic compound, α-amanitin, the active compound in the poisonous mushroom Aminita phalloides, or 'destroying angel.' RNA polymerase I is not inhibited by α-amanitin, RNA polymerase II is inhibited at very low concentrations of the drug, and RNA polymerase III is inhibited at high drug concentrations.

Eukaryotic transcription is dependent on several sequence and structural features. First, actively transcribing genes have a 'looser,' more accessible chromatin structure. The nucleosomes are not as condensed as in other forms of chromatin, especially heterochromatin, and they often do not contain histone H1. The DNA in the promoter region at the 5' end of the gene may not be bound into nucleosomes at all. In this way, the promoter sequences are available for binding to protein transcription factors—proteins that bind to DNA and either repress or stimulate transcription. In addition to promoter sequences, other nucleotide sequences termed enhancers can affect transcription efficiency. Enhancers bind to specialised protein factors and then stimulate transcription. The difference between enhancers and factor-binding promoters depends on their site of action. Unlike promoters, which only affect sequences immediately adjacent to them, enhancers function even when they are located far away (as much as 1,000 base pairs away) from the promoter. Both enhancer-binding and promoter-binding transcription factors recognise their appropriate DNA sequences and then bind to other proteins—for example, RNA polymerase, to help initiate transcription. Because enhancers are located so far from the promoters where RNA polymerase binds, enhancer interactions involve bending the DNA to make a loop so the proteins can interact.

RIBOSOMAL RNA SYNTHESIS

Most of the RNA made in the cell is ribosomal RNA. The large and small subunit RNAs are synthesised by RNA polymerase I. Ribosomal RNA is made in a specialised organelle, the nucleolus, which contains many copies of the rRNA genes, a correspondingly large number of RNA polymerase I molecules, and the cellular machinery that processes the primary transcripts into mature rRNAs. RNA polymerase I is the most abundant RNA polymerase in the cell, and it synthesises RNA at the fastest rate of any of the polymerases. The genes for rRNA are present in many copies, arranged in tandem, one after the other. Each transcript contains a copy of each of three rRNAs: the 28S and 5.8S large subunit RNAs and the small subunit 18S RNA, in that order. The rRNA promoter sequences extend much further upstream than do prokaryotic promoters.

The transcription of rRNA is very efficient. This is necessary because each rRNA transcript can only make one ribosome, in contrast to the large number of proteins that can be made from a single mRNA. The individual ribosomal RNAs must be processed from the large precursor RNA that is the product of transcription. The primary transcript contains small and large subunit RNAs in the order: 28S—5.8S—18S. Processing involves the modification of specific nucleotides in the rRNA, followed by cleavage of the transcript into the individual RNA components (Fig. 12.1).

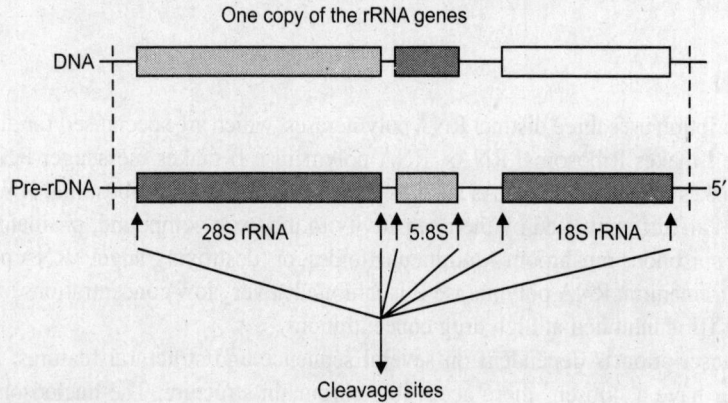

Fig. 12.1: Cleavage of the transcript.

Messenger RNA Transcription

RNA polymerase II transcribes messenger RNA and a few other small cellular RNAs. Class II promoters are usually defined by their sensitivity to α-amanitin. Like prokaryotic promoters, many class II promoters contain two conserved sequences, called the CAAT and TATA boxes. The TATA box is bound by a specialised transcription factor called TBP (for TATA-Binding-Factor). Binding of TBP is required for transcription, but other proteins are required to bind to the upstream (and potentially downstream) sequences that are specific to each gene.

Like prokaryotic transcripts, eukaryotic RNAs are initiated with a nucleoside triphosphate. Termination of eukaryotic mRNA transcription is less well understood than is termination of prokaryotic transcription, because the 3′ ends of eukaryotic mRNAs are derived by processing (Fig. 12.2).

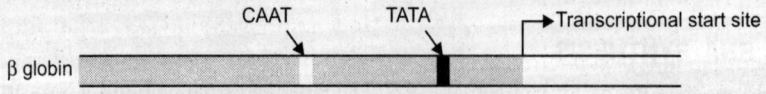

Fig. 12.2: RNA transcription.

Transfer and 5S Ribosomal RNA Transcription

RNA polymerase III transcribes 5S rRNA and tRNA genes. The 'promoter' of these transcripts can actually be located inside the gene itself, in contrast to all the other promoters discussed earlier (Fig. 12.3). The 5′ sequence is not essential for accurate transcription initiation. When the region extending from the 5′ end of the gene (that is, the part that would normally be considered to be the promoter) is deleted, RNA synthesis is carried out just as efficiently as on the native gene. The new 5′ end of the transcript is complementary to whatever sequences take the place of the natural ones. Furthermore, initiation is only affected when sequences within the 5S rRNA gene are disrupted. The molecular explanation for this phenomenon is as follows:

- A protein factor binds to the 5S rRNA gene. Binding is at the internal sequence that is required for accurate initiation.
- The bound factor then interacts with RNA polymerase III, which is then capable of initiation. During transcription, the multiple protein factors (called TFIIIs) remain bound to the transcribing gene.

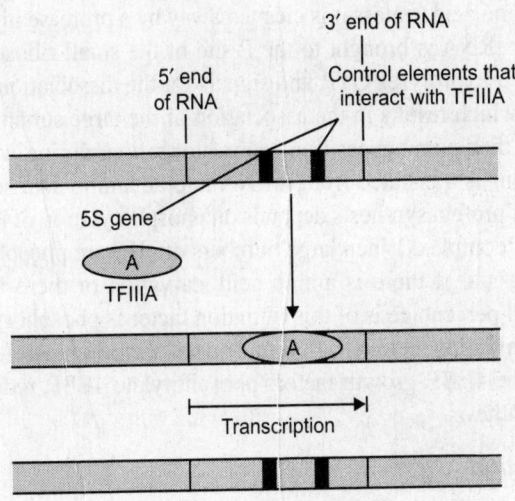

Fig. 12.3: 3′ and 5′ RNA.

EUKARYOTIC TRANSLATION

Eukaryotic translation is the process by which messenger RNA is translated into proteins in eukaryotes. It consists of initiation, elongation, and termination.

Initiation

Cap-dependent initiation

Initiation of translation usually involves the interaction of certain key proteins with a special tag bound to the 5′-end of an mRNA molecule, the 5′ cap, as well as with the 5′ UTR. The protein factors bind the small ribosomal subunit (also referred to as the 40S subunit), and these initiation factors hold the mRNA in place. The eukaryotic Initiation Factor 3 (eIF3) is associated with the small ribosomal subunit, and plays a role in keeping the large ribosomal subunit from prematurely binding. eIF3 also interacts with the eIF4F complex, which consists of three other initiation factors: eIF4A, eIF4E, and eIF4G. eIF4G is a scaffolding protein that directly associates with both eIF3 and the other two components. eIF4E is the cap-binding protein. It is the rate-limiting step of cap-dependent initiation, and is often cleaved from the complex by some viral proteases to limit the cell's ability to translate its own transcripts. This is a method of hijacking the host machinery in favour of the viral (cap-independent) messages. eIF4A is an ATP-dependent RNA helicase, which aids the ribosome in resolving certain secondary structures formed by the mRNA transcript.

There is another protein associated with the eIF4F complex called the Poly(A)-binding protein (PABP), which binds the poly-A tail of most eukaryotic mRNA molecules. This protein has been implicated in playing a role in circularisation of the mRNA during translation. This pre-initiation complex (43S subunit, or the 40S and tRNA) accompanied by the protein factors move along the mRNA chain toward its 3′-end, scanning for the 'start' codon (typically AUG) on the mRNA, which indicates where the mRNA begins coding for the protein. In eukaryotes and archaea, the amino acid encoded by the start codon is methionine. The initiator tRNA charged with Met forms part of the ribosomal complex and, thus, all proteins start with this amino acid (unless it is cleaved away by a protease in subsequent modifications). The Met-charged initiator tRNA is brought to the P-site of the small ribosomal subunit by eukaryotic Initiation Factor 2 (eIF2). It hydrolyses GTP, and signals for the dissociation of several factors from the small ribosomal subunit, which results in the association of the large subunit (or the 60S subunit). The complete ribosome (80S) then commences translation elongation, during which the sequence between the 'start' and 'stop' codons is translated from mRNA into an amino acid sequence—thus, a protein is synthesised. Regulation of protein synthesis depends on phosphorylation of initiation factor eIF2, which is a part of the met-tRNAi complex. When large numbers of eIF2 are phosphorylated, protein synthesis is inhibited. This would occur if there is amino acid starvation or there has been a virus infection. However, naturally a small percentage is of this initiation factor is phosphorylated. Another regulator is 4EBP, which binds to the initiation factor eIF4E found on the 5′ cap on mRNA stopping protein synthesis. To oppose the effects of the 4EBP, growth factors phosphorylate 4EBP, reducing its affinity for eIF4E and permitting protein synthesis.

Cap-independent initiation

The best-studied example of the cap-independent mode of translation initiation in eukaryotes is the Internal Ribosome Entry Site (IRES) approach. What differentiates cap-independent translation from cap-dependent translation is that cap-independent translation does not require the ribosome to start scanning from the 5′ end of the mRNA cap until the start codon. The ribosome can be trafficked to the start site by ITAFs (IRES trans-acting factors) bypassing the need to scan from the 5′ UTR. This method of translation has been recently discovered, and has found important in conditions that require the translation of specific mRNAs, despite cellular stress or the inability to translate most mRNAs. Examples include factors responding to apoptosis, stress-induced responses.

Elongation

Elongation depends on eukaryotic elongation factors. At the end of the initiation step, the mRNA is positioned so that the next codon can be translated during the elongation stage of protein synthesis. The initiator tRNA occupies the P-site in the ribosome, and the A site is ready to receive an aminoacyl-tRNA. During chain elongation, each additional amino acid is added to the nascent polypeptide chain in a three-step microcycle. The steps in this microcycle are: (i) positioning the correct aminoacyl-tRNA in the A site of the ribosome, (ii) forming the peptide bond and (iii) shifting the mRNA by one codon relative to the ribosome. Unlike bacteria, in which translation initiation occurs as soon as the 5′ end of an mRNA is synthesised, in eukaryotes such tight coupling between transcription and translation is not possible because transcription and translation are carried out in separate compartments of the cell (the nucleus and cytoplasm). Eukaryotic mRNA precursors must be processed in the nucleus (e.g. capping, polyadenylation, splicing) before they are exported to the cytoplasm for translation.

Translation can also be affected by ribosomal pausing, which can trigger endo-nucleolytic attack of the mRNA, a process termed mRNA no-go decay. Ribosomal pausing also aids co-translational folding of the nascent polypeptide on the ribosome, and delays protein translation while it is encoding mRNA. This can trigger ribosomal frameshifting.

Termination: Termination of elongation depends on eukaryotic release factors. The process is similar to that of prokaryotic termination.

RNA POLYMERASE I

RNA polymerase I (also called Pol I) is, in higher eukaryotes, the enzyme that only transcribes ribosomal RNA (but not 5S rRNA, which is synthesised by RNA Polymerase III), a type of RNA that accounts for over 50% of the total RNA synthesised in a cell.

Pol I consists of 14 protein subunits (polypeptides) and its crystal structure was recently solved at atomic resolution. Twelve of its subunits have identical or related counterparts in Pol II and Pol III. The additional two subunits are related to Pol II initiation factors and have structural homologues in Pol III. rDNA transcription is confined to the nucleolus where several hundreds of copies of rRNA genes are present, arranged as tandem head-to-tail repeats. Pol I transcribes one large transcript, encoding an rDNA gene over and over again. This gene encodes the 18S, the 5.8S, and the 28S RNA molecules of the ribosome in eukaryotes. The transcripts are cleaved by snoRNA. The 5S ribosomal RNA is transcribed by Pol III. Because of the simplicity of Pol I transcription, it is the fastest-acting polymerase and contributes up to 60% of cellular transcription levels in exponentially growing cells.

Regulation of rRNA Transcription

The rate of cell growth is directly dependent on the rate of protein synthesis, which, itself, is intricately linked to ribosome synthesis and rRNA transcription. Thus, intracellular signals must coordinate the synthesis of rRNA with that of other components of protein translation. Two specific mechanisms have been identified, ensuring proper control of rRNA synthesis and Pol I-mediated transcription. Given the large number of rDNA genes (several hundreds) available for transcription, the first mechanism involves adjustments in the number of genes being transcribed at a specific time. In mammalian cells, the number of active rDNA genes varies between cell types and level of differentiation. In general, as a cell becomes more differentiated, it requires less growth and, therefore, will have a decrease in rRNA synthesis and a decrease in rDNA genes being transcribed. When rRNA synthesis is stimulated, SL1 (selectivity factor 1) will bind to the promoters of rDNA genes that were previously silent, and recruit a pre-initiation complex to which Pol I will bind and start transcription of rRNA. Changes in rRNA transcription can also occur via changes in the rate of transcription. While the exact mechanism through which Pol I increases its rate of transcription is as yet unknown, evidence has shown that rRNA synthesis can increase or decrease without changes in the number of actively transcribed rDNA.

Pol I Transcription Cycle

In the process of transcription (by any polymerase), there are three main stages:

1. Initiation: The construction of the RNA polymerase complex on the gene's promoter with the help of transcription factors.
2. Elongation: The actual transcription of the majority of the gene into a corresponding RNA sequence.
3. Termination: The cessation of RNA transcription and the disassembly of the RNA polymerase complex.

Initiation

Initiation: the construction of the polymerase complex on the promoter. Pol I requires no TATA box in the promoter, instead relying on a UCS (Upstream Control Sequence).

1. UBF (Upstream Binding Factor) binds the UCS.
2. UCS recruits and binds a protein complex incorporating TBP (TATA Binding Protein) and three TAFs (TBP Associated Factors) called SL1 or TIF-IB. The TBP is forced to bind non-sequence specifically.
3. Rrn3/TIF-IA is phosphorylated and binds Pol I.
4. Pol I binds to the UBF/SL1 complex via Rrn3/TIF-IA, and transcription starts.

Elongation

As Pol I escapes and clears the promoter, UBF and SL1 remain-promoter bound, ready to recruit another Pol I. Indeed, each active rDNA gene can be transcribed multiple times simultaneously, as opposed to Pol II-transcribed genes, which associate with only one complex at a time. While elongation proceeds unimpeded *in vitro*, it is unclear at this point whether this process happens in a cell, given the presence of nucleosomes. Pol I does seem to transcribe through nucleosomes, either bypassing or disrupting them, perhaps assisted by chromatin-remodelling activities. In addition, UBF might also act as positive feedback, enhancing Pol I elongation through an anti-repressor function. An additional factor, TIF-IC, can also stimulate the overall rate of transcription and suppress pausing of Pol I. As Pol I proceeds along the rDNA, supercoils form both ahead of and behind the complex. These are unwound by topoisomerase I or II at regular intervals, similar to what is seen in Pol II-mediated transcription. Elongation is likely to be interrupted at sites of DNA damage. Transcription-coupled repair occurs similarly to Pol II-transcribed genes and requires the presence of several DNA repair proteins, such as TFIIH, CSB, and XPG.

Termination

In higher eukaryotes, TTF-I binds and bends the termination site at the 3' end of the transcribed region. This will force Pol I to pause. TTF-I, with the help of transcript-release factor PTRF and a T-rich region, will induce Pol I into terminating transcription and dissociating from the DNA and the new transcript. Evidence suggests that termination might be rate-limiting in cases of high rRNA production. TTF-I and PTRF will then indirectly stimulate the reinitiation of transcription by Pol I at the same rDNA gene. In organisms such as budding yeast the process seems to be much more complicated and is still not completely elucidated.

RNA POLYMERASE II

RNA polymerase II (RNAP II and Pol II) is an enzyme found in eukaryotic cells. It catalyses the transcription of DNA to synthesise precursors of mRNA and most snRNA and microRNA. A 550 kDa complex of 12 subunits, RNAP II is the most studied type of RNA polymerase. A wide range of transcription factors are required for it to bind to upstream gene promoters and begin transcription.

Subunits

The eukaryotic core RNA polymerase II was first purified using transcription assays. The purified enzyme has typically 10–12 subunits (12 in humans and yeast) and is incapable of specific promoter recognition.

Many subunit-subunit interactions are known.

- DNA-directed RNA polymerase II subunit RPB1-an enzyme that in humans is encoded by the POLR2A gene and in yeast is encoded by RPO21. RPB1 is the largest subunit of RNA polymerase II. It contains a carboxy terminal domain (CTD) composed of up to 52 heptapeptide repeats (YSPTSPS) that are essential for polymerase activity. In combination with several other polymerase subunits, it forms the DNA binding domain of the polymerase, a groove in which the DNA template is transcribed into RNA. It strongly interacts with RPB8.

- RPB2 (POLR2B)-the second-largest subunit that in combination with at least two other polymerase subunits forms a structure within the polymerase that maintains contact in the active site of the enzyme between the DNA template and the newly synthesised RNA.

- RPB3 (POLR2C)-the third-largest subunit. Exists as a heterodimer with another polymerase subunit, POLR2J forming a core subassembly. RPB3 strongly interacts with RPB1-5, 7, 10–12.

- RNA polymerase II subunit B4 (RPB4)-encoded by the POLR2D gene is the fourth-largest subunit and may have a stress protective role.

- RPB5-In humans is encoded by the POLR2E gene. Two molecules of this subunit are present in each RNA polymerase II. RPB5 strongly interacts with RPB1, RPB3, and RPB6.

- RPB6 (POLR2F)-forms a structure with at least two other subunits that stabilises the transcribing polymerase on the DNA template.

- RPB7-encoded by POLR2G and may play a role in regulating polymerase function. RPB7 interacts strongly with RPB1 and RPB5.

- RPB8 (POLR2H)-interacts with subunits RPB1-3, 5, and 7.

- RPB9-The groove in which the DNA template is transcribed into RNA is composed of RPB9 (POLR2I) and RPB1.

- RPB10-the product of gene POLR2L. It interacts with RPB1-3 and 5, and strongly with RPB3.

- RPB11-the RPB11 subunit is itself composed of three subunits in humans: POLR2J (RPB11-a), POLR2J2 (RPB11-b), and POLR2J3 (RPB11-c).

- RPB12-Also interacting with RPB3 is RPB12 (POLR2K).

Assembly

RPB3 is involved in RNA polymerase II assembly. A subcomplex of RPB2 and RPB3 appears soon after subunit synthesis. This complex subsequently interacts with RPB1. RPB3, RPB5, and RPB7 interact with themselves to form homodimers, and RPB3 and RPB5 together are able to contact all of the other RPB subunits, except RPB9. Only RPB1 strongly binds to RPB5. The RPB1 subunit also contacts RPB7, RPB10, and more weakly but most efficiently with RPB8. Once RPB1 enters the complex, other subunits such as RPB5 and RPB7 can enter, where RPB5 binds to RPB6 and RPB8 and RPB3 brings in

RPB10, RPB 11, and RPB12. RPB4 and RPB9 may enter once most of the complex is assembled. RPB4 forms a complex with RPB7.

Kinetics

Enzymes can catalyse up to several million reactions per second. Enzyme rates depend on solution conditions and substrate concentration. Like other enzymes POLR2 has a saturation curve and a maximum velocity (Vmax). It has a Km (substrate concentration required for one-half Vmax) and a kcat (the number of substrate molecules handled by one active site per second). The specificity constant is given by kcat/Km. The theoretical maximum for the specificity constant is the diffusion limit of about 10^8 to 10^9 (M^{-1} s^{-1}), where every collision of the enzyme with its substrate results in catalysis. In yeast mutation in the Trigger-Loop domain of the largest subunit can change the kinetics of the enzyme. The turnover number for RNA polymerase II is 0.16 s^{-1} subject to concentration. Bacterial RNA polymerase, a relative of RNA Polymerase II, switches between inactivated and activated states by translocating back and forth along the DNA. Concentrations of [NTP]eq = 10 μM GTP, 10 μM UTP, 5 μM ATP and 2.5 μM CTP, produce a mean elongation rate, turnover number, of ~1 bp $(NTP)^{-1}$ for bacterial RNAP, a relative of RNA polymerase II. RNA Polymerase II is inhibited by α-amanitin.

Holoenzyme

RNA polymerase II holoenzyme is a form of eukaryotic RNA polymerase II that is recruited to the promoters of protein-coding genes in living cells. It consists of RNA polymerase II, a subset of general transcription factors, and regulatory proteins known as SRB proteins. Part of the assembly of the holoenzyme is referred to as the preinitiation complex, because its assembly takes place on the gene promoter before the initiation of transcription. The mediator complex acts as a bridge between RNA polymerase II and the transcription factors.

Control by Chromatin Structure

This is an outline of an example mechanism of yeast cells by which chromatin structure and histone post-translational modification help regulate and record the transcription of genes by RNA polymerase II.

This pathway gives examples of regulation at these points of transcription:

• Pre-initiation (promotion by Bre1, histone modification).
• Initiation (promotion by TFIIH, Pol II modification AND promotion by COMPASS, histone modification).
• Elongation (promotion by Set2, Histone Modification).

Please note that this refers to various stages of the process as regulatory steps. It has not been proven that they are used for regulation, but is very likely they are.

RNA Pol II elongation promoters can be summarised in 3 classes.

1. Drug/sequence-dependent arrest-affected factors (Various interfering proteins).
2. Chromatin structure-oriented factors (Histone post-transcriptional modifiers, e.g. Histone Methyltransferases).
3. RNA Pol II catalysis-improving factors (Various interfering proteins and Pol II cofactors, see RNA polymerase II).

Protein Complexes Involved

Chromatin structure oriented factors:

[HMTs (Histone Methyl Transferases)]:

COMPASS - (Complex of Proteins Associated with Set1) - Methylates lysine 4 of histone H3.

Set2 - Methylates lysine 36 of histone H3.

(interesting irrelevant example: Dot1 Methylates lysine 79 of histone H3.)

(Other): Bre1 - Ubiquinates (adds ubiquitin to) lysine 123 of histone H2B. Associated with pre-initiation and allowing RNA Pol II binding.

N-terminus

The N-terminus (also known as the amino-terminus, NH_2-terminus, N-terminal end or amine-terminus) refers to the start of a protein or polypeptide terminated by an amino acid with a free amine group ($-NH_2$). The convention for writing peptide sequences is to put the N-terminus on the left and write the sequence from N- to C-terminus. When the protein is translated from messenger RNA, it is created from N-terminus to C-terminus.

The N-terminus is the first part of the protein that exits the ribosome during protein biosynthesis. It often contains sequences that act as targeting signals, basically intracellular zip codes, that allow for the protein to be delivered to its designated location within the cell. The targeting signal is usually cleaved off after successful targeting by a processing peptidase. Some proteins are modified post-translationally.

C-terminus

The C-terminus (also known as the carboxyl-terminus, carboxy-terminus, C-terminal end, or COOH-terminus) of a protein or polypeptide is the end of the amino acid chain terminated by a free carboxyl group ($-COOH$). The convention for writing peptide sequences is to put the C-terminal end on the right and write the sequence from N- to C-terminus.

Each amino acid has a carboxyl group and an amine group, and amino acids link to one another to form a chain by a dehydration reaction by joining the amine group of one amino acid to the carboxyl group of the next. Thus polypeptide chains have an end with an unbound carboxyl group, the C-terminus, and an end with an amine group, the N-terminus. Proteins are naturally synthesised starting from the N-terminus and ending at the C-terminus.

The C-terminus can contain retention signals for protein sorting. The most common ER retention signal is the amino acid sequence -KDEL (or -HDEL) at the C-terminus, which keeps the protein in the endoplasmic reticulum and prevents it from entering the secretory pathway.

The C-terminus of proteins can be modified post-translationally, for example, most commonly by the addition of a lipid anchor to the C-terminus that allows the protein to be inserted into a membrane without having a transmembrane domain. With Pol II, the C-terminus of RPB1 is appended to form the C-terminal domain (CTD).

CTD of RNA polymerase

The carboxy-terminal domain of RNA polymerase II typically consists of up to 52 repeats of the sequence Tyr-Ser-Pro-Thr-Ser-Pro-Ser. Other proteins often bind the C-terminal domain of RNA polymerase inorder to activate polymerase activity. It is the protein domain that is involved in the initiation of transcription, the capping of the RNA transcript, and attachment to the spliceosome for RNA splicing.

RNA POLYMERASE III

In eukaryote cells, RNA polymerase III (also called Pol III) transcribes DNA to synthesise ribosomal 5S rRNA, tRNA and other small RNAs. This enzyme complex has a more limited role than the Pol III in prokaryote cells. The genes transcribed by RNA Pol III fall in the category of 'housekeeping' genes whose expression is required in all cell types and most environmental conditions. Therefore the regulation of Pol III transcription is primarily tied to the regulation of cell growth and the cell cycle, thus requiring fewer regulatory proteins than RNA polymerase II. Under stress conditions however, the protein Maf1 represses Pol III activity.

In the process of transcription (by any polymerase) there are three main stages:

1. Initiation, requiring construction of the RNA polymerase complex on the genes promoter.
2. Elongation, the synthesis of the RNA transcript.
3. Termination, the finishing of RNA transcription and disassembly of the RNA polymerase complex.

Initiation

Initiation: the construction of the polymerase complex on the promoter. Pol III is unusual (compared to Pol II) requiring no control sequences upstream of the gene, instead normally relying on internal control sequences - sequences within the transcribed section of the gene (although upstream sequences are occasionally seen, e.g. U6 snRNA gene has an upstream TATA box as seen in Pol II Promoters).

Class I

Typical stages in 5S rRNA (also termed class I) gene initiation:

1. TFIIIA (Transcription Factor for polymerase III A) binds to the intragenic (lying within the transcribed DNA sequence) 5S rRNA control sequence, the C Block (also termed box C).
2. TFIIIA Serves as a platform that replaces the A and B Blocks for positioning TFIIIC in an orientation with respect to the start site of transcription that is equivalent to what is observed for tRNA genes.
3. Once TFIIIC is bound to the TFIIIA-DNA complex the assembly of TFIIIB proceeds as described for tRNA transcription.

Class II

Typical stages in a tRNA (also termed class II) gene initiation:

1. TFIIIC (Transcription Factor for polymerase III C) binds to two intragenic (lying within the transcribed DNA sequence) control sequences, the A and B Blocks (also termed box A and box B).
2. TFIIIC acts as an assembly factor that positions TFIIIB to bind to DNA at a site centered approximately 26 base pairs upstream of the start site of transcription. TFIIIB (Transcription Factor for polymerase III B), consists of three subunits: TBP (TATA Binding Protein), the Pol II transcription factor TFIIB-related protein, BRF1 (or Brf2 for transcription of a subset of Pol III-transcribed genes in vertebrates) and BDP1.
3. TFIIIB is the transcription factor that assembles Pol III at the start site of transcription. Once TFIIIB is bound to DNA, TFIIIC is no longer required. TFIIIB also plays an essential role in promoter opening.
4. TFIIIB remains bound to DNA following initiation of transcription by Pol III (unlike bacterial s factors and most of the basal transcription factors for Pol II transcription). This leads to a high rate of transcriptional reinitiation of Pol III-transcribed genes.

Class III

Typical stages in a U6 snRNA (also termed class III) gene initiation (documented in vertebrates only):

1. SNAPc (SNRNA Activating Protein complex) (also termed PBP and PTF) binds to the PSE (Proximal Sequence Element) centered approximately 55 base pairs upstream of the start site of transcription. This assembly is greatly stimulated by the Pol II transcription factors Oct1 and STAF that bind to an enhancer-like DSE (Distal Sequence Element) at least 200 base pairs upstream of the start site of transcription. These factors and promoter elements are shared between Pol II and Pol III transcription of snRNA genes.

2. SNAPc acts to assemble TFIIIB at a TATA box centered 26 base pairs upstream of the start site of transcription. It is the presence of a TATA box that specifies that the snRNA gene is transcribed by Pol III rather than Pol II.

3. The TFIIIB for U6 snRNA transcription contains a smaller Brf1 paralogue, Brf2.

4. TFIIIB is the transcription factor that assembles Pol III at the start site of transcription. Sequence conservation predicts that TFIIIB containing Brf2 also plays a role in promoter opening.

Termination

Polymerase III terminates transcription at small polyTs stretch (5–6). In Eukaryotes, a hairpin loop is not required, as it is in prokaryotes.

Transcribed RNAs

The types of RNAs transcribed from RNA polymerase III includes:

- Transfer RNAs.
- 5S ribosomal RNA.
- U6 spliceosomal RNA.
- RNase P and RNase MRP RNA.
- 7SL RNA (the RNA component of the signal recognition particle).
- Vault RNAs.
- Y RNA.
- SINEs (short interspersed repetitive elements).
- 7SK RNA.
- Several microRNAs.
- Several small nucleolar RNAs.
- Several gene regulatory antisense RNAs.

TRANSCRIPTION

Transcription is a process in which ribonucleic acid (RNA) is synthesised from DNA. The word gene refers to the functional unit of the DNA that can be transcribed. Thus, the genetic information stored in DNA is expressed through RNA. For this purpose, one of the two strands of DNA serves as a template (non-coding strand or sense strand) and produces working copies of RNA molecules.

The other DNA strand which does not participate in transcription is referred to as coding strand or antisense strand (frequently referred to as coding strand since with the exception of T for U, primary mRNA contains codons with the same base sequence). The entire molecule of DNA is not expressed in transcription. RNAs are synthesised only for some selected regions of DNA. For certain other regions of DNA, there may not be any transcription at all. The exact reason for the selective transcription is not known. This may be due to some in-built signals in the DNA molecule.

The product formed in transcription is referred to as primary transcript. Most often, the primary RNA transcripts are inactive. They undergo certain alterations (splicing, terminal additions, base modifications, etc.) commonly known as post-transcriptional modifications, to produce functionally active RNA molecules. There exist certain differences in the transcription between prokaryotes and eukaryotes. The RNA synthesis in prokaryotes is given in some detail. This is followed by a brief discussion on eukaryotic transcription.

Transcription in Prokaryotes

A single enzyme—DNA dependent RNA polymerase or simply RNA polymerase—synthesises all the RNAs in prokaryotes. RNA polymerase of *E. coli* is a complex holoenzyme (mol wt. 465 kDa) with five polypeptide sub-units—2α, 1β and $1\beta'$ and one sigma(s) factor (Fig. 12.4).

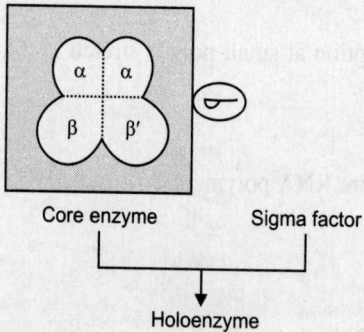

Fig. 12.4: RNA polymerase of *E. coli*.

The enzyme without sigma factor is referred to as core enzyme ($\alpha_2\beta\beta'$). An overview of transcription is shown in Fig. 12.5. Synthesis of RNA from DNA template (transcription) is shown in Fig. 12.6.

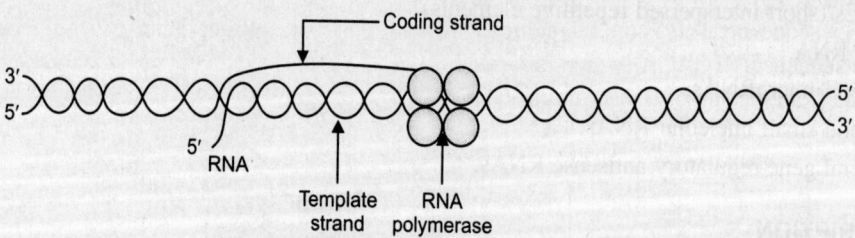

Fig. 12.5: An overview of transcription.

Initiation

The binding of the enzyme RNA polymerase to DNA is the pre-requisite for the transcription to start. The specific region on the DNA where the enzyme binds is known as promoter region.

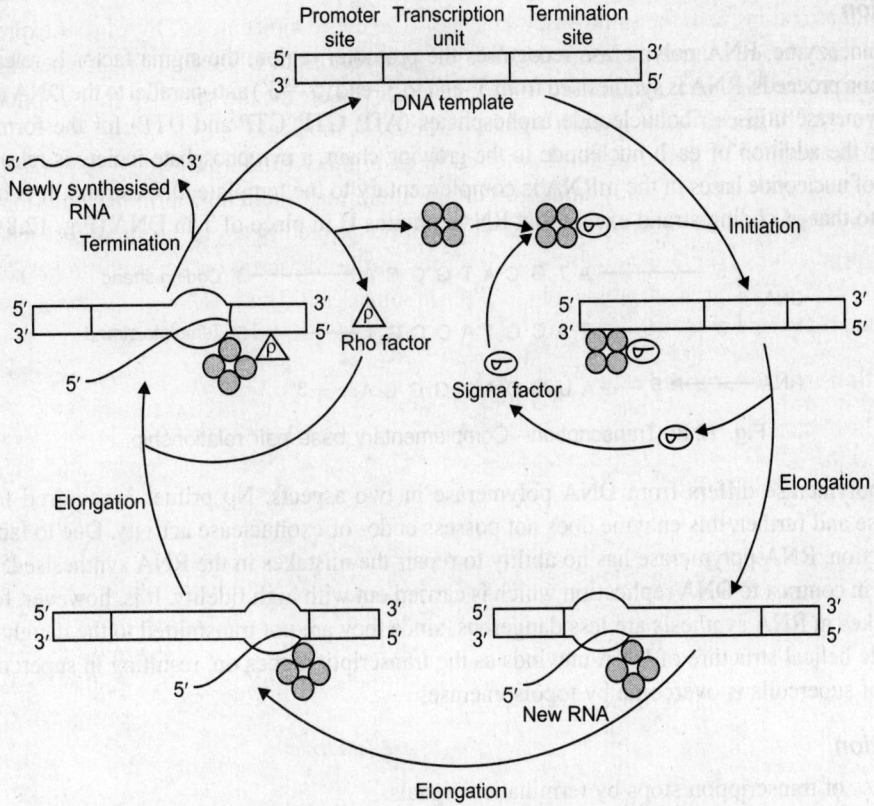

Fig. 12.6: Synthesis of RNA from DNA template (transcription).

There are two base sequences on the coding DNA strand which the sigma factor of RNA polymerase can recognise for initiation of transcription (Fig. 12.7).

1. Pribnow box (TATA box): This consists of 6 nucleotide bases (TATAAT), (Fig. 12.7) about 10 bases away (upstream) from the starting point of transcription.

2. The –35′ sequence: This is the second recognition site in the promoter region of DNA. It contains a base sequence TTGACA, which is located about 35 bases (upstream, hence –35′) away on the left side from the site of transcription start.

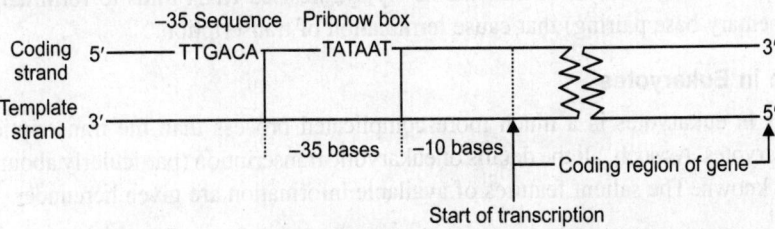

Fig. 12.7: Promoter regions of DNA in prokaryotes.

Elongation

As the holoenzyme, RNA polymerase recognises the promoter region, the sigma factor is released and transcription proceeds. RNA is synthesised from 5'-end to 3'-end (5'→3') anti-parallel to the DNA template. RNA polymerase utilises ribonucleotide triphosphates (ATP, GTP, CTP and UTP) for the formation of RNA. For the addition of each nucleotide to the growing chain, a pyrophosphate moiety is released. The sequence of nucleotide bases in the mRNA is complementary to the template DNA strand. It is however, identical to that of coding strand except that RNA contains U in place of T in DNA (Fig. 12.8).

```
         ┌ 5' ———————— A T G C A T G G C A ———— 3' Coding strand
   DNA ─┤
         └ 3' ———————— T A C G T A C C G T ———— 5' Template strand

   RNA ——————▶ 5' ········ A U G C A U G G C A ········ 3'
```

Fig. 12.8: Transcription—Complementary base pair relationship.

RNA polymerase differs from DNA polymerase in two aspects. No primer is required for RNA polymerase and further, this enzyme does not possess endo- or exonuclease activity. Due to lack of the latter function, RNA polymerase has no ability to repair the mistakes in the RNA synthesised.

This is in contrast to DNA replication which is carried out with high fidelity. It is, however, fortunate that mistakes in RNA synthesis are less dangerous, since they are not transmitted to the daughter cells. The double helical structure of DNA unwinds as the transcription goes on, resulting in supercoils. The problem of supercoils is overcome by topoisomerases.

Termination

The process of transcription stops by termination signals.

Two types of termination are identified:

1. Rho (ρ) dependent termination: A specific protein, named ρ factor, binds to the growing RNA (and not to RNA polymerase) or weakly to DNA and in the bound state it acts as ATPase and terminates transcription and releases RNA. The ρ factor is also responsible for the dissociation of RNA polymerase from DNA.

2. Rho (ρ) independent termination: The termination in this case is brought about by the formation of hairpins of newly synthesised RNA. This occurs due to the presence of palindromes. A palindrome is a word that reads alike forward and backward, e.g. madam, rotor. The presence of palindromes in the base sequence of DNA template (same when read in opposite direction) in the termination region is known. As a result of this, the newly synthesised RNA folds to form hairpins (due to complementary base pairing) that cause termination of transcription.

Transcription in Eukaryotes

RNA synthesis in eukaryotes is a much more complicated process than the transcription described above for prokaryotes. As such, all the details of eukaryotic transcription (particularly about termination) are not clearly known. The salient features of available information are given hereunder.

RNA polymerases

The nuclei of eukaryotic cells possess three distinct RNA polymerases (Fig. 12.9).

1. RNA polymerase I is responsible for the synthesis of precursors for the large ribosomal RNAs.

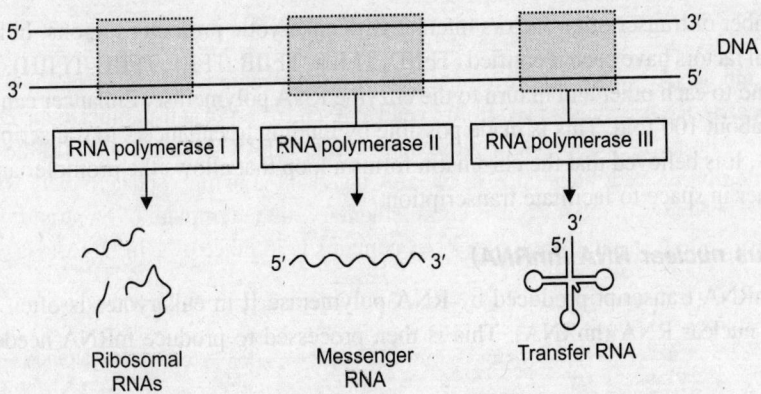

Fig. 12.9: An overview of transcription of eukaryotes.

2. RNA polymerase II synthesises the precursors for mRNAs and small nuclear RNAs.

3. RNA polymerase III participates in the formation of tRNAs and small ribosomal RNAs.

Besides the three RNA polymerases found in the nucleus, there also exists a mitochondrial RNA polymerase in eukaryotes. The latter resembles prokaryotic RNA polymerase in structure and function.

Promoter sites

In eukaryotes, a sequence of DNA bases—which is almost identical to pribnow box of prokaryotes is identified (Fig. 12.10). This sequence, known as Hogness box (or TATA box), is located about 25 nucleotides away (upstream) from the starting site of mRNA synthesis. There also exists another site of recognition between 70 and 80 nucleotides upstream from the start of transcription. This second site is referred to as CAAT box. One of these two sites (or sometimes both) helps RNA polymerase II to recognise the requisite sequence on DNA for transcription.

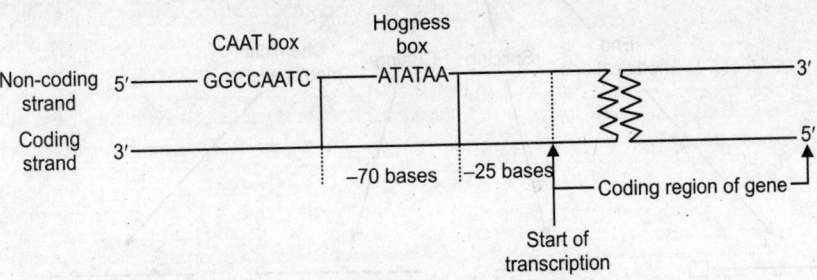

Fig. 12.10: Promoter regions of DNA in eukaryotes.

Initiation of transcription

The molecular events required for the initiation of transcription in eukaryotes are complex and broadly involve three stages:

1. Chromatin containing the promoter sequence made accessible to the transcription machinery.

2. Binding of transcription factors (TFs) to DNA sequences in the promoter region.

3. Stimulation of transcription by enhancers.

A large number of transcription factors interact with eukaryotic promoter regions. In humans, about six transcription factors have been identified (TFIID, TFIIA, TFIIB, TFIIF, TFIIE, TFIIH). It is postulated that the TFs bind to each other and in turn to the enzyme RNA polymerase. Enhancer can increase gene expression by about 100 fold. This is made possible by binding to enhancers to transcription factors to form activators. It is believed that the chromatin forms a loop that allows the promoter and enhancer to be close together in space to facilitate transcription.

Heterogeneous nuclear RNA (hnRNA)

The primary mRNA transcript produced by RNA polymerase II in eukaryotes is often referred to as heterogeneous nuclear RNA (hnRNA). This is then processed to produce mRNA needed for protein synthesis.

Post-Transcriptional Modifications

The RNAs produced during transcription are called primary transcripts. They undergo many alterations— terminal base additions, base modifications, splicing, etc. which are collectively referred to as post-transcriptional modifications. This process is required to convert the RNAs into the active forms. A group of enzymes, namely ribonucleases, are responsible for the processing of tRNAs and rRNAs of both prokaryotes and eukaryotes. The prokaryotic mRNA synthesised in transcription is almost similar to the functional mRNA. In contrast, eukaryotic mRNA (i.e. hnRNA) undergoes extensive post-transcriptional changes. An outline of the post-transcriptional modifications is given in Fig. 12.11 and some highlights are described.

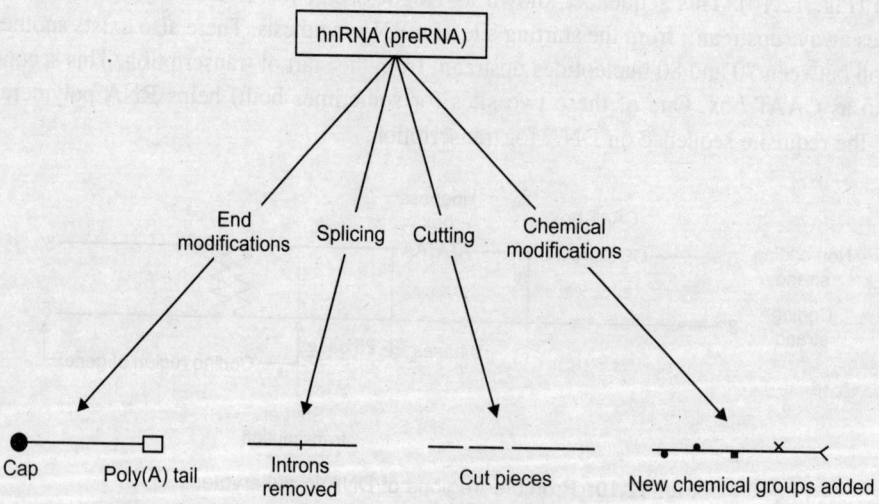

Fig. 12.11: An outline of post-transcriptional modifications of RNA (hnRNA—heterogeneous nuclear RNA).

RNA POLYMERASE

RNA polymerase (ribonucleic acid polymerase), both abbreviated RNAP or RNApol, official name DNA-directed RNA polymerase, is a member of a family of enzymes that are essential to life: they are found in all living organisms and many viruses. RNAP locally opens the double-stranded DNA (usually about four turns of the double helix) so that one strand of the exposed nucleotides can be used as a template for the synthesis of RNA, a process called transcription. A transcription factor and its associated transcription mediator complex must be attached to a DNA binding site called a promoter region before RNAP can initiate the DNA unwinding at that position. RNAP has intrinsic helicase activity, therefore no separate enzyme is needed to unwind the DNA (in contrast to DNA polymerase). RNAP not only initiates RNA transcription, it also guides the nucleotides into position, facilitates attachment and elongation, has intrinsic proofreading and replacement capabilities, and termination recognition capability. In eukaryotes, RNAP can build chains as long as 2.4 million nucleotides.

RNAP produces RNA that functionally is either coding (for protein) (messenger RNA) (mRNA), or non-coding: so-called 'RNA genes'.

At least four functional types of RNA genes exist:

1. Transfer RNA (tRNA): Transfers specific amino acids to growing polypeptide chains at the ribosomal site of protein synthesis during translation.

2. Ribosomal RNA (rRNA): Incorporates into ribosomes.

3. Micro RNA (miRNA): Regulates gene activity.

4. Catalytic RNA (ribozyme): Functions as an enzymatically active RNA molecule.

Eukaryotes have multiple types of nuclear RNAP, each responsible for synthesis of a distinct subset of RNA. All are structurally and mechanistically related to each other and to bacterial RNAP. RNA polymerase I synthesises a pre-rRNA 45S (35S in yeast), which matures and will form the major RNA sections of the ribosome. RNA polymerase II synthesises precursors of mRNAs and most snRNA and microRNAs. RNA polymerase III synthesises tRNAs, rRNA 5S and other small RNAs found in the nucleus and cytosol. RNA polymerase IV synthesises siRNA in plants. RNA polymerase V synthesises RNAs involved in siRNA-directed heterochromatin formation in plants.

Eukaryotic chloroplasts contain an RNAP very highly structurally and mechanistically similar to bacterial RNAP ('plastid-encoded polymerase'). They also contain a second, structurally and mechanistically unrelated, RNAP ('nucleus-encoded polymerase', member of the 'single-subunit RNAP' protein family). Eukaryotic mitochondria contain a structurally and mechanistically unrelated RNAP (member of the 'single-subunit RNAP' protein family).

Given that DNA and RNA polymerases both carry out template-dependent nucleotide polymerisation, it might be expected that the two types of enzymes would be structurally related, but they are not. They seem to have arisen independently twice during the early evolution of cells: one lineage led to the modern DNA polymerases and reverse transcriptases, as well as to a few single-subunit RNA polymerases from viruses, the other lineage formed all of the modern cellular RNA polymerases.

Structure

The 2006 Nobel Prize in Chemistry was awarded to Roger D. Kornberg for creating detailed molecular images of RNA polymerase during various stages of the transcription process. In most prokaryotes, a single RNA polymerase species transcribes all types of RNA. RNA polymerase from *E. coli* consists of five different subunit types. The beta (β) subunit has a molecular weight of 150,000, beta prime (β') 160,000, alpha (α) 40,000, and sigma (σ) 70,000. The σ subunit can dissociate from the rest of the complex, leaving the core enzyme. The complete enzyme with σ is termed the RNA polymerase holoenzyme and is necessary for correct initiation of transcription, whereas the core enzyme can continue transcription after initiation. All RNAPs contain metal cofactors, in particular zinc and magnesium cations which aid in the transcription process.

Function of RNAP

Control of the process of gene transcription affects patterns of gene expression and, thereby, allows a cell to adapt to a changing environment, perform specialised roles within an organism, and maintain basic metabolic processes necessary for survival. Therefore, it is hardly surprising that the activity of RNAP is long, complex, and highly regulated. In *Escherichia coli* bacteria, more than 100 transcription factors have been identified, which modify the activity of RNAP.

RNAP can initiate transcription at specific DNA sequences known as promoters. It then produces an RNA chain, which is complementary to the template DNA strand. The process of adding nucleotides to the RNA strand is known as elongation, in eukaryotes, RNAP can build chains as long as 2.4 million nucleotides (the full length of the dystrophin gene). RNAP will preferentially release its RNA transcript at specific DNA sequences encoded at the end of genes, which are known as terminators.

Products of RNAP include:

1. Messenger RNA (mRNA)—template for the synthesis of proteins by ribosomes.
2. Non-coding RNA or 'RNA genes'—a broad class of genes that encode RNA that is not translated into protein. The most prominent examples of RNA genes are transfer RNA (tRNA) and ribosomal RNA (rRNA), both of which are involved in the process of translation. However, since the late 1990s, many new RNA genes have been found, and thus RNA genes may play a much more significant role than previously thought.
    (a) Transfer RNA (tRNA)—transfers specific amino acids to growing polypeptide chains at the ribosomal site of protein synthesis during translation.
    (b) Ribosomal RNA (rRNA)—a component of ribosomes.
    (c) Micro RNA—regulates gene activity.
    (d) Catalytic RNA (Ribozyme)—enzymatically active RNA molecules

RNAP accomplishes *de novo* synthesis. It is able to do this because specific interactions with the initiating nucleotide hold RNAP rigidly in place, facilitating chemical attack on the incoming nucleotide. Such specific interactions explain why RNAP prefers to start transcripts with ATP (followed by GTP, UTP, and then CTP). In contrast to DNA polymerase, RNAP includes helicase activity, therefore no separate enzyme is needed to unwind DNA.

RNA Polymerase Binding

RNA polymerase binding in bacteria involves the sigma factor recognising the core promoter region containing the -35 and -10 elements (located before the beginning of sequence to be transcribed) and also, at some promoters, the a subunit C-terminal domain recognising promoter upstream elements. There are multiple interchangeable sigma factors, each of which recognises a distinct set of promoters. For example, in *E. coli*, s70 is expressed under normal conditions and recognises promoters for genes required under normal conditions (housekeeping genes), while s32 recognises promoters for genes required at high temperatures (heat-shock genes).

After binding to the DNA, the RNA polymerase switches from a closed complex to an open complex. This change involves the separation of the DNA strands to form an unwound section of DNA of approximately 13 bp, referred to as the transcription bubble. Ribonucleotides are base-paired to the template DNA strand, according to Watson-Crick base-pairing interactions. Supercoiling plays an important part in polymerase activity because of the unwinding and rewinding of DNA. Because regions of DNA in front of RNAP are unwound, there are compensatory positive supercoils. Regions behind

RNAP are rewound and negative supercoils are present. As noted above, RNA polymerase makes contacts with the promoter region. However these stabilising contacts inhibit the enzymes ability to access DNA further downstream and thus the synthesis of the full-length product. Once the open complex is stabilised, RNA polymerase synthesises an RNA strand to establish a DNA-RNA heteroduplex (~8–9 bp) at the active center, which stabilises the elongation complex. In order to accomplish RNA synthesis, RNA polymerase must maintain promoter contacts while unwinding more downstream DNA for synthesis, 'scrunching' more downstream DNA into the initiation complex. During the promoter escape transition, RNA polymerase is considered a 'stressed intermediate.'

Thermodynamically the stress accumulates from the DNA-unwinding and DNA-compaction activities. Once the DNA-RNA heteroduplex is long enough, RNA polymerase releases its upstream contacts and effectively achieves the promoter escape transition into the elongation phase. However, promoter escape is not the only outcome. RNA polymerase can also relieve the stress by releasing its downstream contacts, arresting transcription.

The paused transcribing complex has two options: (i) release the nascent transcript and begin anew at the promoter or (ii) reestablish a new 3'OH on the nascent transcript at the active site via RNA polymerases catalytic activity and recommence DNA scrunching to achieve promoter escape. Scientists have coined the term 'abortive initiation' to explain the unproductive cycling of RNA polymerase before the promoter escape transition. The extent of abortive initiation depends on the presence of transcription factors and the strength of the promoter contacts.

Elongation

Transcription elongation involves the further addition of ribonucleotides and the change of the open complex to the transcriptional complex. RNAP cannot start forming full length transcripts because of its strong binding to the promoter. Transcription at this stage primarily results in short RNA fragments of around 9 bp in a process known as abortive transcription. Once the RNAP starts forming longer transcripts it clears the promoter. At this point, the contacts with the -10 and -35 elements are disrupted, and the s factor falls off RNAP. This allows the rest of the RNAP complex to move forward, as the s factor held the RNAP complex in place.

The 17-bp transcriptional complex has an 8-bp DNA-RNA hybrid, that is, 8 base-pairs involve the RNA transcript bound to the DNA template strand. As transcription progresses, ribonucleotides are added to the 3' end of the RNA transcript and the RNAP complex moves along the DNA. Aspartyl (asp) residues in the RNAP will hold on to Mg^{2+} ions, which will, in turn, coordinate the phosphates of the ribonucleotides. The first Mg^{2+} will hold on to the α-phosphate of the NTP to be added. This allows the nucleophilic attack of the 3'OH from the RNA transcript, adding another NTP to the chain. The second Mg^{2+} will hold on to the pyrophosphate of the NTP. The overall reaction equation is:

$$(NMP)_n + NTP \rightarrow (NMP)_{n+1} + PP_i$$

Fidelity

Unlike the proofreading mechanisms of DNA polymerase those of the RNA variety have only recently been investigated. Proofreading begins with separation of the mis-incorporated nucleotide from the DNA template. This pauses transcription. The polymerase then backtracks by one position and cleaves the dinucleotide that contains the mismatched nucleotide. In the RNA polymerase this occurs at the same active site used for polymerisation and is therefore markedly different from the DNA polymerase where proofreading occurs at a distinct nuclease active site.

Termination

In prokaryotes, termination of RNA transcription can be rho-independent or rho-dependent: Rho-independent transcription termination is the termination of transcription without the aid of the rho protein. Transcription of a palindromic region of DNA causes the formation of a 'hairpin' structure from the RNA transcription looping and binding upon itself. This hairpin structure is often rich in G-C base-pairs, making it more stable than the DNA-RNA hybrid itself. As a result, the 8 bp DNA-RNA hybrid in the transcription complex shifts to a 4 bp hybrid. These last 4 base pairs are weak A-U base pairs, and the entire RNA transcript will fall off the DNA.

Other Organisms

Bacteria

In bacteria, the same enzyme catalyses the synthesis of mRNA and non-coding RNA (ncRNA).

RNAP is a large molecule. The core enzyme has five subunits (~400 kDa):

- β': The β' subunit is the largest subunit, and is encoded by the rpoC gene. The β' subunit contains part of the active center responsible for RNA synthesis and contains some of the determinants for non-sequence-specific interactions with DNA and nascent RNA.

- β: The β subunit is the second-largest subunit, and is encoded by the rpoB gene. The β subunit contains the rest of the active center responsible for RNA synthesis and contains the rest of the determinants for non-sequence-specific interactions with DNA and nascent RNA.

- α: The α subunit is the third-largest subunit and is present in two copies per molecule of RNAP, α^I and α^{II}. Each α subunit contains two domains: αNTD (*N*-Terminal domain) and αCTD (C-terminal domain). αNTD contains determinants for assembly of RNAP. αCTD (C-terminal domain) contains determinants for interaction with promoter DNA, making non-sequence-non-specific interactions at most promoters and sequence-specific interactions at upstream-element-containing promoters, and contains determinants for interactions with regulatory factors.

- The ω subunit is the smallest subunit. The ω subunit facilitates assembly of RNAP and stabilises assembled RNAP.

In order to bind promoters, RNAP core associates with the transcription initiation factor sigma (σ) to form RNA polymerase holoenzyme. Sigma reduces the affinity of RNAP for nonspecific DNA while increasing specificity for promoters, allowing transcription to initiate at correct sites. The complete holoenzyme therefore has 6 subunits: $\beta'\beta\alpha^I$ and $\alpha^{II}\omega\sigma$ (~450 kDa).

Eukaryotes

Eukaryotes have multiple types of nuclear RNAP, each responsible for synthesis of a distinct subset of RNA. All are structurally and mechanistically related to each other and to bacterial RNAP:

- RNA polymerase I synthesises a pre-rRNA 45S (35S in yeast), which matures into 28S, 18S and 5.8S rRNAs which will form the major RNA sections of the ribosome.

- RNA polymerase II synthesises precursors of mRNAs and most snRNA and microRNAs. This is the most studied type, and, due to the high level of control required over transcription, a range of transcription factors are required for its binding to promoters.

- RNA polymerase III synthesises tRNAs, rRNA 5S and other small RNAs found in the nucleus and cytosol.

- RNA polymerase IV synthesises siRNA in plants.
- RNA polymerase V synthesises RNAs involved in siRNA-directed heterochromatin formation in plants.

Eukaryotic chloroplasts contain an RNAP very highly structurally and mechanistically similar to bacterial RNAP (plastid-encoded polymerase). Eukaryotic chloroplasts also contain a second, structurally and mechanistically unrelated, RNAP (nucleus-encoded polymerase, member of the 'single-subunit RNAP' protein family). Eukaryotic mitochondria contain a structurally and mechanistically unrelated RNAP (member of the 'single-subunit RNAP' protein family).

Given that DNA and RNA polymerases both carry out template-dependent nucleotide polymerisation, it might be expected that the two types of enzymes would be structurally related. However, X-ray crystallographic studies of both types of enzymes reveal that, other than containing a critical Mg^{2+} ion at the catalytic site, they are virtually unrelated to each other, indeed template-dependent nucleotide polymerising enzymes seem to have arisen independently twice during the early evolution of cells. One lineage led to the modern DNA Polymerases and reverse transcriptases, as well as to a few single-subunit RNA polymerases from viruses. The other lineage formed all of the modern cellular RNA polymerases.

Archaea

Archaea have a single type of RNAP, responsible for the synthesis of all RNA. *Archaeal* RNAP is structurally and mechanistically similar to bacterial RNAP and eukaryotic nuclear RNAP I-V, and is especially closely structurally and mechanistically related to eukaryotic nuclear RNAP II. The history of the discovery of the archaeal RNA polymerase is quite recent. The first analysis of the RNAP of an archaeon was performed in 1971, when the RNAP from the extreme halophile Halobacterium cutirubrum was isolated and purified. Crystal structures of RNAPs from Sulfolobus solfataricus and Sulfolobus shibatae set the total number of identified archaeal subunits at thirteen.

Viruses

Orthopoxviruses synthesise RNA using a virally encoded RNAP that is structurally and mechanistically related to bacterial RNAP, archaeal RNAP, and eukaryotic nuclear RNAP I-V. Most other viruses that synthesise RNA using a virally encoded RNAP use an RNAP that is not structurally and mechanistically related to bacterial RNAP, archaeal RNAP, and eukaryotic nuclear RNAP I-V. Many viruses use a single-subunit DNA-dependent RNAP that is structurally and mechanistically related to the single-subunit RNAP of eukaryotic chloroplasts and mitochondria and, more distantly, to DNA polymerases and reverse transcriptases. Perhaps the most widely studied such single-subunit RNAP is bacteriophage T7 RNA polymerase. Other viruses use a RNA-dependent RNAP (an RNAP that employs RNA as a template instead of DNA). This occurs in negative strand RNA viruses and dsRNA viruses, both of which exist for a portion of their life cycle as double-stranded RNA. However, some positive strand RNA viruses, such as poliovirus, also contain RNA-dependent RNAP.

Purification of RNA polymerase

RNA polymerase can be isolated in the following ways:

- By a phosphocellulose column.
- By glycerol gradient centrifugation.
- By a DNA column.
- By an ion chromatography column.

Chapter 13

Chromatin and Epigenetics

INTRODUCTION

Epigenetics refers to heritable changes in gene expression that occur without alteration in DNA sequence. These changes may be induced spontaneously, induced by environmental factors or as a consequence of specific mutations.

There are two primary and interconnected epigenetic mechanisms: DNA methylation and covalent modification of histones. In addition, it has become apparent in the last years that non-coding RNA is also intimately involved in this process.

MECHANISMS OF EPIGENETIC

Several types of epigenetic inheritance systems may play a role in what has become known as cell memory, note however that not all of these are universally accepted to be examples of epigenetics.

The different mechanisms that control epigenetic changes do not stand alone, and there is a clear interconnection and interdependency between:

1. DNA methylation
2. Histone modification and incorporation of histone variants
3. Non-coding RNA-mediated epigenetic regulation.

Covalent Modifications

Covalent modifications of either DNA (e.g. cytosine methylation and hydroxymethylation) or of histone proteins (e.g. lysine acetylation, lysine and arginine methylation, serine and threonine phosphorylation, and lysine ubiquitination and sumoylation) play central roles in many types of epigenetic inheritance. Therefore, the word 'epigenetics' is sometimes used as a synonym for these processes. However, this can be misleading. Chromatin remodelling is not always inherited, and not all epigenetic inheritance involves chromatin remodelling. Because the phenotype of a cell or individual is affected by which of its genes are transcribed, heritable transcription states can give rise to epigenetic effects. There are several layers of regulation of gene expression. One way that genes are regulated is through the remodelling of chromatin. Chromatin is the complex of DNA and the histone proteins with which it associates. If the way that DNA is wrapped around the histones changes, gene expression can change as well. Chromatin remodelling is accomplished through two main mechanisms:

1. The first way is post translational modification of the amino acids that make up histone proteins. Histone proteins are made up of long chains of amino acids. If the amino acids that are in the chain are changed, the shape of the histone might be modified. DNA is not completely unwound during replication. It is possible, then, that the modified histones may be carried into each new copy of the DNA. Once there, these histones may act as templates, initiating the surrounding new histones to be shaped in the new manner. By altering the shape of the histones around them, these modified histones would ensure that a lineage-specific transcription programme is maintained after cell division.

2. The second way is the addition of methyl groups to the DNA, mostly at CpG sites, to convert cytosine to 5-methylcytosine. 5-Methylcytosine performs much like a regular cytosine, pairing with a guanine in double-stranded DNA. However, some areas of the genome are methylated more heavily than others, and highly methylated areas tend to be less transcriptionally active, through a mechanism not fully understood. Methylation of cytosines can also persist from the germ line of one of the parents into the zygote, marking the chromosome as being inherited from one parent or the other (genetic imprinting).

Mechanisms of heritability of histone state are not well understood, however, much is known about the mechanism of heritability of DNA methylation state during cell division and differentiation. Heritability of methylation state depends on certain enzymes (such as DNMT1) that have a higher affinity for 5-methylcytosine than for cytosine. If this enzyme reaches a 'hemimethylated' portion of DNA (where 5-methylcytosine is in only one of the two DNA strands) the enzyme will methylate the other half. Although histone modifications occur throughout the entire sequence, the unstructured N-termini of histones (called histone tails) are particularly highly modified. These modifications include acetylation, methylation, ubiquitylation, phosphorylation, sumoylation, ribosylation and citrullination. Acetylation is the most highly studied of these modifications. For example, acetylation of the K14 and K9 lysines of the tail of histone H3 by histone acetyltransferase enzymes (HATs) is generally related to transcriptional competence.

One mode of thinking is that this tendency of acetylation to be associated with 'active' transcription is biophysical in nature. Because it normally has a positively charged nitrogen at its end, lysine can bind the negatively charged phosphates of the DNA backbone. The acetylation event converts the positively charged amine group on the side chain into a neutral amide linkage. This removes the positive charge, thus loosening the DNA from the histone. When this occurs, complexes like SWI/SNF and other transcriptional factors can bind to the DNA and allow transcription to occur. This is the 'cis' model of epigenetic function. In other words, changes to the histone tails have a direct effect on the DNA itself.

Another model of epigenetic function is the 'trans' model. In this model, changes to the histone tails act indirectly on the DNA. For example, lysine acetylation may create a binding site for chromatin-modifying enzymes (or transcription machinery as well). This chromatin remodeler can then cause changes to the state of the chromatin. Indeed, a bromodomain – a protein domain that specifically binds acetyl-lysine – is found in many enzymes that help activate transcription, including the SWI/SNF complex. It may be that acetylation acts in this and the previous way to aid in transcriptional activation.

The idea that modifications act as docking modules for related factors is borne out by histone methylation as well. Methylation of lysine 9 of histone H3 has long been associated with constitutively transcriptionally silent chromatin (constitutive heterochromatin). It has been determined that a chromodomain (a domain that specifically binds methyl-lysine) in the transcriptionally repressive protein

HP1 recruits HP1 to K9 methylated regions. One example that seems to refute this biophysical model for methylation is that tri-methylation of histone H3 at lysine 4 is strongly associated with (and required for full) transcriptional activation. Tri-methylation in this case would introduce a fixed positive charge on the tail. It has been shown that the histone lysine methyltransferase (KMT) is responsible for this methylation activity in the pattern of histones H3 and H4. This enzyme utilises a catalytically active site called the SET domain (Suppressor of variegation, Enhancer of zeste, Trithorax). The SET domain is a 130-amino acid sequence involved in modulating gene activities. This domain has been demonstrated to bind to the histone tail and causes the methylation of the histone. Differing histone modifications are likely to function in differing ways, acetylation at one position is likely to function differently from acetylation at another position. Also, multiple modifications may occur at the same time, and these modifications may work together to change the behaviour of the nucleosome. The idea that multiple dynamic modifications regulate gene transcription in a systematic and reproducible way is called the histone code, although the idea that histone state can be read linearly as a digital information carrier has been largely debunked. One of the best-understood systems that orchestrates chromatin-based silencing is the SIR protein based silencing of the yeast hidden mating type loci HML and HMR.

DNA methylation frequently occurs in repeated sequences, and helps to suppress the expression and mobility of 'transposable elements': Because 5-methylcytosine can be spontaneously deaminated (replacing nitrogen by oxygen) to thymidine, CpG sites are frequently mutated and become rare in the genome, except at CpG islands where they remain unmethylated. Epigenetic changes of this type thus have the potential to direct increased frequencies of permanent genetic mutation. DNA methylation patterns are known to be established and modified in response to environmental factors by a complex interplay of at least three independent DNA methyltransferases, DNMT1, DNMT3A, and DNMT3B, the loss of any of which is lethal in mice. DNMT1 is the most abundant methyltransferase in somatic cells, localises to replication foci, has a 10–40-fold preference for hemimethylated DNA and interacts with the proliferating cell nuclear antigen (PCNA). By preferentially modifying hemimethylated DNA, DNMT1 transfers patterns of methylation to a newly synthesised strand after DNA replication, and therefore is often referred to as the 'maintenance' methyltransferase. DNMT1 is essential for proper embryonic development, imprinting and X-inactivation. To emphasise the difference of this molecular mechanism of inheritance from the canonical Watson-Crick base-pairing mechanism of transmission of genetic information, the term 'Epigenetic templating' was introduced. Furthermore, in addition to the maintenance and transmission of methylated DNA states, the same principle could work in the maintenance and transmission of histone modifications and even cytoplasmic (structural) heritable states.

Histones H3 and H4 can also be manipulated through demethylation using histone lysine demethylase (KDM). This recently identified enzyme has a catalytically active site called the Jumonji domain (JmjC). The demethylation occurs when JmjC utilises multiple cofactors to hydroxylate the methyl group, thereby removing it. JmjC is capable of demethylating mono-, di-, and tri-methylated substrates.

Chromosomal regions can adopt stable and heritable alternative states resulting in bistable gene expression without changes to the DNA sequence. Epigenetic control is often associated with alternative covalent modifications of histones. The stability and heritability of states of larger chromosomal regions are suggested to involve positive feedback where modified nucleosomes recruit enzymes that similarly modify nearby nucleosomes. A simplified stochastic model for this type of epigenetics is found here.

It has been suggested that chromatin-based transcriptional regulation could be mediated by the effect of small RNAs. Small interfering RNAs can modulate transcriptional gene expression via epigenetic modulation of targeted promoters.

RNA transcripts

Sometimes a gene, after being turned on, transcribes a product that (directly or indirectly) maintains the activity of that gene. For example, Hnf4 and MyoD enhance the transcription of many liver- and muscle-specific genes, respectively, including their own, through the transcription factor activity of the proteins they encode. RNA signalling includes differential recruitment of a hierarchy of generic chromatin modifying complexes and DNA methyltransferases to specific loci by RNAs during differentiation and development.

MicroRNAs

MicroRNAs (miRNAs) are members of non-coding RNAs that range in size from 17 to 25 nucleotides. miRNAs regulate a large variety of biological functions in plants and animals. So far, in 2013, about 2000 miRNAs have been discovered in humans and these can be found online in a miRNA database. Each miRNA expressed in a cell may target about 100 to 200 messenger RNAs that it down regulates. Most of the down regulation of mRNAs occurs by causing the decay of the targeted mRNA, while some down regulation occurs at the level of translation into protein.

Prions

Prions are infectious forms of proteins. In general, proteins fold into discrete units that perform distinct cellular functions, but some proteins are also capable of forming an infectious conformational state known as a prion. Although often viewed in the context of infectious disease, prions are more loosely defined by their ability to catalytically convert other native state versions of the same protein to an infectious conformational state. It is in this latter sense that they can be viewed as epigenetic agents capable of inducing a phenotypic change without a modification of the genome.

FUNCTIONS AND CONSEQUENCES OF EPIGENETIC

Developmental epigenetics can be divided into predetermined and probabilistic epigenesis. Predetermined epigenesis is a unidirectional movement from structural development in DNA to the functional maturation of the protein. 'Predetermined' here means that development is scripted and predictable. Probabilistic epigenesis on the other hand is a bidirectional structure-function development with experiences and external molding development. Somatic epigenetic inheritance, particularly through DNA and histone covalent modifications and nucleosome repositioning, is very important in the development of multicellular eukaryotic organisms. The genome sequence is static (with some notable exceptions), but cells differentiate into many different types, which perform different functions, and respond differently to the environment and intercellular signalling.

Thus, as individuals develop, morphogens activate or silence genes in an epigenetically heritable fashion, giving cells a memory. In mammals, most cells terminally differentiate, with only stem cells retaining the ability to differentiate into several cell types ('totipotency' and 'multi-potency'). In mammals, some stem cells continue producing new differentiated cells throughout life, such as in neurogenesis, but mammals are not able to respond to loss of some tissues, for example, the inability to regenerate limbs, which some other animals are capable of. Epigenetic modifications regulate the transition from neural stem cells to glial progenitor cells (for example, differentiation into oligodendrocytes is regulated by the deacetylation and methylation of histones. Unlike animals, plant cells do not terminally differentiate, remaining totipotent with the ability to give rise to a new individual plant. While plants do utilise many of the same epigenetic mechanisms as animals, such as chromatin remodelling, it has been hypothesised that some kinds of plant cells do not use or require 'cellular memories', resetting their gene expression patterns using positional information from the environment and surrounding cells to determine their fate. Epigenetic changes can occur in response to environmental exposure – for example, mice given some dietary supplements have epigenetic changes affecting expression of the agouti gene, which affects their fur colour, weight, and propensity to develop cancer. Controversial results from one study suggested that traumatic experiences might produce an epigenetic signal that is capable of being passed to future generations. Mice were trained, using foot shocks, to fear a cherry blossom odour. The investigators reported that the mouse offspring had an increased aversion to this specific odour. They suggested epigenetic changes that increase gene expression, rather than in DNA itself, in a gene, M71, that governs the functioning of an odour receptor in the nose that responds specifically to this cherry blossom smell. There were physical changes that correlated with olfactory (smell) function in the brains of the trained mice and their descendants.

Several criticisms were reported, including the studys low statistical power as evidence of some irregularity such as bias in reporting results. Due to limits of sample size, there is a probability that an effect will not be demonstrated to within statistical significance even if it exists. The criticism suggested that the probability that all the experiments reported would show positive results if an identical protocol was followed, assuming the claimed effects exist, is merely 0.4%. The researchers also did not indicate which mice were siblings, and treated all of the mice as statistically independent. The original researchers pointed out negative results in the papers appendix that the criticism omitted in its calculations, and undertook to track which mice were siblings in the future.

Transgenerational

Epigenetic mechanisms were a necessary part of the evolutionary origin of cell differentiation. Although epigenetics in multicellular organisms is generally thought to be a mechanism involved in differentiation, with epigenetic patterns 'reset' when organisms reproduce, there have been some observations of transgenerational epigenetic inheritance (e.g. the phenomenon of paramutation observed in maize). Although most of these multigenerational epigenetic traits are gradually lost over several generations, the possibility remains that multigenerational epigenetics could be another aspect to evolution and adaptation. As mentioned above, some define epigenetics as heritable.

EPIGENETICS IN BACTERIA

While epigenetics is of fundamental importance in eukaryotes, especially metazoans, it plays a different role in bacteria. Most importantly, eukaryotes use epigenetic mechanisms primarily to regulate gene expression which bacteria rarely do. However, bacteria make widespread use of postreplicative DNA methylation for the epigenetic control of DNA-protein interactions. Bacteria also use DNA adenine methylation (rather than DNA cytosine methylation) as an epigenetic signal. DNA adenine methylation is important in bacteria virulence in organisms such as *Escherichia coli*, *Salmonella*, *Vibrio*, *Yersinia* (Fig. 13.1), *Haemophilus* (Fig. 13.2), and *Brucella* (Fig. 13.3). In Alphaproteobacteria, methylation of adenine regulates the cell cycle and couples gene transcription to DNA replication. In Gammaproteobacteria, adenine methylation provides signals for DNA replication, chromosome segregation, mismatch repair, packaging of bacteriophage, transposase activity and regulation of gene expression. There exists a genetic switch controlling *Streptococcus pneumoniae* (the *pneumococcus*) that allows the bacterium to randomly change its characteristics into six alternative states that could pave the way to improved vaccines. Each form is randomly generated by a phase variable methylation system.

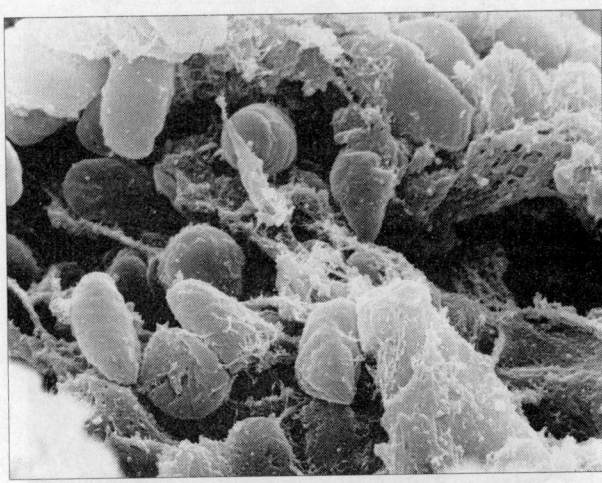

Fig. 13.1: *Yersinia.*

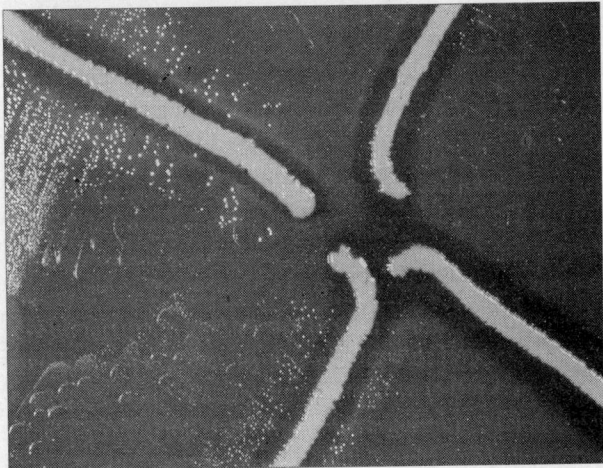

Fig. 13.2: *Haemophilus.*

The ability of the *pneumococcus* to cause deadly infections is different in each of these six states. Similar systems exist in other bacterial genera.

EPIGENETICS IN MEDICINE

Epigenetics has many and varied potential medical applications. In 2008, the National Institutes of Health announced that $190 million had been earmarked for epigenetics research over the next five years. In announcing the funding, government officials noted that epigenetics has the potential to explain mechanisms of ageing, human development, and the origins of cancer, heart disease, mental illness, as well as several other conditions. Some investigators, like Randy Jirtle, PhD, of Duke University Medical Center, think epigenetics may ultimately turn out to have a greater role in disease than genetics.

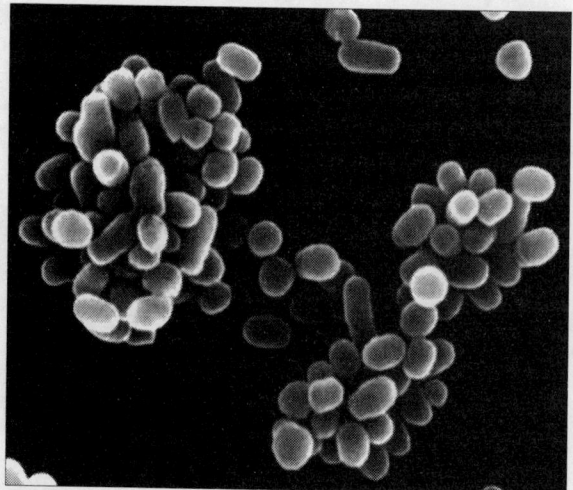

Fig. 13.3: *Brucella.*

TRANSCRIPTION FACTORS

These mechanisms, together with action of transcription factors and ATP-dependent chromatin remodelling, will establish unique epigenetic states resulting in alterations of gene expression that for example can determine cellular diversity with virtually no differences in DNA sequences.

Epigenetic modifications are central to many cellular processes and essential to many organism functions, such as imprinting, X chromosome inactivation, cellular reprogramming and senescence. But if these modifications occur improperly, they can lead to major adverse health effects such as cancer or congenital diseases. Because of their role in cancer development, epigenetic modifications offer promise as potential novel biomarkers for early cancer detection and prognosis. Furthermore, the possibility of reversing epigenetic modifications represents a potential target of novel therapeutic strategies and medication design.

DNA METHYLATION

DNA methylation, the addition of a methyl- group to one of the bases in the deoxyribonucleic acid chain, does not change the primary DNA sequence and it is therefore considered to be an epigenetic modification. DNA methylation is generally repressive to transcription, therefore constituting an important mechanism for gene silencing in embryonic development and inactivation of defined tumour suppressor genes in human cancers. Although cytosine methylation is the most studied modification, adenine has been found to be methylated in prokaryotes and plants. In prokaryotes, DNA methylation is involved in processes such as determination of DNA host specificity, virulence, cell cycle regulation and gene expression. In higher eukaryotes, DNA methylation is involved in the regulation of several cellular processes such as chromatin stability, imprinting, X chromosome inactivation and carcinogenesis.

In mammals, DNA methylation occurs mainly on the fifth carbon of the cytosine base, forming what is known as 5-methylcytosine or 5-methylcytidine (5-mC), and it is almost exclusively found at CpG dinucleotides. 5-mC is a potent epigenetic marker and regulator of gene expression. Methylated CpG clusters – named CpG islands – at gene promoters have been associated with gene inactivation. DNA methylation is catalysed by a family of enzymes called DNA methyltransferase and includes DNMT1,

DNMT3a and DNMT3b. DNMT3a and DNMT3b are known as *de novo* methyltransferases and they are able to methylate previously unmethylated CpG dinucleotides. In contrast, DNMT1, is known as a maintenance methyltransferase, and it methylates hemi-methylated DNA during replication. The reverse reaction - DNA demethylation – is only beginning to be elucidated. It is believed to involve the successive oxidation of 5-mC to 5-hydroxymethyl- (5-hmC), 5-formyl- (5-fC), and 5-carboxy- (5-caC) cytosine in a process that involves the Tet family of enzymes. A glycosylase of the BER (Base Excision Repair) pathway, TDG, was also recently involved in an alternative demethylation pathway, where it can repair the 5-hydroxymethyluracil which can result from deamination of 5-hmC.

Currently, the main approaches to study DNA methylation are:

- Sodium bisulphite modification.
- Sequence-specific enzyme digestion.
- Capture/quantification of methylated DNA.

Sodium Bisulphite Modification

Sodium bisulphite modification, also known as bisulphite conversion, is one of the most useful tools for analysing cytosine methylation. This method is based on treating DNA with sodium bisulphite in order to determine its methylation pattern.

Treatment of DNA with sodium bisulphite leads to the deamination of cytosine residues and converts them to uracil, while 5-mC residues remain the same. The treatment will generate specific changes in the DNA sequence that will depend on the methylation status of individual cytosine residues, potentially providing single-nucleotide resolution information about the methylation status of a DNA region: cytosine residues that have been converted to uracil will be detected as thymidine residues whereas methylated cytosine residues will be detected as cytosines.

Bisulphite-modified DNA can be analysed by PCR methods that can discriminate the methylation state of cytosines in specific genomic regions. Alternatively, bisulphite treatment can be coupled to next generation sequencing to achieve single nucleotide resolution mapping of cytosine methylation across the whole genome.

Sequence-specific Enzyme Digestion

This method involves the use of methylation-sensitive restriction endonucleases to produce DNA fragments based on the methylation status of the sequence. In general, a methylation-sensitive enzyme (i.e. an enzyme that cannot cut methylated DNA) and a methylation-insensitive isoschizomer (i.e. an enzyme which cuts the same DNA sequence regardless of whether this is methylated or not) are used to digest the same DNA sample. Comparison of the sensitive versus insensitive digestion leads to a differentiated band digestion pattern on an agarose gel which indicates the methylation status of the cytosines in the analysed DNA sequence. This technique can also be used in combination with other methods such DNA sequencing, end point and RT-PCR or Southern blotting to provide methylation status information.

Capture/quantification of Methylated DNA

The use of methylated DNA-binding proteins or antibodies that specifically recognise methylated DNA is another common method for studying methylated DNA. Antibodies can be used in an ELISA-type assay to specifically detect the percentage of methylated or hydroxymethylated cytosine residues in the sample: the higher the signal, the higher percentage of methylated DNA. Antibodies can be also used to immunoprecipitate methylated DNA, thereby enriching a DNA sample in methylated DNA. This technique is also known as MeDIP (Methylated DNA Immunoprecipitation) and it can be coupled to locus specific PCR or to whole genome approaches such as microarrays or next generation sequencing. Similar techniques have been developed using methylated DNA-binding proteins instead of antibodies.

CHROMATIN

Chromatin is comprised of histones and DNA: A 147bp of DNA chain wrapped around the 8 core histone forms the basic chromatin unit, the nucleosome. The primary functions of chromatin are to package DNA into a smaller volume to fit in the cell, to strengthen the DNA to allow mitosis and meiosis and prevent chromosome breakage, and to control gene expression and DNA replication. In mammals, chromatin is mainly found as a condensed transcriptionally silent form called heterochromatin, which constitutes telomeres, pericentric regions and areas rich in repetitive sequences. Euchromatin is instead less condensed, and it contains most actively transcribed genes. A vast amount of proteins participate in shaping chromatin structure, including histones and other chromatin interacting proteins such as transcription factors and DNA repair proteins. Chromatin remodelling complexes have the ability of changing the chromatin architecture by modulating the interaction between nucleosomes and DNA, which is often achieved by adding post-translational modifications to histones.

Analysis of Chromatin Associated Factors

In general, heterochromatin is difficult to analyse, not the least because of its condensed state and generally repetitive DNA sequence, whereas euchromatin poses less challenges as it contains active genes and maintains an open and extended structure.

Chromatin Immunoprecipitation (ChIP) has become the optimal technique of choice to study chromatin modifications, as it can be used to dissect the spatial and temporal dynamics of the interactions of chromatin and its associated factors, including transcription factors and histone modifications. This technique allows to map minute-by-minute changes of chromatin associated proteins at a single promoter, or to determine their binding sites over the entire human genome.

The principle of ChIP is simple: the selective enrichment of a chromatin fraction containing a specific antigen. Antibodies that recognise a protein or protein modification of interest can be used to determine the relative abundance of that antigen at one or more locations (loci) in the genome.

Traditionally, end point and/or quantitative PCR are performed after ChIP to verify whether a particular DNA sequence is associated with the protein of interest. Using this classical approach, researchers can evaluate the interaction of a protein of interest with a limited number of targets. However, genome-wide studies are now possible through the use of 'ChIP on chip' and 'ChIP-seq', which couple ChIP with either microarray platforms or next generation sequencing.

Tips for ChIP

Cross-link: necessary or not?

The aim of cross-linking is to fix the antigen of interest to its chromatin binding site, so the further away the interaction of interest lies the less effective ChIP will be without cross-linking. ChIP for histone modifications is unlikely to require cross-linking whereas non-histone proteins such as transcription factors and proteins contained within DNA binding complexes will probably need cross-linking.

If cross-linking is used, ChIP reaction will be known as X-ChIP, whereas a native ChIP reaction will be known as *N*-ChIP.

Chromatin fragmentation

Fragmentation of the chromatin is required to make interactions accessible to antibody reagents. The method chosen for fragmentation will depend on the type of ChIP experiment performed.

N-ChIP: Enzymatic digestion with micrococcal nuclease should be able to generate single monosomes (~175bp). This enzymatic cleavage will not produce 'random' sections of chromatin, as micrococcal nuclease favours certain areas of genome sequence over others and will not digest DNA evenly. Be sure to run a new time course every time you set up an experiment.

X-ChIP: Sonication is necessary as formaldehyde cross-linking restricts the access of enzymes to their targets. Sonication creates randomly sized DNA fragments (average of 500–700 bp), with no preferential cleavage for a section of the genome.

Antibodies for ChIP

If available, use an antibody that has been fully characterised and labelled as ChIP-grade. If there is none available, then an antibody that works in normal immunoprecipitation is a good candidate. A polyclonal antibody is preferable to a monoclonal: monoclonal antibodies recognise only a single epitope, which could be masked during the cross-linking process. As a positive antibody control for the technique, histone H3 (tri methyl K4) is a popular positive control to use when chipping active genes. As a negative control, use an antibody that recognises a non-chromatin epitope such as anti-GFP antibody. Remember though that these antibodies are not positive and negative controls *per se*, as this will depend on the locus you are studying: if there is no histone H3 (tri methyl K4) at the particular locus of interest, the best ChIP antibody in the world will not immunoprecipitate anything from this region and therefore will not be an appropriate positive control.

HISTONES

Histones pack and order the DNA into nucleosomes, the building blocks of chromatin. Each nucleosome contains two subunits each of histones H2A, H2B, H3 and H4, known as the core histones. The linker histone H1 does not form part of the nucleosome itself but seems to act as stabiliser of the internucleosomal DNA. Histones are characterised by a large number of post-translational modifications, which serve to allocate the genome into 'active' regions or euchromatin where DNA is accessible for transcription, and 'inactive' regions or heterochromatin where DNA is more compact and therefore less accessible for transcription. At least nine different types of histone modifications have been described, each catalysed by a specific set of enzymes. The best understood modifications are lysine acetylation, lysine and arginine methylation, serine/threonine/tyrosine phosphorylation, and serine/threonine ubiquitylation. Other modifications include GlcNAcylation, citrullination, krotonilation and proline isomerisation. It is now well established that histone modifications do not stand alone and that there is an intense cross-talk between them, which can occur on the same histone (cross-talk in *cis*), between different histones within the same nucleosome (cross-talk in *trans*), or across different nucleosomes (nucleosome cross-talk).

Histone Acetylation

Acetylation is one of the most widely studied histone modifications, as it was one of the first described and linked to transcriptional regulation. Acetylation on lysine residues leads to relaxation of the chromatin structure and allows the binding of transcription factors and significantly increases gene expression. The enzymes responsible for regulating the acetylation of histone tails are histone acetyltransferases (HAT) and deacetylases (HDAC). While all histones can be acetylated, lysine residues within H3 and

H4 are a preferential target for HAT complexes. Histone acetylation is largely targeted to promoter regions, known as promoter-localised acetylation, however, low levels of global acetylation are also found throughout transcribed genes although the function of this type of acetylation is still unclear.

Histone Methylation

Unlike acetylation, histone methylation does not alter the charge of the modified residues and it is therefore less likely to directly alter nucleosomal interactions required for chromatin folding. This probably explains why histone methylation can either repress or activate transcription depending on location. Arginine methylation of histone H3 and H4 promotes transcriptional activation, whereas lysine methylation of histone H3 and H4 is implicated in both transcriptional activation and repression, depending on the methylation site. In addition, lysine residues can be methylated in the form of mono-, di-, or tri-methylation, providing further functional diversity to each site of lysine methylation. For example, tri-methylation on K4 of Histone H3 (H3K4me3) is generally associated with transcriptional activation, whereas tri-methylation on K9 and K27 of histone H3 (H3K9me3 & H3K27me3) are generally associated with transcriptional repression. For many years, histone methylation was thought to be irreversible as it is a stable mark propagated through multiple cell divisions. However, it was recently shown that, similarly to histone acetylation, methylation is an actively regulated and reversible process.

There are two types of histone methyltransferases: lysine-specific histone methyltransferases, which can be SET-domain containing or non-SET-domain containing, and arginine-specific histone methyl-transferases belonging to the PRMT (protein arginine methyltransferases) family.

Histone demethylases can also be classified based on the residue they modify: KDM1/LSD1 (lysine specific demethylase 1) is involved in demethylation of mono- and di-methylated lysines, while JmjC (Jumonji domain-containing) histone demethylases are able to demethylate mono-, di-, or tri-methylated lysines. Removal of arginine methylation is mediated through conversion of the methylated arginine to citrulline by PAD4/PADI4, and citrullinated histones are then either replaced or converted back to unmodified histone by an unknown mechanism.

Histone Phosphorylation

It has recently been shown that all nucleosome core histones are phosphorylated, and that this modification is critical as intermediate step in chromosome condensation during cell division, transcriptional regulation and DNA damage repair. Contrary to acetylation and methylation, histone phosphorylation seems to function by establishing interactions between other histone modifications and serving as platform for effector proteins, leading to a downstream cascade of events. Known markers for mitosis are phosphorylation of histone H3 at S10, involved in chromatin compaction and phospho-T120 in histone H2A, linked to regulation of chromatin structure and function during mitosis.

On the other hand, phosphorylation of H2AX at S139 (resulting in γH2AX), has been identified as one of the earliest event occurring after DNA double-strand break and serves as recruiting point for DNA damage repair proteins. Histone H2B phosphorylation hasn't been studied as well as H3 and H2A phosphorylation, but recent findings suggest that this modification facilitates apoptosis-related chromatin condensation, DNA fragmentation and cell death.

Histone Ubiquitylation

Histone H2A and H2B are two of the most abundant ubiquitylated proteins found in the nucleus, although ubiquitylated histone H3 and H4 have also been described. The most abundant forms of ubiquitylated histones are monoubiquitylated H2A on K119 and monoubiquitylated H2B on K123 (yeast)/K120 (vertebrates). However, polyubiquitylated histones have also been described, such as K63-linked polyubiquitylation of H2A and H2AX. Monoubiquitylation of H2A is catalysed by Polycomb group proteins, and it is mostly associated with gene silencing. The main enzyme responsible for monoubiquitylated H2B is Bre1 in yeast and its homologues RNF20/RNF40 in mammals. Contrary to H2A, monoubiquitylated H2B is mainly associated with transcription activation.

Like other histone modifications, monoubiquitylation of H2A and H2B is reversible, and it is tightly regulated by histone ubiquitin ligases and deubiquitylating enzymes.

Histone ubiquitylation plays a central role in the DNA damage response: RNF8/RNF168 catalysed K63-linked polyubiquitylation of histone H2A/H2AX provides a recognition site for RAP80 and other DNA repair proteins, and monoubiquitylation of histones H2A, H2B, and H2AX is also found at the sites of DNA DSBs (double strand-breaks).

Chapter 14

Role of Small Nuclear RNAs in Eukaryotic Gene Expression

INTRODUCTION

A fascinating feature of modern eukaryotic genes is the nearly ubiquitous presence of intervening sequences or introns, which interrupt the continuity of the information content of genes. Thus, before primary gene transcripts can be used by the cell, introns must be accurately removed or 'spliced'. In addition, recent research indicates that introns themselves oft en harbour regulatory or otherwise functional sequences, and their accurate and timely removal is often critical for their cellular function. The intronic sequences in higher eukaryotic genes are much longer than the non-intronic sequences, the exons, and the sequence-based information that specifies the intron–exon boundaries is highly complex and poorly understood. Thus, accurately distinguishing these two sets of functional sequences that co-exist in eukaryotic primary transcripts is a highly challenging task for the eukaryotic gene expression machinery.

Although modern mammals have one of the most complex splicing patterns among extant eukaryotes, it is likely that even in primordial eukaryotes splicing was already a highly complex process. On the basis of currently accepted models of evolution of eukaryotes, introns probably originated from self-splicing ribozymes that dated from pre-cellular life and constituted the majority of the genomes of ancient eukaryotes. Later on, probably in order to prevent genomic instability, the introns lost their self-splicing capacity and, instead, the splicing function was delegated to a cellular machine, the spliceosome, which acted *in trans* to remove introns from primary transcripts. Although the origin and evolution of the early spliceosomes is still largely mysterious, several lines of evidence suggest that they probably evolved from self-splicing introns. This hypothesis is partly based on the fact that the mechanism of intron removal by the spliceosome, performed through two consecutive transesterification reactions resulting in removal of a branched lariat intron, is identical with the splicing reaction performed by a class of extant self-splicing introns called the group II introns. These introns, which are found in all three kingdoms of life, are RNA-centric catalytic sequences composed of a number of base-paired RNA structures called 'domains'. Extensive research has elucidated the identity of the catalytically essential sequences in these introns. Intriguingly, the RNA components of the spliceosome, the snRNAs, show unmistakable similarities to fragments of the catalytically essential domains of group II introns in sequence, secondary structure and function. Of the five major spliceosomal snRNAs (U1, U2, U4, U5 and U6), three of them (U2, U5 and U6) have clear structural and functional similarities to critical domains of group II introns. Domain-swapping experiments have indicated that isolated domains of group II introns and U5 and U6 snRNA substructures could functionally replace each other, proving their functional equivalence.

Another set of sequences in group II introns are functionally equivalent to U1 snRNA, despite the lack of structural similarity. Currently there are no known functional or structural equivalents for the U4 snRNA in group II introns and the evolutionary origin of this snRNA is completely unknown. On the other hand, a number of domains of the group II introns do not have an equivalent among the spliceosomal snRNAs and it is likely that, in the spliceosome, these RNA domains are replaced by spliceosomal proteins. While the possibility of convergent evolution cannot be formally ruled out, the above-mentioned similarities strongly suggest that at least a number of snRNAs are evolutionary remnants of primordial self-splicing ribozymes.

ROLES OF snRNAS IN THE SPLICEOSOME

The snRNAs were first discovered in 1970s as small highly abundant nuclear RNAs which formed the core of RNP (ribonucleoprotein) particles which showed strong reactivity with the immune sera from patients with autoimmune disorders. Further analysis indicated the presence of sequence complementarity between one of the snRNAs, U1, and the sequences found at the 52 splice site of primary transcripts, ultimately leading to the discovery of their involvement in splicing. Further research identified a second set of snRNAs, named U11, U12, U4atac and U6atac, which are functional counterparts of U1, U2, U4 and U6 snRNAs respectively, and participate in the formation of a 'minor' spliceosome which is responsible for removal of an atypical subset of introns, most of which have alternative consensus sequences at the splice sites and branch site. U5 snRNA is found in both 'major' and 'minor' spliceosomes. Each of the nine spliceosomal snRNAs are stably associated with a set of proteins, creating the snRNP (small nuclear ribonucleoprotein) particles which form the main functional subunits of the spliceosome. Analysis of the spliceosomal function suggests that snRNPs and several non-snRNP spliceosomal proteins assemble on each intron in a stepwise elaborate fashion through a large number of conformational rearrangements which start from the recognition of the splice junctions and culminate in splicing catalysis, followed by disassembly and recycling of the spliceosomal components.

Recognition of the 52 Splice Site by U1 snRNP

Recognition of introns in primary transcripts is partly mediated by detection of 'consensus' sequences found at the junction of introns and exons, the 5′ and 3′ splice sites. These consensus sequences are rather short: 5′-AG/GURAGU and 5′-YAG/G for 5′ and 3′ splice sites respectively, where R denotes either a G or an A, and Y denotes a C or a U and/marks the location of the splice site. Interestingly, in higher eukaryotes and especially in mammals, the splice site sequences are highly degenerate and, in many cases, significantly deviate from the consensus sequence, thus necessitating an elaborate multi-step recognition mechanism mediated by a combination of RNA–RNA base pairing and RNA–protein interactions.

The association of U1 snRNP and its functional equivalent in the 'minor' spliceosomes, U11, with the 5′ splice site is one of the earliest and arguably most important events in the spliceosomal assembly pathway. The recognition and binding of the 5′ splice site is mediated both by base pairing of a single-stranded sequence at the 5′-end of U1 snRNA to the 5′ splice site and through an intricate web of interactions between the premRNA and U1C, a U1-specific protein. Interestingly, a high–resolution structure of U1 snRNP indicated the presence of a number of interactions between U1C and the nucleotides at the 5′ end of U1 which base pair to the 5′ splice site, thus providing a structural basis for the dual RNA–protein recognition of the 5′ splice site. While this RNA–protein recognition of the 5′ splice site by U1 is functionally critical for the majority of cellular transcripts *in vivo*, several other proteins also contribute to the selection of the 5′ splice site.

Furthermore, at least some primary transcripts can be spliced in the absence of U1 snRNP *in vitro*, pointing to extensive redundancy in the splicing machinery. Finally, the binding of U1 is not necessarily synonymous with productive splicing, since the binding of U1 to sequences involved in negative regulation of splicing has been documented. Current data suggest that the binding of U1 to such elements is important in splicing regulation and exclusion of *pseudo* splice sites, underscoring the importance of sequence context in splicing.

U2 snRNP and Recognition of the Branch Site and 3′ Splice Site

Once bound to the 5′ splice site in a sequence context which is conducive to splicing, U1 helps initiate the spliceosomal assembly by forming a network of interactions with U2 snRNP that plays a dominant role in recognition of the 3′ splice site and the branch site, another region in the introns which is recognised by the spliceosomes. Branch sites, which are typically located ~30 nt from the 32-end of introns, contain the adenosine which acts as the nucleophile of the first transesterification step of splicing and forms the branched lariat structure found in the splicing intermediates and post-splicing introns. In early spliceosomes, U2 snRNP is loosely associated with the end of the intron through protein-mediated interactions. However, in an ATP-dependent step which involves the displacement of intron-bound proteins and remodelling of base-pairing interactions within the U2 snRNA, U2 forms a stable interaction with the branch site and 3′ splice site. This interaction is partly mediated through a base-pairing interaction between U2 and sequences flanking the branch site adenosine, and is stabilised by several RNA–protein interactions. The base pairing between U2 and the branch site leaves the branch site adenosine in an unpaired extrahelical conformation necessary for efficient splicing. In addition, the interaction between U1 and U2 snRNPs generates a loop that brings the 5′ and 3′ splice sites together and helps to 'define' the introns and exons.

Formation of a Catalytically Active Spliceosome

Three of the snRNPs, U4, U5 and U6, form a ternary complex termed the 'tri-snRNP' and collectively integrate into the assembling spliceosomes. Of all of the spliceosomal snRNAs, U6 is the most conserved and contains two invariant domains, the ACAGAGA and AGC boxes, which play a critical functional role in splicing. Furthermore, it contains an ISL (intramolecular stem-loop) which is almost identical with the catalytic domain V of group II introns and, similar to its group II intron counterpart, binds a functionally required divalent cation, pointing to a critical role in splicing catalysis for this snRNA. Perhaps in order to prevent it from prematurely forming a catalytically active structure, within the tri–snRNP U6 is kept in an inactive conformation through a base-pairing interaction with U4 snRNA that prevents the formation of its functionally critical ISL. Current data do not indicate any additional functions for U4 snRNA except acting as a negative chaperon for U6. Once the base paired U4/U6 complex joins the spliceosome in association with U5 within the tri-snRNP, the U4/U6 duplex is unwound in a tightly controlled manner and U2 snRNA replaces U4 as the base-pairing partner of U6. In addition, U6 replaces

U1 at the 5′ splice site, forming canonical and non-canonical base-pairing interactions with this sequence. The base-pairing interactions between U6 and U2 allow the formation of the U6 ISL and, further, serve to juxtapose the branch site, which is bound to the branch-binding sequence in U2, and the 5′ splice site, which is bound by U6. At the same time, U5 snRNA forms non-canonical base-pairing interactions with the exon sequences immediately adjacent to the splice sites and participates in aligning the exons to ensure their optimal positioning for the second step of splicing. These base-pairing rearrangements are accompanied by an extensive rearrangement of protein–protein and protein–RNA interactions, culminating in the formation of catalytically competent spliceosomes. U1 and U4 are not stably associated with fully assembled spliceosomes, thus leaving U2, U5 and U6 snRNAs as the only spliceosomal RNA components required for catalysis. Interestingly, as mentioned above, these three snRNAs have clear structural and functional counterparts in self-splicing group II introns, raising the possibility that the catalytic core of the two splicing systems may be closely similar.

Catalysis of Splicing: The Role of snRNAs

Mutagenesis studies have shown that, at least *in vitro*, the conserved loop of U5, which was previously shown to be the functionally important domain of the molecule, was in fact dispensable for splicing. On the other hand, it has been shown that, under certain conditions, several positions within the branch binding sequence of U2 snRNA can be mistakenly recognised as the 5′ splice site. These results imply that the branch binding sequence of U2, which is functionally the most critical region of this snRNA, is not essential for spliceosomal catalysis, at least under certain conditions. As the rest of U2 seems to mainly fulfill structural roles by forming base-pairing interactions with other U2 sequences or with U6 snRNA, these results suggest that U6 snRNA may be the only RNA that is absolutely crucial for splicing catalysis, at least under the conditions studied so far.

Several additional lines of evidence suggest that U6 may form part of the catalytic domain of the spliceosome. U6 is the most conserved of all spliceosomal snRNAs and several point mutations in its two evolutionarily invariant sequences, the ACAGAGA and AGC boxes, lead to a block in splicing, pointing to a critical function for these two sequences. Cross-linking and mutational complementation analyses have indicated that the first step of splicing occurs in close proximity to the ACAGAGA box, suggesting that this sequence is in the immediate vicinity of or even forms part of the spliceosomal active site. Current data suggest that in group II introns, the active site is formed by juxtaposition of the AGC triad and the asymmetric internal bulge of domain V along with a short purine-rich sequence which is considered functionally equivalent to the ACAGAGA box in U6. Interestingly, U6 contains the equivalent of all of these sequences which form the active site in group II introns, and close similarities in phosphorothioate interference patterns between catalytic domain V of group II introns and U6 suggest that they may be functionally related. Furthermore, hydroxyl radical footprinting and *in vivo* mutagenesis studies have pointed to the proximity of the AGC triad, the ACAGAGA box and the area near the bulged residue in ISL in functional spliceosomes, perhaps in an arrangement similar to or even identical with the one found in group II introns.

Interestingly, analyses on *in-vitro*-transcribed, protein-free U6 and U2 snRNAs indicate that they can efficiently form a base-paired complex *in vitro* which in many respects resembles the one formed in the activated spliceosomes. Furthermore, it has been shown that the *in vitro* assembled human U2–U6 complex can indeed catalyse a two-step splicing reaction which closely resembles the one catalysed by the self-splicing group II introns and the spliceosome. On the basis of the data above, the snRNAs seem to be fully competent to form the majority, if not all, of the spliceosomal active site and to perform catalysis, similar to the self-splicing group II introns, albeit with much lower efficiency. If we assume that the spliceosome is an RNA catalyst, the snRNAs are unusual ribozymes in many respects, perhaps most importantly they are unusually small compared with other natural ribozymes catalysing splicing reactions. The larger size of other natural splicing ribozymes is thought to allow them to fold into complex tertiary structures, which in turn enable them to create sophisticated active sites necessary for such complex reactions. It is conceivable that due to their short length, the U6 and U2 snRNAs at best form an inefficient splicing ribozyme, which requires other spliceosomal factors for stable positioning of the active-site elements and the reacting groups. Although the exact role played by the proteins in the spliceosomal catalytic core is mostly unknown, their possible roles could range from assisting the snRNAs in assuming their functional structure, assisting in or independently co-ordinating critical metal ions and participating in the positioning of the substrates, to independently forming part of the active site and even direct involvement in catalysis.

Other Biological Roles of snRNAs

Although the spliceosomal snRNAs (and their minor spliceosomal counterparts U11, U12, U4atac and U6 atac) play major roles in spliceosomal function, data suggest additional roles in regulation of gene expression for the snRNP particles. The interaction of U1 and the 5′ splice site, in addition to its function in splice-site selection, also seems to play a role in stabilisation of some messages. Both U1 and U2 snRNPs have been implicated in transcriptional regulation through stimulation of the rate of formation of the first phosphodiester bond at transcription initiation and also through interaction with a component of the pre-initiation complex, TFIIH (transcription factor II H) respectively. U1 snRNP seems to also regulate the efficiency of polyadenylation via the interaction of a U1-specific protein, U1A, with a component of the CPSF (cleavage and polyadenylation stimulating factor). In addition, it has been reported that binding of U1 to a 5′ splice site-like sequence in the 3′-UTR (untranslated region) of some mRNAs inhibits their polyadenylation, leading to degradation of the RNA. Thus the snRNAs and their bound proteins seem to act in co- ordination of the various steps in gene expression, in addition to playing the central role in splicing.

Another spliceosomal snRNP, the SL (spliced leader) particle, plays a critical role as the splice donor in a non-canonical *trans*-splicing reaction mainly observed in some protozoa and lower invertebrates. In the *trans*-splicing reaction, SL is treated as a mini exon plus a short intron, with the exonic sequences 'spliced' *in trans* to a 3′ splice site on the primary transcripts of *trans*-splicing organisms. Thus, unlike the other spliceosomal snRNAs, SL is consumed during the *trans*-splicing reaction.

Although the majority of snRNAs play a role in splicing, there are other abundant small nuclear-localised RNAs which play critical roles in other cellular processes. A non-spliceosomal snRNA, U7, functions in 3′-end processing of replication-dependent histone mRNAs, which are not polyadenylated and instead terminate in a conserved stem-loop structure (SL element) generated by endonucleolytic cleavage of the pre-mRNA. Similar to the spliceosomal snRNAs, U7 also forms an snRNP by associating with a set of proteins which together form the so called Sm ring, and is recruited to histone pre-mRNA primarily through base-pairing interactions via its 5′-end with a purine-rich HDE (histone downstream element) which is located in the vicinity of the cleavage site. Together with a protein which binds the SL element, U7 recruits a complex that triggers endonucleolytic cleavage between SL and the HDE by the CPSF73 endonuclease, thus forming the mature histone mRNA.

To sum up, the ability of snRNAs to form strong, specific interactions via base pairing with another RNA is extensively utilised in the spliceosome and during processing of the histone 3′-ends. Base-pairing interactions contribute to substrate recognition (U1, U2 and U7), positioning of the branch site in a strained catalytic bulged conformation (U2), regulation of the activity of another snRNA (U4) and juxtaposition of reactive substrates (U2, U5 and U6). Since RNA–RNA interactions similar to those formed by some of the spliceosomal snRNAs play identical or closely related roles in group II introns, it is conceivable that the robustness of RNA–RNA interactions has led to their preservation throughout the evolution of the spliceosome from group II-like ancient ribozymes. Although RNAs can perform the above-mentioned tasks with ease and even more effectively than proteins, when it comes to catalysis, proteins seem to have an advantage over RNA, at least in the case of natural ribozymes. The evolutionary reason behind the preservation of U6 snRNAs as a constituent of the spliceosomal catalytic core remains an open question.

Another feature of the snRNAs is their participation in multiple sets of base-pairing interactions that at times are mutually exclusive and, thus, act as switches between different functional states. The presence of such interactions underscores the highly complex evolutionary pressures under which the snRNAs have evolved. In addition, most of the snRNAs bind a number of proteins which play important functional roles. While in many cases these proteins complement the function of the snRNA to which they bind, emerging evidence suggests that they can impart a completely novel function on the snRNP. Research in the coming years is likely to provide additional instances of multi-functionality of the snRNPs and further elucidate their contribution to the highly complex network of interactions which regulate eukaryotic gene expression.

RNA-INDUCED SILENCING COMPLEX

The mature miRNA is part of an active RNA-induced silencing complex (RISC) containing Dicer and many associated proteins. RISC is also known as a microRNA ribonucleoprotein complex (miRNP), A RISC with incorporated miRNA is sometimes referred to as a 'miRISC.'

Dicer processing of the pre-miRNA is thought to be coupled with unwinding of the duplex. Generally, only one strand is incorporated into the miRISC, selected on the basis of its thermodynamic instability and weaker base-pairing on the 5′ end relative to the other strand. The position of the stem-loop may also influence strand choice. The other strand, called the passenger strand due to its lower levels in the steady state, is denoted with an asterisk (*) and is normally degraded. In some cases, both strands of the duplex are viable and become functional miRNA that target different mRNA populations.

Members of the Argonaute (Ago) protein family are central to RISC function. Argonautes are needed for miRNA-induced silencing and contain two conserved RNA binding domains: a PAZ domain that can bind the single stranded 3′ end of the mature miRNA and a PIWI domain that structurally resembles ribonuclease-H and functions to interact with the 5′ end of the guide strand. They bind the mature miRNA and orient it for interaction with a target mRNA. Some argonautes, for example human Ago2, cleave target transcripts directly, argonautes may also recruit additional proteins to achieve translational repression. The human genome encodes eight argonaute proteins divided by sequence similarities into two families: AGO (with four members present in all mammalian cells and called E1F2C/hAgo in humans), and PIWI (found in the germ line and hematopoietic stem cells).

Additional RISC components include TRBP [human immunodeficiency virus (HIV) transactivating response RNA (TAR) binding protein], PACT (protein activator of the interferon-induced protein kinase), the SMN complex, fragile X mental retardation protein (FMRP), Tudor staphylococcal nuclease-domain-containing protein (Tudor-SN), the putative DNA helicase MOV10, and the RNA recognition motif containing protein TNRC6B.

Mode of Silencing and Regulatory Loops

Gene silencing may occur either via mRNA degradation or preventing mRNA from being translated. For example, miR16 contains a sequence complementary to the AU-rich element found in the 3′UTR of many unstable mRNAs, such as TNF alpha or GM-CSF. It has been demonstrated that given complete complementarity between the miRNA and target mRNA sequence, Ago2 can cleave the mRNA and lead to direct mRNA degradation. In the absence of complementarity, silencing is achieved by preventing translation. The relation of miRNA and its target mRNA(s) can be based on the simple negative regulation of a target mRNA, but it seems that a common scenario is the use of a 'coherent feed-forward loop', 'mutual negative feedback loop' (also termed double negative loop) and 'positive feedback/feed-forward loop'. Some miRNAs work as buffers of random gene expression changes arising due to stochastic events in transcription, translation and protein stability. Such regulation is typically achieved by the virtue of negative feedback loops or incoherent feed-forward loop uncoupling protein output from mRNA transcription.

SECTION IV

Protein Synthesis, Processing and Regulation

Chapter 15

Protein Synthesis and Degradation

INTRODUCTION

The regulation of protein synthesis is an important part of the regulation of gene expression. Regulation of mRNA translation controls the levels of particular proteins that are synthesised upon demand, such as synthesis of the different chains of globin in haemoglobin, or the production of insulin from stored insulin mRNAs in response to blood glucose levels, to name a few. The control of the cell cycle and cell proliferation also involves regulation of protein synthesis, and malignant transformation of cells involves loss of certain translational regulatory controls. In fact, several translation initiation factors are over-expressed in certain cancers and play key roles in tumour development and progression. The process of protein synthesis and important examples of its regulation are now understood at the molecular level. We will discuss the mechanism and regulation of protein synthesis, elucidating this complex area of gene regulation with specific examples. Many viruses compete with their infected host cell and often dominate the protein synthetic machinery to maintain viral production and thwart innate (intracellular) anti-viral responses. For many viruses, the inhibition of host cell protein synthesis is an important component of their ability to propagate and destroy the infected cell. The infected cell, in turn, responds by enacting antiviral activities that include the production of potent biological molecules such as α-interferon that function, in part, to inhibit protein synthesis. Finally, a large proportion of antibiotics currently in use or under development inhibit protein synthesis in bacteria but not animal cells by exploiting differences in the structure of prokaryotic and eularyotic ribosomes.

BASICS OF GENETIC CODE

The genetic code is the set of rules by which information encoded in genetic material (DNA or mRNA sequences) is translated into proteins (amino acid sequences) by living cells. The code defines a mapping between trinucleotide sequences, called codons, and amino acids. With some exceptions, a triplet codon in a nucleic acid sequence usually specifies a single amino acid. Because the vast majority of genes are encoded with exactly the same code, this particular code is often referred to as the canonical or standard genetic code or simply the genetic code, though in fact there are many variant codes. Thus the canonical genetic code is not universal. In humans, for example, protein synthesis in mitochondria relies on a genetic code that varies from the standard genetic code. Not all genetic information is stored using the genetic code. All organisms' DNA contains regulatory sequences, intergenic segments, and chromosomal structural areas that can contribute greatly to phenotype. Those higher-level or epigenetic elements operate under sets of rules that are distinct from the codon-to-amino acid paradigm underlying the genetic code.

Cracking the Genetic Code

After the structure of DNA was deciphered by James Watson, Francis Crick, Maurice Wilkins and Rosalind Franklin, serious efforts to understand the nature of the encoding of proteins began. George Gamow postulated that a three-letter code must be employed to encode the 20 standard amino acids used by living cells to encode proteins (because 3 is the smallest integer n such that 4^n is at least 20).

The fact that codons consist of three DNA bases was first demonstrated in the Crick and Brenner experiment. They used a cell-free system to translate a polyuracil RNA sequence (e.g. UUUUU...) and discovered that the polypeptide that they had synthesised consisted of only the amino acid phenylalanine. They thereby deduced from this polyphenylalanine that the codon UUU specified the amino acid phenylalanine. Extending this work, Nirenberg and Philip Leder revealed the triplet nature of the genetic code and allowed the codons of the standard genetic code to be deciphered. In these experiments various combinations of mRNA were passed through a filter which contained ribosomes, the components of cells that translate RNA into protein. Unique triplets promoted the binding of specific tRNAs to the ribosome. Leder and Nirenberg were able to determine the sequences of 54 out of 64 codons in their experiments.

Transfer of Information via the Genetic Code

The genome of an organism is inscribed in DNA, or in the case of some viruses, RNA. The portion of the genome that codes for a protein or an RNA is referred to as a gene. Those genes that code for proteins are composed of trinucleotide units called codons, each coding for a single amino acid. Each nucleotide subunit consists of a phosphate, deoxyribose sugar and one of the four nitrogenous nucleotide bases. The purine bases adenine (A) and guanine (G) are larger and consist of two aromatic rings. The pyrimidine bases cytosine (C) and thymine (T) are smaller and consist of only one aromatic ring. In the double-helix configuration, two strands of DNA are joined to each other by hydrogen bonds in an arrangement known as base pairing.

These bonds almost always form between an adenine base on one strand and a thymine on the other strand and between a cytosine base on one strand and a guanine base on the other. This means that the number of A and T residues will be the same in a given double helix, as will the number of G and C residues. In RNA, thymine (T) is replaced by uracil (U), and the deoxyribose is substituted by ribose.

Each protein-coding gene is transcribed into a template molecule of the related polymer RNA, known as messenger RNA or mRNA. This, in turn, is translated on the ribosome into an amino acid chain or polypeptide. The process of translation requires transfer RNAs specific for individual amino acids with the amino acids covalently attached to them, guanosine triphosphate as an energy source, and a number of translation factors. tRNAs have anticodons complementary to the codons in mRNA and can be 'charged' covalently with amino acids at their 3′ terminal CCA ends. Individual tRNAs are charged with specific amino acids by enzymes known as aminoacyl tRNA synthetases, which have high specificity for both their cognate amino acids and tRNAs. The high specificity of these enzymes is a major reason why the fidelity of protein translation is maintained.

There are $4^3 = 64$ different codon combinations possible with a triplet codon of three nucleotides, all 64 codons are assigned for either amino acids or stop signals during translation. If, for example, an RNA sequence, UUUAAACCC is considered and the reading-frame starts with the first U (by convention, 5′ to 3′), there are three codons, namely, UUU, AAA and CCC, each of which specifies one amino acid. This RNA sequence will be translated into an amino acid sequence, three amino acids long. A comparison may be made with computer science, where the codon is similar to a word, which is the standard 'chunk' for handling data (like one amino acid of a protein), and a nucleotide is similar to a bit, in that it is the smallest unit.

Salient Features

Sequence reading frame

A codon is defined by the initial nucleotide from which translation starts. For example, the string GGGAAACCC, if read from the first position, contains the codons GGG, AAA and CCC, and, if read from the second position, it contains the codons GGA and AAC, if read starting from the third position, GAA and ACC. Every sequence can thus be read in three reading frames, each of which will produce a different amino acid sequence (in the given example, Gly-Lys-Pro, Gly-Asn, or Glu-Thr, respectively). With double-stranded DNA there are six possible reading frames, three in the forward orientation on one strand and three reverse on the opposite strand.

The actual frame in which a protein sequence is translated is defined by a start codon, usually the first AUG codon in the mRNA sequence. Mutations that disrupt the reading frame by insertions or deletions of a non-multiple of 3 nucleotide bases are known as frameshift mutations. These mutations may impair the function of the resulting protein, if it is formed, and are thus rare in *in vivo* protein-coding sequences. Such misformed proteins are often targeted for proteolytic degradation. In addition, a frame shift mutation is very likely to cause a stop codon to be read, which truncates the creation of the protein. One reason for the rareness of frame-shifted mutations being inherited is that, if the protein being translated is essential for growth under the selective pressures the organism faces, absence of a functional protein may cause death before the organism is viable.

Start/stop codons

Translation starts with a chain initiation codon (start codon). Unlike stop codons, the codon alone is not sufficient to begin the process. Nearby sequences (such as the Shine-Dalgarno sequence in *E. coli*) and initiation factors are also required to start translation. The most common start codon is AUG which is read as methionine or, in bacteria, as formylmethionine.

Alternative start codons (depending on the organism), include 'GUG' or 'UUG', which normally code for valine or leucine, respectively. However, when used as a start codon, these alternative start codons are translated as methionine or formylmethionine.

The three stop codons have been given names: UAG is amber, UGA is opal (sometimes also called umber), and UAA is ochre. 'Amber' was named by discoverers Richard Epstein and Charles Steinberg after their friend Harris Bernstein, whose last name means 'amber' in German. The other two stop codons were named 'ochre' and 'opal' in order to keep the 'colour names' theme. Stop codons are also called termination or nonsense codons and they signal release of the nascent polypeptide from the ribosome due to binding of release factors in the absence of cognate tRNAs with anticodons complementary to these stop signals.

Effect of mutations

Frameshift mutations altering the sequence reading frame, and nonsense mutations causing a stop codon are examples of point mutations. In addition, there may be missense mutations that cause exchange of one amino acid for another. Clinically important missense mutations generally change the properties of the coded amino acid residue between being basic, acidic polar or nonpolar, while nonsense mutations result in a stop codon.

Degeneracy of the genetic code

The genetic code has redundancy but no ambiguity. For example, although codons GAA and GAG both specify glutamic acid (redundancy), neither of them specifies any other amino acid (no ambiguity). The codons encoding one amino acid may differ in any of their three positions. For example the amino acid glutamic acid is specified by GAA and GAG codons (difference in the third position), the amino acid leucine is specified by UUA, UUG, CUU, CUC, CUA, CUG codons (difference in the first or third position), while the amino acid serine is specified by UCA, UCG, UCC, UCU, AGU, AGC (difference in the first, second or third position).

A position of a codon is said to be a four-fold degenerate site if any nucleotide at this position specifies the same amino acid. For example, the third position of the glycine codons (GGA, GGG, GGC, GGU) is a fourfold degenerate site, because all nucleotide substitutions at this site are synonymous, i.e. they do not change the amino acid. Only the third positions of some codons may be fourfold degenerate. A position of a codon is said to be a twofold degenerate site if only two of four possible nucleotides at this position specify the same amino acid. For example, the third position of the glutamic acid codons (GAA, GAG) is a twofold degenerate site. In twofold degenerate sites, the equivalent nucleotides are always either two purines (A/G) or two pyrimidines (C/U), so only transversional substitutions (purine to pyrimidine or pyrimidine to purine) in two-fold degenerate sites are nonsynonymous. A position of a codon is said to be a non-degenerate site if any mutation at this position results in amino acid substitution. There is only one threefold degenerate site where changing three of the four nucleotides may have no effect on the amino acid (depending on what it is changed to), while changing the fourth possible nucleotide always results in an amino acid substitution. This is the third position of an isoleucine codon: AUU, AUC or AUA all encode isoleucine, but AUG encodes methionine. In computation this position is often treated as a twofold degenerate site.

There are three amino acids encoded by six different codons: serine, leucine, arginine. Only two amino acids are specified by a single codon, one of these is the amino-acid methionine, specified by the codon AUG, which also specifies the start of translation, the other is tryptophan, specified by the codon UGG. The degeneracy of the genetic code is what accounts for the existence of synonymous mutations.

Degeneracy results because a triplet code designates 20 amino acids and a stop codon. Because there are four bases, triplet codons are required to produce at least 21 different codes. For example, if there were two bases per codon, then only 16 amino acids could be coded for ($4^2 = 16$). Because at least 21 codes are required, then 4^3 gives 64 possible codons, meaning that some degeneracy must exist.

These properties of the genetic code make it more fault-tolerant for point mutations. For example, in theory, four-fold degenerate codons can tolerate any point mutation at the third position, although codon usage bias restricts this in practice in many organisms, twofold degenerate codons can tolerate one out of the three possible point mutations at the third position. Since transition mutations (purine to purine or pyrimidine to pyrimidine mutations) are more likely than transversion (purine to pyrimidine or vice-versa) mutations, the equivalence of purines or that of pyrimidines at two-fold degenerate sites adds a further fault-tolerance. A practical consequence of redundancy is that some errors in the genetic code only cause a silent mutation or an error that would not affect the protein because the hydrophilicity or hydrophobicity is maintained by equivalent substitution of amino acids, for example, a codon of NUN (where N = any nucleotide) tends to code for hydrophobic amino acids. NCN yields amino acid residues that are small in size and moderate in hydropathy, NAN encodes average size hydrophilic residues. These tendencies may result from that the aminoacyl tRNA synthetases related the such codons share a common ancestry (Fig. 15.1).

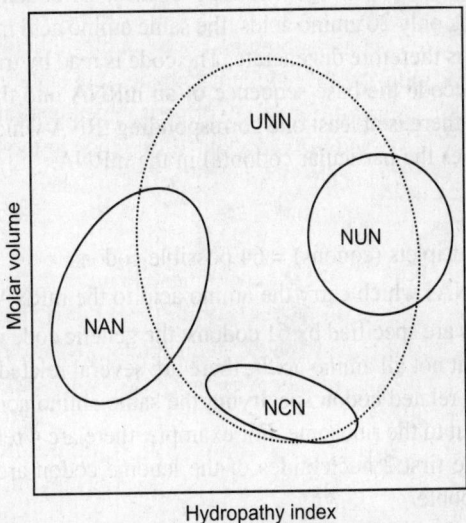

Fig. 15.1: Grouping of codons by amino acid residue molar volume and hydropathy.

Even so, single point mutations can still cause dysfunctional proteins. For example, a mutated haemoglobin gene causes sickle-cell disease. In the mutant haemoglobin a hydrophilic glutamate (Glu) is substituted by the hydrophobic valine (Val), that is, GAA or GAG becomes GUA or GUG. The substitution of glutamate by valine reduces the solubility of β-globin which causes haemoglobin to form linear polymers linked by the hydrophobic interaction between the valine groups causing sickle-cell deformation of erythrocytes. Sickle-cell disease is generally not caused by a *de novo* mutation. Rather it is selected for in malarial regions (in a way similar to thalassemia), as heterozygous people have some resistance to the malarial *Plasmodium* parasite (heterozygote advantage). These variable codes for amino acids are allowed because of modified bases in the first base of the anticodon of the tRNA, and the base-pair formed is called a wobble base pair. The modified bases include inosine and the Non-Watson-Crick U-G basepair.

Variations to the Standard Genetic Code

While slight variations on the standard code had been predicted earlier, none were discovered until 1979, when researchers studying human mitochondrial genes discovered they used an alternative code. Many slight variants have been discovered since, including various alternative mitochondrial codes, as well as small variants such as Mycoplasma translating the codon UGA as tryptophan and Candida species translating CUG as a serine rather than a leucine. In bacteria and archaea, GUG and UUG are common start codons. However, in rare cases, certain specific proteins may use alternative initiation (start) codons not normally used by that species. In certain proteins, nonstandard amino acids are substituted for standard stop codons, depending upon associated signal sequences in the messenger RNA: UGA can code for selenocysteine and UAG can code for pyrrolysine as discussed in the relevant articles. Selenocysteine is now viewed as the 21st amino acid, and pyrrolysine is viewed as the 22nd.

Not-with-standing these differences, all known codes have strong similarities to each other, and the coding mechanism is the same for all organisms: three-base codons, tRNA, ribosomes, reading the code in the same direction and translating the code three letters at a time into sequences of amino acids.

Since the genetic code is read in triplets (codons) comprising three of the four bases, there are 4^3 or 64 possible triplets encoding the 20 amino acids. All but 3 of these 64 codons specify amino acids. Since there are 61 codons specifying only 20 amino acids, the same amino acid may be encoded by more than one codon. The genetic code is therefore degenerate. The code is read by transfer RNAs (tRNAs) which are adapter molecules that decode the base sequence of an mRNA into the amino acid sequence of a protein. For each amino acid there is at least one corresponding tRNA which transports that amino acid to the ribosome and recognises the particular codon(s) in the mRNA.

Code Facts

1. Genetic code is read in triplets (codons) = 64 possible codons.

2. Codons are read by tRNAs which carry the amino acid to the mRNA.

3. Because 20 amino acids are specified by 61 codons, the genetic code is said to be degenerate. This means that for many, but not all amino acids, there are several related codons that can specify the same amino acid. Each related codon specifying the same amino acid corresponds to a different tRNA which transports it to the ribosome. For example, there are 4 related codons that specify the amino acid leucine. The first 2 nucleotides of the leucine codon are invariant, whereas the 3rd position can vary or wobble.

4. AUG specifies methionine, which almost always initiates polypeptide synthesis.

5. UAA, UAG, UGA specify translation termination. There are no corresponding tRNAs for termination. Rather, termination is carried out by protein factors during translation.

Wobble pairing refers to relaxed rules for basepairing that occur between the anticodon of the tRNA and the codon within families of tRNAs, such as the 4 different leucine tRNAs.

1. Wobble pairing indicates that the 3rd codon position recognises multiple pairing partners leucine: 4 related codons

$$(5') -1 - 2 - 3 - (3')$$

```
C U U
C U C
C U A
C U G
```

2. Most 3rd positions of codons wobble, and can therefore bind to 2 or 3 different nucleotides in the anticodon, with the following rules for pairing.

Codon 3rd position	Anticodon 1st position
C	G, I
G	C, U
A	U, I
U	A, G, I

3. Wobble pairing provides for multiple ways to specify a single amino acid in the genetic code.

tRNAs

1. Short molecules, 70–90 nts long.
2. All terminate with CCA_{OH}-3′ to which an amino acid can be covalently attached.
3. Contain unusual nucleotides, which are modifications of the purine/pyrimidine bases or ribose sugar, such as methylations, reductions, altered site of sugar linking to base examples include:
   - Thymidine (uridine with C5 methyl).
   - Methylated guanosines, methylated adenosines.
   - Inosine and methylinosine (modified purines).
   - *Pseudouridine* (ribose sugar attached to uridine in the C-5 rather than C-1 position).
   - Dihydrouridine (uridine reduced at the C5-C6 double bond).
4. Function of modifications
   - Control specific folding of the tRNAs.

Some modifications are universal, and are therefore found in all tRNAs. These modifications contribute to the secondary structure (cloverleaf) shape of tRNAs, and the tertiary (L-shape) structure as well. Other modifications are specific to members of a family of tRNAs, and define them as such to the molecular machinery that covalently attaches a specific amino acid. Family specific modifications often serve as recognition signals for aminoacyl tRNA synthetases. All tRNAs possess a common secondary and tertiary stem-loop structure that is critical for their function. A typical tRNA has the following secondary structure: A T-*pseudouridine*-C-G loop (TψCG loop), a dihydrouracil or D-loop, and an anticodon loop. The anticodon loop contains the three complementary nucleotides that basepair with a specific codon in the mRNA. A given tRNA interacts with different codons that specify a given amino acid due to nonstandard or wobble basepairing in the 3rd position of the codon with the 1st position of the anticodon (Fig. 15.2).

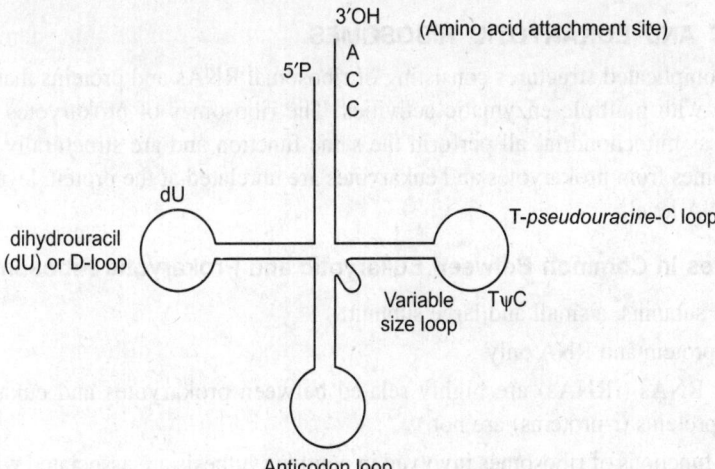

Fig. 15.2: Anticodon loop contains three complementary nucleotides.

Anticodon Facts

1. 1st anticodon position wobbles as does codon 3rd position, but with fewer choices for pairing.

1st position anticodon	3rd position codon pair
C	G
A	U
G	C, U
U	A, G
I	C, A, U

2. Inosine found in anticodon

3. Genetic code is almost universal:
   - Same for prokaryotes and eukaryotes.
   - In mitochondria, the codon AUA encodes methionine rather than isoleucine, and AGA/G signals stop rather than arginine.

AMINOACYL-tRNA SYNTHETASES COUPLE AMINO ACIDS TO tRNAS

Synthetase Facts

1. Aminoacyl tRNA synthetases are enzymes that covalently attach a specific amino acid to a specific tRNA.

2. There are 20 different tRNA synthetases that recognise the 20 different amino acids. For example: synthetase for Ala attaches it to all 4 Ala tRNAs, in a reaction that utilises ATP.

3. Attachment of the amino acid is to the 3'OH of the A residue ribose sugar in the conserved CCA sequence on tRNA.

4. Energy in this bond utilised later for polypeptide synthesis.

5. Synthetases recognise different characteristics of tRNAs: unusual bases and anticodon, tertiary structure.

PROKARYOTIC AND EUKARYOTIC RIBOSOMES

Ribosomes are complicated structures consisting of ribosomal RNAs and proteins that associate into a precise structure with multiple enzymatic activities. The ribosomes of prokaryotes, eukaryotes and organelles (such as mitochondria) all perform the same function and are structurally quite similar. In evolution, ribosomes from prokaryotes and eukaryotes are unrelated at the protein level, but are highly related at the rRNA level.

General Features in Common Between Eukaryotic and Prokaryotic Ribosomes

- 2 ribosome subunits, a small and large subunit.
- Consist of protein and RNA only.
- Ribosomal RNAs (rRNAs) are highly related between prokaryotes and eukaryotes, whereas ribosomal proteins (r-proteins) are not.
- Enzymatic functions of ribosomes involved in peptide synthesis are associated with rRNAs rather than r-proteins. r-proteins are thought to fine tune and enhance function of rRNAs under physiological conditions.

Bacterial ribosomes	*Eukaryotic ribosomes*
30S and 50S subunits	40S and 60S subunits
30S:21 proteins and 16S rRNA	40S:30 proteins and 18S rRNA
50S:32 proteins and 2 rRNAs	60S:40 proteins and 3 rRNAs
23S and 5S rRNA	28S, 5S and 5.8S rRNA

The functions of ribosomes in translation are primarily associated with rRNAs rather than r-protiens. The rRNAs:

- Function to bring ribosome subunits together.
- Interact with, and position mRNAs (in prokaryotes).
- Bind most translation factors and create enzymatic centers.
- Catalyse peptide bond formation.

Ribosome Structure

Ribosome structure is shown in Fig. 15.3.

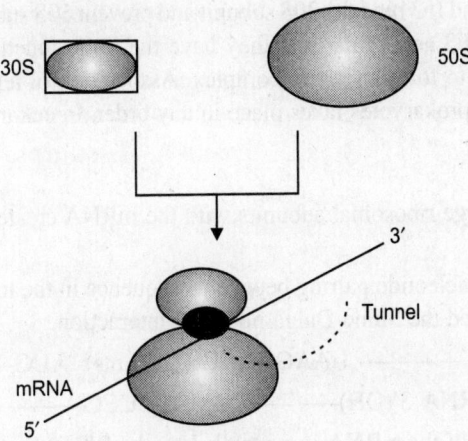

Fig. 15.3: Ribosome structure.

MECHANISM OF PROTEIN SYNTHESIS-OVERVIEW

Protein synthesis can be divided into 6 stages:

1. Amino acid activation: tRNA is charged by covalently linking it to its cognate amino acid.
2. Formation of initiation complexes: Association of mRNA, ribosomal subunits and initiation factors.
3. Initiation of translation: Assembly of stable ribosome complex at the initiation codon.
4. Chain elongation: Polypeptide synthesis by repetitive addition of amino acids to the nascent (growing) chain.
5. Chain termination: Release of nascent polypeptide.
6. Ribosome dissociation: Subunits separate before initiating new round of translation.

INITIATION COMPLEX FORMATION

Initiating tRNA

1. Translation generally initiates with a Met encoded by AUG (prokaryotes and eukaryotes).
2. Special initiating tRNA carries Met to AUG codon.
   - In bacteria the initiating Met is modified, while attached to the tRNA, to contain an N-formyl group. It is referred to as N-formylMet (tRNAf^{met}).
   - The formyl group blocks acceptance of a growing peptide chain.
   - Elongating met-tRNA is distinct (tRNA^{met}), and the Met is not modified. The formyl group is always removed from bacterial proteins.
   - In eukaryotes the initiating Met is not modified (tRNAi^{met}).
   - The initiating Met is removed from roughly half of bacterial proteins, and from some eukaryotic proteins.

Initiation Complex Formation in Prokaryotes

Anti-association factors IF1 and IF3 bind the 30S subunit and prevent 50S subunit association. Eukaryotic initiation factors eIF1 and eIF3 are similar and they have the same functions. 30S subunit associates with tRNAf^{met}, GTP and IF2 to form a ternary complex. Association of ternary complex components, 30S ribosome and mRNA in prokaryotes takes place in any order. In eukaryotes it is highly ordered.

Initiation of Translation

- Joining of small and large ribosomal subunits with the mRNA creates a 70S ribosome initiation complex.
- Initiation is guided by nucleotide pairing between a sequence in the mRNA and the 3′ end of 16S rRNA, in a process called the Shine-Dalgarno (S/D) interaction.

$$mRNA5′——— UAAGGAGG\text{-}(5–10 \text{ nts})\text{-} AUG———$$
$$16S \text{ rRNA } 3′(OH)————\text{-}AUUCCUCC————$$

- The level of translation of the mRNA is controlled by the S/D interaction, which is the extent of complementarity between mRNA:rRNA, and the most optimal AUG position (5-10 nts downstream of the S/D element). This explains why prokaryotic ribosomes can initiate protein synthesis internally. As a consequence, prokaryotic mRNAs are generally multicistronic, encoding more than one polypeptide. This also explains why the ternary complex can form on ribosomes after the subunits associate in prokaryotes, because there is no need for tRNAf^{met} to provide anticodon identification of the initiating AUG.
- In eukaryotes there is no such sequence or S/D interaction (at least routinely). In fact, the Shine Dalgarno sequence is specifically missing from the 3′ end of eukaryotic 18S rRNA. As covered later, eukaryotes initiate translation quite differently.
- The joining of the two ribosome subunits on the mRNA creates two enzymatic regions which direct protein synthesis. This is similar in both eukaryotes and prokaryotes. (i) aminoacyl (A) site: contains IF2-GTP but will contain the incoming tRNA, (ii) peptidyl (P) site: contains tRNAf^{met} but will contain the growing nascent chain.

Specific segments of 16S and 23S rRNAs have been identified that correspond to the A and P sites. Many antibiotics act by binding or blocking rRNA activity within these enzymatic sites.

- Thiostrepton- binds 23S rRNA (residue A1067) and prevents 50S subunit association. Methylation of A1067 provides resistance.
- Puromycin (aminoacyl-tRNA analogue)- blocks domain V of 23S rRNA responsible for peptidyl transferase activity, blocks peptide bond formation.
- Tetracycline- probably binds 16S rRNA at A892, same site that tRNA binds in the A-site.
- Streptomycin- probably binds and blocks activity of 16S rRNA near nt 900. Activity is similar to tetracycline.
- Aminoglycosides (neomycin, gentamicin, kanamycin, hygromycin)- bind specific sites in the A-site contributed by 16S rRNA, prevents translocation of the ribosome along the mRNA. Resistance is associated with mutation of sites in this region.
- Edeine-binds P-site within 16S rRNA, prevents tRNA association with 30S subunit.
- Chloramphenicol and carbomycin- bind domain V loop in 23S rRNA, inhibit peptidyl transferase activity. Resistance is associated with mutation in this region.

Elongation

Elongation is a repetition of these events to form additional peptide bonds while charged tRNAs 'read' the codons. Elongation utilises a charged tRNA and 3 elongation factors, known as EF-Tu, EF-Ts and EF-G.

- The charged tRNA to the A-site as a complex with EF-Tu-GTP.
- GTP hydrolysis releases EF-Tu-GDP, and deposits the charged tRNA at the ribosome.
- EF-TS then recycles EF-Tu-GDP to EF-Tu-GTP.

- A similar GTP recycling scheme appears in eukaryotes for recharging initiation factor eIF2. In eukaryotes, this is the most highly regulated step in protein synthesis and it is a primary site of antiviral action of interferon-α. This is covered below.

Termination and Ribosome Dissociation

- Termination is specified by protein factors, not tRNAs.
- The growing nascent polypeptide is in the P-site.
- The termination codon is in the A-site.
- Several protein releasing factors bind to A-site in the presence of the stop codon (UAA, UGA or UAG), then activate a peptidyl-tRNA hydrolase.
- This activity cleaves the amino acid from the tRNA and releases the polypeptide chain.
- The post-translational ribosome can proceed on the mRNA for an unknown distance, but is thought to ultimately be dissociated by factors IF1/IF3.

EUKARYOTIC INITIATION OF TRANSLATION

There are major differences between prokaryotic and eukaryotic initiation, which leads to different mechanisms for the regulation of protein synthesis. One difference is that in eukaryotes, there is no 'Shine-Dalgarno' interaction typically between the mRNA and 18S rRNA to select the proper protein coding region. Consequently:

- Prokaryotic mRNAs are usually multicistronic. Ribosomes bind prokaryotic mRNAs internally, specified solely by Shine-Dalgarno interactions.
- Eukaryotic mRNAs are generally monocistronic. Eukaryotic ribosomes usually (but not always) initiate translation through a precisely regulated process by scanning from the 5′ end of mRNA, surveying the mRNA for the initiating AUG codon in a nucleotide by nucleotide manner which is highly ordered.

In prokaryotes the components comprising the initiation complex can be individually assembled on the small ribosomal subunit (30S subunit) in any order. In eukaryotes this process follows a precise ordering and is highly regulated.

1. A ternary complex is formed prior to 40S ribosome subunit binding to mRNA:

$$tRNAi^{met} + GTP + eIF2$$

2. The ternary complex binds to the 40S ribosome subunit.
3. Ribosomal 40S subunit binds to a complex of proteins at the 5′ end of capped mRNA.
   - Almost all eukaryotic mRNAs are capped, i.e. contain an inverted ^{7}MethylGTP (m^7GTP) attached to the first nucleotide.
   - The cap is a signal to ribosomes that an mRNA is to be translated.
   - Most uncapped mRNAs are poorly translated, if at all.

A group of initiation factor proteins binds the capped end of the mRNA and directs 40S ribosome-mRNA interaction in eukaryotes. They are collectively known as the cap-initiation complex or factor eIF4F.

- 40S ribosome cannot recognise mRNA without these proteins.
- eIF4F acts as a molecular bridge, bringing the mRNA and the 40S subunit together.
- eIF4F acts as a cap-dependent mRNA helicase, promoting ribosome binding while unwinding the 5′ end of mRNA, permitting the 40S ribosome subunit to search for the initiating AUG codon.

The protein complex eIF4F consists of the cap binding protein eIF4E, the ATP-dependent helicase eIF4A, and the adapter protein eIF4G upon which the complex assembles. Also associated with eIF4F is a protein kinase, Mnk1, that phosphorylates eIF4E, activating initiation of translation. The large initiation factor eIF3 is also associated. eIF3 has many functions in translation, one of which is to bind the 40S ribosome and add the ternary complex. Thus, the 40S ribosome associates with the mRNA through eIF3. Also associated with the eIF4F complex are poly(A) binding protein (PABP), which coats the poly(A) tail on the mRNA, protecting the mRNA from degradation. Interaction of PABP with eIFG is also thought to stimulate initiation. The eIF4F complex, with associated polypeptides, binds the cap, unwinds the 5′ end of the mRNA to promote 40S ribosome loading, and probably propels the 40S ribosome subunit on its scanning search for the initiating AUG codon. The functional implications of the interaction of PABP with the complex are not established, but it is thought to provide a mechanism by which only fully intact mRNAs, processing a cap and polyA tail are translated. The PABP-eIF4G interaction may also facilitate ribosome reinitiation on the mRNA, possibly by tethering the initiation complex and thereby functionally circularising mRNAs during translation. 40S ribosomes normally 'scan' processively from the 5' capped end of the mRNA to the first appropriate AUG, directed by the eIF4F complex. Scanning involves a nucleotide by nucleotide search for the initiation codon (AUG), beginning at the cap of the mRNA. In eukaryotes, the nucleotides flanking the initiation codon contribute to recognition of the start codon by the 40S ribosome and the anticodon of the inititating tRNA. This is known as the AUG context. Poor context is associated with usage of downstream AUGs in better context.

Codon context	Frequency of initiation at AUG
-3 -2 -1 +1 +2 +3 +4	100%
A c c A U G G	
G G	50%
C A/C/U	0-5%
U A/C/U	0-5%

60S large ribosome subunit joins at the AUG

As in prokaryotes, upon 60S ribosome subunit joining, the hydrolysis of GTP and release of eIF2:GDP prepares the ribosome for an incoming aminoacylated tRNA.

Recycling of eIF2:GDP to eIF2:GTP is a highly controlled step in eukaryotic protein synthesis and a primary site of antiviral action of α-interferon. Recycling of GDP to GTP on eIF2 occurs catalytically using recycling factor (RCF) (also called guanine nucleotide exchange factor or GEF). RCF exchanges GDP for GTP on eIF2 (eIF2-GDP $\rightarrow$ eIF2-GTP).

INITIATION OF TRANSLATION IN EUKARYOTES IS HIGHLY REGULATED

The regulation of mRNA translation has evolved in many cell types and tissues to coordinate the levels of different protein products that assemble to form biologically active molecules, and which are required in precise amounts. One of the best studied examples is the regulation of α and β-globin synthesis in red blood cells, which assemble with the molecule heme in the ratio of 2:2:4. This same mechanism of regulation has been exploited by non-red blood cells as the basis for protection against many infecting viruses by the antiviral agent α-interferon.

Regulation of Haemoglobin Synthesis

Red blood cells (RBCs) synthesise large amounts of globin proteins, which account for ~90% of RBC protein synthesis. When heme is in excess of globin proteins, protein synthesis in the RBC is stimulated (which corresponds largely to globin synthesis). When heme levels are low, protein synthesis is inhibited. Under conditions of inhibition, about 30% of the pool of eIF2 is phosphorylated on the alpha subunit (eIF2 contains 3 subunits, α, β, γ). The phosphorylated eIF2(αP) that accumulates is associated with GDP rather than GTP. This indicates that eIF2 is phosphorylated after it participates in protein synthesis, but before the GDP can be exchanged for GTP, which is essential for the participation of eIF2 in translation. The phosphorylation of eIF2 is not the direct cause of inhibition. Rather, eIF2(αP) inactivates the GTP exchange factor RCF. Phosphorylated eIF2(αP)-GDP has a 10-fold higher binding affinity for RCF than non-phosphorylated eIF2(α)-GDP. RCF is only ~1/10-1/20 as abundant as eIF2 in most cells. Therefore, RCF is rapidly sequestered by eIF2(αP)-GDP into inactive complexes, blocking GTP recycling on eIF2 and preventing translation initiation. Thus, the total increase in eIF2 phosphorylation needs to rise by only 30% to shut-off all protein synthesis in the RBC. The kinase that phosphorylates eIF2α is called the heme controlled repressor (HCR). As heme synthesis catches up to globin levels, heme becomes abundant enough to suppress the HCR activity. eIF2(αP) is constitutively dephosphorylated by a phosphatase. The loss of eIF2(αP) liberates RCF which converts eIF2-GDP to eIF2-GTP for protein synthesis once again.

Regulation by Interferon

The same mechanism used to regulate globin synthesis underlies the antiviral action of α-interferon. Non-red blood cells contain a kinase related to HCR, that targets eIF2α as its substrate. The HCR related kinase is not regulated by heme, but is activated by double-stranded RNA (dsRNA). Hence, it is known as protein kinase double-strand RNA regulated, or PKR.

Cells infected by different viruses often synthesise and secrete α-interferon, which in turn stimulates synthesis of PKR in uninfected cells. Activation of PKR is mediated by low levels of dsRNA. Why dsRNA? Most viruses containing DNA genomes have opposing transcription units that are simultaneously active at some point in their life cycles, and therefore generate dsRNA. Other viruses use RNA as a genome, and therefore must generate dsRNA to replicate. Formation of dsRNA is therefore a signal to cells that they are infected by a virus. In uninfected cells, dsRNA is quite rare so the PKR kinase is not activated. Activation of the kinase inhibits all protein synthesis in the cell, both host and virus. Although the cell may die, it destroys the virus in the process. In other cases, the viral RNA or infecting genome may be degraded, removing the source of dsRNA and permitting recovery of the cell. The activity of PKR kinase is such an important control point in translation, and a critical marker of infection to the cell, that many viruses have evolved mechanisms to prevent its activation. PKR activation is inhibited by adenoviruses, pox viruses (Vaccinia virus), influenza viruses, and reoviruses, in some cases utilising similar mechanisms. A great many viruses, however, do not possess mechanisms to inhibit the activation of PKR and remain acutely sensitive to the antiviral effects of interferon α.

Inhibition of PKR by Viruses

Adenovirus has a dsDNA genome with many opposing transcription units. Adenovirus synthesises a small RNA called Virion Associated (VA) RNA I. VA RNA I is a highly structured RNA that lacks a cap, AUG, and polyA tail. VA RNA I binds to PKR and prevent its activation by dsRNA. Vaccinia virus produces two proteins called E3L and K3L. E3L binds dsRNA, scavenging and removing the low levels of dsRNA that are present in a Vaccinia virus infected cell, preventing activation of PKR kinase. The K3L protein mimics the site of eIF2α subunit phosphorylation, binding and sequestering PKR. Vaccinia has evolved a two-pronged strategy for inhibition of PKR activity.

Other eIF2 Kinases

Nutrient deprivation of cells has been shown to inhibit protein synthesis by activation of a third eIF2 kinase known as GCN2. GCN2 is activated by low levels of the amino acid histidine, and in turn phosphorylates eIF2 in the α-subunit, blocking protein synthesis as described above. Oxidative and Other Stresses can activated an eIF2 kinase that resides in the endoplasmic reticulum (ER) known as PERK. PERK detects changes in ER status, including the unfolding of proteins, and inhibits protein synthesis by phosphorylation of the eIF2 α-subunit.

Regulators of Translation Acting on Cap Binding Protein eIF4E

The activity of eIF4E is tightly regulated in cells by distinct mechanisms. The available cellular pool of eIF4E is controlled by inhibitory eIF4E-binding proteins (4EBPs). These proteins bind to the eIF4G binding site of eIF4E, removing eIF4E from eIF4G and blocking initiation of translation. The activity of the 4EBPs (i.e. the ability to bind and sequester eIF4E) is in turn regulated by phosphorylation in response to growth factors including insulin, IGF-1, and angiotensin II (signalling occurs by the PI3-kinase/Akt/mTOR signal transduction pathway). In the presence of activating growth factors, 4EBP phosphorylation increases, thereby lowering the amount bound to eIF4E and therefore stimulating translation.

Regulation of eIF4E Activity

eIF4E is the mRNA 5′ cap-binding component of the eIF4F cap-complex. Its availability is limited by sequestration via the eIF4E binding proteins (4EBPs), which prevent eIF4E interaction with the eIF4G scaffold component. The affinity of 4EBP for eIF4E is greatly diminished by mphosphorylation mediated by mTOR kinase via the cell growth signallingPI3K-Akt pathway. In addition theIF4E kinase, Mnk, activated undconditions of cellular growth, interactswith the eIF4G scaffold and can phosphorylate eIF4E, which may potentiate cap-dependent initiation. The cap-binding activity of eIF4E is also thought to be regulated, although less stringently, by phosphorylation, which occurs on Ser-209. The phosphorylation is catalised by the serine/threonine kinase, Mnk1, which is associated with eIF4G. Generally, increased eIF4E phosphorylation correlates with increased translational activity.

Cellular Transformation and the Control of Protein Synthesis

During malignant transformation, a cell accumulates characteristics necessary for unchecked proliferation and enhanced survivability by means of up-regulation of oncogenes and down-regulation of tumour suppressor genes. One means of control of proto-oncogene and tumour suppressor gene expression is regulation of protein synthesis. Modifications in the translational apparatus of cells, particularly changes in several initiation and elongation factors, are associated with malignant transformation and the acquisition of transformed and oncogenic properties of tumour cells. Cells that are highly transformed generally show higher rates of protein synthesis as compared with non-transformed, quiescent cells. Up-regulation of protein synthesis may promote critical aspects of tumour progression, such as angiogenesis (induced growth of new blood vessels and revascularisation to tumours), metabolic adaptation, and invasiveness, or there may be specific components or pathways that are selectively up-regulated to achieve these responses. Initiation factor related to Cancer is shown in Table 15.1.

Table 15.1: Initiation factor related to cancer.

Initiation factor	Cancer
eIF4E	Up-regulated in some invasive ductal breast cancers, head and neck carcinomas, lymphomas, bladder carcinomas, colon carcinomas
eIF4A	Up-regulated in some melanomas, hepatocellular carcinomas
eIF4G	Up-regulated in squamous cell lung carcinomas, breast cancers
eIF2α	Up-regulated in lymphomas, gastro-intestinal carcinomas
eIF2B	Up-regulated in breast carcinomas

Several specific components of the protein synthesis machinery have been significantly associated with malignant transformation of cells. Elevated cellular levels of protein synthesis initiation factors, particularly eIF4E and eIF4G, have been implicated as promoters of malignancy and suppression of apoptosis (programmed cell death) which generally limit tumour invasiveness. In addition to the components of the eIF4F-cap dependent initiation complex, other key components of translational initiation have been cited for potential roles in transformation.

PROTEIN DEGRADATION

The newly synthesised proteins are folded and glycosylated in the ER in preparation for their transport to other organelles. However, life is not always perfect in the ER: proteins may turn out to have mutations that prevent proper folding, or poisonous compounds may inhibit glycosylation. Similarly, some of the proteins in the cytoplasm may also be misfolded, or damaged by oxygen radicals or other compounds, and aggregate. If all this junk is allowed to accumulate, the cell would die. Therefore, the cell rapidly breaks such protein down. Hence a need for a proteolysis pathway. In addition to removal of misfolded proteins, proteolysis is also important in recycling or turnover of proteins and amino acids, as well as regulation of processes such as cell cycle, transcription, cell signalling, and apoptosis.

Proteolysis takes place primarily in the cytoplasm. So why don't 'normal' cytosolic proteins get chewed up? The first reason is that protein degradation occurs in defined compartments that are excluded from the cytosol. Secondly, proteins that are destined to be degraded are often marked. We'll look at the organelles or machines involved in protein degradation, and then see how ER proteins, which are excluded from the cytosol, get degraded.

Lysosomes

The lysosome is a membrane bound organelle that contains enzymes involved in the degradation of a variety of substances. Lysosomes are the main organelle for the degradation of extracellular materials, which are collected by endocytosis, which will be discussed in detail in later lectures. Lysosomes also digest entire organelles or parts of the cytoplasm that are engulfed in a process known as autophagy. There is yet a third, more specific process. During stress situations such as starvation, there is a large turnover of proteins in the cell. Studies have shown that RNase A, and other cytosolic proteins bearing the amino acids sequence KFERQ, are directly and selectively transported to the lysosome for degradation.

About 40–50 acid hydrolases reside in the lysosome. In addition to proteases, there are nucleases, glycosylases, lipases, phospholipases, etc. They are acid hydrolases because their optimal pH for activity is about 5, which is the pH inside lysosomes. The cell is smart in that if a lysosome accidentally ruptures and releases its contents to the cytosol, the cell won't be chewed up, because the enzymes will not be active. If you isolate lysosomes, and put them in a test tube with solution that has ADP and Pi, ATP is made and the pH of the solution goes up. What does this tell you? As you could guess by now, the internal pH is maintained by a proton pump that derives its energy through ATP hydrolysis. This pump is formally known as the vesicular ATPase, or VATPase. A variety of proteases exists inside the lysosome. These include carboxypeptidase, aminopeptidase, and endopeptidase. Most of them belong to the class they also have a catalytic triad, this time consisting of Cys-His-Asn. Lysosome is also discussed in detail in Chapter 22.

Ubiquitin-Proteasome Pathway

This is the major pathway by which cytosolic proteins are selectively degraded during normal metabolic growth. As mentioned, it is also very important for regulation of processes such as cell cycle control and cell signalling.

Ubiquitination

The first step is the attachment of a signal/flag to the protein that is to be degraded. In this case the signal is a polyubiquitin chain. Ubiquitin is a 72 amino acids polypeptide that is very abundant, as its name suggests.

Linkage of ubiquitin to the 'condemned' protein occurs in 3 enzyme-catalysed steps.

1. E1- ubiquitin – a thioester bond is formed between the C-terminal amino acids of ubiquitin and an internal Cys residue of E1, the ubiquitin activating enzyme. This is an ATP dependent process.

2. E2- ubiquitin – an exchange reaction occurs, and the ubiquitin is transferred to a sulphydryl group on E2, the ubiquitin-conjugating enzyme. The thioester bond is preserved and no ATP is required in this reaction.

3. E2-ubiquitin then interacts with E3, to which the substrate is specifically bound. E3 is known as the ubiquitin-protein ligase. It transfers the activated ubiquitin to the ε-NH_2 group on a lysine residue in the protein substrate, thus establishing an amide linkage. In subsequent reactions, additional ubiquitin molecules are added to an ε-NH2 group on a lysine residue of the previously conjugated ubiquitin molecule to form a multiubiquitin chain linked by isopeptide bonds.

The specificity of the system is conferred primarily by E3. To date there are 4 main classes that have been identified.

1. *N*-end rule E3s. The residue at the N-terminus of proteins affect their half-lives. E3a is one of the E3s that have been identified. It has two distinct sites that recognise either basic (type1) or bulky-hydrophobic (type 2) residues. It also recognises other non-*N*-end rule substrates via its 'body site'.

2. HECT-domain E3s. (Homologous to the E6-AP C-terminus). E6-AP is a cellular protein that forms a complex with the human papillomavirus protein E6 (thus AP=associated protein). Together they act like an E3 to target p53, a tumour suppressor protein in the cell, for degradation. The conserved HECT domain is in the C-terminus of these E3s, and has catalytic function, and an invariable Cys residue. The *N*-terminus of HECT-domain E3s is not highly conserved. Rsp5 is an example of a HECT-domain E3. It contains a calcium-binding domain, C2, and 3 WW domains in the amino-terminal two-thirds of the protein. The WW domains are in part responsible for substrate recognition.

3. Cyclosome/APC (anaphase promoting complex). Cyclosomes are inactive during interphase. They are activated by a mitotic kinase. When phosphorylated, they specifically recognise cell-cycle regulators such as mitotic cyclins that contain a 9 amino acids motif termed the destruction box. While *N*-end rule and HECT-domain E3s are single polypeptides, the cyclosome has several subunits. Cells that have mutations in any of these subunits fail to degrade B-type cyclins, cannot complete or exit from mitosis.

4. Phosphoprotein-ubiquitin ligase complexes. These complexes also degrade cell cycle regulators. However, their substrates need to be phosphorylated before these E3s will recognise them. While certain subunits in these complexes are invariant, others can be swapped to alter the substrate specificity.

Proteasome

Structure: The core of the proteasome is a 20S complex composed of 4 stacked rings. There are 2β rings on the inside and 2 α rings on the outside. Each ring is composed of 7 subunits. A central channel is present in the 20S complex. This arrangement is reminiscent of GroEL. The opening at the top created by the alpha subunits is about 13 Å and is just big enough for an unfolded chain to enter. The 19S Cap complex normally sits on top of the alpha ring, rather like GroES. The 19S cap consists of more than 15 subunits, including ATPases. The functions of the 19S complex includes recognition of condemned proteins via the ubiquitin chain (another way to prevent the accidental degradation of cytoplasmic proteins), release and subsequent hydrolysis of the ubiquitin chain, unfolding of the condemned polypeptide, and translocation of the unfolded protein into 20S. It may also control the exit of degradation products. The step(s) that require energy has not been clearly demonstrated, though it is highly likely that both unfolding of the protein and its translocation are coupled to ATP hydrolysis. Even though the α and β subunits are closely related in sequence, only the β subunits have protease activity. Chymotrypsin-like, trypsin-like protease activity, and an activity that cleaves after glutamate residues have been identified. As the polypeptide is fed through the 20S complex, it gets degraded by the β subunits, and peptides of 7–10 amino acids are released from the proteasome. Thus, the architecture of the proteasome machine segregates the proteolytic component from the cytoplasm, and also prevents cytosolic proteins from accidentally falling in and getting degraded. An inhibitor of the proteasome has been identified. It is called lactacystin. Studies using this inhibitor showed that most cytosolic proteins are degraded by the proteasome.

ER Proteins

So far we've seen that proteolysis in the cell takes place in the cytoplasm, albeit in structurally confined spaces. Are there proteases in the ER that degrade misfolded proteins? If so, how are they separated from resident and newly synthesised proteins? Are there proteasomes in the ER? These large structures have never been observed in the ER. Studies of human cytomegalovirus (HCMV) suggest that proteins that aren't properly folded, or not glycosylated correctly are secreted out of the ER by retrograde transport. When most viruses infect a cell, the cell responds by putting some of the foreign protein on a flagpole on the surface of the cell to tell T cells to come kill it. These flagpoles are known as major histocompatibility (MHC) antigens. MHC class I heavy chains bind to peptides of about 7–9 amino acids (yes, you guessed it, produced by the proteasome) and its partner β2-microglobulin. This complex is transported to the surface of the cell. In HCMV infected cells, the heavy chains are co-translationally transported into the ER and glycosylated, as in normal uninfected cells, but then are quickly deglycosylated, transported back to the cytoplasm and degraded. This degradation is inhibited by lactacystin, suggesting the proteasome is involved. Furthermore, researchers have been able to detect an association between Sec61p and the heavy chain. Since proteasomes have also been observed to be closely associated with ER membranes, one model is that retrograde transport of errant polypeptides from the ER is tightly coupled to degradation by the proteasome. How the ER distinguishes a protein that is in the process of folding from those that are not able to fold, and how these errant proteins are delivered to the translocation machinery to be exported back to the cytoplasm is not known.

Unfolded Protein Response

What we do know is an interesting phenomenon known as the unfolded protein response (UPR). When a lot of 'junk' proteins accumulate in the cell, for example by treating cells with reducing agents, or by preventing glycosylation, the ER sends out a signal that upregulates resident ER proteins. These include BiP, protein disulphide isomerase, and peptidyl-prolyl isomerase, which as you learnt last time, help proper folding of proteins. The mechanism by which this response is mediated is very interesting. All the genes that are upregulated in the UPR have a *cis*-acting element in their control region that is bound by the transcription factor HAC1. During normal growth, HAC1 is produced but quickly degraded by the ubiquitin/proteasome pathway. However, during UPR, the mRNA of HAC1 is spliced and produces a stable protein that can then upregulate the response genes. It turns out that an ER transmembrane protein, Ire1p, somehow senses the abundance of junk in the ER. The cytosolic side of this protein is partly a serine/threonine kinase, and partly an endoribonuclease. Ire1p is responsible for cleaving the HAC1 mRNA, which is then ligated by RLG1, a tRNA ligase.

Chapter 16

Translation of mRNA

INTRODUCTION

The control of mRNA translation plays a key role in regulating gene expression under a wide range of circumstances in eukaryotic cells, and to a lesser extent in bacteria. The field has grown enormously in recent years. This chapter discusses a general overview of the types of translational regulation which occur, discuss some of the situations in which it is important and outline some of the mechanisms by which it is achieved. Controlling translation offers advantages over other levels of control of gene expression under particular conditions, as follows.

REGULATION OF mRNA TRANSLATION

Rapidity of Response

Where cells need to increase rapidly the synthesis of particular proteins, the ability to up-regulate the translation of pre-existing mRNAs clearly allows the cell to start to make the corresponding protein without a requirement to activate transcription, process the resulting transcript and transport it to the cytoplasm. Such situations include stimulation by mitogens, growth factors and hormones, and also responses to nutrient availability and to certain stressful conditions. Examples of these kinds of control are discussed in detail later.

Independence from Transcription

The ability to control translation is essential where there is little or no ongoing transcription, for example, in early development of a number of organisms, where transcription is essentially switched off, and in cells which have no functional nucleus. One example of the latter is the mammalian reticulocyte. Globin production is regulated by haemin, but since reticulocytes lack a functional nucleus, regulation of transcription is not an option and translation is the control point.

Localised Protein Expression

If a protein is only required at a specific location in the cell, this can be achieved in various ways. Firstly, the mRNA can be localised within the cell. Secondly, the protein can be made throughout the cell and

223

then transported to its destination. A third option is to localise the translation of the mRNA, which may itself be present widely in the cell. Important examples of the first and third options play key roles in controlling gene expression during development, e.g. to generate intracellular gradients of proteins involved in specifying cell polarity.

Protein Synthesis as an Anabolic Process

Activation of protein synthesis is also an important response to stimuli which regulate cell growth. For example, insulin promotes protein synthesis and anabolic processes such as glycogen storage in a variety of tissues and cell types. The effect of such stimuli on protein metabolism is, of course, a balance between its effects on protein synthesis and degradation.

BIOLOGICAL ROLES OF ncRNA

Noncoding RNAs belong to several groups and are involved in many cellular processes. These range from ncRNAs of central importance that are conserved across all or most cellular life through to more transient ncRNAs specific to one or a few closely related species. The more conserved ncRNAs are thought to be molecular fossils or relics from LUCA and the RNA world, some suggest a viral origin.

ncRNAs in Translation

Many of the conserved, essential and abundant ncRNAs are involved in translation. Ribonucleoprotein (RNP) particles called ribosomes are the 'factories' where translation takes place in the cell. The ribosome consists of more than 60 per cent ribosomal RNA, these are made up of 3 ncRNAs in prokaryotes and 4 ncRNAs in eukaryotes. Ribosomal RNAs catalyse the translation of nucleotide sequences to protein. Another set of ncRNAs, Transfer RNAs, form an 'adaptor molecule' between mRNA and protein. The H/ACA box and C/D box snoRNAs are ncRNAs found in archaea and eukaryotes, RNase MRP is restricted to eukaryotes, both groups of ncRNA are involved in the maturation of rRNA. The snoRNAs guide covalent modifications of rRNA, tRNA and snRNAs, RNase MRP cleaves the internal transcribed spacer 1 between 18S and 5.8S rRNAs. The ubiquitous ncRNA, RNase P, is an evolutionary relative of RNase MRP. RNase P matures tRNA sequences by generating mature 5′-ends of tRNAs through cleaving the 5′-leader elements of precursor-tRNAs. Another ubiquitous RNP called SRP recognises and transports specific nascent proteins to the endoplasmic reticulum in eukaryotes and the plasma membrane in prokaryotes. In bacteria transfer-messenger RNA (tmRNA) is an RNP involved in rescuing stalled ribosomes, tagging incomplete polypeptides and promoting the degradation of aberrant mRNA (Fig. 16.1).

ncRNAs in RNA Splicing

In eukaryotes the spliceosome performs the splicing reactions essential for removing intron sequences, this process is required for the formation of mature mRNA. The spliceosome is another RNP often also known as the snRNP or tri-snRNP. There are two different forms of the spliceosome, the major and minor forms. The ncRNA components of the major spliceosome are U1, U2, U4 and U5. The ncRNA components of the minor spliceosome are U11, U12, U5, U4atac and U6atac. Another group of introns can catalyse their own removal from host transcripts, these are called self-splicing RNAs. There are two main groups of self-splicing RNAs, these are the group I catalytic intron and group II catalytic intron. These ncRNAs catalyse their own excision from mRNA, tRNA and rRNA precursors in a wide range of organisms. In mammals it has been found that snoRNAs can also regulate the alternative splicing of mRNA, for example snoRNA HBII-52 regulates the splicing of serotonin receptor 2C. In nematodes the SmY ncRNA appears to be involved in mRNA *trans*-splicing.

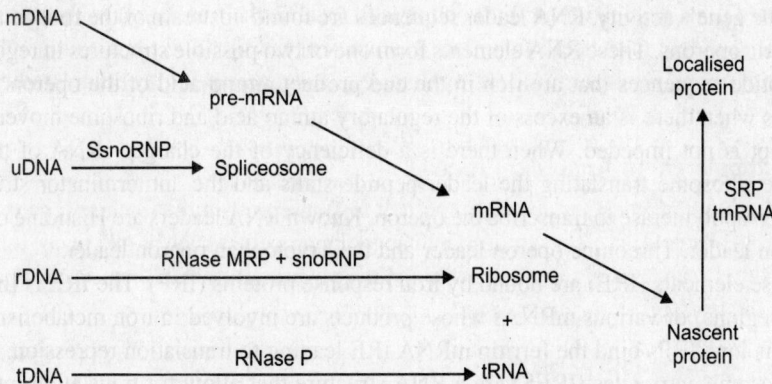

Fig. 16.1: An illustration of the central dogma of molecular biology annotated with the processes ncRNAs are involved in.

ncRNAs in Gene Regulation

The expression of many thousands of genes are regulated by ncRNAs. This regulation can occur in *trans* or in *cis*.

Trans-acting ncRNAs

In higher eukaryotes MicroRNAs regulate gene expression. A single miRNA can reduce the expression levels of hundreds of genes. The mechanism by which mature miRNA molecules act is through partial complementary to one or more messenger RNA (mRNA) molecules, generally in 3′ UTRs. The main function of miRNAs is to down-regulate gene expression.

The ncRNA RNase P has also been shown to influence gene expression. In the human nucleus RNase P is required for the normal and efficient transcription of various ncRNAs transcribed by RNA polymerase III. These include tRNA, 5S rRNA, SRP RNA and U6 snRNA genes. RNase P exerts its role in transcription through association with Pol III and chromatin of active tRNA and 5S rRNA genes.

It has been shown that 7SK RNA, a metazoan ncRNA, acts as a negative regulator of the RNA polymerase II elongation factor P-TEFb, and that this activity is influenced by stress response pathways.

The bacterial ncRNA, 6S RNA, specifically associates with RNA polymerase holoenzyme containing the sigma70 specificity factor. This interaction represses expression from a sigma70-dependent promoter during stationary phase. Another bacterial ncRNA, OxyS RNA represses translation by binding to Shine-Dalgarno sequences thereby occluding ribosome binding. OxyS RNA is induced in response to oxidative stress in *Escherichia coli*. The B2 RNA is a small noncoding RNA polymerase III transcript that represses mRNA transcription in response to heat shock in mouse cells. B2 RNA inhibits transcription by binding to core Pol II. Through this interaction, B2 RNA assembles into preinitiation complexes at the promoter and blocks RNA synthesis. A recent study has shown that just the act of transcription of ncRNA sequence can have an influence on gene expression. RNA polymerase II transcription of ncRNAs is required for chromatin remodelling in the *Schizosaccharomyces pombe*. Chromatin is progressively converted to an open configuration, as several species of ncRNAs are transcribed.

Cis-acting ncRNAs

A number of ncRNAs are embedded in the 5′ UTRs of protein coding genes and influence their expression in various ways. For example, a riboswitch can directly bind a small target molecule, the binding of the target affects the gene's activity. RNA leader sequences are found upstream of the first gene of in amino acid biosynthetic operons. These RNA elements form one of two possible structures in regions encoding very short peptide sequences that are rich in the end product amino acid of the operon. A terminator structure forms when there is an excess of the regulatory amino acid and ribosome movement over the leader transcript is not impeded. When there is a deficiency of the charged tRNA of the regulatory amino acid the ribosome translating the leader peptide stalls and the antiterminator structure forms. This allows RNA polymerase to transcribe the operon. Known RNA leaders are Histidine operon leader, Leucine operon leader, Threonine operon leader and the Tryptophan operon leader.

Iron response elements (IRE) are bound by iron response proteins (IRP). The IRE is found in UTRs (untranslated regions) of various mRNAs whose products are involved in iron metabolism. When iron concentration is low, IRPs bind the ferritin mRNA IRE leading to translation repression.

Internal ribosome entry sites (IRES) are a RNA structure that allow for translation initiation in the middle of a mRNA sequence as part of the process of protein synthesis.

ncRNAs and Genome Defense

Piwi-interacting RNAs (piRNAs) expressed in mammalian testes and somatic cells, they form RNA-protein complexes with Piwi proteins. These piRNA complexes (piRCs) have been linked to transcriptional gene silencing of retrotransposons and other genetic elements in germ line cells, particularly those in spermatogenesis. Clustered Regularly Interspaced Short Palindromic Repeats (CRISPR) are repeats found in the DNA of many bacteria and archaea. The repeats are separated by spacers of similar length. It has been demonstrated that these spacers can be derived from phage and subsequently help protect the cell from infection.

ncRNAs and Chromosome Structure

Telomerase is an RNP enzyme that adds specific DNA sequence repeats ('TTAGGG' in vertebrates) to telomeric regions, which are found at the ends of eukaryotic chromosomes. The telomeres contain condensed DNA material, giving stability to the chromosomes. The enzyme is a reverse transcriptase that carries telomerase RNA, which is used as a template when it elongates telomeres, which are shortened after each replication cycle. Xist (X-inactive-specific transcript) is a long ncRNA gene on the X chromosome of the placental mammals that acts as major effector of the X chromosome inactivation process forming Barr bodies. An antisense RNA, Tsix, is a negative regulator of Xist. X chromosomes lacking Tsix expression (and thus having high levels of Xist transcription) are inactivated more frequently than normal chromosomes. In drosophilids, which also use an XY sex-determination system, the roX (RNA on the X) RNAs are involved in dosage compensation. Both Xist and roX operate by epigenetic regulation of transcription through the recruitment of histone-modifying enzymes.

Bifunctional RNA

Bifunctional RNAs are RNAs that have two distinct functions, these are also known as dual function RNAs. The majority of the known bifunctional RNAs are both mRNAs that encode a protein and ncRNAs. However there are also a growing number of ncRNAs that fall into two different ncRNA categories, e.g. H/ACA box snoRNA and miRNA. Two well known examples of bifunctional RNAs are SgrS RNA and RNAIII. However, a handful of other bifunctional RNAs are known to exist, e.g. SRA (Steroid Receptor Activator), VegT RNA, Oskar RNA and enod40.

ncRNAs and Disease

As with proteins, mutations or imbalances in the ncRNA repertoire within the body can cause a variety of diseases.

Cancer

Many ncRNAs show abnormal expression patterns in cancerous tissues. These include miRNAs, long mRNA-like ncRNAs, GAS5, SNORD50, telomerase RNA and Y RNAs. The miRNAs are involved in the large scale regulation of many protein coding genes, the Y RNAs are important for the initiation of DNA replication, telomerase RNA that serves as a primer for telomerase, an RNP that extends telomeric regions at chromosome ends (see telomeres and disease for more information). The direct function of the long mRNA-like ncRNAs is less clear.

Germ-line mutations in miR-16-1 and miR-15 primary precursors have been shown to be much more frequent in patients with chronic lymphocytic leukemia compared to control populations.

It has been suggested that a rare SNP (rs11614913) that overlaps hsa-mir-196a2 has been found to be associated with non-small cell lung carcinoma. Likewise, a screen of 17 miRNAs that have been predicted to regulate a number of breast cancer associated genes found variations in the microRNAs miR-17 and miR-30c-1, these patients were noncarriers of BRCA1 or BRCA2 mutations, lending the possibility that familial breast cancer may be caused by variation in these miRNAs.

Prader–Willi syndrome

The deletion of the 48 copies of the C/D box snoRNA SNORD116 has been shown to be the primary cause of Prader–Willi syndrome. Prader–Willi is a developmental disorder associated with overeating and learning difficulties. SNORD116 has potential target sites within a number of protein-coding genes, and could have a role in regulating alternative splicing.

Autism

The chromosomal locus containing the small nucleolar RNA SNORD115 gene cluster has been duplicated in approximately 5 per cent of individuals with autistic traits. A mouse model engineered to have a duplication of the SNORD115 cluster displays autistic-like behaviour.

Cartilage-hair hypoplasia

Mutations within RNase MRP have been shown to cause cartilage-hair hypoplasia, a disease associated with an array of symptoms such as short stature, sparse hair, skeletal abnormalities and a suppressed immune system that is frequent among Amish and Finnish. The best characterised variant is an A-to-G transition at nucleotide 70 that is in a loop region two bases 5' of a conserved pseudoknot. However, many other mutations within RNase MRP also cause CHH.

The antisense RNA, BACE1-AS is transcribed from the opposite strand to BACE1 and is upregulated in patients with Alzheimer's disease. BACE1-AS regulates the expression of BACE1 by increasing BACE1 mRNA stability and generating additional BACE1 through a post-transcriptional feed-forward mechanism. By the same mechanism it also raises concentrations of beta amyloid, the main constituent of senile plaques. BACE1-AS concentrations are elevated in subjects with Alzheimer's disease and in amyloid precursor protein transgenic mice.

miR-96 and hearing loss

Variation within the seed region of mature miR-96 has been associated with autosomal dominant, progressive hearing loss in humans and mice. The homozygous mutant mice were profoundly deaf, showing no cochlear responses. Heterozygous mice and humans progressively lose the ability to hear.

Distinction between Functional RNA (fRNA) and ncRNA

Several publications have started using the term functional RNA (fRNA), as opposed to ncRNA, to describe regions functional at the RNA level that may or may not be stand-alone RNA transcripts. Therefore, every ncRNA is a fRNA, but there exist fRNA (such as riboswitches, SECIS elements, and other *cis*-regulatory regions) that are not ncRNA. Yet the term fRNA could also include mRNA as this is RNA coding for protein and hence is functional. Additionally artificially evolved RNAs also fall under the fRNA umbrella term. Some publications state that the terms ncRNA and fRNA are nearly synonymous.

Localised mRNA Translation during Development

During early development, embryos must begin to define crucial developmental features such as their anterior and posterior poles. The regulation of the translation of certain maternal mRNAs is known to play a key role in this process, which has been studied most intensively in the fruit fly, *Drosophila melanogaster*. Nanos protein is required for specification of the anterior–posterior axis in *Drosophila* embryos. Prior to fertilisation of the egg, Nanos mRNA is present but is not translated. Translation of Nanos requires another protein, Oskar, which both localises the Nanos mRNA to the posterior pole and permits its localised translation (Fig. 16.2). Oskar protein is made prior to fertilisation and this depends on localisation of Oskar mRNA to the posterior pole. Nanos regulates the translation of another mRNA (for Hunchback) by binding, together with a further protein Pumilio, to sequences in the 3′-UTR of the Hunchback mRNA and repressing its translation. Since levels of Nanos protein are higher towards the posterior pole of the embryo, Hunchback translation occurs primarily towards the anterior pole of the developing embryo. This leads to the accumulation of Nanos and Hunchback proteins in opposing concentration gradients (Fig. 16.2), with Hunchback protein accumulating at the anterior end of the embryo, where it represses transcription of abdomen-specific genes.

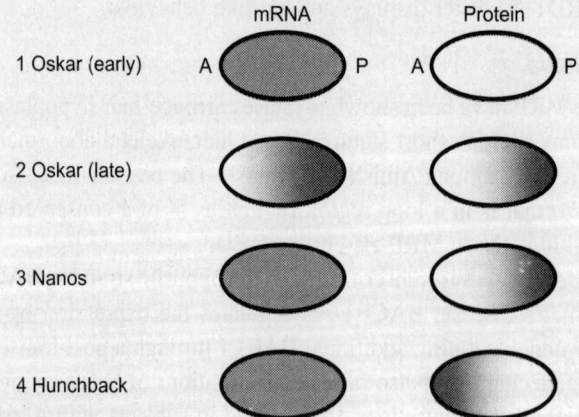

Fig. 16.2: Translational control during early development: localised translation of specific mRNAs creates concentration gradients of proteins involved in determining cell polarity. Intensity of shading indicates the absence or presence of a concentration gradient and its polarity. A, anterior pole, P, posterior pole.

These translation control mechanisms underlie the acquisition of anterior–posterior polarity. Their importance for normal development of the embryo is underlined by the observation that disruption of the control of Nanos translation, for example, results in abnormal patterning of the embryo, resulting, in the most severe cases, in the formation of two complete posterior abdomens in mirror-image with each other.

Other Types of Translational Control during Development

Two further ways in which the translation of specific mRNAs is regulated during development involve unmasking and cytoplasmic polyadenylation. Unmasking refers to the fact that some mRNAs, whose translation is turned on at specific stages during gametogenesis or embryonic development, appear to be sequestered as inactive messenger ribonucleoprotein complexes at earlier times. In other words, their translation is repressed by binding to proteins which dissociate at the appropriate time, thus allowing the mRNA to be translated. How is the association of these proteins with their mRNA partners regulated? Little is known about this beyond the fact that several such proteins are phosphoproteins suggesting that changes in their phosphorylation states may regulate mRNA binding.

It is widely accepted that the 3'-poly(A) tail plays a key role in controlling the translation of certain mRNAs during gametogenesis and embryogenesis. Increased poly(A) tail length favours translation. The tails of a number of mRNAs are lengthened when they become translationally active, and when mRNAs with different tail lengths were microinjected into cells, those with long tails were found to be translated better. Tail length is regulated through the opposing actions of adenylating and deadenylating enzymes. How this is controlled is unclear, but sequences in the 3'-UTR are important in modulating tail length. How do longer tails facilitate mRNA translation? Recent data show that the 3'- and 5'-ends of mRNAs are brought together by the interaction of the poly(A)-binding protein (PABP) with eIF4F. This may explain how tail length (and indeed proteins bound to the 3'-UTR) can influence the translation initiation events occurring at the 5' end of the mRNA.

To sum up, many mechanisms exist to regulate mRNA translation in eukaryotic organisms, and that control of mRNA translation plays an important role in regulating gene expression in response to varied stimuli and in diverse physiological situations. These mechanisms involve control of translation factors or components of the ribosome, or of proteins which interact with the 5'- or 3'-UTRs of the mRNA. A common feature of these mechanisms is that many, if not most, involve protein phosphorylation/dephosphorylation. Many aspects still require clarification. How do the proteins which interact with the 3'-UTR exert their varied effects upon translation and poly(A) tail length (and on also mRNA stability, not discussed here)? How do the protein factors and RNA molecules really function at the molecular level in the process of mRNA translation and its control? An understanding of this requires knowledge of their three-dimensional structures and it is thus highly significant that the last 2–3 years have seen the determination of the structures of several translation factors. The signalling pathways linking the control of translation factors to cellular cues also remain to be elucidated in many cases, especially for the regulation by nutrients such as amino acids. Thirdly, there are undoubtedly many more mRNA-binding proteins awaiting discovery, for example those that interact with the 5'-UTR.

ALZHEIMER'S DISEASE

Alzheimer's disease (Fig. 16.3) is an irreversible, progressive brain disorder that slowly destroys memory and thinking skills and, eventually, the ability to carry out the simplest tasks. In most people with Alzheimer's, symptoms first appear in their mid-60s. Estimates vary, but experts suggest that more than 5 million Americans may have Alzheimer's. Alzheimer's disease is currently ranked as the sixth leading

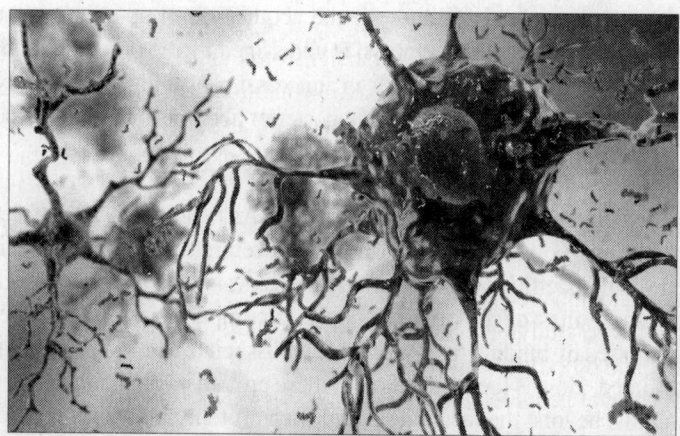

Fig. 16.3: Alzheimer's disease.

cause of death in the United States, but recent estimates indicate that the disorder may rank third, just behind heart disease and cancer, as a cause of death for older people.

Alzheimer's is the most common cause of dementia among older adults. Dementia is the loss of cognitive functioning—thinking, remembering, and reasoning—and behavioural abilities to such an extent that it interferes with a person's daily life and activities. Dementia ranges in severity from the mildest stage, when it is just beginning to affect a person's functioning, to the most severe stage, when the person must depend completely on others for basic activities of daily living. The causes of dementia can vary, depending on the types of brain changes that may be taking place. Other dementias include Lewy body dementia, frontotemporal disorders, and vascular dementia. It is common for people to have mixed dementia—a combination of two or more disorders, at least one of which is dementia. For example, some people have both Alzheimer's disease and vascular dementia. Alzheimer's disease is named after Dr. Alois Alzheimer. In 1906, Dr. Alzheimer noticed changes in the brain tissue of a woman who had died of an unusual mental illness. Her symptoms included memory loss, language problems, and unpredictable behaviour. After she died, he examined her brain and found many abnormal clumps (now called amyloid plaques) and tangled bundles of fibres (now called neurofibrillary, or tau, tangles). These plaques and tangles in the brain are still considered some of the main features of Alzheimer's disease. Another feature is the loss of connections between nerve cells (neurons) in the brain. Neurons transmit messages between different parts of the brain, and from the brain to muscles and organs in the body.

Changes in the Brain

Scientists continue to unravel the complex brain changes involved in the onset and progression of Alzheimer's disease. It seems likely that damage to the brain starts a decade or more before memory and other cognitive problems appear. During this preclinical stage of Alzheimer's disease, people seem to be symptom-free, but toxic changes are taking place in the brain. Abnormal deposits of proteins form amyloid plaques and tau tangles throughout the brain. Once healthy neurons stop functioning and lose connections with other neurons, they die. The damage initially appears to take place in the hippocampus, the part of the brain essential in forming memories. As more neurons die, additional parts of the brain are affected, and they begin to shrink. By the final stage of Alzheimer's, damage is widespread, and brain volume has shrunk significantly.

Signs and symptoms

Memory problems are typically one of the first signs of cognitive impairment related to Alzheimer's disease. Some people with memory problems have a condition called mild cognitive impairment (MCI). In MCI, people have more memory problems than normal for their age, but their symptoms do not interfere with their everyday lives. Movement difficulties and problems with the sense of smell have also been linked to MCI. Older people with MCI are at greater risk for developing Alzheimer's, but not all of them do. Some may even go back to normal cognition. The first symptoms of Alzheimer's vary from person to person. For many, decline in non-memory aspects of cognition, such as word-finding, vision/spatial issues, and impaired reasoning or judgment, may signal the very early stages of Alzheimer's disease. Researchers are studying biomarkers (biological signs of disease found in brain images, cerebrospinal fluid, and blood) to see if they can detect early changes in the brains of people with MCI and in cognitively normal people who may be at greater risk for Alzheimer's disease. Studies indicate that such early detection may be possible, but more research is needed before these techniques can be relied upon to diagnose Alzheimer's disease in everyday medical practice.

Mild Alzheimer's disease

As Alzheimer's disease progresses, people experience greater memory loss and other cognitive difficulties. Problems can include wandering and getting lost, trouble handling money and paying bills, repeating questions, taking longer to complete normal daily tasks, and personality and behaviour changes. People are often diagnosed at this stage.

Moderate Alzheimer's disease

In this stage, damage occurs in areas of the brain that control language, reasoning, sensory processing, and conscious thought. Memory loss and confusion grow worse, and people begin to have problems recognising family and friends. They may be unable to learn new things, carry out multistep tasks such as getting dressed, or cope with new situations. In addition, people at this stage may have hallucinations, delusions, and paranoia and may behave impulsively.

Severe Alzheimer's disease

Ultimately, plaques and tangles spread throughout the brain, and brain tissue shrinks significantly. People with severe Alzheimer's cannot communicate and are completely dependent on others for their care. Near the end, the person may be in bed most or all of the time as the body shuts down.

Causes of Alzheimer's Disease

Scientists don't yet fully understand what causes Alzheimer's disease in most people. In people with early-onset Alzheimer's, a genetic mutation is usually the cause. Late-onset Alzheimer's arises from a complex series of brain changes that occur over decades. The causes probably include a combination of genetic, environmental, and lifestyle factors. The importance of any one of these factors in increasing or decreasing the risk of developing Alzheimer's may differ from person to person.

Basics of Alzheimer's Disease

Scientists are conducting studies to learn more about plaques, tangles, and other biological features of Alzheimer's disease. Advances in brain imaging techniques allow researchers to see the development and spread of abnormal amyloid and tau proteins in the living brain, as well as changes in brain structure and function. Scientists are also exploring the very earliest steps in the disease process by studying changes in the brain and body fluids that can be detected years before Alzheimer's symptoms appear. Findings from these studies will help in understanding the causes of Alzheimer's and make diagnosis easier. One of the great mysteries of Alzheimer's disease is why it largely strikes older adults. Research on normal brain aging is shedding light on this question. For example, scientists are learning how age-related changes in the brain may harm neurons and contribute to Alzheimer's damage. These age-related changes include atrophy (shrinking) of certain parts of the brain, inflammation, production of unstable molecules called free radicals, and mitochondrial dysfunction (a breakdown of energy production within a cell).

Genetics

Most people with Alzheimer's have the late-onset form of the disease, in which symptoms become apparent in their mid-60s. The apolipoprotein E (APOE) gene is involved in late-onset Alzheimer's. This gene has several forms. One of them, APOE e4, increases a person's risk of developing the disease and is also associated with an earlier age of disease onset. However, carrying the APOE e4 form of the gene does not mean that a person will definitely develop Alzheimer's disease, and some people with no APOE e4 may also develop the disease.

Also, scientists have identified a number of regions of interest in the genome (an organism's complete set of DNA) that may increase a person's risk for late- onset Alzheimer's to varying degrees.

Early-onset Alzheimer's disease occurs in people age 30 to 60 and represents less than 5 per cent of all people with Alzheimer's. Most cases are caused by an inherited change in one of three genes, resulting in a type known as early-onset familial Alzheimer's disease, or FAD. For others, the disease appears to develop without any specific, known cause, much as it does for people with late-onset disease.

Most people with Down syndrome develop Alzheimer's. This may be because people with Down syndrome have an extra copy of chromosome 21, which contains the gene that generates harmful amyloid.

Health, Environmental, and Lifestyle Factors

Research suggests that a host of factors beyond genetics may play a role in the development and course of Alzheimer's disease. There is a great deal of interest, for example, in the relationship between cognitive decline and vascular conditions such as heart disease, stroke, and high blood pressure, as well as metabolic conditions such as diabetes and obesity. Ongoing research will help us understand whether and how reducing risk factors for these conditions may also reduce the risk of Alzheimer's.

A nutritious diet, physical activity, social engagement, and mentally stimulating pursuits have all been associated with helping people stay healthy as they age. These factors might also help reduce the risk of cognitive decline and Alzheimer's disease. Clinical trials are testing some of these possibilities.

Diagnosis and Treatment of Alzheimer's Disease

Doctors use several methods and tools to help determine whether a person who is having memory problems has 'possible Alzheimer's dementia' (dementia may be due to another cause) or 'probable Alzheimer's dementia' (no other cause for dementia can be found).

To diagnose Alzheimer's, doctors may:

- Ask the person and a family member or friend questions about overall health, past medical problems, ability to carry out daily activities, and changes in behaviour and personality.
- Conduct tests of memory, problem solving, attention, counting, and language.

- Carry out standard medical tests, such as blood and urine tests, to identify other possible causes of the problem.
- Perform brain scans, such as computed tomography (CT), magnetic resonance imaging (MRI), or positron emission tomography (PET), to rule out other possible causes for symptoms.

These tests may be repeated to give doctors information about how the person's memory and other cognitive functions are changing over time. Alzheimer's disease can be definitively diagnosed only after death, by linking clinical measures with an examination of brain tissue in an autopsy. People with memory and thinking concerns should talk to their doctor to find out whether their symptoms are due to Alzheimer's or another cause, such as stroke, tumor, Parkinson's disease, sleep disturbances, side effects of medication, an infection, or a non-Alzheimer's dementia.

Some of these conditions may be treatable and possibly reversible. If the diagnosis is Alzheimer's, beginning treatment early in the disease process may help preserve daily functioning for some time, even though the underlying disease process cannot be stopped or reversed.

An early diagnosis also helps families plan for the future. They can take care of financial and legal matters, address potential safety issues, learn about living arrangements, and develop support networks. In addition, an early diagnosis gives people greater opportunities to participate in clinical trials that are testing possible new treatments for Alzheimer's disease or other research studies.

Treatment of Alzheimer's Disease

Alzheimer's disease is complex, and it is unlikely that any one drug or other intervention will successfully treat it. Current approaches focus on helping people maintain mental function, manage behavioural symptoms, and slow or delay the symptoms of disease. Researchers hope to develop therapies targeting specific genetic, molecular, and cellular mechanisms so that the actual underlying cause of the disease can be stopped or prevented.

Maintaining mental function

Several medications are approved by the US Food and Drug Administration to treat symptoms of Alzheimer's. Donepezil (Aricept®), rivastigmine (Exelon®), and galantamine (Razadyne®) are used to treat mild to moderate Alzheimer's (donepezil can be used for severe Alzheimer's as well). Memantine (Namenda®) is used to treat moderate to severe Alzheimer's. These drugs work by regulating neurotransmitters, the brain chemicals that transmit messages between neurons. They may help maintain thinking, memory, and communication skills, and help with certain behavioural problems. However, these drugs don't change the underlying disease process. They are effective for some but not all people and may help only for a limited time.

Managing behaviour

Common behavioural symptoms of Alzheimer's include sleeplessness, wandering, agitation, anxiety, and aggression. Scientists are learning why these symptoms occur and are studying new treatments—drug and nondrug—to manage them. Research has shown that treating behavioural symptoms can make people with Alzheimer's more comfortable and makes things easier for caregivers.

Looking for new treatments

Alzheimer's disease research has developed to a point where scientists can look beyond treating symptoms to think about addressing underlying disease processes. In ongoing clinical trials, scientists are developing and testing several possible interventions, including immunisation therapy, drug therapies, cognitive training, physical activity, and treatments used for cardiovascular disease and diabetes.

Support for families and caregivers

Caring for a person with Alzheimer's disease can have high physical, emotional, and financial costs. The demands of day-to-day care, changes in family roles, and decisions about placement in a care facility can be difficult. There are several evidence-based approaches and programmes that can help, and researchers are continuing to look for new and better ways to support caregivers. Becoming well-informed about the disease is one important strategy. Programmes that teach families about the various stages of Alzheimer's and about ways to deal with difficult behaviours and other caregiving challenges can help. Good coping skills, a strong support network, and respite care are other ways that help caregivers handle the stress of caring for a loved one with Alzheimer's disease. For example, staying physically active provides physical and emotional benefits. Some caregivers have found that joining a support group is a critical lifeline. These support groups allow caregivers to find respite, express concerns, share experiences, get tips, and receive emotional comfort. Many organisations sponsor in-person and online support groups, including groups for people with early-stage Alzheimer's and their families.

SECTION V

Importance of Cell Structure and Function

Chapter 17

Nucleus and Nuclear Bodies

INTRODUCTION

The nucleus is the most obvious organelle in any eukaryotic cell. It is a membrane-bound organelle and is surrounded by a double membrane. It communicates with the surrounding cytosol, via., numerous nuclear pores. Within the nucleus is the DNA responsible for providing the cell with its unique characteristics. The DNA is similar in every cell of the body, but depending on the specific cell type, some genes may be turned on or off-mitotic spindle that's why a liver cell is different from a muscle cell and a muscle cell is different from a fat cell. When a cell is dividing, the DNA and surrounding protein condense into chromosomes that are visible by microscopy.

STRUCTURES OF NUCLEUS

The nucleus is the largest cellular organelle in animals. In mammalian cells, the average diameter of the nucleus is approximately 6 micrometers (μm), which occupies about 10% of the total cell volume. The viscous liquid within it is called nucleoplasm and is similar in composition to the cytosol found outside the nucleus. It appears as a dense, roughly spherical organelle.

Function of Cell Nucleus

The main function of the cell nucleus is to control gene expression and mediate the replication of DNA during the cell cycle. The nucleus provides a site for genetic transcription that is segregated from the location of translation in the cytoplasm, allowing levels of gene regulation that are not available to prokaryotes. Nucleus of eukaryotic cell is shown in Fig. 17.1.

Cell compartmentalisation

The nuclear envelope allows the nucleus to control its contents and separate them from the rest of the cytoplasm where necessary. This is important for controlling processes on either side of the nuclear membrane. In some cases where a cytoplasmic process needs to be restricted, a key participant is removed to the nucleus, where it interacts with transcription factors to downregulate the production of certain enzymes in the pathway. This regulatory mechanism occurs in the case of glycolysis, a cellular pathway

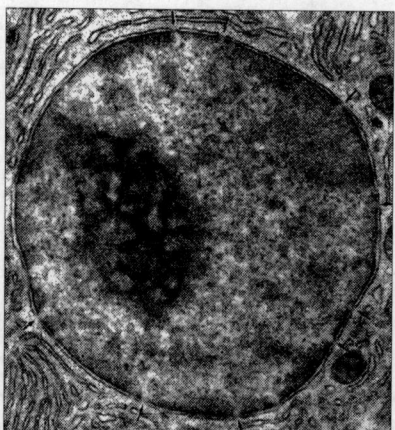

Fig. 17.1: Nucleus of eukaryotic cell.

for breaking down glucose to produce energy. Hexokinase is an enzyme responsible for the first step of glycolysis, forming glucose-6-phosphate from glucose. At high concentrations of fructose-6-phosphate, a molecule made later from glucose-6-phosphate, a regulator protein removes hexokinase to the nucleus, where it forms a transcriptional repressor complex with nuclear proteins to reduce the expression of genes involved in glycolysis. In order to control which genes are being transcribed, the cell separates some transcription factor proteins responsible for regulating gene expression from physical access to the DNA until they are activated by other signaling pathways. This prevents even low levels of inappropriate gene expression. For example in the case of NF-κB-controlled genes, which are involved in most inflammatory responses, transcription is induced in response to a signal pathway such as that initiated by the signaling molecule TNF-α, binds to a cell membrane receptor, resulting in the recruitment of signalling proteins and eventually activating the transcription factor NF-κB. A nuclear localisation signal on the NF-κB protein allows it to be transported through the nuclear pore and into the nucleus, where it stimulates the transcription of the target genes.

INTERPHASE NUCLEUS

A body cell that is not undergoing cell division is said to be in interphase and it is during this time that the cell carries out its specialised functions. The nucleus of such a cell consists of several components, each of which will be discussed it turn. Components of the nucleus: (i) nuclear envelope, (ii) chromatin, (iii) nucleolus, and (iv) nuclear matrix

Nuclear Envelope

The nuclear envelope, as indicated by its name, surrounds the contents of the nucleus and demarcates them from those of the cytoplasm. It consists of two unit membranes separated by a space about 25 nm wide called the perinuclear space. The outer nuclear membrane is studded with ribosomes and is continuous with the rough endoplasmic reticulum in the cytoplasm. The cisternal lumen of the RER is therefore in direct continuity with the perinuclear space. At numerous places on the nuclear envelope are openings called nuclear pores, which are thought to regulate the passage of large molecules to and from the nucleus. Nuclear pores range in size from 30 to 100 nm in diameter, depending on the cell type, and the number of pores reflects the transcriptional activity of the nucleus. Nuclear pores are not just simple openings in the envelope, but exhibit a complex substructure when viewed in the EM. At the rim of each pore, the inner and outer membranes are continuous and a thin diaphragm, which presumably controls passage through the pore, covers the aperture. On both the cytoplasmic and nuclear sides of the pore is a thickened annulus composed of eight protein subunits (nucleoporins) situated around the pore perimeter. The entire affair is termed a nuclear pore complex.

Chromatin

During interphase, the genetic material is extended in the form of chromatin. It is in interphase that DNA replication and transcription occur. During cell division, however, the chromatin is tightly organised into compact chromosomes.

Chromatin structure

Because chromatin contains DNA, it stains with basic dyes and is also Feulgen-positive. DNA or deoxyribonucleic acid constitutes the chemical basis of genes. A molecule of DNA consists of two strands wound about each other in the form of a double helix. Each strand has a backbone of alternating phosphate and deoxyribose groups, and a side chain of nitrogenous bases arranged in a specific sequence. This sequence of bases determines the composition of a polypeptide chain, each triplet (codon) coding for a particular amino acid. Bonding between nitrogenous base pairs holds the two strands together: adenine bonds with thymine, and cytosine bonds with guanine. During replication of DNA, the two strands separate and new strands are formed by complimentary base pairing with the original strands. This is called semiconservative replication. In addition to DNA, chromatin also contains five types of basic proteins called histones, as well as some non-histone proteins that are thought to have a regulatory role in gene expression. Four of the histones (H2A, H2B, H3, and H4) associate into a spherical core around which is wrapped a couple of turns of DNA. This is termed a nucleosome. A series of many such nucleosomes leads to the appearance of evenly spaced 'beads on a string' separated by regions of linker DNA. The fifth histone (H1) is found on the surface of the nucleosome. This nucleoprotein thread is then supercoiled to form a 20 to 30 nm diameter chromatin fibre.

Chromatin classification

Heterochromatin: This is condensed chromatin and is therefore genetically inactive, that is, transcription is not occurring. Heterochromatin is seen associated with the nuclear envelope (peripheral chromatin), with the nucleolus (nucleolar associated chromatin), and scattered throughout the nucleus (chromatin granules). There are two types of heterochromatin:

1. Constitutive heterochromatin, which is permanently inactive (e.g. centromere region of chromosome).
2. Facultative heterochromatin, which may have been active in the past and may be so again in the future. It represents inactivated genes. The amount of facultative heterochromatin depends on the cell type and stage of development.

Euchromatin: This is extended chromatin and is therefore genetically active, that is, transcription is occurring. At the EM level, euchromatin appears as electronlucent regions interspersed among clumps of electron-dense heterochromatin.

Chromatin function

During transcription, the genetic information encoded in the base sequence of DNA is copied onto a molecule of messenger RNA or ribonucleic acid. RNA differs from DNA in two fundamental ways.

First, it contains ribose instead of 2-deoxyribose and, second, it contains uracil in place of thymine. Using one strand of DNA as a template, a single molecule of mRNA is constructed by complimentary base pairing, incorporating uracil in place of thymine. The precursor mRNA molecule thus formed contains transcripts not only for sequences of DNA that contain genetic instructions (exons), but also for sequences of irrelevant DNA interposed in between (introns). Before the genetic instructions encoded in the mRNA can be translated, however, the irrelevant sequences must be excised and the exon-coded regions spliced back together. This is called RNA processing and it also occurs in the nucleus.

Afterwards, the mature mRNA molecule passes through a pore out of the nucleus and into the cytoplasm. Once in the cytoplasm, the information encoded in the mRNA molecule is translated into a polypeptide chain. As you recall from our discussion of the cytoplasm, this requires the participation of two other forms of RNA: transfer RNA and ribosomal RNA. Each molecule of tRNA contains a specific attachment site for one of twenty amino acids, as well as a base triplet called an anticodon that matches a specific codon on the mRNA molecule. As the molecule of mRNA passes between the large and small subunits of a ribosome, molecules of tRNA insert amino acids into a polypeptide chain in a specific order that is determined by the base sequence of the mRNA. After each amino acid is inserted into the growing end of the polypeptide chain, the ribosome shifts to the next codon sequence and another tRNA carrying an amino acid moves into place.

Nucleolus

Ribosomal RNA is a structural component of ribosomes and is synthesised in the nucleolus. The nucleolus is a separate entity within the nucleus consisting largely of rRNA and protein. It is intensely basophilic but Feulgen-negative. Moreover, treatment with RNAase abolishes most of the staining, suggesting that it is due primarily to the presence of rRNA. The nucleolus is very prominent in cells that are active in protein synthesis. Often, two or more nucleoli are present in the same nucleus. Ribosomal RNA is transcribed from multiple copies of nucleolar genes. These genes are located along the nucleolar organising regions of five different chromosomes (13,14,15,21,22). During active transcription, each nucleolar gene has the appearance of a 'lamp brush' as viewed in the EM. Each stand of the 'brush' represents a molecule of precursor rRNA at various stages of completion.

The completed molecules of precursor rRNA are then cleaved into two smaller pieces, which will be incorporated into the large (60s) and small (40s) ribosomal subunits. The mature rRNA quickly associates with basic protein that enters the nucleus from the cytoplasm and forms ribonucleoprotein particles. These subunits leave the nucleus through the pores and are assembled into ribosomes in the cytoplasm.

At the ultrastructural level, the nucleolus displays a characteristic organisation:

- Fibrillar centers, which represent the nucleolar organising regions of the chromosomes carrying the nucleolar genes.
- Pars fibrosa, which represents the newly transcribed precursor molecules of rRNA.
- Pars granulosa, which represents the ribonucleoprotein particles after the rRNA has complexed with protein.

Nuclear Matrix

The nuclear matrix is analogous to the cytoplasmic matrix. It consists of a protein skeletal framework surrounded by a fluid nucleoplasm. The nuclear matrix supports and organises the nucleus. It is also involved in the regulation of DNA replication and transcription. The main component of the nuclear matrix is the fibrous lamina, which is seen attached to the inner surface of the nuclear envelope. It is composed of lamins (a type of intermediate filament) and associated proteins. Extending from the fibrous lamina into the interior of the nucleus is a fibrogranular network that supports the chromatin and nucleolus.

Nuclear indicators of cell death

Alterations in nuclear morphology are often the best indicators of cell death. There are three types:

1. Pyknosis—the nucleus shrinks to a dark-staining homogeneous mass.
2. Karyorrhexis—the nucleus fragments.
3. Karyolysis—the nucleus dissolves away.

DIVIDING NUCLEUS

It is well know that body cells carry out their specialised functions while in interphase. We now need to consider how body cells divide to increase their numbers. This process is called mitosis. Mitosis and interphase together comprise the cell cycle.

Cell Cycle

Prior to mitosis, the cell must replicate its DNA in order to distribute the genetic information equally to both daughter cells. This occurs during interphase and is given a special term called the S phase (for synthesis). Both before and after the S period are two gaps: G1 between the end of mitosis and the beginning of S phase, and G2 between the end of S phase and the beginning of mitosis. Thus, interphase is subdivided into three periods: G1, S, G2. The duration of the entire cell cycle (generation time) depends on the cell type and usually exceeds 24 hr, however, the period of mitosis generally lasts only 1 to 1.5 hr. In general, specialised functions are carried out by interphase cells with an extended G1 period, or by cells that have exited the cell cycle permanently during G1 (i.e. end cells). Some nonspecialised interphase cells exit the cell cycle during G1 for an indefinite period termed the G0 stage. These cells are thought to be in sort of a standby mode, and can re-enter the cell cycle at G1 after the appropriate stimulus. At each stage in the cell cycle, there are one or more 'checkpoints' that control the transition from one stage to the next. These checkpoints assure that the cycle does not to progress to the next stage until the previous stage has been successfully completed and the DNA is undamaged. Regulation of the cell cycle is under the control of proteins called cyclins and cyclin-dependent kinases, which act in concert to activate enzymes and other proteins needed for phase-specific functions.

Populations of Renewing Cells

The body contains essentially three populations of cells that differ in their ability to divide:

1. Non-renewing populations: These are highly specialised end cells that have lost all ability to divide. There is no way to replace such cells when they are worn out or destroyed, so their numbers decline over time. Examples of this cell type include neurons and cardiac muscle cells.
2. Continuously renewing populations: In this case, less differentiated progenitor cells that still have the capacity for division replace the more highly specialised end cells that do not divide. Examples of this type include intestinal epithelial cells and blood cells. Within this context, there are two cell types that need to be defined:
   (a) Progenitor cells: These are dividing cells that are restricted to specific lines of differentiation. When progenitor cells divide, they give rise only to daughter cells that further differentiate to become end cells. Thus, progenitor cells lack the capacity for self-renewal.

(b) Stem cells: These are usually non-dividing cells that can be triggered to re-enter the cell cycle when there is a critical shortage of end cells (i.e. cells in G0 stage). When stem cells divide, they give rise to daughter cells that either differentiate further to become committed progenitor cells, or do not differentiate further and remain as stem cells. Thus, stem cells have the capacity for self-renewal. Stem cells are said to be pluripotent if their progeny have the potential to differentiate into more than one kind of end cell, or unipotent if they are restricted to producing only one type of end cell.

3. Potentially renewable populations: These are highly differentiated cells that retain the capacity to divide, but do so only under conditions of critical cell depletion. Examples of this type include liver cells and certain hormone-producing cells.

Mitosis

Mitosis is the process whereby a somatic cell divides to produce two daughter cells with identical genetic endowment. It involves both division of the nucleus (karyokinesis) and division of the cytoplasm (cytokinesis). Although both processes usually occur together, it is possible to have nuclear division without accompanying cytoplasmic division. This leads to the development of multinucleated cells.

Human somatic cells contain 46 chromosomes, which is referred to as the diploid number. During G1, prior to DNA synthesis in S phase, each chromosome consists of a single thread. During G2, however, each chromosome consists of two identical threads called chromatids held together at the centromere. During this same time, before the start of mitosis, two new centrioles are formed adjacent to the two preexisting centrioles so that the cell now has two pairs of centrioles.

Mitosis itself consists of four sequential stages, each characterising particular aspects of this continuous process.

Prophase

The first stage is prophase, which is characterised by the following events: Each centriole pair migrates to opposite poles of the cell. Around each pair, microtubules start growing outward in a radiating pattern called an aster. Microtubules between the two asters (called interpolar microtubules) continue to grow, pushing the centriole pairs apart, and eventually form the mitotic spindle. The nuclear envelope fragments, the nucleolus disappears, and the chromosomes start to condense.

Metaphase

During metaphase, the chromosomes finish condensing and become attached to chromosomal microtubules. These microtubules attach to the centromere region at specific sites called kinetochores, each chromatid is attached to a group of microtubules from the corresponding pole. Traction on the microtubules aligns the chromosomes along the equatorial plane of the cell (metaphase plate), so that their long axes are perpendicular to the spindle fibres.

Anaphase

During anaphase, the chromatids separate at the centromere and are moved to opposite poles. At this time they are referred to as daughter chromosomes, each of which is an exact genetic duplicate of the other. This movement is accomplished through the action of molecular motors (dyneins) sliding along the chromosomal microtubules toward the MTOC.

Telophase

Telophase is the final stage. During this stage, a cleavage furrow forms around the middle of the cell and constricts, eventually cleaving the cell in two. This is due to contraction of a ring-shaped band of microfilaments associated with the inner side of the cell membrane. The chromosomes decondense and the nuclear envelope and nucleoli reform, thereby restoring the cell to its interphase state. Because the spindle is composed of microtubules, mitosis can be blocked with drugs that inhibit microtubule assembly. As mentioned earlier, these drugs include: (i) colchicine, (ii) vinblastine, and (iii) vincristine.

These drugs are sometimes used in the treatment of cancer, as well as for a variety of experimental purposes. Ionising radiation also interferes with mitosis largely by damaging DNA, which results in altered or fragmented chromosomes.

Meiosis

In contrast to the division of somatic cells discussed above, another form of cell division, termed meiosis, involves germ cells. During meiosis, the diploid ($2n$) chromosome number of 46 is reduced by one half to 23, which is called the haploid ($1n$) number and is characteristic of spermatozoa and ova. The specifics of germ cell development will be detailed in a later lecture. Before we get into the details of meiosis, however, we need to learn a little more about the chromosomes.

The typical somatic cell, contains 46 chromosomes, 44 of which are termed autosomes, and the remaining 2 are the sex chromosomes. All of the autosomes exist in what are called homologous pairs. Each member of the pair (homologues) carries alternate forms of the same genes, termed alleles. The sex chromosomes, however, come in two microscopically distinguishable forms, the X chromosome and the Y chromosome. Males possess an XY combination, whereas females possess an XX homologous pair. Since the XY combination is not considered a homologous pair, males are considered to have only 22 homologous pairs, whereas females have 23. After meiosis, germ cells contain one autosome from each homologous pair and one sex chromosome for a total of 23 chromosomes. Spermatozoa contain either an X or a Y chromosome, but ova contain only an X. Thus, once fertilisation is achieved, the diploid number of 46 chromosomes is restored and the sex of the resulting zygote is determined by whether the ova was fertilised by a spermatozoon carrying an X or a Y chromosome. Meiosis consists of two divisions. In the first meiotic division, chromosomes from each homologous pair are separated to form two haploid daughter cells. This is therefore termed a reductional division because the number of chromosomes is reduced by half. In the second meiotic division, chromatids are separated from the intact chromosomes as in mitosis. This is therefore termed an equational division since no further reduction in chromosome number occurs. The net result is the formation of four haploid daughter cells.

First meiotic division

The first meiotic division consists of the following stages: Prophase I, which is divided into five periods:

1. Leptotene: The chromosomes, each consisting of two chromatids, begin to condense and become visible as slender threads. The chromosomes show bead-like thickenings called chromomeres along their length.
2. Zygotene: Homologous chromosomes pair up along side each other and form a bivalent. This process is called synapsis. The alignment between the two chromosomes is very precise and involves the formation of a special structure called a synaptonemal complex that is visible in EM.

3. Pachytene: The chromosomes in the bivalent continue to condense and thicken. Individual chromatids become visible. During this time, adjacent chromatids within a bivalent exchange segments in a process called crossing over. In this way, genetic material of paternal and maternal origin is recombined.

4. Diplotene: The chromosomes of the bivalent begin to pull apart revealing chiasmata, which are the visible manifestations of the crossing over started during pachytene.

5. Diakinesis: The chromosomes reach their maximal condensation. Due to partial separation of the homologues during this period, the bivalents exhibit various ring and cross configurations. The nuclear envelope and nucleoli disappear.

Metaphase I: The bivalents align along the equatorial plane (random assortment).

Anaphase I: The homologues separate and move to opposite ends of the cell (segregation).

Telophase I: The chromosomes decondense and the nuclear envelope and nucleoli reform. This is then followed by a brief interphase similar to that of mitosis, except that there is no replication of DNA. We now have two haploid daughter cells. Remember that the chromosomes in these cells consist of two chromatids connected at the centromere.

Second meiotic division

The second meiotic division is essentially the same as mitosis:

- Prophase II: The chromosomes recondense.
- Metaphase II: The chromosomes align on the equatorial plane.
- Anaphase II: The chromatids separate at the centromere and move to opposite poles.
- Telophase II: The daughter chromosomes, each consisting of a single fibre, decondense.

The four resultant cells each contain the haploid number of 23 chromosomes. Equally important, the processes of recombination, random assortment, and segregation have produced cells that are genetically unique, each containing a different mixture of parental genes.

Chromosomes

Now that we have discussed cell division, we need to turn our attention to the chromosomes. When we think of chromosomes, we generally think of their appearance during metaphase when they are in a state of maximal condensation and consist of two chromatids connected at the centromere.

Chromosome morphology

In general, metaphase chromosomes are classified according to the position of their centromere.

Metacentric: The centromere is in the middle of the chromosome so that the arms are of equal length.

Submetacentric: The centromere is closer to one end of the chromosome than the other so that the arms are of unequal length.

Acrocentric: The centromere is very close to one end of the chromosome. On some acrocentric chromosomes, secondary constrictions on the short arms form small satellites. These secondary constrictions are the sites of nucleolar genes in certain chromosomes.

Chromosome banding

In addition to centromere position and overall length, each pair of chromosomes can also be identified by a unique banding pattern that is produced by special staining techniques.

Some of the more common bands include:

Q-bands: These bands are seen after staining with the fluorescent dye quinacrine. They are thought to represent chromatin regions particularly rich in adenine-thymine base pairs.

G-bands: These bands are similar to the Q-bands but can be visualised in an ordinary light microscope. The staining procedure involves denaturation of chromosomal proteins followed by Giemsa stain.

C-bands: These bands are very different from the Q- and G-bands. The staining procedure involves harsh treatment to extract DNA followed by Giemsa stain. Regions containing constitutive heterochromatin are those that stain (e.g. the centromere region and much of the Y chromosome).

With the advent of fluorescent *in situ* hybridisation (FISH) techniques, unique banding patterns can now be revealed using a variety of DNA probes that bind to specific regions of the chromosome.

Chromosome number

Cells are characterised according to the number of chromosomes they contain.

Haploid: As we have seen, a haploid cell is one that contains 23 chromosomes or one complete set (n). This is characteristic of germ cells.

Diploid: Most normal somatic cells contain 46 chromosomes or two complete sets ($2n$) and are therefore diploid.

Polyploid: A few normal somatic cells contain three or more complete sets of chromosomes (Xn) and are therefore polyploid. Liver cells and blood cells called megakaryocytes are a couple of examples.

Aneuploid: Cells that have an irregular number of chromosomes (45 or 47) are said to be aneuploid. This usually means that one member of a homologous pair is missing (monosomy, 45 chromosomes) or that an extra chromosome is present in addition to the usual pair (trisomy, 47 chromosomes). Such conditions arise when there is an incomplete segregation of chromosomes during meiosis (non-disjunction), thereby forming germ cells with either an excess or a deficiency of a particular chromosome. Aneuploidy results when fertilisation occurs and can cause a variety of congenital defects depending on the particular chromosome involved. Aneuploidy is also a frequent finding in cancer cells.

Karyotyping

To karyotype an individual, a photomicrograph is taken of the metaphase chromosomes obtained from a dividing cell. After 'cutting out' the individual chromosomes with imaging software, the 23 pairs of chromosomes are arranged in order of decreasing length and assigned to one of 7 groups (A through G). In doing so, abnormalities in the morphology or number of chromosomes become readily apparent.

Sex chromatin

In normal somatic cells, only one X chromosome is expressed during interphase. Any additional X chromosomes are permanently inactivated and appear as small basophilic masses called Barr bodies or sex chromatin. In most cell types, Barr bodies appear at the periphery of the nucleus, attached to the inner aspect of the nuclear envelope. The total number of X chromosomes is equal to the number of Barr bodies plus one. Thus, normal human females have one Barr body, whereas normal males have none.

Telomeres

The terminal ends of chromosomes are called telomeres. Studies have shown that telomeres gradually shorten over time as cells repeatedly divide, and that telomere length reflects the cell lifespan, i.e. the shorter the telomere, the shorter the remaining lifespan. In cells transformed into malignant cells (effectively immortal), telomere lengths are maintained through the action of telomerase, which repeatedly adds nucleotide sequences to the telomere ends.

Cell Death

There are two major mechanisms of cell death.

Necrosis

Cell injury and associated damage to the plasma membrane results in swelling and lysis, which releases the cellular contents including hydrolytic enzymes into the extracellular environment. This causes damage to surrounding tissues and an intense inflammatory reaction.

Apoptosis

Apoptosis results when programmed physiological responses are activated by certain internal or external triggering events. Apoptosis has been referred to as 'programed cell death' or 'cellular suicide'. During apoptosis, the integrity of the plasma membrane is maintained and there is no consequent inflammation. Apoptosis is regulated by the Blc-2 family of proteins, which induce the release of cytochrome C from mitochondria. Cytochrome C, in turn, activates a cascade of proteolytic enzymes called caspases, which degrade proteins throughout the cell. Apoptosis has several characteristic features:

- Fragmentation of DNA by endonucleases.
- Shrinkage in cell volume.
- Alterations to the plasma membrane resulting in membrane blebbing without loss of membrane integrity.
- Formation of apoptotic bodies, which are small membrane-bound vesicles containing organelles and nuclear fragments.
- Removal of apoptotic bodies by phagocytic cells.

Cellular Differentiation and Proliferation

Differentiation

The term potentiality refers to a cell's ability to give rise to other types of cells. For example, a fertilised ovum is said to be totipotent because it has the capacity to produce all of the different kinds of cells in the body. However, as cell division proceeds during development, this capacity declines and the cells become increasingly different from one another. Such cells are said to have undergone some degree of differentiation, that is, they have lost some of their former potentiality and now possess new characteristics that are different from their cells of origin. The distinctive structural and functional attributes of a differentiated cell, referred to as the phenotype, usually remain fairly stable. Some types of cells, however, can undergo limited changes in phenotypic expression (e.g. the response to steroid hormones). This is called phenotypic modulation.

Cell differentiation occurs because certain genes remain transcriptionally active while other genes are selectively inactivated. There is also evidence that cytoplasmic factors play a role in cellular differentiation. For example, when a cell divides, the chromosomes are segregated equally so that each daughter cell receives an identical genetic complement. However, the cytoplasm often does not divide equally, which results in daughter cells that receive different portions of the original cytoplasm. In early development, such unequal division often results in daughter cells that differentiate into different types of cells. This suggests that certain cytoplasmic conditions are conducive to particular lines of differentiation. In fact, it is thought that a given line of differentiation is maintained from one cell generation to the next due to specific generegulatory proteins that are passed in the cytoplasm.

Proliferation

In general, the more highly differentiated a cell becomes, the less it retains the capacity to proliferate. If this intrinsic regulation is lost, however, a cell will continue to divide unchecked and give rise to a tumor or neoplasm. A neoplasm that has the ability to spread into healthy tissues is said to be malignant. Neoplasms are usually less differentiated than their normal counterparts and their proliferative ability is unrestricted. This malignant transformation is thought to be the consequence of critical genetic changes, such as the rearrangement of certain genes or the occurrence of critical point mutations.

Another cause of malignant transformation is infection with tumor viruses, which insert their genetic material into the host cell genome. Recent attention has focused on certain RNA-containing viruses that carry transforming genetic material known as oncogenes. These oncogenes appear to have originated from cells infected with the virus at some time in the distant past. In other words, the oncogenes found in RNA tumor viruses are derived from ancestral genes, termed proto-oncogenes, which were present in early vertebrate cells. These proto-oncogenes are also present in modern vertebrate cells, where they are thought to be important in regulating cell division. Under certain conditions, however, these same genes can cause malignant transformation. For example, mutation of a proto-oncogene might change the structure and function of its gene product. Alternatively, the transcriptional activity of a proto-oncogene might be increased, leading to elevated levels of gene product. This could happen if the protooncogene were translocated to the vicinity of a gene undergoing active transcription. Because the gene products of proto-oncogenes are involved in the control of mitosis, it is easy to see how alterations in the functions or levels of these products could lead to uncontrolled cellular proliferation. When this occurs, the 'proto-oncogene' responsible for the malignant transformation is referred to as an 'oncogene'. In addition to the intrinsic regulation discussed above, cellular proliferation is also subject to extrinsic regulation. For example, there are several growth factors that influence cell division. These substances (usually proteins) are released from certain cells in the body and exert their effects on other kinds of cells located some distance away. Most of the known growth factors stimulate mitosis (mitogenic), although a few inhibit cell division. Among those that act as mitogens are epidermal growth factor, nerve growth factor, platelet-derived growth factor, fibroblast-derived growth factor, and the insulin-like growth factors, to name a few. When these factors bind to specific cell surface receptors on certain cells, they initiate a sequence of biochemical events affecting genetic transcription and inducing cell division. Moreover, it is of interest that several of the oncogenes code for proteins that closely resemble growth factors or their receptors.

NUCLEAR BODIES

Nuclear bodies, (NBs) (also known as nuclear dots, or nuclear domains, are structures found in the cell nuclei of some cells. Nuclear bodies include Cajal bodies the nucleolus and PML nuclear bodies also called PML oncogenic dots. Nuclear bodies also include ND10s (Fig. 17.2). ND stands for nuclear domain, and 10 refers to the number of dots seen. Nuclear bodies were first seen as prominent interchromatin structures in the nuclei of malignant or hyperstimulated animal cells identified using anti-sp100 auto-antibodies from primary biliary cirrhosis and subsequently the promyelocytic leukemia (PML) factor, but appear also to be elevated in many autoimmune and cancerous diseases. Nuclear dots are metabolically stable and resistant to nuclease digestion and salt extraction.

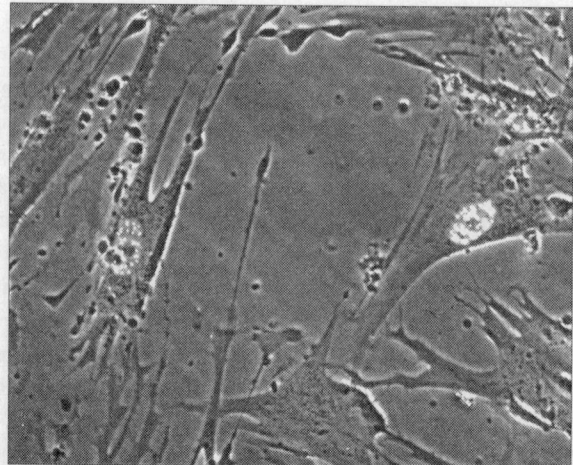

Fig. 17.2: ND10s in human embryonic lung cells.

Structure of Nuclear Bodies

Simple nuclear bodies (types I and II) and the shells of complex NB (types III, IVa and V) consist of a non-chromatinic fibrillar material which is most likely proteinaceous. That nuclear bodies co-isolated with the nuclear matrix, and were linked to the fibrogranular nuclear matrix component by projections from the surface of the nuclear bodies (Fig. 17.3). The primary components of the nuclear dots are the proteins sp100 nuclear antigen, LYSP100(a homolog of sp100), ISG20, PML antigen, NDP55 and 53kDa protein associated with the nuclear matrix. Other proteins, such as PIC1/SUMO-1, which are associated with nuclear pore complex also associate with nuclear dots. The proteins can reorganise in the nucleus, by increasing number of dispersion in response to different stress (stimulation or heat shock, respectively).

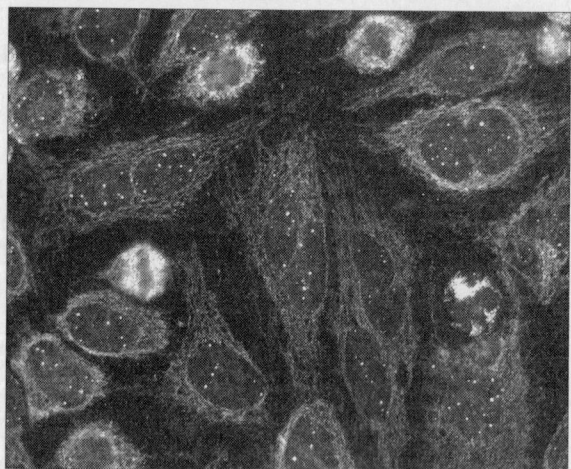

Fig. 17.3: Immunofluorescence staining pattern of sp100 antibodies. Nuclear dots can be seen in the nucleus of the cells. Produced using serum from a patient with primary biliary cirrhosis on HEp-20-10 cells with a FITC conjugate.

Function of Nuclear Bodies

One of the nuclear body proteins appears to be involved in transcriptional active regions. Expression of PML antigen and sp100 is responsive to interferons. Sp100 seems to have transcriptional transactivating properties. PML protein was reported to suppress growth and transformation, and specifically inhibits the infection of vesicular stomatitis virus (VSV) (a rhabdovirus) and influenza A virus, but not other types of viruses. The SUMO-1 ubiquitin like protein is responsible for modifying PML protein such that it is targeted to dots, whereas overexpression of PML results in programmed cell death.

One hypothesised function of the dots is as a 'nuclear dump' or 'storage depot'. The nuclear bodies may not all perform the same function. Sp140 associates with certain bodies and appears to be involved in transcriptional activation. ND10 nuclear bodies have been shown to play a major role in chromatin regulation.

Pathology

These, or similar, bodies have been found increased in the presence of lymphoid cancers and SLE (lupus). They are also observed at higher frequencies in subacute sclerosing panencephalitis, in this instance, antibodies to measles show expression in and localisation to the nuclear bodies.

- In Promyelocytic Leukemia (PML), the oncogenic PML-RARalpha chimera disrupts the normal concentration of PML in nuclear bodies. Administraton of As_2O_3 plus all-trans retinoic acid causes remission of this leukemia by triggering the bodies reorganisation. As_2O_3 destroys the chimera, allowing new SUMO-1 ubiquitinated PML to relocalise to nuclear bodies. Retinoic acid induces a caspase-3 mediated degradation of the same chimera.
- In HHV, ICP0 disrupts nuclear dots in the early stage of infection.

Chapter 18

Nuclear Lamina Diseases

INTRODUCTION

The nuclear lamina is a proteinaceous structure located underneath the inner nuclear membrane (INM), where it associates with the peripheral chromatin. It contains lamins and lamin-associated proteins, including many integral proteins of the INM, chromatin modifying proteins, transcriptional repressors and structural proteins.

A fraction of lamins is also present in the nucleoplasm, where it forms stable complexes and is associated with specific nucleoplasmic proteins. The lamins and their associated proteins are required for most nuclear activities, mitosis and for linking the nucleoplasm to all major cytoskeletal networks in the cytoplasm. Mutations in nuclear lamins and their associated proteins cause about 20 different diseases that are collectively called 'laminopathies'.

This chapter discusses mainly lamins, their structure and their roles in DNA replication, chromatin organisation, adult stem cell differentiation, ageing.

LAMIN MOLECULES IN EVOLUTION

Lamins are detected in all metazoan cells. In contrast, lamins are absent in single cell organisms or in plants. Although lamins from vertebrates and invertebrates differ significantly in their primary sequence, the general structural organisation of lamins is evolutionarily conserved with a few exceptions. Tunicate lamins are the only known lamins that have a deletion of 90 amino acids in the region of the Ig fold. Caenorhabditis elegans single lamin protein (Ce-lamin) contains a Coil 2B that is shorter by 14 amino acids (two heptads), a tail domain that is shorter by ~25 amino acids as compared to Drosophila and vertebrate lamins. It also lacks the conserved CDK1 sites.

Lamin-binding Proteins

The many roles of lamins are mediated by interactions with numerous lamin-binding proteins both at the nuclear periphery and in the nucleoplasm. There is increasingly growing number of mammalian inner nuclear membrane (INM) proteins, and most of these proteins probably bind lamins either directly or indirectly.

NUCLEAR LAMINA

The nuclear lamina is a dense (~30 to 100 nm thick) fibrillar network inside the nucleus of most cells. It is composed of intermediate filaments and membrane associated proteins. Besides providing mechanical support, the nuclear lamina regulates important cellular events such as DNA replication and cell division. Additionally, it participates in chromatin organisation and it anchors the nuclear pore complexes embedded in the nuclear envelope. The nuclear lamina is associated with the inner face of the double bilayer nuclear envelope, whereas the outer face is continuous with the endoplasmic reticulum. The nuclear lamina is similar in structure to the nuclear matrix, but the latter extends throughout the nucleoplasm.

Role and Interaction Aspects

The nuclear lamina is assembled by interactions of two lamin polypeptides in which the α-helical regions are wound around each other to form a two stranded α-helical coiled-coil structure, followed by a head-to-tail association of the multiple dimers. The linearly elongated polymer is extended laterally by a side-by-side association of polymers, resulting in a 2D structure underlying the nuclear envelope. Next to providing mechanical support to the nucleus, the nuclear lamina plays an essential role in chromatin organisation, cell cycle regulation, DNA replication, DNA repair, cell differentiation and apoptosis.

Chromatin organisation

The non-random organisation of the genome strongly suggests that the nuclear lamina plays a role in chromatin organisation. It has been shown that lamin polypeptides have an affinity for binding chromatin through their a-helical (rod like) domains at specific DNA sequences called matrix attachment regions (MAR). A MAR has a length of approximately 300–1000 bp and has a high A/T content. Lamin A and B can also bind core histones through a sequence element in their tail domain. Chromatin that interacts with lamina forms lamina-associated domains (LADs). The average length of human LADs is 0.1–10 MBp. LADs are flanked by CTCF-binding cites.

Cell cycle regulation

At the onset of mitosis (prophase, prometaphase), the cellular machinery is engaged in the disassembly of various cellular components including structures such as the nuclear envelope, the nuclear lamina and the nuclear pore complexes. This nuclear breakdown is necessary to allow the mitotic spindle to interact with the (condensed) chromosomes and to bind them at their kinetochores.

These different disassembly events are initiated by the cyclin B/Cdk1 protein kinase complex (MPF). Once this complex is activated, the cell is forced into mitosis, by the subsequent activation and regulation of other protein kinases or by direct phosphorylation of structural proteins involved in this cellular reorganisation. After phosphorylation by cyclin B/Cdk1, the nuclear lamina depolymerises and B-type lamins stay associated with the fragments of the nuclear envelope whereas A-type lamins remain completely soluble throughout the remainder of the mitotic phase.

The importance of the nuclear lamina breakdown at this stage is underlined by experiments where inhibition of the disassembly event leads to a complete cell cycle arrest.

At the end of mitosis, (anaphase, telophase) there is a nuclear reassembly which is highly regulated in time, starting with the association of 'skeletal' proteins on the surface of the still partially condensed chromosomes, followed by nuclear envelope assembly.

Novel nuclear pore complexes are formed through which nuclear lamins are actively imported by use of their NLS. This typical hierarchy raises the question whether the nuclear lamina at this stage has a stabilising role or some regulative function, for it is clear that it plays no essential part in the nuclear membrane assembly around chromatin.

Embryonic development and cell differentiation

The presence of lamins in embryonic development is readily observed in various model organisms such as Xenopus laevis, the chick and mammals. In Xenopus laevis, five different types were identified which are present in different expression patterns during the different stages of the embryonic development. The major types are LI and LII, which are considered homologs of lamin B1 and B2. LA are considered homologous to lamin A and LIII as a B-type lamin. A fourth type exists and is germ cell specific.

In the early embryonic stages of the chick, the only lamins present are B-type lamins. In further stages, the expression pattern of lamin B1 decreases and there is a gradual increase in the expression of lamin A. Mammalian development seems to progress in a similar way. In the latter case as well it is the B-type lamins that are expressed in the early stages. Lamin B1 reaches the highest expression level, whereas the expression of B2 is relatively constant in the early stages and starts to increase after cell differentiation. With the development of the different kinds of tissue in a relatively advanced developmental stage, there is an increase in the levels of lamin A and lamin C. These findings would indicate that in its most basic form, a functional nuclear lamina requires only B-type lamins.

DNA replication

Various experiments show that the nuclear lamina plays a part in the elongation phase of DNA replication. It has been suggested that lamins provide a scaffold, essential for the assembly of the elongation complexes, or that it provides an initiation point for the assembly of this nuclear scaffold. Not only nuclear lamina associated lamins are present during replication, but free lamin polypeptides are present as well and seem to have some regulative part in the replication process.

DNA repair

Repair of DNA double-strand breaks can occur by either of two processes, non-homologous end joining (NHEJ) or homologous recombination (HR). A-type lamins promote genetic stability by maintaining levels of proteins that have key roles in NHEJ and HR. Mouse cells deficient for maturation of prelamin A show increased DNA damage and chromosome aberrations and are more sensitive to DNA damaging agents.

Apoptosis

Apoptosis (cellular suicide) is of the highest importance in homeostasis of tissue and in defending the organism against invasive entry of viruses or other pathogens. Apoptosis is a highly regulated process in which the nuclear lamina is disassembled in an early stage. In contrast to the phosphorylation-induced disassembly during mitosis, the nuclear lamina is degraded by proteolytic cleavage, and both the lamins and the nuclear lamin-associated membrane proteins are targeted. This proteolytic activity is performed by members of the caspase-protein family who cleave the lamins after aspartic acid (Asp) residues.

Laminopathies

Defects in the genes encoding for nuclear lamin (such as lamin A and lamin B1) have been implicated in a variety of diseases (laminopathies) such as:

- Emery - Dreifuss muscular dystrophy: A muscle wasting disease.

- Progeria: Premature ageing.
- Restrictive dermopathy: A disease associated with extremely tight skin and other severe neonatal abnormalities.

Emery–Dreifuss muscular dystrophy

Emery–Dreifuss muscular dystrophy (EDMD) is a condition that mainly affects muscles used for movement, such as skeletal muscles and also affects the cardiac muscle, it is named after Alan Eglin H. Emery and Fritz E. Dreifuss.

Symptoms/signs of EDMD

Symptoms of EDMD begin in teenage years with toe-walking, rigid spine, face weakness, hand weakness and calf hypertrophy. Among other signs/symptoms of Emery–Dreifuss muscular dystrophy are:

- Muscle weakness EDMD can affect the shoulders and lower legs.
- Cardiac involvement can affect an individuals heart rate (bradycardia, palpitations).
- Contractures of the muscles occurs slowly, eventually leading to the need for orthopedics (walker, cane).

Genetics of EDMD: Mutations in the EMD, LMNA, and several other genes cause the various types of Emery–Dreifuss muscular dystrophy. The EMD and LMNA genes provide instructions for making proteins that are components of the nuclear envelope, which surrounds the nucleus in cells. The nuclear envelope regulates the movement of molecules into and out of the nucleus, and researchers believe it may play a role in regulating the activity of certain genes.

Diagnosis of EDMD: The diagnosis of Emery–Dreifuss muscular dystrophy can be established via single-gene testing or genomic testing, and clinically diagnosed via the following exams/methods:

- CAT scan
- Serum CK analysis
- EKG
- Echocardiogram
- Electromyogram
- Immunodetection

Treatment of EDMD

The treatment (management) of Emery–Dreifuss muscular dystrophy can be done via several methods, however secondary complications should be consider in terms of the progression of EDMD, therefore cardiac defibrillators may be needed at some point by the affected individual. Other possible forms of management and treatment are the following:

- Orthopaedics.
- Surgery.
- Monitor/treat any cardiac issues:
    Medication (beta-blockers, ACE inhibitors).
- Respiratory aid.
- Physical therapy

Progeria

Progeria is an extremely rare autosomal dominant genetic disorder in which symptoms resembling aspects of ageing are manifested at a very early age. Progeria is one of several progeroid syndromes. Those born with progeria typically live to their mid-teens to early twenties. It is a genetic condition that occurs as a new mutation, and is rarely inherited, as carriers usually do not live to reproduce children. Although the term progeria applies strictly speaking to all diseases characterised by premature ageing symptoms, and is often used as such, it is often applied specifically in reference to Hutchinson–Gilford progeria syndrome (HGPS).

Signs and symptoms of Progeria

Children with progeria usually develop the first symptoms during their first few months of life. The earliest symptoms may include a failure to thrive and a localised scleroderma-like skin condition. As a child ages past infancy, additional conditions become apparent usually around 18–24 months. Limited growth, full-body alopecia (hair loss), and a distinctive appearance (a small face with a shallow recessed jaw, and a pinched nose) are all characteristics of progeria. Signs and symptoms of this progressive disease tend to become more marked as the child ages. Later, the condition causes wrinkled skin, atherosclerosis, kidney failure, loss of eyesight, and cardiovascular problems. Scleroderma, a hardening and tightening of the skin on trunk and extremities of the body, is prevalent. People diagnosed with this disorder usually have small, fragile bodies, like those of elderly people. The face is usually wrinkled, with a larger head in relation to the body, a narrow face and a beak nose. Prominent scalp veins are noticeable (made more obvious by alopecia), as well as prominent eyes. Musculoskeletal (Fig. 18.1) degeneration causes loss of body fat and muscle, stiff joints, hip dislocations, and other symptoms generally absent in the non-elderly population. Individuals usually retain typical mental and motor development.

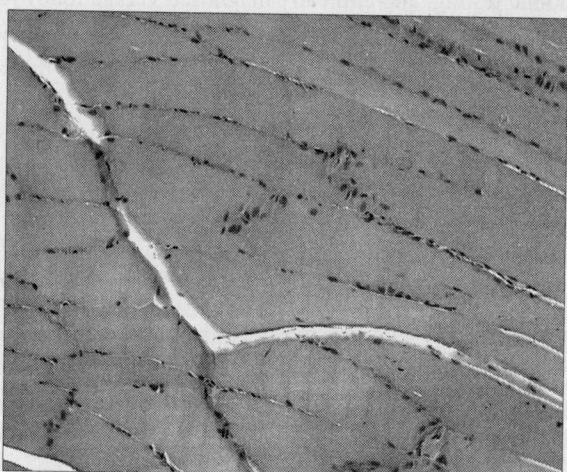

Fig. 18.1: Musculoskeletal.

Cause of Progeria

Progeria is caused by mutations that weaken the structure of the cell nucleus, making normal cell division difficult. In normal conditions, the LMNA gene codes for a structural protein called prelamin A, which undergoes a series of processing steps before attaining its final form, called lamin A. In one of these steps, after prelamin A is made in the cytoplasm, an enzyme called farnesyl transferase attaches a farnesyl functional group to the protein's carboxyl-terminus. The farnesylated prelamin A is then transported through a nuclear pore to the interior of the nucleus. The farnesyl group allows prelamin A to attach temporarily to the nuclear rim. Once the protein is attached, it is cleaved by a protease, which removes the farnesyl group along with a few adjacent amino acids. Failure to remove this farnesyl group permanently attaches the protein to the nuclear rim. After cleavage by the protease, prelamin A is referred to as lamin A. Lamin A, along with lamin B and lamin C, makes up the nuclear lamina, which provides structural support to the nucleus. Before the late 20th century, research on progeria yielded very little information about the syndrome. In 2003, the cause of progeria was discovered to be a point mutation in position 1824 of the LMNA gene, which replaces a cytosine with thymine. This mutation creates a 5' cryptic splice site within exon 11, resulting in a shorter than normal mRNA transcript. When this shorter mRNA is translated into protein, it produces an abnormal variant of the prelamin A protein, referred to as progerin. Progerin's farnesyl group cannot be removed, so the abnormal protein is permanently attached to the nuclear rim, and it cannot become incorporated as a structural part of the nuclear lamina. Without lamin A protein, the nuclear lamina does not provide the nuclear envelope with enough structural support, causing it to take on an abnormal shape. Since the support that the nuclear lamina normally provides is necessary for the organising of chromatin during mitosis, weakening of the nuclear lamina limits the ability of the cell to divide.

Diagnosis of Progeria

Diagnosis is suspected according to signs and symptoms, such as skin changes, abnormal growth, and loss of hair. A genetic test for LMNA mutations can confirm the diagnosis of progeria.

Treatment of Progeria

No treatment has yet proven effective. Most treatment options have focused on reducing complications (such as cardiovascular disease) with coronary artery bypass surgery and low-dose aspirin. Growth hormone treatment has been attempted. The use of Morpholinos has also been attempted in mice and cell cultures in order to reduce progerin production. Antisense Morpholino oligonucleotides specifically directed against the mutated exon 11–exon 12 junction in the mutated pre-mRNAs were used.

A type of anticancer drug, the farnesyltransferase inhibitors (FTIs), has been proposed, but their use has been mostly limited to animal models. A Phase II clinical trial using the FTI lonafarnib began in May 2007. In studies on the cells another anti-cancer drug, rapamycin, caused removal of progerin from the nuclear membrane through autophagy. It has been proved that pravastatin and zoledronate are effective drugs when it comes to the blocking of farnesyl group production.

Farnesyltransferase inhibitors (FTIs) are drugs that inhibit the activity of an enzyme needed in order to make a link between progerin proteins and farnesyl groups. This link generates the permanent attachment of the progerin to the nuclear rim. In progeria, cellular damage can occur because that attachment takes place and the nucleus is not in a normal state. Lonafarnib is an FTI, which means it can avoid this link, so progerin can not remain attached to the nucleus rim and it now has a more normal state. Studies of sirolimus, an mTOR Inhibitor, demonstrate that it can minimise the phenotypic effects of progeria fibroblasts. Other observed consequences of its use are: abolishment of nuclear blebbing, degradation of progerin in affected cells and reduction of insoluble progerin aggregates formation. These results have been observed only in vitro and are not the results of any clinical trial, although it is believed that the treatment might benefit HGPS patients.

The delivery of lonafarnib is not approved by the US Food and Drug Administration (FDA). Therefore, it can only be used in certain clinical trials. Until treatment with FTIs is thoroughly tested in progeria children in clinical trials, its effects on humans cannot be known, although its effects on mice seem to be positive. A 2012 clinical trial found that it improved weight gain and other symptoms of progeria.

Prognosis of Progeria

As there is no known cure, few people with progeria exceed 13 years of age. At least 90 per cent of patients die from complications of atherosclerosis, such as heart attack or stroke. Mental development is not adversely affected; in fact, intelligence tends to be average to above average. With respect to the features of ageing that progeria appears to manifest, the development of symptoms is comparable to ageing at a rate eight to ten times faster than normal. With respect to features of ageing that progeria does not exhibit, patients show no neurodegeneration or cancer predisposition. They also do not develop conditions that are commonly associated with ageing, such as cataracts (caused by UV exposure) and osteoarthritis. Although there may not be any successful treatments for progeria itself, there are treatments for the problems it causes, such as arthritic, respiratory, and cardiovascular problems. Sufferers of progeria have normal reproductive development and there are known cases of women with progeria who had delivered healthy offspring.

Epidemiology of Progeria

A study from the Netherlands has shown an incidence of 1 in 4 million births. Currently, there are about 100 known cases in the world. Approximately 140 cases have been reported in medical history. However, the Progeria Research Foundation believes there may be as many as 150 undiagnosed cases worldwide.

Classical Hutchinson–Gilford progeria syndrome is usually caused by a sporadic mutation taking place during the early stages of embryo development. It is almost never passed on from affected parent to child, as affected children rarely live long enough to have children themselves.

There have been only two cases in which a healthy person was known to carry the LMNA mutation that causes progeria. These carriers were identified because they passed it on to their children. One family from India has five children with progeria, though not the classical HGPS type. This family was the subject of a 2005 Bodyshock documentary titled The 80 Year Old Children. The Vandeweert family of Belgium has two children, Michiel and Amber, with classic HGPS.

Restrictive dermopathy

Restrictive dermopathy is a rare, lethal autosomal recessive skin condition characterised by syndromic facies, tight skin, sparse or absent eyelashes, and secondary joint changes.

Mechanism of Restrictive dermopathy

Restrictive dermopathy (RD) is caused either by the loss of the gene ZMPSTE24, which encodes a protein responsible for the cleavage of farnesylated prelamin A into mature non-farnesylated lamin, or by a mutation in the LMNA gene. This results in the accumulation of farnesyl-prelamin A at the nuclear membrane. Mechanistically, restrictive dermopathy is somewhat similar to Hutchinson–Gilford progeria syndrome (HGPS), a disease where the last step in lamin processing is hindered by a mutation that causes the loss of the ZMPSTE24 cleavage site in the lamin A gene.

NUCLEAR LOCALISATION SIGNALS

A nuclear localisation signal or sequence (NLS) is an amino acid sequence that 'tags' a protein for import into the cell nucleus by nuclear transport. Typically, this signal consists of one or more short sequences of positively charged lysines or arginines exposed on the protein surface. Different nuclear localised proteins may share the same NLS. An NLS has the opposite function of a nuclear export signal (NES), which targets proteins out of the nucleus.

Types of Signals

Classical signals

These types of NLSs can be further classified as either monopartite or bipartite. The major structural differences between the two is that the two basic amino acid clusters in bipartite NLSs are separated by a relatively short spacer sequence (hence bipartite - 2 parts), while monopartite NLSs are not. The first NLS to be discovered was the sequence PKKKRKV in the SV40 Large T-antigen (a monopartite NLS). The NLS of nucleoplasmin, KR[PAATKKAGQA]KKKK, is the prototype of the ubiquitous bipartite signal: two clusters of basic amino acids, separated by a spacer of about 10 amino acids. Both signals are recognised by importin a.

Importin a contains a bipartite NLS itself, which is specifically recognised by importin β. The latter can be considered the actual import mediator. Chelsky and others proposed the consensus sequence K-K/R-X-K/R for monopartite NLSs. A Chelsky sequence may, therefore, be part of the downstream basic cluster of a bipartite NLS. Makkerh and others carried out comparative mutagenesis on the nuclear localisation signals of SV40 T-Antigen (monopartite), C-myc (monopartite), and nucleoplasmin (bipartite), and showed amino acid features common to all three.

The role of neutral and acidic amino acids was shown for the first time in contributing to the efficiency of the NLS. Rotello and others compared the nuclear localisation efficiencies of eGFP fused NLSs of SV40 Large T-Antigen, nucleoplasmin (AVKRPAATKKAGQAKKKKLD), EGL-13 (MSRRRKANPT KLSEN AKKLAKEVEN), c-Myc (PAAKRVKLD) and TUS-protein (KLKIKRPVK) through rapid intracellular protein delivery. They found significantly higher nuclear localisation efficiency of c-Myc NLS compared to that of SV40 NLS.

Non-classical

There are many other types of NLS, such as the acidic M9 domain of hnRNP A1, the sequence KIPIK in yeast transcription repressor Mata2, and the complex signals of U snRNPs. Most of these NLSs appear to be recognised directly by specific receptors of the importin β family without the intervention of an importin α-like protein.

A signal that appears to be specific for the massively produced and transported ribosomal proteins, seems to come with a specialised set of importin β-like nuclear import receptors. Recently a class of NLSs known as PY-NLSs has been proposed, originally by Lee and others. This PY-NLS motif, so named because of the proline-tyrosine amino acid pairing in it, allows the protein to bind to Importin β2 (also known as transportin or karyopherin β2), which then translocates the cargo protein into the nucleus. The structural basis for the binding of the PY-NLS contained in Importin β2 has been determined and an inhibitor of import designed.

Discovery

The presence of the nuclear membrane that sequesters the cellular DNA is the defining feature of eukaryotic cells. The nuclear membrane, therefore, separates the nuclear processes of DNA replication and RNA transcription from the cytoplasmic process of protein production. Proteins required in the nucleus must be directed there by some mechanism. The first direct experimental examination of the ability of nuclear proteins to accumulate in the nucleus were carried out by John Gurdon when he showed that purified nuclear proteins accumulate in the nucleus of frog (Xenopus) oocytes after being micro-injected into the cytoplasm. These experiments were part of a series that subsequently led to studies of nuclear reprogramming, directly relevant to stem cell research.

The presence of several million pore complexes in the oocyte nuclear membrane and the fact that they appeared to admit many different molecules (insulin, bovine serum albumin, gold nanoparticles) led to the view that the pores are open channels and nuclear proteins freely enter the nucleus through the pore and must accumulate by binding to DNA or some other nuclear component. In other words, there was thought to be no specific transport mechanism.

Using a protein called nucleoplasmin, the archetypal 'molecular chaperone', they identified a domain in the protein that acts as a signal for nuclear entry. This work stimulated research in the area, and two years later the first NLS was identified in SV40 Large T-antigen (or SV40, for short). However, a functional NLS could not be identified in another nuclear protein simply on the basis of similarity to the SV40 NLS. In fact, only a small percentage of cellular (non-viral) nuclear proteins contained a sequence similar to the SV40 NLS. A detailed examination of nucleoplasmin identified a sequence with two elements made up of basic amino acids separated by a spacer arm. One of these elements was similar to the SV40 NLS but was not able to direct a protein to the cell nucleus when attached to a non-nuclear reporter protein. Both elements are required. This kind of NLS has become known as a bipartite classical NLS. The bipartite NLS is now known to represent the major class of NLS found in cellular nuclear proteins and structural analysis has revealed how the signal is recognised by a receptor (importin a) protein (the structural basis of some monopartite NLSs is also known). Many of the molecular details of nuclear protein import are now known. This was made possible by the demonstration that nuclear protein import is a two-step process, the nuclear protein binds to the nuclear pore complex in a process that does not require energy. This is followed by an energy-dependent translocation of the nuclear protein through the channel of the pore complex. By establishing the presence of two distinct steps in the process the possibility of identifying the factors involved was established and led on to the identification of the importin family of NLS receptors and the GTPase Ran.

Mechanism of Nuclear Import

Proteins gain entry into the nucleus through the nuclear envelope. The nuclear envelope consists of concentric membranes, the outer and the inner membrane. The inner and outer membranes connect at multiple sites, forming channels between the cytoplasm and the nucleoplasm. These channels are occupied by nuclear pore complexes (NPCs), complex multiprotein structures that mediate the transport across the nuclear membrane. A protein translated with a NLS will bind strongly to importin (aka karyopherin), and, together, the complex will move through the nuclear pore. At this point, Ran-GTP will bind to the importin-protein complex, and its binding will cause the importin to lose affinity for the protein. The protein is released, and now the Ran-GTP/importin complex will move back out of the nucleus through the nuclear pore. A GTPase-activating protein (GAP) in the cytoplasm hydrolyses the Ran-GTP to GDP, and this causes a conformational change in Ran, ultimately reducing its affinity for importin. Importin is released and

Ran-GDP is recycled back to the nucleus where a Guanine nucleotide exchange factor (GEF) exchanges its GDP back for GTP.

Nuclear Export Signal

A nuclear export signal (NES) is a short amino acid sequence of 4 hydrophobic residues in a protein that targets it for export from the cell nucleus to the cytoplasm through the nuclear pore complex using nuclear transport. It has the opposite effect of a nuclear localisation signal, which targets a protein located in the cytoplasm (Fig. 18.2) for import to the nucleus. The NES is recognised and bound by exportins. In silico analysis of known NESs found the most common spacing of the hydrophobic residues to be LxxxLxxLxL, where 'L' is a hydrophobic residue (often leucine) and 'x' is any other amino acid, the spacing of these hydrophobic residues may be explained by examination of known structures that contain an NES, as the critical residues usually lie in the same face of adjacent secondary structures within a protein, which allows them to interact with the exportin. Ribonucleic acid (RNA) is composed of nucleotides, and thus, lacks the nuclear export signal to move out of the nucleus. As a result, most forms of RNA will bind to a protein molecule to form a ribonucleoprotein complex to be exported from the nucleus.

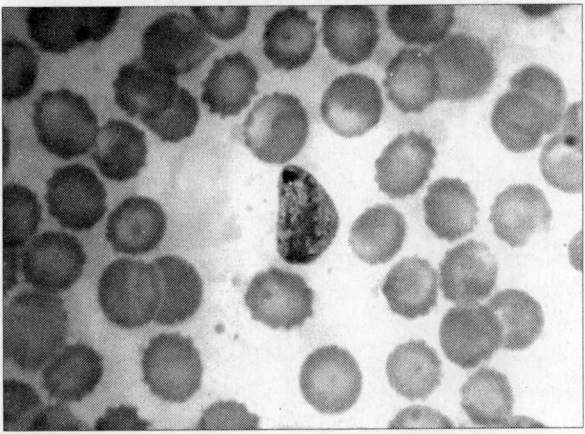

Fig. 18.2: Cytoplasm.

Nuclear export first begins with the binding of Ran-GTP (a G-protein) to exportin. This causes a shape change in exportin, increasing its affinity for the export cargo. Once the cargo is bound, the Ran-exportin-cargo complex moves out of the nucleus through the nuclear pore. GTPase activating proteins (GAPs) then hydrolyse the Ran-GTP to Ran-GDP, and this causes a shape change and subsequent exportin release. Once no longer bound to Ran, the exportin molecule loses affinity for the nuclear cargo as well, and the complex falls apart. Exportin and Ran-GDP are recycled to the nucleus separately, and guanine exchange factor (GEF) in the nucleus switches the GDP for GTP on Ran. NES signals were first discovered in the human immunodeficiency virus type 1 (HIV-1) Rev protein and cAMP-dependent protein kinase inhibitor (PKI). The karyopherin receptor CRM1 has been identified as the export receptor for leucine-rich NESs in several organisms and is an evolutionarily conserved protein. The export mediated by CRM1 can be effectively inhibited by the fungicide leptomycin B (LMB), providing excellent experimental verification of this pathway.

Other proteins of various functions have also been experimentally inhibited of the NES signal such as the cyto-skeletal protein actin, which functions include cell motility and growth. The use of LBM as a NES inhibitor proved successful for actin resulting in accumulation of the protein within the nucleus, concluding universal functionality of NES throughout various protein functional groups. Not all NES substrates are constitutively exported from the nucleus, meaning that CRM1-mediated export is a regulated event. Several ways of regulating NES-dependent export have been reported. These include masking/unmasking of NESs, phosphorylation and even disulphide bond formation as a result of oxidation. The binding of NES to the export receptor of a protein gives the universal export function of NES an individually specified activation of export to each protein. Studies of specified NES amino acid sequences for particular proteins show the possibility of blocking the NES activation of one protein with an inhibitor for that amino acid sequence while other proteins of the same nucleus remain unaffected.

NESbase

NESbase is a database of proteins, experimentally authenticated leucine-rich nuclear export signals (NES). A study was conducted by Center for Biological Sequence Analysis, Technical University of Denmark, and Department of Protein Chemistry, University of Copenhagen to validate NESbase version 1.0. Every entry in its database includes information whether nuclear export signals were sufficient for export or if it was only mediated transport by CRM1, the export receptor.

SECTION VI

Protein Sorting and Transport: Golgi Apparatus and Lysosomes

Chapter 19

Protein Sorting and Transport

INTRODUCTION

The protein sorting and translocation is a complex task involving multiple decision makings at multiple stages. Various proteins are involved in the translocation process. As described, no hard and fast rules can be derived for any locations. The address signals do not share common features in many cases. These difficulties can be addressed by computational prediction techniques. For making a computational prediction, biological features which have qualitative impact on the biological process have to be observed and quantified. The biology discussed in this chapter serves towards this purpose.

Cell is the basic unit of life and proteins are the biological workhorses in the cell. For a protein to perform its function correctly, it should be located into its intended organelle. This chapter, in brief, discusses the biology of protein localisation, protein sorting and translocation. A background knowledge of cell, its organelles and amino acids are essential to comprehend the protein sorting. The beginning part of the chapter presents this background information. The chapter then progresses with a general discussion on proteins and how they are synthesised in the cell. This is followed by a detailed description of protein sorting and translocation. This section deals with the major organelles of protein localisation and how the organelles recognise their native proteins. In addition to these, the chapter also mentions about the wetlab techniques employed for identifying protein localisation. The chapter is ended by highlighting the need for the computational prediction of protein subcellular localisation.

BACKGROUND BIOLOGY OF CELL

Knowledge of cell, different types of cells and amino acids are indispensable in understanding protein sorting and translocation. Proteins localise to various organelles or locations in the cell or moves out of the cell as secretory proteins. The organelles include nucleus, chloroplast, mitochondrion, Endoplasmic Reticulum (ER), Golgi apparatus, peroxisome, etc.

Cell and its Organelles

According to cell theory, one of the basic principles of biology, a cell is the fundamental unit of structure, function and organisation in living organisms. The hereditary information is contained within the cell in the form of deoxyribonucleic acid (DNA) and this information is passed from cell to cell during cell division. A typical human cell is of size 10 m and humans have around 100 trillion cells.

Different types of cell

Life on earth can be classified into prokaryotes and eukaryotes according to the difference in their cell structure. Prokaryotes are unicellular organisms like bacteria whereas eukaryotes are often multicellular organisms like plants and animals. A prokaryotic cell is simpler than an eukaryotic and the main difference is the lack of a well defined nucleus in the prokaryotes. Eukaryotic cells are called so because of the presence of a true nucleus. The nucleus has a well defined boundary defined by the nuclear membrane. In prokaryotes, the genetic material DNA is concentrated in a region called nucleoid, which do not have a membrane bound structure. The eukaryotic DNA is linear and complexes with proteins called histones. The DNA of prokaryotes is always circular. The DNA content of prokaryotes is only around 1×10^2 to 5×10^6 base pairs. Eukaryotes have much more DNA content and the number of base pairs ranges from 1.5×10^7 to 5×10^9. The cytoplasm of eukaryotic cells contains many large and compound collections of organelles. An organelle has its own boundary of lipid membrane which separates it from the rest of the cell and there by allowing to perform a special function. The prokayotes lack these membrane bound organelles like Golgi, lysosome, peroxisome, mitochondria and chloroplast. The presence of the membrane bound organelles makes eukaryotic cell more complex. The membrane bound structure of the organelles enhances the efficiency of functions by restricting them to occur within well defined boundary, thus limiting the span of communication and movement within the organelle itself. The eukaryote cell is much bigger, typically 10–100 micrometers in diameter, compared to the prokaryotic cell which is typically 1 micrometer in diameter. The size of the ribosomes present in the prokaryotic cell is smaller than that of eukaryotic cell. Cytoskeleton, the organelle responsible for giving structure to the cell, is not found in the prokaryotes. In prokayotes, the cell division happens in simple steps by binary fission or simple fission. In eukaryotes the cell division is of two types called mitosis and meiosis, which are complex multi-stage process. Within the eukaryotes, there is difference in cell structure between plant and animal cell. Plant cell has a cell wall which is made of cellulose and is intricately cross-linked with fibres of other carbohydrate molecules. This structural pattern allows each cell to withstand the increased internal pressure from osmosis, when the plant absorbs water. Animal cells do not have rigid cell walls like plant cells and this allows them to take up a variety of shapes. The chloroplasts in the plant cell are the site of photosynthesis. This is absent in the animal cells. In chloroplast, carbon dioxide is turned into sugar as part of photosynthesis. This is in opposite to energy production in animal through mitochondria where sugar is broken down to carbon dioxide to make energy. The vacuole present in plant cells are large compared to animal cells. The plant cell communicates by linking pores in their cell wall to connect to each other and pass information. The communication in animal cell is by an analogous system of gap-junctions.

Organelles in the Cell

Organelles are membrane bound subunits, which can perform specific functions. The most important organelle in a eukaryotic cell is the nucleus. Organelles are membrane bound subunits, which can perform a specific function. The most important organelle in a eukaryotic cell is the nucleus. It is the store house of hereditary information, the DNA. Nucleus is surrounded by a double membrane and the communication to the cytosol happens through nuclear pores present in the membrane. The DNA present in the cell is the same for all cells in the body of an organism. The genes in the DNA of each cell are expressed only according to the requirement of that cell. Depending on the specific cell type, some genes may be turned on or off. At the time of cell division the DNA condense into chromosomes. The nucleolus of the nucleus builds ribosomes, which move out of the nucleus to cytoplasm. Ribosomes are the site of protein synthesis. The mRNA which is copied from the DNA sequence of the gene comes out of the nucleus through the nuclear pores and bind to the ribosome.

At ribosome, the mRNA is translated according to the genetic codons with the help of tRNA. The amino acids corresponding to the genetic codons are brought in by the tRNA. Peptide bonds are formed between these amino acids linearly to build up the protein. Depending on the translocation pathway of the protein being synthesised, ribosomes attach themselves to ER. The ER is of two types, rough ER and smooth ER. The ribosome attach to rough ER which is involved in protein translocation and sorting. The ER is a network of membranes extending through out the cytoplasm of eukaryotic cell. The ER consists of tubular membranes and flattened sacs or cisternae, which appear to be interconnected. The internal space enclosed by the ER is called the lumen. The ER is continuous with the outer membrane of the nuclear envelope. The smooth ER is involved in the synthesis of lipids and steroids. The Golgi apparatus is a stack of flattened vesicles and is closely related to ER in performing the function of protein sorting. Vescicles that arise by budding off the ER are accepted by the Golgi complex. These are further processed at the Golgi and are packaged for further translocation by means of vesicles that arise by budding off the Golgi complex.

Lysosomes store hydrolase, the enzyme capable of digesting molecules like proteins, carbohydrates and fats. Lysosomes are common in animal cells but rare in plant cells. Peroxisome, which is present in both plant and animal cell, resembles lysosome in size but differ in internal structure. Peroxisome is responsible for protecting the cell from its own production of toxic hydrogen peroxide. Vacuoles are membrane bound organelles used for temporary storage and transportation of molecules. In plant cell, the central vacuole maintains the turgor pressure. Mitochondria and chloroplasts have double-membrane boundary and their own DNA. Mitochondrion is the power house in the cell generating the ATP molecules. In muscle cells, number of mitochondrion are present as there is a high demand for energy. Chloroplast is found only in plant cells and is the site of photosynthesis. The cytoskeleton is the cellular skeleton that provides a dynamic structure to the cell. The cytoskeleton has important role in maintaining cell shape, enabling cellular motion and intracellular transport. In all the above discussed organelles, the biological functions are performed by the proteins.

Amino Acids

All proteins are polymers of alpha-amino acids. Alpha-amino acids have the general formula $H_2NCHRCOOH$, where R is an organic substituent. The carbon atom next to the carbonyl group is called the alpha carbon. In the alpha amino acids, the amino and carboxylate groups are attached to the alpha carbon. The various alpha amino acids differ in the side chain (R group) attached to their alpha carbon. The physico-chemical properties of the amino acids are defined by the side chain. The physico-chemical properties of the amino acid influence its interactions with other amino acids, within a single protein and between proteins which in turn determines the biological activity of the protein. An example of the physico-chemical property is hydrophobicity, the molecule's affinity to water. The hydrophobicity of an amino acid is determined by the polarity of the side chain. Hydrophobic amino acids are incapable of forming hydrogen bonds with water and are buried within the hydrophobic core of the protein, or within the lipid portion of the membrane. The distribution of hydrophilic and hydrophobic amino acids plays important role in determining the tertiary and quaternary structure of the protein. The amino acids that are encoded by the standard genetic code and are used for protein synthesis is called proteinogenic amino acids or standard amino acids. The proteinogenicnic amino acids are alanine, cysteine, aspartic acid, glutamic acid, phenylalanine, glycine, histidine, isoleucine, lysine, leucine, methionine, asparagine, proline, glutamine, arginine, serine, threonine, valine, tryptophan and tyrosine. Alanine is very abundant and versatile. It is not particularly hydrophobic and is non-polar. Since it is neutral, it can be located in both hydrophilic and hydrophobic regions on the protein. The alanine side chain is inert, and is thus rarely directly involved in protein function. Cysteine is usually classified as a hydrophobic amino acid. Within extracellular proteins, it is frequently involved in disulphide bonds. Aspartic acid and glutamic acid are negatively charged, polar amino acids. Being charged and polar, they prefer to be on the surface of proteins, when exposed to an aqueous environment. When buried within the protein they are frequently involved in salt-bridges, where they pair with a positively charged amino acid to create stabilising hydrogen bonds, that can be important for protein stability. Phenylalanine is an aromatic, hydrophobic amino acid and prefers to be buried in protein hydrophobic cores.

The aromatic side chain makes phenyalanine to be involved in stacking interactions with other aromatic side-chains. Phenylalanine side chain is fairly non-reactive, and is thus rarely directly involved in protein function. Glycine has only one hydrogen as its side chain and has good conformational flexibility. It can reside in parts of protein structures like tight turns in structures, that are not possible for other amino acids. Histidine is a polar amino acid and is the most common amino acids in protein active sites. Isoleucine is an aliphatic, hydrophobic, amino acid. The isoleucine side chain is very non-reactive, and is thus rarely directly involved in protein function. Lysine is a positively charged, polar amino acid and is involved in salt-bridges. Leucine is an aliphatic, hydrophobic amino acid and prefers to be buried in protein hydrophobic cores. It is found more common in alpha-helices than in beta strands of protein secondary structure. As methionine is a hydrophobic and aliphatic amino acid, it prefers to be buried in protein hydrophobic cores. Asparagine is a polar amino acid and prefers generally to be on the surface of proteins. It is frequently present in protein active or binding sites. Proline plays important roles in molecular recognition, particularly in intracellular signalling. Glutamine is a polar amino acid and prefers generally to be on the surface of proteins, exposed to an aqueous environment. Glutamines are frequently found in protein active or binding sites. The polar side-chain is good for interactions with other polar or charged atoms. Arginine is a positively charged, polar amino acid and involve in salt-bridges. Serine is a polar amino acid. It can reside both within the interior of a protein, or on the protein surface. Its small size makes it a good candidate for turns on the protein surface, where it is possible for the serine side-chain hydroxyl oxygen to form a hydrogen bond with the protein backbone.

Serines are quite common in protein functional centres. The hydroxyl group is fairly reactive, being able to form hydrogen bonds with a variety of polar substrates. Threonine is a slightly polar amino acid. Threonine can reside both within the interior of a protein, or on the protein surface and are frequently found in protein functional centres. The hydroxyl group is fairly reactive, being able to form hydrogen bonds with a variety of polar substrates. Valine is an aliphatic, hydrophobic amino acid and is often buried in protein hydrophobic cores. Tryptophan is an aromatic, hydrophobic amino acid. Tryptophan prefers to be buried in protein hydrophobic cores. Being aromatic, it is involved in stacking interactions with other aromatic side chains.

Among these twenty amino acids, a subset of amino acids are called essential amino acids because they cannot be synthesised by the human body. These essential amino acids must be taken in with food. In humans, the essential amino acids are lysine, isoleucine, phenylalanine, leucine, methionine, tryptophan, threonine, valine, arginine and histidine. The remaining standard amino acids are nonessential in the sense that the body can synthesise them as needed. There are a large number of non-standard or non-proteinogenic amino acids which are not found in proteins or not coded in the standard genetic code.

PROTEINS

Proteins are the most abundant macromolecules in the cell. They are the workhorses, carrying out vital biological functions. They perform critical roles in growth, giving structure to cell, maintenance in tissues, etc. Proteins have a wide range of functions as enzymes, hormones, antibodies, structural protein, storage protein and transport protein to name a few. Enzymes facilitate biochemical reactions and are vital to metabolism. Hormones like insulin, oxytocin and somatotropin are messenger proteins, giving signals to coordinate various activities. Antibodies are proteins that defend the body from antigens. Structural proteins like keratin, collagen, actin and elastin are fibrous and stringy which help in providing structure, stiffness and rigidity to otherwise-fluid biological components. Storage proteins like ovalbumin and casein store amino acids. Transport proteins like haemoglobin and cytochromes are carrier proteins which move molecules from one place to another around the body.

Proteins are made of amino acids, connected together by the peptide bonds between the carboxyl and amino groups of adjacent amino acid residues. One end of this amino acid chain has a free amino group and is called amino terminal or *N*-terminal. The other end, with a free carboxyl group, is called the carboxyl terminal or C-terminal. The amino acid sequence is the order in which amino acid residues appear in the protein. The amino acid sequence is written in the order, starting from *N*-terminal and ending in C-terminal. The linear order of the amino acids in a protein or peptide constitutes the primary structure of the protein. Proteins cannot perform its intended function in the primary structure level. They fold to form secondary, tertiary and quaternary structure.

Secondary structure is formed by the hydrogen bonds between the amino acids in the polypeptide. Secondary structures are regularly repeating local structures. Multiple secondary structures can be present in a single protein. Alpha-helix and beta sheets are examples of secondary structure. Tertiary structure is the three-dimensional structure of the polypeptide chain into which it folds naturally or with the assistance of chaperones. The function of a protein depends on its tertiary structure. When denatured, the protein tertiary structure is disrupted and the protein loses its activity. The tertiary structure is the spatial arrangement of secondary structures interacting through hydrophobicity, salt bridges, hydrogen bonds, disulphide bonds, and post-translational modifications. In quaternary structure, separate peptide chain, known as subunits join together to form a complex.

The sequence of amino acids in a protein is decided by the three letter codons in the messenger RNA (mRNA) from which the protein was translated. The sequence of codons in the mRNA is, in turn, decided by the sequence of codons in the DNA from which the mRNA was transcribed. The coding portion of DNA is known as genes. Thus, the instructions to define a protein are written in the genes which reside in the nucleus.

PROTEIN BIOSYNTHESIS

Protein synthesis is the process in which cells build proteins. It is a multistep process of transcribing the genetic information in the gene to mRNA and translating the information with help of tRNA to generate protein at the ribosome. Protein biosynthesis differs in prokaryotes and eukaryotes. The nucleus stores the genetic information which is the instruction to generate the protein. The genetic information is written in deoxyribo nucleic acid (DNA) a long molecule, made up of nucleotides. There are four nucleotides Adenine, Thymine, Cytosine and Guanine. The long DNA molecule is packed as chromosomes which are the carriers of the hereditary information. Certain parts of the DNA contains biologically meaningful instruction to form biomolecules. These parts are known as genes. When a protein is needed in the cell, the gene which encodes for that particular protein has to be expressed. In gene expression, the double helix of the DNA open up and the gene is copied to mRNA.

This is possible because of the complementarities of the nucleotides. This mRNA undergoes several processing like splicing of introns, the inter non-coding areas in the gene. The mRNA travels outside of the nucleus to the ribosomes which are in the cytoplasm. The proteins are made in the ribosome with the help of tRNAs. Ribosomes are made of a small and large subunit which can surround the mRNA. The first step in translation is the initiation, the binding of ribosome to mRNA. The information in the mRNA is decoded to amino acid by the rules of the trinucleotide genetic code. In the next step called elongation, the triplet code is sensed by the tRNA which has a matching anticodon, and the corresponding amino acid is added to the growing polypeptide chain. When the triplet codon which acts as the stop codon is sensed, the translation stops and the polypeptide chain is ready.

PROTEIN SORTING AND TRANSPORT

For a cell to function properly, each of its numerous proteins must be localised to the correct organelle like chloroplast, mitochondria, lysosome. Hormone receptor proteins must be delivered to the plasma membrane for the cell to recognise hormones, and specific ion-channel and transporter proteins are needed in the membrane, for the cell to import or export the corresponding ions and small molecules. Enzymes such as RNA and DNA polymerases must be targeted to the nucleus for gene expression and protein synthesis. Proteolytic enzymes or catalase, must go to lysosomes or peroxisomes, respectively for proper functioning. Hormones must be directed to the cell surface and secreted. The process of directing each newly made protein to its particular destination is critical to the organisation and functioning of eukaryotic cells and this is referred to as protein targeting or protein sorting.

Protein Sorting

Except for a small number of proteins, coded in the genomes of mitochondria and chloroplasts, most of the proteins in a cell are encoded by nuclear DNA and are synthesised on ribosomes in the cytosol. For proper functioning, these proteins are to be distributed to their correct destinations in the cell. In 1999, Gunter Blobel was awarded Nobel Prize in Physiology or Medicine for the discovery that 'proteins have intrinsic signals that govern their transport and localisation in the cell.' The sorting signals are present in the primary amino acid sequence levels mostly at its N-terminal. For further sorting within the organelle, additional targeting information may be located in a secondary targeting sequence, either placed adjacent to the original targeting sequence or in other regions of the protein.

Proteins are translocated to their targeted location either cotranslationaly or post-translationaly. In cotranslational translocation, the translocation starts while the protein is still being synthesised on the ribosome. Proteins targeted for ER, Golgi apparatus, plasma membrane, lysosome, vacuole and extra-cellular space uses the SRP-dependent pathway and are translocated cotranslationally. The N-terminal signal sequence of these proteins, is recognised by a signal recognition particle (SRP), while the proteins being translated in the free ribosome. The ribosome-protein complex is transferred to a SRP receptor on the ER and the synthesis pauses. There, the nascent protein is inserted into the translocon that passes through the ER membrane. Transfer of the ribosome-mRNA complex from the SRP to the translocon opens the gate on the translocon and allows the translation to resume. The signal sequence is immediately cleaved from the polypeptide once it has been translocated into the ER by signal peptidase in secretory proteins. Within the ER, chaperone helps protein to fold correctly. From ER, proteins are transported in vescicles to the Golgi apparatus where they are further processed and sorted for transport to endosomes, lysosomes, plasma membrane or secretion from the cell. The proteins for ER will have various ER retention signals to keep them in the ER itself.

Most of the proteins targeted for mitochondria, chloroplast, nucleus and peroxisome are translocated post-translationaly. In contrast to the cotranslationaly translocated proteins, these proteins are translated in the free ribosomes in the cytosol. Once the translation is complete, they are released into the cytosol. These proteins which enter the non-secretory pathway are sorted to their destination site based on the presence of the targeting signal. Once the protein has reached its destination, the targeting signals are cleaved off. The targeting sequence for mitochondrial proteins, mitochondrial transfer peptide (mTP), will have 3–5 nonconsecutive Arg or Lys residues, often with Ser and Thr, at the *N*-terminal of the polypeptide chain. No Glu or Asp residues are generally found here. In the case of chloroplast, chloroplast transit peptide (cTP), no common sequence motifs are found but the *N*-terminal is generally rich in Ser, Thr, and small hydrophobic amino acid residues and the region is poor in Glu and Asp residues. For peroxisome proteins, the sorting signal is generally found at extreme C-terminal usually as Ser-Lys-Leu and these signals are not cleaved off after reaching the destination.

Proteins destined for nucleus have a distributed sorting signal which is not cleaved off after sorting. One cluster of 5 basic amino acids or two smaller clusters of basic residues, separated by around 10 amino acids are usually found as nuclear localisation signal.

Major Locations

Proteins are sorted to their locations with the help of an address signal present in the primary structure level. Each organelle has a mechanism to identify its own proteins. In this section, important protein localisation sites like nucleus, mitochondrion, chloroplast, peroxisome, and secretory proteins are explained.

Endoplasmic reticulum

The Endoplasmic Reticulum (ER) is the first branching point in protein sorting. Most of the proteins targeted for secretion, Golgi apparatus, plasma membrane, vacuole, lysosome are translated on the ribosomes bounded to the endoplasmic reticulum and they enter into the ER cotranslationally. Only a few proteins enter the ER post-translationally. The protein translation starts at the free ribosomes in the cytosoL The synthesis continues till the sorting signal which is present in the *N*-terminal emerges. This sorting signal is recognised by signal recognition particle. The SRP binds to the sorting signal and the translation pauses. The complex of SRP, ribosome, polypeptide chain and mRNA moves to the ER and the polypeptide chain enters the ER through translocon. The translocon is a protein complex containing various components used for protein translocation. The SRP receptor of the translocon binds with the SRP, the ribosome receptor binds with the ribosme and hold it in the correct position, the pore protein forms the channel through which the growing polypetide enter the ER lumen, the signal peptidase cut the signal once it enters the ER. After the SRP and ribosomes are bound by SRP receptor and ribosme receptor respectively, GTP binds to the complex of SRP and SRP receptor and the translation resumes. This causes the transfer of the signal sequence into the channel of pore protein. Then the GTP is hydrolysed and the SRP is released. While the sorting signal remains bound at the pore protein, the polypeptide grows into a loop and translocates into the ER lumen. When the polypetide synthesis is finished, the signal peptidase cleaves off the sorting signal, releasing the polypeptide into the ER lumen. After this, the ribosome detaches from the ER and dissociate into its subunits, and the mRNA is released. Inside the ER, the polypeptide chains are folded into their native forms usually with the help of molecular chaperones, which controls the quality of protein folding.

Integral membrane proteins of the plasma membrane or the membranes of the ER, Golgi apparatus, and lysosome are first inserted into the membrane of ER. These proteins do not enter the lumen cotranslationally but anchored to the ER membrane by membrane spanning α helices that stop transfer of the growing polypeptide chain across the membrane.

Proteins travel along the secretory pathway in transport vesicle, which bud from the membrane of one organelle and then fuse with the membrane of another. The proteins are exported from the ER in vesicles that bud from the transitional ER and carry their cargo through the ER-Golgi intermediate compartment and then to Golgi apparatus. The proteins targeted for the ER has a retention signal in their C terminal that makes them come back to the ER even if they are exported from the ER. Two such retention signals are KDEL (Lys-Asp-Glu-Leu) and KKXX (two lysine residues followed by any two amino acids) present in the C-terminal of the sequences. If the signal is removed from the ER proteins, they are transported to Golgi and then move out of the cell. The ER retention signals do not prevent the ER proteins from being packaged and exported from the ER. Instead these signals retrieve the ER proteins from Golgi apparatus or ER-Golgi intermediate compartments and put them back to ER using a recycling pathway. Specific recycling receptors bind to these retention signals and bring them back to ER. There are many retention signals other than KDEL and KKXX but they are not well characterised. Endoplasmic reticulum is discussed in details in Chapter 20.

Golgi apparatus

Golgi apparatus is composed of flattened membrane-enclosed sacs called cisternae and associated vesicles. The Golgi apparatus is a main center for protein sorting. It receives proteins from the ER and further process them and sort them to their targeted location: lysosomes, endosomes, plasma membrane, or extracellular. The proteins from the ER enter the *cis* face of the ER which is convex in shape and is oriented towards the nucleus. They are transported through the Golgi and exit from its concave shaped *trans* face. The proteins that function within the Golgi has to be retained from export. All proteins known to be retained in the Golgi complex are associated with the Golgi membrane and their retention signals are present in the transmembrane domain. This prevents these proteins from being packaged in the transport vesicle that leave trans Golgi network. Golgi apparatus is discussed in details in Chapter 21.

Membranes

Most of the eukaryotic membrane proteins are inserted into the ER membrane using the translocon complex used for protein secretion. They are inserted into the membrane by translocation, until the process is interrupted by a stop-transfer sequence, also called a membrane anchor sequence. These membrane proteins are understood to be using the same model of targeting for secretory proteins. In contrast to secretory proteins, the first transmembrane domain acts as the first signal sequence and targets them to the ER membrane. This results in the translocation of the amino terminus of the protein into the ER membrane lumen.

Transmembrane proteins span the entire membrane. The transmembrane regions of the proteins are either α-helical or β-barrels. α-helical proteins are the major category of membrane proteins and are often found in the inner membranes of bacterial cells, the plasma membrane of eukaryotes and in the outer membranes. β-barrels proteins are found in outer membranes of Gram-negative bacteria, cell wall of Gram-positive bacteria, and outer membranes of mitochondria and chloroplasts. No common localisation signal was observed for membrane proteins. Helical transmembrane proteins are usually identified from the distribution of the hydrophobic amino acids. The transmembrane regions are significantly more hydrophobic than an average piece of sequence. The length of the transmembrane region varies depending on the angle between the helix and the membrane and the kind of membrane the protein resides in. Usually transmembrane region is of 14 to 36 residues in length. Cell membrane proteins are usually identified by the skewed distribution of charges between inner and outer loops.

Extracellular proteins

Extracellular proteins or secreted proteins are fundamental to intercellular communications in multicellular organisms. The extracellular accessibility of these proteins makes them ideal targets for protein therapeutics. Virtually all protein-based therapeutic drugs in the market target these secreted and cell-surface proteins. Secreted proteins and a majority of cell-surface proteins possess an *N*-terminal address signal known as signal peptide.

The signal peptide (SP) has a length of nearly 20–25 residues. The enzyme, signal peptidase (SPase) cleaves off the signal peptide during the export process. Small and apolar residues like alanine are found at positions -1 and -3 relative to the cleavage site. The *N*-terminal domain of the signal peptide is usually positively charged. The central region will be hydrophobic and leucines are the most common amino acids in this region. The cleavage site region is usually populated with small residues. Secretion happens through different pathways and most important among them are SRP-dependent (Signal Recognition Particle) pathway and the SRP independent pathway. In SRP-dependent pathway, the nascent polypeptide chain is recognised by SRP and the translation is paused and the translation complex is brought to the SRP receptor. The polypeptide chain is translocated through the Sec machinery and the translocation resumes. The SRP-independent pathway (know as Sec-dependent pathway in prokaryotes) involves post-translational translocation and employs many proteins and the hydrolysis of ATP, for identification of the signal peptide and translocation. In prokaryotes, the deltapH or TAT (twin-arginine translocation) pathway is also used for secretion. It needs no ATP but requires a pH-gradient over the membrane. Proteins transported via this route contain a twinarginine motif in the *N*-terminal part of the signal peptide, and the signal peptide is longer than others.

Nucleus

Nucleus is known as the control centre of the cell and is the largest organelle in animal cell. It is the storage place of the genetic material, DNA. A eukaryote nucleus and subnuclear locations. Proteins are transported into the nucleus post-translationally and in a folded state. Most of the nuclear proteins are imported to nucleus with the help of carrier proteins (e.g. importins). These carrier proteins form a complex with the proteins that are to be imported into the nucleus, and this complex is translocated through the nuclear pore. Inside the nucleus, the complex is dissociated and the importin is shuttled back to the cytoplasm and reused.

The address signal for nucleus is known as nuclear localisation signal (NLS) and is a short stretch of amino acids. The deletion of the NLS from a nuclear protein disrupts nuclear import and the addition of NLS to a non-nuclear protein facilitate nuclear import. These details have been widely used to experimentally unravel NLS motifs. The nuclear localisation signals can be present anywhere in the protein sequence. Since NLSs do not have any particular consensus sequence, it is difficult to differentiate an NLS from a non-NLS region. Usually NLS is rich with positively charged residues, since some of these positive residues bind to carrier proteins like importins. Mutating these positively charged amino acids will disrupt nuclear import. However, there are Glycine-rich NLS motifs with few positive charges like monopartite and bipartite motifs. Monopartite consists of four basic and one helixbreaking residues, and the bipartite consists of two clusters of basic residues with a spacer of 9–12 amino acids in between. But these patterns also are not at all unique to nuclear proteins and may well be observed in many other proteins. Other observed NLS includes, the 38 amino acid long M9 sequence and the repeated G-R motif. However, these signals are in general significantly less frequent than the monopartite and bipartite NLS. There are also signals for nuclear protein export and retention. Nucleus is discussed in details in Chapter 17.

Mitochondrion

Mitochondria is known as the power house of the cell as they generate most of the cell's supply of adenosine triphosphate (ATP) in the process of cellular respiration by breaking down carbohydrates and fatty acids. Mitochondria consist of a smooth outer membrane and an inner membrane separated by an intermembrane space. The inner membrane forms numerous folds known as cristae. The space inside the inner membrane is called the mitochondrial matrix and contains the genetic material of mitochondria.

The matrix and inner membrane represents the major working compartments of the mitochondria. As sugar is burned for fuel, a mitochondrion shunts various chemicals back and forth across the inner membrane. Even though mitochondrion has a genome of its own, it does not code for the proteins necessary for DNA replication, transcription and translation. All these proteins, the proteins required for oxidative phosphorylation and the proteins to act as enzymes has to be generated from nuclear.

DNA is imported into the mitochondria. The double membrane structure of the mitochondrion makes the protein import a difficult task. The proteins for the matrix of mitochondria have to cross two membranes. The proteins for other location have to be resorted with a secondary targeting signal, once they reach mitochondria. The sorting signal of mitochondrion is known as mitochondrial transfer peptide (mTP) and is on average 35 amino acids long. The mTP binds to the receptors on the surface of mitochondria. These receptors are part of TOM (Translocase of the Outer Membrane) complex that directs translocation across the outer membrane. The individual receptors, on the TOM complex are TOM20, TOM22 and TOM5. From these receptors, proteins are transferred to the TOM40 pore protein and translocated across the outer membrane. The protein is transported, via the GIP complex (general import pore), in an ATP-requiring process through the outer mitochondrial membrane. The proteins are then transferred to a second protein complex in the inner membrane, the TIM (Ttanslocase of the Inner Membrane) complex for translocation into the matrix. The translocation is through a process that requires an electrochemical hydrogen ion gradient across the inner membrane. After entering mitochondrial matrix, the mTP is cleaved off by the mitochondrial processing peptidase, MPP (Matrix Processing Peptidase) by proteolytic cleavage. Some mitochondrial matrix proteins are then cleaved again by the mitochondrial intermediate peptidase (MIP) which removes an additional eight or nine residues from the *N*-terminus. For some proteins, a second adjacent targeting signal that resembles the signal peptide for secretion is exposed after MPP cleavage. These proteins are re-exported from the matrix to the intermembrane space (IMS), or inserted into the inner membrane, in a process very similar to bacterial protein secretion. Alternatively, the translocation over either of the membranes is halted by a stop-transfer signal, which is specifically recognised by a TOM or TIM component, and the protein is subsequently inserted into the outer or inner membrane, respectively. The inner membrane metabolite carrier proteins of mitochondria contain internal localisation signals. In mitochondrial targeting peptides (mTPs), Arg, Ala and Ser are over-represented while negatively charged amino acid residues (Asp and Glu) are rare. Other than this, there is no obvious features that distinguish the mTP from other N-terminal sequences. The degree of sequence conservation around the cleavage site is also poor. Many mTPs have an arginine in position -2 or 3 relative to the MPP cleavage site. It is reported that, the mTP forms an amphipathic alpha-helix when bound to the receptor protein but adopts an extended structure, when processed by the MPP. Mitochondria is discussed in details in Chapter 23.

Chloroplast

The chloroplast is double membrane bound organelle present in photosynthetic plants and algae. In addition to the inner and outer membranes of the envelope, chloroplasts have a third internal membrane system, called the thylakoid membrane. The thylakoid membrane forms a network of flattened discs called thylakoids, which are frequently arranged in stacks called grana. Because of this three-membrane structure, the internal organisation of chloroplasts is more complex than that of mitochondria. In particular, the three membranes divide chloroplasts into three distinct internal compartments: the intermembrane space between the two membranes of the chloroplast envelope, the stroma, which lies inside the envelope but outside the thylakoid membrane, and the thylakoid lumen.

Stroma is the site of the dark reactions, more properly called the Calvin cycle. Stacks of thylakoids are called granum. Even though it has a small genome of its own in stroma, the majority of chloroplast proteins are encoded in the nuclear genome and post-translationally imported into the organelle.

Protein import into chloroplasts generally resembles mitochondrial protein import. Proteins are targeted for import into chloroplasts by N-terminal sequences of 30 to 100 amino acids, called chloroplast transit peptides (cTP), which direct protein translocation across the two membranes of the chloroplast envelope and are then removed by proteolytic cleavage. The transit peptides are recognised by the translocation complex of the chloroplast outer membrane (the Toc complex), and proteins are transported through this complex across the membrane. They are then transferred to the translocation complex of the inner membrane (the Tic complex) and transported across the inner membrane to the stroma. As in mitochondria, the translocation requires energy in the form of ATP. In contrast to the mTP, transit peptides are not positively charged and the translocation of polypeptide chains into chloroplasts does not require an electric potential across the membrane.

Inside the chloroplast, the cTP is cleaved off by the stromal processing peptidase (SPP). cTPs are rich in hydroxylated residues, especially serines, and have a low content of acidic residues. The cTPs from different proteins varies from 20 to 120 residues in length. At the N-terminus of cTP, there is a conserved alanine next to the initial methionine. A semiconserved motif, V-R-A-(:)-A-A-V, around the SPP cleavage site has also been recognised. The signal is not very strong and there are several proteins that are located to both mitochondria and chloroplasts using identical sorting signals.

Proteins designated for the lumen of the intra-chloroplastic thylakoid compartment normally have a bipartite targeting sequence composed of an N-terminal stroma targeting cTP followed by a thylakoid lumen transfer peptide (LTP). There are two different pathways from the chloroplast stroma into the thylakoid lumen, the Sec-dependent pathway and the delta-pH or twin arginine translocation (TAT) pathway. The signals for the two pathways are very similar, the only significant difference being that the TAT pathway proteins contain a twin-arginine (RR) motif in the LTP (KR and RK may also be accepted). The -3, -1 motif found at the SP cleavage site in secreted proteins is present also in LTPs, and more strongly conserved. Many proteins are needed in both mitochondria and chloroplasts. In general the targeting peptide is of intermediate character to the two specific ones. The targeting peptides of these proteins have a high content of basic and hydrophobic amino acids, a low content of negatively charged amino acids. They have a lower content of alanine and a higher content of leucine and phenylalanine. The dual targeted proteins have a more hydrophobic targeting peptide than both mitochondrial and chloroplastic ones. Chloroplast is discussed in details in Chapter 24.

PEROXISOME

Peroxisomes were discovered as biochemical entities by De Duve's group. They were identified as small sedimentable particles containing marker enzymes that distinguished them from other known organelles. The presence of hydrogen-peroxide-producing oxidases and catalase inspired the name peroxisomes and focused attention on their role in oxidative metabolic transactions. Despite having appeared in the literature for almost half a century, peroxisomes have yet to find their rightful place in biochemical and cell-biological textbooks. There are a number of reasons for this. First, we do not understand why they exist in the first place. Are they remnants of early symbionts that have completely lost their DNA? Attempts to find homologies among evolutionarily conserved proteins do not overtly support a bacterial origin.

The remarkable variability in enzyme content in different species is also not consistent with this concept. Second, there are no good reasons for peroxisomal metabolism to be compartmentalised and separated from the remainder of the cell. Many reactive oxygen species arising within peroxisomes are membrane permanent. Indeed, a particular *Hansenula polymorpha* mutant can grow without peroxisomes, using the peroxisomal enzymes located in the cytosol. Finally, the variability of protein content in different species hindered early recognition of microbodies as one well-defined group of cellular organelles. Microbodies comprise peroxisomes, glycosomes, glyoxysomes and possibly (some) hydrogenosomes. The recent recognition that the proper functioning of peroxisomes is important for human health and the observation that central processes such as import of proteins into peroxisomes are not simply reiterations of established principles are contributing to a renewed interest in the organelle. As is often the case in a rapidly developing field, contradictory experimental findings and differences of opinion abound.

Thus, peroxisome is a type of organelle known as a microbody, found in virtually all eukaryotic cells. They are involved in catabolism of very long chain fatty acids, branched chain fatty acids, D-amino acids, and polyamines, reduction of reactive oxygen species – specifically hydrogen peroxide – and biosynthesis of plasmalogens, i.e., ether phospholipids critical for the normal function of mammalian brains and lungs. They also contain approximately 10% of the total activity of two enzymes in the pentose phosphate pathway, which is important for energy metabolism. It is vigorously debated whether peroxisomes are involved in isoprenoid and cholesterol synthesis in animals. Other known peroxisomal functions include the glyoxylate cycle in germinating seeds (glyoxysomes), photorespiration in leaves, glycolysis in trypanosomes (glycosomes), and methanol and/or amine oxidation and assimilation in some yeasts.

Peroxisome Metabolism

Isolated peroxisomes are permeable to small molecules such as sucrose. During isolation, they often lose proteins that are normally confined to the peroxisomal matrix. This loss of peroxisomal content was initially taken as evidence for the permeability of the peroxisomal membrane *in vivo*, but is now known to be an isolation artifact.

Metabolic Functions

A major function of the peroxisome is the breakdown of very long chain fatty acids through beta oxidation. In animal cells, the long fatty acids are converted to medium chain fatty acids, which are subsequently shuttled to mitochondria where they are eventually broken down to carbon dioxide and water. In yeast and plant cells, this process is carried out exclusively in peroxisomes.

The first reactions in the formation of plasmalogen in animal cells also occur in peroxisomes. Plasmalogen is the most abundant phospholipid in myelin. Deficiency of plasmalogens causes profound abnormalities in the myelination of nerve cells, which is one reason why many peroxisomal disorders affect the nervous system. Peroxisomes also play a role in the production of bile acids important for the absorption of fats and fat-soluble vitamins, such as vitamins A and K. Skin disorders are features of genetic disorders affecting peroxisome function as a result.

Peroxisomes can be derived from the endoplasmic reticulum and replicate by fission. Peroxisome matrix proteins are translated in the cytoplasm prior to import. Specific amino acid sequences (PTS or peroxisomal targeting signal) at the C-terminus (PTS1) or N-terminus (PTS2) of peroxisomal matrix proteins signals them to be imported into the organelle. There are at least 32 known peroxisomal proteins, called peroxins, which participate in the process of peroxisome assembly. Proteins do not have to unfold to be imported into the peroxisome. The protein receptors, the peroxins PEX5 and PEX7, accompany their cargoes (containing a PTS1 or a PTS2 amino acid sequence, respectively) all the way into the peroxisome where they release the cargo and then return to the cytosol – a step named recycling. A model describing the import cycle is referred to as the extended shuttle mechanism. There is now evidence that ATP hydrolysis is required for the recycling of receptors to the cytosol. Also, ubiquitination appears to be crucial for the export of PEX5 from the peroxisome, to the cytosol.

Associated medical conditions: Peroxisomal disorders are a class of medical conditions that typically affect the human nervous system as well as many other organ systems. Two common examples are X-linked adrenoleukodystrophy and peroxisome biogenesis disorders.

Protein content of peroxisomes: The protein content of peroxisomes varies across species or organism, but the presence of proteins common to many species has been used to suggest an endosymbiotic origin, that is, peroxisomes evolved from bacteria that invaded larger cells as parasites, and very gradually evolved a symbiotic relationship. However, this view has been challenged by recent discoveries. For example, peroxisome-less mutants can restore peroxisomes upon introduction of the wild-type gene.

WETLAB TECHNIQUES

A wide range of experimental methods are used in the wetlabs to identify protein subellular localisation. Immunofluorescence and immunoelectron microscopy, PhoA protein fusions, fluorescent-protein tagging, and Western/SDS-PAGE analysis of subcellular fractions are used for this purpose. Even though the output of these methods are highly accurate, they have several limitations like only a few proteins can be tested at a time and they are costly, time-consuming, and the number of proteins for which it can be used is relatively low. One of the laboratory techniques for subcellular localisation identification is transposon-mediated random epitope tagging and plasmid based expression of epitope-tagged proteins followed by immunofluorescence. This method had been used for comprehensive global analysis of protein localisation performed in the budding yeast, *Saccharomyces cerevisiae*. The disadvantage is that these techniques can introduce potential errors in localisation by interfering with localisation signals via random insertion of tags or saturation of binding sites by over expression of proteins.

In addition, the immunofluorescence adds a cumbersome and costly step to the analysis that may introduce non-specific staining. A study of subcellular localisation on yeast employed oligonucleotide-directed homologous recombination to insert GFP preceding the stop codon of open reading frames (ORFs) and generate yeast strains with proteins tagged at the carboxy terminus. The proteins were expressed under the control of their endogenous promoters and presumably at relatively normal levels. On the other hand, the carboxyl terminal tagging interfered in some cases with protein localisation signals such as palmitoylation and farnesylation that direct proteins to the plasma membrane.

Techniques such as two-dimensional gel electrophoresis and mass spectrometry have been frequently used to analyse localisation for a variety of bacterial genomes, including pathogenic organisms. A major disadvantage of subproteome analysis is that the fractionation of a complex structure like the cell into several subcellular compartments is not a trivial task, because of the contamination from other cellular compartments and the multiple localisation of several proteins. Computational methods for subcellular localisation prediction solve these problems to a great extend.

NEED FOR COMPUTATIONAL PREDICTION

Although the subcellular localisation of a protein can be determined by conducting various biochemical experiments they have many practical limitations and are costly and time consuming. High throughput genomic techniques in the past decade have resulted in rapid accumulation of genomic and proteomic data in the biological databases. For example, in 1986 the total sequence entries in Swiss-Prot was only 3,939 while the number was increased to 514789 sequence entries as of Swiss-Prot release 57.14 of 9-Feb-10. This explosive growth of the biological databases demands development of automated methods with high accuracy to reliably annotate the subcellular attributes of uncharacterised proteins.

For proteins, that are only predicted from the sequenced genome and not extracted as biological molecule, the only available data will be the predicted amino acid sequence. In such cases, the features of proteins, including subcellular localisation can be predicted using the computational methods. These annotation will bring out the importance of that particular protein. Proteins which are isolated and sequenced often lack the *N*-terminal signal in it, as the import machinery of the compartments cleave off the address signal in the protein. Even this information loss will not affect prediction, because most of the tools use a wide range of biological information that are derived from the sequence for making prediction. Most of the computational prediction tools are available in the Internet. They are publicly accessible and free of cost. Since a wide range of tools are available, the biologist can make prediction using different methods to increase the reliability of the prediction. Even organism specific tools are available, providing greater accuracy for the prediction. Performing the prediction prior to experimental confirmation will save valuable resources. Most of the tools accept multiple amino acid sequence as input and allows high throughput perdition.

Chapter 20

Endoplasmic Reticulum

INTRODUCTION

The endoplasmic reticulum (ER) is a continuous membrane system but consists of various domains that perform different functions. Structurally distinct domains of this organelle include the nuclear envelope (NE), the rough and smooth ER, and the regions that contact other organelles. The establishment of these domains and the targeting of proteins to them are understood to varying degrees. Despite its complexity, the ER is a dynamic structure. In mitosis it must be divided between daughter cells and domains must be re-established, and even in interphase it is constantly rearranged as tubules extend along the cytoskeleton. Throughout these rearrangements the ER maintains its basic structure. How this is accomplished remains mysterious, but some insight has been gained from *in vitro* systems.

The endoplasmic reticulum (ER) has many different functions. These include the translocation of proteins (such as secretory proteins) across the ER membrane, the integration of proteins into the membrane, the folding and modification of proteins in the ER lumen, the synthesis of phospholipids and steroids on the cytosolic side of the ER membrane, and the storage of calcium ions in the ER lumen and their regulated release into the cytosol. These functions have been studied extensively. Here, we concentrate on structural and other aspects of the ER that are less well understood.

ER SHAPE

At the light microscopy level, when stained by fluorescent dyes, or with antibodies, when marked with GFP-tagged proteins, the interphase ER can be divided into nuclear and peripheral ER. The nuclear ER, or nuclear envelope (NE), consists of two sheets of membranes with a lumen. The NE surrounds the nucleus, with the inner and outer membranes connecting only at the nuclear pores. It is underlaid by a network of lamins. The peripheral ER is a network of interconnected tubules that extends throughout the cell cytoplasm. In some cell types, such as sea urchin eggs, flat sheets are also abundant. The lumenal space of the peripheral ER is continuous with that of the nuclear envelope and together they can comprise >10% of the total cell volume. In *Saccharomyces cerevisiae*, the peripheral, tubular ER network is located exclusively underneath the plasma membrane, and about a dozen large tubules connect it to the membrane sheets of the NE. The ultrastructure of the ER has been visualised by electron microscopy in a number of cell types. The most obvious difference seen is between rough, i.e. ribosome-studded, and smooth regions of the ER. The RER often has a tubular appearance, whereas the SER is often more dilated and convoluted. The relative abundance of RER and SER found among different cell types correlates with their functions. For example, cells that secrete a large percentage of their synthesised proteins contain mostly RER.

ER IS A SINGLE COMPARTMENT

Several approaches have provided evidence that the ER is a single membrane system with a continuous intralumenal space. In one experiment, a fluorescent dye that cannot exchange between discontinuous membranes was injected into cells in an oil droplet. The dye diffused throughout the cell in a membrane network that, based on morphological criteria, was the ER. This was observed in a number of different cell types including sea urchin eggs, starfish oocytes and Purkinje neurons. Because the dye spread in fixed as well as live cells it must be diffusing through a continuous network rather than being transported by active trafficking. In another type of experiment, GFP-tagged proteins were targeted either to the lumen or membrane of the ER, and then one region of the cell was repeatedly bleached (fluorescence loss in photobleaching, FLIP). All fluorescence was rapidly lost from the entire cell.

Creating Domains in the ER — The Nuclear Envelope

How can different ER domains, such as the NE or the RER, be generated in a continuous membrane system? For the NE, domain establishment is attributed to a set of proteins that is concentrated within the inner membrane. In mammalian cells, these include the lamin B receptor (LBR), lamin-associated proteins 1 and 2 (LAP1 and 2), emerin, MAN1, nurim, LUMA and a murine protein related to UNC-84. The property that unites all of these proteins is direct or indirect attachment to nuclear structures, like the lamina or chromatin, as indicated by either resistance to detergent extraction or slow fluorescence recovery after photobleaching (FRAP). The only sequence or structural features these proteins share is an *N*-terminal nucleoplasmic domain of >200 amino acids found in LBR, LAP1 and 2, emerin and MAN1, and a short stretch of sequence similarity within this domain in LAP2, emerin and MAN1 (LEM domain). Inner NE proteins are synthesised on the RER. The classical nuclear localisation sequences (NLSs) that target soluble nuclear proteins to the nucleus are unable to target membrane proteins to the NE. Instead, these proteins appear to travel through the continuous outer NE and enter into the inner NE membrane by diffusion through the pore membrane. It is believed that once the proteins arrive in the inner membrane, they are retained by their association with lamins and/or chromatin. In support of this hypothesis, the *N*-terminal region of LBR that is responsible for its accumulation in the inner membrane contains lamin- and chromatin-binding determinants. The inner NE membrane proteins that bind directly to lamins or chromatin are likely to be responsible for establishing and maintaining NE structure. This is supported by their involvement in NE assembly *in vitro*.

Rough and Smooth ER

The morphological differences between RER and SER allow these two regions of the ER to be distinguished visually, for example, the SER is often more convoluted than RER, and the RER tends to be more granular in texture. These differences in appearance may be directly related to the presence of bound ribosomes on the RER as there is some evidence that this affects ER structure. Ultimately, however, the distinction between the two must be explained by differences in membrane protein composition. Most membrane proteins are shared between RER and SER (general ER proteins), but several proteins involved in translocation or processing of newly synthesised proteins are enriched in RER, as shown by the fractionation of liver cells. Since protein translocation is essential for all eukaryotic cells, they all have RER. One type of SER that is also found in all cells is the transitional ER. It is involved in packaging proteins for transport from the ER to the Golgi and is enriched in proteins required for this process.

However, SER is abundant only in certain cell types, such as in steroid-synthesising cells, liver cells, neurons and muscle cells. The primary activities of the SER are very different in each of these cell types. In liver, the SER is important for detoxification of hydrophobic substances. In steroid producing cells, it is the site of many of the synthesis steps. In muscle, it is called sarcoplasmic reticulum (SR) and is primarily involved in calcium release and uptake for muscle contraction and in neurons, although less well established, it is also probably required for calcium handling. Thus, the SER acts as an overflow site to house upregulated enzymes, and as these enzymes vary, it is also a cell type-specific suborganelle. Why are bound ribosomes concentrated in the RER and excluded from SER, rather than being found at lower levels throughout the ER? One proposed explanation is that the functions associated with bound ribosomes (translocation and modification of newly synthesised proteins) are more efficient if the proteins performing them are concentrated in one part of the membrane.

It is not known how the RER and SER maintain distinct protein compositions. Perhaps, like inner NE proteins, RER membrane proteins are localised by tight binding to a fixed substrate. In this case, the best candidate substrate would be ribosomes as they are essentially fixed and, at least in one system, co-localise with RER membrane proteins. The parallel between RER and NE protein targeting is not, however, complete, as FRAP experiments show that localised RER membrane proteins are not immobilised like NE membrane proteins. Other mechanisms, for example, active retrieval from the SER, may play a role in the concentration of RER membrane proteins.

ER Contacts Other Organelles

The ER is closely associated with essentially all other organelles in the cell. These include the plasma membrane, Golgi, vacuoles, mitochondria, peroxisomes, late endosomes and lysosomes. The contact sites may establish separate ER domains. In skeletal muscle (Fig. 20.1), the SR abuts either the plasma membrane or the T-tubules, specialised extensions of the plasma membrane that invaginate into the

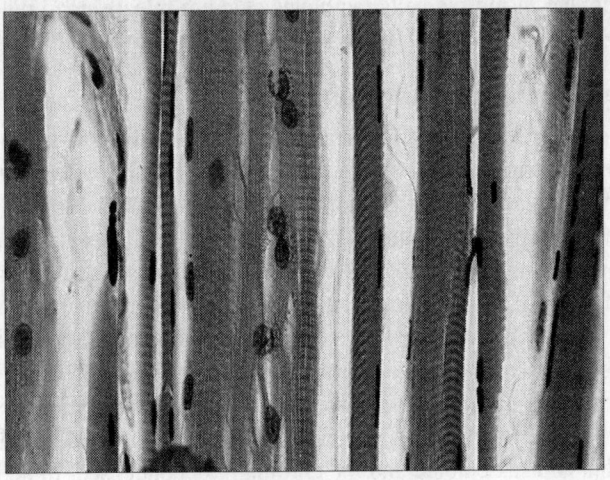

Fig. 20.1: Skeletal muscle.

muscle cell, thereby forming junctional membranes. Several proteins including ryanodine receptors (RyRs), which are ER calcium release channels, localise to these structures. The junctophilin (JP) family members contribute to the formation of these structures, transfection of cells with at least one of the junctophilin proteins (JP-1) establishes regions of proximity between the plasma membrane and SR, and its elimination in mice disrupts the junctional membrane structure. The JP proteins are proposed to reside in the SR membrane and to bind an unidentified plasma membrane component to establish the contact. It is not clear how the other membrane proteins, for example the RyRs, are targeted to junctional membranes once these structures are established.

The most complete story of how contact between the ER and another organelle is established is that of the nucleus–vacuole junction in yeast. It has been observed by electron microscopy that the nuclei and vacuoles of yeast are often in close contact and two proteins that mediate this contact have been identified. Nvj1p localises to regions of the NE adjacent to vacuoles and binds to the vacuolar membrane protein Vac8p. The absence of either of these proteins reduces the number of junctions. At least one other protein, Osh1p, also localises to this domain. Peroxisomes and mitochondria are also in close contact with the ER. A portion of the ER can be isolated with mitochondria and is enriched in some enzymes involved in lipid synthesis, such as phosphatidylserine (PS) synthase. Some of the PS synthesised in the ER is transferred to mitochondria where it is decarboxylated to phosphatidylethanolamine (PE) and then transported back to the ER. Peroxisomes and ER are similarly intertwined by the synthesis of complex lipids, which requires both ER and peroxisomal enzymes.

Microscopy has linked the ER to two other classes of organelle. Electron microscopy tomography shows that the contact between an ER domain and the *trans*-Golgi is as intimate as that between the stacks of the Golgi itself. In addition, one class of late endosomes/lysosomes has been observed to move in coordination with ER tubules, and to perhaps be deformed by the force of this interaction. Why is the ER close to other organelles in the cell? Most likely, the major reason is that all organelles need lipids that are made in the ER, close contact may allow their direct transfer to these other membranes. Some organelles, like mitochondria, have no connection with the ER via vesicular trafficking, and therefore direct transfer of lipids seems to be the only way they could receive lipids from the ER. Another reason for the close proximity of the ER with other organelles is calcium signalling. The connection between ER and plasma membrane in muscle cells facilitates calcium release upon membrane depolarisation, and the proximity between ER and mitochondria may also contribute to calcium signalling and regulation.

Propagation of the ER during Cell Division

All components of the cell are dramatically rearranged during cell division. In the face of this turbulence, does the ER maintain its structure as a single tubular network, and do its domains remain distinct? Accumulating evidence suggests that the ER network does not disassemble into vesicles during the cell cycle, but that it is divided between daughter cells by cytokinesis. The strongest support for maintenance of ER continuity comes from FLIP and FRAP experiments demonstrating that ER markers retain interphase patterns of motility during mitosis. In addition, both light and electron microscopy show that ER networks can be visualised during cell division. Are domain-specific proteins still concentrated in subregions of the mitotic network? Of the domain-specific ER proteins, the inner NE membrane proteins are the only ones whose fates during mitosis have been examined. The NE disassembles during mitosis in most eukaryotic cells: the scaffolds to which NE membrane proteins are bound in interphase are reorganised, the lamina is disassembled and the chromatin is condensed. In addition, phosphorylation of many NE proteins reduces their affinity for these partners and imaging of these proteins suggests that once freed, they diffuse throughout the ER network. However, biochemical fractionation of mitotic or meiotic cells has shown that vesicles are enriched in NE proteins, particularly in egg cells. It is not clear whether this result reflects a portion of the ER that maintains a distinct composition because it is not part of the bulk ER network, or whether domains are somehow retained in the absence of scaffolds like the lamina.

ER is Dynamic and Connected to the Cytoskeleton

In interphase cells, the peripheral ER is a dynamic network consisting of cisternal sheets, linear tubules, polygonal reticulum and three-way junctions. Several basic movements contribute to its dynamics: elongation and retraction of tubules, tubule branching, sliding of tubule junctions and the disappearance of polygons. These movements are constantly rearranging the ER network while maintaining its characteristic structure.

The dynamics of the ER network depend on the cytoskeleton. In mammalian tissue culture cells, goldfish scale cells, and *Xenopus* and sea urchin embryos the ER tubules often co-align with microtubules. Microtubule-based ER dynamics were studied with time-lapse microscopy and appear to be based on three different mechanisms. First, new ER tubules can be pulled out of existing tubules by motor proteins migrating along microtubules. Secondly, new tubules may be dragged along by the tips of polymerising microtubules. Finally, ER tubules may associate with the sides of microtubules, via motor proteins, as they slide along other microtubules. Each of these mechanisms can lead to tubule extension and, when tubules intersect, they fuse and create three-way junctions. In yeast and plants, the actin cytoskeleton, rather than the microtubule network, is required for ER dynamics.

The cytoskeleton contributes to ER dynamics, but it is not necessary for the maintenance of the existing ER network. Although depolymerisation of microtubules by nocodazole in mammalian tissue culture cells inhibits new tubule growth and causes some retraction of ER tubules from the cell periphery, the basic tubular-cisternal structure of the ER remains intact. Similarly, actin depolymerisation in yeast blocks ER movements but does not disrupt its structure.

Formation of ER Tubules

The cytoskeleton is also not necessary for the formation of a tubular network *in vitro*. In *Xenopus* egg extracts, ER networks can form *de novo* and this process is not affected by the addition of inhibitors of microtubule polymerisation, by the depletion of tubulin from the extract or by inhibitors of actin polymerisation.

If the ER network is not formed along a cytoskeleton, how is it generated? The answer is not known, but some properties of ER formation have been elucidated using *in vitro* systems. ER network formation in extracts requires ATP and GTP, and is NEM (*N*-ethyl maleimide)-sensitive. In a *Xenopus in vitro* system, incubation of membranes in the absence of cytosol leads to the formation of large vesicles that cannot subsequently be converted into networks by the addition of cytosol, and it is thought that cytosolic factors convert a basic fusion reaction into a regulated process that produces tubular networks.

Inhibition of network formation by GTPγS and NEM, suggests that a Rab protein and/or a factor similar to the NEM-sensitive fusion protein (NSF) may be involved. There is some evidence that a homolog of NSF, p97, and its co-factor p47, contribute to efficient ER network formation in *Xenopus* egg extracts and the yeast homolog of p97, Cdc48, has been shown to be involved in homotypic ER fusion. A role for p97/p47 in the *in vitro* formation of the transitional ER has also been suggested. Surprisingly, however, a mutant of Cdc48 does not affect ER structure in yeast.

Possible Mechanisms behind Tubulation

Membrane tubules are a structural feature of both the ER and the Golgi complex. Both types of tubule have similar diameters (50–100 nm), whether formed *in vitro* or *in vivo*, and in the case of the ER, tubule diameter is conserved from yeast to mammalian cells, suggesting that their formation is a regulated and fundamental process. The mechanism behind tubulation is mysterious. The simplest model is that tubules form along a cytoskeletal scaffold, although the *in vitro* experiments do not support a role for the cytoskeleton. Perhaps a different scaffold within or around the membrane is used. Regulation of lumenal volume could also contribute to tubule shape. If lumenal volume is restricted during vesicle fusion, the shape that the fused membrane could adopt would also be restricted. For example, a sphere has a different ratio of surface area to volume than a tubule. The most obvious way to control lumenal volume would be with an ion pump to maintain an ion gradient, resulting in expulsion of solution from the lumen, however, no such mechanism has been identified. Tubules also have a unique curvature of the lipid bilayer. The regulation of this curvature, by flippases or by the modification of lipids on one side of the membrane, could be another mechanism by which tubulation could be promoted. For example, modifications that change the ratio of cone-shaped to inverted cone-shaped phospholipids in one leaflet of the membrane bilayer relative to the other leaflet will alter membrane curvature. Studies on Golgi tubule formation indicate a potential role for a lipid modification reaction in tubule formation, several inhibitors of phospholipase A2 inhibit Golgi tubule formation *in vitro*.

Perspectives of ER

Exciting progress has been made in understanding ER structure and function, but some of the most interesting questions remain to be answered. How are proteins concentrated in the RER? What are the molecules that link the ER to other organelles? How are lipids transported between the ER and other organelles? How are membrane tubules generated and maintained? Some of these problems can probably be addressed by genetic experiments and with *in vitro* assays that reproduce these complex cellular events. In addition, visual methods employing fluorescent protein fusions will help to understand the dynamics of ER components. We are clearly at the beginning of a new era in understanding how biological membrane structures are generated and maintained.

Plasma membrane

The plasma membrane is a phospholipid bilayer membrane that separates the cell from its environment and regulates the transport of molecules and signals into and out of the cell. Embedded in the membrane are proteins that perform the functions of the plasma membrane. Both prokaryotic and eukaryotic cells have a plasma membrane, a double layer of lipids that separates the cell interior from the outside environment. This double layer consists largely of specialised lipids called phospholipids. A phospholipid is made up of a hydrophilic, water-loving, phosphate head, along with two hydrophobic, water-fearing, fatty acid tails. Phospholipids spontaneously arrange themselves in a double-layered structure with their hydrophobic tails pointing inward and their hydrophilic heads facing outward. This energetically favorable two-layer structure, called a phospholipid bilayer, is found in many biological membranes.

In addition to these universal functions, the plasma membrane has a more specific role in multicellular organisms. Glycoproteins on the membrane assist the cell in recognising other cells, in order to exchange metabolites and form tissues. Other proteins on the plasma membrane allow attachment to the cytoskeleton and extracellular matrix; a function that maintains cell shape and fixes the location of membrane proteins. Enzymes that catalyse reactions are also found on the plasma membrane.

Receptor proteins on the membrane have a shape that matches with a chemical messenger, resulting in various cellular responses. The plasma membrane is not fixed or rigid structure, the molecules that compose the membrane are capable of laterally movement. This movement and the multiple components of the membrane are why it is referred to as a fluid mosaic. Smaller molecules such as carbon dioxide, water, and oxygen can pass through the plasma membrane freely by diffusion or osmosis. Larger molecules needed by the cell are assisted by proteins through active transport.

The plasma membrane of a cell has multiple functions. These include transporting nutrients into the cell, allowing waste to leave, preventing materials from entering the cell, averting needed materials from leaving the cell, maintaining the pH of the cytosol, and preserving the osmotic pressure of the cytosol. Transport proteins which allow some materials to pass through but not others are used for these functions. These proteins use ATP hydrolysis to pump materials against their concentration gradients.

Structure of plasma membrane

- The plasma membrane (also known as the cell membrane or cytoplasmic membrane) is a biological membrane that separates the interior of a cell from its outside environment.
- It is a fluid mosaic of lipids, proteins and carbohydrate.
- The plasma membrane is impermeable to ions and most water-soluble molecules.
- They cross the membrane only through transmembrane channels, carriers, and pumps.
- These transmembrane proteins provide the cell with nutrients, control internal ion concentrations, and establish a transmembrane electrical potential.
- A single amino acid change in one plasma membrane pump and Cl^- channel causes the human disease cystic fibrosis.
- The cell membrane is primarily composed of a mix of proteins and lipids.
- Depending on the membrane's location and role in the body, lipids can make up anywhere from 20 to 80 per cent of the membrane, with the remainder being proteins.
- While lipids help to give membranes their flexibility, proteins monitor and maintain the cell's chemical climate and assist in the transfer of molecules across the membrane.
- The fundamental structure of the membrane is the phospholipid bilayer, which forms a stable barrier between two aqueous compartments.
- The plasma membrane is composed of a phospholipid bilayer, which is two layers of phospholipids back-to-back.
- Phospholipids are lipids with a phosphate group attached to them.
- The phospholipids have one head and two tails.
- The head is polar and hydrophilic, or water-loving.
- The tails are nonpolar and hydrophobic, or water-fearing.

Functions of plasma membrane

- The primary function of the plasma membrane is to protect the cell from its surroundings.
- The plasma membrane also plays a role in anchoring the cytoskeleton to provide shape to the cell, and in attaching to the extracellular matrix and other cells to help group cells together to form tissues.
- The membrane also maintains the cell potential.

- The cell membrane interacts with the cell membrane of adjacent cells, e.g. to form plant and animal tissues.
- The cell membrane is primarily composed of proteins and lipids. While lipids help to give membranes their flexibility and proteins monitor and maintain the cell's chemical climate and assist in the transfer of molecules across the membrane.
- The lipid bilayer is semi-permeable, which allows only selected molecules to diffuse across the membrane.

Components of the plasma membrane

Component	Location
Phospholipids	Main fabric of the membrane
Cholesterol	Tucked between the hydrophobic tails of the membrane phospholipids
Integral protein	Embedded in the phospholipid bilayer, may or may not extend through both layers
Peripheral proteins	On the inner or outer surface of the phospholipid bilayer, but not embedded in its hydrophobic core
Carbohydrates	Attached to proteins or lipids on the extracellular side of the membrane (forming glycoproteins and glycolipids)

ENDOCYTIC PATHWAY

Two basic processes are discussed in this section of chapter, endocytosis and phagocytosis.

Endoeytosis

Endoeytosis (Fig. 20.2) is a widespread cellular function that regulates the quantal uptake of exogenous molecules from the cell's environment via plasmamembrane-derived vesicles and vacuoles. Both soluble (pinocytosis) and particulate (phagocytosis) substances may be interiorised, destined either for the vacuolar apparatus and intracellular digestion or transport through the cytoplasm and subsequent exocytosis. Although most, if not all, eukaryotic cells demonstrate these primitive functions, they are particularly prominent in leucocytes, macrophages, capillary endothelial and thyroid epithelial cells, yolk sac, and

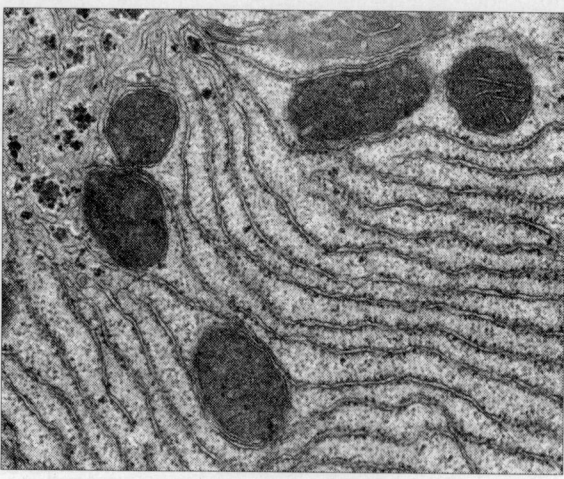

Fig. 20.2: Endoeytosis.

oocytes. Here they are involved in host defense, immunological reactions, macromolecular transport, hormone transformations, and the regulation of metabolic pathways, and perhaps in cellular nutrition as well. Many cells generate pinocytic vesicles at constant but different rates, enclosing fluid and solutes at the concentration at which they are found in the extracellular milieu.

Endocytosis is the process by which cells absorb molecules (such as proteins) from outside the cell by engulfing it with their cell membrane. It is used by all cells of the body because most substances important to them are large polar molecules that cannot pass through the hydrophobic plasma membrane or cell membrane. The process opposite to endocytosis is exocytosis.

Types of endoeytosis

There are three main types of endocytosis that are distinguished by the size of the vesicle formed and the organelle machinery involved.

1. Phagocytosis (literally, cell-eating) is the process by which cells ingest solids, such as bacteria, viruses, or the remnants of cells which have undergone apoptosis. The membrane invaginates enclosing the wanted particles in a pocket, then engulfs the object by pinching it off, and the object is sealed off into a large vacuole known as a phagosome.

2. Pinocytosis (literally, cell-drinking). This process is how cells take in liquids. Both phagocytosis and pinocytosis are non-receptor-mediated forms of endocytosis, and may result in the cell engulfing non-specific or unwanted particles.

3. Receptor-mediated endocytosis is a more specific active event where the cytoplasm membrane folds inward to form coated pits. In this case, proteins or other trigger particles lock into receptors/ligands in the cell's plasma membrane. It is then, and only then that the particles are engulfed. These inward budding vesicles bud to form cytoplasmic vesicles. This process may also result in engulfing of unwanted particles, however not to the extent of pino/phagocytosis.

Function of endocytosis

Endocytosis is required for a vast number of functions that are essential for the well-being of cell. It intimately regulates many processes, including nutrient uptake, cell adhesion and migration, receptor signalling, pathogen entry, neurotransmission, receptor downregulation, antigen presentation, cell polarity, mitosis, growth and differentiation, and drug delivery.

Endocytosis pathways

Endocytosis pathways could be subdivided into four categories: Namely, clathrin-mediated endocytosis, caveolae, macropinocytosis, and phagocytosis:

1. Clathrin-mediated endocytosis is mediated by small (approximately 100 nm in diameter) vesicles that have a morphologically characteristic crystalline coat made up of a complex of proteins that mainly associated with the cytosolic protein clathrin. Clathrin-coated vesicles (CCVs) are found in virtually all cells and from domains of the plasma membrane termed clathrin-coated pits.

2. Caveolae are the most common reported non-clathrin coated plasma membrane buds, which exist on the surface of many, but not all cell types. They consist of the cholesterol-binding protein caveolin (Vip21) with a bilayer enriched in cholesterol and glycolipids. Caveolae are small (approximately 50 nm in diameter) flask-shape pits in the membrane that resemble the shape of a cave (hence the name caveolae).

3. Macropinocytosis, which usually occurs from highly ruffled regions of the plasma membrane, is the invagination of the cell membrane to form a pocket, which then pinches off into the cell to form a vesicle (0.5–5 μm in diameter) filled with large volume of extracellular fluid and molecules within it.

4. Phagocytosis is the process by which cells bind and internalise particulate matter larger than around 0.75 μm in diameter, such as small-sized dust particles, cell debris, micro-organisms and even apoptotic cells, which only occurs in specialised cells.

Principal components of endocytic pathway

The endocytic pathway of mammalian cells consists of distinct membrane compartments that internalise molecules from the plasma membrane and recycle them back to the surface (early endosomes and recycling endosomes) or sort them to degradation (late endosomes and lysosomes). The principle components of endocytic pathway are:

1. Early endosomes are the first station on the endocytic pathway. Early endosomes are often located in the periphery of the cell and receive most of types of vesicles coming from the cell surface. They have a characteristic tubulo-vesicular morphology (vesicles up to 1 μm in diameter with connected tubules of approximately 50 nm diameter) and a mildly acid pH.

2. Late endosomes receive internalised material en route to lysosomes, usually from early endosomes in the endocytic pathway, from *trans*-Golgi network (TGN) in the biosynthetic pathway, and from phagosomes in the phagocytic pathway. Late endosomes often contain many membrane vesicles or membrane lamellae and proteins characteristic of lysosomes, including lysosomal membrane glycoproteins and acid hydrolases.

3. Lysosomes are the last compartment of the endocytic pathway. They are acidic (approximately pH 4.8) and by EM usually appear as large vacuoles (1–2 μm in diameter) containing electron dense material.

Clathrin-mediated endocytosis

The major route for endocytosis in most cells, and the best-understood, is that mediated by the molecule clathrin. This large protein assists in the formation of a coated pit on the inner surface of the plasma membrane of the cell. This pit then buds into the cell to form a coated vesicle in the cytoplasm of the cell. Coats function to deform the donor membrane to produce a vesicle, and they also function in the selection of the vesicle cargo. Coat complexes have been well characterised so far including: coat protein-I (COP-I), COP-II, and clathrin. Clathrin coats are involved in two crucial transport steps: (i) receptor-mediated and fluid-phase endocytosis from the plasma membrane to early endosome, and (ii) transport from the TGN to endosomes. Vesicles selectively concentrate and exclude certain proteins during formation and are not representative of the membrane as a whole. AP2 adaptors are multisubunit complexes that perform this function at the plasma membrane. The best-understood receptors that are found concentrated in coated vesicles of mammalian cells are the LDL receptor (which removes LDL from circulating blood), the transferrin receptor (which brings ferric ions bound by transferrin into the cell) and certain hormone receptors (such as that for EGF). LDL receptor discussed in the end of this chapter.

Phagocytosis

Phagocytosis is the cellular process of phagocytes and protists of engulfing solid particles by the cell membrane to form an internal phagosome. Phagocytosis is a specific form of endocytosis involving the vesicular internalisation of solid particles, such as bacteria, and is therefore distinct from other forms of endocytosis such as the vesicular internalisation of various liquids. Phagocytosis is involved in the acquisition of nutrients for some cells, and in the immune system it is a major mechanism used to remove pathogens and cell debris.

Bacteria, dead tissue cells, and small mineral particles are all examples of objects that may be phagocytosed (Fig. 20.3). The process is only homologous to eating at the level of single-celled organisms; in multicellular animals, the process has been adapted to eliminate debris and pathogens, as opposed to taking in fuel for cellular processes, except in the case of the Trichoplax.

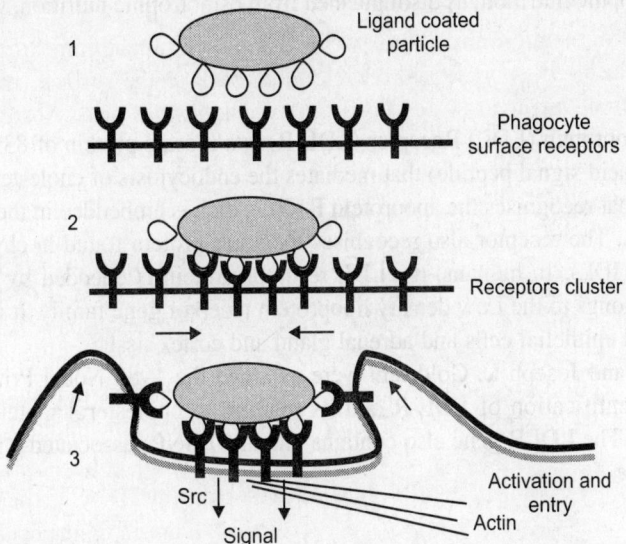

Fig. 20.3: Phagocytosis in three steps: 1. Unbound phagocyte surface receptors do not trigger phagocytosis. 2. Binding of receptors causes them to cluster. 3. Phagocytosis is triggered and the particle is taken-up by the phagocyte.

Phagocytosis is in immune system

Phagocytosis in mammalian immune cells is activated by attachment to Pathogen-associated molecular patterns (PAMPS), which leads to NF-κB activation. Opsonins such as C3b and antibodies can act as attachment sites and aid phagocytosis of pathogens. Engulfment of material is facilitated by the actin-myosin contractile system. The phagosome of ingested material is then fused with the lysosome, leading to degradation.

Degradation can be oxygen-dependent or oxygen-independent:

1. Oxygen-dependent degradation depends on NADPH and the production of reactive oxygen species. Hydrogen peroxide and myeloperoxidase activate a halogenating system which leads to the destruction of bacteria.

2. Oxygen-independent degradation depends on the release of granules, containing proteolytic enzymes such as defensins, lysozyme and cationic proteins. Other antimicrobial peptides are present in these granules, including lactoferrin which sequesters iron to provide unfavourable growth conditions for bacteria.

It is possible for cells other than dedicated phagocytes (such as dendritic cells) to engage in phagocytosis.

Phagocytosis in apoptosis

Following apoptosis, the dying cells need to be taken up into the surrounding tissues by macrophages in a process called Efferocytosis. One of the features of an apoptotic cell is the presentation of a variety of intracellular molecules on the cell surface, such as calreticulin, phosphatidylserine (from the inner layer of the plasma membrane), Annexin A1 and oxidised LDL.

Phagocytosis in protists

In many protists, phagocytosis is used as a means of feeding, providing part or all of their nourishment. This is called phagotrophic nutrition, as distinguished from osmotrophic nutrition, which takes place by absorption.

LDL RECEPTOR

The Low-Density Lipoprotein (LDL) Receptor (LDL-R) is a mosaic protein of 839 amino acids (after removal of 21-amino acid signal peptide) that mediates the endocytosis of cholesterol-rich LDL. It is a cell-surface receptor that recognises the apoprotein B100, which is embedded in the outer phospholipid layer of LDL particles. The receptor also recognises the apoE protein found in chylomicron remnants and VLDL remnants (IDL). In humans, the LDL receptor protein is encoded by the LDLR gene on chromosome 19. It belongs to the Low density lipoprotein receptor gene family. It is most significantly expressed in bronchial epithelial cells and adrenal gland and cortex tissue.

Michael S. Brown and Joseph L. Goldstein were awarded the 1985 Nobel Prize in Physiology or Medicine for their identification of LDL-R and its relation to cholesterol metabolism and familial hypercholesterolemia. The LDLR gene also contains one of 27 SNPs associated with increased risk of coronary artery disease.

Structure of LDLR

Gene

The LDLR gene resides on chromosome 19 at the band 19p13.2 and is split into 18 exons. Exon 1 contains a signal sequence that localises the receptor to the endoplasmic reticulum for transport to the cell surface. Beyond this, exons 2–6 code the ligand binding region; 7–14 code the epidermal growth factor (EGF) domain, 15 codes the oligosaccharide rich region; 16 (and some of 17) code the membrane spanning region; and 18 (with the rest of 17) code the cytosolic domain. This gene produces 6 isoforms through alternative splicing.

Protein

This protein belongs to the LDLR family and is made up of a number of functionally distinct domains, including 3 EGF-like domains, 7 LDL-R class A domains, and 6 LDL-R class B repeats.

The *N*-terminal domain of the LDL receptor, which is responsible for ligand binding, is composed of seven sequence repeats (~50% identical). Each repeat, referred to as a class A repeat or LDL-A, contains roughly 40 amino acids, including 6 cysteine residues that form disulfide bonds within the repeat. Additionally, each repeat has highly conserved acidic residues which it uses to coordinate a single calcium ion in an octahedral lattice. Both the disulfide bonds and calcium coordination are necessary for the structural integrity of the domain during the receptors repeated trips to the highly acidic interior of the endosome. The exact mechanism of interaction between the class A repeats and ligand (LDL) is unknown, but it is thought that the repeats act as 'grabbers' to hold the LDL. Binding of ApoB requires repeats 2–7 while binding ApoE requires only repeat 5 (thought to be the ancestral repeat).

Next to the ligand binding domain is an EGF precursor homology domain (EGFP domain). This shows approximately 30% homology with the EGF precursor gene. There are three 'growth factor' repeats, A, B and C. A and B are closely linked while C is separated by the YWTD repeat region, which adopts a beta-propeller conformation (LDL-R class B domain). It is thought that this region is responsible for the pH-dependent conformational shift that causes bound LDL to be released in the endosome.

A third domain of the protein is rich in *O*-linked oligosaccharides but appears to show little function. Knockout experiments have confirmed that no significant loss of activity occurs without this domain. It has been speculated that the domain may have ancestrally acted as a spacer to push the receptor beyond the extracellular matrix.

The single transmembrane domain of 22 (mostly) non-polar residues crosses the plasma membrane in a single alpha helix.

The cytosolic C-terminal domain contains ~50 amino acids, including a signal sequence important for localizing the receptors to clathrin-coated pits and for triggering receptor-mediated endocytosis after binding. Portions of the cytosolic sequence have been found in other lipoprotein receptors, as well as in more distant receptor relatives.

Mutations

Mutations in the gene encoding the LDL receptor are known to cause familial hypercholesterolaemia.

There are 5 broad classes of mutation of the LDL receptor:

- Class 1 mutations affect the synthesis of the receptor in the endoplasmic reticulum (ER).
- Class 2 mutations prevent proper transport to the Golgi body needed for modifications to the receptor, e.g. a truncation of the receptor protein at residue number 660 leads to domains 3,4 and 5 of the EGF precursor domain being missing. This precludes the movement of the receptor from the ER to the Golgi, and leads to degradation of the receptor protein.
- Class 3 mutations stop the binding of LDL to the receptor, e.g. repeat 6 of the ligand binding domain (*N*-terminal, extracellular fluid) is deleted.
- Class 4 mutations inhibit the internalisation of the receptor-ligand complex, e.g. JD mutant results from a single point mutation in the NPVY domain (C-terminal, cytosolic; C residue converted to a Y, residue number 807). This domain recruits clathrin and other proteins responsible for the endocytosis of LDL, therefore this mutation inhibits LDL internalisation.
- Class 5 mutations give rise to receptors that cannot recycle properly. This leads to a relatively mild phenotype as receptors are still present on the cell surface (but all must be newly synthesised).

Function of LDL Receptor

LDL receptor mediates the endocytosis of cholesterol-rich LDL and thus maintains the plasma level of LDL. This occurs in all nucleated cells, but mainly in the liver which removes ~70% of LDL from the circulation. LDL receptors are clustered in clathrin-coated pits, and coated pits pinch off from the surface to form coated endocytic vesicles that carry LDL into the cell. After internalisation, the receptors dissociate from their ligands when they are exposed to lower pH in endosomes. After dissociation, the receptor folds back on itself to obtain a closed conformation and recycles to the cell surface. The rapid recycling of LDL receptors provides an efficient mechanism for delivery of cholesterol to cells. It was also reported that by association with lipoprotein in the blood, viruses such as hepatitis C virus, Flaviviridae viruses and bovine viral diarrheal virus could enter cells indirectly via LDLR-mediated endocytosis. LDLR has been identified as the primary mode of entry for the Vesicular stomatitis virus in mice and humans. In addition, LDLR modulation is associated with early atherosclerosis-related lymphatic dysfunction. Synthesis of receptors in the cell is regulated by the level of free intracellular cholesterol; if it is in excess for the needs of the cell then the transcription of the receptor gene will be inhibited. LDL receptors are translated by ribosomes on the endoplasmic reticulum and are modified by the Golgi apparatus before travelling in vesicles to the cell surface.

Clinical Significance

In humans, LDL is directly involved in the development of atherosclerosis,which is the process responsible for the majority of cardiovascular diseases, due to accumulation of LDL-cholesterol in the blood. Hyperthyroidism may be associated with hypocholesterolemia via upregulation of the LDL receptor, and hypothyroidism with the converse. A vast number of studies have described the relevance of LDL receptors in the pathophysiology of atherosclerosis, metabolomics syndrome, and steatohepatitis Previously, rare mutations in LDL-genes have been shown to contribute to myocardial infarction risk in individual families, whereas common variants at more than 45 loci have been associated with myocardial infarction risk in the population. When compared with non-carriers, LDLR mutation carriers had higher plasma LDL cholesterol, whereas APOA5 mutation carriers had higher plasma triglycerides. Recent evidence has connected MI risk with coding-sequence mutations at two genes functionally related to APOA5, namely lipoprotein lipase and apolipoprotein C-III. Combined, these observations suggest that, as well as LDL cholesterol, disordered metabolism of triglyceride-rich lipoproteins contributes to MI risk. Overall, LDLR has a high clinical relevance in blood lipids.

Clinical marker

A multi-locus genetic risk score study based on a combination of 27 loci, including the LDLR gene, identified individuals at increased risk for both incident and recurrent coronary artery disease events, as well as an enhanced clinical benefit from statin therapy. The study was based on a community cohort study (the Malmo Diet and Cancer study) and four additional randomised controlled trials of primary prevention cohorts (JUPITER and ASCOT) and secondary prevention cohorts (CARE and PROVE IT-TIMI 22).

Chapter 21

Golgi Apparatus

INTRODUCTION

Golgi apparatus is a complex network of smooth membrane enclosed organelle which helps in collection, packaging, distribution and secretion of biomolecules.

Location: The Golgi apparatus occurs in all eukaryotic cells except male gametes of bryophytes and pteridophytes, mature sieve tubes, some fungal cells, and mature sperms and RBCs of animals. It is also absent in prokaryotic cells.

Distribution: In most animal cells Golgi apparatus is single and localised near nucleus and often close to the centrosome. But in most invertebrate cells, it is diffused in form of two or more interconnected units. However in most plant cells, liver and nerve cells of vertebrate the Golgi apparatus consists of many independent units called dictyosomes or Golgi bodies or Golgi stacks. Their number is highly variable – from one in simple alga like Micromonas to 25000 in rhizoidal cell of aquatic alga chara. A liver cell may have up to 50 dictyosomes. The Golgi apparatus constitutes about 2% of total cell volume.

STRUCTURE OF GOLGI APPARATUS

Golgi apparatuses are extremely dynamic and pleomorphic structure because of its variable shape and form in different cell types. The Golgi apparatus of plant cells consists of about 10–20 individual subunits that found scattered throughout the cytoplasm. Each individual subunit is called a dictyosome or Golgi body or Golgi stack. The zone of clear cytoplasm surrounding a Golgi body is called zone of exclusion. The Golgi apparatus is one of the important organelles of eukaryotic cells. Structure of Golgi apparatus is shown in Fig. 21.1. Each dictyosome is about 1–5 μm in diameter. Under EM a Golgi body seen to consist of a stack of 3–10 flatted sacs or cisternae with a complex irregular network of tubules vesicles and vacuoles on the outer edges. The adjacent cisternae are separated by an intercisternal space of 10–30 nm. The intercisternal space contains protein cross-links that hold the cisternae together. The cisternae maybe flat, but often curved to give a definite polarity to the Golgi body. Thus, a Golgi body has 2 distinct faces: a convex forming or *cis* face and a concave maturing or transface. So a *cis* face always facing toward nucleus while the trans face facing towards plasma membrane contains a tubular reticulum called trans Golgi network (TGN). The membranes of the maturing face are thicker (7–8 μm) while

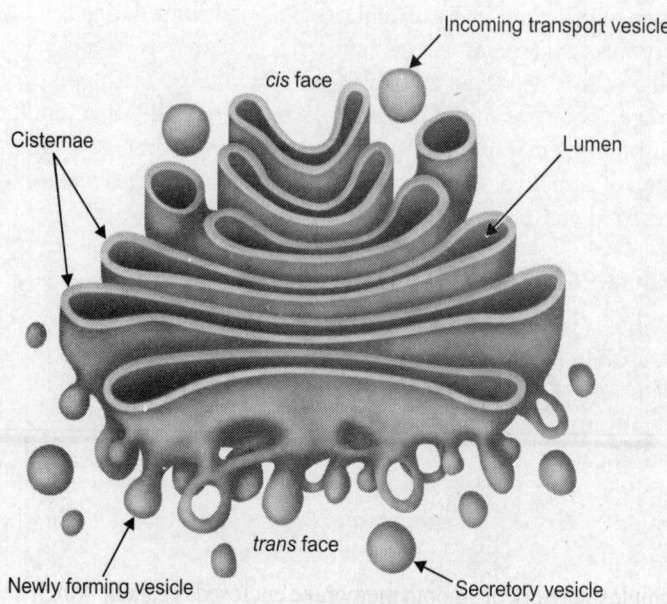

Fig. 21.1: Structure of Golgi apparatus.

those of forming face are thinner (about 4 μm). Many small Golgi vesicles (20–80 μn in diameter) are found associated with the Golgi body. These vesicles are thought to transport proteins and lipids between the cisternae and tubules. The transitional vesicles pinched off from the rough ER and fuse with the *cis* face of the Golgi. The transport or shuttle vesicles that keep budding off from the cisternal edges tubules transport materials between the cisternae in *cis* – to – *trans* direction. The secretary vesicles that derive from TGN carry glycoproteins, glycolipids and polysaccharides to different destinations in the cell or outside the cell. The secretary vesicles are of 2 types: smooth secretary vesicles and coated vesicles. The coated vesicles are covered by a basketlike network of protein complex consists of clathrin triskelions. The larger secretary vesicles are called Golgian vacuoles. Some of them function as lysosomes.

FUNCTIONS OF GOLGI APPARATUS

Secretion is the major function of Golgi apparatus, which help in collection, storage condensation, modification and packaging of various materials into secretary vesicles. These release the contents to the exterior through exocytosis, e.g. secretion of mucilage by root cap cells, secretion of hormones, gum, wax, cell wall material, ground matrix of connective tissue, etc.

Secretory proteins are seen emerging from the maturing face contained in a membranous dilation termed a prosecretory granule. The prosecretory granule buds off to become a condensing vacuole, which, after the removal of fluid, is termed a secretory granule or secretory vesicle. Secretory granules containing digestive enzymes are specifically referred to as zymogen granules. Under the appropriate conditions, the secretory granule moves to the cell surface and fuses with the membrane, thereby releasing its contents to the outside. This Ca^{++} dependent process is called exocytosis or secretion.

There are two kinds of secretion:

1. Constitutive secretion: Secretory products are produced and released continuously.
2. Regulated secretion: Secretory products are released in response to specific stimuli.

It helps in formation of cell plate, cell wall and new plasma lemma during cell division. It also helps in the formation of primary lysosomes, sperm acrosome, nematocysts in coelenterates and root hairs. In oocytes of animals, yolk is deposited around Golgi apparatus by the process called vitellogenesis. Golgi apparatus brings about transformation of membrane (e.g. ER) into another such as plasma membrane and lysosomal membrane. It also participate in recycling of membranes. It facilitates glycosylation (addition of carbohydrates to proteins), liposylation (formation of lipoprotein) sulphation (addition of sulphates) and phosphorylation (addition of phosphates).

ORIGIN OF GOLGI APPARATUS

There are two prevailing theories as to the formation of the Golgi apparatus. The vesicular shuttle model postulates that Golgi cannot be made from scratch and that the vesicles of the endoplasmic reticulum are sent to the pre-existing Golgi. On the other hand, the cisternae maturation model suggests that vesicles from the ER fuse together to form the Golgi and as proteins are processed and mature they create the next Golgi compartment. Intriguing new data suggest that perhaps neither model is completely correct. This will likely lead to yet another model. You may not see what all the fuss is about, but the differing Golgi theories say very different things about how cells function. Understanding basic cellular processes, such as how the Golgi works, ultimately can have a profound impact on the development of methods to diagnose, treat and prevent diseases that involve those processes. Here's an example of the Golgi apparatus as it is seen in the electron microscope. The complex arrangements of stacked cisternae, with their associated vesicles, is obvious. The Golgi apparatus has a convex forming face (at the bottom of this image) to which proteins to be packaged and/or modified are brought, and a concave maturing face from which the vesicles containing the modified product are pinched off. Golgi apparatus as seen in electron microscope is shown in Fig. 21.2. For many years, the existence of this organelle was controversial and it was considered by some people to be an artifact of preparation, but its demonstrability in unstained preparations (using phase contrast microscopy) and in the transmission electron microscope settled the question. The Golgi apparatus is found in most cell types, though it's sometimes inconspicuous. The Golgi Apparatus or Golgi Body, appears in both plant and animal cells. It's function is to receive food from the Endoplasmic Reticulum, package it and send it to organelles throughout the cell. The Golgi also plays an important role in the synthesis of proteoglycans, molecules present in the extracellular matrix of animals and it is a major site of carbohydrate synthesis. Golgi apparatus process and packages

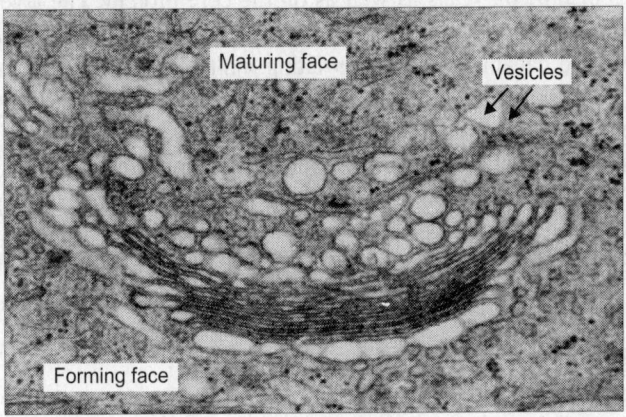

Fig. 21.2: Golgi apparatus as seen in electron microscope.

proteins for deliver to other organelles in the cell after they have been synthesised. Figure 21.3 shows Chief (peptic) in the gastric gland of a monkey. The basal cytoplasm is filled with parallel cisternae of the rough ER (see inset). The cell apex contains zymogenic secretory granules and elements of the Golgi complex.

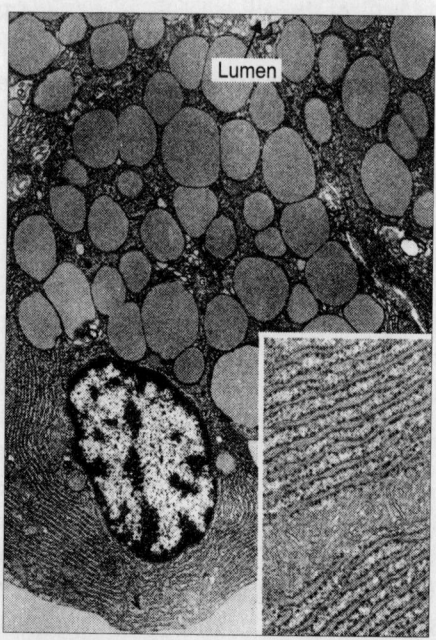

Fig. 21.3: Chief (peptic) in the gastric gland of a monkey. The basal cytoplasm is filled with parallel cisternae of the rough ER (see inset). The cell apex contains zymogenic secretory granules and elements of the Golgi complex.

This includes the productions of glycosaminoglycans or GAGs, long unbranched polysaccharides which the Golgi then attaches to a protein synthesised in the endoplasmic reticulum to form the proteoglycan. Enzymes in the Golgi will polymerise several of these GAGs via a xylose link onto the core protein. Another task of the Golgi involves the sulphation of certain molecules passing through its lumen via sulphotranferases that gain their sulphur molecule from a donor called PAPs. This process occurs on the GAGs of proteoglycans as well as on the core protein. The level of sulphation is very important to the proteoglycans' signalling abilities as well as giving the proteoglycan its overall negative charge. The Golgi is also capable of phosphorylating molecules. To do so it transports ATP into the lumen. The Golgi itself contains resident kinases, such as casein kinases. One molecule that is phosphorylated in the Golgi is Apolipoprotein, which forms a molecule known as VLDL that is a constitute of blood serum. It is thought that the phosphorylation of these molecules is important to help aid in their sorting of secretion into the blood serum. The Golgi also has a putative role in apoptosis, with several Bcl-2 family members localised there, as well as to the mitochondria. In addition a newly characterised anti-apoptotic protein, GAAP (Golgi anti-apoptotic protein), which almost exclusively resides in the Golgi, protects cells from apoptosis by an as-yet undefined mechanism.

Vesicular Transport

Vesicles which leave the rough endoplasmic reticulum are transported to the *cis* face of the Golgi apparatus, where they fuse with the Golgi membrane and empty their contents into the lumen. Once inside they are modified, sorted and shipped towards their final destination. As such, the Golgi apparatus tends to be more prominent and numerous in cells synthesising and secreting many substances: plasma B cells, the antibody-secreting cells of the immune system, have prominent Golgi complexes.

Those proteins destined for areas of the cell other than either the endoplasmic reticulum or Golgi apparatus are moved towards the *trans* face, to a complex network of membranes and associated vesicles known as the *trans*-Golgi network (TGN). This area of the Golgi is the point at which proteins are sorted and shipped to their intended destinations by their placement into one of at least three different types of vesicles, depending upon the molecular marker they carry.

Type of vesicular transport

Exocytotic vesicles (continuous): Vesicle contains proteins destined for extracellular release. After packaging the vesicles bud off and immediately move towards the plasma membrane, where they fuse and release the contents into the extracellular space in a process known as constitutive secretion. Antibody release by activated plasma B cells.

Secretory vesicles (regulated): Vesicle contains proteins destined for extracellular release. After packaging the vesicles bud off and are stored in the cell until a signal is given for their release. When the appropriate signal is received they move towards the membrane and fuse to release their contents. This process is known as regulated secretion. Neurotransmitter release from neurons.

Lysosomal vesicles: Vesicle contains proteins destined for the lysosome, an organelle of degradation containing many acid hydrolases or to lysosome-like storage organelles. These proteins include both digestive enzymes and membrane proteins. The vesicle first fuses with the late endosome and the contents are then transferred to the lysosome via unknown mechanisms. Digestive proteases destined for the lysosome.

CISTERNAE MATURATION MODEL

According to this model, packages of processing enzymes and newly made proteins that originate in the ER fuse together to form the Golgi. As the proteins are processed and mature, they create the next Golgi compartment. This is called the cisternae maturation model. In this model, the cisternae of the Golgi apparatus move by being built at the *cis* face and destroyed at the *trans* face.

The vesicles from the endoplasmic reticulum fuse together to form a cisterna at the *cis* face and this cisternae would appear to move through the Golgi stack when a new cisterna is formed at the *cis* face. This model is supported by the fact that structures larger than the transport vesicles were observed microscopically to progress through the Golgi apparatus. In summary, packages of processing enzymes and new proteins originating in the ER fuse together to form the Golgi and as the proteins are processed and mature, the next Golgi compartment is created. Vesicular transport is one of models of Golgi apparatus that says that Golgi cannot make from scratch and that vesicles in the ER are sent to pre-existing Golgi.

VESICULAR SHUTTLE MODEL

According to this model newly made proteins are packaged in the rough ER and are sent for further processing to a pre-existing structure (the Golgi) that is made up of different compartments. This is called the vesicular shuttle model. This model views the Golgi apparatus as a very stable organelle that is divided into compartments in the *cis* to *trans* direction. Membrane bound carriers transport material between the endoplasmic reticulum and the different compartments of the Golgi. Experimental evidence shows the abundance of small vesicles in close proximity to the Golgi apparatus. Actin filaments direct the vesicles by connecting packaging proteins to the membrane to ensure that they fuse with the correct compartment. To summarise, newly made proteins are packaged in the rough ER and are sent for processing to a pre-existing structure known as the Golgi which is made up of different compartments.

PROTEIN GLYCOSYLATION WITHIN THE GOLGI

Protein processing within the Golgi involves the modification and synthesis of the carbohydrate portions of glycoproteins. One of the major aspects of this processing is the modification of the N-linked oligosaccharides that were added to proteins in the ER. As discussed earlier in this chapter, proteins are modified within the ER by the addition of an oligosaccharide consisting of 14 sugar residues. Three glucose residues and one mannose are then removed while the polypeptides are still in the ER. Following transport to the Golgi apparatus, the N-linked oligosaccharides of these glycoproteins are subject to extensive further modifications. N-linked oligosaccharides are processed within the Golgi apparatus in an ordered sequence of reactions (Fig. 21.4). The first modification of proteins destined for secretion or for the plasma membrane is the removal of three additional mannose residues. This is followed by the sequential addition of an N-acetylglucosamine, the removal of two more mannoses and the addition of a fucose and two more N-acetylglucosamines. Finally, three galactose and three sialic acid residues are added and different glycoproteins are modified to different extents during their passage through the Golgi, depending on both the structure of the protein and on the amount of processing enzymes that are present within the Golgi complexes of different types of cells. Consequently, proteins can emerge from the Golgi with a variety of different N-linked oligosaccharides. The processing of the N-linked oligosaccharide of lysosomal proteins differs from that of secreted and plasma membrane proteins. Rather than the initial removal of three mannose residues, proteins destined for incorporation into lysosomes are modified by mannose phosphorylation. In the first step of this reaction, N-acetylglucosamine phosphates are added to specific mannose residues, probably while the protein is still in the *cis* Golgi network (Fig. 21.5). This is followed by removal of the N-acetyl-glucosamine group, leaving mannose-6-phosphate residues

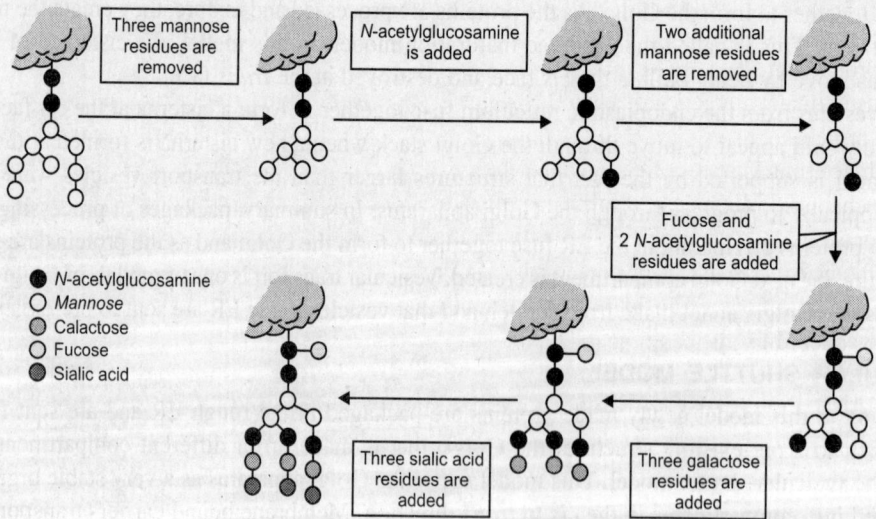

Fig. 21.4: Processing of N-linked oligosaccharides in the Golgi. The N-linked oligo-saccharides of glycoproteins transported from the ER are further modified by an ordered sequence of reactions in the Golgi.

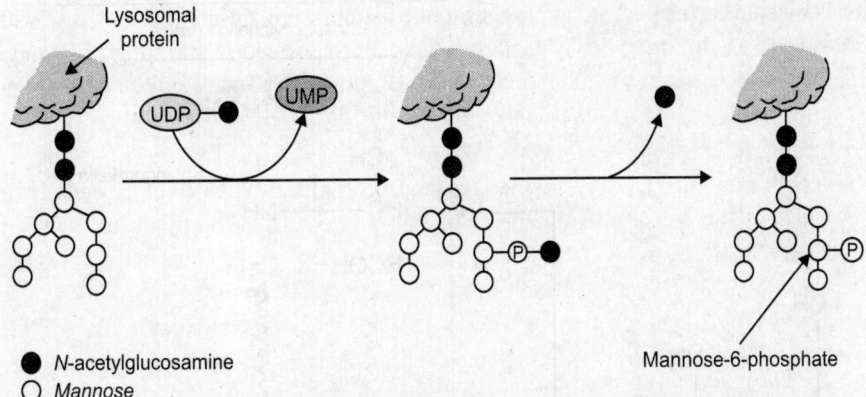

Fig. 21.5: Targeting of lysosomal proteins by phosphorylation of mannose residues. Proteins destined for incorporation into lysosomes are specifically recognised and modified by the addition of phosphate groups to the 6 position of mannose residues. In the first step of the reaction, N-acetylglucosamine phosphates are transferred to mannose residues from UDP-N-acetylglucosamine. The N-acetylglucosamine groups are then removed, leaving mannose-6-phosphates.

on the N-linked oligosaccharide. Because of this modification, these residues are not removed during further processing. Instead, these phosphorylated mannose residues are specifically recognised by a mannose-6-phosphate receptor in the *trans* Golgi network, which directs the transport of these proteins to lysosomes. The phosphorylation of mannose residues is thus a critical step in sorting lysosomal proteins to their correct intracellular destination. The specificity of this process resides in the enzyme that catalyses the first step in the reaction sequence—the selective addition of N-acetylglucosamine phosphates to lysosomal proteins. This enzyme recognises a structural determinant that is present on lysosomal proteins but not on proteins destined for the plasma membrane or secretion. This recognition determinant is not a simple sequence of amino acids, rather, it is formed in the folded protein by the juxtaposition of amino acid sequences from different regions of the polypeptide chain. In contrast to the signal sequences that direct protein translocation to the ER, the recognition determinant that leads to mannose phosphorylation and thus ultimately targets proteins to lysosomes, depends on the three-dimensional conformation of the folded protein.

Such determinants are called signal patches, in contrast to the linear targeting signals discussed earlier in this chapter. Proteins can also be modified by the addition of carbohydrates to the side chains of acceptor serine and threonine residues within specific sequences of amino acids (O-linked glycosylation). These modifications take place in the Golgi apparatus by the sequential addition of single sugar residues. The serine or threonine is usually linked directly to N-acetylgalactosamine, to which other sugars can then be added. In some cases, these sugars are further modified by the addition of sulphate groups.

LIPID AND POLYSACCHARIDE METABOLISM IN THE GOLGI

In addition to its activities in processing and sorting glycoproteins, the Golgi apparatus functions in lipid metabolism—in particular, in the synthesis of glycolipids and sphingomyelin. As discussed earlier, the glycerol phospholipids, cholesterol and ceramide are synthesised in the ER. Sphingomyelin and glycolipids are then synthesised from ceramide in the Golgi apparatus (Fig. 21.6). Sphingomyelin (the only nonglycerol phospholipid in cell membranes) is synthesised by the transfer of a phosphorylcholine

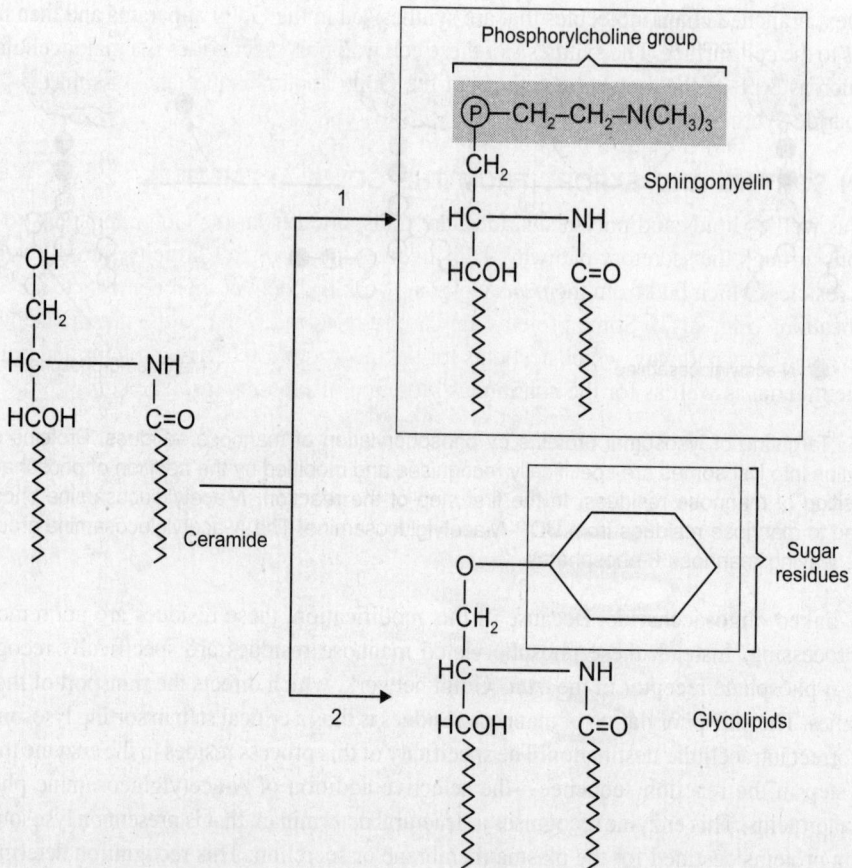

Fig. 21.6: Synthesis of sphingomyelin and glycolipids. Ceramide, which is synthesised in the ER, is converted either to sphingomyelin (a phospholipid) or to glycolipids in the Golgi apparatus. In the first reaction, a phosphorylcholine group is transferred from phosphatidyl-choline to ceramide. Alternatively, a variety of different glycolipids can be synthesised by the addition of one or more sugar residues (e.g. glucose).

group from phosphatidylcholine to ceramide. Alternatively, the addition of carbohydrates to ceramide can yield a variety of different glycolipids. Sphingomyelin is synthesised on the lumenal surface of the Golgi, but glucose is added to ceramide on the cytosolic side. Glucosylceramide then apparently flips, however and additional carbohydrates are added on the lumenal side of the membrane.

Neither sphingomyelin nor the glycolipids are then able to translocate across the Golgi membrane, so they are found only in the lumenal half of the Golgi bilayer. Following vesicular transport, they are correspondingly localised to the exterior half of the plasma membrane, with their polar head groups exposed on the cell surface. The oligosaccharide portions of glycolipids are important surface markers in cell-cell recognition. In plant cells, the Golgi apparatus has the additional task of serving as the site where complex polysaccharides of the cell wall are synthesised.

The plant cell wall is composed of three major types of polysaccharides. Cellulose, the predominant constituent, is a simple linear polymer of glucose residues. It is synthesised at the cell surface by enzymes in the plasma membrane. The other cell wall polysaccharides (hemicelluloses and pectins), however, are complex, branched chain molecules that are synthesised in the Golgi apparatus and then transported in vesicles to the cell surface. The synthesis of these cell wall polysaccharides is a major cellular function and as much as 80% of the metabolic activity of the Golgi apparatus in plant cells may be devoted to polysaccharide synthesis.

PROTEIN SORTING AND EXPORT FROM THE GOLGI APPARATUS

Proteins, as well as lipids and polysaccharides, are transported from the Golgi apparatus to their final destinations through the secretory pathway. This involves the sorting of proteins into different kinds of transport vesicles, which bud from the *trans* Golgi network and deliver their contents to the appropriate cellular locations (Fig. 21.7). Some proteins are carried from the Golgi to the plasma membrane by a constitutive secretory pathway, which accounts for the incorporation of new proteins and lipids into the plasma membrane, as well as for the continuous secretion of proteins from the cell.

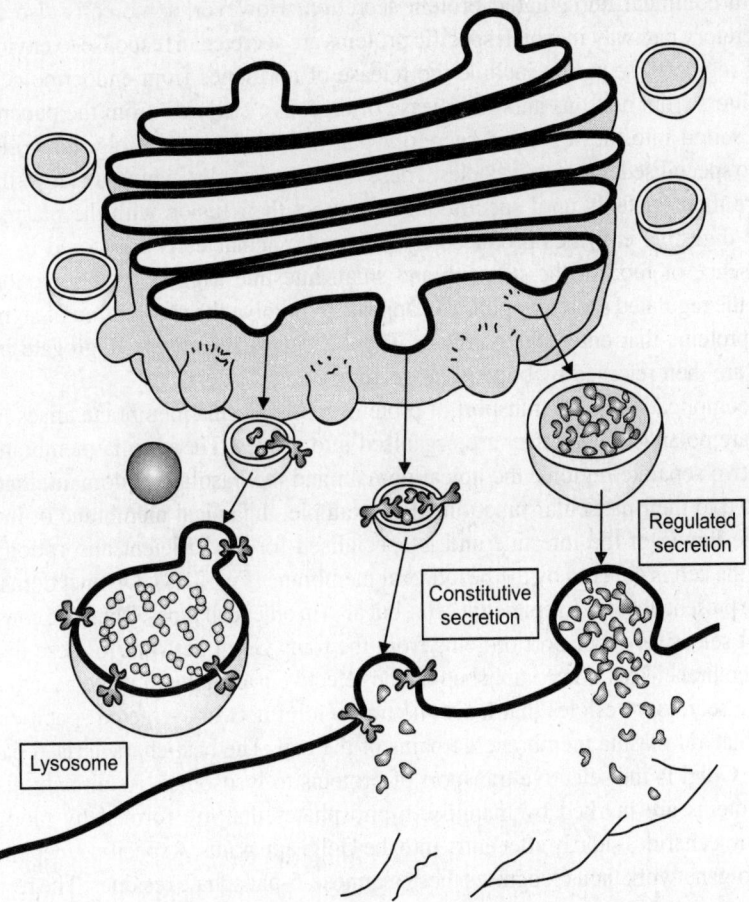

Regulated secretion

Constitutive secretion

Lysosome

Fig. 21.7: Transport from the Golgi apparatus. Proteins are sorted in the *trans* Golgi network and transported in vesicles to their final destinations. In the absence of specific targeting signals, proteins are carried to the plasma membrane by constitutive secretion. Alternatively, proteins can be diverted from the constitutive secretion pathway and targeted to other destinations, such as lysosomes or regulated secretion from the cells.

Other proteins are transported to the cell surface by a distinct pathway of regulated secretion or are specifically targeted to other intracellular destinations, such as lysosomes in animal cells or vacuoles in yeast.

Proteins that function within the Golgi apparatus must be retained within that organelle, rather than being transported along the secretory pathway. In contrast to the ER, all of the proteins retained within the Golgi complex are associated with the Golgi membrane rather than being soluble proteins within the lumen. The signals responsible for retention of some proteins within the Golgi have been localised to their trans membrane domains, which retain proteins within the Golgi apparatus by preventing them from being packaged in the transport vesicles that leave the trans Golgi network. In addition, like the KKXX (are short carboxy-terminal signals) sequences of resident ER membrane proteins, signals in the cytoplasmic tails of some Golgi proteins mediate the retrieval of these proteins from subsequent compartments along the secretory pathway. The constitutive secretory pathway, which operates in all cells, leads to continual unregulated protein secretion. However, some cells also possess a distinct regulated secretory pathway in which specific proteins are secreted in response to environmental signals. Examples of regulated secretion include the release of hormones from endocrine cells, the release of neurotransmitters from neurons and the release of digestive enzymes from the pancreatic acinar cells. Proteins are sorted into the regulated secretory pathway in the trans Golgi network, where they are packaged into specialised secretory vesicles. These secretory vesicles, which are larger than other transport vesicles, store their contents until specific signals direct their fusion with the plasma membrane. For example, the digestive enzymes produced by pancreatic acinar cells are stored in secretory vesicles until the presence of food in the stomach and small intestine triggers their secretion. The sorting of proteins into the regulated secretory pathway appears to involve the recognition of signal patches shared by multiple proteins that enter this pathway. These proteins selectively aggregate in the trans Golgi network and are then released by budding as secretory vesicles.

A further complication in the transport of proteins to the plasma membrane arises in many epithelial cells, which are polarised when they are organised into tissues. The plasma membrane of such cells is divided into two separate regions, the apical domain and the basolateral domain, that contain specific proteins related to their particular functions. For example, the apical membrane of intestinal epithelial cells faces the lumen of the intestine and is specialised for the efficient absorption of nutrients, the remainder of the cell is covered by the basolateral membrane (Fig. 21.8). Distinct domains of the plasma membrane are present not only in epithelial cells, but also in other cell types. Thus, the constitutive secretory pathway must selectively transport proteins from the trans Golgi network to these distinct domains of the plasma membrane. This is accomplished by the selective packaging of proteins into at least two types of constitutive secretory vesicles that leave the trans Golgi network targeted specifically for either the apical or basolateral plasma membrane domains of the cell. The best-characterised pathway of protein sorting in the Golgi is the selective transport of proteins to lysosomes. As already discussed, lumenal lysosomal proteins are marked by mannose-6-phosphates that are formed by modification of their N-linked oligosaccharides shortly after entry into the Golgi apparatus. A specific receptor in the membrane of the trans Golgi network then recognises these mannose-6-phosphate residues. The resulting complexes of receptor plus lysosomal enzyme are packaged into transport vesicles destined for lysosomes. Lysosomal membrane proteins are targeted by sequences in their cytoplasmic tails, rather than by mannose-6-phosphates. In yeasts and plant cells, which lack lysosomes, proteins are transported from the Golgi apparatus to an additional destination: the vacuole. Vacuoles assume the functions of lysosomes in these cells as well as performing a variety of other tasks, such as the storage of nutrients and the maintenance of

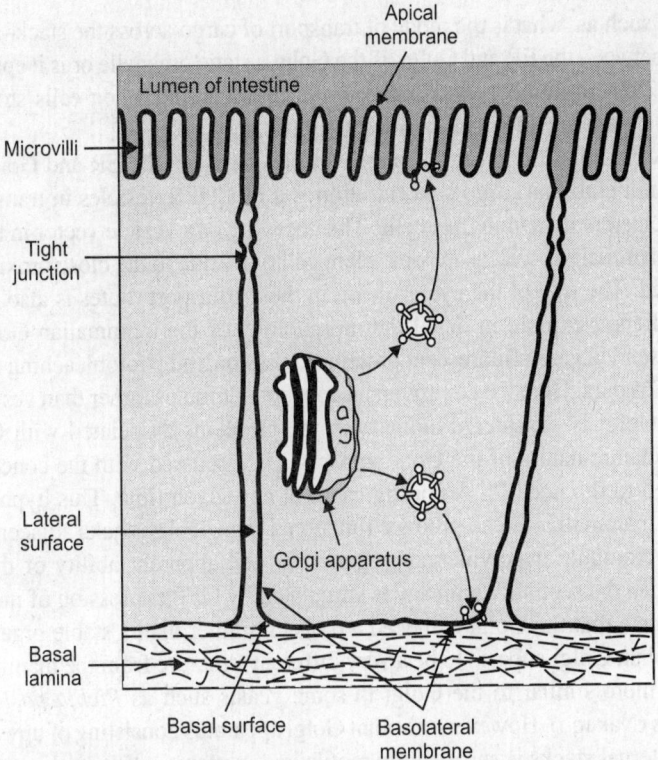

Fig. 21.8: Transport to the plasma membrane of polarised cells. The plasma membranes of polarised epithelial cells are divided into apical and basolateral domains. In this example (intestinal epithelium), the apical surface of the cell faces the lumen of the intestine, the lateral surfaces are in contact with neighboring cells, and the basal surface rests on a sheet of extracellular matrix (the basal lamina). The apical membrane is characterised by the presence of microvilli, which facilitate the absorption of nutrients by increasing surface area. Specific proteins are targeted to either the apical or basolateral membranes in the trans Golgi network. Tight junctions between neighbouring cells maintain the identity of the apical and basolateral membranes by preventing the diffusion of proteins between these domains.

turgor pressure and osmotic balance. In contrast to lysosomal targeting, proteins are directed to vacuoles by short peptide sequences instead of carbohydrate markers.

SORTING PROBLEMS FACED BY GOLGI APPARATUS

The Golgi apparatus lies at the very heart of the secretory pathway, which is composed of a series of organelles involved in the production, processing, storage and secretion of a hugely diverse range of complex carbohydrates, proteins and lipids. The Golgi is unique in that not only can it receive, package and send material (cargo) to and from organelles such as the endoplasmic reticulum (ER), the vacuolar and endosomal system and the cell surface (exocytosis and endocytosis), but it also has considerable biosynthetic capability. It is therefore not surprising that huge efforts have been directed at elucidating its structure, molecular dynamics and modes of action in a range of cell types in different kingdoms. By the very nature of the different experimental approaches pursued by different laboratories, this has resulted in a very considerable controversy about the nature and mechanics of the various secretory organelles. Questions such as, what is the mode of transport of cargo across the stack–are vesicles really involved in transport between the ER and Golgi–is the Golgi a static organelle or is it ephemeral in nature, increasing in size or even in number when needed and disappearing when cells stop secreting–have stimulated robust debate amongst the cell biological community.

Murshid and Presley discuss the recent data on transport between the ER and Golgi and the role of COPII coat proteins in membrane cargo concentration and of COPII vesicles in transport to the Golgi via vesicular-tubular clusters in mammalian cells. The necessity of a vesicle vector in transport between the ER and Golgi in mammals as well as in some plant cell types due to the close proximity of the Golgi to the ER is questioned. The role of the cytoskeleton in these transport routes is also considered.

Polishchuk and Miranov explore in detail the morphology of the mammalian Golgi stack and the new data that have arisen via green fluorescent protein expression and photobleaching studies combined with analysis of new EM data. Here the controversial concept of tubules rather than vesicles for transport between the ER and Golgi is considered along with the problems associated with COPI vesicles as cargo carriers. The dynamic nature of the Golgi apparatus is discussed with the concept of the size of the Golgi being related to the need for exporting cargo at any given time. This hypothesis, combined with the ability of the mammalian ER to produce functional mini-Golgi stacks adjacent to ER exit sites in the presence of microtubule depolymerising agents and the apparent ability of the plant Golgi to increase in number when the secretory pathway is stimulated by GFP expression of membrane proteins may lead one to postulate that the Golgi is indeed a transient rather than a stable organelle.

At first glance the plant Golgi appears to be a very different structure from the mammalian ribbonlike organelle and maybe more similar to the Golgi in some yeasts such as *Pichia pastoris,* which have distinct cisternal stacks (Nakano). However, the plant Golgi apparatus consisting of upwards of a hundred or more individual cisternal stacks is surprisingly motile and in many cells travels over the cortical ER network driven by the actin/myosin cytoskeleton. Thus, how cargo is transferred from the ER to the Golgi is still a matter for debate. Various researchers also consider the various mechanisms by which transferases are targeted to and are held in the Golgi stack along with vacuolar sorting receptors, as well as the role of the plant Golgi as a major factory for the production of non-cellulosic cell wall material.

The power of fluorescent protein technology combined with FRAP (fluorescent recovery after photobleaching) in analysing protein transport in the secretory pathway is addressed by Ward and Brandizzi. By photobleaching specific regions of the Golgi apparatus or ER, transport of new protein into the bleached area can be measured. Any recovery of fluorescence, however, not only reveals transport into the bleached region but also indicates a corresponding transport of equivalent molecules out of the region. Thus, for example, it has been shown that Golgi transferases continually cycle between the Golgi and ER in mammalian cells and likely in plant cells. Thus, the concept of retention of such enzymes within the Golgi by some form of oligomerisation now seems unlikely. Whether the development of photoactivatable fluorescent proteins will be able to shed more light on Golgi function remains to be tested. Finally, Nakano considers the yeast Golgi complex in comparison with its mammalian and plant counterparts. With these organisms we can address the question of why or why not to stack. In *Saccharomyces cerevisiae* the Golgi can function perfectly adequately as a series of dispersed cisternae, each having equivalent function of *cis, medial* or *trans* cisternae of a stacked Golgi. The power of genetic screening has revealed new proteins such as Emp46p and Emp47p, which function as receptors for packaging cargo into COPII vesicles and the development of high-resolution real-time imaging systems may permit us to at last resolve putative COPII and COPI vesicles in yeast cells. A final thought here addresses the apparent fundamental differences in the nature of the Golgi among the yeasts, mammals and plants. Do the different morphologies and patterns of Golgi distribution in different cells reflect fundamental differences in the organelle or do they just reflect the exceedingly pleiomorphic nature of a structure that is ever changing, ever dynamic but operates under the guidance of a basic fundamental set of rules governing cargo and membrane transport out of and back to the ER?

CELL-SPECIFIC FUNCTIONS OF GOLGI APPARATUS

Formation of Cell Plate and Cell Wall in Plant Tissues

Cell plate

Cytokinesis in terrestrial plants occurs by cell plate formation. This process entails the delivery of Golgi-derived and endosomal vesicles carrying cell wall and cell membrane components to the plane of cell division and the subsequent fusion of these vesicles within this plate. After formation of an early tubulo-vesicular network at the center of the cell, the initially labile cell plate consolidates into a tubular network and eventually a fenestrated sheet. The cell plate grows outward from the center of the cell to the parental plasma membrane with which it will fuse, thus completing cell division. Formation and growth of the cell plate is dependent upon the phragmoplast, which is required for proper targeting of Golgi-derived vesicles to the cell plate (Fig. 21.9).

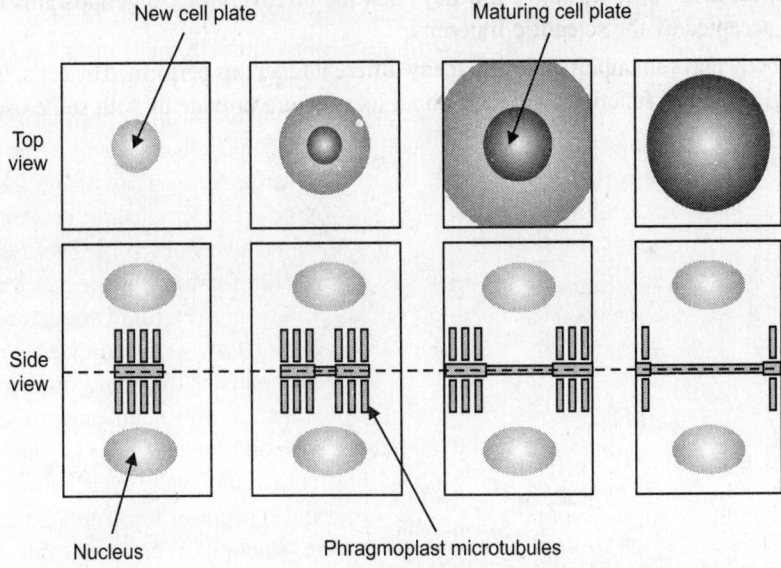

Fig. 21.9: Phragmoplast and cell plate formation in a plant cell during cytokinesis. Left side: Phragmoplast forms and cell plate starts to assemble in the center of the cell. Towards the right: Phragmoplast enlarges in a donut-shape towards the outside of the cell, leaving behind mature cell plate in the center. The cell plate will transform into the new cell wall once cytokinesis is complete.

As the cell plate matures in the central part of the cell, the phragmoplast disassembles in this region and new elements are added on its outside. This process leads to a steady expansion of the phragmoplast and, concomitantly, to a continuous retargeting of Golgi-derived vesicles to the growing edge of the cell plate. Once the cell plate reaches and fuses with the plasma membrane the phragmoplast disappears.

This event not only marks the separation of the two daughter cells, but also initiates a range of biochemical modifications that transform the callose-rich, flexible cell plate into a cellulose-rich, stiff primary cell wall. The heavy dependence of cell plate formation on active Golgi stacks explains why plant cells, unlike mammalian cells, do not disassemble their secretion machinery during cell division.

INTERESTING FACTS ABOUT GOLGI APPARATUS

1. Earlier, the Golgi apparatus was known by different names like Golgi-Kopsch apparatus, Golgi-Holmgren apparatus and Golgi-Holmgren ducts. Eventually, it was agreed upon that this cell organelle be called the Golgi apparatus.

2. In animal cells, the Golgi body undergoes disintegration at the time of mitosis, it is again formed at the time of telophase. In plant cells, the Golgi body does not undergo this kind of transformation and thus, remains intact.

3. Functioning of the Golgi apparatus is often compared to working of a 'post-office'. The reason behind this is that proteins in the Golgi body are modified, sorted and then packaged before they are secreted.

4. Earlier, Camillo Golgi's claim of discovering the Golgi body was not given due consideration by few researchers. They considered the Golgi body, as identified by Camillo Golgi, nothing more than an optical illusion. It was after few days that the discovery of Golgi apparatus by Camillo Golgi was accepted by the scientific fraternity.

5. The Golgi body plays an important role in many different functions performed by cells. Information about Golgi apparatus functions and facts about its structure provide us with some useful details on the cell organelle.

Chapter 22

Lysosomes

INTRODUCTION

Lysosomes are large, spherical organelles that contain enzymes (acid hydrolases). They break up food so it is easier to digest. They are found in animal cells, while in plant cells the same roles are performed by the vacuole. They digest excess or worn-out organelles, food particles, and engulfed viruses or bacteria. The membrane around a lysosome allows the digestive enzymes to work at the 4.5 pH they require. Lysosomes fuse with vacuoles and dispense their enzymes into the vacuoles, digesting their contents.

Lysosomes are created by the addition of hydrolytic enzymes to early endosomes from the Golgi apparatus. The name *lysosome derives* from the Greek words *lysis*, which means dissolution or destruction, and *soma*, which means body. They are frequently nicknamed 'suicide-bags' or 'suicide-sacs' by cell biologists due to their role in autolysis. Lysosomes were discovered by the Belgian cytologist Christian de Duve in 1949.

STRUCTURE OF LYSOSOMES

Lysosomes are single membrane bound organelle. They are round dense bodies filled with large number of hydrolytic enzymes and lytic components. Lysosomes are so called because they contain lytic enzymes. The enzymes are kept inside by the lysosomal membrane. These enzymes remain inactive inside the lysosomes. When the pH of the interior lysosomes changed to acidic pH 4.8, enzymes become active. At pH 4.8, the interior of the lysosomes is acidic compared to the slightly alkaline cytosol (pH 7.2). The lysosome maintains this pH differential by pumping protons (H^+ ions) from the cytosol across the membrane via proton pumps and chloride ion channels. The lysosomal membrane protects the cytosol, and therefore the rest of the cell, from the degradative enzymes within the lysosome. The cell is additionally protected from any lysosomal acid hydrolases that leak into the cytosol as these enzymes are pH-sensitive and function less well in the alkaline environment of the cytosol.

FUNCTIONS OF LYSOSOMES

Lysosomes are the cells garbage disposal system. They are used for the digestion of macromolecules from phagocytosis (ingestion of other dying cells or larger extracellular material, like foreign invading microbes) endocytosis (where receptor proteins are recycled from the cell surface). And autophagy (wherein old or unneeded organelles or proteins, or microbes that have invaded the cytoplasm are delivered to the lysosome). Autophagy may also lead to autophagic cell death, a form of programmed self-destruction, or autolysis, of the cell, which means that the cell is digesting itself. Lysosomes have the following functions namely, heterophagy, autophagy, autolysis, extracellular digestion, fertilisation and chromosomal damage (Fig. 22.1a and b).

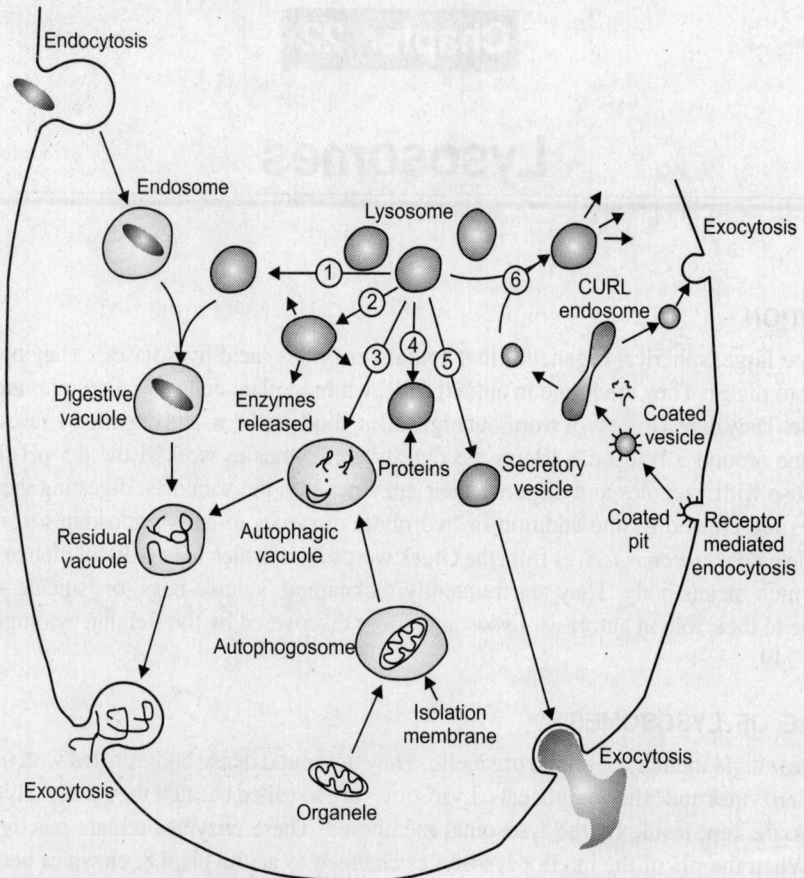

Fig. 22.1a: Functions of lysosomes. (1) digestion of ingested material, (2) cell death, (3) autophogy, (4) molecular turnover, (5) extracellular functions and (6) receptor recycling.

ENZYMES

Some important enzymes found within lysosomes include:

- Lipase, which digests lipids.
- Amylase, which digest carbohydrates (e.g. sugars).
- Proteases, which digest proteins.
- Nucleases, which digest nucleic acids.
- Phosphoric acidmonoesters.

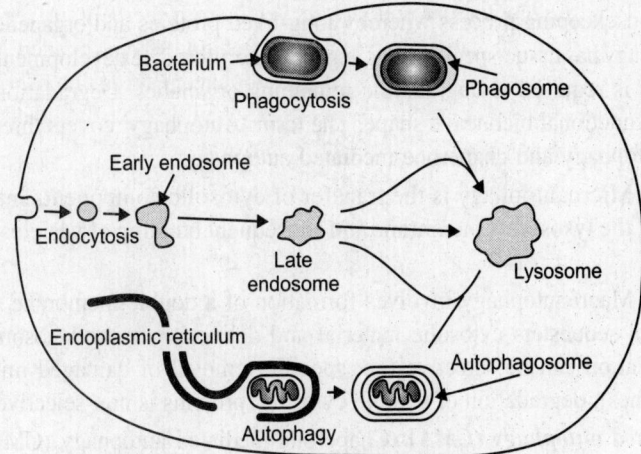

Fig. 22.1b: Three pathways leading to lysosomes.

- Lysosomal enzymes are synthesised in the cytosol and the endoplasmic reticulum, where they receive a mannose-6-phosphatetag that targets them for the lysosome

Lysosomal Enzymes

The lysosomal enzymes are collectively called as hydrolases. The hydrolases bring about the cleavage of substrates by the addition of a water molecules. Most of the lysosomal enzymes function in the acid medium. Hence they are called as acid hydrolases. The lysosomes may contain about 40 varieties of enzymes. Lytic component present in lysosome include lactoferrin which act as iron chelators, i.e. it removes iron from the lysoendosomal vesicle during the lytic function of lysosome. Lysosomes might be differentiated into four types depending upon their content during their function namely, primarily lysosome, secondary lysosome, residual body and autophagic vacuoles.

Primary lysosome are small saclike structures enclosing enzymes synthesised by the ribosomes. Since they store enzymes, they are also said to be storage granules.

Secondary lysosome are formed by the fusion of primary lysosome with phagosomes. They contain engulfed materials and enzymes. The materials are progressively digested by the enzymes. So it is also otherwise called as digestive vacuole.

Residual bodies are nothing but secondary lysosomes with undigested wastes. The digested materials are diffused into the cell cytoplasm through the lysosomal membrane. Autophagic lysosomes are special type of lysosmes, which are formed when the cells feed on their own intracellular organelles and they digest them ultimately. This happens only during starvation of organisms.

Autophagy

Autophagy is essential in helping to maintain the balance between the increase and decrease in the number of a cell population. It is undoubtedly active at a basal level in most cells and contributes to the routine turnover of cytoplasmic components. Three predominant cellular functions can be assigned to autophagy. Autophagy is a response to nutrient starvation. Decreased levels of amino acids can induce the autophagic response in numerous cell types and situations, e.g. the neonatal period, when the supply of nutrients via the milk has not yet replaced the nutrients via the placenta.

Autophagy is a housekeeping process whereby long-lived proteins and organelles are recycled, e.g. Mitochondria. Autophagy has tissue-specific roles, e.g. during erythrocyte development, following nucleus expulsion, autophagy is required to degrade the remaining organelles. Degradation of the autophagic vesicle results in the functional biconcave shape. The term 'Autophagy' covers three processes, micro-autophagy, macro-autophagy and chaperone-mediated autophagy:

Microautophagy: Microautophagy is the transfer of cytosolic components into the lysosome by direct invagination of the lysosomal membrane and subsequent budding of vesicles into the lysosomal lumen.

Macroautophagy: Macroautophagy involves formation of a double-membrane structure called the autophagosome which sequesters cytosolic material and delivers it to the lysosome for degradation. Although this degradation can be selective (i.e. specific removal of damaged mitochondria sparing normal functioning ones), degradation of soluble cytosolic proteins is non-selective.

Chaperone-mediated autophagy (CMA): Chaperone-mediated autophagy (CMA) is characterised by its selectivity regarding the specific substrates (cytosolic proteins) degraded.

Autolysis

Autolysis refers to the digestion of own cells by the lysosomes. Auto means self and lysis means digestion. It is self digestion. It is also otherwise known as programmed cell death or apoptopic lysis. In autolysis, the lysosome digests its own cell. Hence autolysis is also called as cellular autophagy. In this process, the lysosome ruptures inside its cell and the released enzymes digest and degrade the cell. As lysosome kills its own cell, it is called as sucidal bag. Autolysis occurs during amphibian metamorphosis, insect meta-morphosis, mensuration, etc. During amphibiam metamorphosis, the cells in tail, gills, etc. are digested by autolysis. Similarly during menstruation the cells in the uterine epithelium are lysed by autolysis.

Extracellular digestion

Digestion of materials outside the cell is called extracellular digestion. In certain occasions lysosomes release enzymes outside the cell by exocytosis and bring out digestion. Extracellular digestion takes place during bone erosion process. Osteoclast cell (Fig. 22.2) of bone contain more number of lysosomes.

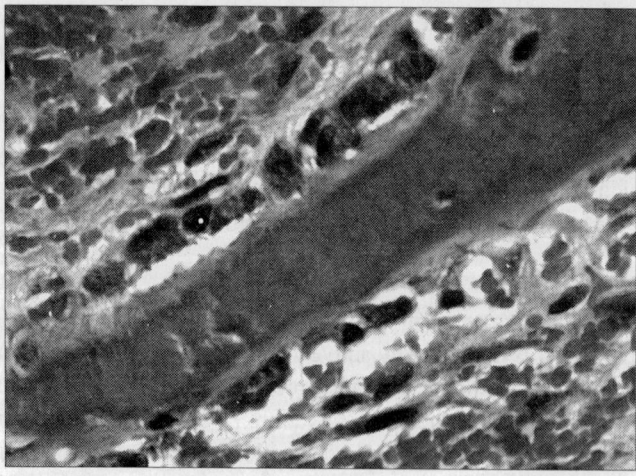

Fig. 22.2: Osteoclast cell.

These cells when release their lysosomal content on the surface of the bone, lysosomal enzymes bring about the extracellular digestion of bone and it result in bone desorption.

Fertilisation

During fertilisation process, acrosome (giant lysosome) of sperm head ruptures and releases enzymes on the surface of the egg. These enzymes digest the egg membrane and provide way for the entry of sperm nucleus into the egg. This action also activates the egg for the developmental processes.

Chromosomal damage

Due to the presence of DNase enzyme, lysosome had an ability to attacks chromosome and cause chromosomal breakages. These breakages can leads to diseases like cancer, etc.

PLANT VACUOLE

A vacuole is a membrane bound organelle which is present in all plant and fungal cells and some protist, animal and bacterial cells. Vacuoles are essentially enclosed compartments which are filled with water containing inorganic and organic molecules including various enzymes in solution, though in certain cases they may contain solids which have been engulfed. Plant vacuole (Fig. 22.3) are formed by the fusion of multiple membrane vesicles and are effectively just larger forms of these. The organelle has no basic shape or size, its structure varies according to the needs of the cell.

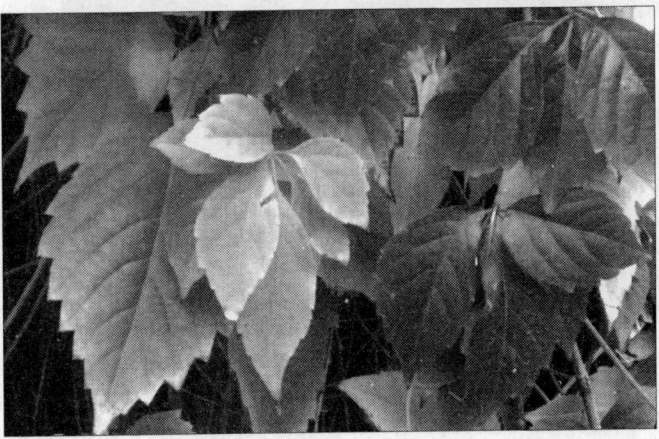

Fig. 22.3: Plant vacuole.

The function and importance of vacuoles varies greatly according to the type of cell in which they are present, having much greater prominence in the cells of plants, fungi and certain protists than those of animals and bacteria. In general, the functions of the vacuole include:

1. Isolating materials that might be harmful or a threat to the cell.
2. Containing waste products.
3. Maintaining internal hydrostatic pressure or turgor within the cell.
4. Maintaining an acidic internal pH.
5. Containing small molecules.
6. Exporting unwanted substances from the cell.

7. Allows plants to support structures such as leaves and flowers due to the pressure of the central vacuole.

Vacuoles also play a major role in autophagy, maintaining a balance between biogenesis (production) and degradation (or turnover), of many substances and cell structures in certain organisms. They also aid in destruction of invading bacteria or of misfolded proteins that have begun to build up within the cell. In protists, vacuoles have the additional function of storing food which has been absorbed by the organism, and assist in the digestive and waste management process for the cell. Large central vacuoles are found in three genera of filamentous sulphur bacteria, the *Thioploca* (Fig. 22.4), *Beggiatoa* (Fig. 22.5) and *Thiomargarita*. The cytoplasm is extremely reduced in these genera and the vacuole can occupy between 40–98 per cent of the cell. The vacuoles contain high concentrations of nitrate ions and is therefore thought to be a storage organelle.

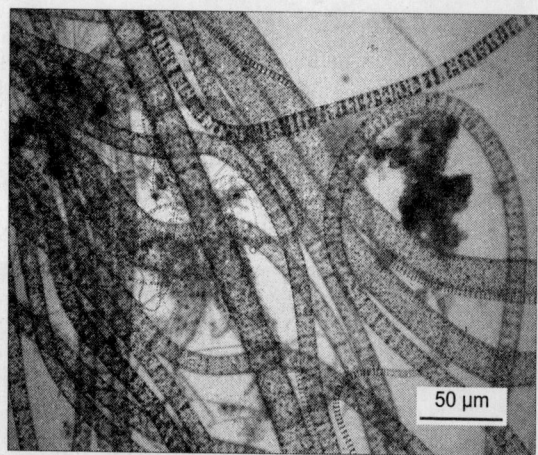

50 μm

Fig. 22.4: *Thioploca.*

Genetic Disorders

A group of genetic disorders caused by defective lysosomal enzymes demonstrates the importance of lysosomes. Called lysosomal storage diseases, these disorders are characterised by the harmful accumulation of undigested substances. The accumulated materials impair or kill the affected cells, resulting in skeletal or muscular defects, mental retardation, or even death.

Formation of Lysosomes

Many components of animal cells are recycled by transferring them inside or embedded in sections of membrane. For instance, in endocytosis (more specifically, macropinocytosis), a portion of the cell's plasma membrane pinches off to form vesicles that will eventually fuse with an organelle within the cell. Without active replenishment, the plasma membrane would continuously decrease in size. It is thought that lysosomes participate in this dynamic membrane exchange system and are formed by a gradual maturation process from endosomes. The production of lysosomal proteins suggests one method of lysosome sustainment. Lysosomal protein genes are transcribed in the nucleus. mRNA transcripts exit the nucleus into the cytosol, where they are translated by ribosomes. The nascent peptide chains are translocated into the rough endoplasmic reticulum, where they are modified. Lysosomal soluble proteins exit the endoplasmic reticulum via CLN8-mediated recruitment in COPII-coated vesicles and enter the

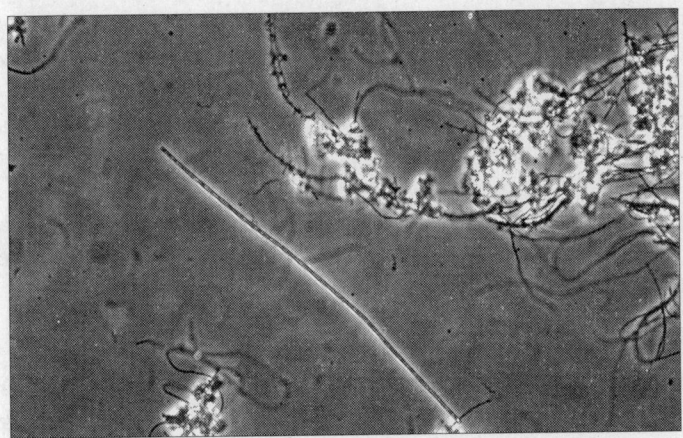

Fig. 22.5: *Beggiatoa.*

Golgi apparatus, where a specific lysosomal tag, mannose 6-phosphate, is added to the peptides. The presence of these tags allow for binding to mannose 6-phosphate receptors in the Golgi apparatus, a phenomenon that is crucial for proper packaging into vesicles destined for the lysosomal system.

Upon leaving the Golgi apparatus, the lysosomal enzyme-filled vesicle fuses with a late endosome, a relatively acidic organelle with an approximate pH of 5.5. This acidic environment causes dissociation of the lysosomal enzymes from the mannose 6-phosphate receptors. The enzymes are packed into vesicles for further transport to established lysosomes. The late endosome itself can eventually grow into a mature lysosome, as evidenced by the transport of endosomal membrane components from the lysosomes back to the endosomes.

Pathogen Entry

As the endpoint of endocytosis, the lysosome also acts as a safeguard in preventing pathogens from being able to reach the cytoplasm before being degraded. Pathogens often hijack endocytotic pathways such as pinocytosis in order to gain entry into the cell. The lysosome prevents easy entry into the cell by hydrolysing the biomolecules of pathogens necessary for their replication strategies, reduced Lysosomal activity results in an increase in viral infectivity, including HIV. In addition, AB5 toxins such as cholera hijack the endosomal pathway while evading lysosomal degradation.

Clinical Significance

Lysosomes are involved in a group of genetically inherited deficiencies, or mutations called lysosomal storage diseases (LSD), inborn errors of metabolism caused by a dysfunction of one of the enzymes. The rate of incidence is estimated to be 1 in 5000 births, and the true figure expected to be higher as many cases are likely to be undiagnosed or misdiagnosed. The primary cause is deficiency of an acid hydrolase. Other conditions are due to defects in lysosomal membrane proteins that fail to transport the enzyme, non-enzymatic soluble lysosomal proteins. The initial effect of such disorders is accumulation of specific macromolecules or monomeric compounds inside the endosomal–autophagic–lysosomal system. This results in abnormal signalling pathways, calcium homeostasis, lipid biosynthesis and degradation and intracellular trafficking, ultimately leading to pathogenetic disorders. The organs most affected are brain, viscera, bone and cartilage.

There is no direct medical treatment to cure LSDs. The most common LSD is Gaucher's disease, which is due to deficiency of the enzyme glucocerebrosidase. Consequently, the enzyme substrate, the fatty acid glucosylceramide accumulates, particularly in white blood cells, which in turn affects spleen, liver, kidneys, lungs, brain and bone marrow. The disease is characterised by bruises, fatigue, anaemia, low blood platelets, osteoporosis, and enlargement of the liver and spleen. As of 2017, enzyme replacement therapy is available for treating 8 of the 50–60 known LDs.

The most severe and rarely found, lysosomal storage disease is inclusion cell disease. Metachromatic leukodystrophy is another lysosomal storage disease that also affects sphingolipid metabolism. Gaucher disease is discussed in end of this chapter.

Lysosomotropism

Weak bases with lipophilic properties accumulate in acidic intracellular compartments like lysosomes. While the plasma and lysosomal membranes are permeable for neutral and uncharged species of weak bases, the charged protonated species of weak bases do not permeate biomembranes and accumulate within lysosomes. The concentration within lysosomes may reach levels 100 to 1000 fold higher than extracellular concentrations. This phenomenon is called lysosomotropism, 'acid trapping' or 'proton pump' effect. The amount of accumulation of lysosomotropic compounds may be estimated using a cell-based mathematical model.

A significant part of the clinically approved drugs are lipophilic weak bases with lysosomotropic properties. This explains a number of pharmacological properties of these drugs, such as high tissue-to-blood concentration gradients or long tissue elimination half-lifes, these properties have been found for drugs such as haloperidol, levomepromazine, and amantadine. However, high tissue concentrations and long elimination half-lives are explained also by lipophilicity and absorption of drugs to fatty tissue structures. Important lysosomal enzymes, such as acid sphingomyelinase, may be inhibited by lysosomally accumulated drugs. Such compounds are termed FIASMAs (functional inhibitor of acid sphingomyelinase) and include for example fluoxetine, sertraline, or amitriptyline. Ambroxol is a lysosomotropic drug of clinical use to treat conditions of productive cough for its mucolytic action. Ambroxol triggers the exocytosis of lysosomes via neutralisation of lysosomal pH and calcium release from acidic calcium stores. Presumably for this reason, Ambroxol was also found to improve cellular function in some disease of lysosomal origin such as Parkinson's or lysosomal storage disease.

Systemic lupus erythematosus

Impaired lysosome function is prominent in systemic lupus erythematosus preventing macrophages and monocytes from degrading neutrophil extracellular traps and immune complexes. The failure to degrade internalised immune complexes stems from chronic mTORC2 activity, which impairs lysosome acidification. As a result, immune complexes in the lysosome recycle to the surface of macrophages causing an accumulation of nuclear antigens upstream of multiple lupus-associated pathologies.

GAUCHER'S DISEASE

Gaucher's disease is one of the most common lysosomal storage disorder with defects in the enzyme glucosylceramidase (glucocerebrosidase). The disease is caused by mutations in the GBA gene on chromosome 1, (autosomal recessive) and affects both sexes. Gaucher's disease (Fig. 22.6) or Gaucher disease is a genetic disorder in which glucocerebroside (a sphingolipid, also known as glucosylceramide) accumulates in cells and certain organs. The disorder is characterized by bruising, fatigue, anemia, low blood platelet count and enlargement of the liver and spleen, and is caused by a hereditary deficiency of the enzyme glucocerebrosidase (also known as glucosylceramidase), which acts on glucocerebroside. When the enzyme is defective, glucocerebroside accumulates, particularly in white blood cells and especially in macrophages (mononuclear leukocytes). Glucocerebroside can collect in the spleen, liver, kidneys, lungs, brain, and bone marrow.

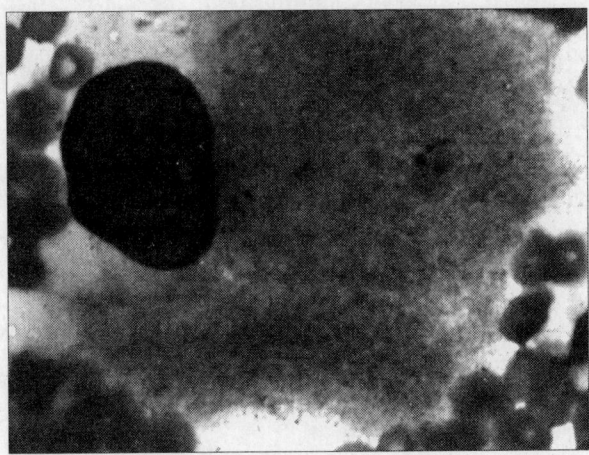

Fig. 22.6: Gaucher's disease.

Signs and Symptoms of Gaucher's Disease

- Painless hepatomegaly and splenomegaly: the size of the spleen can be 1500–3000 ml, as opposed to the normal size of 50–200 ml. Splenomegaly may decrease the affected individuals capacity for eating by exerting pressure on the stomach. While painless, enlargement of spleen increases the risk of splenic rupture.

- Hypersplenism and pancytopenia, the rapid and premature destruction of blood cells, leads to anemia, neutropenia, leukopenia, and thrombocytopenia (with an increased risk of infection and bleeding).

- Cirrhosis of the liver is rare.

- Severe pain associated with joints and bones occurs, frequently presenting in hips and knees.

- Neurological symptoms occur only in some types of Gaucher's:

  Type I: Impaired olfaction and cognition.

  Type II: Serious convulsions, hypertonia, intellectual disability, and apnea.

  Type III: Muscle twitches known as myoclonus, convulsions, dementia, and ocular muscle apraxia.

  Parkinson's disease is recognized as being more common in Gaucher's disease patients and their heterozygous carrier relatives.

- Osteoporosis: 75% of patients develop visible bony abnormalities due to the accumulated glucosylceramide. A deformity of the distal femur in the shape of an Erlenmeyer flask is commonly described (aseptic necrosis of the femur joint).

- Yellowish-brown skin pigmentation.

Fig. 12.6. Gaucher's disease.

Signs and Symptoms of Gaucher's Disease

SECTION VII

Mitochondria, Chloroplasts and Peroxisomes

Chapter 23

Mitochondria

INTRODUCTION

Mitochondria are now known to be more than the hub of energy metabolism. They are the central executioner of cells, and control cellular homeostasis through involvement in nearly all aspects of metabolism. As our understanding of mitochondria has expanded it has become clear that the structure, function and pathology of the organelle are so intimately connected that it is difficult, if not impossible, to study any one area without context of the others. Here is presented a relatively brief overview of the diverse areas of mitochondrial research to provide the background and stimulate the broad thinking that is needed to understand the role that mitochondria play in some of the more common and devastating human conditions including genetic mitochondrial cytopathies and neuropathies, Parkinsons and Alzheimers disease, diabetes and cancer.

STRUCTURE OF MITOCHONDRIA

Morphology and Organelle Interactions

The classic picture of cellular mitochondria based on low-resolution electron micrographs is of a set of relatively small bean shaped particles scattered around the cytosol. However, our understanding of the morphology of the organelle has changed with the advent of higher resolution electron microscopes and cryopreservation of samples. Foremost, mitochondria are now known to be highly dynamic and can be punctate as previously proposed, but can also be organised as a continuum or reticulum under some cell conditions. Further, the organelle moves within the cell in the punctate state or as a reticular unit to provide foci of energy production such as at the nucleus during cell division, or to synapses in neuronal cells at times of high information transfer. This movement is along microtubules in one direction and along actin filaments in the other. Several important studies have established that the switching between punctate and reticulum forms is physiologically important. For example it is cell cycle dependent, being reticular in the G1 phase but then converting to the punctate form for cell division. The transitioning of mitochondria between punctate and reticulum states through alternating fission and fusion is now known to be critical to maintaining mitochondrial quality control. Fission allows separation of the healthy mitochondrial segments from the defective ones. Not surprising then, failure to transition between the different morphological forms is thought to contribute to several diseases, e.g. Parkinson's disease (Fig. 23.1). Another aspect of mitochondrial organisation that is now known to be important is the interaction between this and other cellular organelles including, endoplasmic reticulum, lysosomes and peroxisomes. These interactions are labile and occur through contact sites involving proteins of the two organelles. Among key functions is the movement of Ca^{++} between mitochondria and ER and the co-ordination of the unfolded protein response by these two organelles.

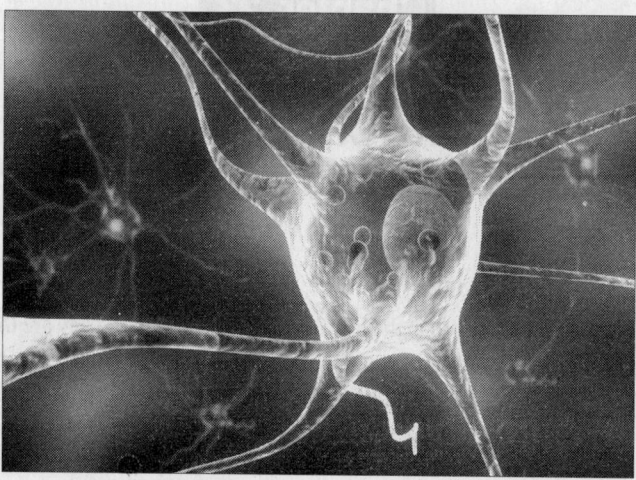

Fig. 23.1: Parkinson's disease.

Fusion Fission Cycle of Mitochondria

Mitochondrial fusion can be divided into two processes, the fusion of the mitochondrial outer membrane followed by that of the inner membrane. The outer membrane fusion requires proteins known as mitofusins, (Mfn1 and Mfn2). Inner membrane fusion mainly involves an inner membrane-localised protein (Opa1). The mitofusins are transmembrane dynamin-related GTPases, which induce the joining of 2 mitochondrial 'fragments' by forming dimers across the interface. The tethering of mitochondria together is followed by GTP hydrolysis, which induces conformation changes to cause mitochondrial fusion. The activity of mitofusins is regulated by ubiquitination, which causes their degradation in response to stress. The control of this degradation involves several proteins (PINK1, Parkin, E3 ligase Huwe1, MULAN and Bcl-2 family members). The inner membrane protein Opa1 is named based on its identification as a mutated gene in optic atrophy. It is a dynaminrelated GTPase that interacts with cardiolipin, a mitochondrial inner membrane lipid, and is mostly found in cristae, consistent with its role in maintaining cristae morphology. Opa 1 is also found in the cytosol in lipid droplets.

Opa1 activity involves the coordinated action of a long isoform of protein and its cleaved short isoform. The long isoform is located in the mitochondrial cristae membrane, while the short isoform is soluble in the intermembrane space. Opa1 proteolytic cleavage is regulated by the mitochondrial membrane potential, apoptosis, ATP level and mtDNA stability. Mitochondrial fission involves another GTPase called Drp1. On translocation from cytosol to mitochondria, this protein oligomerises into an X-shaped dimer on mitochondrial outer membranes. The binding sites for Drp1 association include endoplasmic reticulum (ER)-mitochondria contact points. When localised to the mitochondrial outer membrane, Drp1 rims the mitochondria in multimeric spirals at the constriction site, with the GTPase domain pointing away from the membrane. Formation of a complete spiral is thought to activate the GTPase domain causing GTP hydrolysis leading to a spiral constriction.

In apoptosis, Drp1 is also involved in Bax oligomerisation on the outer membrane and in cytochrome c release. Functioning of Drp1 is controlled by post-translational modifications including phosphorylation by a signalling kinase (GSK3) and the post-translational modifications S-nitrosylation, ubiquitination, SUMOylation and O-linked-N-acetyl-glucosamine glycosylation.

A second protein important for mitochondrial fission is human fission protein 1 homologue (Fis1). This protein binds to the mitochondrial outer membrane with the help of C-terminal trans-membrane domain. Unlike Drp1, Fis1 is distributed evenly on the outer mitochondrial membrane surface, and appears as punctate complexes. Functionally it is involved in binding of Drp1 (at least in yeast). Fis1 overexpression amplifies mitochondrial fragmentation, suggesting that it is a limiting factor for mitochondrial fission. Its expression is regulated via ubiquitination by a mitochondrial ubiquitin ligase (Mitol). Several other proteins have been identified as important to the fission process (Mff ,trap1, MiD49 and Mid51). Interestingly, the levels of one of these (trap1) are related to ROS production, suggesting that this protein signals the mitochondrial stress that initiates fission for subsequent mitophagy of damaged organelle segments. Sensing of ATP levels (by the AMP kinase) can activate fission by phosphorylating the protein Mff to recruit the fission apparatus.

Note that two of the proteins involved in maintaining the mitochondrial reticulum are Pink 1 and Parkin. Mutations of either of these two proteins along with DRP1 each cause early onset Parkinsons disease, hence the great interest in mitochondrial dynamics of those interested in neurological diseases.

Internal Structure

A typical low-resolution electron micrograph of bovine heart mitochondria is shown in Fig. 23.2. Such images led to a model in which there was a distinct outer membrane and a convoluted inner membrane surrounding the matrix space. These convolutions were called cristae. The space between the inner and outer membranes was called the intracristal space. Improved electron microscopy techniques have provided a more complex.

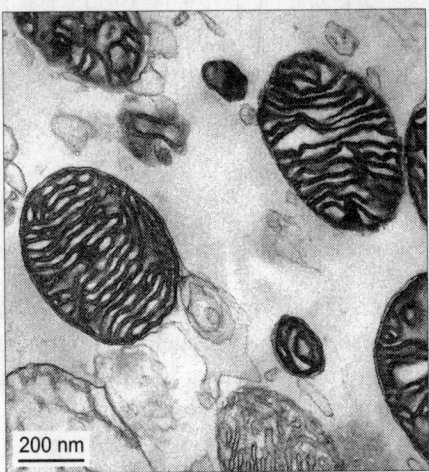

200 nm

Fig. 23.2: A typical low-resolution electron micrograph of bovine heart mitochondria.

There are 3 distinct membranes, the outer membrane, an inner boundary membrane and cristae membrane(s) which are attached to the inner boundary membrane by a specific structure now called MICOS. This means that a mitochondrion contains three separated spaces each with different protein content, the inter-membrane space, the intracristal space and the matrix space.

The protein composition of the outer membrane, boundary membrane and cristae membrane are very different. The cristae membrane is the major seat of the OXPHOS complexes, the inner membrane contains the majority of the translocases such as the ATP/ADP transporter and ion transport proteins, while the outer membrane houses the key proteins involved in apoptosis.

In addition to the morphology changes discussed already, there are other physiologically relevant changes in mitochondrial structure. The relative volume of the intracristal space and matrix space changes with organelle functioning. Under conditions of OXPHOS the volume of the intracristal space is greatly increased to generate what has been called the orthodox state of the mitochondrion. With reduced levels of OXPHOS, as when cells are using glycolysis for the bulk of their ATP, the cristae are much thinner, more regular and this is called the condensed state. Schematic showing the mitochondrial compartments are shown in Fig. 23.3.

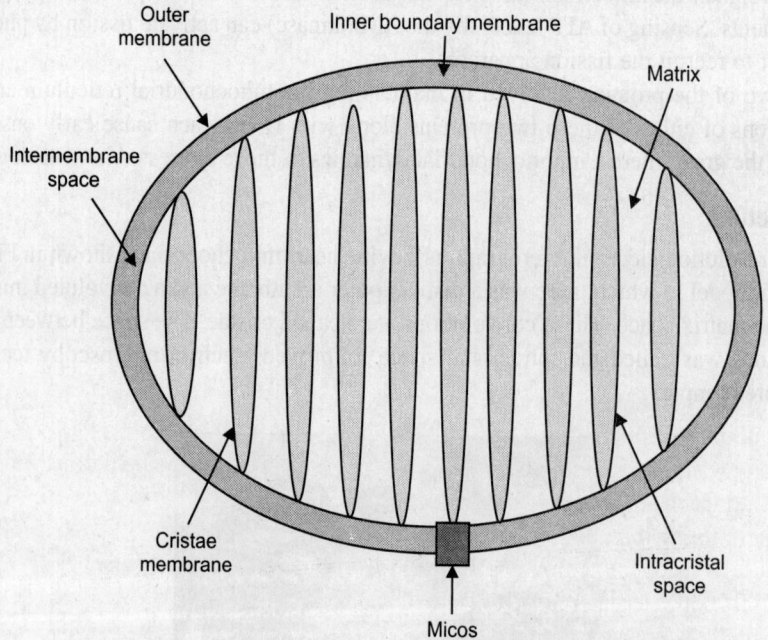

Fig. 23.3: Schematic showing the mitochondrial compartments.

A result of these volume changes is that the protein concentration within the matrix in the orthodox state is very high to the point that it is essentially a thick gel. The implication is that under such conditions free diffusion of proteins is seriously limited, arguing that proteins of a specific pathway, e.g. Krebs cycle enzymes are arranged in complexes so that the product of each reaction is passed directly as substrate to the next protein in the pathway.

Protein analysis has identified recently the structural complex that links the outer membrane, inner boundary membrane, and this is now called MICOS for mitochondrial contact site and cristae organising system. This complex contains a number of different subunits (including Mic10 and Mic60 also called mitofilin, and Fcj1 respectively), along with three further subunits, which are all integral inner membrane proteins (Mic12, Mic26, and Mic27). Also involved is a peripheral membrane protein (Mic19) that is an important organising factor. In addition, an inner membrane protein (called Aim24) is required for the integrity of MICOS and several recent studies add other proteins (apolipoprotein O, ApoO-like andQIL1 proteins) to the MICOS complex.

The MICOS complex also interacts with several protein complexes of the outer membrane (TOM and SAM complexes), with the outer membrane channel protein porin (VDAC), and with a component of the mitochondrial fusion machinery. It is evident that the MICOS complex participates in protein translocation into mitochondria although the precise role remains to be worked out.

MtDNA, Structure and Packaging

It came as a surprise in the1960s to find that mitochondria have their own DNA (mtDNA). In humans mtDNA is 16kb and encodes 13 protein- encoding genes (all components of the OXPHOS complexes) along with information for several tRNAs. Other organisms have mtDNAs with as few as two protein-coding genes, and as big as that of the mitochondrial genome of *Saccharomyces cerevisiae* with 85,779 bp and encoding two rRNAs and 30 proteins. The mtDNA encoded proteins are made on ribosomes within the organelle that have many of the characteristics of those found in bacteria, and are different from the cytosolic ribosomes that convert the nuclear genes to proteins.

The DNA strands in mitochondria are not well protected, e.g. by chromatin as in the nucleus, but instead are bundled with several DNA-binding proteins into so-called nucleoids. These nucleoids are irregular ellipsoidal in shape and typically contain a single copy of mtDNA encased in the mitochondrial transcription factor TFAM. The average nucleoid diameter is around 220 nm in HepG2 cells. On fragmentation of the mitochondrial reticulum there is one nucleoid per minimal sized fragment. The crystal structure of TFAM shows that it bends mtDNA in a sharp U-turn. Several other proteins are a part, often transiently, of the nucleoid including prohibitin, single-stranded DNA-binding protein, mtSSB,, twinkle, pol G, ATAD3 and Lon.

There is very limited repair of mtDNA with the result that mutations readily accumulate. Of considerable importance, unlike the nuclear genome which consists of a paternal and a maternal copy of each, there are anywhere from 20 to several thousand copies of mtDNA in mammalian cells, all maternal in origin. This leads to the concept of heteroplasmy, which typifies many diseases caused by mutations in mtDNA. Heteroplasmy can arise from *de novo* mutations of the mtDNA but is much more often inherited by the cells receiving a mixture of normal and mutant mtDNA copies from the egg.

Penetrance as it applies to inheritance of the mitochondrial genome thus depends on the copy number of 'wild type' mtDNA required to make the needed mitochondrially -encoded proteins for adequate functioning. This threshold is different in different cells depending on their energetic need and extent of reliance on oxidative phosphorylation.

Note that damaged mtDNA copies can and are removed as part of the process of mitophagy, the process in which cells remove mitochondria using the autophagic pathway.

Recent studies show that the ERMES complex, which links mitochondria to the ER, localises with a subset of actively replicating mitochondrial nucleoids and that mitochondrial division is spatially linked to nucleoids. The implication is that ER-associated division serves to link the distribution of mitochondria and mitochondrial nucleoids in cells. Both twinkle and ATAD3 are attached at or close to the mitochondria-ER contact sites with interaction with mitochondrial cholesterol.

Import of Proteins into Mitochondria

The biogenesis of mitochondria involves the coordinated transcription and translation of two genomes: one inside mitochondria and the other the nuclear genome. The vast majority of mitochondrial proteins are encoded by nuclear genes and synthesised on cytosolic ribosomes. These must be targeted to the organelle and then taken up and sorted to the correct compartment. Proteins destined for mitochondria are made as precursors that have both a targeting signal to direct them to receptors on the mitochondrial surface and intramitochondrial sorting signals. At present five major classes of precursor proteins have been identified, each of which uses a different pathway of translocation into mitochondria. The protein translocase of the outer membrane (TOM) is the major mitochondrial entry site. Around 60% of all mitochondrial precursor proteins are synthesised with amino- terminal presequences that form positively charged amphipathic alphahelices. These are translocated through an outer membrane channel formed by Tom40 and are transferred to the pre- sequence translocase of the inner membrane (TIM23 complex). Hydrophilic preproteins are imported into the matrix with the help of the presequence translocase-associated motor (PAM). Preproteins destined for the inner membrane have a hydrophobic sorting signal behind the positively charged matrix-targeting signal and are released into the lipid phase of the inner membrane. Once properly located the targeting signal is cleaved off by the mitochondrial processing peptidase (MPP). Some multi-spanning inner membrane proteins have an internal targeting signal rather than the N-terminal one, which is not removed during import, but remain part of the mature mitochondrial protein. Such proteins are initially translocated by the TOM complex and bind to soluble TIM chaperones present in the intermembrane space. These guide them to the carrier translocase of the inner membrane (TIM22 complex) that inserts them driven by the membrane potential. Proteins destined for the intermembrane space have their own import machinery. They are recognised by the TOM apparatus and then handed to the so-called mitochondrial intermembrane space import and assembly apparatus (MIA), which can recognise a cysteine containing signal and insert disulphide bonds into the protein.

The mitochondrial outer membrane contains two types of transmembrane proteins, beta barrel proteins and those with alphahelical transmembrane segments. The precursors of beta-barrel proteins are initially recognised and translocated by the TOM complex before being transferred to the intermembrane space side where they bind to the small TIM chaperones. The insertion of proteins into the outer membrane is mediated by a sorting and assembly machinery called SAM. As yet the insertion of the alpha helical transmembrane proteins is only poorly understood but also appears to involved the SAM complex.

As polypeptides as delivered to their residence sites in the different mitochondrial compartments, many associate with partner polypeptides and with prosthetic groups to produce complexes. In the case of the respiratory chain complexes and ATP there is the added complication in that these are made up not only of nuclear encoded proteins but ones coded on mtDNA and made on mitochondrial ribosomes. The mitochondrially-made polypeptides are for the most part transferred into the cristae membrane by the cytochrome oxidase activity associated translocase (OXA). The assembly of complexes I,III and IV as well as the ATP synthase is orchestrated by multiple assembly factors that are specific for each complex. These maintain polypeptides in partly folded states during insertion of prosthetic group and stabilise partly assembled complexes to ensure correct protein-protein interactions.

FUNCTION OF MITOCHONDRIA

Energy production is the important function of mitochondria. The food is broken into simpler molecules like carbohydrates, fats, etc. These are entered to mitochondrion where they are further processed to produce charged molecules that combine with oxygen and produce ATP molecules. This process is known as oxidative phosphorylation. The maintainance of proper concentration of calcium ions present in the various compartments of the cell is achieved by mitochondria by serving as storage tanks of calcium ions. Mitochondria has a role for the building of certain parts of the blood and hormones like testosterone and estrogen. The ammonia in the liver cells that detoxified by the presence of mitochondria.

Mitochondrial membranes contain numerous transport systems for the import of metabolites and high energy intermediates, export of ATP which is utilised in the cytosol and inorganic phosphate, which is returned to the matrix via a phosphate-proton symport that is driven by the chemiosmotic gradient. Thus some of the gradient energy is always used for purposes other than synthesis of ATP. It is in the inner mitochondrial membrane where the three enzyme complexes (NADH dehydrogenase, b-c1 cytochrome and cytochrome oxidase) and the three electron carriers (iron-sulphur centers, ubiquinone, cytochrome c) of the respiratory chain are located. The electron transfer through this chain creates a high proton concentration in the outer mitochondrial compartment, resulting in an electro-chemical gradient. The passage of these protons to the inner mitochondrial compartment through the ATP synthase complex drives the synthesis of ATP. This is a very efficient energy obtaining machinery that results in fifteen times more ATP molecules than anaerobic glycolysis.

Mitochondrial Plasticity

Mitochondria are able to modify their structure to meet the changing requirements of the cell. Some of these changes are typical of specialised cells, i.e. tubulo-vesicular cristae in steroid-producing cells. In other instances, there is an increase in the number of cristae or a change in their shape that results in a larger active surface for energy conversion, such as in zigzag, longitudinal or prismatic cristae, the latter resulting in a 75% increase in active membrane surface. Mitochondria may fuse or increase in size to form giant mitochondria or megamitochondria and they are also able to divide in a sequence that morphologically resembles bacterial division. Thus, increased number of mitochondria are generated in situations with high metabolic activity.

Isolation of Mitochondria

Isolation of mitochondria involves cell disruption and centrifugation. The process of cell disruption involves breaking open of cell so as to spill out the contents within the cell. Centrifugation is the process by which mixtures of cell components are separated by centrifugal force. The more dense particles migrate away from the axis, while less dense components of the mixture migrates towards the axis of centrifuge. The centrifugal technique which is used to separate the cell components from whole cell is called differential centrifugation. Differential centrifugation gives only a crude extract.

Cell Disruption Method

The process by which cell contents are spilled out of the plasma membrane barrier is called cell disruption. The cell disruption step should be gentle enough not as to mutilate the structure of the organelles. There are several techniques involved in cell disruption.

The cell disruption method used in the experiment is grinding:

1. Grinding.
2. Cutting.
3. Ultrasonic vibrations.
4. High pressure.
5. Enzymatic method.

Mitochondria Functioning in Intermediary Metabolism

Post-translational control of mitochondrial metabolism

Mitochondria are integral in the metabolism of carbohydrates, fats and amino acids in that they house all of the components of oxidative phosphorylation, Krebs cycle, urea cycle, fatty acid oxidation and key proteins of ketogenesis, triacylglycerol synthesis and gluconeogenesis. The basic enzymology of all of these pathways is now well understood and can be found in standard textbooks. Issues that are the focus of more recent study relate to the detailed mechanisms of several specific proteins in the pathways, particularly in oxidative phosphorylation, and to the regulation of intermediary metabolism in response to cellular events. Intermediary metabolism as a whole is integrated to match the overall energy production and cell constituent synthesis with the prevailing cell conditions such as substrate availability, hormonal action and stress events. This integration involves feedback by metabolites and control by a set of signalling pathways that change the levels of specific proteins and/or induce post-translational modifications such as phosphorylation/dephosphorylation and acetylation/deacteylation.

ATP, NAD and acetyl CoA each can stimulate or inhibit cellular processes either by direct effect on an enzyme of a particular pathway, or by modulating signalling pathways. For example the levels of ATP are constantly monitored by the AMP kinase, which in turn regulates glucose utilisation and energy dependent processes via the AKT/mTor signalling pathway. All three metabolites also directly affect the levels of metabolic enzymes and components of other cellular processes by inducing epigenetic effects in the nucleus.

Many proteins in mitochondria are subject to phosphorylation/dephosphorylation reactions at Thr, Ser and Tyr residues via mitochondrial kinases and phosphatases. The phosphoproteome of the organelle in humans has been extensively characterised. Such modifications are particularly important in the control of oxidative phosphorylation as well as in lipid metabolism. The acetylation of lysine residues by several acetylases in the organelle and deacetylation by a set of proteins, collectively called sirtuins, also regulates oxidative phosphorylation, as well as controlling the enzymes of the urea cycle, fatty acid oxidation and antioxidant proteins. At least 3 of the 7 well-defined sirtuins, i.e. 3, 4 and 5, are mitochondrial in location. These deacetylases has drawn widespread attention because of suggestions that their modulation may alter longevity. For example there is considerable work on the natural product resveratrol, an inhibitor of sirtuins, as an anti-ageing compound. The brief descriptions below of selected metabolic enzymes of mitochondria shows both the complexity and yet the progress made recently toward understanding structure function relationships.

Pyruvate dehydrogenase complex

Pyruvate dehydrogenase complex (PDH) is central to glucose metabolism, converting pyruvate to acetylCoA (from a 3 carbon to two carbon compound) with release of CO_2 and production of NADH. This large 8KDa complex links and regulates the flow of energy in cells by determining when pyruvate should be used for oxidative phosphorylation versus 'neutralised' to lactic acid to allow continued glycolysis. At the same time the control of acetyl Co-A directly influences fatty acid oxidation and production of ketone bodies.

The PDH complex is an example of the way that enzymes of a metabolic pathway are often organised in mitochondria. In this case the 3 enzymes required to complete the conversion of pyruvate to acetyl coA are together in a tight complex. These enzymes, pyruvate dehydrogenase, dihydrolipoyl transacetylase and dihydrolipoyl dehydrogenase respectively, work in sequence within the complex so that the product of the first reaction is handed off as substrate of the second etc. There is evidence of tight association of enzymes in other metabolic pathways as tight complexes. This includes the Krebs cycle enzymes the urea cycle enzymes, the enzymes of fatty acid oxidation and even the 4 respiratory chain complexes, which are now thought to exist in the mitochondrial inner membrane as supercomplexes.

PDH also provides an example of the control of intermediary metabolism by multiple post-translational modifications. The enzyme undergoes reversible phosphorylation by PDH kinases (PDK). There are four known isoforms of PDKs that are distributed differently in tissues. Their expressions are regulated differently by factors such as starvation, hypoxia, glucose utilisation and oxidation of fatty acids in various tissues. In addition, transcription regulators such as PGC-1α, retinoic acid and the glucocorticoid receptor are involved. De-phosphorylation to restore the activity of PDH is catalysed by PDH phosphatases (PDP). There are two known isoforms of PDPs, which are expressed differently in various tissues, PDP1 is present in high levels in skeletal muscle and PDP2 in liver and adipocytes. PDH is also acetylated by an as yet unknown acetylase and deacetylated by sirtuin 3 as part of the control of reactivity. This acetylation/deacetylation is different in different tissues, further optimising pyruvate conversion to acetyl CoA in response to cell conditions. Finally, PDH is one of most often causes of so-called mitochondrial diseases. It is an X-linked disease. Most of the mutations in PDH detected to date prevent proper assembly of the complex, and present as encephalopathies or myopathies with lactic acidosis.

Succinate dehydrogenase

Succinate dehydrogenase (SDH), complex II of the respiratory chain and a component enzyme of the Krebs cycle, shows similar features to PDH in terms of associations with other proteins (Krebs cycle enzymes) to facilitate substrate/product interchange, in terms of control of functioning by post–translational modifications, and in terms of mutations of the enzyme causing disease.

In addition, studies of SDH have provided important insight into the role of energy metabolites in causing cell transformation. SDH deficiencies along with those of fumarase, both Krebs cycle enzymes, leading to increased concentrations of succinate or fumarate, cause paragangliomas and adrenal or extra-adrenal phaeochromocytomas. The mechanism of this cell transformation is now understood. Accumulation of fumarate and succinate (so called oncometabolites) in mitochondria and in the cytosol impairs the enzymatic activity of several alpha ketoglutarate-dependent dioxygenases. These include JMJd3, which regulates chromatin structure, PHD3 which is involved in promoting neuronal apoptosis in response to NGF withdrawal, and PHD2 which primarily regulates HIFa stability.

ATP synthase

The ATP synthase is ubiquitous to all organisms. It is in the plasma membrane of prokaryotes along with respiratory chain proteins. In eukaryotes it is located predominantly in the mitochondrial cristae (but in some circumstances it is also found in the plasma membrane as discussed later). This enzyme can be seen in electron micrographs and more recently in X ray structural studies to be organised in 3 parts, and F1 part in the matrix of mitochondria attached to an F0 part in the cristae membrane by a stalk region now known to contain 2 distinct stalks. In all forms of the enzyme, the F1 part contains 5 different subunits, alpha3, beta3, gamma, delta and epsilon. The F0 part contains 3 different subunits a, b2 and c12 respectively in mammals. There are 3 catalytic sites per F1part, at the interfaces of the 3alpha/beta pairs respectively. The c subunits are arranged as a ring. The F1 part and F0 parts are connected by two stalks, one (the rotor includes gamma and epsilon, the other the stator contains the b subunit pair). The eukaryote ATP synthase is more complex than that of prokaryotes. The mammalian enzyme has the additional subunits F6, d, e, A6L, f, g and OSCP with most of these in the so-called stalk region of the complex. The full X ray structure of the yeast ATP synthase has been obtained, while the structure of most of the individual segments of the ATP synthase of mammals have been determined and modelled into the unit complex.

The structure of the ATP synthase is an important clue to the workings of this complex as first recognised by Boyer in his alternating site hypothesis, and made clearer as the detailed X-ray data emerged. First the three catalytic sites are in three different conformations. These are specified by the different interaction of the alpha-beta pairs with the central gamma subunit. Remarkably, the gamma subunit rotates through 120 degree steps driven by ATP hydrolysis in one direction and by proton translocation in the reverse direction, i.e. during ATP synthesis. This rotation has been shown elegantly in real time by the studies of Yoshida, Kinosita and their groups. The delta subunit and additional subunits in mammalian ATP synthase act as a stator or second stalk to facilitate this rotation.

There are additional features of the ATP synthase that have changed thinking about mitochondrial functioning and broader cell homeostasis. First it is now clear that this enzyme is involved in programmed cell death or apoptosis as the mitochondrial permeability transition pore. At one time the MPT was considered to be complex of the VDAC, adenylate kinase in the intermembrane space, the peripheral benzodiazepine receptor, cyclophilin D and the adenine nucleotide translocator. It now seems that the MPT is the dimeric form of the ATP synthase. The evidence comes from reconstitution experiments with purified ATP synthase (free of the other components above). In lipid bilayers, and on addition of a benzodiazepine derivative known to induce MPT, the enzyme dimer forms a channel with many of the same features seen on MPT opening in vitro including Ca^{++} sensitivity. Additionally, it has been shown that the c subunit ring of the complex alone forms a channel that is Ca^{++} sensitive and partly blocked by the beta subunit of the F1 part.

As would be expected, the functioning of the mitochondrial ATP synthase in under tight control. An inhibitor protein, IF1, controls whether the enzyme acts as an ATP synthase or an ATP hydrolase. IF1 binds to the F1 part of the ATP synthase. It is a small, predominantly alpha helical, polypeptide that interacts at the interface of an alpha and a beta subunit by associations with 5 subunits of the enzyme in total. IF1 is a dimer at pH below 6.5 when it binds to the ATP synthase to inhibit ATP hydrolysis. At higher pH the inhibitor progressively aggregates into a tetramer, which can no longer bind to the enzyme. In this way IF1 responds to the electron transfer-derived proton gradient that turns the matrix space acidic when OXPHOS is favoured, thereby preventing wasteful ATP hydrolysis and indirectly promoting glycolysis. Interestingly, IF1 is highly expressed in cancer cells, a feature that is now considered a part of the Warburg effect. In forming a dimer, IF1 helps to stabilise the ATP synthase dimer in the cristae membranes. Down regulation of IF1 levels by RNAi induces increased apoptosis in response to cell stressors.

One further and surprising finding related to the ATP synthase is that it is not exclusive to mitochondria but can be found under some conditions on the plasma membrane of cells. It may be that other mitochondrial enzymes can occupy the plasma membrane, e.g. the respiratory chain complexes but the ectopic location of the ATP synthase is the most studied example.

The presence of the 'mitochondrial' ATP synthase on the plasma membrane raises the interesting, and as yet unanswered question, of how it gets there. Assembly of a functional complex requires subunits encoded on mtDNA and synthesised in mitochondria. The most likely way is that there is fusion of mitochondria with the cell membrane and some resorting of proteins during this process.

MITOCHONDRIA IN APOPTOSIS

As well as acting in intermediary metabolism, mitochondria have a second key cellular function: they are the central executioners in the process of programmed cell death or apoptosis. Key proteins in apoptosis (Fig. 23.4) can be signalled from outside the cell by signalling molecules and growth factors as in development of tissues and organs (extrinsic), or from within the cell in response to various cell stress events (intrinsic). Intrinsic apoptosis can be a response to ER stress or from mitochondrial dysfunction, DNA modifications, loss of energy or other substrate molecules.

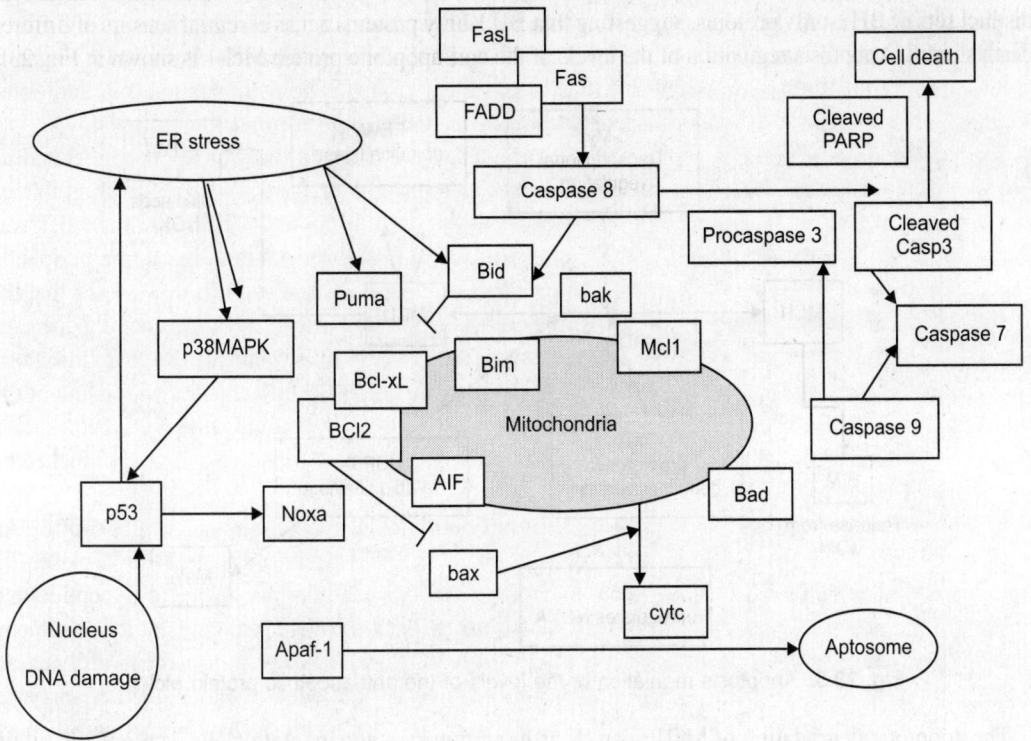

Fig. 23.4: Key proteins in apoptosis.

Mitochondria play an important role in the cell death process when initiated externally or internally. The key is that in healthy cells the mitochondrial outer membrane contains or has attached a set of antiapoptotic proteins that protect the cell from death. During apoptosis these are neutralised via altered interactions and/or proteolytic digestion by a set of pro-apoptotic proteins. The outcome of this is release of molecules from mitochondria, specifically cytochrome *c*, AIF, endonuclease G, Smac and OMI/HtrA2. The release of cytochrome *c* induces formation of the aptosome, which in turn activates a caspase cascade that leads to cleavage of proteins and DNA and further degradation of these fragments for uptake into macrophages and other inflammatory cells. The key proteins orchestrating apoptosis belong to the Bcl-2 family. The prototype member of this family, Bcl-2 itself, was initially identified in a common form of B-cell lymphoma, where a chromosome translocation causes overproduction of the Bcl-2 protein. The high levels of Bcl-2 promote cancer by inhibiting apoptosis, thereby prolonging cell survival.

More than 20 members of the Bcl-2 family have been identified, some pro-apoptotic and some anti-apoptotic, all defined by the presence of one to four Bcl-2 homology (BH) domains. The proapoptotic Bcl-2 proteins can be further subdivided into two subfamilies based on the sharing of BH domains. BH multidomain proteins, such as Bax and Bak, are the triggers of apoptosis, most likely as a result of their ability to form pores in the outer mitochondrial membrane. The other subfamily, the BH3-only proteins, which contain only the BH3 domain, act as upstream regulators by controlling the allosteric activation of the gatekeepers Bax and Bak. In healthy cells, BH3-only proteins are either not expressed or are inactive, until rapidly activated following exposure to cellular stresses. Different types of stresses activate distinct sets of BH3-only proteins, suggesting that BH3-only proteins act as essential sensors of different death stimuli. Apoptosis regulation of the levels of the anti-apoptotic protein Mcl-1 is shown in Fig. 23.5.

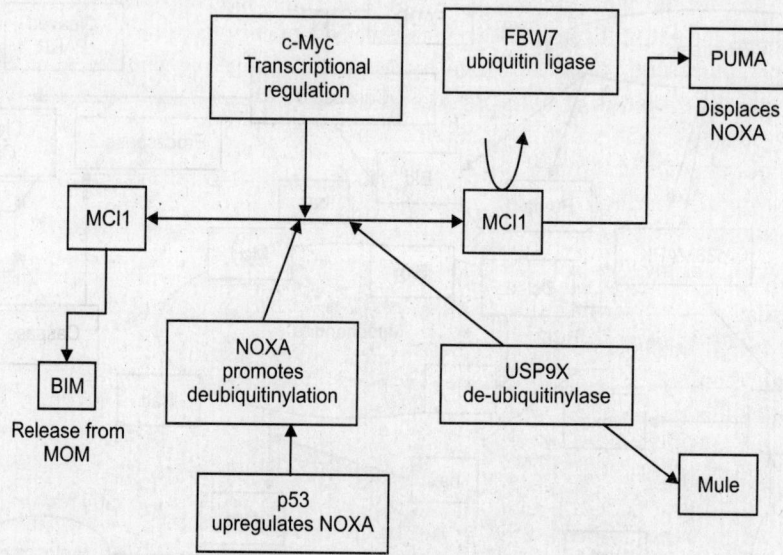

Fig. 23.5: Apoptosis regulation of the levels of the anti-apoptotic protein Mcl-1.

The apoptotic degradation of Mcl1, as well as its turnover in nonapoptotic cells, is regulated by the counteracting activities of the Ub ligase ARF-BP1/Mule and the deubiquitinase Usp9x. Expression levels of ARF- BP1/Mule and Usp9x appears to be critical for the maintenance of proper cellular balance of anti- and pro- apoptotic proteins, and contributes to cell sensitivity to apoptosis. Turnover of other mitochondria-associated Bcl-2 family proteins, including Bax and Bcl-2 is also under Ub/proteasome control. Bax, a pro-apoptotic Bcl-2 family protein, is mainly localised in the cytosol in an apoptotically inactive form, but moves to mitochondria upon proapoptotic trigger- induced change in its conformation. Proteasomedependent degradation of Bax occurs specifically on mitochondria, suggesting that the apoptotic conformation of Bax might be recognised by the Ub conjugation machinery, and serve as a degradation signal preventing the accumulation of potentially dangerous apoptotically-active Bax in healthy cell mitochondria. The protein Omi/HtrA2, once released from mitochondria along with cytochrome *c*, promote apoptosis by counteracting the inhibitor-of-apoptosis proteins (IAPs), which comprise a family of endogenous caspase inhibitors. Other proteins released from mitochondria, i.e. apoptosis-inducing factor (AIF) and endonuclease G promote cell death in a caspase-independent manner by inducing chromatin condensation and DNA degradation. Thus, if for some reason cells do not activate caspases after MOMP, these mediators might still ensure that cell death proceeds. Phagocytic uptake of apoptotic cells, the last step of apoptosis, is identified by a phospholipid asymmetry and externalisation of phosphatidylserine on the surface of apoptotic cells.

CONTROL OF MITOCHONDRIAL LEVELS: PRODUCTION VERSUS DESTRUCTION

The total level of mitochondria in a cell is continually balanced by competing biosynthesis and mitophagy. Addition of proteins and lipids during biosynthesis uses existing mitochondria as a template.

Biogenesis

Multiple intrinsic cellular signalling pathways monitor mitochondrial functioning and trigger organelle biogenesis. These include the AMPkinase pathway which monitors ATP levels, the calcium/calmodulin-dependent kinase and p38 mitogen-activated kinase which monitors Ca^{++} homeostasis, mTOR a moderator of overall cell homeostasis, the cAMP/PKA pathway, ROS signalling and NO and CO_2 levels. These stimuli activate the synthesis of mitochondrial genes, both on mtDNA and nuclear DNA through a series of transcription factors mostly under control of a family of coactivators. (PGC-1alpha, PGC-1beta and PRC). Signalling through PGC-1α and PGC-1β is sufficient to increase total mitochondrial mass, reactive oxygen species scavenging enzymes, oxidative phosphorylation components, mitochondrial metabolic pathways, protein import complexes, proteins involved in fission and fusion, and the levels of mitochondrial sirtuins. Control of mitochondrial biogenesis by PGC-1alpha is shown in Fig. 23.6.

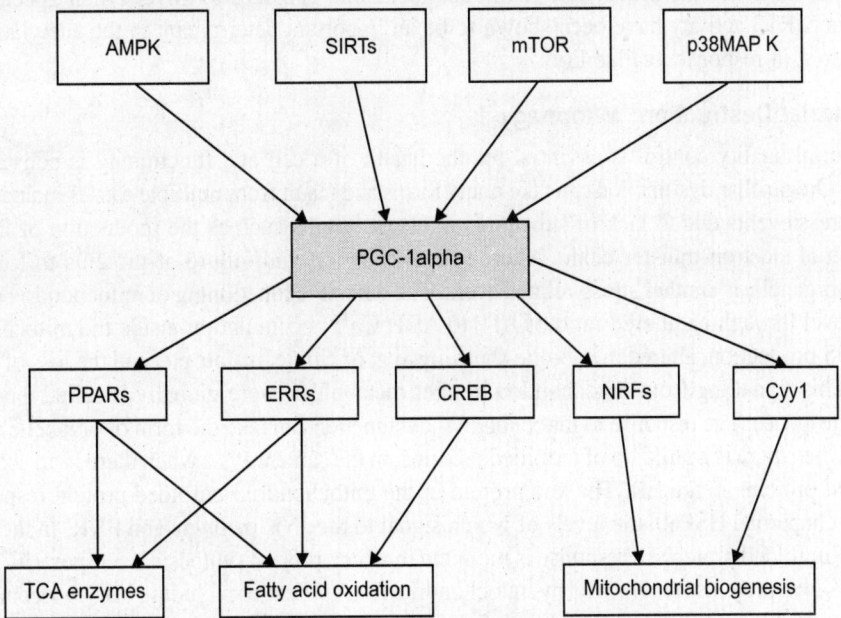

Fig. 23.6: Control of mitochondrial biogenesis by PGC-1alpha.

NRF-1 controls the expression of a significant number of the proteins that make up the five respiratory complexes, as well as proteins integral to mitochondrial import and heme biosynthesis. NRF-1 is also able to integrate nuclear control of the transcriptional and replicative activity of the mitochondrial genome through the direct modulation of transcription factor A mitochondrial (TFAM) and transcription factor B proteins (TFBs) gene expression. NRF-2 is also able to regulate the expression of proteins in the electron transport chain. The differential regulation of NRF1 and NRF2 is not completely understood but phosphorylation of these factors can alter their transcriptional activities. Thyroid hormone receptors (THRs) are another set of factors that promote mitochondrial biogenesis in relation to tissue-specific function. This includes mitochondrial-driven thermogenesis that occurs in brown fat during the adaptation to lower temperatures In some instances, THRs directly drive the transcription of nuclearencoded genes, whereas, in others, the effects can occur indirectly through the thyroid hormone-mediated up-regulation of NRF-1 Also involved are estrogen-related receptors ERR-α, ERR-β, and ERR-γ. These receptors have no known endogenous ligands and are primary expressed in tissues with high oxidative metabolism capacities They are involved in transcriptional control of enzymes of oxidative phosphorylation, fatty acid oxidation, TCA cycle, and factors regulating mitochondrial fusion/fission.

Two other transcription factors that orchestrate mitochondrial biogenesis are CREB, a cAMP activated transcription factor that can promote the expression of several mitochondrial genes, including those for complex IV and enzymes involved in the β-oxidation pathway. Finally the overall process is regulated by a set of NAD^+-dependent protein deacylases, the sirtuins. Mammals have 7 sirtuins, SIRT1, SIRT6, and SIRT7 are nuclear proteins, SIRT3, SIRT4, and SIRT5 are imported into mitochondria, and SIRT2 is principally cytoplasmic. Through their deacylation activities, SIRT1, SIRT3, SIRT4, and SIRT5 have profound effects on mitochondrial function. SIRT1 deacetylates several key transcription factors that result in the upregulation of numerous genes involved in mitochondrial respiration. In addition, as discussed already, sirtuins deacetylate numerous metabolic enzymes to govern their specific activity. Changes in SIRT3 activity have been shown to be an important determinant in the acetylation state of mitochondrial in response availability.

Mitochondrial Destruction: Mitophagy

Mitochondrial quality control is essential for the health of a cell and functioning is constantly being evaluated. Oreganellar dysfunction can take many forms and result from multiple causes including genetic defects, stress events due to lack of substrate, and toxic insults such as the production of ROS by the mitochondrial electron transfer chain. Altered protein import and failure of proteins to fold properly within the organelle is another stress-related event. The defective functioning of mitochondria is signalled to the cytosol through an altered ratio of ATP to ADP, Ca^{++} accumulation inside the mitochondria, the excess ROS production, altered metabolite shuttling, e.g. of citrate, malate etc. and the loss of membrane potential This signalling from mitochondria to alter metabolism more globally is called the retrograde signalling response. The response to mitochondrial dysfunction can take the form of organelle repair such as occurs when there is a build up of unfolded proteins, in the same way as when there is an accumulation of unfolded proteins in the ER. The key protein in the mitochondrial unfolded protein response is the molecular chaperone HSP60, the levels of which signal to the JNK pathway and PKR. In the event of a build up of unfolded proteins, a response is mounted in which protein synthesis is temporarily suspended and the unfolded proteins are removed by mitochondrial AAA proteases including Lon. A second cleansing mechanism involves vesicular transport of defective mitochondrial proteins to the lysosome for degradation. Mitochondrial retrograde signalling are shown in Fig. 23.7.

Finally, whole mitochondria (fragmented form) can be removed. This degradation of mitochondria by a process called mitophagy is of particular importance in the removal of male sperm mitochondria on fertilisation of an egg. Mitophagy is also involved in the generation of erythrocytes, which lose their mitochondria before maturation. Cellular unfolded protein response are shown in Fig. 23.8.

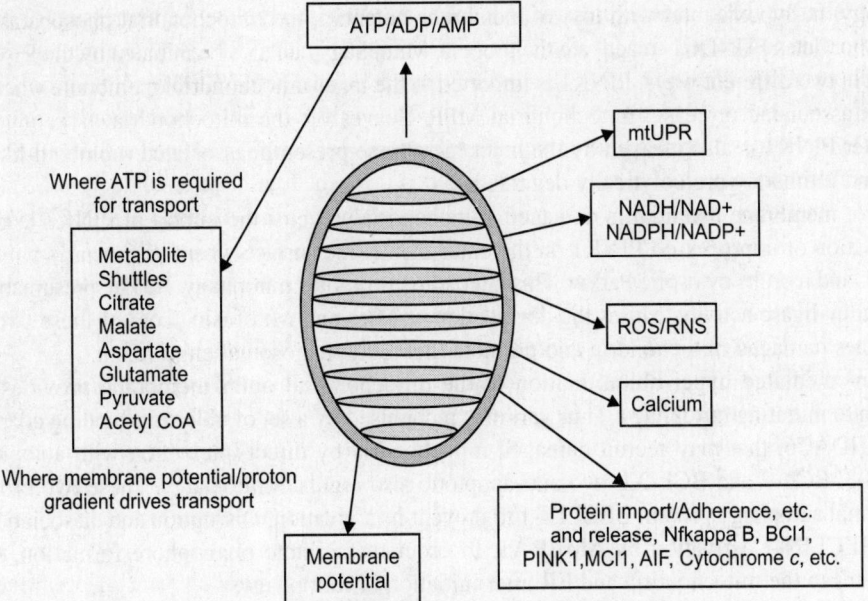

Fig. 23.7: Mitochondrial retrograde signalling.

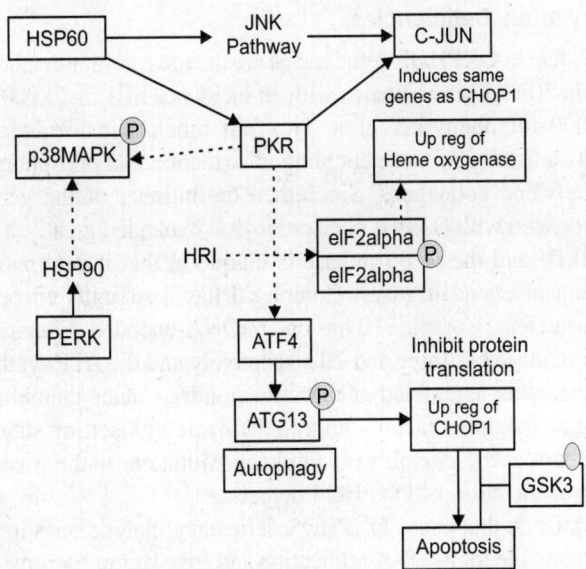

Fig. 23.8: Cellular unfolded protein response.

Mitophagy can be triggered by a receptor response involving several outer membrane receptor proteins including NIX/BNIP3L, BNIP3 and FUNDC1 in mammalian systems. These proteins have a classic motif to bind directly to LC3 and initiate mitophagy. This receptormediated mitophagy is regulated by reversible protein phosphorylation. Thus phosphorylation of FUNDC1 by Src kinase, ULK1, and CK2 prevent mitophagy. In hypoxia, and with loss of membrane potential, the mitochondrial phosphatase PGAM5 dephosphorylates FUNDC1 to activate the process. Mitophagy can also be initiated by the PINK1/parkin reaction in two different ways. PINK1 is imported to the inner mitochondrial membrane where the TIM complex-associated protease, mitochondrial MPP, cleaves off the mitochondrial targeting sequence. Thereafter PINK1 is also cleaved by the inner membrane presenilinassociated rhomboid-like protease PARL and ultimately proteolytically degraded.

Loss of membrane potential in damaged mitochondria prevents the import of PINK1 leading to the accumulation of unprocessed PINK1 on the outer membrane surface where it associates with the TOM complex, and recruits cytosolic Parkin. This interaction promotes mitophagy. Parkin, presumably through its ubiquitin–ligase activity, causes the degradation of Miro and Mitofusin. Loss of these two proteins, quarantines damaged mitochondria and promote their autophagosomal engulfment.

Parkin- mediated hyper-ubiquitination of the mitochondrial outer membrane provides a second approach to initiating mitophagy. Thus parkin is recognised by a set of ubiquitin-binding adaptors, such as p62, HDAC6, that may recruit damaged mitochondria by direct interaction with autophagosomal protein L3. BCL-2 and BCL-XL two anti-apoptotic also regulate mitophagy. These two proteins bind the essential autophagy protein BECLIN-1 to prevent its activation, Disruption and dissociation of BCL allows BECLIN-1 activation by AMBRA1. In order to facilitate phagophore formation, AMBRA1 translocates to the mitochondria and ER after initiation of mitophagy.

MITOCHONDRIAL IN DISEASE

Oxidative Phosphorylation Deficiencies

Mitochondrial disorders due to OXPHOS deficiencies are the most common inborn errors of metabolism with an incidence of 1 in 5000. This compares with an incidence of 1 in 10,000 for fatty acid oxidation disorders and 1in 15000 for phenylketourea. The first biochemical evidence of a mitochondrial dysfunction: specifically a finding of loose coupling of oxidation and phosphorylation in a patient, was reported in 1962 by Luft and colleagues. Since then the number of the genotypes and breadth of phenotypes that are associated with OXPHOS disorders has expanded greatly. The genotype of electron transfer complexes I,III,IV and the ATP synthase is unique in that it can involve mutations in either mtDNA encoded or nuclear encoded genes. Complex I has 7 subunits encoded on mtDNA and 38 subunits encoded in the nucleus. Complex III has one mtDNA-encoded subunit and 10 nuclear encoded subunits, cytochrome c oxidase has three and 10 respectively and the ATP synthase has 2 and 14. Each of the OXPHOS complexes is assembled at the mitochondrial inner membrane by a set of nuclear encoded proteins acting as assembly factors through their role in inserting subunits in a specific order and adding prosthetic groups as the assembly is completed. Mutations in these assembly factors represent a significant proportion of the cases of OXPHOS defects.

Other mutations in mtDNA that cause OXPHOS deficiency include ones in the tRNAs encoded on mtDNA, in proteins responsible for mtDNA replication and translation, for protein folding and transport into the organelle, in lipid biosynthesis and specifically in a protein called tafazzin (which encodes an enzyme involved in cardiolipin synthesis and produces Barth syndrome).

The common biochemical phenotype induced by all of these different mutations is reduced ATP synthesis, increased oxidative stress, and often, uncoupling of the membrane potential. The physiological phenotype is much more varied. Among the conditions described are Lebers hereditary optic neuropathy (LHON), mitochondrial encephalopathy, lactic acidosis and stroke like episodes (MELAS),

Kearn-Sayre syndrome, Leighs disease, progressive external opthalmoplegia, and neuropathy, ataxia and retinitis pigmentosa (NARP). Some mutations induce cardiomyopathy and diabetes. It is not uncommon for the same mutation to cause different conditions in different patients. Even when the same condition is diagnosed there is variability of phenotype. A recent study of over 300 patients with the mtDNA mutation 8344A>G gave a diverse clinical picture with myoclonus, muscle weakness and ataxia in around 40% of patients, generalised seizures and hearing loss in around 30%, cognitive impairment, multiple lipomatosis, neuropathy, and exercise intolerance in 20%, and increased creatine kinase levels, ptosis/ophthalmoparesis, optic atrophy, cardiomyopathy, muscle wasting, respiratory impairment, diabetes, muscle pain, tremor, migraine in about 10%.

There are 2 key reasons for this diversity of physiological phenotype. First is the combination of maternal inheritance of mtDNA (mitochondria from the sperm are destroyed in the fertilised egg as discussed already) along with the so-called bottleneck in which the number of copies of mtDNA is dramatically reduced and then segregated stochastically during embryogenesis. In this way the distribution of mutant mDNA in different tissues is random and depends on the position of normal and mutant copies with respect to cleavage patterns in the embryo. The second consideration is the threshold for dysfunction. The phenotype is dependent on the level of oxidative phosphorylation needed for a particular tissue. Thus the percent mutation mtDNA at which cells are unable to generate sufficient energy is a determinant of cell maintainance.

Fatty Acid Oxidation Disorders

The degradation of fatty acids by mitochondrial fatty acid β-oxidation (FAO) is a key metabolic pathway for energy homoeostasis in organs such as the liver, heart and skeletal muscle. During fasting, when glucose supply becomes limited, FAO is of particular importance. Under this condition, most tissues, except the brain, can use fatty acids directly to generate energy. Furthermore, the liver converts fatty acids into ketone bodies, a process for which FAO is indispensable. Ketone bodies serve as an additional energy source that is used by all tissues including the brain.

Beta-oxidation defects are potentially fatal disorders. Symptoms are usually seen during fasting or prolonged exercising. Often, but not always, the patients have hypoketotic hypoglycaemia along with alterations in liver, heart, muscular and nervous systems. There are three different presentations. First is the hepatic presentation, which is a severe, often lethal, disease in infancy or the neonatal period with hypoketotic hypoglycaemia and Reye-like syndrome. During infancy, patients may also present with cardiac symptoms such as dilated or hypertrophic cardiomyopathy and/or arrhythmias. Alternatively, FAO defects might present as a milder, later ('adult') onset disease. This form is characterised by exercise-induced myopathy and rhabdomyolysis. To date, FAO defects have been found inglutaric aciduria type 2, primary carnitine deficiency and deficiencies of CPT1a, CACT, CPT2, VLCAD, MTP (including isolated LCHAD or thiolase), MCAD, M/SCHAD, SCAD and 2,4-dienoyl CoA reductase (DECR).

Mitochondria and Cancer

As the cells of various tissues transform into cancer they undergo a multitude of changes that have been elegantly summarised as the 6 hallmarks of cancer. These include sustaining proliferative signalling, evading growth suppression, inducing angiogenesis, enabling replicative immortality, activating invasion and metastasis and preventing cell death. Added to these changes, cancer cells alter energy metabolism to use glycolysis more readily and utilise substrates other than glucose for oxidative phosphorylation, and they have mechanisms to avoid immune detection.

The altered metabolism of cancer cells was first noted by Warburg and is now called the Warburg Effect. Warburg found that cancer cells tend to make the energy for their growth and replication by glycolysis in the cytosol rather than oxidative phosphorylation even when oxygen is plentiful. More recent studies have established that this is an oversimplification as some cancer cells use oxidative phosphorylation as well as glycolysis. It is now evident that cancer cannot be defined by a single effect on energy metabolism but is heterogeneous depending on tissue, stage of the cancer growth and environmental conditions under which the transformation is occurring. There is considerable variation within solid tumours as well as between them. Nevertheless there are sufficient differences between the energy metabolism of cancerous tissue and normal tissue to believe that practical treatments that attack these differences can be effective cancer treatments. Of particular importance, in transformation the stabilising of HIF1alpha induces switching of isoforms of several of the glycolytic enzymes including transporters (GLUT1, GLUT3) and enzymes (HKI, HKII, PFK-L, ALD-A, ALD-C, PGK1, ENO-alpha, PYKM2, LDH-A, PFKFB-3). These are now being exploited as targets for drug therapy.

More specific to transformed cells than the mode of energy generation is the substrates used. Amino acids and fatty acids are a major source of both energy production and generation of intermediates for biosynthesis of cell components. Cancer cells are particularly adept at using glutamine and also glycine and serine as sources of carbon and nitrogen. The oncogene, Cmyc, facilitates this through the coordinate enhanced expression of the genes responsible for amino acid catabolism. Thereby, glutaminolysis not only serves for ATP production in some situations, but also provides the needed metabolites such as glucose-6-phosphate, ammonia and aspartate for the synthesis of purine and pyrimidine nucleotides.

Another significant feature of cancer metabolism is the high level of free radicals produced in mitochondria mainly generated by complexes I and III of the respiratory chain, but also produced by cytosolic NADH oxidase. At low levels, free radicals such as superoxide act as signalling molecules, but at high levels they are toxic. Mitochondria of cancer cells show high levels of damage from oxidative stress both in mtDNA and in the organellar proteins. This has led to the proposal that mtDNA damage is oncogenic. The strongest evidence of mitochondrial dysfunction leading directly to transformation is for the defects in the Krebs cycle enzymes succinate dehydrogenase and fumarase discussed already, along with mutations in isocitrate dehydrogenase, which causes glial tumours. These defects generate what are now called oncometabolites.

Also, given that mitochondria are the central executioners of the cell, it is not surprising that many of the mitochondrial proteins involved in apoptosis and in mitophagy are oncogenes. The dysfunction of such proteins, e.g. BCl2 proteins, can affect induction of the mitochondrial permeability pore. Additionally these proteins are required for fission and fragmentation, necessary steps in the cell death process, which if blocked, lead to cell proliferation and cancer induction.

Mitochondria in the Innate Immune Response

Mitochondria are now known to play a critical role in the fight against viral infections. So called innate immunity against RNA viral infection involves the activation of multiple signalling steps that culminate in the rapid production of type I interferons, such as IFN-α and -β, and other pro-inflammatory cytokines. Two distinct pathways initiate signal transduction, one involves the endosomal Toll- like receptor 3 which targets RNA viruses entering the cell by endocytosis, the other is prompted by retinoic acid-inducible gene I (RIG-I)-like receptors (RLRs), which recognise cytoplasmic viral- derived double-stranded (ds)RNA. RIG-1 and a second RNA helicase, MDA-5, recognise distinct types of cytosolic RNA species and are recruited to the mitochondrial outer membrane where they interact with the protein, mitochondrial antiviral signalling protein (MAVS): also called IPS-1, VISA and CARDIF. This protein of 56Kd contains an *N*-terminal caspase activation and recruitment domain (CARD) comprising six helices. The same structure is found in both RIG-1 and MDA-5. MAVS also contains a transmembrane domain that anchors it to the mitochondrial outer membrane. Activation of immunity. MAVS leads to downstream translational activation of NF kappaB and/or IRF3/7, inducing rapid production of the interferons and cytokines. It also activates autophagy or apoptosis to rid the cell of viral elements or remove the infected cell from tissue. Other mitochondrial outer membrane proteins are involved in the antiviral response, e.g. TOM70 which acts as a viral receptor including for the hepatitis C virus. HIV infection leads to induction of TOM70 expression, which in turn induces resistance to tumour necrosis factoralpha (TNF-α)-mediated apoptosis but not to Fas-induced apoptosis in HepG2 cells. TOM70 was found to be induced by the HCV nonstructural protein (NS)3/4A protein, and silencing of TOM70 decreased the levels of the NS3 and Mcl-1 proteins.

While much is known about the upregulation of MAVS, less is known about its degradation after viral infection. However two proteins have been shown to play such a role recently. These are the poly c-binding proteins (PCBP-1 and PCBP-2). Overexpression of PCBP1 impairs MAVS-mediated antiviral response while knockdown of this protein has the opposite effect. PCBP1 is abundantly expressed while PCBP2 shows low basal expression but rapid induction after infection several recent studies show how viruses can get the better of a cell. For example, murine gamma herpes virus 68 subverts cytokine production by modifying upstream signalling to MAVS. Further, HIV tat protein can react with mitochondria to induce permeabilisation of the organelle and to inactivate cytcochrome *c*.

Mitochondria Neurodegeneration

It has long been thought that mitochondria play a critical role in a variety of diseases characterised by neuro-degeneration. Early on the focus was on oxidative stress and the effect this had on energy production. More recently emphasis has shifted to disease-causing alterations in mitochondrial trafficking and/or removal of defective organelle by mitophagy, although as yet there is no definitive evidence in any of the diseases below.

The proposal that mitochondrial dysfunction played a role in Parkinsons disease originated with the observation that the Complex I inhibitors rotenone and MTTP caused Parkinsonian symptoms. More recent work has identified Complex I protein changes in patients with the disease. Proteomic studies showed that complex I of brains from Parkinsons patients had an average decrease of 34% in the 8 kDa subunit, and contained 47% more protein carbonyls in catalytic subunits coded for by mitochondrial and nuclear genomes. Further, NADH-driven electron transfer rates through complex I inversely correlate with complex I protein subunit modifications. Similar patterns were observed when the mitochondria from brains of control subjects were incubated with NADH in the presence of rotenone, but not with exogenous oxidant, indicating that the oxidative damage is induced from within the complex and not by exogenous free radicals.

The damage caused by Complex I dysfunction and consequent superoxide production is broader than just in this complex, and is found in DNA, lipids and proteins of PD brains, particularly in the substancia nigra which has low concentrations of anti-oxidant proteins. Oxidative damage is also seen in peripheral tissues. Importantly, these broad oxidative effects are observed in animals treated with rotenone, confirming that the initial free radical generator is Complex I.

One way in which reduced respiratory chain activity and build up of oxidative damage can cause death of neurons in PD is through reduced ATP production. Alternatively, based on recent work, it is the failure to identify and excise damage mitochondria by mitophagy that is central to the disease. Several genes have been linked to early onset Parkinsons including Pink 1, Parkin, DJ1, LRRK2 and alpha synuclein. Structure and function studies of pink1 and parkin proteins, two essential components of mitophagy signalling in neurons, have provided the link between the disease and mitochondria. As discussed already, pink1 and parkin are direct participants in the process of mitophagy.

The link between mitochondrial dysfunction and PD is more tenuous with respect to forms caused by mutation of DJI. DJ1 functions to protect cells against oxidative stress. It protects neurons from oxidative stress by scavenging H_2O_2 from the neuronal environment and thus it also protects mitochondrial integrity in these cells. The role of LRRK2 is less clear. This ubiquitous protein has GTPase and kinase activity. Similarly the role of alpha synuclein in cells is not well known. The link with mitochondria for both proteins is their association with the organelle. Both associate with microtubules. Thus they may after mitochondrial transport and/or the fussion/fission process when defective in PD.

Amiotrophic lateral sclerosis or ALS has been shown to involve the misfolding of the predominantly cytosolic antioxidant protein superoxide dismutase (SOD1). Mitochondria also contain SOD1 as well as a second form of this enzyme SOD2, which is not affected by the disease. Wild type SOD1, and a copper chaperone for SOD1 (CCS), are localised to the intermembrane space (IMS) in normal mitochondria. It has been proposed that the nascent SOD1 polypeptide with no metal ion bound can efficiently enter mitochondria and that the maturation of SOD1 including metal ion binding and intra-molecular disulphide bond formation inside mitochondria and the subsequent retention in IMS involve the SOD1-CCS interaction. The ALS-related mutant SOD1 proteins have also been found in the IMS, but also in the matrix and outer membrane of mitochondria. Once associated with mitochondria, the mutant SOD1 is seen to cause impaired respiratory complexes, disrupted redox homeostasis and decreased ATP production. However, the primary effect could be altered mitochondrial cell transport. As in Parkinsons disease, the reason that mitochondrial dysfunction is observed predominantly in neurons may relate to altered mitochondrial cell transport in these extended cells. Thus it has been shown that primary neurons isolated from G93A SOD1 transgenic mice and cortical neurons transfected with G93A SOD1, have reduced antegrade mitochondrial transport.

In Alzheimer's disease (AD), as in PD, membrane-associated oxidative stress, increased free radical production, and perturbed Ca^{2+} homeostasis have been observed. Increased mitochondrial permeability and cyt c release, which is promoted by Aβ oligomerisation and polymerisation, is thought to trigger the opening of MPTP leading to apoptosis. Different from PD there is evidence of reduced cytochrome c oxidase activity. This is at least in part due to oxidative damage of mtDNA that is beyond that seen in normal age controls. Complex I down regulation is also seen in AD brains. As in PD, the primary insult leading to AD is not known. Most likely this is a heterogeneous disease, with altered mitochondrial function leading to reduced ATP production, increased free radical production, and increased apoptosis.

Huntingtons disease is linked to the presence of an elongated polyglutamine (polyQ) stretch in huntingtin protein (Htt). This mutation in Htt correlates with neuronal dysfunction in the striatum and cerebral cortex and eventually leads to neuronal cell death. How this happens remains unclear but like PD and AD focus is now on anomalous mitochondrial dynamics, and trafficking along with disrupted mitophagy. In addition, deficiency in oxidative metabolism and defects in mitochondrial Ca^{2+} handling are considered essential contributing factors to neuronal dysfunction in HD.

Chapter 24

Chloroplasts and Others Plastids

INTRODUCTION

The word chloroplast is derived from the Greek words *chloros*, which means green, and *plast*, which means form or entity. Chloroplasts are members of a class of organelles known as plastids. Chloroplasts are organelles found in plant cells and other eukaryotic organisms that conduct photo-synthesis. Chloroplasts capture light energy to conserve free energy in the form of ATP and reduce NADP to NADPH through a complex set of processes called photosynthesis.

Chloroplasts are the food producers of the cell. They are only found in plant cells and some protists. Animal cells do not have chloroplasts. Every green plant you see is working to convert the energy of the sun into sugars. Plants are the basis of all life on earth. They create sugars and the by-product of that process is the oxygen that we breathe. That process happens in the chloroplast. Mitochondria work in the opposite direction and break down the sugars and nutrients that the cell receives. Chloroplasts are structures in which photosynthesis takes place. In each cell, there are 40–50 of these disk shaped organelles. Chloroplasts are surrounded in two membranes and contain a ground substances called the stroma, which is crossed by connected sacs called lamelles.

In green plants, chloroplasts are surrounded by two lipid-bilayer membranes. They are believed to correspond to the outer and inner membranes of the ancestral cyanobacterium. Chloroplasts have their own genome, which is considerably reduced compared to that of free-living cyanobacteria, but the parts that are still present show clear similarities with the cyanobacterial genome. Plastids may contain 60–100 genes whereas cyanobacteria often contain more than 1500 genes. Many of the missing genes are encoded in the nuclear genome of the host. The transfer of nuclear information has been estimated in tobacco plants at one gene for every 16000 pollen grains.

In some algae (such as the heterokonts and other protists such as Euglenozoa and Cercozoa), chloroplasts seem to have evolved through a secondary event of endosymbiosis, in which a eukaryotic cell engulfed a second eukaryotic cell containing chloroplasts, forming chloroplasts with three or four membrane layers. In some cases, such secondary endosymbionts may have themselves been engulfed by still other eukaryotes, thus forming tertiary endosymbionts. In the alga *Chlorella*, there is only one chloroplast, which is bell-shaped. In some groups of mixotrophic protists such as the dinoflagellates, chloroplasts are separated from a captured alga or diatom and used temporarily. These klepto chloroplasts may only have a lifetime of a few days and are then replaced.

STRUCTURE AND FUNCTION OF CHLOROPLASTS

Plant chloroplasts (Fig. 24.1) are large organelles (5 to 10 μm long) that, like mitochondria, are bounded by a double membrane called the chloroplast envelope. In addition to the inner and outer membranes of the envelope, chloroplasts have a third internal membrane system, called the thylakoid membrane. The thylakoid membrane forms a network of flattened discs called thylakoids, which are frequently arranged in stacks called grana. Because of this three-membrane structure, the internal organisation of chloroplasts is more complex than that of mitochondria. In particular, their three membranes divide chloroplasts into three distinct internal compartments: (i) the intermembrane space between the two membranes of the chloroplast envelope, (ii) the stroma, which lies inside the envelope but outside the thylakoid membrane and (iii) the thylakoid lumen.

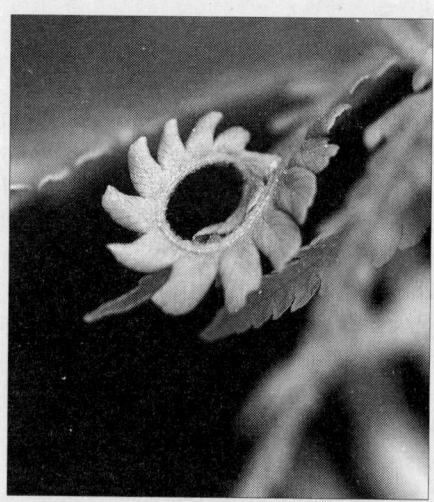

Fig. 24.1: Plant chloroplasts.

Despite this greater complexity, the membranes of chloroplasts have clear functional similarities with those of mitochondria—as expected, given the role of both organelles in the chemiosmotic generation of ATP. The outer membrane of the chloroplast envelope, like that of mitochondria, contains porins and is therefore freely permeable to small molecules. In contrast, the inner membrane is impermeable to ions and metabolites, which are therefore able to enter chloroplasts only, via., specific membrane transporters. These properties of the inner and outer membranes of the chloroplast envelope are similar to the inner and outer membranes of mitochondria. In both cases the inner membrane restricts the passage of molecules between the cytosol and the interior of the organelle. The chloroplast stroma is also equivalent in function to the mitochondrial matrix. It contains the chloroplast genetic system and a variety of metabolic enzymes, including those responsible for the critical conversion of CO_2 to carbohydrates during photosynthesis. The major difference between chloroplasts and mitochondria, in terms of both structure and function, is the thylakoid membrane. This membrane is of central importance in chloroplasts, where it fills the role of the inner mitochondrial membrane in electron transport and the chemiosmotic generation of ATP (Fig. 24.2). The inner membrane of the chloroplast envelope (which is not folded into cristae) does not

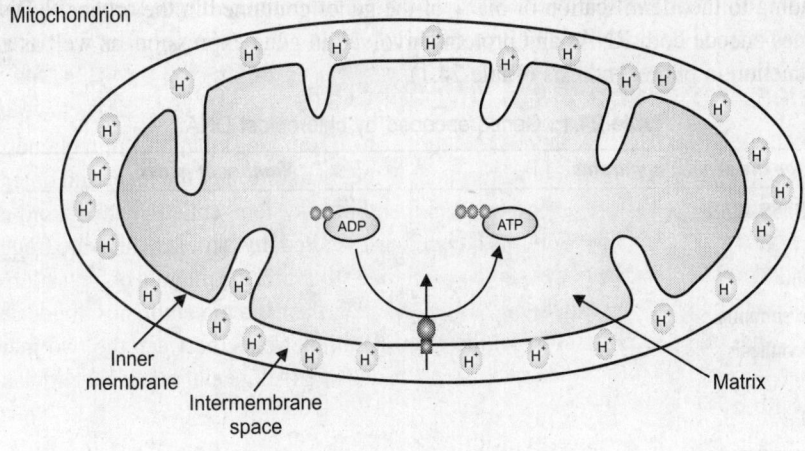

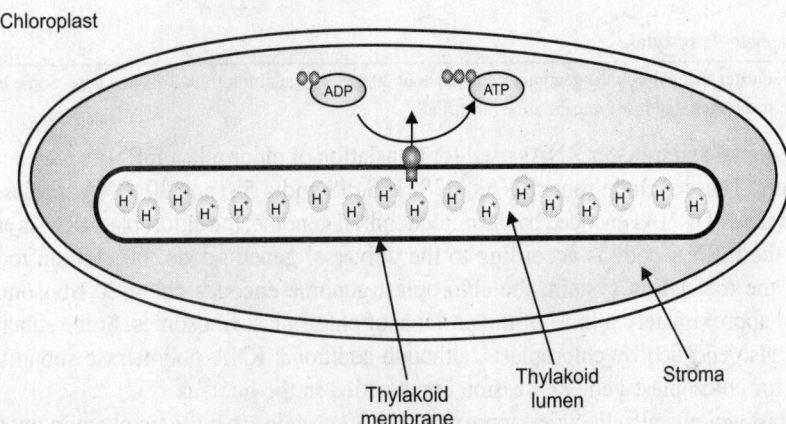

Fig. 24.2: Chemiosmotic generation of ATP in chloroplasts and mitochondria. In mitochondria, electron transport generates a proton gradient across the inner membrane, which is then used to drive ATP synthesis in the matrix. In chloroplasts, the proton gradient is generated across the thylakoid membrane and used to drive ATP synthesis in the stroma.

function in photo-synthesis. Instead, the chloroplast electron transport system is located in the thylakoid membrane and protons are pumped across this membrane from the stroma to the thylakoid lumen. The resulting electrochemical gradient then drives ATP synthesis as protons cross back into the stroma. In terms of its role in generation of metabolic energy, the thylakoid membrane of chloroplasts is thus equivalent to the inner membrane of mitochondria.

CHLOROPLAST GENOME

Like mitochondria, chloroplasts contain their own genetic system, reflecting their evolutionary origins from photosynthetic bacteria. The genomes of chloroplasts are similar to those of mitochondria in that they consist of circular DNA molecules present in multiple copies per organelle. However, chloroplast genomes are larger and more complex than those of mitochondria, ranging from 120 to 160 kb and containing approximately 120 genes. The chloroplast genomes of several plants have been completely sequenced, leading to the identification of many of the genes contained in the organelle DNAs. These chloroplast genes encode both RNAs and proteins involved in gene expression, as well as a variety of proteins that function in photosynthesis (Table 24.1).

Table 24.1: Genes encoded by chloroplast DNA.

Function genes for the genetic apparatus	Number of genes
rRNAs (23S, 16S, 5S, 4.5S)	4
tRNAs	30
Ribosomal proteins	21
RNA polymerase subunits	4
Genes for photosynthesis	
Photosystem I	5
Photosystem II	12
Cytochrome *bf* complex	4
ATP synthase	6
Ribulose *bis*-phosphate carboxylase	1

Sequence analysis indicates that chloroplast genomes contain about 30 genes in addition to those listed here. Some of these encode proteins involved in respiration, but most remain to be identified.

Both the ribosomal and transfer RNAs used for translation of chloroplast mRNAs are encoded by the organelle genome. These include four rRNAs (23S, 16S, 5S and 4.5S) and 30 tRNA species. In contrast to the smaller number of tRNAs encoded by the mitochondrial genome, the chloroplast tRNAs are sufficient to translate all the mRNA codons according to the universal genetic code. In addition to these RNA components of the translation system, the chloroplast genome encodes about 20 ribosomal proteins, which represent approximately a third of the proteins of chloroplast ribosomes. Some subunits of RNA polymerase are also encoded by chloroplasts, although additional RNA polymerase subunits and other factors needed for chloroplast gene expression are encoded in the nucleus.

The chloroplast genome also encodes approximately 30 proteins that are involved in photosynthesis, including components of photosystems I and II, of the cytochrome bf complex and of ATP synthase. In addition, one of the subunits of ribulose bisphosphate carboxylase (*rubisco*) is encoded by chloroplast DNA. Rubisco is the critical enzyme that catalyses the addition of CO_2 to ribulose-1,5-bisphosphate during the Calvin cycle. Not only is it the major protein component of the chloroplast stroma, but it is also thought to be the single most abundant protein on earth, so it is noteworthy that one of its subunits is encoded by the chloroplast genome.

Import and Sorting of Chloroplast Proteins

Although chloroplasts encode more of their own proteins than mitochondria, about 90% of chloroplast proteins are still encoded by nuclear genes. As with mitochondria, these proteins are synthesised on cytosolic ribosomes and then imported into chloroplasts as completed polypeptide chains. They must then be sorted to their appropriate location within chloroplasts—an even more complicated task than protein sorting in mitochondria, since chloroplasts contain three separate membranes that divide them into three distinct internal compartments. Protein import into chloroplasts generally resembles mitochondrial protein import (Fig. 24.3). Proteins are targeted for import into chloroplasts by N-terminal sequences of 30 to 100 amino acids, called transit peptides, which direct protein translocation across the

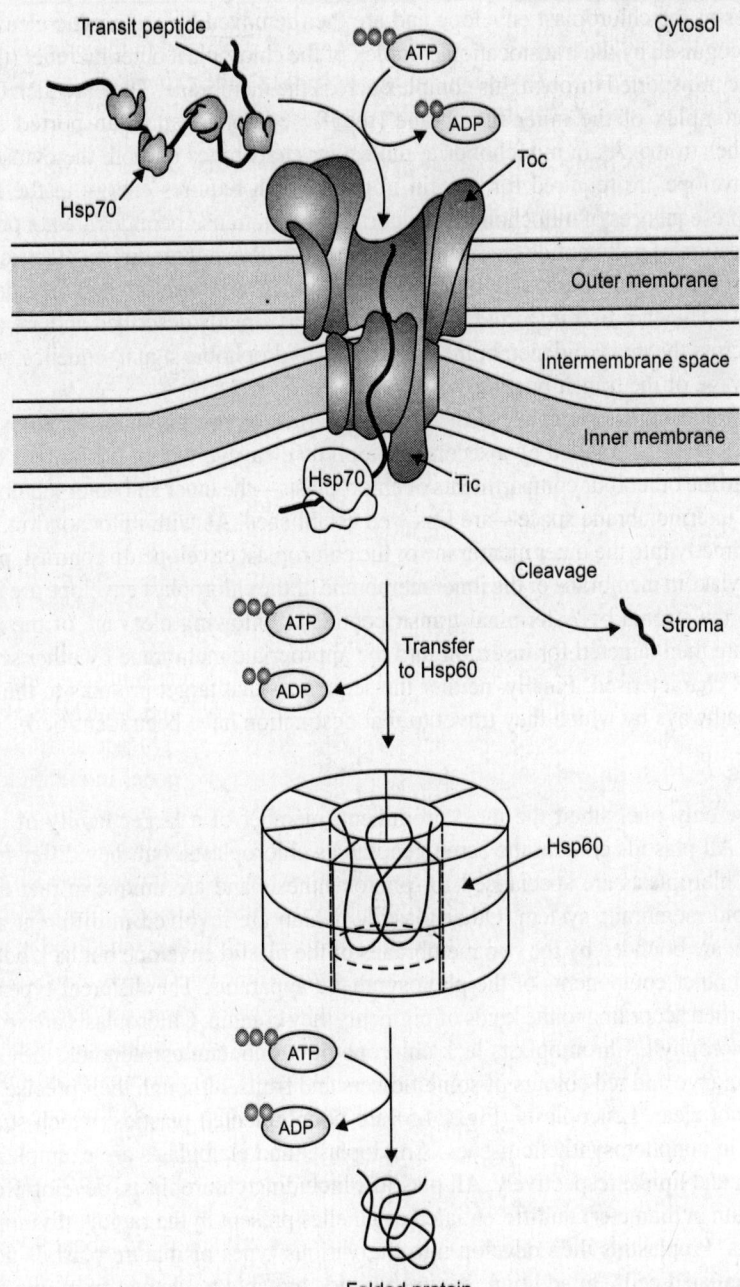

Fig. 24.3: Protein import into the chloroplast stroma. Proteins are targeted for import into chloroplasts by a transit peptide at their amino terminus. The transit peptide directs polypeptide translocation through the Toc complex in the chloroplast outer membrane and the Tic complex in the chloroplast inner membrane. This peptide is then removed by proteolytic cleavage within the stroma. Both cytosolic and chloroplast chaperones (Hsp60 and Hsp70) are required for protein import.

two membranes of the chloroplast envelope and are then removed by proteolytic cleavage. The transit peptides are recognised by the translocation complex of the chloroplast outer member (the Toc complex) and proteins are transported through this complex across the membrane. They are then transferred to the translocation complex of the inner membrane (the Tic complex) and transported across the inner membrane to the stroma. As in mitochondria, molecular chaperones on both the cytosolic and stromal sides of the envelope are required for protein import, which requires energy in the form of ATP. In contrast to the presequences of mitochondrial import, however, transit peptides are not positively charged and the translocation of polypeptide chains into chloroplasts does not require an electric potential across the membrane. Proteins incorporated into the thylakoid lumen are transported to their destination in two steps (Fig. 24.4). They are first imported into the stroma, as already described and are then targeted for translocation across the thylakoid membrane by a second hydrophobic signal sequence, which is exposed following cleavage of the transit peptide.

The hydrophobic signal sequence directs translocation of the polypeptide across the thylakoid membrane and is finally removed by a second proteolytic cleavage within the lumen. The pathways of protein sorting to the other four compartments of chloroplasts—the inner and outer membranes, thylakoid membrane and intermembrane space—are less well established. As with mitochondria, proteins appear to be inserted directly into the outer membrane of the chloroplast envelope. In contrast, proteins destined for either the thylakoid membrane or the inner membrane of the chloroplast envelope are initially targeted for import into the stroma by N-terminal transit peptides. Following cleavage of the transit peptides, these proteins are then targeted for insertion into the appropriate membrane by other sequences, which are not yet well characterised. Finally, neither the sequences that target proteins to the intermembrane space nor the pathways by which they travel to that destination have been identified.

Other Plastids

Chloroplasts are only one, albeit the most prominent, member of a larger family of plant organelles called plastids. All plastids contain the same genome as chloroplasts, but they differ in both structure and function. Chloroplasts are specialised for photosynthesis and are unique in that they contain the internal thylakoid membrane system. Other plastids, which are involved in different aspects of plant cell metabolism, are bounded by the two membranes of the plastid envelope but lack both the thylakoid membranes and other components of the photosynthetic apparatus. The different types of plastids are frequently classified according to the kinds of pigments they contain. Chloroplasts are so named because they contain chlorophyll. Chromoplasts lack chlorophyll but contain carotenoids, they are responsible for the yellow, orange and red colours of some flowers and fruits, although their precise function in cell metabolism is not clear. Leucoplasts (Fig. 24.5) are nonpigmented plastids, which store a variety of energy sources in nonphotosynthetic tissues. Amyloplasts and elaioplasts are examples of leucoplasts that store starch and lipids, respectively. All plastids, including chloroplasts, develop from proplastids, small (0.5 to 1 μm in diameter) undifferentiated organelles present in the rapidly dividing cells of plant roots and shoots. Proplastids then develop into the various types of mature plastids according to the needs of differentiated cells. In addition, mature plastids are able to change from one type to another. Chromoplasts develop from chloroplasts, for example, during the ripening of fruit (e.g. tomatoes). During this process, chlorophyll and the thylakoid membranes break down, while new types of carotenoids are synthesised. An interesting feature of plastids is that their development is controlled both by environmental signals and by intrinsic programs of cell differentiation. In the photosynthetic cells of leaves, for example, proplastids develop into chloroplasts (Fig. 24.6).

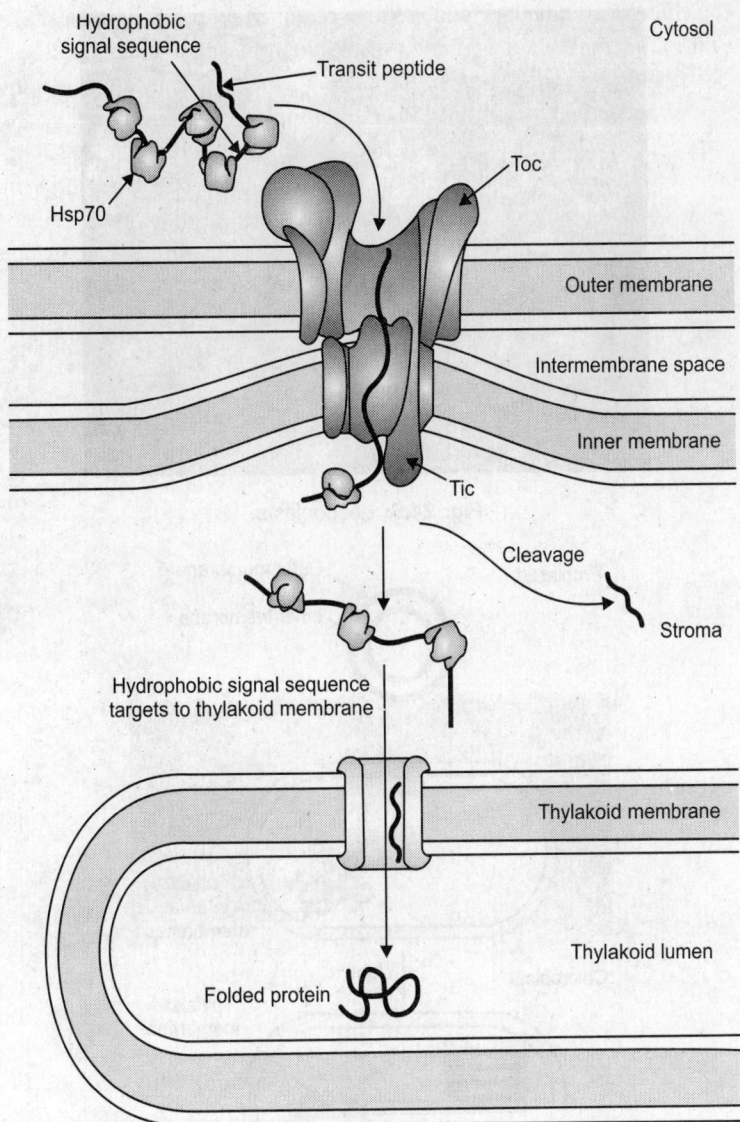

Fig. 24.4: Import of proteins into the thylakoid lumen. Proteins are imported into the thylakoid lumen in two steps. The first step is import into the chloroplast stroma, as illustrated in Fig. 24.3. Cleavage of the transit peptide then exposes a second hydrophobic signal sequence, which directs protein translocation across the thylakoid membrane.

During this process, the thylakoid membrane is formed by vesicles budding from the inner membrane of the plastid envelope and the various components of the photosynthetic apparatus are synthesised and assembled. However, chloroplasts develop only in the presence of light. If plants are kept in the dark, the development of proplastids in leaves is arrested at an intermediate stage (called etioplasts), in which a semicrystalline array of tubular internal membranes has formed but chlorophyll has not been synthesised.

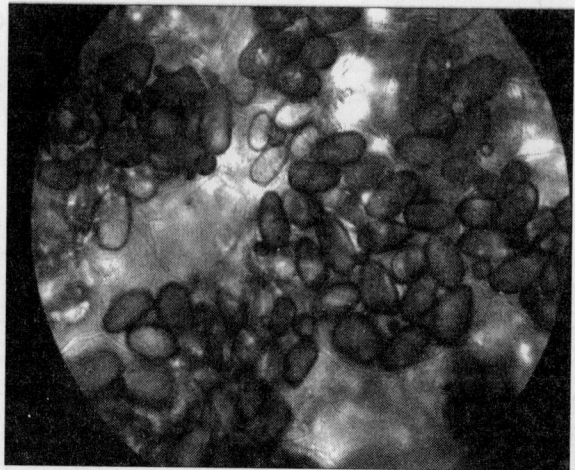

Fig. 24.5: Leucoplasts.

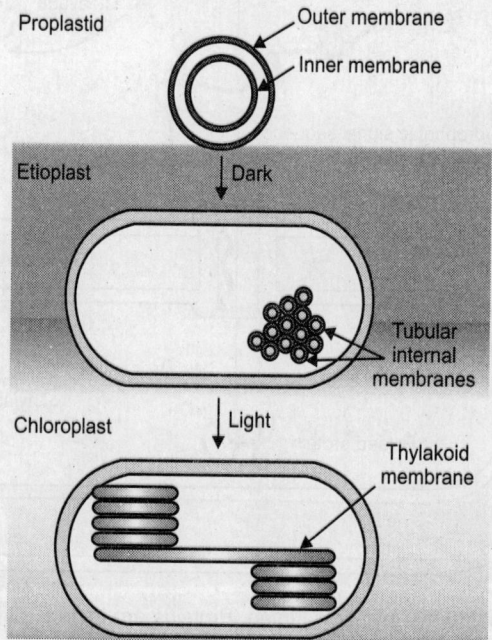

Fig. 24.6: Development of chloroplasts. Chloroplasts develop from proplastids in the photo-synthetic cells of leaves. Proplastids contain only the inner and outer envelope membranes; the thylakoid membrane is formed by vesicle budding from the inner membrane during chloroplast development. If the plant is kept in the dark, chloroplast development is arrested at an intermediate stage (etioplasts). Etioplasts lack chlorophyll and contain semicrystalline arrays of membrane tubules. In the presence of light, they continue their development to chloroplasts.

If dark-grown plants are then exposed to light, the etioplasts continue their development to chloroplasts. It is noteworthy that this dual control of plastid development involves the coordinated expression of genes within both the plastid and nuclear genomes. The mechanisms responsible for such coordinated gene expression are largely unknown and their elucidation represents a challenging problem in plant molecular biology.

CHLOROPLAST RNA PROCESSING AND STABILITY

In the chloroplast, just as in the nucleus, the process of gene expression is a cascade in which each phase is of importance and is regulated. RNA longevity is of major importance for gene expression. Transcription rate and the transcript stability are both involved in determining availability of transcripts for the translation machinery. Chloroplasts have a rather constant pattern of relative transcription rates, and while it is regulated by environmental and developmental signals, it retains its relative transcription rates. This pattern is maintained despite transcription rate changes in response to environmental and developmental signals. The search for differential regulation of gene expression leads therefore further down the gene expression cascade to RNA stability and translatability, which have been shown to be determined by elements in the RNA molecules themselves.

RNA sequence and structure are crucial for its function since they interact with other elements active in the gene expression process. Messenger RNAs consist of a coding region surrounded by non-coding sequences called untranslated regions (UTRs). The 5'UTR and the 3'UTR play a major role in RNA stability, translatability and degradation. The structure of the untranslated regions depends largely on the maturation process of the RNA molecule. This section aims to present the maturation process of RNA in the chloroplast and its significance for gene expression in the chloroplast, as well as examine the final product, mature RNA, what defines its fate and how this affects gene expression.

RNA Processing

Plastid RNA may undergo several types of processing before reaching its mature form, including RNA editing, RNA splicing, intercistronic-endonucleolytic cleavage, 5'-end maturation and 3'-end maturation. The results of this processing affect the stability, translatability and degradation of mature RNA. In many cases, specific nuclear loci are found that are involved in chloroplast RNA processing, suggesting potential differential regulation of chloroplast gene expression.

RNA editing

RNA editing is a process in which individual nucleotides in the sequence of a transcript are changed and no longer coincide with the genomic sequence from which they were transcribed. This process was found in the chloroplast mRNA of land plants, but not of cyanobacteria and algae. The most common editing event in chloroplasts is the conversion of a genomic-encoded C residue into a U residue, though examples for the opposite conversion (U→C), also called 'reverse editing', have also been found. While some editing events are silent ones, many are known to have functional significance. Editing sites have been found to create initiation (ACG→AUG) and termination (CGA→UGA) codons and are also involved in restoring conserved amino-acids in proteins and conserved elements in untranslated regions of RNAs.

The mechanism in which editing occurs in the chloroplast appears to be a base conversion mechanism that involves both *cis*-acting elements flanking the editing sites and site-specific *trans*-acting factors. No consensus in sequence or secondary structure is known for the *cis*-acting elements, and none of the *trans*-acting factors involved in this conversion have been identified, but some chloroplast-encoded site-specific RNA-binding proteins have been found to interact with the *cis*-elements. Editing appears to occur early in RNA processing, prior to other RNA processing events like splicing and intercistronic cleavage. At the same time, evidence for the dependence of editing on translation is varying. While many editing sites show complete independence from translation, others exhibit complete or partial dependence of editing efficiency on translation. This, however, is likely to be the result of a possible effect of ribosome-binding on secondary structures that may be obscuring editing sites from *trans*-acting factors, and does not contradict the early occurrence of editing in the processing of mRNA. As with other stages in chloroplast gene expression, RNA editing and also responds to environmental and developmental signals and changes in editing efficiency in response to such signals have been observed. In light of its role in transcript translatability, and the evidence of non-functional proteins and mutant phenotype resulting from translation of unedited transcripts, it can be assumed that editing has a functional role in the regulation of gene expression in the chloroplast. However, differential editing in response to various cues has not been proven. Recent evidence shows that other parameters, such as transcript abundance, play a more significant role than editing in adapting gene expression in the chloroplast according to developmental signals. This points towards a mutation-correction role for editing, rather than a role in regulating gene expression.

Intron splicing

A number of chloroplast genes, including rRNA-, tRNA- and mRNA-coding genes, contain introns, which must be spliced during the maturation process of the RNA molecule. Splicing can connect between different exons in the same transcript ('*cis*-splicing'), or between exons on different transcripts ('*trans*-splicing'). Plastid introns are divided into three major classes known as Groups I, II and III, based on their structural elements and splicing fashion. Organelle introns differ from nuclear introns in structure and function, although similarities are found between group II plastid introns and nuclear introns. It is suggested that organelle introns may have been the origin of nuclear introns. At least some introns of groups I and II exhibit self-splicing *in vitro*. However, it is likely that even self-splicing introns require *trans*-acting factors for their splicing *in vivo*. Nuclear loci, chloroplasts RNAs and chloroplast proteins are known to be involved in intron splicing in the chloroplast. There is evidence for the regulation of splicing by developmental and environmental cues. Some group II introns in land plants exhibit tissue-specific differences in their splicing, and the splicing of several group I introns in *C. reinhardtii* is stimulated by light, via photosynthetic electron transport. In addition, functional significance of splicing has been found, as in the case of the *Chlamydomonas psb*A transcripts, in which splicing efficiency is linked to the organism's ability to grow photosynthetically. It therefore seems that intron splicing is of importance in chloroplast gene expression.

Intercistronic processing

Many plastid genes are organised in operons and transcribed as polycistronic RNAs, which are then cleaved into monocistronic transcripts. Intercistronic cleavage is of importance for gene expression in chloroplasts, since its absence can prevent the translation of proteins encoded by the polycistronic transcript. Several known examples show different ways in which intercistronic processing can affect chloroplast gene expression.

The translation of *psa*C and *ndh*D in tobacco depends on the cleavage of the dicistronic *psa*C-*ndh*D transcript because in its dicistronic form, a base pairing between an element in the coding region of *psa*C and an element in the 5′UTR of *ndh*D forms a structure that inhibits ribosome access to the initiation codons of both *psa*C and *ndh*D. A similar structural barrier occurs in the dicistronic transcript of *pet*D and *pet*B in maize, but in this case a site-specific nuclear-encoded factor, *crp*1, allows the cleavage and translation of the transcripts. The involvement of nuclear gene products in intercistronic cleavage opens up a possibility for differential regulation of gene expression through this type of processing. Examples for intercistronic cleavage of rRNA show how this type of RNA processing can control the availability of the translation machinery. In these examples nuclear loci are responsible for this processing, which allows ribosome assembly. In addition, intercistronic processing can affect chloroplast gene expression is through its role in the maturation of the 3′UTR and 5′UTR, which contain stability and instability elements.

5′end maturation

The maturation of chloroplast transcripts requires in some cases 5′end processing. Two types of processing are known – endoribonuclease cleavage and 5′→3′ exonuclease trimming. Ribonucleolytic cleavage is often observed by the finding of two transcript populations for the same gene, one with a 5′end corresponding to transcription initiation site and the other shorter and with a 5′end corresponding to a processing site. Studies show a correlation between transcript processing and translation. In *Chlamydomonas*, the processed transcript was found to be the only translatable transcript form. Ribonucleolytic cleavage may be followed by 5′→3′ exonuclease trimming. Exonuclease trimming may also follow intercistronic cleavage, which makes the 5′end of a transcript available for it. Nuclear-encoded factors are involved in the 5′end processing of transcripts and are important for the translatability of the transcripts. It has also been established that 5′end maturation responds to environmental signals.

3′end maturation

The 3′UTRs of chloroplast mRNAs usually contain inverted repeats (IRs) that can form stem-loop structures, which stabilise the transcript). These IRs protect from transcript degradation by preventing exonuclease progress, or by binding proteins that protect from degradation. Transcription of chloroplast genes is not efficiently terminated by the 3′UTR. The process of 3′end maturation is made of endonucleolytic cleavage downstream of the IRs, followed by 3′→5′ exonuclease trimming until the first encountered IR stem. However, it seems that the endonucleolytic cleavage site is not always necessary for 3′end maturation and that alternative maturation pathways may exist, as in the case of 3′ends generated through the cleavage of polycistronic transcripts. A number of proteins, mostly nuclear-encoded, are involved in 3′end processing. As with 5′end maturation, 3′end maturation appears to modulate translatability of chloroplast mRNAs and promote polysome association.

RNA Stability

As mentioned before, RNA is characterised by both sequence and secondary structure. Intrinsic elements of both sequence and secondary structure have been found that affect transcript stability.

5′UTR mRNA stability elements

RNA stability elements have been found in the chloroplasts of higher plants and of algae. Extensive research on the role of 5′UTR in chloroplast mRNA has been done in Chlamydomonas. 5′UTR stability elements have been well defined in the rbcL and atpB genes of Chlamydomonas. In addition, examples of nuclear mutations have been found that affect mRNA stability through the interaction of the nuclear gene products with the 5′UTRs of chloroplast mRNAs. Interestingly, the 5′UTRs of different genes provide different degrees of stability to transcripts. Transcript stability has been shown to compensate for changes in transcription rate in response to environmental stimuli and transcripts coding for products with different roles may need to be stabilised to a different degree under different conditions.

5'UTR mRNA instability elements

While in most cases elements in the 5'UTRs are found to confer transcript stability, some examples of the opposite effect have been found. Such examples are the AU-motif of cyanobacterial *psb*A2 5'UTR, which confers instability in the dark and the +21 to +41 sequence of *Chlamydomonas rbc*L 5'UTR, ·which is required for photo-accelerated degradation.

3'UTR mRNA stability elements

As mentioned above, most chloroplast 3'UTRs contain inverted repeats (IRs) that fold into stem-loops. The IRs are known in some cases to be transcript-stabilising. The IRs function as a protection from 3'→5' exoribonuclease.

Some examples of orientation-dependent IR function suggest that the orientation may determine the formation of 3'ends or the binding of proteins, which prevent ribonuclease degradation. Site-specific RNA-binding proteins that bind to 3'UTRs have been identified. At the same time, there is also evidence of IRs being unnecessary for mRNA stabilisation. Moreover, the IR sequence itself does not appear to be required for mRNA stabilising. The 3'IRs sequences of the rbcL gene of non-flowering land plants and algae have not been found to be conserved.

mRNA stability/instability elements in the coding region

Stability determinants have been found also inside the coding region of mRNAs. These were found to function in different ways, such as stalling ribosomes and interacting with determinants in the 5'UTR, possibly blocking endonuclease attack. Instability determinants have been found in the coding region of spinach psbA mRNA, where degradation that is initiated by endonucleolytic cleavage in the coding region is probably directed by structural sequences at the cleavage sites. The cleavage of these sites is regulated by magnesium ions, which block the site and stabilise the mRNA.

CHLOROPLAST TRANSFORMATION

A revolutionary method for plant cells transformation was reported in 1987. Using microprojectiles shot at high velocity nucleic acids could be delivered into living cells. In 1988, it was reported that the method, also referred to as 'biolistics', could be used to transform organelles. Due to a homologous recombination mechanism in the organelles, stable transformation was accomplished when using DNA with sequences homologous to organelle genome sequences. Foreign DNA could also be incorporated into an organelle genome if flanked by homologous sequences.

Mutation complementation is commonly used for transformant screening. In *Chlamydomonas*, a working method was developed for the selection of transformants using a non-photosynthetic mutant *Chlamydomonas* strain for the transformation and complementing its mutation with the inserted DNA, using restored photosynthetic-ability as a selection marker for transformants.

The *rbc*L gene is a chloroplast gene that codes for the large subunit of ribulose-1,5-biphosphate carboxylase/oxygenase (RUBISCO). This enzyme is a part of the photosynthesis apparatus and is responsible for CO_2 fixation. RNA secondary structure is of importance for RNA stability. The Chlamydomonas *rbc*L 5'UTR has been extensively studied for its role in *rbc*L transcript stability. The location of a restriction enzyme site that allows cutting the transcribed sequence from the DNA exactly at +1 (transcription start site) position makes this gene particularly ideal for 5'UTR research.

The secondary structure of the *Chlamydomonas rbc*L 5'UTR has been deduced and is predicted to consist of a large stem-loop (nucleotides +1 to +41) followed by a smaller stem-loop (nucleotides +49 to +63) downstream of it. In this work, the importance of the sequence of the large stem-loop is examined by introducing two different changes to it. Work on the *rbc*L 5′UTR was done with constructs made of the changed *rbc*L 5′UTR, followed by the *E. coli uid*A gene and *Chlamydomonas psa*B 3′region downstream of it. The constructs were incorporated into the chloroplast genome between the *atp*B gene and the IR.

The first change tested reverses the nucleotide sequence in positions +5 to +37, while the second change examined is a complete change of sequence, in which nucleotides +6 to +36 are changed so that each purine is replaced by another purine (A→G, G→A), and each pyrimidine by another pyrimidine (C→T, T→C). Both of these introduced changes affect only the sequence of the predicted large stem-loop, but not its structure.

CHLOROPLAST EVOLUTION

Primary Endosymbiosis

New evidence implies that primary endosymbiosis might have been more complex than has been envisaged hitherto, possibly involving a 'ménage à trois'. Members of the genus *Chlamydia* are obligate intracellular bacteria, which include important pathogens of humans and other animals, and are found as endosymbionts in amoebae and insects. Although *Chlamydiae* (Fig. 24.7)are not found in plants, an unexpected number of *chlamydial* genes share significant similarities with plant genes, and these often contain a plastid-targeting signal. In several studies, between 21 and 55 genes were shown to be transferred between *Chlamydiae* and primary photosynthetic eukaryotes. This suggests that a protist lineage that could enter into a symbiosis with a particular cyanobacterium was routinely infected by an ancestor of extant *Chlamydia* that facilitated the establishment of the cyanobacterial endosymbiont by Chlamydia-to-protist lateral gene transfer. Recent studies suggest that the chlamydial symbiont compartment was probably not the site of any essential biochemical pathway and was maintained only until all possible chlamydial genes had been transferred to the host. Thus, the two critical steps in primary plastid endosymbiosis might have been the secretion of effector proteins into the host cytosol by intracellular chlamydial pathogens, together with the maintenance of the afflicted host by the cyanobiont, which

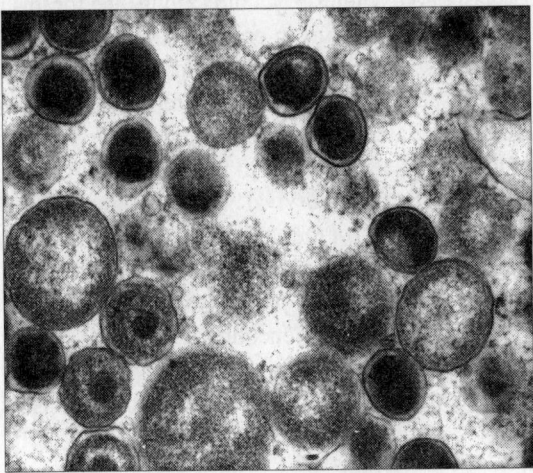

Fig. 24.7: *Chlamydiae.*

supplied photosynthetic carbon to a *chlamydia*-controlled assimilation pathway. If such complex interactions were indeed necessary for the establishment of the primary endosymbiotic relationship between plastid and host cytoplasms, this could explain why endosymbiotic relationships between heterotrophs and photoautotrophs were so rarely successful in the long term.

Second Primary Endosymbiosis

Evidence has also emerged for an independent instance of the primary endosymbiotic acquisition of a cyanobacterium—by the rhizarian amoeba *Paulinella chromatophora* about 60 million years ago. This organism contains stably transmitted cyanobacterium-like photosynthetic organelles termed 'chromatophores', the genome of which encodes about a quarter of the protein-coding genes that can be found in its free-living relative *Synechococcus* WH5701. Eleven putative *pseudogenes* were identified, indicating that reductive genome evolution is ongoing. More than 30 expressed genes have been transferred from the chromatophore to the nuclear genome of the host. In the case of three photosynthetic genes that now reside in the nucleus, biochemical evidence indicates that their products are synthesised in the amoeba cytoplasmand delivered to the chromatophores, where they form complexes with chromatophore-encoded subunits. This highlights *P. chromatophora* as an exceptional model for the study of early events in the generation of an organelle, and suggests that protein import into bacterial endosymbionts might be more widespread than is currently assumed.

Basis for the Longevity of Kleptoplasts

Kleptoplasts are a special case of transient internal photosynthetic symbionts in otherwise non-photosynthetic eukaryotes. In contrast to some lineages, in which the cells of photosynthetic symbionts are retained in their entirety (photosymbionts), other eukaryotes collect and retain only the chloroplasts of photosynthetic species, generating structures termed 'kleptoplasts'. The most dramatic kleptoplast association known to date occurs in the sacoglossan sea slug *Elysia chlorotica*, which can maintain photosynthetically active kleptoplasts derived from ingested xanthophyte algae for up to 10 months. This gives these animals their distinctive green colour, which is why they are also called 'leaves that crawl', 'solar-powered slugs' or 'photosynthetic slugs'. It is widely assumed that the slugs survive starvation by means of kleptoplast photosynthesis, yet direct evidence for this is lacking. Moreover, the inference that kleptoplasts require many proteins in order to support a photosynthetic lifestyle implies that essential genes for photosynthesis have been transferred by lateral gene transfer (LGT) from the alga to the slug, and in fact one instance of a tentative transfer has been reported so far. However, no evidence for massive LGT has been obtained, and genome- and transcriptome-wide approaches actually argue against it. Recently, doubts have been raised as to whether these molluscs are actually dependent upon photosynthesis, and the role of light in the survival of the sea slugs was reinvestigated. Surprisingly, photosynthesis was found not to be essential for the slugs to survive months of starvation, which explains the lack of LGT from alga to animal in these species. A possible explanation for the longevity of the sacoglossan kleptoplast was suggested previously: plastids that remain photosynthetically active within slugs for periods of months share the property of encoding FtsH, a D1 quality-control protease that is essential for photosystem II repair. A replenishable supply of chloroplast-encoded FtsH could, in principle, rescue kleptoplasts from D1 photodamage, thereby influencing plastid longevity in sacoglossan slugs.

SECTION VIII

Cytoskeleton and Cell Movement

Chapter 25

Cytoskelton

INTRODUCTION

When a eukaryotic cell is taken out of its physiological context and placed in a plastic or glass *Petri dish*, it is generally seen to flatten out to some extent. On a precipice, it would behave like a Salvador Dali watch, oozing over the edge. The immediate assumption, particularly in light of the fact that the cell is known to be mostly water by mass and volume, is that the cell is simply a bag of fluid. However, the cell actually has an intricate microstructure within it, framed internally by the components of the cytoskeleton (Fig. 25.1). As the name implies, the cytoskeleton acts much like our own skeletons in supporting the general shape of a cell. Unlike our skeletons though, the cytoskeleton is highly dynamic and internally motile, shifting and rearranging in response to the needs of the cell. It also has a variety of purposes beyond simply providing the shape of the cell. Generally, these can be categorised as structural and transport. While all three major components of the cytoskeleton perform each of these functions, they do not do so

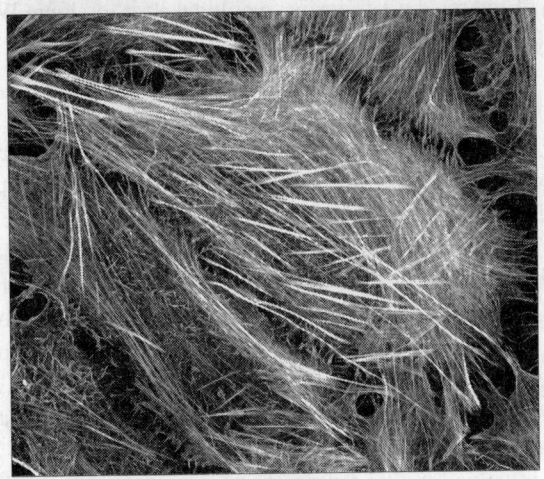

Fig. 25.1: Cytoskeleton.

equally, as their biophysical characteristics are quite different. With respect to structure, at some point in the life of every cell, it must change shape, whether simply increasing or decreasing in size, or a more drastic alteration like the super-elongated form of neurons with axons, the cytoskeleton must be able to respond by dynamically increasing and decreasing the size of the internal structures as needed. Structure also applies to the relative position of internal cellular elements, such as organelles or proteins, to one another. In many highly specialised cells, the segregation of particular structures within certain parts of the cell is crucial for it to function.

Transport refers to the movement of molecules and organelles within the cell as well as movement of the cell as a whole. It is well know that intracellular movement of proteins and lipids is by way of vesicles in the last chapter. These vesicles, as we will see in this chapter, are not just floating from one place to another, they are moved purposefully and directionally along the cytoskeleton like cargo on highways or railroad tracks. With respect to whole cell movement, this can range from paddling or swimming by single-celled organisms to the stereotyped and highly coordinated crawling of many cells from their point of origin to their eventual destination during the development of a metazoan organism or the movement of fibroblasts to heal a cut in your skin.

The three major components of the cytoskeleton are microtubules, microfilaments, and intermediate filaments. Each of these are polymers composed of repeating subunits in specific arrangements. With just a quick glance, it is very clear that the intermediate filaments will likely play a significantly different role from either microtubules or microfilaments. Because the IF's are made of long fibrous subunits that coil around one another to form the filament, there is clearly a great deal of contact (which facilitates formation of hydrogen bonds, aka molecular velcro™) between subunits providing great tensile strength. It is very difficult to break these subunits apart, and thus the IF's are primarily used for long-term or permanent load-bearing purposes. Looking at the other two components of the cytoskeleton, one can see that with the globular instead of fibrous shape of the subunits, the maximum area of contact between subunits is greatly limited (think of the contact area when you push two basketballs together), making it easier to separate the subunits or break the microfilament or microtubule. The cell can use this characteristic to its advantage, by utilising these kinds of cytoskeletal fibres in dynamic situations where formation or destruction of intermediate filaments would take far too long. We now address these three groups of cytoskeletal elements in more detail.

INTERMEDIATE FILAMENTS

'Intermediate filaments' is actually a generic name for a family of proteins (grouped into 6 classes based on sequence and biochemical structure) that serve similar functions in protecting and shaping the cell or its components. Interestingly, they can even be found inside the nucleus. The nuclear lamins, which constitute class V intermediate filaments, form a strong protective mesh attached to the inside face of the nuclear membrane. Neurons have neurofilaments (class IV), which help to provide structure for axons — long, thin, and delicate extensions of the cell that can potentially run meters long in large animals. Skin cells have a high concentration of keratin (class I), which not only runs through the cell, but connects almost directly to the keratin fibres of neighbouring cells through a type of cellular adhesion structure called a desmosome. This allows pressure that might be able to burst a single cell to be spread out over many cells, sharing the burden, and thus protecting each member. In fact, malformations of either keratins or of the proteins forming the desmosomes can lead to conditions collectively termed *epidermolysis bullosa*, in which the skin is extraordinarily fragile, blistering and breaking down with only slight contact, compromising the patient's first line of defense against infection. Structurally, as mentioned previously, all intermediate filaments start from a fibrous subunit (Fig. 25.2). This then coils around another filamentous subunit to form a coiled-coil dimer, or protofilament. These protofilaments then interact to form tetramers, which are considered the basic unit of intermediate filament construction. Using proteins called *plectins*, the intermediate filaments can be connected to one another to form sheets and meshes. Plectins can also connect the intermediate filaments to other parts of the cytoskeleton, while other proteins can help to attach the IF cytoskeleton to the cell membrane (e.g. desmoplakin). The most striking characteristic of intermediate filaments is their relative longevity. Once made, they change and move very slowly. They are very stable and do not break down easily. They are not usually completely inert, but compared to microtubules and microfilaments, they sometimes seem to be.

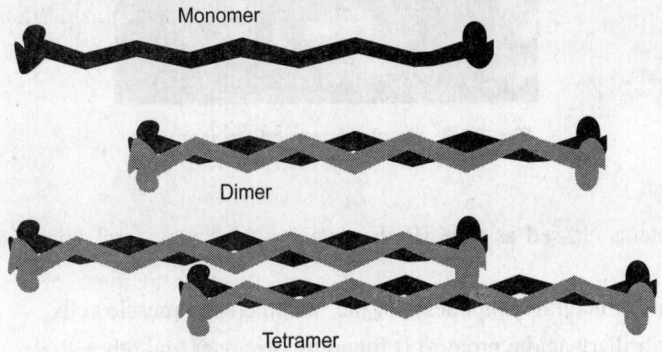

Fig. 25.2: Structure of intermediate filament.

Biomechanical Properties

IFs are extremely stretchy proteins that can be deformed several times their initial length. The key to facilitate this large deformation is due to their hierarchical structure, which facilitates a cascaded activation of deformation mechanisms at different levels of strain.

Types of Intermediate Filament Proteins

There are about 70 different genes coding for various intermediate filament proteins. However, different kinds of IFs share basic characteristics: they are all polymers that generally measure between 9–11 nm in diameter when fully assembled. IF are subcategorised into six types based on similarities in amino acid sequence and protein structure.

Types I and II—acidic and basic keratins

These proteins are the most diverse among IFs and constitute type I (acidic) and type II (basic) IF proteins. The many isoforms are divided in two groups:

1. Epithelial keratins (about 20) in epithelial cells .
2. Trichocytic keratins (about 13) (hair keratins) which make up hair, nails, horns and reptilian scales.

Regardless of the group, keratins are either acidic or basic. Acidic and basic keratins bind each other to form acidic-basic heterodimers and these heterodimers then associate to make a keratin filament (Fig. 25.3).

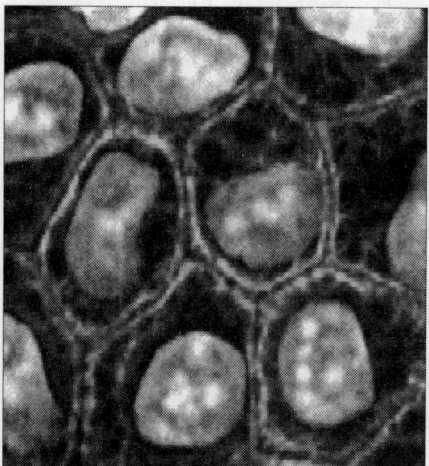

Fig. 25.3: Keratin intermediate filaments.

Type III

There are four proteins classed as type III IF proteins which may form homo- or hetero-polymeric proteins.

1. Desmin IFs are structural components of the sarcomeres in muscle cells.
2. GFAP (glial fibrillary acidic protein) is found in astrocytes and other glial.
3. Peripherin found in peripheral neurons.
4. Vimentin, the most widely distributed of all IF proteins, can be found in fibroblasts, leukocytes, and blood vessel endothelial cells. They support the cellular membranes and keep some organelles in a fixed place within the cytoplasm.

Type IV

1. α-Internexin.
2. Neurofilaments—the type IV family of intermediate filaments that is found in high concentrations along the axons of vertebrate neurons.
3. Synemin.
4. Syncoilin.

Type V—Nuclear lamins

Lamins: Lamins are fibrous proteins having structural function in the cell nucleus. In metazoan cells there are A and B type lamins which differ in their length and pI. Human cells have three differentially regulated genes. B-type lamins are present in every cell. B type lamins, B1 and B2, are expressed from the LMNB1 and LMNB2 genes on 5q23 and 19q13, respectively. A-type lamins are only expressed following gastrulation. Lamin A and C are the most common A-type lamins and are splice variants of the LMNA gene found at 1q21. These proteins localise to two regions of the nuclear compartment, the nuclear lamina—a proteinaceous structure layer subjacent to the inner surface of the nuclear envelope and throughout the nucleoplasm in the nucleoplasmic 'veil'.

Comparison of the lamins to vertebrate cytoskeletal IFs shows that lamins have an extra 42 residues (six heptads) within coil 1b. The c-terminal tail domain contains a nuclear localisation signal (NLS), an Ig-fold like domain, and in most cases a carboxy-terminal CaaX box that is isoprenylated and carboxymethylated (lamin C does not have a CAAX box). Lamin A is further processed to remove the last 15 amino acids and its farnesylated cysteine. During mitosis, lamins are phosphorylated by MPF which drives the disassembly of the lamina and the nuclear envelope.

Type VI

Nestin.

Cell adhesion

At the plasma membrane, some keratins interact with desmosomes (cell-cell adhesion) and hemidesmosomes (cell-matrix adhesion) via adapter proteins.

Associated Proteins

Filaggrin binds to keratin fibres in epidermal cells. Plectin links vimentin to other vimentin fibres, as well as to microfilaments, microtubules, and myosin II. Keratin filaments in epithelial cells link to desmosomes (desmosomes connect the cytoskeleton together) through plakoglobin, desmoplakin, desmogleins and desmocollins, desmin filaments are connected in a similar way in heart muscle cells.

Diseases Arising from Mutations in IF Genes

1. Epidermolysis bullosa simplex, K5 or K14 mutation.
2. Laminopathies are a family of diseases caused by mutations in nuclear lamins and include Hutchinson Gilford Progeria Syndrome and various lipodystrophies and cardiomyopathies among others.
3. Human intermediate filament database (HIFD), a comprehensive database of human intermediate filament proteins, their associated variations and diseases.

MICROFILAMENT

Microfilaments (or actin filaments) are the thinnest filaments of the cytoskeleton found in the cytoplasm of all eukaryotic cells. These linear polymers of actin subunits are flexible and relatively strong, resisting buckling by multi-piconewton compressive forces and filament fracture by nanonewton tensile forces.

Microfilaments are highly versatile, functioning in: (i) cell crawling, amoeboid movement, and changes in cell shape, where one end of the actin filament elongates while the other end contractile, presumably by myosin II molecular motors (though an alternative 'actoclampin'-driven expansile molecular motors exists), and (ii) actomyosin-driven contractile molecular motors, where the thin filaments serve as tensile platforms for myosin's ATP hydrolysis-dependent pulling action in muscle contraction and uropod advancement.

Microfilaments are also known as actin filaments: Filamentous actin, and f-actin, and they are the cytoskeletal opposites of the intermediate filaments. These strands are made up of small globular actin (γ-actin) subunits that stack on one another with relatively small points of contact. You might envision two tennis balls, one fuzzy and the other covered in velcro hooks. Even if you push hard to mush them together, the area of contact between the balls (i.e. the area available for H-bonding between subunits) is fairly small compared to the overall surface area, or to the area of contact between IF subunits. They will hold together, but they can also fall apart with relatively little force. Contrast this with intermediate filaments, which might be represented as two ribbons of velcro hooks or loops. Considerably more work is required to take them apart. Because there are fewer H-bonds to break, the microfilaments can be deconstructed very quickly, making it suitable for highly dynamic applications. Actin filaments are assembled in two general types of structures: bundles and networks. Bundles can be composed of polar (all barbed ends point to the same end of the bundle) or non-polar (barbed ends point towards both ends) arrays of filaments.

A class of actin-binding proteins, called cross-linking proteins, dictate the formation of these structures. Cross-linking proteins determine filament orientation and spacing in the bundles and networks. These structures are regulated by many other classes of actin-binding proteins (motor proteins, branching proteins, severing proteins, polymerisation promoters, capping proteins, etc.).

In vitro Self-assembly

The thinnest fibres of the cytoskeleton (measuring approximately 6 nm in diameter), microfilaments are formed by the head-to-tail polymerisation of actin monomers (also known as globular or G-actin). Actin subunits as part of a fibre are referred to as filamentous actin (or F-actin). Each microfilament is made up of two helical interlaced strands of subunits. Much like microtubules, actin filaments are polarised, with their fast-growing barbed-ends (because of their appearance in electron micrographs after binding of myosin S1 sub-fragments) and a slow-growing pointed-end (again based on the pattern created by S1 binding). The pointed end is sometimes referred to as the minus (−) end and the barbed end is sometimes referred to as the plus (+) end because of the growth rates, but this is nomenclature adapted from the microtubule field, and is not generally accepted in the actin field.

In vitro actin polymerisation, nucleation, starts with the self-association of three G-actin monomers to form a trimer. ATP-actin then binds the barbed end, and the ATP is subsequently hydrolysed with a half time of about 2 seconds and the inorganic phosphate released with a half-time of about 6 minutes, which reduces the binding strength between neighbouring units and generally destabilises the filament. *In vivo* actin polymerisation is catalysed by a new class of filament end-tracking molecular motors known as actoclampins.

Recent evidence suggests that ATP hydrolysis can be prompt in such cases (i.e. the rate of monomer incorporation is matched by the rate of ATP hydrolysis). ADP-actin dissociates slowly from the pointed end, but this process is greatly accelerated by ADP-cofilin, which severs ADP-rich regions nearest the (−)-ends. Upon release, ADP-actin undergoes exchange of its bound ADP for solution-phase ATP, thereby forming the ATP-actin monomeric units needed for further barbed-end filament elongation. This rapid turnover is important for the cell's movement. End-capping proteins such as CapZ prevent the addition or loss of monomers at the filament end where actin turnover is unfavourable like in the muscle apparatus.

Mechanism of Force Generation

As a result of the ATP hydrolysis, filaments elongate approximately 10 times faster at their barbed ends than their pointed ends. At steady-state, the polymerisation rate at the barbed end matches the depolymerisation rate at the pointed end, and microfilaments are said to be treadmilling. Treadmilling results in elongation in the barbed end and shortening in the pointed-end, so that the filament in total moves. Since both processes are energetically favourable, this means force is generated, and the energy ultimately comes from the NTP hydrolisation.

Actin in Cells

Intracellular actin cytoskeletal assembly and disassembly are tightly regulated by cell signalling mechanisms. Many signal transduction systems use the actin cytoskeleton as a scaffold holding them at or near the inner face of the peripheral membrane. This subcellular location allows immediate and exquisite responsiveness to transmembrane receptor action and signal-processing enzyme cascades. Because actin monomers must be recycled to sustain high rates of actin-based motility during chemotaxis, cell signalling is believed to activate cofilin, an actin-filament depolymerising protein which binds to ADP-rich actin subunits nearest the filament's pointed-end and promotes filament fragmentation, with concomitant depolymerisation to liberate actin monomers. The protein profilin enhances the ability of monomers to assemble by stimulating the exchange of actin-bound ADP for solution-phase ATP to yield Actin-ATP and ADP. In most animal cells, monomeric actin is bound to profilin and thymosin-beta4, both of which preferentially bind with one-to-one stoichiometry to ATP-containing monomers. Although thymosin-beta4 is strictly a monomer-sequestering protein, the behaviour of profilin is far more complex.

Profilin is transferred to the leading edge by virtue of its PIP2 binding site, and profilin also employs its poly-L-proline binding site to dock onto end-tracking proteins. Once bound, profilin-actin-ATP is loaded into the monomer-insertion site of actoclampin motors. Another important component in filament formation is the Arp2/3 complex, which binds to the side of an already existing filament (or 'mother filament'), where it nucleates the formation of a new actin filament and creates a fan-like branched filament network. In non-muscle cells, actin filaments are formed at/near membrane surfaces.

MICROTUBULES

Microtubules are made up of two equally distributed, structurally similar, globular subunits: α and α tubulin. Like microfilaments, microtubules are also dependent on a nucleotide triphosphate for polymerisation, but in this case, it is GTP. Another similarity is that microtubules have a polarity in which the (–) end is far less active than the (+) end. However, unlike the twisted-pair microfilaments, the microtubules are mostly found as large 13-stranded (each strand is called a protofilament) hollow tube structures. Also, the α and β tubulin used for building the microtubules not only alternate, but they are actually added in pairs. Both the α-tubulin and β-tubulin must bind to GTP to associate, but once bound, the GTP bound to α-tubulin does not move. On the other hand, GTP bound in the β-tubulin may be hydrolysed to GDP. GDP-bound $\alpha\beta$-dimers will not be added to a microtubule, so similar to the situation with ATP and γ-actin, if the tubulin has GDP bound to it, it must first exchange it for a GTP before it can be polymerised. Although the affinity of tubulin for GTP is higher than the affinity for GDP, this process is usually facilitated by a GEF, or guanine nucleotide exchange factor. As the signal transduction chapter will show in more detail, this type of nucleotide exchange is a common mechanism for activation of various biochemical pathways.

Again like actin, the tubulin itself has enzymatic activity, and over time, the GTPase activity hydrolyses the GTP to GDP and phosphate. This changes the attachment between β-tubulin of one dimer and the α-tubulin of the dimer it is stacked on because the shape of the subunit changes. Even though it isn't directly loosening its hold on the neighbouring tubulin, the shape change causes increased stress as that part of the microtubule tries to push outward. This is the basis of a property of microtubules known as *dynamic instability*. If there is nothing to stabilise the microtubule, large portions of it will fall apart. However, as long as new tubulin (which will have GTP bound) is being added at a high enough rate to keep a section of low-stress 'stable'-conformation microtubule (called the GTP cap) on top of the older

GDP-containing part, then it stabilises the overall microtubule. When new tubulin addition slows down, and there is only a very small or nonexistent cap, then the microtubule undergoes a *catastrophe* in which large portions rapidly break apart. Note that this is a very different process than breakdown by depolymerisation, which is the gradual loss of only a few subunits at a time from an end of the microtubule. Depolymerisation also occurs, and like with actin, is determined partially by the relative concentrations of free tubulin and microtubules. From a physical standpoint, the microtubule is fairly strong, but not very flexible. A microfilament will flex and bend when a deforming force is applied (imagine the filament anchored at the bottom end standing straight up, and something pushing the tip to one side). The microtubule in the same situation will bend only slightly, but break apart if the deforming force is sufficient. There is, of course, a limit to the flexibility of the microfilament and eventually, it will also break. Intermediate filaments are slightly less flexible than the microfilaments, but can resist far more force that either microfilaments or microtubules.

MICROTUBULE ORGANISING CENTERS

Microtubules, like microfilaments, are dynamic structures, changing in length and interactions to react to intra- and extra-cellular changes. However, the general placement of microtubules within the cell is significantly different from microfilaments, although there is some overlap as well as interaction. Microfilaments do not have any kind of global organisation with respect to their polarity. They start and end in many areas of the cell. On the other hand, almost all microtubules have their (–) end in a perinuclear area known as the Microtubule Organising Centers (MTOC), or microtubule organising center and they radiate outward from that center. Since the microtubules all radiate outward from the MTOC, it is not surprising that they are concentrated more centrally in the cell than the microfilaments which, as mentioned above, are more abundant around the periphery of the cell. In some cell types (primarily animal), the MTOC contains a structure known as the *centrosome*. This consists of a centriole (two short barrel-shaped microtubulebased structures positioned perpendicular to each other) and a poorly defined concentration of pericentriolar material (PCM). The centriole is composed of nine fibrils, all connected to form a cylinder, and each also connected by radial spokes to a central axis.

However, in each triplet, only one is a complete microtubule (designated the A tubule), while the B and C tubules do not form complete tubes (they share a wall with the A and B tubules, respectively). Interestingly, the centrioles do not appear to be connected to the cellular microtubule network. However, whether there is a defined centrosome or not, the MTOC region is the point of origin for all microtubule arrays. This is because the MTOC contains a high concentration of γ-tubulin. Why is this important? With all of the cytoskeletal elements, though it is most pronounced with microtubules, the rate of nucleation, or starting a microtubule is significantly slower than the rate of elongating an existing structure. Since it is the same biochemical interaction, the assumption is that the difficulty lies in getting the initial ring of dimers into position. The γ-tubulin facilitates this process by forming a γ-tubulin ring complex that serves as a template for the nucleation of microtubules. This is true both in animal and fungal cells with a single defined MTOC, as well as in plant cells, which have multiple, dispersed sites of microtubule nucleation.

TRANSPORT ON THE CYTOSKELETON

While it can be useful to think of these cytoskeletal structures as analogous to an animal skeleton, perhaps a better way to remember the relative placement of the microtubules and microfilaments is by their function in transporting intracellular cargo from one part of the cell to another. By that analogy, we might consider the microtubules to be a railroad track system, while the microfilaments are more like the streets. By the same analogy, we can suggest that the microtubule network and microfilament network are connected at certain points so that when cargo reaches its general destination by microtubule (rail), then it can be taken to its specific address by microfilament. Let's extend this analogy a bit further. If the microtubules and microfilaments are the tracks and streets, then what are the trains and trucks? On the microtubules, the 'trains' are one of two families of molecular motors: the kinesins and the dyneins.

We can generalise somewhat and say that the kinesins drive towards the (+) end (toward periphery of cell) while the dyneins go toward the (–) end (toward the MTOC). On actin microfilaments, the molecular motors are proteins of the myosin family. At this point, the analogies end, as the functioning of these molecular motors is very different from locomotion by train or truck. Finally, one might question the biological need for such a transport system. Again, if we analogise to human transport, then we could say that transport via simple diffusion is akin to people carrying packages randomly about the cell. That is to say, the deliveries will eventually be made, but you wouldn't want to count on this method for time-critical materials. Thus a directed, high-speed system is needed to keep cells (particularly larger, eukaryotic cells) alive. All of the kinesins and dyneins have a few key commonalities. There is a catalytic energy-releasing 'head' connected to a hinge or neck region allowing the molecule to flex or 'step', and there is a cargo-carrying tail beyond that. The head of a kinesin or dynein catalyses the hydrolysis of ATP, releasing energy to change its conformation relative to the neck and tail of the molecule, allowing it to temporarily release its grip on the microtubule, swivel its 'hips' around to plant itself a 'step' away, and rebind to the microtubule. On the actin microfilaments, the myosins, of which there are also many types are the molecular motors.

Their movement is different from dyneins and kinesins, as will be described in the next section, but also uses the energy of ATP hydrolysis to provide energy for the conformational changes needed for movement. We have introduced the motors, but considering the enormous diversity in the molecules that need to be transported around a cell, it would be impossible for the motors to directly bind to all of them. In fact, the motors bind to their cargo via adapter molecules that bind the motor on one side, and a cargo molecule or vesicle on the other. Further examination of the cargo and the routing of the cargo by address markers (SNAREs) was discussed in the vesicular transport chapter.

ACTIN - MYOSIN STRUCTURES IN MUSCLE

The motor proteins that transport materials along the acting microfilaments are similar in some ways, such as the globular head group that binds and hydrolyses ATP, yet different in other ways, such as the motion catalysed by the ATP hydrolysis. Much of the f-actin and myosin in striated and cardiac muscle cells is found in a peculiar arrangement designed to provide a robust contractile response over the entire length of the cell. The sarcomere is an arrangement of alternating fibres of f-actin (also known as 'thin fibres' based on their appearance in electron micrographs) and myosin II (or 'thick fibres'). Although we do not normally think of the motor protein as a fibre, in this case the tails of the myosin II molecules intertwine to form a continuous fibre of myosin molecules. As the contractile cycle proceeds, the myosin molecules grip the adjacent actin fibres, and move them. Sarcomere is constructed so that the stationary myosin fibres are located centrally, with two parallel sets of actin fibres interspersed between the myosin fibres, to the left and the right of the center. Note that the actin fibres do not cross the center line, and that at the center, the myosin molecules switch orientation. The physiological effect of this is that the actin filaments are all pulled inwards toward the center of the sarcomere. The sarcomere in turn, is merely one of many connected together to form a myofibril. The myofibrils extend the length of the muscle cell. When the myosin head is in its resting state, it is tightly attached to the actin filament. In fact, *rigor mortis* occurs in dead animals because there is no more ATP being made, and thus the sarcomeres are locked into place. Rigor begins approximately 2–3 hr after death in humans, after reserves of ATP are depleted. When the body relaxes again in about 3 days, it is due to the decomposition and breakdown of the actin and myosin proteins. However, while they are still living animals, ATP is generally available, and it can bind to the myosin head, causing it to lose affinity for the f-actin, and let go. At this point, no significant movement has occurred. Once the ATP is hydrolysed though, the myosin head can reattach to the f-actin a little further down the filament than it had originally. The energy released is stored in the neck region. The ADP and Pi are still attached to the myosin head as well. The next step is for the Pi to drop off the myosin, leading to the power stroke. The neck of the myosin swivels around, leading to a translocation of the head by approximately 10 nm for myosin II. The distance of translocation varies depending on the type of myosin, but it is not yet clear whether the length of the neck is proportional to the displacement of the head. Finally, the ADP drops off the myosin head, increasing the affinity of the head for the f-actin.

The sarcomere structure described in the first paragraph was incomplete in order to place the major players clearly in their roles. There are other proteins in the sarcomere with important structural and regulatory functions. One of the key regulatory components is tropomyosin. This is a fibrous protein that lies in the groove of an actin microfilament and blocks access to the myosin binding site.

Tropomyosin attaches to the microfilament in conjunction with a multi-subunit troponin complex. When Ca^{++} is available, it can bind to troponin-C, leading to a conformational change that shifts the position of tropomyosin to reveal the myosin binding site. This is the primary point of control for muscle contraction: recall that intracellular Ca^{++} levels are kept extremely low because its primary function is in intracellular signalling. One way that the Ca^{++} levels are kept that low is to pump it into a reservoir, such as the endoplasmic reticulum.

In muscle cells, there is a specialisation of the ER called the sarcoplasmic reticulum (SR) that is rich in Ca^{++} pumps and Ca^{++}. When a signal is sent from a controlling nerve cell to the muscle cell, it causes a depolarisation of the muscle cell membrane. This consequently depolarises a set of membranes called the transverse tubules (T-tubules) that lie directly on parts of the sarcoplasmic reticulum. There are proteins on the t-tubule surface that directly interact with a set of Ca^{++} channel proteins, holding the channel closed normally. When the t-tubule is depolarised, the proteins change shape, which changes the interaction with the Ca^{++} channels on the SR, and allows them to open. Ca^{++} rushes out of the SR where it is available to troponin-c. Troponin-C bound to Ca^{++} shifts the tropomyosin away from the actin filament, and the myosin head can bind to it. ATP can bind the myosin head to start the power stroke cycle, and voila, we have controlled muscle cell contraction.

In addition to the 'moving parts', there are also more static, structural, proteins in the sarcomere. *Titin* is a gigantic protein (the largest known, at nearly 3 MDa), and can be thought of as something of a bungee cord tether to the myosin fibre. Its essential purpose is to prevent the forces generated by the myosin from pulling the fibre apart. Titin wraps around the myosin fibre and attaches at multiple points, with the most medial just near the edge of the H zone. At the Z-line, titin attaches to a telethonin complex, which attach to the Z-disk proteins (antiparallel α-actinin). Titin also interacts with obscurin in the I-band region, where it may link myofibrils to the SR, and in the M-band region it can interact with the Ca^{++}-binding protein calmodulin-1 and TRIM63, thought to acts as a link between titin and the microtubule cytoskeleton. There are multiple isoforms of titin from alternative splicing, with most of the variation coming in the I-band region. Of course in an actual muscle, what happens is that nerves grow into the muscle and make synaptic connections with them. At these synaptic connections, the nerve cell releases neurotransmitters such as acetylcholine (ACh), which bind to receptors (AChR) on the muscle cell. This then opens ion channels in the muscle cell membrane, triggering a voltage change across that membrane, which also happens to affect the nearby membrane of the transverse tubules subsequently opening Ca^{++} channels in the SR. The contraction of sarcomeres can then proceed as already described above.

MUSCLE CONTRACTILITY

Skeletal muscles derive their name from the fact that most of them are anchored to bones that they move. They are under voluntary control and can be consciously commanded to contract. Skeletal muscle cells have a highly unorthodox structure. A single, cylindrically shaped muscle cell is typically 10 to 100 μm thick, over 100 mm long, and contains hundreds of nuclei. Because of these properties, a skeletal muscle cell is more appropriately called a muscle fibre. Muscle fibres have multiple nuclei because each fibre is a product of the fusion of large numbers of mononucleated myoblasts (premuscle cells) in the embryo.

Skeletal muscle cells may have the most highly ordered internal structure of any cell in the body. A longitudinal section of a muscle fibre (Fig. 25.4) reveals a cable made up of hundreds of thinner, cylindrical strands, called myofibrils. Each myofibril consists of a repeating linear array of contractile units, called sarcomeres. Each sarcomere in turn exhibits a characteristic banding pattern, which gives the muscle fibre a striped or striated appearance.

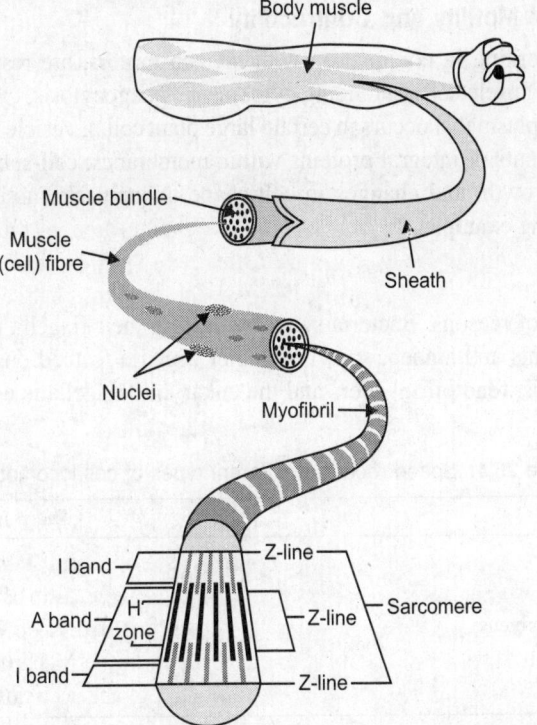

Fig. 25.4: The structure of skeletal muscle: levels of organisation of a skeletal muscle.

Examination of stained muscle fibres in the electron microscope shows the banding pattern to be the result of the partial overlap of two distinct types of filaments, thin filaments and thick filaments.

NONMUSCLE MOTILITY

Skeletal muscle cells are an ideal system for the study of contractility and movement because the interacting contractile proteins are present in high concentration and are part of defined cellular structures. The study of nonmuscle motility is more challenging, because the critical components tend to be present in less ordered, more labile, transient arrangements. Moreover, they are typically restricted to a thin cortex just beneath the plasma membrane. The cortex is an active region of the cell, responsible for such processes as the ingestion of extracellular materials, the extension of processes during cell movement, and the constriction of a single animal cell into two cells during cell division. All of these processes are dependent on the assembly of microfilaments in the cortex. In the following section we will consider a number of examples of nonmuscle contractility and motility that depend on actin filaments and, in some cases, members of the myosin superfamily. First, however, it is important to survey the factors that govern the rates of assembly, numbers, lengths, and spatial patterns of actin filaments.

Actin-binding Proteins

Actin-binding proteins (also known as ABP) are proteins that bind to actin. This may mean ability to bind actin monomers or polymers or both. Many actin-binding proteins, including α-actinin, β-spectrin, dystrophin, utrophin and fimbrin, do this through the actin-binding calponin homology domain.

Example of Nonmuscle Motility and Contractility

Actin filaments, often working in conjunction with myosin motors, are responsible for a variety of dynamic activities in nonmuscle cells, including cytokinesis, phagocytosis, cytoplasmic streaming (the directed bulk flow of cytoplasm that occurs in certain large plant cells), vesicle trafficking, blood platelet activation, lateral movements of integral proteins within membranes, cell-substratum interactions, cell locomotion, axonal outgrowth, and changes in cell shape. Nonmuscle motility and contractility are illustrated by the following examples.

Cell locomotion

Cells move for a variety of reasons. Bacteria swim by beating their flagella in order to exploit newly created micro environments and amoeba crawl to gather bacteria to feed on. The cells of vertebrates must move to heal wounds, fend off invaders and the eukaryotic flagella is used to propel sperm cells toward eggs (Table 25.1).

Table 25.1: Speed record of different types of cell locomotion.

Cell type	Speed (mm/sec)
Bacteria	10
Ciliate	1000
Amoeba proteus	3
Neutrophil	0.1
Fibroblast	0.01

Prokaryotic flagellum: Bacteria invented the wheel. The bacterial flagellum is a helical structure that drives the cell through the media like a propeller. The structure is rigid and turned by a rotatory motor at the base where it connects to the bacteria's body. The rotary motor consist of several wheel-like discs one of which the M-ring (and/or possibly the S-ring) interact with the C-ring and studs to rotate the whole structure. The rotary motor is very like a stepping motor. The flagella is composed of a protein called flagellin which is synthesised in the cell body and transported through the narrow lumen of the growing flagella itself to polymerise at the tip as it is about to exit the bacteria. This system has evolved into a syringe-like mechanism to inject toxins into the cells of vertebrates during infection (this is called 'type 3 secretion'). There are two main type of prokaryotic flagella, those belonging to Gram-positive (one membrane) and Gram-negative (two membranes) bacteria (Fig. 25.5). The bacterial flagellum is driven by a proton motive force resulting from a gradient of protons. Bacterial chemotaxis is brought about by alterations in the direction that the motor rotates in, this in turn is controlled by phosphorylation.

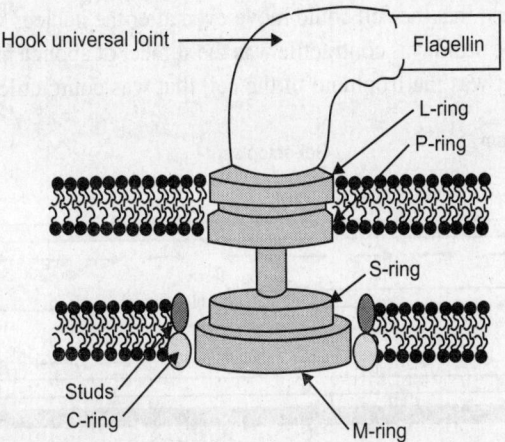

Fig. 25.5: Prokaryotic flagella, belonging to gram-positive (one membrane) and gram-negative (two membranes) bacteria.

Eukaryotic flagellum: Although at first sight the flagella of eukaryotes is similar to the flagella of prokaryotes, our flagella are completely dissimilar in structure, function and in the genes that encode their components. The principle component of the eukaryotic flagella is the microtubule, a tubular array of proteins of the tubulin family. Instead of rotating as the prokaryotic flagella does, the eukaryotic flagella produces contortions in shape that travel around the structure like a Mexican wave.

The term cilia is generally used to describe small grouped structures less than 10 µm, and flagella tend to be single structures about 40 µm. Our cilia are considered to be a cellular organelle and are almost certain to be derived from a primitive protist cell in the distant past. In the human body they are used in mucus membranes to driven mucus around (out of the lungs), to drive sperm cells, but bizarrely, in development a single cilium is responsible for setting up the asymmetry of our internal organs (heart slightly to the left, etc.) rare mutations in the genes encoding this structure cause *situs inversus*. Like many small things, the eukaryotic flagella was first seen by Anton van Leuwenhoek. The outer doublets are composed of microtubules and the outer and inner arms are dynein. Dynein is a motor protein that works with microtubules much like myosin works on actin so that the whole flagellum is sent into spiral motions as each set of arms (dynein) walks up the microtubules.

Crawling locomotion of cells: It has been suggested that the primary driving force behind the evolution of the actin cytoskeleton was to permit the equal division of components at cytokinesis. If this is so, then a close second must have been the ability to move. The subject of cell locomotion has been a very long one. As far back as primitive microscopes were available scientists have been studying the so called 'Giant amoeba' (Amoeba proteus and Chaos carolinensis). At 1-mm in length, these cells are enormous and so were ideal subject for the early studies. The fact that these cells moved in 'real time' (3–10 µM/sec) meant that no time lapse photography was necessary either. The large size of these amoebae made it possible to perform 'Micrurgy', such as enucleation and tactile stimulation. It was concluded from such tactile studies that prodding the front of the cell caused the cell to change direction, whereas a gentle prod in the rear made the cell accelerate transiently (as it would any sensible creature). It was found that the uroid was contractile and that the cell could move even after the nucleus was removed with fine glass needle. The finding that the uroid was contractile was the subject of about a hundred years of controversy as others suggested that it was the front end of the cell that was contractile and active (Fig. 25.6).

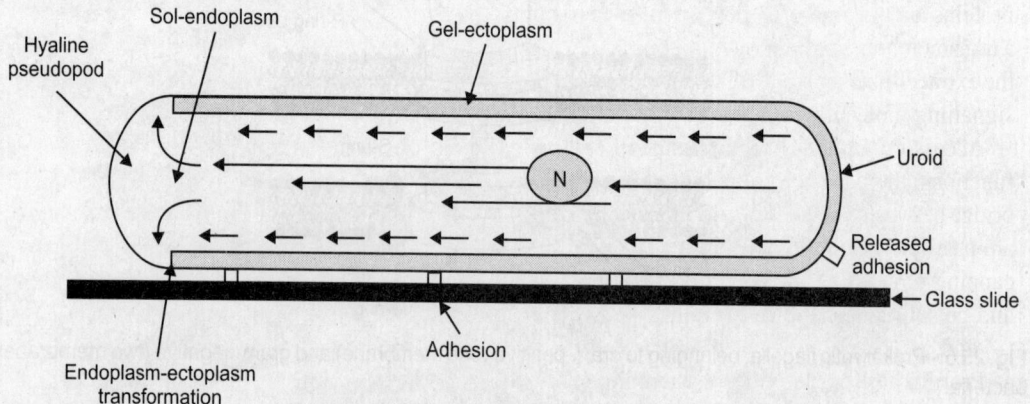

Fig. 25.6: Crawling locomotion of cells.

Observations on the amoeba revealed that there were two convertible states of cytoplasm, endoplasm and ectoplasm. Endoplasm (seen at the cell center, thus the name) was fluid, while ectoplasm under the cell membrane is gellated and comparatively static. During active locomotion, endoplasm flows forwards faster than the speed of the cell. As the fluid endoplasm reaches the 'hyaloplasm', a special optically clear form of ectoplasm, the flow diverted toward the membrane whereupon the endoplasm gelled to form ectoplasm. Vesicles, crystals, and other visible cytoplasmic inclusions are seen to become suddenly immobile having previously been seen to vibrate in Brownian motion.

These transformations also take place in other cell types but are less visible because of the much smaller scale and because they take place over a much longer time scale. However, these transformations are quite clearly visible in small amoeba such as *Acanthamoeba*, *Dictyostelium* and *Naegleria*, and also in highly motile human cells such as macrophages and neutrophils.

CYTOSKELETAL DYNAMICS

In the early development of animals, there is a huge amount of cellular rearrangement and migration as the roughly spherical blob of cells called the blastula starts to differentiate and form cells and tissues with specialised functions. These cells need to move from their point of birth to their eventual positions in the fully developed animal. Some cells, like neurons, have an additional type of cell motility - they extend long processes (axons) out from the cell body to their target of innervation. In both neurite extension and whole cell motility, the cell needs to move first its attachment points and then the bulk of the cell from one point to another.

This is done gradually, and uses the cytoskeleton to make the process more efficient. The major elements in cell motility are changing the point of forward adhesion, clearing of internal space by myosin-powered rearrangement of actin microfilaments and the subsequent filling of that space with microtubules. For force to be transmitted, the membrane must be attached to the cytoskeleton. In fact, signalling from receptors in the membrane can sometimes directly induce rearrangements or movements of the cytoskeleton via adapter proteins that connect actin (or other cytoskeletal elements) to transmembrane proteins such as integrin receptors.

One of the earliest experimental systems for studies of cytoskeletonmembrane interaction was the erythrocyte (red blood cell). Ankyrin and spectrin are important linkage proteins between the transmembrane proteins and the microfilaments. This idea of building a protein complex around the cytoplasmic side of a transmembrane protein is ubiquitous, and scaffolding (linking) proteins are used not only in connecting the extracellular substrate (via transmembrane protein) to the cytoskeleton, but also to physically connect signalling molecules and thus increase the speed and efficiency of signal transduction.

Accessory proteins to actin filaments and microtubules were briefly mentioned earlier. Among other functions, they can control polymerisation and depolymerisation, form bundles, arrange networks, and bridge between the different cytoskeletal networks. For actin, the primary polymerisation control proteins are profilin, which promotes polymerisation and thymosin β_4, which sequesters γ-actin. The minus end capping proteins Arp 2/3 complex and tropomodulin, and the plus end capping proteins CapZ, severin, and gelsolin can stabilise the ends of f-actin. Finally, cofilin can increase depolymerisation from the (–) end.

Profilin has two activities that promote polymerisation. First, it is a nucleotide exchange factor that removes ATP bound to γ-actin, and replaces it with ADP. This sounds counterintuitive, but keep reading through to the next paragraph. Second, when bound to a γ-actin, it increases the rate of addition to actin microfilaments. It does so by binding to the end opposite the ATP-binding site, leaving that site and that side open to binding both ATP and the (+) end of a microfilament. Profilin can be found both in the cytoplasm at large, and associated with phospholipids (PIP2) and membrane proteins, to control such processes as leading edge remodelling of f-actin cytoskeletal structures.

Thymosin β_4 regulates microfilament assembly by controlling the available pool of gactin. We already stated that greater concentrations of γ-actin can increase polymerisation rates. However, because of the highly dynamic nature of the actin cytoskeleton, the time constraints of degrading and producing new actin would prevent the fastresponse control necessary. Therefore, the optimal mechanism is to maintain a large pool of γ-actin monomers, but regulate its availability by tying it up with a sequestering protein - thymosin β_4. Thymosin β_4 has a 50x higher affinity for γ-actin-ATP than for γ-actin-ADP, so here is where profilin comes back into the picture. Profilin exchanges the ATP of a Tβ_4-γ-actin-ATP complex for an ADP. The result is that the Tβ_4 releases the γ-actin-ADP, allowing it to enter the general pool for building up filaments. Increased depolymerisation and slowing or cessation of polymerisation can gradually break down f-actin structures, but what if there is a need for rapid breakdown? Two of the capping proteins previously mentioned, gelsolin and severin, have an alternate mode of action that can sever actin microfilaments at any point by binding alongside an actin filament and altering the conformation of the subunit to which it is bound. The conformational change forces the actin-actin interaction to break, and the gelsolin or severin then remains in place as a (+) end capping protein.

On the microtubule side of things, due to dynamic instability, one might think that a severing enzyme is not needed, but in fact, spastin and katanin are microtubulesevering proteins found in a variety of cell types, particularly neurons. There is also a $T\beta_4$-like protein for tubulin: Op18, or stathmin, which binds to tubulin dimers (not monomers), acting to sequester them and lower the working concentration. It is regulated by phosphorylation (which turns off its tubulin binding). Microtubule-associated proteins MAP1, MAP2, and tau (β_4) each work to promote assembly of microtubules, as well as other functions. MAP1 is the most generally distributed of the three, with tau being found mostly in neurons, and MAP2 even more restricted to neuronal dendrites. These and some other MAPs also act to stabilise microtubules against catastrophe by binding alongside the microtubule and reinforcing the tubulin-tubulin interactions.

Finally, with respect to microfilament and microtubule accessory proteins, there are the linkers. Some of the aforementioned MAPs can cross-link microtubules either into parallel or mesh arrays, as can some kinesins and dyneins, although they are conventionally considered to be motor proteins. On the microfilament side, there are many known proteins that cross-link f-actin, many of which are in the calponin homology domain superfamily, including fimbrin, a-actinin, b-spectrin, dystrophin, and filamin. Although they all can bind to actin, the shape of the protein dictates different types of interaction: for example, fimbrin primarily bundles f-actin in parallel to form bundles, while filamin brings actin filaments together perpendicularly to form mesh networks.

CELL MOTILITY

There are a number of ways in which a cell can move from one point in space to another. In a liquid medium, that method may be some sort of swimming, utilising ciliary or flagellar movement to propel the cell. On solid surfaces, those mechanisms clearly will not work efficiently, and the cell undergoes a crawling process. In this section, we begin with a discussion of ciliary/flagellar movement, and then consider the more complicated requirements of cellular crawling.

Cilia and flagella, which differ primarily in length rather than construction, are microtubule-based organelles that move with a back-and-forth motion. This translates to 'rowing' by the relatively short cilia, but in the longer flagella, the flexibility of the structure causes the back-and-forth motion to be propagated as a wave, so the flagellar movement is more undulating or whiplike (consider what happens as you waggle a garden hose quickly from side to side compared to a short piece of the same hose). The core of either structure is called the axoneme, which is composed of 9 microtubule doublets connected to each other by *ciliary dynein* motor proteins, and surrounding a central core of two separate microtubules.

This is known as the 9+2 formation, although the nine doublets are not the same as the two central microtubules. The A tubule is a full 13-protofilaments, but the B tubule fused to it contains only 10 protofilaments. Each of the central microtubules is a full 13 protofilaments. The 9+2 axoneme extends the length of the cilium or flagellum from the tip until it reaches the base, and connects to the cell body through a *basal body*, which is composed of 9 microtubule triplets arrange in a short barrel, much like the centrioles from which they are derived. The ciliary dyneins provide the motor capability, but there are two other linkage proteins in the axoneme as well. There are *nexins* that join the A-tubule of one doublet to the B-tubule of its adjacent doublet, thus connecting the outer ring. And, there are *radial spokes* that extend from the A tubule of each doublet to the central pair of microtubules at the core of the axoneme. Neither of these has any motor activity. However, they are crucial to the movement of *cilia* and *flagella* because they help to transform a sliding motion into a bending motion. When ciliary dynein (very similar to cytoplasmic dyneins but has three heads instead of two) is engaged, it binds an A microtubule on one side, a B microtubule from the adjacent doublet, and moves one relative to the other. A line of these dyneins moving in concert would thus slide one doublet relative to the other, if (and it's a big if) the two doublets had complete freedom of movement. However, since the doublets are interconnected by the nexin proteins, what happens as one doublet attempts to slide is that it bends the connected structure instead. This bend accounts for the rowing motion of the cilia, which are relatively short, as well as the whipping motion of the long flagella, which propagate the bending motion down the axoneme.

Although we think of ciliary and flagellar movement as methods for the propulsion of a cell, such as the flagellar swimming of sperm towards an egg, there are also a number of important places in which the cell is stationary, and the *cilia* are used to move fluid past the cell. In fact, there are cells with *cilia* in most major organs of the body. Several ciliary dyskinesias have been reported, of which the most prominent, primary ciliary dyskinesia (PCD), which includes *Kartagener syndrome* (KS), is due to mutation of the DNAI1 gene, which encodes a subunit (intermediate chain 1) of axonemal (ciliary) dynein. PCD is characterised by respiratory distress due to recurrent infection, and the diagnosis of KS is made if there is also *situs inversus*, a condition in which the normal left-right asymmetry of the body (e.g. stomach on left, liver on right) is reversed. The first symptom is due to inactivity of the numerous cilia of epithelial cells in the lungs. Their normal function is to keep mucus in the respiratory track constantly in motion. Normally the mucus helps to keep the lungs moist to facilitate function, but if the mucus becomes stationary, it becomes a breeding ground for bacteria, as well as becoming an irritant and obstacle to proper gas exchange.

Situs inversus is an interesting malformation because it arises in embryonic development, and affects only 50% of PCD patients because the impaired ciliary function causes randomisation of left-right asymmetry, not reversal. In very simple terms, during early embryonic development, left-right asymmetry is due in part to the movement of molecular signals in a leftward flow through the embryonic node. This flow is caused by the coordinated beating of cilia, so when they do not work, the flow is disrupted and randomisation occurs.

Other symptoms of PCD patients also point out the work of cilia and flagella in the body. Male infertility is common due to immotile sperm. Female infertility, though less common, can also occur, due to dysfunction of the cilia of the oviduct and fallopian tube that normally move the egg along from ovary to uterus. Interestingly there is also a low association of hydrocephalus internus (overfilling of the ventricles of the brain with cerebrospinal fluid, causing their enlargement which compresses the brain tissue around them) with PCD. This is likely due to dysfunction of cilia in the ependymal cells lining the ventricles, and which help circulate the CSF, but are apparently not completely necessary. Since CSF bulk flow is thought to be driven primarily by the systole/diastole change in blood pressure in the brain, some hypothesise that the cilia may be involved primarily in flow through some of the tighter channels in the brain.

Cell crawling requires the coordinated rearrangement of the leading edge microfilament network, extending (by both polymerisation and sliding filaments) and then forming adhesions at the new forwardmost point. This can take the form of *filopodia* or *lamellipodia*, and often both simultaneously. *Filopodia* are long and very thin projections with core bundles of parallel microfilaments and high concentrations of cell surface receptors. Their purpose is primarily to sense the environment.

Lamellipodia (Fig. 25.7) often extend between two filopodia and is more of a broad ruffle than a finger. Internally the actin forms more into meshes than bundles, and the broader edge allows for more adhesions to be made to the substrate. The microfilament network then rearranges again, this time opening a space in the cytoplasm that acts as a channel for the movement of the microtubules towards the front of the cell. This puts the transport network in place to help move intracellular bulk material forward. As this occurs, the old adhesions on the tail end of the cell are released. This release can happen through two primary mechanisms: endocytosis of the receptor or deactivation of the receptor by signalling/conformational change. Of course, this over simplification belies the complexities in coordinating and controlling all of these actions to accomplish directed movement of a cell.

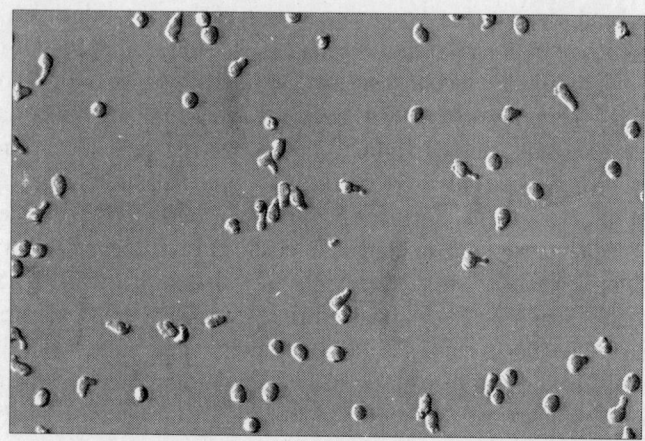

Fig. 25.7: *Lamellipodia.*

Once a cell receives a signal to move, the initial cytoskeletal response is to polymerise actin, building more microfilaments to incorporate into the leading edge. Depending on the signal (attractive or repulsive), the polymerisation may occur on the same or opposite side of the cell from the point of signal-receptor activation. Significantly, the polymerisation of new f-actin alone can generate sufficient force to move the membrane forward, even without involvement of myosin motors! Models of force generation are being debated, but generally start with the incorporation of new γ-actin into a filament at its tip, that is, at the filament-membrane interface. Even if that might technically be enough, in a live cell, myosins are involved, and help to push and arrange filaments directionally in order to set up the new leading edge. In addition, some filaments and networks must be quickly severed, and new connections made, both between filaments and between filaments and other proteins such as adhesion molecules or microtubules.

How is the polymerisation and actin rearrangement controlled? The receptors that signal cell locomotion may initiate somewhat different pathways, but many share some commonalities in activating one or more members of the Ras-family of small GTPases. These signalling molecules, such as Rac, Rho, and cdc42 can be activated by receptor tyrosine kinases. Each of these has a slightly different role in cell motility: cdc42 activation leads to filopodia formation, Rac activates a pathway that includes Arp2/3 and cofilin to lamellipodia formation, and Rho activates myosin II to control focal adhesion and stress fibre formation. A different type of receptor cascade, the G-protein signalling cascade, can lead to activation of PLC and subsequent cleavage of PIP2 and increase in cytosolic Ca^{++}. These changes, as noted earlier, can also activate myosin II, as well as the remodelling enzymes gelsolin, cofilin, and profilin.

This breaks down existing actin structures to make the cell more fluid, while also contributing more γ-actin to form the new leading edge cytoskeleton. *In vitro* experiments show that as the membrane pushes forward, new adhesive contacts are made through adhesion molecules or receptors that bind the substrate (often cell culture slides or dishes are coated with collagen, laminin, or other extracellular matrix proteins). The contacts then recruit cytoskeletal elements for greater stability to form a focal adhesion. However, the formation of focal adhesions appears to be an artifact of cell culture, and it is unclear if the types of adhesions that form in vivo recruit the same types of cytoskeletal components.

The third step to cell locomotion is the bulk movement of the cellular contents forward. The mechanisms for this phase are unclear, but there is some evidence that using linkages between the actin cytoskeleton at the leading edge and forward parts of the microtubule cytoskeleton, the microtubules are rearranged to form an efficient transport path for bulk movement. Another aspect to this may be a 'corralling' effect by the actin networks, which directionally open up space towards the leading edge.

The microtubules then enter that space more easily than working through a tight actin mesh, forcing flow in the proper direction. Finally, the cell must undo its old adhesions on the trailing edge. This can happen in a number of different ways. In vitro, crawling cells have been observed to rip themselves off of the substrate, leaving behind tiny bits of membrane and associated adhesion proteins in the process. The force generated is presumed to come from actin-myosin stress fibres leading from the more forward focal adhesions. However, there are less destructive mechanisms available to the cells. In some cases, the adhesivity of the cellular receptor for the extracellular substrate can be regulated internally, perhaps by phosphorylation or dephosphorylation of a receptor. Another possibility is endocytosis of the receptor, taking it off the cell surface. It could simply recycle up to the leading edge where it is needed (i.e. transcytosis), or if it is no longer needed or damaged, it may be broken down in a lysosome.

Chapter 26

Motor Protein Kinesin

INTRODUCTION

Cell is the basic unit of life. A typical cell measures few microns in diameter. Most molecules in the cell are few nanometers. There is an immense need to transport materials from one part of the cell to another. The need is all the more pronounced in cells like neurons which can be many centimeters long.

The task of transportation is carried out by a complex machinery of proteins. Tubulin molecules in cells assemble themselves into structures known as *microtubules* which provide highways for this transport to take place. A kinesin attaches to microtubules and moves along the microtubule in order to transport cellular cargo, such as vesicles.

Nature, through millions of years of evolution, has taken these molecular motors to near perfection, in the process, making them very complex. Various mathematical models have been proposed to account for the observed properties of kinesins. Understanding the structure and functioning of these molecules will help us mimic their efficiency and functionality and design systems which will have applications ranging from medical sciences to space exploration.

MOLECULAR MOTORS

Eukaryotic cells are organised into membrane bound organelles viz. the nucleus, the Golgi complex, the endoplasmic reticulum etc. The products of these have to be transported to other parts of the cell. The distribution system is complex, and uses three sets of molecular transporters: myosin, kinesin and dynein motors. Dozens of different motor proteins coexist in every eukaryotic cell.

Intracellular transport occurs along two sets of paths: the more or less randomly oriented actin filaments, used by myosin, and the often radially organised microtubules, used by both kinesin and dynein. Transport occurs along each of these when the appropriate motor binds to a cargo through its 'tail' and simultaneously binds to its filament through one of its 'heads'. The motor then moves along the filament by using repeated cycles of coordinated binding and unbinding of its two heads, powered by energy derived from hydrolysis of ATP.

The identity of the track and the direction of movement along it are determined by the motor domain (head), while the identity of the cargo is determined by the tail of the motor protein. Some of them also cause cytoskeletal filaments to slide against each other, generating the force that drives phenomena such as muscle contraction, ciliary beating, and cell division. Each dimer in protofilament has directionality as the β-tubulin and α-tubulin are not identical. The protofilaments arrange themselves in such a way that the directionality is retained in the microtubule. Thus one end of the microtubule (Fig. 26.1) is called the plus end and the other end is called the minus end. In a free microtubule, the tubulin dimers keep adding at the plus end and keep falling off at the minus end. This is called *treadmilling*. Most kinesin-related proteins move toward the plus end of the microtubule, as does kinesin itself, but some move toward the minus end.

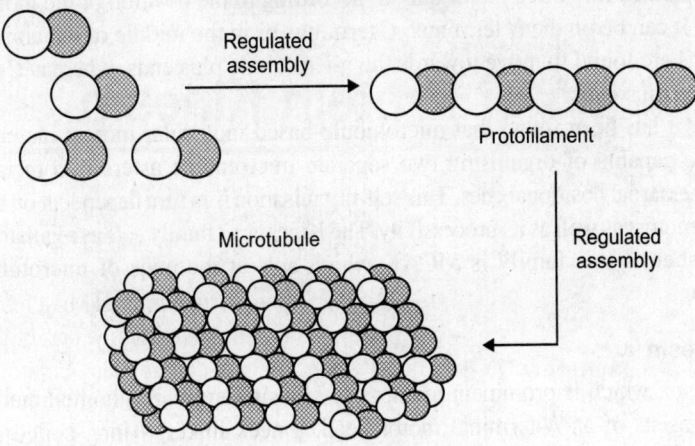

Fig. 26.1: Microtubule.

Dynamic Instability

While formation of the protofilament of the microtubule, the GTP attached to the β-tubulin undergoes hydrolysis to form GDP. β-tubulin is more stable when it is associated with a GTP molecule than when it is associated with a GDP molecule. So the formation of microtubule which is driven by GTP hydrolysis leads to destabilisation of its own self. This makes microtubule capable of undergoing catastrophic destruction by converting GDP to GTP and stabilising β-tubulin monomers. Thus microtubules in the cell keep undergoing random cycles of polymerisation and depolymerisation.

Functions of Microtubule

Microtubule is part of the cytoskeleton of the cell. It helps maintain the structure of the cell by providing support. It is especially important for transport of organelles and vesicles in the cells as motor proteins use them as tracks to move from one part of the cell to another. As microtubules are radially aligned in the cell they play an important role in pigment translocation. The flagella in many bacterial cells are made of microtubules. Microtubule also plays an important role in cell division.

Microtubule Associated Proteins

There are proteins which can bind to microtubules and affect their length, formation, rate of treadmilling, and stability. These proteins, which may widely differ in function and structure, are collectively called microtubule-associated proteins. Examples of such proteins are *tau* and MAP1.

KINESIN: MICROTUBULE ASSOCIATED MOTOR PROTEIN

Kinesins constitute a large motor-protein super-family that transports cargoes within a cell by moving on microtubule filaments. There are at least ten families of *kinesin-related proteins,* or KRPs, in the kinesin super-family. It was first identified in the giant axon of the squid, where it carries membrane-enclosed organelles away from the neuronal cell body toward the axon terminal by walking toward the plus end of microtubules. It is classified as one among the microtubule-binding proteins, owing to its attachment to microtubules for carrying out the transportation of cargo in cells. They are called motor proteins because they convert chemical energy into mechanical energy.

Kinesins are separated into three major classes according to the position of the motor domain on the peptide sequence. It can be on the *N* terminus, *C* terminus or in the middle of the amino acid sequence. *N*-terminal kinesins are found to move towards the microtubule plus ends, whereas *C*-terminal kinesins move towards the minus ends.

In recent years, it has been found that microtubule-based molecular motors including a number of kinesin motors are capable of organising two separate microtubule asters into metastable structures independent of any external positional cues. This self-organisation is in turn dependent on the directionalities of these molecular motors as well as its processivity. The Kinesin 13 family acts as regulators of microtubule dynamics. A member of this family is MCAK which acts at the ends of microtubule polymers to depolymerise them.

Structure of Kinesin

Conventional kinesin, which is prominent member of kinesin family, is a homodimeric motor protein. Each monomer consists of an *N*-terminal motor head, a neck linker, a long coiled-coil dimerisation region and a globular tail domain. The motor heads bind to microtubules and ATP. Each head is connected to a flexible neck linker that enables motor stepping. The neck linker is connected to a 70-nm long coiled-coil stalk (body) that holds two heads together. At the end of the stalk, kinesin has a cargo-binding domain that recognises membranous organelles and vesicles. The distance between the heads is 8.3 nm which is approximately the distance between adjacent tubulins. Conventional kinesin has two heavy chains and two light chains per active motor. Motor domain is the only common among all members of kinesin superfamily

All kinesins share the conserved catalytic core, which consists of a central β-sheet sandwiched between six alpha-helices and a topologically conserved smaller lobe (called the β-domain here) with three additional alpha-strands which have both the nucleotide- and microtubule-binding sites. Each head is connected to a neck linker, which is a mechanical element that undergoes nucleotide-dependent conformational changes. Neck-linker docking and undocking creates the powerstroke and determines the directionality of the motor movement. The neck linker is, in-turn, connected to a common stalk that leads to the globular tail domain. Kinesin tail domains are highly diverse and not so well conserved even within a sub-family. They are responsible for cargo association in certain motors. The kinesin may self assemble to form dimer and a coiled coil structure etc. One of the most striking features of the molecular self-assembly is the asymmetric nature of the association between the klc and khc subunits. Two coiled coil domains of khc always form a parallel or head-to head assembly with each other and two additional klc subunits associated with the dimeric coiled coil stalk of khc in yet another parallel assembly. All these suggest that the helical interaction plays a key role in motor subunit assembly *in vivo*. It is also evident that almost all the kinesin complexes contain at least two motor subunits, which is essential for proper kinesin functions *in vivo*.

Function of Kinesin

The function of kinesin in a cell is to carry out organelle and vesicle transport to various parts of the cell. This is clearly visible in the fast axonal transport mediated by kinesin-1 sub-family in which it transports mitochondria, secretory vesicles and various types of synaptic components to the axons. During interphase, kinesin translating along the microtubules organises the position of different organelles in the daughter cells. This is best exemplified by the organisation of endoplasmic reticulum and Golgi apparatus, whose orientation in the cells helps in their proper functioning.

Vesicular transport is best demonstrated in highly polarised and differentiated cells such as epithelial cells and neurons, this transport is very important for the proper targeting of proteins, packed into vesicles, to distinct parts of cells. Kinesin 2 sub-family also play role in dispersion of pigment carrying granules known as melanosomes.

They are also involved in intraflagellar transport, which is responsible for formation and maintenance of *cilia* and *flagella*. Some types of kinesins are tightly associated with the microtubular central pair apparatus of motile 9+2 flagella, though the function of the central pair is unknown.

They play important role in mitosis and meiosis also. They are proposed to generate force required for assembly and maintenance of spindles, attachment of chromosomes to the spindles and movement of chromosomes to opposite ends. They have also been shown to play an important role in establishing spindle bipolarity, i.e. separation of spindle pole body and also arrangement of chromosomes on the metaphase plate. Discovery of kinesin involved in depolymerising microtubules suggest their role in microtubule kinetics during mitosis.

Regulation

The kinesincargo interaction is likely to be controlled by altering the phosphorylation state of the protein, i.e., addition/removal of covalently attached phosphates (PO_4) form certain regions of the protein. Some observations suggest that the same motor complex could independently interact with two different cargoes at the same time and space inside the cell, and deliver them to different destinations controlled by the molar concentrations of the cargoes. The cargo association may also regulate the speed of the motor. A recent study using kinesins attached to the quantum dots showed that though a single kinesin molecule is capable of processive movement on the MT, the run lengths of the dot were proportionally increased with increasing number of motors attached. Certain experimental evidence from cultured neurons indicates that organisation and structure of MT could influence the process to select their direction of transport within the cell. Processivity of the walk and run lengths are controlled by the sequences in the hinge neck region of the motor subunits. For the kinesin-1 family members, the motor activity is regulated by cargo interactions. Free khc dimers assumes a folded and compact form as a part of their tail domain binds the motor domain, thus, preventing the motor from interacting with MT. The light chain subunit (klc) associates with the C-terminal half of the coiled coil stalk and this could prevent the khc tail from interacting with the motor domain.

HOW DOES KINESIN MOVE?

The kinesins are processive motors having a duty ratio = 0.5. The *duty ratio* indicates the relative time a motor domain remains bound on the filament as fraction of the entire ATP hydrolysis cycle. The conformational change in the motor region caused by ATP hydrolysis is converted to a net displacement. In the past decade, single-molecule studies have revealed that kinesin takes 8.3-nm steps per ATP hydrolysed, which is equal to the distance between adjacent tubulins. The motor can complete approx

100 ATP turnovers and walk 800 nm per sec. A single powerstroke of the motor can generate a force of around 6 pN. Biochemical studies show that the two heads are strongly coordinated so that binding of the second head accelerates dissociation of the already bound head. The kinesin head binds to a microtubule in its ATP-bound state and detaches in the ADP-bound state. ATP binding causes the neck linker to be docked pointing towards the plus end of microtubules.

To transport cargos for a sufficiently long distance, kinesins would need to do the following: (i) associate with the cargo at the beginning of the run, (ii) maintain a sufficiently long run length while associated with the cargo, and (iii) release the cargo at an appropriate site at the end of the run or transfer it to another motor complex. The mechanism of initial docking and dissociation is still unclear. However a lot of work has been done on kinesin propogation.

Hand-over-hand Model

In the hand-over-hand model, kinesin moves in much the same way as humans walk. The rear head (head 1) takes a step while the front head (head 2) remains stationary on the microtubule. Head 1 attaches to the next tubulin-binding site and becomes the leading head. Thus, kinesin moves along the microtubule by alternating the positions of the heads. This means that, if the centroid position of the motor moves 8.3 nm, the rear head must move 16.6 nm and the front head must not move at all In the next step, head 2 moves forward and becomes the leading head again while head 1 stays fixed to the track. Therefore, each of the heads alternately takes 0-nm (i.e. it is stationary) and 16.6-nm steps, and the cargo is moved 8.3 nm in each case. In the first, the rear head always passes the stalk from the same side, presuming that the stalk rotates 180° along the same direction every step. Because the tail region is fixed when kinesin is attached to the cargo, rotation along one direction would overwind the stalk. After several steps, the torsional barrier would prevent kinesin from walking. In the second, the rear head alternately passes the stalk from the right side and then the left side, presuming that the stalk is rotated 180° back and forth every other step.

Inchworm Mechanism

The inchworm mechanism suggests that only one head is catalytically active. In this model, one head always leads and the other head follows. It is a symmetric model in which the motor can revert to the same state after each step without rotating the stalk.

Kaseda and others performed a motility experiment with a heterodimeric construct in which one head catalysed ATP 18 times slower than the other head did. The experiment was designed to test whether both of the heads catalyse ATP, as in the hand-over-hand model, or whether only a single head does so, as in the inchworm model. The authors observed alternating short and long dwell periods during which the kinesin stalk took 8.3-nm steps. The overall speed of the motor decreased nine times compared with the speed of wild-type kinesin. The data are completely consistent with the hand-over-hand model.

Asbury and others performed an optical-trap assay with homodimeric kinesins that had stalks truncated at different positions. Under high load (around 4.5 pN), kinesins truncated near the motor domain limped, the motor alternated between fast and slow motion, much like the observations that Kaseda and others made. The limping behaviour shows that kinesin uses its heads alternately, which is in agreement with the hand-over-hand model. According to the Hoenger model, the neck linker first wraps around the stalk and then unwraps during the second step. When the neck linker wraps around the stalk, it is harder for the trailing head to move forward because of the torsional barrier. As the neck linker unwraps, this barrier is removed and the motor can take a faster step. Consequently, switching between wrapped and unwrapped states implies that kinesin, despite having two identical heads, moves by alternating slow and fast steps The experiment indicates that the limping is caused by the difference in geometry between the even and odd steps.

Surprisingly, kinesins with a full-length tail did not limp to a significant degree. It is more difficult and, hence, slower to take a step when the stalk is over wound. For this reason, the bead can bias the motor asymmetrically, particularly when the tail is too short. In full-length kinesin, however, the rotation of the stalk can average out on the long coiled coil region. Therefore, no limping should be observed. Such asymmetric models are attractive because the motor does not need to rotate its cargo within the cytoplasm, and many motors can work together more easily using this mechanism. Many kinesins must carry the cargo cooperatively and prevent its detachment from the microtubule. However, many motors could also work together using the symmetric mechanism if the 180° rotation were averaged out by twisting the long stalk instead of rotating the cargo.

Coordination between Motor Domains in Processive Kinesins

Stability of the neck coiled coil, which does not unwind during movement of kinesin, keeps the two motor domains in register. At the same time, flexibility of the neck linker allows the motor domains to propel over each other, optimising their positions while searching for the new binding site.

Cooperatively between Motor Domains Drives Processive Movement of Kinesin that at a critical point of its movement conventional kinesin adopts a configuration on the microtubule with both motor domains bound to the track. In this bridged state , the trailing motor is firmly attached to the microtubule, has ATP/ADP-Pi in its nucleotide site, and adopts the ATP-like conformation with the neck linker docked alongside the core and pointing (from N to C termini) toward the plus end of the microtubule. This configuration allows the leading motor to attach to the next site on the protofilament, releasing ADP and adopting the nucleotide-free conformation with the neck linker pointing in the opposite direction leading motor cannot bind ATP until the trailing motor hydrolyses ATP and releases one of the hydrolysis products, Pi. This release weakens attachment of the motor core to the microtubule, and the trailing motor detaches from the track, loosing constraints placed onto the leading motor and allowing it to bind ATP and enter its nucleotide hydrolysis cycle. Note that, in the absence of bound nucleotide, the neck linker is distributed between forward (+125°) and backward (−30°) pointing states that are separated by 50A.On the basis of these two positions, it was predicted that the neck linker is able to pivot about a point that lies near the C terminus of a6. Subsequent binding of ATP analogues to the catalytic core locks the neck linker into a second forward pointing position at +50°. After phosphate release, however, the neck linker is again mobile and weakly interacts with two sites on the catalytic core. This dimer configuration is translated toward the minus end of the microtubule (by 3Å) and rotated clockwise relative to the position of the trailing core bound to the equivalent tubulin dimer. The mechanism underlying this changed orientation has been explained by the compensatory countermovement of the motor relative to its switch II cluster, which changes its position relative to the core between the nucleotide-free and ATP-bound states. In a sense, the extended leading neck linker in the constrained, bridged state of kinesin acts as a structural sensor that coordinates work of the enzymatic active sites in two kinesin cores keeping them out of phase.

In its newly proposed role for conventional kinesin, β-domain would function similar to the extended alpha-strands of the central core, stabilising and pointing the neck linker either toward plus or minus end directions in the ATP/ADP-Pi and nucleotide-free states of the motor, respectively. The transition between two alternative docked conformations of the neck linker would not rely on Brownian motion only but would be forced by the countermovement of the core, placement of the detached trailing motor toward the new site on the track could be achieved more efficiently. Importantly, the countermovement of the leading motor upon binding ATP would also prevent the trailing motor from rebinding to the same site on the microtubule. The free-energy gain would come from favourable enthalpy changes balancing out unfavourable entropy changes associated with straightening of the leading neck linker during forward stepping.

Kinesin Steps Back

A single kinesin molecule attached to a plastic bead was probed using optical tweezer. When it was pulled strongly enough, kinesin could be made to walk backwards in a sustained manner. This dramatic result could provide the basis for developing a motor to drive nanoscale molecular machines it has been shown that the two kinesin heads move in hand-over-hand in a coordinated fashion and that movement stalls when the backward load exceeds about 7 piconewtons. But still two scenarios arose. First is about the presence of substeps or a single rapid step powered by the articulations of the molecule. Second suggests that kinesin can be made to step backwards.

Carter and Cross reported that sudden application of super stall force causes the motion to revert, whereby phasing of the ATP hydrolysis cycles on the lead and trailing heads seems to be swapped during backwards movement. If true, kinesin would use the same amount of ATP fuel when it walks forwards as it does staggering backwards under load. Carter and Cross suggested an underlying mechanism in which, once ATP has bound to the microtubule-attached head, the other head undergoes a diffusional search for its next site, the outcome of which can be biased by an applied load.

They did not observe sub-steps, so kinesin movements must be completed within the (excellent) time resolution of their measurements (less than 50 μs). The absence of substeps within the 8-nm kinesin step indicates that load transfers from one head to the other in a single mechanical event.

Backwards mechanical strain counteracts the intrinsic forward bias in the diffusional search, thus increasing the probability that the tethered head will bind behind the holdfast head. Probability of a forward step decreases exponentially with increasing load, whereas the probability of a backward step is constant. At stall (7.2 pN), the probability of forward stepping is equal to that of backward stepping. Above stall, Carter and Cross model predicts that efficiency goes negative as backward steps begin to predominate. There are previous reports of substeps, and several current models predict substeps. But their data also rule out substeps that take longer than 30 ms. This indicates that the appearance of substantial substeps in previous analyses might have been an artefact. However according to the recent experiments it is shown that the 8-nm step can be resolved into fast and slow substeps, each corresponding to a displacement of approximately 4 nm. The substeps are most probably generated by structural changes in one head of kinesin, leading to rectified forward thermal motions of the partner head. It is also possible that the kinesin steps along the 4-nm repeat of tubulin monomers. Thus Processive stepping (walking) can usefully be thought of as the outcome of a race between lead head attachment and trail head detachment: if lead head attachment is faster than trail head detachment, then the motor is processive.

Finally the data indicate that stepping by kinesin-1 absolutely requires a functional (dockable) neck linker, and it was originally proposed that neck linker docking is the force-generating engine of kinesin. However, this view was revised in light of calculations showing that the free energy change on docking is too small to account for the ability of kinesin to step 8 nm against a 7 pN load. Strong possibility is that it biases the attachment position of the leading head.

The neck plays a very important role in the function. Our findings indicate that a stiff Kinesin-1 neck coiled-coil impedes force generation. First, the average velocity is reduced under load and second, the run length of the stable neck mutant is severely affected by external forces. After the kinesin neck linker has docked to the rear head upon the binding of ATP, the leading head faces in the forward direction. Driven by Brownian motion it undergoes a diffusive search for the next microtubule binding site.

In a loaded state the head has to borrow a part of the necessary coverage to reach this binding site from a flexible element in the molecule, presumably the kinesin neck coiled-coil. They found no difference in velocities of the cross-linked and non-cross-linked motor under load, and only a subtle effect on the run length.

PROBING OF KINESIN

The most common techniques employed in probing kinesin for modeling purposes include optical trapping and video imaging. Since Optical trapping is often used to manipulate and study single molecules by interacting with a bead that has been attached to that molecule, it finds heavy application in the quantitative mathematical derivations of kinesin models while video imaging exploits the potential of a fluorophor in fluorescence microscopy. The basic principle in optical trapping is the momentum transfer associated with the bending light.

In a typical 2D *optical force clamp setup* the incoming light comes from a laser which has a Gaussian intensity profile. Because the intensity of ray 'a' is higher than that of ray 'b,' the force F_a is greater than F_b. Adding all such symmetrical pairs of rays striking the sphere, one sees that the net force can be resolved into two components, F_{scat}, called the scattering force component pointing in the direction of the incident light, and F_{grad}, a gradient component arising from the gradient in light intensity and pointing transversely toward the high intensity region of the beam.

The restoring force of the optical trap works like an optical spring: the force is proportional to the displacement out of the trap. In practice, the bead is constantly moving with Brownian motion. But whenever it leaves the center of the optical trap the restoring force pulls it back to the center. If the kinesin attached to the bead were to pull the bead away from the center of the trap, a restoring force would be imparted to the bead and thus to the kinesin. Advanced sensitive position detectors, based on interferometry or quadrant photodiodes (QPDs), are used to track bead motion and the interaction forces of the kinesin with the microtubule, with subnanometer accuracy and high bandwidth.

A drawback of optical trapping has been the damage induced by the intense trapping light, resulting in opticution-death by light. This was avoided by changing from the previous green (5145Å) argon laser to an infrared yttrium/aluminum garnet laser at 1.06 m.

The tweezers technique in combination with the so called 'microbeam' technique of pulsed laser cutting (sometimes called laser scissors or scalpel) is employed for cutting and moving cells, organelles and manipulation of pieces of chromosomes for gene isolation.

Imaging can be simply done using a fluorophore attached to kinesin to determine its mechanochemical properties. However, when these molecules are excited and detected with a conventional fluorescence microscope, the resulting fluorescence from those fluorophores bound to the surface is often overwhelmed by the background fluorescence due to the much larger population of non-bound molecules. Hence, Total Internal Reflection Fluoroscence Microcscopy (TIRFM) is employed.

TIRFM, also called evanescent wave microscopy, selectively excites the fluorophores by impeding the beam at a high angle causing it to totally internally reflect (TIR). TIR generates a very thin electromagnetic field in the liquid with the same frequency as the incident light, exponentially decaying in intensity with distance from the surface. This field is capable of exciting fluorophores near the surface while avoiding excitation of a possibly much larger number of fluorophores farther out in the liquid possibly much larger number of fluorophores farther out in the liquid. More importantly, the fluorescence excitation energy of the evanescent wave is the same as the energy of the wavelength of the light that was totally internally reflected. Some of the most commonly used fluorophores for biological systems include the Green fluorescent protein (GFP), luciferin and quantum dots (2–10 nm dia, 100–100,000 atoms). Quantum dots are widely preferred because they reduce the effect of photobleaching, are photostable fluorophores and highly bright to facilitate effective tracking down of individual single molecules. Kinesin molecules labeled with GFP and streptavidin-coated quantum dots (585nm), and the microbtubules labeled with Texas red have been used to study its mechanochemical properties. Qdots-Kinesin is linked through streptavidin-biotin linkage.

KINETICS OF KINESIN

The kinetic mechanism of Kinesin evolved from results obtained from various experiments. These results includes: microtubules increase the rate of ATP turnover, the non-hydrolysable analogue AMPPNP (5′-adenylylimido-diphosphate) which is presumed to mimic ATP, induces a tightly bound (stable) microtubule kinesin complex, and ADP release is the rate-limiting step of ATP turnover in the absence of microtubules.

Kinesin dimers moving at a low load take approximately 50–200 steps per second, requires one molecule of ATP in each step and the two heads step alternatively. Mg•ADP acts as a competitive inhibitor of Mg•ATP binding to Kinesin with an inhibition constant of 150 M. One of the possible reasons is the allosteric stabilisation by microtubules of the catalytically active Kinesin conformation. Another important observation is that the rate of phosphate release from kinesin monomers is not greatly affected by microtubule binding. This leads to the conclusion that K•ADP•Pi is strongly bound and therefore that phosphate release occurs from a microtubule-attached closed state.

The first major breakthrough in this respect came when it was discovered that ADP is released sequentially from Kinesin dimers. When K%ADP dimers are mixed with microtubules, only one of the two trapped ATPs is released. Release of the second ADP depends on the binding of an ATP to the first head. That is ATP dependent conformational change in the trail head works as a trigger for microtubule-activated release of ADP from the lead head. The key aspects of kinesins forward (plus-end) cycle have been elucidated through a varied multitude of experiments, including cryo-EM, X-ray structural, force bead, and others. This can be explained by the following Fig. 26.2.

In the diagram T labels the ATP nucleotide state, D the ADP nucleotide state, 'the no-nucleotide state, and P the phosphate after ATP hydrolysis.

Frames 1, 2: The free head weakly binds to the plus-end binding site, leading to strong binding once ADP is released.

Frames 3, 5: Hydrolysis of ATP in the minus-end head leads to an intermediate ADP-phosphate state, D.P, and phosphate release alters the binding of the minus-end head into weak binding, which allows rapid release of the minus-end head from tubulin.

Frame 6: The free head tends not to strongly bind until ATP binds to the microtubule-bound head. ATP binding initiates zippering of the microtubule-bound heads neck linker, coinciding with a large acceleration of the rate for the free head to bind onto microtubule. This entire forward cycle consumes one ATP and moves the center of mass of the system by approximately 8 nm.

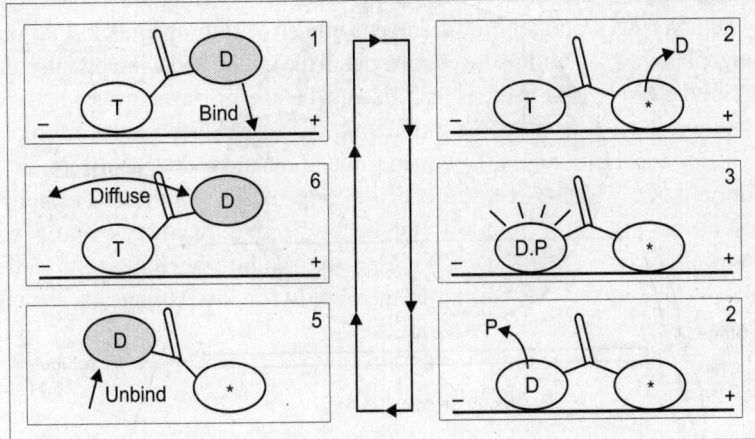

Fig 26.2: The diagram above depicts the six stages in Kinesin.

BROWNIAN DYNAMICS MODEL OF KINESIN

The basic aim of any model made on Kinesin is to understand mathematically how the protein converts chemical energy to mechanical work. Among the various models, which have been proposed for Kinesin movement, one has been discussed here. It is a three dimensional Brownian Dynamics model that takes into account excluded volume interactions. The two homologous globular domains, referred to as heads are joined together by a long coiled-coil alpha-helix structure, which extends to attach like a tether to cargo transported by the motor. The motor moves along the track laid by the microtubule by binding and unbinding its heads from interaction sites on the microtubule surface. The binding sites are spaced at approximately 8-nm increments. The main aim of this model is to calculate the force that the tether provides and the potential energy of the entire system.

The heads have special binding site for ATP hydrolysis and separate sites for interaction with the microtubules. The microtubule binding sites are modelled by hemispherical regions as shown in Fig. 26.2. The internal geometry of the two heads is neglected in the model and is represented by two spherical excluded volumes. The neck linker is a sequence of 15 amino acid residues joining the heads to the hinge point. The coiled-coil tether transmits the forces acting on the cargo to the motor and hence when the cargo is transmitted subject to a load force the tether elasticity plays an important role. The tether is actually modelled as a nonlinear spring with a force-extension relationship derived from experimental data (optical trap data).

It was shown that depending on the model of the motor protein different tether stiffness were optimal in the velocity attained by the motor. A nomenclature used in this model is that when both the heads of the Kinesin are bound to the microtubule, the one closer to plus end will be referred to as the leading head and the one away from it will be referred to as the trailing head.

The detailed geometry of the stage-mounted microtubule is also neglected since it is too small to make significant contribution to bead-diffusion dynamics. Figure 26.3 illustrate the point further.

Optical traps are capable of manipulating nanometer and micrometer sized dielectric particles by exerting extremely small forces by a highly focused laser beam. The narrowest point on the beam is known as beam waist (as shown in the diagram below) which contains a very strong electric field gradient and hence particles are attracted to the centre of the beam (region of strongest electric field).

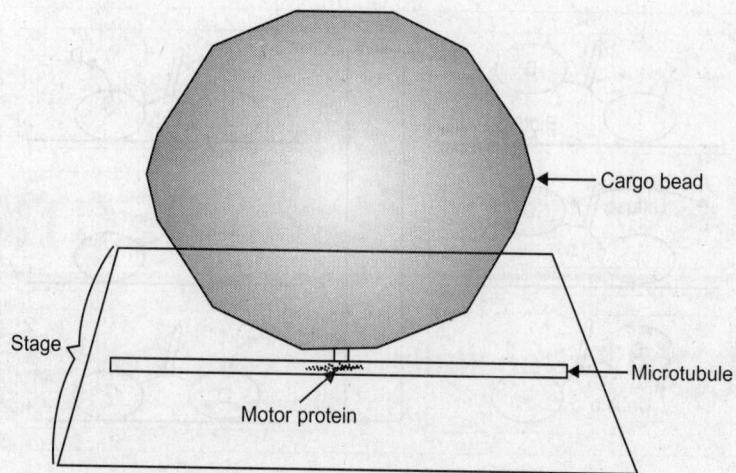

Fig. 26.3: Illustration of the model plotted according to scale.

The particle to be observed experiences a force even when it moves slightly away from the centre of the trap. This force is linear with respect to its displacement from the center of the trap as long as the displacement is small. So for small displacements an optical trap turns out to be a simple linear spring following Hookes law.

FUTURE APPLICATIONS OF KINESIN

Designing of nanomachines based on the mechanism of Kinesin still proves to be a challenge in this field of Kinesin research. These nanomachines will help us in scanning surfaces and studying microscopic objects in greater detail than is possible with microscopes. Another major advantage of these proposed nanorobots is their specificity in action. For example they might be used for precise drug delivery to specific cells in need of repair. Some researchers believe this might even cause a shift from treatment to prevention in medical sciences. The backward movement of Kinesin is also an increasingly growing research interest in this field. On increasing the force on the bead in opposite direction Kinesin can be made to move backwards. This dramatic result could provide the basis for developing a motor to drive nanoscale molecular machines. The mechanism of interaction of more than two heads in Kinesin movement also remains to be elucidated.

SECTION IX

Cell Walls, the Extracellular Matrix and Cell Interactions

Chapter 27

Cell Walls

INTRODUCTION

The cell wall is the tough, usually flexible but sometimes fairly rigid layer that surrounds some types of cells. It is located outside the cell membrane and provides these cells with structural support and protection, in addition to acting as a filtering mechanism. A major function of the cell wall is to act as a pressure vessel, preventing over-expansion when water enters the cell. Cell walls are found in plants, bacteria, fungi, algae and some *archaea*. Animals and protozoa do not have cell walls.

The material in the cell wall varies between species and can also differ depending on cell type and developmental stage. In bacteria, peptidoglycan forms the cell wall. *Archaean* cell walls have various compositions and may be formed of glycoprotein S-layers, pseudopeptidoglycan or polysaccharides. Fungi possess cell walls made of the glucosamine polymer chitin and algae typically possess walls made of glycoproteins and polysaccharides. Unusually, diatoms have a cell wall composed of biogenic silica. Often, other accessory molecules are found anchored to the cell wall.

The cell wall serves a similar purpose in those organisms that possess them. The wall gives cells rigidity and strength, offering protection against mechanical stress. In multicellular organisms, it permits the organism to build and hold its shape (morphogenesis). The cell wall also limits the entry of large molecules that may be toxic to the cell. It further permits the creation of a stable osmotic environment by preventing osmotic lysis and helping to retain water. The composition, properties and form of the cell wall may change during the cell cycle and depend on growth conditions.

Rigidity of cell walls: The rigidity of the cell walls is often overestimated. In most cells, the cell wall is flexible, meaning that it will bend rather than holding a fixed shape, but has considerable tensile strength. The apparent rigidity of primary plant tissues is enabled by cell walls, but not due to the walls' stiffness. Hydraulic turgor pressure creates this rigidity, along with the wall structure. The flexibility of the cell walls is seen when plants wilt, so that the stems and leaves begin to droop or in seaweeds that bend in water currents. As John Howland states it: 'Think of the cell wall as a wicker basket in which a balloon has been inflated so that it exerts pressure from the inside. Such a basket is very rigid and resistant to mechanical damage. Thus does the prokaryote cell (and eukaryotic cell that possesses a cell wall) gain strength from a flexible plasma membrane pressing against a rigid cell wall'.

The rigidity of the cell wall thus results in part from inflation of the cell contained. This inflation is a result of the passive uptake of water. In plants, a secondary cell wall is a thicker additional layer of cellulose which increases wall rigidity. Additional layers may be formed containing lignin in xylem cell walls or containing suberin in cork cell walls. These compounds are rigid and waterproof, making the secondary wall stiff. Both wood and bark cells of trees have secondary walls. Other parts of plants such as the leaf stalk may acquire similar reinforcement to resist the strain of physical forces.

Certain single-cell protists and algae also produce a rigid wall. Diatoms build a frustule from silica extracted from the surrounding water, radiolarians also produce a test from minerals. Many green algae, such as the *Dasycladales* (Fig. 27.1) encase their cells in a secreted skeleton of calcium carbonate. In each case, the wall is rigid and essentially inorganic.

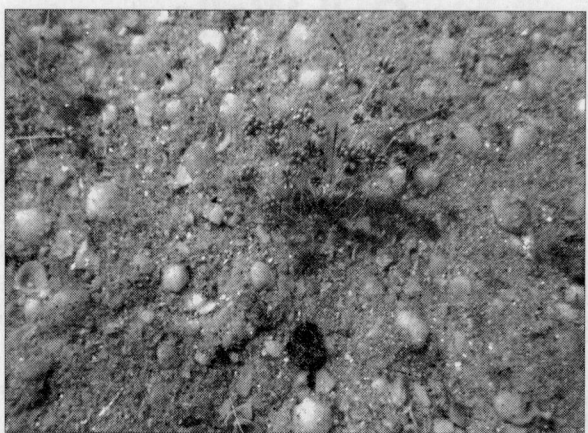

Fig. 27.1: Dasycladales.

Permeability: The primary cell wall of most plant cells is semi-permeable and permits the passage of small molecules and small proteins, with size exclusion estimated to be 30–60 kDa. Key nutrients, especially water and carbon dioxide, are distributed throughout the plant from cell wall to cell wall in apoplastic flow. The pH is an important factor governing the transport of molecules through cell walls.

TYPES OF CELL WALLS

Plant Cell Walls

The major carbohydrates making up the primary (growing) plant cell wall are cellulose, hemicellulose and pectin. The cellulose microfibrils are linked via hemicellulosic tethers to form the cellulose-hemicellulose network, which is embedded in the pectin matrix. The most common hemicellulose in the primary cell wall is xyloglucan. In grass cell walls, xyloglucan and pectin are reduced in abundance and partially replaced by glucuronarabinoxylan, a hemicellulose. Primary cell walls characteristically extend (grow) by a mechanism called acid growth, which involves turgor-driven movement of the strong cellulose microfibrils within the weaker hemicellulose/pectin matrix, catalysed by expansin proteins. The outer part of the primary cell wall of the plant epidermis is usually impregnated with cutin and wax, forming a permeability barrier known as the plant cuticle.

Secondary cell walls contain a wide range of additional compounds that modify their mechanical properties and permeability. The major polymers that make up wood (largely secondary cell walls) include cellulose (35 to 50 per cent), xylan, a type of hemicellulose, (20 to 35 per cent) and a complex phenolic polymer called lignin (10 to 25 per cent).

Lignin penetrates the spaces in the cell wall between cellulose, hemicellulose and pectin components, driving out water and strengthening the wall. The walls of cork cells in the bark of trees are impregnated with suberin, and suberin also forms the permeability barrier in primary roots known as the Casparian strip. Secondary walls—especially in grasses—may also contain microscopic silica crystals, which may strengthen the wall and protect it from herbivores.

Plant cells walls also contain numerous enzymes, such as hydrolases, esterases, peroxidases, and transglycosylases, that cut, trim and cross link wall polymers. Small amounts (1–5 per cent) of structural proteins are found in most plant cell walls, they are classified as hydroxyproline-rich glycoproteins (HRGP), arabinogalactan proteins (AGP), glycine-rich proteins (GRPs), and proline-rich proteins (PRPs). Each class of glycoprotein is defined by a characteristic, highly repetitive protein sequence. Most are glycosylated, contain hydroxyproline (Hyp) and become cross-linked in the cell wall. These proteins are often concentrated in specialised cells and in cell corners. Cell walls of the epidermis and endodermis may also contain suberin or cutin, two polyester-like polymers that protect the cell from herbivores.

The relative composition of carbohydrates, secondary compounds and protein varies between plants and between the cell type and age.

Up to three strata or layers may be found in plant cell walls:

- The middle lamella, a layer rich in pectins. This outermost layer forms the interface between adjacent plant cells and glues them together.
- The primary cell wall, generally a thin, flexible and extensible layer formed while the cell is growing.
- The secondary cell wall, a thick layer formed inside the primary cell wall after the cell is fully grown. It is not found in all cell types. Some cells, such as the conducting cells in xylem, possess a secondary wall containing lignin, which strengthens and waterproofs the wall.

Cell walls in some plant tissues also function as storage depots for carbohydrates that can be broken down and resorbed to supply the metabolic and growth needs of the plant. For example, endosperm cell walls in the seeds of cereal grasses, nasturtium, and other species, are rich in glucans and other polysaccharides that are readily digested by enzymes during seed germination to form simple sugars that nourish the growing embryo. Cellulose microfibrils are not readily digested by plants, however.

The middle lamella is laid down first, formed from the cell plate during cytokinesis, and the primary cell wall is then deposited inside the middle lamella. The actual structure of the cell wall is not clearly defined and several models exist—the covalently linked cross model, the tether model, the diffuse layer model and the stratified layer model. However, the primary cell wall, can be defined as composed of cellulose microfibrils aligned at all angles. Microfibrils are held together by hydrogen bonds to provide a high tensile strength. The cells are held together and share the gelatinous membrane called the middle lamella, which contains magnesium and calcium pectates (salts of pectic acid).

Cells interact though plasmodesma (ta), which are interconnecting channels of cytoplasm that connect to the protoplasts of adjacent cells across the cell wall. In some plants and cell types, after a maximum size or point in development has been reached, a secondary wall is constructed between the plant cell and primary wall. Unlike the primary wall, the microfibrils are aligned mostly in the same direction, and with each additional layer the orientation changes slightly. Cells with secondary cell walls are rigid. Cell to cell communication is possible through pits in the secondary cell wall that allow plasmodesma to connect cells through the secondary cell walls.

Algal Cell Walls

Like plants, algae have cell walls. Algal cell walls contain either polysaccharides [such as cellulose (a glucan)] or a variety of glycoproteins (Volvocales) or both. The inclusion of additional polysaccharides in algal cells walls is used as a feature for algal taxonomy.

- *Mannans:* They form microfibrils in the cell walls of a number of marine green algae including those from the genera, *Codium, Dasycladus* and *Acetabularia* as well as in the walls of some red algae, like *Porphyra* (Fig. 27.2) and *Bangia.*
- *Xylans.*
- *Alginic acid:* It is a common polysaccharide in the cell walls of brown algae.
- *Sulphonated polysaccharides:* They occur in the cell walls of most algae, those common in red algae include *agarose, carrageenan, porphyran, furcelleran* and *funoran.*

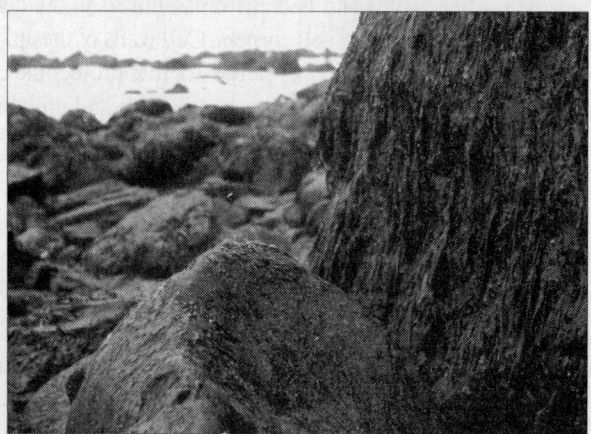

Fig. 27.2: *Porphyra.*

Other compounds that may accumulate in algal cell walls include sporopollenin and calcium ions. The group of algae known as the diatoms synthesise (Fig. 27.3) their cell walls (also known as frustules or valves) from silicic acid (specifically orthosilicic acid, H_4SiO_4). The acid is polymerised intra-cellularly, then the wall is extruded to protect the cell. Significantly, relative to the organic cell walls produced by other groups, silica frustules require less energy to synthesise (approximately 8%), potentially a major saving on the overall cell energy budget and possibly an explanation for higher growth rates in diatoms. In brown algae, phlorotannins may be a constituent of the cell walls.

Fungal Cell Walls

There are several groups of organisms that may be called 'fungi'. Some of these groups have been transferred out of the Kingdom Fungi, in part because of fundamental biochemical differences in the composition of the cell wall. Most true fungi have a cell wall consisting largely of chitin and other polysaccharides. True fungi do not have cellulose in their cell walls, but some fungus-like organisms do.

True fungi: Not all species of fungi have cell walls but in those that do, the plasma membrane is followed by three layers of cell wall material. From inside out these are:

- A chitin layer (polymer consisting mainly of unbranched chains of *N*-acetyl-*D*-glucosamine).

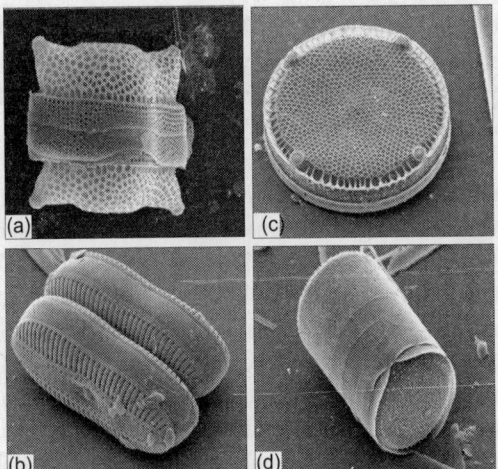

Fig. 27.3: Scanning electron micrographs of diatoms showing the external appearance of the cell wall.

- A layer of β-1,3-glucan (zymosan).
- A layer of mannoproteins (mannose-containing glycoproteins) which are heavily glycosylated at the outside of the cell.

Cell walls of water and slime molds

The group Oomycetes, also known as water molds, are saprotrophic plant pathogens like fungi. Until recently they were widely believed to be fungi, but structural and molecular evidence has led to their reclassification as heterokonts, related to autotrophic brown algae and diatoms. Unlike fungi, oomycetes typically possess cell walls of cellulose and glucans rather than chitin, although some genera (such as *Achlya* and *Saprolegnia*) do have chitin in their walls. The fraction of cellulose in the walls is no more than 4 to 20%, far less than the fraction comprised by glucans. Oomycete cell walls also contain the amino acid hydroxyproline, which is not found in fungal cell walls. The dictyostelids are another group formerly classified among the fungi. They are slime molds that feed as unicellular amoebae, but aggregate into a reproductive stalk and sporangium under certain conditions. Cells of the reproductive stalk, as well as the spores formed at the apex, possess a cellulose wall. The spore wall has been shown to possess three layers, the middle of which is composed primarily of cellulose and the innermost is sensitive to cellulase and pronase.

Prokaryotic Cell Walls

Around the outside of the cell membrane is the bacterial cell wall. Bacterial cell walls are made of peptidoglycan (also called murein), which is made from polysaccharide chains cross-linked by unusual peptides containing D-amino acids. Bacterial cell walls are different from the cell walls of plants and fungi which are made of cellulose and chitin, respectively. The cell wall of bacteria is also distinct from that of *Archaea*, which do not contain peptidoglycan. The cell wall is essential to the survival of many bacteria, although L-form bacteria can be produced in the laboratory that lack a cell wall. The antibiotic penicillin is able to kill bacteria by preventing the cross-linking of peptidoglycan and this causes the cell wall to weaken and lyse.

The matrix of cell wall is composed of three types of macromolecules (Fig. 27.4).

1. A hemicellulose can be any of several heteropolymers (matrix polysaccharides), such as arabinoxylans present in almost all plant cell walls along with cellulose. While cellulose is crystalline, strong, and resistant to hydrolysis, hemicellulose has a random, amorphous structure with little strength. It is easily hydrolysed by dilute acid or base as well as myriad hemicellulase enzymes. Hemicellulose contains many different sugar monomers. In contrast, cellulose contains only anhydrous glucose. For instance, besides glucose, sugar monomers in hemicellulose can include xylose, mannose, galactose, rhamnose, and arabinose. Hemicelluloses contain most of the D-pentose sugars, and occasionally small amounts of L-sugars as well. Xylose is always the sugar monomer present in the largest amount, but mannuronic acid and galacturonic acid also tend to be present. Unlike cellulose, hemicellulose (also a polysaccharide) consists of shorter chains 500–3000 sugar units as opposed to 7000–15,000 glucose molecules per polymer seen in cellulose. In addition, hemicellulose is a branched polymer, while cellulose is unbranched. Hemicelluloses are embedded in the cell walls of plants, sometimes in chains that form a 'ground' —they bind with pectin to cellulose to form a network of cross-linked fibres. Hemicelluloses are synthesised from sugar nucleotides in the Golgi. Two models explain their synthesis: (i) a '2 component model' where modification occurs at two transmembrane proteins, and (ii) a '1 component model' where modification occurs only at one transmembrane protein. After synthesis, hemicelluloses are transported to the plasma membrane via Golgi vesicles. As per cent content of hemicellulose increases in animal feed, the voluntary feed intake decreases. Hemicelluloses include xylan, glucuronoxylan, arabinoxylan, glucomannan, and xyloglucan.

2. Pectin is a structural heteropolysaccharide contained in the primary cell walls of terrestrial plants. It was first isolated and described in 1825 by Henri Braconnot. It is produced commercially as a white to light brown powder, mainly extracted from citrus fruits, and is used in food as a gelling agent particularly in jams and jellies. It is also used in fillings, sweets, as a stabiliser in fruit juices and milk drinks and as a source of dietary fibre. In plant cells, pectin consists of a complex set of polysaccharides that are present in most primary cell walls and particularly abundant in the non-woody parts of terrestrial plants. Pectin is present throughout primary cell walls but also in the middle lamella between plant cells where it helps to bind cells together. The amount, structure and

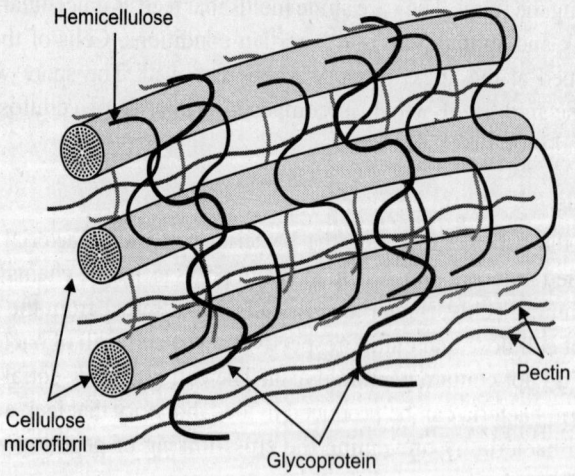

Fig. 27.4: Schematic diagram of a model of a generalised plant cell wall.

chemical composition of the pectin differs between plants, within a plant over time and in different parts of a plant. During ripening, pectin is broken down by the enzymes pectinase and pectinesterase, in this process the fruit becomes softer as the middle lamella breaks down and cells become separated from each other. A similar process of cell separation caused by pectin breakdown occurs in the abscission zone of the petioles of deciduous plants at leaf fall. Pectin is a natural part of human diet, but does not contribute significantly to nutrition. The daily intake of pectin from fruit and vegetables can be estimated to be around 5 g (assuming consumption of approximately 500 g fruit and vegetable per day). In human digestion, pectin goes through the small intestine more or less intact. Pectin is thus a soluble dietary fibre. Consumption of pectin has been shown to reduce blood cholesterol levels. The mechanism appears to be an increase of viscosity in the intestinal tract, leading to a reduced absorption of cholesterol from bile or food. In the large intestine and colon, micro-organisms degrade pectin and liberate short-chain fatty acids that have positive influence on health (prebiotic effect). Pectins are a family of complex polysaccharides that contain 1,4-linked α-D-galactosyluronic acid residues. Three pectic polysaccharides have been isolated from plant primary cell walls and structurally characterised. These are: (i) homogalacturonans, (ii) substituted galacturonans, and (iii) rhamnogalacturonans. Homogalacturonans are linear chains of α-(1-4)-linked D-galacturonic acid. Substituted galacturonans are characterised by the presence of saccharide appendant residues (such as D-xylose or D-apiose in the respective cases of xylogalacturonan and apiogalacturonan) branching from a backbone of D-galacturonic acid residues. Rhamnogalacturonan I pectins (RG-I) contain a backbone of the repeating disaccharide: 4-α-D-galacturonic acid-(1,2)-α-L-rhamnose-1. From many of the rhamnose residues, sidechains of various neutral sugars branch off. The neutral sugars are mainly D-galactose, L-arabinose and D-xylose, the types and proportions of neutral sugars varying with the origin of pectin. Another structural type of pectin is rhamnogalacturonan II (RG-II), which is a less frequent complex, highly branched polysaccharide. Rhamnogalacturonan II is classified by some authors within the group of substituted galacturonans since the rhamnogalacturonan II backbone is made exclusively of D-galacturonic acid units. Isolated pectin has a molecular weight of typically 60–1,30,000 g/mol, varying with origin and extraction conditions. In nature, around 80 per cent of carboxyl groups of galacturonic acid are esterified with methanol. This proportion is decreased more or less during pectin extraction. The ratio of esterified to nonesterified galacturonic acid determines the behaviour of pectin in food applications. This is why pectins are classified as high- vs. low-ester pectins—or in short HM- vs. LM-pectins, with more or less than half of all the galacturonic acid esterified. The nonesterified galacturonic acid units can be either free acids (carboxyl groups) or salts with sodium, potassium or calcium. The salts of partially esterified pectins are called pectinates, if the degree of esterification is below 5 per cent the salts are called pectates, the insoluble acid form, pectic acid. Some plants like sugar beet, potatoes and pears contain pectins with acetylated galacturonic acid in addition to methyl esters. Acetylation prevents gel-formation but increases the stabilising and emulsifying effects of pectin. Amidated pectin is a modified form of pectin. Here, some of the galacturonic acid is converted with ammonia to carboxylic acid amide. These pectins are more tolerant of varying calcium concentrations that occur in use. To prepare a pectin-gel, the ingredients are heated, dissolving the pectin. Upon cooling below gelling temperature, a gel starts to form. If gel formation is too strong, syneresis or a granular texture are the result, whilst weak gelling leads to excessively soft gels. In high-ester pectins at soluble solids content above 60 per cent and a pH-value between 2.8 and 3.6, hydrogen bonds and hydrophobic interactions bind the individual pectin chains together. These bonds form as water is bound by sugar and forces pectin strands to stick together. These form a 3-dimensional molecular net that creates the macromolecular gel. The gelling-mechanism is called a low-water-activity gel or sugar-acid-pectin gel. In low-ester pectins, ionic bridges are formed between calcium ions and the ionised carboxyl groups of the galacturonic acid. This is idealised in the so-called 'egg box-model'. Low-ester pectins need calcium to form a gel, but can do so at lower soluble solids and higher pH-values than high-ester pectins. Amidated pectins behave like low-ester pectins but need less calcium and are more tolerant of excess calcium. Also, gels from amidated pectin are thermoreversible—they can be heated and after cooling solidify again, whereas conventional pectin-gels will afterwards remain liquid. High-ester pectins set at higher temperatures than low-ester pectins. However, gelling reactions with calcium increase as the degree of esterification falls. Similarly, lower pH-values or higher soluble solids (normally sugars) increase gelling speed. Suitable pectins can therefore be selected for jams and for jellies or for higher sugar confectionery jellies.

3. Proteins, whose functions are not well understood, mediate dynamic activities. One class, the expansins, facilitate cell growth. These proteins cause localised relaxation of the cell wall, which allows the cell to elongate at that site in response to the turgor pressure generated within the cell. Cell wall-associated protein kinases span the plasma membrane and are thought to transmit signals from the cell wall to the cytoplasm.

Sources and production

Apples, guavas, quince, plums, gooseberries, oranges and other citrus fruits contain good amounts of pectin, while soft fruits like cherries, grapes and strawberries contain small amounts pectin. Typical levels of pectin in plants are (fresh weight):

1. Apples, 1–1.5 per cent.
2. Apricot, 1 per cent.
3. Cherries, 0.4 per cent.
4. Oranges 0.5–3.5 per cent.
5. Carrots approximately 1.4 per cent.
6. Citrus peels, 30 per cent.

The main raw-materials for pectin production are dried citrus peel or apple pomace, both by-products of juice production. Pomace from sugar-beet is also used to a small extent. From these materials, pectin is extracted by adding hot dilute acid at pH-values from 1.5–3.5. During several hours of extraction, the protopectin loses some of its branching and chain-length and goes into solution. After filtering, the extract is concentrated in vacuum and the pectin then precipitated by adding ethanol or isopropanol. An old technique of precipitating pectin with aluminium salts is no longer used (apart from alcohols and polyvalent cations, pectin also precipitates with proteins and detergents).

Alcohol-precipitated pectin is then separated, washed and dried. Treating the initial pectin with dilute acid leads to low-esterified pectins. When this process includes ammonium hydroxide, amidated pectins are obtained. After drying and milling pectin is usually standardised with sugar and sometimes calcium-salts or organic acids to have optimum performance in a particular application.

Uses

The main use for pectin is as a gelling agent, thickening agent and stabiliser in food. The classical application is giving the jelly-like consistency to jams or marmalades, which would otherwise be sweet juices. For household use, pectin is an ingredient in gelling sugar (also known as 'jam sugar') where it is diluted to the right concentration with sugar and some citric acid to adjust pH. In some countries, pectin is also available as a solution or an extract, or as a blended powder, for home jam making. For conventional jams and marmalades that contain above 60 per cent sugar and soluble fruit solids, high-ester pectins are used. With low-ester pectins and amidated pectins less sugar is needed, so that diet products can be made. Pectin can also be used to stabilise acidic protein drinks, such as drinking yogurt, and as a fat substitute in baked goods.

Typical levels of pectin used as a food additive are between 0.5–1.0 per cent this is about the same amount of pectin as in fresh fruit. In medicine, pectin increases viscosity and volume of stool so that it is used against constipation and diarrhea. Until 2002, it was one of the main ingredients used in Kaopectate, along with kaolinite. Pectin is also used in throat lozenges as a demulcent. In cosmetic products, pectin acts as stabiliser. Pectin is also used in wound healing preparations and speciality medical adhesives, such as colostomy devices. Also, it is considered a natural remedy for nausea. Pectin rich foods are proven to help nausea. In ruminant nutrition, depending on the extent of lignification of the cell wall, pectin is up to 90 per cent digestible by bacterial enzymes. Ruminant nutritionists recommend that the digestibility and energy concentration in forages can be improved by increasing pectin concentration in the forage.

In the cigar industry, pectin is considered an excellent substitute for vegetable glue and many cigar smokers and collectors will use pectin for repairing damaged tobacco wrapper leaves on their cigars.

Chapter 28

Extracellular Matrix

INTRODUCTION

In cell biology, molecular biology and related fields, the word extracellular (or sometimes extracellular space) means 'outside the cell'. This space is usually taken to be outside the plasma membranes, and occupied by fluid. The term is used in contrast to intracellular (inside the cell). The composition of the extracellular space includes metabolites, ions, proteins, and many other substances that might affect cellular function. For example, hormones act by travelling the extracellular space towards biochemical receptors on cells. Other proteins that are active outside the cell are the digestive enzymes. The term 'extracellular' is often used in reference to the extracellular fluid (ECF) compartment which composes about 15 litres of an average adult 70 kg human body which is assumed to contain a total of about 50 litres of water (thus, about 30 per cent of the body's water is in the ECF compartment). The cell membrane (and, in plants and fungi, the cell wall) is the barrier between the two, and chemical composition of intra- and extracellular milieu can be radically different. In most organisms, for example, a Na^+/K^+-ATPase pump maintains a high concentration of sodium ions outside cells while keeping that of potassium low, leading to chemical excitability. Many cold-tolerant plants force water into the extracellular space when the temperature drops below 0°C, so that when it freezes, it does not lyse the plants' cells.

EXTRACELLULAR SPACE

Two compartments comprise the extracellular space: the vascular space and the interstitial space. This extracellular material is very prominent in some types of cells, such as the epithelial cells that line the mammalian digestive tract. The glycocalyx is thought to mediate cell–cell and cell–substratum interactions, provide mechanical protection to cells, serve as a barrier to particles moving toward the plasma membrane, and bind important regulatory factors that act on the cell surface.

Extracellular Matrix

In biology, the extracellular matrix (ECM) is the extracellular part of animal tissue that usually provides structural support to the animal cells in addition to performing various other important functions. The extracellular matrix is the defining feature of connective tissue in animals.

Extracellular matrix includes the interstitial matrix and the basement membrane. Interstitial matrix is present between various animal cells (i.e. in the intercellular spaces). Gels of polysaccharides and fibrous proteins fill the interstitial space and act as a compression buffer against the stress placed on the ECM. Basement membranes are sheet-like depositions of ECM on which various epithelial cells rest.

Due to its diverse nature and composition, the ECM can serve many functions, such as providing support and anchorage for cells, segregating tissues from one another, and regulating intercellular communication. The ECM regulates a cell's dynamic behaviour. In addition, it sequesters a wide range of cellular growth factors, and acts as a local depot for them. Changes in physiological conditions can trigger protease activities that cause local release of such depots. This allows the rapid and local growth factor-mediated activation of cellular functions, without *de novo* synthesis.

Formation of the extracellular matrix is essential for processes like growth, wound healing and fibrosis. An understanding of ECM structure and composition also helps in comprehending the complex dynamics of tumour invasion and metastasis in cancer biology as metastasis often involves the destruction of extracellular matrix by enzymes such as serine and threonine proteases and matrix metalloproteinase.

Components of the ECM are produced intracellularly by resident cells, and secreted into the ECM via exocytosis. Once secreted they then aggregate with the existing matrix. The ECM is composed of an interlocking mesh of fibrous proteins and glycosaminoglycans (GAGs).

Proteoglycans

GAGs are carbohydrate polymers and are usually attached to extracellular matrix proteins to form proteoglycans (hyaluronic acid is a notable exception). Proteoglycans have a net negative charge that attracts water molecules, keeping the ECM and resident cells hydrated. Proteoglycans may also help to trap and store growth factors within the ECM. Described below are the different types of proteoglycan found within the extracellular matrix.

Heparan sulphate: Heparan sulphate (HS) is a linear polysaccharide found in all animal tissues. It occurs as a proteoglycan (PG) in which two or three HS chains are attached in close proximity to cell surface or extracellular matrix proteins. It is in this form that HS binds to a variety of protein ligands and regulates a wide variety of biological activities, including developmental processes, angiogenesis, blood coagulation and tumour metastasis.

In the extracellular matrix, especially basement membranes, the multi-domain proteins perlecan, agrin and collagen XVIII are the main proteins to which heparan sulphate is attached.

Chondroitin sulphates: Chondroitin sulphates contribute to the tensile strength of cartilage, tendons, ligaments and walls of the aorta. They have also been known to affect neuroplasticity.

Keratan sulphates: Keratan sulphates have a variable sulphate content and unlike many other GAGs, do not contain uronic acid. They are present in the cornea, cartilage, bones and the horns of animals.

Hyaluronic acid: Hyaluronic acid (or hyaluronan) is a polysaccharide consisting of alternative residues of D-glucuronic acid and *N*-acetylglucosamine, and unlike other GAGs is not found as a proteoglycan. Hyaluronic acid in the extracellular space confers upon tissues the ability to resist compression by providing a counteracting turgor (swelling) force by absorbing a lot of water. Hyaluronic acid is thus found in abundance in the ECM of load-bearing joints. It is also a chief component of the interstitial gel. Hyaluronic acid is found on the inner surface of the cell membrane and is translocated out of the cell during biosynthesis. Hyaluronic acid acts as an environmental cue that regulates cell behaviour during embryonic development, healing processes, inflammation and tumour development. It interacts with a specific transmembrane receptor, CD44.

Elastins: Elastins, in contrast to collagens, give elasticity to tissues, allowing them to stretch when needed and then return to their original state. This is useful in blood vessels, the lungs, in skin, and the ligamentum nuchae, and these tissues contain high amounts of elastins. Elastins are synthesised by fibroblasts and smooth muscle cells. Elastins are highly insoluble, and tropoelastins are secreted inside a chaperone molecule, which releases the precursor molecule upon contact with a fibre of mature elastin. Tropoelastins are then deaminated to become incorporated into the elastin strand. Diseases such as cutis laxa and Williams syndrome are associated with deficient or absent elastin fibres in the ECM.

Laminins: Laminins are proteins found in the basal laminae of virtually all animals. Rather than forming collagen-like fibres, laminins form networks of web-like structures that resist tensile forces in the basal lamina. They also assist in cell adhesion. Laminins bind other ECM components such as collagens, nidogens and entactins.

Cell adhesion to the ECM

Many cells bind to components of the extracellular matrix. Cell adhesion can occur in two ways, by focal adhesions, connecting the ECM to actin filaments of the cell, and hemidesmosomes, connecting the ECM to intermediate filaments such as keratin. This cell-to-ECM adhesion is regulated by specific cell surface cellular adhesion molecules (CAM) known as integrins. Integrins are cell surface proteins that bind cells to ECM structures, such as fibronectin and laminin, and also to integrin proteins on the surface of other cells. Fibronectins bind to ECM macromolecules and facilitate their binding to transmembrane integrins. The attachment of fibronectin to the extracellular domain initiates intracellular signalling pathways as well as association with the cellular cytoskeleton via a set of adaptor molecules such as actin.

Cell types involved in ECM formation

There are many cell types that contribute to the development of the various types of extracellular matrix found in plethora of tissue types. The local components of ECM determine the properties of the connective tissue. Fibroblasts are the most common cell type in connective tissue ECM, in which they synthesise, maintain and provide a structural framework, fibroblasts secrete the precursor components of the ECM, including the ground substance. Chondrocytes are found in cartilage and produce the cartilagenous matrix. Osteoblasts (Fig. 28.1) are responsible for bone formation.

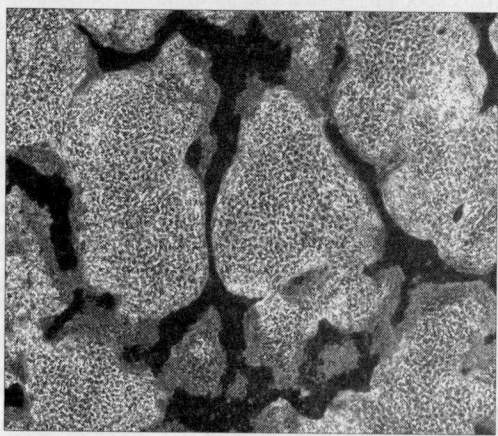

Fig. 28.1: Osteoblasts.

Extracellular matrix in plants

Plant cells are tessellated to form tissues. The cell wall is the relatively rigid structure surrounding the plant cell. The cell wall provides lateral strength to resist osmotic turgor pressure, but is flexible enough to allow cell growth when needed, it also serves as a medium for intercellular communication. The cell wall comprises multiple laminate layers of cellulose microfibrils embedded in a matrix of glycoproteins such as hemicellulose, pectin, and extensin. The components of the glycoprotein matrix help cell walls of adjacent plant cells to bind to each other. The selective permeability of the cell wall is chiefly governed by pectins in the glycoprotein matrix. Plasmodesmata (singular: plasmodesma) are pores that traverse the cell walls of adjacent plant cells. These channels are tightly regulated and selectively allow molecules of specific sizes to pass between cells.

Medical applications of extracellular matrix cells

Extracellular matrix cells have been found to cause regrowth and healing of tissue. In human fetuses, for example, the extracellular matrix works with stem cells to grow and regrow all parts of the human body, and fetuses can regrow anything that gets damaged in the womb. Scientists have long believed that the matrix stops functioning after full development. It has been used in the past to help horses heal torn ligaments, but it is being researched further as a device for tissue regeneration in humans.

In terms of injury repair and tissue engineering, the extracellular matrix serves two main purposes. First, it prevents the immune system from triggering from the injury and responding with inflammation and scar tissue. Next, it facilitates the surrounding cells to repair the tissue instead of forming scar tissue. For medical applications, the cells required are usually extracted from pig bladders, an easily accessible and relatively unused source. It is currently being used regularly to treat ulcers by closing the hole in the tissue that lines the stomach, but further research is currently being done by many universities as well as the US government for wounded soldier applications.

Collagen

Collagen is a group of naturally occurring proteins. In nature, it is found exclusively in animals. It is the main protein of connective tissue. It is the most abundant protein in mammals, making up about 25 to 35 per cent of the whole-body protein content. In muscle tissue it serves as a major component of endomysium. Collagen constitutes 1 to 2 per cent of muscle tissue, and accounts for 6 per cent of the weight of strong, tendinous muscles. Gelatine, which is used in food and industry, is derived from collagen.

Molecular structure: The tropocollagen or 'collagen molecule' is a subunit of larger collagen aggregates such as fibrils. It is approximately 300 nm long and 1.5 nm in diameter, made up of three polypeptide strands (called alpha chains), each possessing the conformation of a left-handed helix (its name is not to be confused with the commonly occurring alpha helix, a right-handed structure). These three left-handed helices are twisted together into a right-handed coiled coil, a triple helix or 'super helix', a cooperative quaternary structure stabilised by numerous hydrogen bonds. With type I collagen and possibly all fibrillar collagens if not all collagens, each triple-helix associates into a right-handed super-super-coil that is referred to as the collagen microfibril. Each microfibril is interdigitated with its neighbouring microfibrils to a degree that might suggest that they are individually unstable although within collagen fibrils they are so well ordered as to be crystalline. A distinctive feature of collagen is the regular arrangement of amino acids in each of the three chains of these collagen subunits. The sequence often follows the pattern Gly-Pro-Y or Gly-X-Hyp, where X and Y may be any of various other amino acid residues. Proline or hydroxyproline constitute about 1/6 of the total sequence. With glycine accounting for the 1/3 of the sequence, this means that approximately half of the collagen sequence is not glycine, proline or hydroxyproline, a fact often missed due to the distraction of the unusual GXY character of collagen alpha-peptides.

Uses: Collagen is one of the long, fibrous structural proteins whose functions are quite different from those of globular proteins such as enzymes. Tough bundles of collagen called collagen fibres are a major component of the extracellular matrix that supports most tissues and gives cells structure from the outside, but collagen is also found inside certain cells. Collagen has great tensile strength, and is the main component of fascia, cartilage, ligaments, tendons, bone and skin. Along with soft keratin, it is responsible for skin strength and elasticity, and its degradation leads to wrinkles that accompany ageing. It strengthens blood vessels and plays a role in tissue development. It is present in the cornea and lens of the eye in crystalline form. It is also used in cosmetic surgery and burns surgery. Hydrolysed collagen can play an important role in weight management, as a protein, it can be advantageously used for its satiating power.

Medical uses: The cardiac valve rings, the central body and the cardiac skeleton of the heart summarily represent a unique and moving collagen anchor to the fluid mechanics of the heart. Individual valvular leaflets are arguably held in shape by collagen under great extremes of pressure. Calcium deposition within collagen occurs as a natural consequence of ageing. These fixed points in an otherwise static display of blood and muscle enable current cardiac imaging technology to arrive at ratios essentially stating blood in cardiac input and blood out cardiac output. Specified imaging such as calcium scoring illustrates the utility of this methodology, especially in an ageing patient subject to pathology of the collagen underpinning. Collagen has been widely used in cosmetic surgery, as a healing aid for burn patients for reconstruction of bone and a wide variety of dental, orthopedic and surgical purposes.

Proteoglycan

Proteoglycans are glycoproteins that are heavily glycosylated. They have a core protein with one or more covalently attached glycosaminoglycan (GAG) chain(s). The chains are long, linear carbohydrate polymers that are negatively charged under physiological conditions, due to the occurrence of sulphate and uronic acid groups. Proteoglycans occur in the connective tissue.

Proteoglycans can be categorised depending upon the nature of their glycosaminoglycan chains. These chains may be:

1. Chondroitin sulphate and dermatan sulphate.
2. Heparin and heparan sulphate.
3. Keratan sulphate.

Proteoglycans can also be categorised by size. Examples of large proteoglycans are aggrecan (Fig. 28.2), the major proteoglycan in cartilage, and versican, present in many adult tissues including blood vessels and skin. The small leucine-rich repeat proteoglycans (SLRPs) include decorin, biglycan, fibromodulin (Fig. 28.3) and lumican. Proteoglycans are a major component of the animal extracellular matrix, the 'filler' substance existing between cells in an organism. Here they form large complexes, both to other proteoglycans, to hyaluronan and to fibrous matrix proteins (such as collagen). They are also involved in binding cations (such as sodium, potassium and calcium) and water, and also regulating the movement of molecules through the matrix. Evidence also shows they can affect the activity and stability of proteins and signalling molecules within the matrix. Individual functions of proteoglycans can be attributed to either the protein core or the attached GAG chain and serve as lubricants. The protein component of proteoglycans is synthesised by ribosomes and translocated into the lumen of the rough endoplasmic

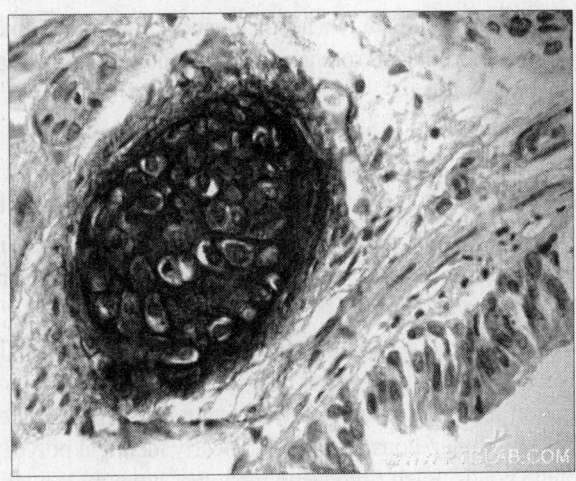

Fig. 28.2: Aggrecan.

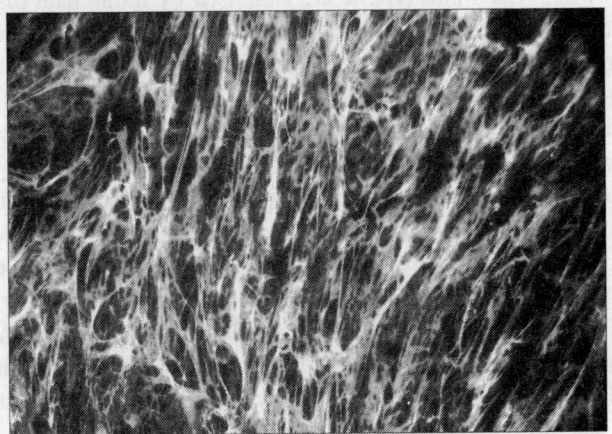

Fig. 28.3: Fibromodulin.

reticulum. Glycosylation of the proteoglycan occurs in the Golgi apparatus in multiple enzymatic steps. First a special link tetrasaccharide is attached to a serine side chain on the core protein to serve as a primer for polysaccharide growth. Then sugars are added one at a time by glycosyl transferase. The completed proteoglycan is then exported in secretory vesicles to the extracellular matrix of the cell.

An inability to break down proteoglycans is characteristic of a group of genetic disorders, called mucopolysaccharidoses. The inactivity of specific lysozomal enzymes that normally degrade glyco-saminoglycans leads to the accumulation of proteoglycans within cells. This leads to a variety of disease symptoms, depending upon the type of proteoglycan that is not degraded.

Fibronectin

Fibronectin is a high-molecular weight (~440 kDa) extracellular matrix glycoprotein that binds to membrane-spanning receptor proteins called integrins. In addition to integrins, fibronectin also binds extracellular matrix components such as collagen, fibrin and heparan sulphate proteoglycans (e.g. syndecans).

Fibronectin exists as a dimer, consisting of two nearly identical monomers linked by a pair of disulphide bonds. The fibronectin protein is produced from a single gene, but alternative splicing of its pre-mRNA leads to the creation of several isoforms.

Two types of fibronectin are present in vertebrates:

1. Soluble plasma fibronectin (formerly called 'cold-insoluble globulin', or CIg) is a major protein component of blood plasma (300 µg/ml) and is produced in the liver by hepatocytes.
2. Insoluble cellular fibronectin is a major component of the extracellular matrix. It is secreted by various cells, primarily fibroblasts, as a soluble dimer and is then assembled into an insoluble matrix in a complex cell-mediated process.

Fibronectin plays a major role in cell adhesion, growth, migration and differentiation, and it is important for processes such as wound healing and embryonic development. Altered fibronectin expression, degradation, and organisation has been associated with a number of pathologies, including cancer and fibrosis. Fibronectin exists as a dimer, consisting of two nearly identical polypeptide chains linked by a pair of C-terminal disulphide bonds. Each fibronectin monomer has a molecular weight of 230–250 kDa and contains three types of modules: type I, II, and III. All three modules are composed of two anti-parallel β-sheets, however, type I and type II are stabilised by intra-chain disulphide bonds, while type III modules do not contain any disulphide bridges. The absence of disulphide bonds in type III modules allows them to partially unfold under applied force. Fibronectin has numerous functions that ensure the normal functioning of vertebrate organisms. It is involved in cell adhesion, growth, migration and differentiation. Cellular fibronectin is assembled into the extracellular matrix, an insoluble network that separates and supports the organs and tissues of an organism.

Fibronectin plays a crucial role in wound healing. Along with fibrin, plasma fibronectin is deposited at the site of injury, forming a blood clot that stops bleeding and protects the underlying tissue. As repair of the injured tissue continues, fibroblasts and macrophages begin to remodel the area, degrading the proteins that form the provisional blood clot matrix and replacing them with a matrix that more resembles the normal, surrounding tissue. Fibroblasts secrete proteases, including matrix metalloproteinases, that digest the plasma fibronectin, and then the fibroblasts secrete cellular fibronectin and assemble it into an insoluble matrix. Fragmentation of fibronectin by proteases has been suggested to promote wound contraction, a critical step in wound healing.

Fragmenting fibronectin further exposes its V-region, which contains the site for α4β1 integrin-binding. These fragments of fibronectin are believed to enhance α4β1 integrins-expressing cell binding, allowing them to adhere to and forcefully contract the surrounding matrix. Fibronectin is necessary for embryogenesis, and inactivating the gene for fibronectin results in early embryonic lethality. Fibronectin is important for guiding cell attachment and migration during embryonic development. In mammalian development, the absence of fibronectin leads to defects in mesodermal, neural tube, and vascular development. Similarly, the absence of a normal fibronectin matrix in developing amphibians causes defects in mesodermal patterning and inhibits gastrulation. Fibronectin is also found in normal human saliva, which helps prevent colonisation of the oral cavity and pharynx by potentially pathogenic bacteria.

Matrix assembly: Cellular fibronectin is assembled into an insoluble fibrillar matrix in a complex cell-mediated process. Fibronectin matrix assembly begins when soluble, compact fibronectin dimers are secreted from cells, often fibroblasts. These soluble dimers bind to α5β1 integrin receptors on the cell surface and aide in clustering the integrins. The local concentration of integrin-bound fibronectin increases, allowing bound fibronectin molecules to more readily interact with one another. Short fibronectin fibrils then begin to form between adjacent cells. As matrix assembly proceeds, the soluble fibrils are converted into larger insoluble fibrils that comprise the extracellular matrix. Fibronectin's shift from soluble to insoluble fibrils proceeds when cryptic fibronectin-binding sites are exposed along the length of a bound fibronectin molecules. Cells are believed to stretch fibronectin by pulling on their fibronectin-bound integrin receptors. This force partially unfolds the fibronectin ligand, unmasking cryptic fibronectin-binding sites and allowing nearby fibronectin molecules to associate. This fibronectin–fibronectin interaction enables the soluble, cell-associated fibrils to branch and stabilise into an insoluble fibronectin matrix.

Role in cancer: Several of the morphological changes observed in tumours and tumour-derived cell lines have been attributed to decreased fibronectin expression, increased fibronectin degradation, and/ or decreased expression of fibronectin-binding receptors, such as $\alpha5\beta1$ integrins.

Fibronectin has been implicated in carcinoma development. In lung carcinoma, fibronectin expression is increased, especially in non-small cell lung carcinoma. The adhesion of lung carcinoma cells to fibronectin enhances tumorigenicity and confers resistance to apoptosis-inducing chemotherapeutic agents. Fibronectin has been shown to stimulate the gonadal steroids that interact with vertebrate androgen receptors, which are capable of controlling the expression of cyclin D and related genes involved in cell cycle control. These observations suggest that fibronectin may promote lung tumour growth/survival and resistance to therapy, and it could represent a novel target for the development of new anticancer drugs.

Laminin

Laminins are major proteins in the basal lamina (formerly improperly called basement membrane), a protein network foundation for most cells and organs. The laminins are an important and biologically active part of the basal lamina, influencing cell differentiation, migration, adhesion as well as phenotype and survival. Laminins are large trimeric proteins that contain an α-chain, a β-chain and a γ-chain, found in five, three and three genetic variants, respectively. The laminin molecules are named according to their chain composition. Thus, laminin-511 contains $\alpha5$, $\beta1$ and $\gamma1$ chains. Fourteen other chain combinations have been identified *in vivo*. The trimeric proteins form a cross, giving a structure that can bind to other cell membrane and extracellular matrix molecules. The three shorter arms are particularly good at binding to other laminin molecules, which allows them to form sheets. The long arm is capable of binding to cells, which helps anchor organised tissue cells to the membrane.

The laminins are a family of glycoproteins that are an integral part of the structural scaffolding in almost every tissue of an organism. They are secreted and incorporated into cell-associated extracellular matrices. Laminin is vital for the maintenance and survival of tissues. Defective laminins can cause muscles to form improperly, leading to a form of muscular dystrophy, lethal skin blistering disease (junctional epidermolysis bullosa) and defects of the kidney filter (nephrotic syndrome).

Fifteen laminin trimmers have been identified. The laminins are combinations of different alpha-, beta-, and gamma-chains.

1. There are five forms of alpha-chains: LAMA1, LAMA2, LAMA3, LAMA4, LAMA5.
2. There are four of beta-chains: LAMB1, LAMB2, LAMB3, LAMB4.
3. There are three of gamma-chains: LAMC1, LAMC2, LAMC3.

Laminins form independent networks and are associated with type IV collagen networks via entactin, and perlecan. They also bind to cell membranes through integrin receptors and other plasma membrane molecules, such as the dystroglycan glycoprotein complex and Lutheran blood group glycoprotein. Through these interactions, laminins critically contribute to cell attachment and differentiation, cell shape and movement, maintenance of tissue phenotype, and promotion of tissue survival. Some of these biological functions of laminin have been associated with specific amino-acid sequences or fragments of laminin. For example, the peptide sequence [GTFALRGDNGDNGQ], which is located on the alpha-chain of laminin, promotes adhesion of endothelial cells.

Laminins can be used to culture cells, such as pluripotent stem cells, that are difficult to culture on other substrates. Mostly two types of laminins have been used. Laminin-111 extracted from mouse sarcomas is one popular laminin type, as well as a mixture of laminins 511 and 521 from human placenta. Various laminin isoforms are practically impossible to isolate from tissues in pure form due to extensive cross-linking and the need for harsh extraction conditions such as proteolytic enzymes or low pH that cause degradation. In 2008, two groups independently showed that mouse embryonic stem cell can be grown for months on top of recombinant laminin-511.

Laminin-111 is a major substrate along which nerve axons will grow, both *in vivo* and *in vitro*. For example, it lays down a path that developing retinal ganglion cells follow on their way from the retina to the tectum. It is also often used as a substrate in cell culture experiments. Interestingly, the presence of laminin-1 can influence how the growth cone responds to other cues. For example, growth cones are repelled by netrin when grown on laminin-111, but are attracted to netrin when grown on fibronectin. This effect of laminin-111 probably occurs through a lowering of intracellular cyclic AMP.

INTERACTIONS OF CELLS WITH EXTRACELLULAR MATERIAL

The most important family of receptors that attach cells to their extracellular microenvironment is the integrins.

Integrin

Integrins are receptors that mediate attachment between a cell and the tissues surrounding it, which may be other cells or the extracellular matrix (ECM). They also play a role in cell signalling and thereby define cellular shape, mobility, and regulate the cell cycle. Typically, receptors inform a cell of the molecules in its environment and the cell evokes a response. Not only do integrins perform this outside-in signalling, but they also operate an inside-out mode. Thus, they transduce information from the ECM to the cell as well as reveal the status of the cell to the outside, allowing rapid and flexible responses to changes in the environment, for example to allow blood coagulation by platelets.

There are many types of integrin, and many cells have multiple types on their surface. Integrins are of vital importance to all animals and have been found in all animals investigated, from sponges to mammals. Integrins have been extensively studied in humans. Integrins work alongside other proteins such as cadherins, cell adhesion molecules and selectins to mediate cell–cell and cell–matrix interaction and communication. Integrins bind cell surface and ECM components such as fibronectin, vitronectin, collagen, and laminin. Integrins are obligate heterodimers containing two distinct chains, called the α (alpha) and β (beta) subunits. In mammals, 18α and 8β subunits have been characterised, whereas the *Drosophila* genome encodes only five α and two β subunits, and the *Caenorhabditis* nematodes possess two α and one β genes. Both the α and β subunits contain two separate tails, both of which penetrate the plasma membrane and possess small cytoplasmic domains.

There are various ways of categorising the integrins. For example, a subset of the α chains has an additional structural element (or domain) inserted toward their *N*-terminal, the so-called alpha-A domain (because it has a similar structure to the A-domains found in the protein von Willebrand factor: it is also termed the α-I domain). Integrins carrying this domain either bind to collagens (e.g. integrins α1β1, and α2β1) or act as cell–cell adhesion molecules (integrins of the β2 family). This α-I domain is the binding site for ligands of such integrins. Those integrins that do not carry this inserted domain, also have an A-domain in their ligand binding site, but this A-domain is found on the β subunit.

Function of Integrin

Integrins have two main functions:

1. Attachment of the cell to the ECM.
2. Signal transduction from the ECM to the cell.

However, they are also involved in a wide range of other biological activities, including immune patrolling, cell migration, and binding to cells by certain viruses, such as adenovirus, echovirus, hantavirus, and foot and mouth disease viruses.

A prominent function of the integrins is seen in the molecule GPIIbIIIa, an integrin on the surface of blood platelets (thrombocytes) responsible for cross-linking platelets in fibrin within a developing blood clot. This switches its adhesiveness for fibrin/fibrinogen from being non-adhesive to being intensely sticky, in a fast and precisely controlled manner. As such it provides a thought-model for how many integrins are believed to be regulated. As you may have noted, although blood is normally very rich in platelets, we do not spontaneously clot. This is clearly good news. On the other side, and equally positively, even minor wounds are rapidly blocked by the mass of fibrin, platelets and erythrocytes in a blood clot. A primary event in clot formation is the binding of platelets to exposed collagen in the wound site, which leads to their 'activation', and a clotting cascade. Among the many molecular events during activation, is the switching of GPIIbIIIa integrin from a quiescent state, unable to bind to fibrinogen/fibrin, to an active state, able to bind strongly to fibrinogen/fibrin. This is a remarkable event: first it involves all the GPIIbIIIa on a single platelet (some 50000 molecules), second it is completed within 5 seconds, third, it increases the affinity of the integrin concerned over several orders of magnitude. Fourth, it involves widespread changes in the molecular structure of the GPIIbIIIa molecule, as resolved by LIBS antibodies, which gain the ability to bind GPIIbIIIa only following activation of the platelets. Finally, it is intensely localised to the precise region of the damage, be it a couple of square micrometres, or the results of falling off a mountain bike at high speed.

Attachment of cell to the ECM: Integrins couple the ECM outside a cell to the cytoskeleton (in particular the microfilaments) inside the cell. Which ligand in the ECM the integrin can bind to is mainly decided by which α and β subunits the integrin is made of. Among the ligands of integrins are fibronectin, vitronectin, collagen, and laminin. The connection between the cell and the ECM may help the cell to endure pulling forces without being ripped out of the ECM. The ability of a cell to create this kind of bond is also of vital importance in ontogeny.

Cell attachment to the ECM is a basic requirement to build a multicellular organism. Integrins are not simply hooks, but give the cell critical signals about the nature of its surroundings. Together with signals arising from receptors for soluble growth factors like VEGF, EGF, and many others, they enforce a cellular decision on what biological action to take, be it attachment, movement, death, or differentiation. Thus integrins lie at the heart of many cellular biological processes. The attachment of the cell takes place through formation of cell adhesion complexes, which consist of integrins and many cytoplasmic proteins such as talin, vinculin, paxillin, and alpha-actinin. These act by regulating kinases such as FAK (focal adhesion kinase) and Src kinase family members to phosphorylate substrates such as p130CAS thereby recruiting signalling adaptors such as CRK. These adhesion complexes attach to the actin cytoskeleton. The integrins thus serve to link across the plasma membrane two networks: the extracellular

ECM and the intracellular actin filamentous system. One of the most important functions of surface integrins is their role in cell migration. Cells adhere to a substrate through their integrins. During movement, the cell makes new attachments to the substrate at its front and concurrently releases those at its rear. When released from the substrate, integrin molecules are taken back into the cell by endocytosis, they are transported through the cell to its front by the endocytic cycle where they are added back to the surface. In this way they are cycled for reuse, enabling the cell to make fresh attachments at its leading front.

Signal transduction: Integrins play an important role in cell signalling. Connection with ECM molecules can cause a signal to be relayed into the cell through protein kinases that are indirectly and temporarily connected with the intracellular end of the integrin molecule, likely following shape changes directly stimulated by ECM binding.

The signals the cell receives through the integrin can have relation to: (i) cell growth, (ii) cell division, (iii) cell survival, (iv) cellular differentiation, and (v) apoptosis (programmed cell death).

Focal Adhesion

In cell biology, focal adhesions (also cell-matrix adhesions or FAs) are specific types of large macro-molecular assemblies through which both mechanical force and regulatory signals are transmitted. More precisely, they can be considered as subcellular macromolecules that mediate the regulatory effects (e.g. cell anchorage) of extracellular matrix (ECM) adhesion on cell behaviour. Focal adhesions serve as the mechanical linkages to the ECM, and as a biochemical signalling hub to concentrate and direct numerous signalling proteins at sites of integrin binding and clustering.

Focal adhesions are large, dynamic protein complexes through which the cytoskeleton of a cell connects to the extracellular matrix, or ECM. They are limited to clearly defined ranges of the cell, at which the plasma membrane closes to within 15 nm of the ECM substrate. Focal adhesions are in a state of constant flux: proteins associate and disassociate with it continually as signals are transmitted to other parts of the cell, relating to anything from cell motility to cell cycle. Focal adhesions can contain over 100 different proteins, which suggests a considerable functional diversity. They actually serve for not only the anchorage of the cell, but can function beyond that as signal carriers (sensors), which inform the cell about the condition of the ECM and thus affect their behaviour. In sessile cells, focal adhesions are quite stable under normal conditions, while in moving cells their stability is diminished. This is because in motile cells, focal adhesions are being constantly assembled and disassembled as the cell establishes new contacts at the leading edge, and breaks old contacts at the trailing edge of the cell. One example of their important role is in the immune system, in which white blood cells migrate along the connective endothelium following cellular signals and to damaged biological tissue.

Connection between focal adhesions and proteins of the extracellular matrix generally involves integrins. Integrins bind to extracellular proteins via short amino acid sequences, such as the R-G-D sequence motif (found in proteins such as fibronectin, laminin or vitronectin) or the DGEA and GFOGER motifs found in collagen. Integrins are heterodimers which are formed from one beta and one alpha subunit. These subunits are present in different forms, which differ in their specificity and affinity to the different ECM proteins. Within the cell, the intracellular domain of integrin binds to the cytoskeleton via adapter proteins such as talin, α-actinin, filamin and vinculin. Many other intracellular signalling proteins, such as focal adhesion kinase, bind to and associate with this integrin-adapter protein-cytoskeleton complex, and this forms the basis of a focal adhesion.

The dynamic assembly and disassembly of focal adhesions plays a central role in cell migration. During cell migration, both the composition and the morphology of the focal adhesion changes. Initially, small (0.25 µm²) focal adhesions called 'focal complexes' are formed at the leading edge of the cell in lamellipodia: they consist of integrin, and some of the adapter proteins, such as talin and paxilin. Many of these focal complexes fail to mature and are disassembled as the lamellipodia withdraws. However, some focal complexes mature into larger and stable focal adhesions, and recruit many more proteins such as zyxin. Focal adhesion components are amongst the known calpain substrates, and it is possible that calpain degrades these components to aid in focal adhesion disassembly.

INTERACTIONS OF CELLS WITH OTHER CELLS

It is presumed that this process depends heavily on selective interactions between cells of the same type, as well as between cells of different type. Evidence indicates that cells can recognise the surfaces of other cells, interacting with some and ignoring others.

Selectin

Selectins are a family of cell adhesion molecules (or CAMs). All selectins are single-chain transmembrane glycoproteins that share similar properties to C-type lectins due to a related amino terminus and calcium-dependent binding. Selectins bind to sugar moieties and so are considered to be a type of lectin, cell adhesion proteins that bind sugar polymers.

There are three subsets of selectins:

1. E-selectin (in endothelial cells).
2. L-selectin (in leukocytes).
3. P-selectin (in platelets and endothelial cells).

During an inflammatory response, stimuli such as histamine and thrombin cause endothelial cells to mobilise P-selectin from stores inside the cell to the cell surface. In addition, cytokines such as TNF-alpha stimulate the expression of E-selectin and additional P-selectin a few hours later.

As the leukocyte rolls along the blood vessel wall, the distal lectin-like domain of the selectin binds to certain carbohydrate groups presented on proteins (such as PSGL-1) on the leukocyte, which slows the cell and allows it to leave the blood vessel and enter the site of infection. The low-affinity nature of selectins is what allows the characteristic 'rolling' action attributed to leukocytes during the leukocyte adhesion cascade. The best characterised ligand for the three selectins is P-selectin glycoprotein ligand-1 (PSGL-1), which is a mucin-type glycoprotein expressed on all white blood cells.

Immunoglobulin Superfamily

The immunoglobulin superfamily (IgSF) is a large group of cell surface and soluble proteins that are involved in the recognition, binding or adhesion processes of cells. Molecules are categorised as members of this superfamily based on shared structural features with immunoglobulins (also known as antibodies), they all possess a domain known as an immunoglobulin domain or fold. Members of the IgSF include cell surface antigen receptors, co-receptors and co-stimulatory molecules of the immune system, molecules involved in antigen presentation to lymphocytes, cell adhesion molecules, certain cytokine receptors and intracellular muscle proteins. They are commonly associated with roles in the immune system.

Proteins of the IgSF possess a structural domain known as an immunoglobulin (Ig) domain. Ig domains are named after the immunoglobulin molecules. They contain about 70–110 amino acids and are categorised according to their size and function. Ig-domains possess a characteristic Ig-fold, which has a sandwich-like structure formed by two sheets of antiparallel beta strands. Interactions between hydrophobic amino acids on the inner side of the sandwich and a highly conserved disulphide bonds formed between cysteine residues in the B and F strands, stabilise the Ig-fold. One end of the Ig domain has a section called the complementarity determining region that is important for the specificity of antibodies for their ligands.

Members of the immunoglobulin superfamily

The Ig domain was reported to be the most populous family of proteins in the human genome with 765 members identified. Members of the family can be found even in the bodies of animals with a simple physiological structure such as poriferan sponges. They have also been found in bacteria which presumably moved inside the micro-organisms through horizontal gene transfer.

Antigen receptors and ligands: Antigen receptors found on the surface of T and B lymphocytes in all jawed vertebrates belong to the IgSF. Immunoglobulin molecules (the antigen receptors of B cells) are the founding members of the IgSF. In humans, there are five distinct types of immunoglobulin molecule all containing a heavy chain with four Ig domains and a light chain with two Ig domains. The antigen receptor of T cells is the T cell receptor (TCR), which is composed of two chains, either the TCR-alpha and -beta chains or the TCR-delta and gamma chains. All TCR chains contain two Ig domains in the extracellular portion, one IgV domain at the N-terminus and one IgC1 domain adjacent to the cell membrane. The ligands for TCRs are major histocompatibility complex (MHC) proteins. These come in two forms, MHC class I forms a dimer with a molecule called beta-2 microglobulin (β2M) and interacts with the TCR on cytotoxic T-cells and MHC class II has two chains (alpha and beta) that interact with the TCR on helper T cells. MHC class I, MHC class II and β2M molecules all possess Ig domains and are therefore also members of the IgSF.

Co-receptors and accessory molecules: Other molecules on the surfaces of T cells also interact with MHC molecules during TCR engagement. These are known as co-receptors. In lymphocyte populations, the co-receptor CD4 is found on helper T cells and the co-receptor CD8 is found on cytotoxic T cells. CD4 has four Ig domains in its extracellular portion and functions as a monomer. CD8, in contrast, functions as a dimer with either two identical alpha chains or, more typically, with an alpha and beta chain. CD8-alpha and CD8-beta each has one extracellular IgV domain in its extracellular portion.

Co-stimulatory or inhibitory molecules: Co-stimulatory and inhibitory signalling receptors and ligands control the activation, expansion and effector functions of cells. One major group of IgSF co-stimulatory receptors are molecules of the CD28 family, CD28, CTLA-4, program death-1 (PD-1), the B- and T-lymphocyte attenuator (BTLA, CD272), and the inducible T-cell co-stimulator (ICOS, CD278), and their IgSF ligands belong to the B7 family, CD80 (B7-1), CD86 (B7-2), ICOS ligand, PD-L1 (B7-H1), PD-L2 (B7-DC), B7-H3, and B7-H4 (B7x/B7-S1).

Adherens Junctions and Desmosomes

The cells of certain tissues, particularly epithelia and cardiac muscle, are notoriously difficult to separate from one another because they are held together tightly by specialised calcium-dependent adhesive junctions. There are two main types of adhesive junction: adherens junctions and desmosomes. In addition to adhesive junctions, epithelial cells often contain other types of cell junctions that are also located along their lateral surfaces near the apical lumen. When these junctions are arranged in a specific array, this assortment of surface specialisations is called a junctional complex.

Adherens junctions (or zonula adherens) are protein complexes that occur at cell–cell junctions in epithelial tissues, usually more basal than tight junctions. An adherens junction is defined as a cell junction whose cytoplasmic face is linked to the actin cytoskeleton. They can appear as bands encircling the cell (zonula adherens) or as spots of attachment to the extracellular matrix (adhesion plaques).

A similar cell junction in nonepithelial cells is the fascia adherens. It is structurally the same, but appears in ribbon-like patterns that do not completely encircle the cells. One example is in cardiomyocytes. Adherens junctions are composed of the following proteins:

1. Cadherins: The cadherins are a family of transmembrane proteins that form homodimers in a calcium-dependent manner with other cadherin molecules on adjacent cells.
2. P120 (sometimes called delta catenin) binds the juxtamembrane region of the cadherin.
3. β-Catenin or γ-catenin (plakoglobin) binds the catenin-binding region of the cadherin.
4. α-Catenin binds the cadherin indirectly via β-catenin or plakoglobin.

Adherens junctions were, for many years, thought to share the characteristic of anchor cells through their cytoplasmic actin filaments. Adherens junctions may serve as a regulatory module to maintain the actin contractile ring with which it is associated in microscopic studies. A desmosome, also known as macula adherens, is a cell structure specialised for cell-to-cell adhesion. A type of junctional complex, they are localised spot-like adhesions randomly arranged on the lateral sides of plasma membranes.

Desmosomes help to resist shearing forces and are found in simple and stratified squamous epithelium. The intercellular space is very wide (about 30 nm). Desmosomes are also found in muscle tissue where they bind muscles cells to one another. Desmosomes are molecular complexes of cell adhesion proteins and linking proteins that attach the cell surface adhesion proteins to intracellular keratin cytoskeletal filaments. The cell adhesion proteins of the desmosome, desmoglein and desmocollin, are members of the cadherin family of cell adhesion molecules. They are transmembrane proteins that bridge the space between adjacent epithelial cells by way of homophilic binding of their extracellular domains to other desmosomal cadherins on the adjacent cell. Both have five extracellular domains, and have calcium-binding motifs.

The extracellular domain of the desmosome is called the extracellular core domain (ECD) or the Desmoglea, and is bisected by an electron-dense midline where the desmoglein and desmocollin proteins bind to each other. These proteins can bind in a W, S or λ manner.

On the cytoplasmic side of the plasma membrane, there are two dense structures called the outer dense plaque (ODP) and the inner dense plaque (IDP). These are spanned by the desmoplakin protein. The outer dense plaque is where the cytoplasmic domains of the cadherins attach to desmoplakin via plakoglobin and plakophillin. The inner dense plaque is where desmoplakin attaches to the intermediate filaments of the cell.

TIGHT JUNCTIONS: SEALING EXTRACELLULAR SPACE

A simple epithelium, like the lining of the intestine or lungs, is composed of a layer of cells that adhere tightly to one another to form a thin cellular sheet. Biologists have known for decades that when certain types of epithelia, such as frog skin or the wall of the urinary bladder, are mounted between two compartments containing different solute concentrations, very little diffusion of ions or solutes is observed across the wall of the epithelium from one compartment to the other. Given the impermeability of plasma membranes, it is not surprising that solutes cannot diffuse freely through the cells of an epithelial layer. Tight junctions or zonula occludens, are the closely associated areas of two cells whose membranes join together forming a virtually impermeable barrier to fluid. It is a type of junctional complex present only in vertebrates. The corresponding junctions that occur in invertebrates are septate junctions.

Tight junctions are composed of a branching network of sealing strands, each strand acting independently from the others. Therefore, the efficiency of the junction in preventing ion passage increases exponentially with the number of strands. Each strand is formed from a row of transmembrane proteins embedded in both plasma membranes, with extracellular domains joining one another directly. Although more proteins are present, the major types are the claudins and the occludins. These associate with different peripheral membrane proteins located on the intracellular side of plasma membrane, which anchor the strands to the actin cytoskeleton. Thus, tight junctions join together the cytoskeletons of adjacent cells.

They perform three vital functions:

1. They hold cells together.

2. They help to maintain the polarity of cells by preventing the lateral diffusion of integral membrane proteins between the apical and lateral/basal surfaces, allowing the specialised functions of each surface (for example receptor-mediated endocytosis at the apical surface and exocytosis at the basolateral surface) to be preserved. This aims to preserve the transcellular transport.

3. They prevent the passage of molecules and ions through the space between cells. So materials must actually enter the cells (by diffusion or active transport) in order to pass through the tissue. This pathway provides control over what substances are allowed through. (Tight junctions play this role in maintaining the blood-brain barrier).

GAP JUNCTIONS AND PLASMODESMATA

A gap junction or nexus is a specialised intercellular connection between a multitude of animal cell-types. It directly connects the cytoplasm of two cells, which allows various molecules and ions to pass freely between cells. One gap junction is composed of two connexons (or hemichannels) which connect across the intercellular space. Gap junctions are analogous to the plasmodesmata that join plant cells.

A notable use of gap junctions is in the electrical synapse found in some neurons. In vertebrates, gap junction hemichannels are primarily homo- or hetero-hexamers of connexin proteins. Invertebrate gap junctions comprise proteins from the hypothetical innexin family. However, the recently characterised pannexin family, which was originally thought to form intercellular channels (based on similar amino acid sequence similarity to innexins), in fact functions as single-membrane channels that communicate with the extracellular environment, and have been shown to pass calcium and ATP.

At gap junctions, the intercellular space is 4 nm and unit connexons in the membrane of each cell are lined up with one another. Gap junctions formed from two identical hemichannels are called homotypic, while those with differing hemichannels are heterotypic. In turn, hemichannels of uniform connexin composition are called homomeric, while those with differing connexins are heteromeric. Channel composition is thought to influence the function of gap junction channels.

Levels of Organisation

1. DNA to RNA to connexin protein.

2. One connexin protein has four transmembrane domains.

3. Six connexins create one connexon (hemichannel). When different connexins join together to form one connexon, it is called a heteromeric connexon.

4. Two hemichannels, joined together across a cell membrane comprise a gap junction. When two identical connexons come together to form a gap junction, it is called a homotypic GJ. When one

homomeric connexon and one heteromeric connexon come together, it is called a heterotypic gap junction. When two heteromeric connexons join, it is also called a heteromeric gap junction.

5. Several gap junctions (hundreds) assemble into a macromolecular complex called a plaque.

Properties

1. Allows for direct electrical communication between cells, although different connexin subunits can impart different single channel conductances, from about 30 to 500 pS.

2. Allows for chemical communication between cells, through the transmission of small second messengers, such as inositol triphosphate (IP_3) and calcium (Ca^{2+}), although different connexin subunits can impart different selectivity for particular small molecules.

3. Generally allows molecules smaller than 1000 Daltons to pass through, although different connexin subunits can impart different pore sizes and different charge selectivity. Large biomolecules, for example, nucleic acid and protein, are precluded from cytoplasmic transfer between cells.

4. Ensures that molecules and current passing through the gap junction do not leak into the intercellular space.

Up-to-date, five different functions have been ascribed to gap junction protein: (i) electrical and metabolic coupling between cells, (ii) electrical and metabolic exchange through hemichannels, (iii) tumour suppressor genes (Cx43, Cx32 and Cx36), (iv) adhesive function independent of conductive gap junction channel (neural migration in neocortex), and (v) role of carboxyl-terminal in signalling cytoplasmic pathways (Cx43).

Areas of electrical coupling

Gap junctions are particularly important in cardiac muscle: the signal to contract is passed efficiently through gap junctions, allowing the heart muscle cells to contract in tandem. Gap junctions are expressed in virtually all tissues of the body, with the exception of mobile cell types such as sperm or erythrocytes. Several human genetic disorders are associated with mutations in gap junction genes. Many of those affect the skin because this tissue is heavily dependent upon gap junction communication for the regulation of differentiation and proliferation.

Few locations have been discovered where there is significant coupling between neurons in the brain. Structures in the brain that have been shown to contain electrically coupled neurons include the vestibular nucleus, the nucleus of trigeminal nerve, the inferior olivary nucleus, and the Ventral Tegmental Area. There has been some observation of weak neuron to glial cell coupling in the locus coeruleus, and in the cerebellum between Purkinje neurons and Bergmann glial cells. It now seems that astrocytes are strongly coupled by gap junctions. Experimental data show strong gap junction expression in astrocytes.

Plasmodesma

Plasmodesmata (singular: plasmodesma) are microscopic channels which traverse the cell walls of plant cells and some algal cells enabling transport and communication between them. Species that have plasmodesmata include members of the *Charophyceae* (Fig. 28.4), Charales and Coleochaetales (which are all algae), as well as all embryophytes, better known as land plants. Unlike animal cells, every plant cell is surrounded by a polysaccharide cell wall. Neighbouring plant cells are therefore separated by a pair of cell walls and the intervening middle lamella, forming an extracellular domain known as the apoplast. Although cell walls are permeable to small soluble proteins and other solutes, plasmodesmata enable

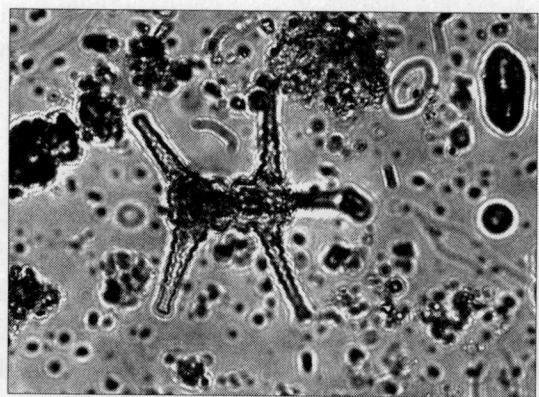

Fig. 28.4: *Charophyceae.*

direct, regulated, symplastic intercellular transport of substances between cells (Fig. 28.5). There are two forms of plasmodesmata, primary ones are formed during cell division and secondary ones can form between mature cells. Similar structures, called gap junctions and membrane nanotubes, interconnect animal cells and stromules form between plastids in plant cells.

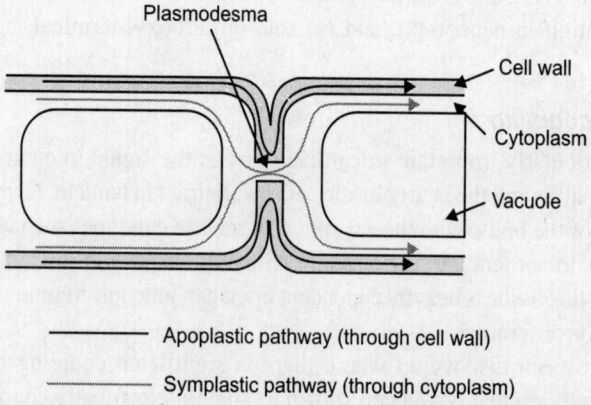

Fig. 28.5: Plasmodesma allow molecules to travel between plant cells through the symplastic pathway.

Plasmodesmata are formed when portion of the endoplasmic reticulum are trapped across the middle lamella as new cell wall is laid down between two newly divided plant cells and these eventually become the cytoplasmic connections between cells (primary plasmodesmata). Here the wall is not thickened further, and depressions or thin areas known as pits are formed in the walls. Pits normally pair up between adjacent cells. Alternatively, plasmodesmata can be inserted into existing cell walls between nondividing cells (secondary plasmodesmata).

A typical plant cell may have between 10^3 and 10^5 plasmodesmata connecting it with adjacent cells equating to between 1 and 10 per μm^2. Plasmodesmata are approximately 50–60 nm in diameter at the midpoint and are constructed of three main layers, the plasma membrane, the cytoplasmic sleeve, and the desmotubule. They can transverse cell walls that are up to 90 nm thick.

SECTION X

Cell Signalling and Cancer: Signal Transduction and Oncogenes

Chapter 29

Cell Signalling

INTRODUCTION

Cell signalling is part of any communication process that governs basic activities of cells and co-ordinates all cell actions. The ability of cells to perceive and correctly respond to their micro environment is the basis of development, tissue repair, and immunity, as well as normal tissue homeostasis. Errors in signalling interactions and cellular information processing are responsible for diseases such as cancer, autoimmunity, and diabetes. By understanding cell signalling, diseases may be treated more effectively and, theoretically, artificial tissues may be created.

Systems biology studies the underlying structure of cell signalling networks and how changes in these networks may affect the transmission and flow of information (signal transduction). Such networks are complex systems in their organisation and may exhibit a number of emergent properties including bistability and ultrasensitivity. Analysis of cell signalling networks requires a combination of experimental and theoretical approaches including the development and analysis of simulations and modeling. Long-range allostery is often a significant component of cell signalling events.

In biology, signal transduction refers to any process by which a cell converts one kind of signal or stimulus into another. Most processes of signal transduction involve ordered sequences of biochemical reactions inside the cell, which are carried out by enzymes and activated by second messengers, resulting in a signal transduction pathway. Such processes are usually rapid, lasting on the order of milliseconds in the case of ion flux or minutes for the activation of protein- and lipid-mediated kinase cascades, but some can take hours, and even days (as is the case with gene expression), to complete. The number of proteins and other molecules participating in the events involving signal transduction increases as the process emanates from the initial stimulus, resulting in a signal cascade, beginning with a relatively small stimulus that elicits a large response. This is referred to as amplification of the signal.

Essential to the survival of every cell is to monitor the environment and to respond to external stimuli. For most cells this includes appropriate communication with neighbouring cells. Cell signalling (or signal transduction) involves:

- Detection of the stimulus (in most cases a molecule secreted by another cell) on the surface of the plasma membrane.

413

- Transfer of the signal to the cytoplasmic side.
- Transmission of the signal to effector molecules and down a signalling pathway where every protein typically changes the conformation of the next down the path, most commonly by phosphorylation (by kinases) or dephosphorylation (by phosphatases).

The final effect is to trigger a cells response, such as the activation of gene transcription.

Cell signalling has been most extensively studied in the context of human diseases and signalling between cells of a single organism. However, cell signalling may also occur between the cells of two different organisms. In many mammals, early embryo cells exchange signals with cells of the uterus. In the human gastrointestinal tract, bacteria exchange signals with each other and with human epithelial and immune system cells. For the yeast *Saccharomyces cerevisiae* during mating, some cells send a peptide signal (mating factor pheromones) into their environment. The mating factor peptide may bind to a cell surface receptor on other yeast cells and induce them to prepare for mating.

CLASSIFICATION OF CELL SIGNALLING

Cell signalling can be classified as either mechanical or biochemical based on the type of the signal. Mechanical signals are the forces exerted on the cell and the forces produced by the cell. These forces can both be sensed and responded to by the cells. Biochemical signals are the biochemical molecules such as proteins, lipids, ions and gases. These signals can be categorised based on the distance between signalling and responder cells. Signalling within, between, and amongst cells is subdivided into the following classifications:

- Intracrine signals are produced by the target cell that stay within the target cell.
- Autocrine signals are produced by the target cell, are secreted, and affect the target cell itself via receptors. Sometimes autocrine cells can target cells close by if they are the same type of cell as the emitting cell. An example of this are immune cells.
- Juxtacrine signals target adjacent (touching) cells. These signals are transmitted along cell membranes via protein or lipid components integral to the membrane and are capable of affecting either the emitting cell or cells immediately adjacent.
- Paracrine signals target cells in the vicinity of the emitting cell. Neurotransmitters represent an example.
- Endocrine signals target distant cells. Endocrine cells produce hormones that travel through the blood to reach all parts of the body.

Cells communicate with each other via direct contact (juxtacrine signalling), over short distances (paracrine signalling), or over large distances and/or scales (endocrine signalling).

Some cell–cell communication requires direct cell–cell contact. Some cells can form gap junctions that connect their cytoplasm to the cytoplasm of adjacent cells. In cardiac muscle, gap junctions between adjacent cells allows for action potential propagation from the cardiac pacemaker region of the heart to spread and coordinate contraction of the heart.

The notch signalling mechanism is an example of juxtacrine signalling (also known as contact-dependent signalling) in which two adjacent cells must make physical contact in order to communicate. This requirement for direct contact allows for very precise control of cell differentiation during embryonic development. In the worm Caenorhabditis elegans, two cells of the developing gonad each have an equal chance of terminally differentiating or becoming a uterine precursor cell that continues to divide. The choice of which cell continues to divide is controlled by competition of cell surface signals. One cell will happen to produce more of a cell surface protein that activates the Notch receptor on the adjacent cell. This activates a feedback loop or system that reduces Notch expression in the cell that will differentiate and that increases Notch on the surface of the cell that continues as a stem cell.

Many cell signals are carried by molecules that are released by one cell and move to make contact with another cell. Endocrine signals are called hormones. Hormones are produced by endocrine cells and they travel through the blood to reach all parts of the body. Specificity of signalling can be controlled if only some cells can respond to a particular hormone. Paracrine signals such as retinoic acid target only cells in the vicinity of the emitting cell. Neurotransmitters represent another example of a paracrine signal. Some signalling molecules can function as both a hormone and a neurotransmitter. For example, epinephrine and norepinephrine can function as hormones when released from the adrenal gland and are transported to the heart by way of the blood stream. Norepinephrine can also be produced by neurons to function as a neurotransmitter within the brain. Estrogen can be released by the ovary and function as a hormone or act locally via paracrine or autocrine signalling. Active species of oxygen and nitric oxide can also act as cellular messengers. This process is dubbed redox signalling.

SIGNALLING MOLECULES

Most signal transduction involves the binding of extracellular signalling molecules (and ligands) to cell-surface receptors that face outward from the plasma membrane and trigger events inside the cell. Intracellular signalling cascades can also be triggered through cell-substratum interactions, as in the case of integrins, which bind ligands found within the extracellular matrix. Steroids represent another example of extracellular signalling molecules that may cross the plasma membrane due to their lipophilic or hydrophobic nature. Many, but not all, steroids have receptors within the cytoplasm, and usually act by stimulating the binding of their receptors to the promoter region of steroid-responsive genes. Within multicellular organisms, numerous small molecules and polypeptides serve to coordinate a cell's individual biological activity within the context of the organism as a whole. These molecules have been functionally classified as:

1. Hormones (e.g. melatonin).
2. Growth factors (e.g. epidermal growth factor).
3. Extracellular matrix components (e.g. fibronectin).
4. Cytokines (Fig. 29.1) (e.g. interferon-gamma).
5. Chemokines (e.g. RANTES).
6. Neurotransmitters (e.g. acetylcholine).
7. Neurotrophins (e.g. nerve growth factor).
8. Active oxygen species.

Most of these classifications do not take into account the molecular nature of each class member. For example, as a class, neurotransmitters consist of neuropeptides such as endorphins and small molecules such as serotonin and dopamine. Hormones, another generic class of molecules capable of initiating signal transduction, include insulin (a polypeptide), testosterone (a steroid), and epinephrine (an amino acid derivative, in essence a small organic molecule).

The classification of one molecule into one class or another is not exact. For example, epinephrine and norepinephrine secreted by the central nervous system act as neurotransmitters. However, epinephrine when secreted by the adrenal medulla acts as a hormone.

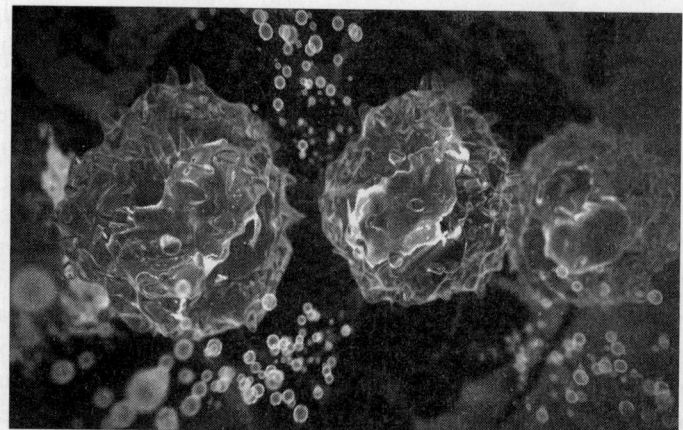

Fig. 29.1: Cytokines.

Environmental Stimuli

In bacteria and other single-cell organisms, the variety of a signal transduction processes of which the cell is capable, influences how many ways it can react and respond to its environment. In multicellular organisms, numerous signal transduction processes are required for co-ordinating the behaviour of individual cells to support the function of the organism as a whole. The complexity of an organism's signal transduction processes tends to increase with the complexity of the organism itself. Sensing of both the external and internal environments at the cellular level relies on signal transduction. Many disease processes, such as diabetes, heart disease, autoimmunity, and cancer arise from defects in signal transduction pathways, further highlighting the critical importance of signal transduction to biology, as well as medicine.

Various environmental stimuli in addition to many of the regular signal transduction stimuli listed above initiate signal transmission processes in complex organisms. Environmental stimuli may also be molecular in nature or more physical, such as light striking cells in the retina of the eye, odourants binding to odourant receptors in the nasal epithelium, and bitter and sweet tastes stimulating taste receptors in the taste buds.

Certain microbial molecules, e.g. viral nucleotides, bacterial lipopolysaccharides, and protein antigens, are able to elicit an immune system response against invading pathogens, mediated by signal transduction processes. An immune response may occur independent of signal transduction stimulation by other molecules, as is the case for signal transduction by way of the Toll-like receptor or with help from stimulatory molecules located at the cell surface of other cells, as is the case for T-cell receptor signalling.

Unicellular organisms may also respond to environmental stimuli through the activation of signal transduction pathways. For example, slime molds secrete cyclic-AMP upon starvation, which stimulates individual cells in the immediate environment to aggregate. Yeast use mating factors to determine the mating types of other yeast and to participate in sexual reproduction.

Cellular Responses

Activation of genes, alterations in metabolism, the continued proliferation and death of the cell, and the stimulation or suppression of locomotion, are some of the cellular responses to extracellular stimulation that require signal transduction. Gene activation leads to further cellular effects, since the protein products of many of the responding genes include enzymes and transcription factors themselves. Transcription factors produced as a result of a signal transduction cascade can, in turn, activate yet more genes. Therefore an initial stimulus can trigger the expression of an entire cohort of genes, and this, in turn, can lead to the activation of any number of complex physiological events. These events include the increased uptake of glucose from the blood stream stimulated by insulin and the migration of neutrophils to sites of infection stimulated by bacterial products. The set of genes and the order in which they are activated in response to stimuli are often referred to as a genetic programme. Most mammalian cells require stimulation to control not only cell division but also survival. In the absence of growth factor stimulation, programmed cell death ensues in most cells.

Such requirements for extracellular stimulation are necessary for controlling cell behaviour in the context of both unicellular and multicellular organisms. Signal transduction pathways are perceived to be so central to biological processes that it is not surprising that a large number of diseases have been attributed to their disregulation. Discussed below are how signal transduction via various classes of receptor may lead to the above cellular responses.

Types of Receptors

There are a number of receptor classes that are used in different signalling pathways. The two more predominant are:

1. G-protein-coupled receptors.
2. Cell-surface receptors.

G-protein-coupled receptors

G-protein-coupled receptors (GPCRs) are a family of integral membrane proteins that possess seven membrane-spanning domains, and are linked to a guanine nucleotide-binding protein (or heterotrimeric G-protein). Many receptors make up this family, including adrenergic receptors, neurotransmitter receptors, olfactory receptors, opioid receptors, chemokine receptors, and rhodopsin.

The total strength of signal amplification by a GPCR is determined by:

1. The lifetime of the ligand-receptor-complex.
2. The amount and lifetime of the receptor-effector protein-complex.
3. Deactivation of the activated receptor.
4. Deactivation of effectors through intrinsic enzymatic activity.

The idea that G-protein-coupled receptors, to be specific, chemokine receptors, participate in cancer development is suggested by a study wherein a point mutation was inserted into the gene encoding the chemokine receptor CXCR2. Cells transfected with the CXCR2 mutant underwent a malignant transformation. The result of the point mutation was the expression of CXCR2 in an active conformation, despite the absence of chemokine-binding (the CXCR2 mutant is said to be 'constitutively active').

Cell-surface receptors

Cell-surface receptors are integral transmembrane proteins and recognise the vast majority of extracellular signalling molecules. Transmembrane receptors span the plasma membrane of the cell, with one part of the receptor on the outside of the cell (the extracellular domain), and the other on the inside of the cell (the intracellular domain).

Signal transduction occurs as a result of stimulatory molecule or the binding of a ligand to its extracellular domain, the ligand itself does not pass through the plasma membrane prior to receptor-binding.

Receptor tyrosine kinases

Receptor tyrosine kinases (RTKs) are transmembrane proteins with an intracellular kinase domain and an extracellular domain that binds ligand. There are many RTK proteins that are classified into subfamilies depending on their structural properties and ligand specificity. These include many growth factor receptors such as insulin receptor and the insulin-like growth factor receptors, and many others receptors. To conduct their biochemical signals, RTKs need to form dimers in the plasma membrane. The dimer is stabilised by ligand binding by the receptor. Interaction between the two cytoplasmic domains of the dimer is thought to stimulate autophosphorylation of tyrosines within the cytoplasmic tyrosine kinase domains of the RTKs causing their conformational changes. The kinase domain of the receptors is subsequently activated, initiating signalling cascades of phosphorylation of downstream cytoplasmic molecules. These signals are essential to various cellular processes, such as control of cell growth, differentiation, metabolism, and migration.

Integrins

Integrins are produced by a wide variety of cell types, and play a role in the attachment of a cell to the extracellular matrix (ECM) and to other cells, and in the signal transduction of signals received from extracellular matrix components such as fibronectin, collagen, and laminin. Ligand-binding to the extracellular domain of integrins induces a conformational change within the protein and a clustering of the protein at the cell surface to initiate signal transduction.

Important differences exist between integrin-signalling in circulating blood cells and that in non-circulating blood cells such as epithelial cells. Integrins at the cell-surface of circulating cells are inactive under normal physiological conditions.

For example, cell-surface integrins on circulating leukocytes are maintained in an inactive state to avoid epithelial cell attachment. Only in response to appropriate stimuli are leukocyte integrins converted into an active form, such as those received at the site of an inflammatory response. In a similar manner, it is important that integrins at the cell surface of circulating platelets are kept in an inactive state under normal conditions to avoid thrombosis. Epithelial cells, in contrast, have active integrins at their cell surface under normal conditions, which help maintain their stable adhesion to underlying stromal cells, which provide appropriate signals to maintain their survival and differentiation.

Toll-like receptors

When activated, Toll-like receptors (TLRs) recruit adapter molecules within the cytoplasm of cells in order to propagate a signal. Four adapter molecules are known to be involved in signalling. These proteins are known as MyD88, Tirap (also called Mal), Trif, and Tram.

Ligand-gated ion channel receptors

A ligand-activated ion channel will recognise its ligand, and then undergo a structural change that opens a gap (channel) in the plasma membrane through which ions can pass. These ions will then relay the signal. An example for this mechanism is found in the receiving cell or postsynaptic cell of a neural synapse. By contrast, other ion channels open in response to a change in cell potential, that is, the difference of the electrical charge across the membrane. In neurons, this mechanism underlies the action potentials that travel along nerves.

Intracellular receptors

Intracellular receptors include nuclear receptors and cytoplasmic receptors, and are soluble proteins localised within the nucleoplasm or the cytoplasm, respectively. The typical ligands for nuclear receptors are lipophilic hormones, with steroid hormones (for example, testosterone, progesterone, and cortisol) and derivatives of vitamin A and D among them. To reach its receptor and initiate signal transduction, the hormone must pass through the plasma membrane, usually by passive diffusion. The nuclear receptors are ligand-activated transcription activators, on binding with the ligand (the hormone), the ligands will pass through the nuclear membrane into the nucleus and enable the transcription of a certain gene and, thus, the production of a protein.

The nuclear receptors that were activated by the hormones attach at the DNA at receptor-specific hormone-responsive elements (HREs), DNA sequences that are located in the promoter region of the genes that are activated by the hormone-receptor complex. As this enables the transcription of the according gene, these hormones are also called inductors of gene expression.

The activation of gene transcription is much slower than signals that directly affect existing proteins. As a consequence, the effects of hormones that use nucleic receptors are usually long-term. Although the signal transduction via these soluble receptors involves only a few proteins, the details of gene regulation are yet not well understood.

The nucleic receptors all have a similar, modular structure:

N-AAAABBBBCCCCDDDDEEEEFFFF-C

where, CCCC is the DNA-binding domain that contains zinc fingers, and EEEE the ligand-binding domain. The latter is also responsible for dimerisation of most nuclearic receptors prior to DNA binding. As a third function, it contains structural elements that are responsible for transactivation, used for communication with the translational apparatus. The zinc fingers in the DNA-binding domain stabilise DNA binding by holding contact to the phosphate backbone of the DNA. The DNA sequences that match the receptor are usually hexameric repeats, either normal, inverted or everted. The sequences are quite similar, but their orientation and distance are the parameters by which the DNA-binding domains of the receptors can tell them apart.

Steroid receptors are a subclass of nuclear receptors, located primarily within the cytosol. In the absence of steroid hormone, the receptors cling together in a complex called an aporeceptor complex, which also contains chaperone proteins (also known as heatshock proteins or Hsps). The Hsps are necessary to activate the receptor by assisting the protein to fold in a way such that the signal sequence that enables its passage into the nucleus is accessible. Steroid receptors can also have a repressive effect on gene expression, when their transactivation domain is hidden so it cannot activate transcription. Furthermore, steroid receptor activity can be enhanced by phosphorylation of serine residues at their N-terminal end, as a result of another signal transduction pathway, for example, by a growth factor. This behaviour is called cross-talk.

RXR- and orphan-receptors

These nuclear receptors can be activated by:

1. A classic endocrine-synthesised hormone that entered the cell by diffusion.
2. A hormone that was built within the cell (for example, retinol) from a precursor or prohormone, which can be brought to the cell through the bloodstream.
3. A hormone that was completely synthesised within the cell, for example, prostaglandin.

These receptors are located in the nucleus and are not accompanied by chaperone proteins. In the absence of hormone, they bind to their specific DNA sequence, repressing the gene. Upon activation by the hormone, they activate the transcription of the gene that they were repressing.

Certain intracellular receptors of the immune system are examples of cytoplasmic receptors. Recently-identified NOD like receptors (NLRs) reside in the cytoplasm of specific eukaryotic cells and interact with particular ligands, such as microbial molecules, using a leucine-rich repeat (LRR) motif that is similar to the ligand-binding motif of the extracellular receptors known as TLRs. Some of these molecules (e.g. NOD1 and NOD2) interact with an enzyme called RICK kinase (or RIP2 kinase) that activates NF-κB signalling, whereas others (e.g. NALP3) interact with inflammatory caspases (e.g. caspase 1) and initiate processing of particular cytokines (e.g. interleukin-1β). Similar receptors exist inside plant cells and are called plant R-proteins. Another type of cytoplasmic receptor also has a role in immune surveillance. These receptors are known as RNA Helicases and include RIG-I, MDA5, and LGP2.

G-PROTEIN-COUPLED RECEPTOR AND THEIR SECOND MESSENGERS

G-protein-coupled receptors (GPCRs), also known as seven-transmembrane (7TM) domain receptors, 7TM receptors, heptahelical receptors, serpentine receptor, and G-protein-linked receptors (GPLR), comprise a large protein family of transmembrane receptors that sense molecules outside the cell and activate inside signal transduction pathways and, ultimately, cellular responses. G-protein-coupled receptors are found only in eukaryotes, including yeast, choanoflagellates (Fig. 29.2), and animals.

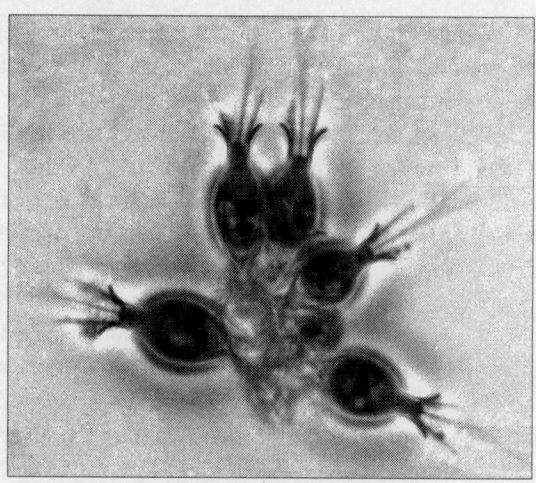

Fig. 29.2: Choanoflagellates.

The ligands that bind and activate these receptors include light-sensitive compounds, odours, pheromones, hormones, and neurotransmitters, and vary in size from small molecules to peptides to large proteins. G-protein-coupled receptors are involved in many diseases, and are also the target of approximately 30 per cent of all modern medicinal drugs.

There are two principal signal transduction pathways involving the G-protein-coupled receptors: the cAMP signal pathway and the Phosphatidylinositol signal pathway. When a ligand binds to the GPCR it causes a conformational change in the GPCR, which allows it to act as a guanine nucleotide exchange factor (GEF). The GPCR can then activate an associated G-protein by exchanging its bound GDP for a

GTP. The G-protein's α subunit, together with the bound GTP, can then dissociate from the β and γ subunits to further affect intracellular signalling proteins or target functional proteins directly depending on the a subunit type ($G_{\alpha s}$, $G_{\alpha i}$, $G_{\alpha q/11}$, $G_{\alpha 12/13}$).

Classification of GPCRs

GPCRs can be grouped into six classes based on sequence homology and functional similarity:

1. Class A (or 1) (Rhodopsin-like).
2. Class B (or 2) (Secretin receptor family).
3. Class C (or 3) (Metabotropic glutamate/pheromone).
4. Class D (or 4) (Fungal mating pheromone receptors).
5. Class E (or 5) (Cyclic AMP receptors).
6. Class F (or 6) (Frizzled/Smoothened).

The very large rhodopsin A group has been further subdivided into 19 subgroups (A1-A19). More recently, an alternative classification system called GRAFS (glutamate, rhodopsin, adhesion, frizzled/taste2, secretin) has been proposed. The human genome encodes thousands of G-protein-coupled receptors, about 350 of which detect hormones, growth factors, and other endogenous ligands. Approximately 150 of the GPCRs found in the human genome have unknown functions.

Physiological roles

GPCRs are involved in a wide variety of physiological processes. Some examples of their physiological roles include:

1. The visual sense: The opsins use a photoisomerisation reaction to translate electromagnetic radiation into cellular signals. Rhodopsin, for example, uses the conversion of 11-*cis*-retinal to all-*trans*-retinal for this purpose.
2. The sense of smell: Receptors of the olfactory epithelium bind odourants (olfactory receptors) and pheromones (vomeronasal receptors).
3. Behavioural and mood regulation: Receptors in the mammalian brain bind several different neurotransmitters, including serotonin, dopamine, GABA, and glutamate.
4. Regulation of immune system activity and inflammation: Chemokine receptors bind ligands that mediate intercellular communication between cells of the immune system, receptors such as histamine receptors bind inflammatory mediators and engage target cell types in the inflammatory response.
5. Autonomic nervous system transmission: Both the sympathetic and parasympathetic nervous systems are regulated by GPCR pathways, responsible for control of many automatic functions of the body such as blood pressure, heart rate, and digestive processes.
6. Cell density sensing: A novel GPCR role in regulating cell density sensing.

Receptor structure

GPCRs are integral membrane proteins that possess seven membrane-spanning domains or transmembrane helices. The extracellular parts of the receptor can be glycosylated. These extracellular loops also contain two highly-conserved cysteine residues that form disulphide bonds to stabilise the receptor structure. Some seven-transmembrane helix proteins (channel rhodopsin) that resemble GPCRs may contain ion channels, within their protein. Early structural models for GPCRs were based on their weak analogy to bacterio rhodopsin, for which a structure had been determined by both electron diffraction. This human β_2-adrenergic receptor GPCR structure, proved to be highly similar to the bovine rhodopsin in terms of the relative orientation of the seven-transmembrane helices. However, the conformation of the second extracellular loop is entirely different between the two structures. Since this loop constitutes the 'lid' that covers the top of the ligand binding site, this conformational difference highlights the difficulties in constructing homology models of other GPCRs based only on the rhodopsin structure.

Mechanism

The G-protein-coupled receptor is activated by an external signal in the form of a ligand or other signal mediator. This creates a conformational change in the receptor, causing activation of a G-protein. Further effect depends on the type of G-protein.

Ligand binding: GPCRs include receptors for sensory signal mediators (e.g. light and olfactory stimulatory molecules), adenosine, bombesin, bradykinin, endothelin, γ-aminobutyric acid (GABA), hepatocyte growth factor, melanocortins, neuropeptide Y, opioid peptides, opsins, somatostatin, tachykinins, vasoactive intestinal polypeptide family, and vasopressin, biogenic amines [e.g. dopamine, epinephrine, norepinephrine, histamine, glutamate (metabotropic effect), glucagon, acetylcholine (muscarinic effect), and serotonin], chemokines, lipid mediators of inflammation (e.g. prostaglandins, prostanoids, platelet-activating factor, and leukotrienes), and peptide hormones [e.g. calcitonin, C5a anaphylatoxin, follicle-stimulating hormone (FSH), gonadotropic-releasing hormone (GnRH), neurokinin, thyrotropin-releasing hormone (TRH), and oxytocin]. GPCRs that act as receptors for stimuli that have not yet been identified are known as orphan receptors.

Conformational change: The transduction of the signal through the membrane by the receptor is not completely understood. It is known that the inactive G-protein is bound to the receptor in its inactive state. Once the ligand is recognised, the receptor shifts conformation and, thus, mechanically activates the G-protein, which detaches from the receptor. The receptor can now either activate another G-protein or switch back to its inactive state. This is an overly simplistic explanation, but suffices to convey the overall set of events.

It is believed that a receptor molecule exists in a conformational equilibrium between active and inactive biophysical states. The binding of ligands to the receptor may shift the equilibrium toward the active receptor states. Three types of ligands exist: Agonists are ligands that shift the equilibrium in favour of active states, inverse agonists are ligands that shift the equilibrium in favour of inactive states, and neutral antagonists are ligands that do not affect the equilibrium. It is not yet known how exactly the active and inactive states differ from each other.

GPCR signalling without G-proteins: In the late 1990s, evidence began accumulating to suggest that some GPCRs are able to signal without G-proteins. The ERK2 mitogen-activated protein kinase, a key signal transduction mediator downstream of receptor activation in many pathways, has been shown to be activated in response to cAMP-mediated receptor activation in the slime mold *D. discoideum* despite the absence of the associated G protein α- and β-subunits. In mammalian cells, the much-studied β_2-adrenoceptor has been demonstrated to activate the ERK2 pathway after arrestin-mediated uncoupling of G-protein-mediated signalling. Therefore it seems likely that some mechanisms previously believed to be purely related to receptor desensitisation are actually examples of receptors switching their signalling pathway rather than simply being switched off. In kidney cells, the bradykinin receptor B2 has been shown to interact directly with a protein tyrosine phosphatase.

The presence of a tyrosine-phosphorylated ITIM (immunoreceptor tyrosine-based inhibitory motif) sequence in the B2 receptor is necessary to mediate this interaction and subsequently the antiproliferative effect of bradykinin.

Two principal pathways

There are two principal signal transduction pathways involving the G-protein-linked receptors: cAMP signal pathway and phosphatidylinositol signal pathway.

cAMP signal pathway

The cAMP signal transduction contains five main characters: stimulative hormone receptor (Rs) or inhibitory hormone receptor (Ri), stimulative regulative G-protein (Gs) or inhibitory regulative G-protein (Gi), adenylyl cyclase, protein kinase A (PKA), and cAMP phosphodiesterase.

Stimulative hormone receptor (Rs) is a receptor that can bind with stimulative signal molecules, while inhibitory hormone (Ri) is a receptor that can bind with inhibitory signal molecules. Dissociation/association of the G-protein is shown in Fig. 29.3.

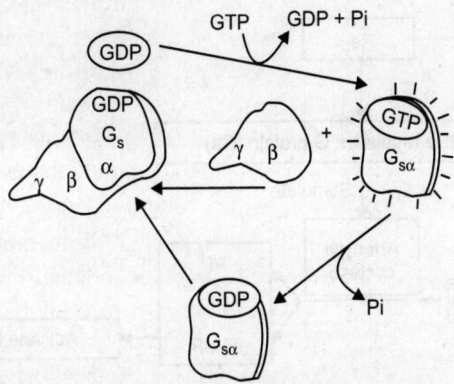

Fig. 29.3: Dissociation/association of the G-protein.

Stimulative regulative G-protein is a G-protein-linked to stimulative hormone receptor (Rs) and its α subunit upon activation could stimulate the activity of an enzyme or other intracellular metabolism. On the contrary, inhibitory regulative G-protein is linked to an inhibitory hormone receptor and its α subunit upon activation could inhibit the activity of an enzyme or other intracellular metabolism.

The adenylyl cyclase is a 12-transmembrane glucoprotein that catalyses ATP to form cAMP with the help of cofactor Mg^{2+} or Mn^{2+}. The cAMP produced is a second messenger in cellular metabolism and is an allosteric activator to protein kinase A (Fig. 29.4).

Protein kinase A is an important enzyme in cell metabolism due to its ability to regulate cell metabolism by phosphorylating specific committed enzymes in the metabolic pathway. It can also regulate specific gene expression, cellular secretion, and membrane permeability. The protein enzyme contains two catalytic subunits and two regulatory subunits. When there is no cAMP, the complex is inactive. When cAMP binds to the regulatory subunits, their conformation is altered, causing the dissociation of the regulatory subunits, which activates protein kinase A and allows further biological effects (Fig. 29.5). cAMP phosphodiesterase is an enzyme that can degrade cAMP to 5′-AMP, which will terminate the signal. Figure 29.6 shows the effect of Ri and Gs in cAMP signal pathway.

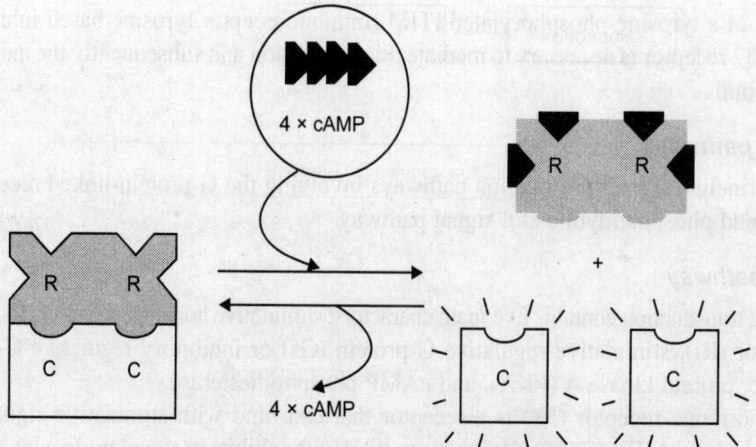

Fig. 29.4: Activation effects of cAMP on protein kinase A.

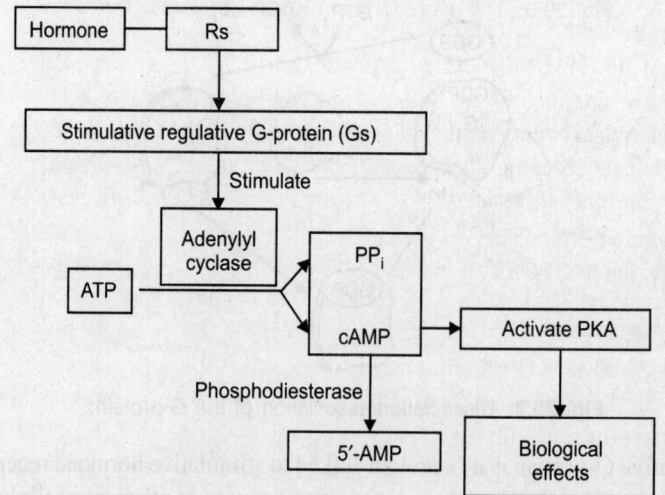

Fig. 29.5: The effect of Rs and Gs in cAMP signal pathway.

Phosphatidylinositol signal pathway: In the phosphatidylinositol signal pathway, the extracellular signal molecule binds with the G-protein receptor (G_q) on the cell surface and activates phospholipase C, which is located on the plasma membrane. The lipase hydrolyses phosphatidylinositol 4,5-bisphosphate (PIP2) into two second messengers: Inositol 1,4,5-triphosphate (IP3) and diacylglycerol (DAG).

Receptor regulation

GPCRs become desensitised when exposed to their ligand for a prolonged period of time. There are two recognised forms of desensitisation: (i) homologous desensitisation, in which the activated GPCR is downregulated, and (ii) heterologous desensitisation, wherein the activated GPCR causes downregulation of a different GPCR.

The key reaction of this downregulation is the phosphorylation of the intracellular (or cytoplasmic) receptor domain by protein kinases.

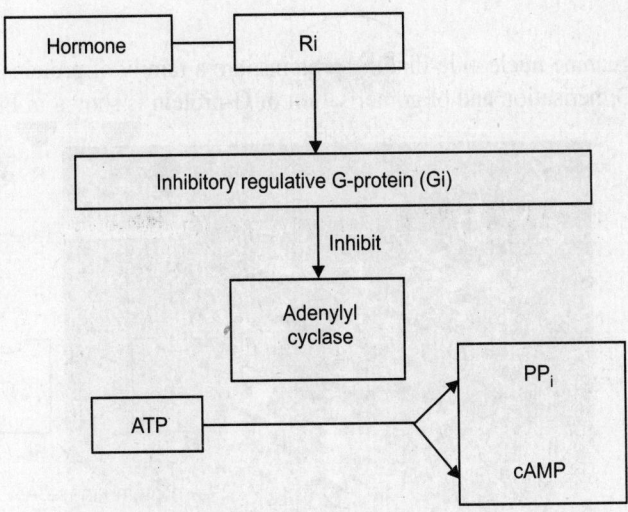

Fig. 29.6: The effect of Ri and Gs in cAMP signal pathway.

Phosphorylation by cAMP-dependent protein kinases: Cyclic AMP-dependent protein kinases (protein kinase A) are activated by the signal chain coming from the G-protein (that was activated by the receptor) via adenylate cyclase and cyclic AMP (cAMP). In a feedback mechanism, these activated kinases phosphorylate the receptor. The longer the receptor remains active, the more kinases are activated, the more receptors are phosphorylated.

Phosphorylation by GRKs: The G-protein-coupled receptor kinases (GRKs) are protein kinases that phosphorylate only active GPCRs.

Receptor oligomerisation

It is generally accepted that G-protein-coupled receptors can form heteromers such as homo- and heterodimers as well as more complex oligomeric structures, and indeed heterodimerisation has been shown to be essential for the function of receptors such as the metabotropic GABA(B) receptors. However, it is presently unproven that true heterodimers exist. Present biochemical and physical techniques lack the resolution to differentiate between distinct homodimers assembled into an oligomer or true 1:1 heterodimers. It is also unclear what the functional significance of oligomerisation might be, although it is thought that the phenomenon may contribute to the pharmacological heterogeneity of GPCRs in a manner not previously anticipated. This is an actively-studied area in GPCR research.

The best-studied example of receptor oligomerisation are the metabotropic GABA$_B$ receptors. These receptors are formed by heterodimerisation of GABA$_B$R1 and GABA$_B$R2 subunits. Expression of the GABA$_B$R1 without the GABA$_B$R2 in heterologous systems leads to retention of the subunit in the endoplasmic reticulum. Expression of the GABA$_B$R2 subunit alone, meanwhile, leads to surface expression of the subunit, although with no functional activity (i.e. the receptor does not bind agonist and cannot initiate a response following exposure to agonist). Expression of the two subunits together leads to plasma membrane expression of functional receptor. It has been shown that GABA$_B$R2 binding to GABA$_B$R1 causes masking of a retention signal of functional receptors.

Dictyostelium: A novel GPCR containing a lipid kinase domain has recently been identified in *Dictyostelium* that regulates cell density sensing.

G-Protein

G-proteins, short for guanine nucleotide-binding proteins, are a family of proteins involved in second messenger cascades. Dimerisation and oligomerisation of G-protein is shown in Fig. 29.7.

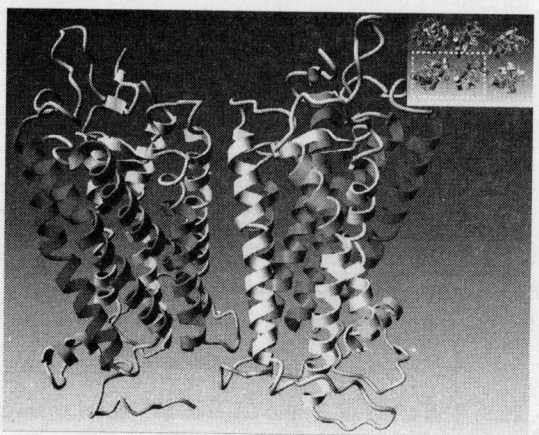

Fig. 29.7: Dimerisation and oligomerisation of G-protein.

G-proteins are so-called because they function as 'molecular switches'. They alternate from 'inactive' guanosine diphosphate (GDP) (Fig. 29.8) to 'active' guanosine triphosphate (GTP) (Fig. 29.9), which is a binding state, and which proceeds to regulate downstream cell processes.

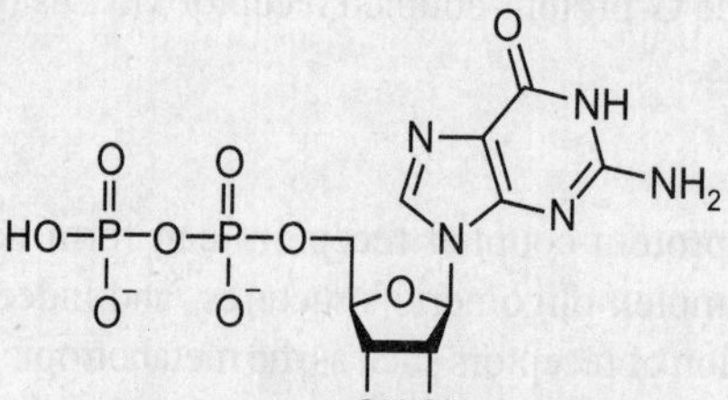

Fig. 29.8: Guanosine diphosphate.

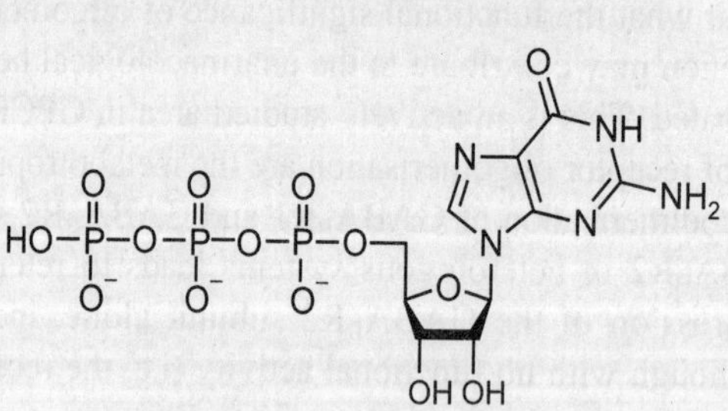

Fig. 29.9: Guanosine triphosphate.

G-proteins were discovered when Alfred G. Gilman and Martin Rodbell investigated stimulation of cells by adrenaline. They found that, when adrenaline binds to a receptor, the receptor does not stimulate enzymes directly. Instead, the receptor stimulates a G-protein, which stimulates an enzyme, for example, adenylate cyclase, which produces a second messenger, cyclic AMP. For this discovery they won the 1994 Nobel prize in physiology or medicine. G-proteins belong to the larger group of enzymes called GTPases.

Function of G-protein

G-proteins are important signal transducing molecules in cells. In fact, diseases such as diabetes, blindness, allergies, depression, cardiovascular defects, and certain forms of cancer, among other pathologies, are thought to arise due to derangement of G-protein signalling. The human genomes encodes roughly 950 G-protein-coupled receptors, which detect photons (light), hormones, growth factors, drugs, and other endogenous ligands. Approximately 150 of the GPCRs found in the human genome have unknown functions.

Types of G-protein signalling

G-protein can refer to two distinct families of proteins. Heterotrimeric G-proteins, sometimes referred to as the large G-proteins that are activated by G-protein-coupled receptors and made up of alpha (α), beta (β), and gamma (γ) subunits. There are also small G-proteins (20–25 kDa) that belong to the Ras superfamily of small GTPases. These proteins are homologous to the alpha (α) subunit found in heterotrimers, and are in fact monomeric. However, they also bind GTP and GDP and are involved in signal transduction.

Heterotrimeric G-proteins: Different types of heterotrimeric G-proteins share a common mechanism. They are activated in response to a conformation change in the G-protein-coupled receptor, exchange GDP for GTP, and dissociate to activate other proteins in the signal transduction pathway. The specific mechanisms, however, differ among the types.

Common mechanism: Receptor-activated G-proteins are bound to the inside surface of the cell membrane. They consist of the G_α and the tightly associated $G_{\beta\gamma}$ subunits. There are four classes of G_α subunits: $G_{\alpha s}$, $G_{\alpha i}$, $G_{\alpha q/11}$, and $G_{\alpha 12/13}$. They behave differently in the recognition of the effector, but share a similar mechanism of activation.

Activation: When a ligand activates the G-protein-coupled receptor, it induces a conformational change in the receptor that allows the receptor to function as a guanine nucleotide exchange factor (GEF) that exchanges GDP for GTP on the G_α subunit. In the traditional view of heterotrimeric protein activation, this exchange triggers the dissociation of the G_α subunit, bound to GTP, from the $G_{\beta\gamma}$ dimer and the receptor. However, models that suggest molecular rearrangement, reorganisation, and pre-complexing of effector molecules are beginning to be accepted. Both G_α-GTP and $G_{\beta\gamma}$ can then activate different signalling cascades (or second messenger pathways) and effector proteins, while the receptor is able to activate the next G-protein.

Termination: The G_α subunit will eventually hydrolyse the attached GTP to GDP by its inherent enzymatic activity, allowing it to re-associate with $G_{\beta\gamma}$ and starting a new cycle. A group of proteins called RBMs or RGSs, act as GTPase-activating proteins (GAPs), specific for G_α subunits. These proteins act to accelerate hydrolysis of GTP to GDP and terminate the transduced signal. In some cases, the effector itself may possess intrinsic GAP activity, which helps deactivate the pathway. This is true in the case of phospholipase C beta, which possesses GAP activity within its C-terminal region. This is an alternate form of regulation for the G_α subunit.

Specific mechanisms

1. $G_{\alpha s}$ activates the cAMP-dependent pathway by stimulating the production of cAMP from ATP. This is accomplished by direct stimulation of the membrane-associated enzyme adenylate cyclase.

cAMP acts as a second messenger that goes on to interact with and activate protein kinase A (PKA). PKA can then phosphorylate a myriad of downstream targets.

2. $G_{\alpha i}$ inhibits the production of cAMP from ATP.

3. $G_{\alpha q/11}$ stimulates membrane-bound phospholipase C beta, which then cleaves PIP_2 (a minor membrane phosphoinositol) into two second messengers, IP3 and diacylglycerol (DAG).

4. $G_{\alpha 12/13}$ are involved in Rho family GTPase signalling (through RhoGEF superfamily) and control cell cytoskeleton remodelling, thus regulating cell migration.

5. $G_{\beta\gamma}$ sometimes also have active functions, e.g. coupling to L-type calcium channels.

Small GTPases: Small GTPases also bind GTP and GDP and are involved in signal transduction. These proteins are homologous to the alpha (α) subunit found in heterotrimers, but exist as monomers. They are small (20-kDa to 25-kDa) proteins that bind to guanosine triphosphate (GTP). This family of proteins is homologous to Ras GTPases and is also called the Ras superfamily GTPases.

Lipidation

In order to associate with the inner leaflet of the plasma membrane, many G-proteins and small GTPases are lipidated, that is, covalently modified with lipid extensions. They may be myristolated, palmitoylated or prenylated.

Bacterial toxin

A bacterial toxin is a type of toxin that is generated by bacteria. Toxinosis is pathogenesis caused by the bacterial toxin alone, not necessarily involving bacterial infection (e.g. when the bacteria have died, but have already produced toxin, which becomes ingested). It can be caused by *Staphylococcus aureus* toxins.

One primary classification used is to distinguish between exotoxin and endotoxin.

1. Exotoxins are generated by the bacteria and actively secreted.

2. Endotoxins are part of the bacteria itself. Usually, endotoxin is part of the bacterial outer membrane, and it is not released until the bacteria is killed by the immune system. The body's response to endotoxin can involve severe inflammation. In general, the inflammation process is usually considered beneficial to the infected host, but if the reaction is severe enough, it can lead to sepsis.

Some bacterial toxins can be used in the treatment of tumours.

Second Messengers

Intracellular signal transduction is largely carried out by second messenger molecules.

Calcium: Ca^{2+} concentration is usually maintained at a very low level in the cytosol by sequestration in the smooth endoplasmic reticulum and the mitochondria. Ca^{2+} release from the endoplasmic reticulum into the cytosol results in the binding of the released Ca^{2+} to signalling proteins that are then activated.

There are two combined receptor/ion channel proteins that perform the task of controlled transport of Ca^{2+}:

1. The $InsP_3$-receptor will transport Ca^{2+} upon interaction with inositol triphosphate (thus the name) on its cytosolic side. It consists of four identical subunits.

2. The ryanodine receptor is named after the plant alkaloid ryanodine. It is similar to the $InsP_3$ receptor and stimulated to transport Ca^{2+} into the cytosol by recognising Ca^{2+} on its cytosolic side, thus establishing a feedback mechanism, a small amount of Ca^{2+} in the cytosol near the receptor

will cause it to release even more Ca^{2+}. It is especially important in neurons and muscle cells. In heart and pancreas cells, another second messenger (cyclic-ADP ribose) takes part in the receptor activation. The localised and time-limited activity of Ca^{2+} in the cytosol is also called a Ca^{2+} wave. Once released into the cytosol from intracellular stores or extracellular sources, Ca^{2+} acts as a signal molecule within the cell. This works by tightly limiting the time and space when Ca^{2+} is free (and thus active). Therefore, the concentration of free Ca^{2+} within the cell is usually very low, it is stored within organelles, usually the endoplasmic reticulum (sarcoplasmic reticulum in muscle cells), where it is bound to molecules like calreticulin.

Ca^{2+} is used in a multitude of processes, among them muscle contraction, release of neurotransmitter from nerve endings, vision in retina cells, proliferation, secretion, cytoskeleton management, cell migration, gene expression, and metabolism. The three main pathways that lead to Ca^{2+} activation are:

1. G-protein-regulated pathways.
2. Pathways regulated by receptor-tyrosine kinases.
3. Ligand- or current-regulated ion channels.

There are two different ways by which Ca^{2+} can regulate proteins:

1. A direct recognition of Ca^{2+} by the protein.
2. Binding of Ca^{2+} in the active site of an enzyme.

One of the best-studied interactions of Ca^{2+} with a protein is the regulation of calmodulin by Ca^{2+}. Calmodulin itself can regulate other proteins or be part of a larger protein (for example, phosphorylase kinase). The Ca^{2+}/calmodulin complex plays an important role in proliferation, mitosis, and neural signal transduction.

Lipophilic: Lipophilic second messenger molecules are derived from lipids that normally reside in cellular membranes. Enzymes stimulated by activated receptors modify the lipids, converting them into second messengers. Diacylglycerol is a lipophilic second messenger, required for the activation of protein kinase C. Ceramide, the eicosanoids, and lysophosphatidic acid are also lipophilic second messengers.

Nitric oxide: Nitric oxide (NO) can act as a second messenger. Nitric oxide gas is a free radical that diffuses through the plasma membrane and affects nearby cells. NO is made from arginine and oxygen by the enzyme NO synthase, with citrulline as a by-product. NO works mainly through activation of its target receptor, the enzyme soluble guanylate cyclase, which, when activated, produces the second messenger cyclic-guanosine monophosphate (cGMP). NO can also act through covalent modification of proteins or their metal co-factors.

Some of these modifications are reversible and work through a redox mechanism. NO is toxic in high concentrations, and is thought to cause damages caused by stroke. NO is involved in a number of functions, including relaxation of blood vessels, regulation of exocytosis of neurotransmitters, cellular immune response, modulation of the hair cycle, production and maintenance of penile erections, and activation of apoptosis by initiating signals that lead to H2AX phosphorylation.

Major pathway examples

1. cAMP-dependent pathway: In humans, cAMP works by activating protein kinase A (PKA, cAMP-dependent protein kinase), and thus, further effects mainly depend on cAMP-dependent protein kinase, which vary based on the type of cell.

2. MAPK/ERK pathway: A pathway that couples intracellular responses to the binding of growth factors to cell surface receptors. This pathway is very complex and includes many protein components. In many cell types, activation of this pathway promotes cell division.

3. IP_3/DAG pathway: PLC cleaves the phospholipid phosphatidylinositol 4,5-bisphosphate (PIP_2) yielding diacyl glycerol (DAG) and inositol 1,4,5-triphosphate (IP_3). DAG remains bound to the membrane, and IP_3 is released as a soluble structure into the cytosol. IP_3 then diffuses through the cytosol to bind to IP_3 receptors, particular calcium channels in the endoplasmic reticulum (ER). These channels are specific to calcium and only allow the passage of calcium to move through. This causes the cytosolic concentration of calcium to increase, causing a cascade of intracellular changes and activity. In addition, calcium and DAG together works to activate PKC, which goes on to phosphorylate other molecules, leading to altered cellular activity. End effects include taste, manic depression, tumour promotion, etc.

Phosphatidylinositol

Phosphatidylinositol (abbreviated PtdIns or PI) is a negatively charged phospholipid and a minor component in the cytosolic side of eukaryotic cell membranes. The inositol can be phosphorylated to form phosphatidylinositol phosphate (PIP), phosphatidylinositol bisphosphate (PIP_2) and phosphatidylinositol trisphosphate (PIP_3). PIP, PIP_2 and PIP_3 are collectively called phosphoinositides.

Biosynthesis: The synthesis of phosphatidylinositol is catalysed by phosphatidylinositol synthase and involves CDP-diacylglycerol and L-*myo*-inositol.

Chemistry: PI has a polar and nonpolar region, making the lipid an amphiphile. Amphiphatic lipids demonstrate polymorphic behaviour, a current academic research topic. Phosphatidylinositol is classified as a glycerophospholipid that contains a glycerol backbone, two nonpolar fatty acid tails, a phosphate group substituted with an inositol polar head group. The most common fatty acids of phosphoinositides are stearic acid in the SN_1 position and arachidonic acid, in the SN_2 position. Hydrolysis of phosphoinositides yield one mole of glycerol, two moles of fatty acids, one mole of inositol and one, two, or three moles of phosphoric acids, depending on the number of phosphates on the inositol rings. Phosphoinositides are regarded as the most acidic phospholipid.

Phosphoinositides: Phosphorylated forms of phosphatidylinositol are called phosphoinositides and play important roles in lipid signalling, cell signalling and membrane trafficking. The inositol ring can be phosphorylated by a variety of kinases on the three, four and five hydroxyl groups in seven different combinations. However, the two and six hydroxyl group is typically not phosphorylated due to steric hindrance.

Phospholipase C

Phospholipase C is a class of enzymes that cleave phospholipids just before the phosphate group. It is most commonly taken to be synonymous with the human forms of this enzyme, which plays an important role in eukaryotic cell physiology, in particular signal transduction pathways. Thirteen kinds of mammalian phospholipase C are classified into six models (β, γ, δ, ε, ζ, η) according to structure.

Human variant: The human variant has EC. 3.1.4.11.

Activation: Receptors that activate this pathway are mainly G-protein-coupled receptors coupled to the $G_{\alpha q}$ subunit, including:

1. 5-HT_2 serotonergic receptors.

2. α_1 (alpha-1) adrenergic receptors.

3. Calcitonin receptor.

4. H_1 histamine receptor.

5. Metabotropic glutamate receptor, Group I.

6. M_1, M_3, and M_5 muscarinic receptors.

Other, minor, activators than $G_{\alpha q}$ are:

1. MAP kinase. Activators of this pathway include PDGF and FGF.

2. $\beta\gamma$-complex of heterotrimeric G-proteins, as in a minor pathway of growth hormone release by growth hormone-releasing hormone.

Effects: PLC cleaves a phospholipid. In the process, phosphatidylinositol 4,5-bisphosphate (PIP_2) is cleaved into diacyl glycerol (DAG) and inositol 1,4,5-trisphosphate (IP_3). DAG remains bound to the membrane, and IP_3 is released as a soluble structure into the cytosol. IP_3 then diffuses through the cytosol to bind to IP_3 receptors, particular calcium channels in the endoplasmic reticulum (ER). This causes the cytosolic concentration of calcium to increase, causing a cascade of intracellular changes and activity. In addition, calcium and DAG together work to activate protein kinase C, which goes on to phosphorylate other molecules, leading to altered cellular activity. End effects include taste, tumour promotion, etc.

In other organisms: Other phospholipase C enzymes have been identified in bacteria and in trypanosomes, each with its own EC number.

1. Phosphoinositide phospholipase C EC 3.1.4.11. The main form found in eukaryotes, especially mammals.

2. Zinc-dependent phospholipase C family of bacterial enzymes EC 3.1.4.3 that includes alpha toxins.

3. Phosphatidylinositol diacylglycerol-lyase EC 4.6.1.13. Another related bacterial enzyme.

4. Glycosylphosphatidylinositol diacylglycerol-lyase EC 4.6.1.14. A trypanosomal enzyme.

Blood Sugar

The blood sugar concentration or blood glucose level is the amount of glucose (sugar) present in the blood of a human or animal. Normally, in mammals the body maintains the blood glucose level at a reference range between about 3.6 and 5.8 mM (mmol/l). It is tightly regulated as a part of metabolic homeostasis. Glucose is the primary source of energy for body's cell, lipids (in the form of fats and oils) being primarily a compact energy store. It is transported from the intestines or liver to body cells via the bloodstream, and is absorbed by body cells with the intervention of the hormone insulin normally produced by the body. The mean normal blood glucose level in humans is about 4 mM (4 mmol/l or 72 mg/dl). However, the glucose level fluctuates during the day. It rises after meals for an hour or two by a few grams and is usually lowest in the morning, before the first meal of the day (termed 'the fasting level'). When a blood sugar level is outside the normal range, it may be an indicator of a medical condition. A persistently high level is referred to as hyperglycemia or if low as hypoglycemia.

Diabetes mellitus is characterised by persistent hyperglycemia from any of several causes, and is the most prominent disease related to failure of blood sugar regulation. A temporary elevated blood sugar level may also result from severe stress, such as trauma, stroke, heart attack or surgery, and also from illness. Alcohol, after an initial surge in blood sugar, tends to cause blood sugar to fall. Also, certain drugs can increase or decrease glucose levels.

Blood glucose measurement units

In most countries, blood glucose levels are reported in terms of a molar concentration, measured in mmol/l (millimoles per litre, or millimolar, abbreviated mM). In the United States, and in other places, mass concentration, measured in mg/dl (milligrams per decilitre), is typically used. Since the molecular weight of glucose $C_6H_{12}O_6$ is about 180 g/mol, for the measurement of glucose, the difference between the two scales is a factor of 18, so that 1 mmol/l of glucose is equivalent to 18 mg/dl.

Normal values

Many factors affect a person's blood sugar level. A body's homeostatic mechanism, when operating normally, restores the blood sugar level to a narrow range of about 4.4 to 6.1 mmol/l (82 to 110 mg/dl). Despite widely variable intervals between meals or the occasional consumption of meals with a substantial carbohydrate load, human blood glucose levels normally remain within the normal range. However, shortly after eating the blood glucose level may rise temporarily up to 7.8 mmol/l (140 mg/dl) or a bit more in non-diabetics. The American Diabetes Association recommends a post-meal glucose level less than 10 mmol/l (180 mg/dl) and a pre-meal plasma glucose of 5 to 7.2 mmol/l (90–130 mg/dl).

The actual amount of glucose in the blood and body fluids is very small. The control mechanism in the human body works on very small quantities of glucose. In a healthy adult male of 75 kg (165 lb) with a blood volume of 5 litres (1.3 gal), a blood glucose level of 100 mg/dl or 5.5 mmol/l corresponds to about 5 g (0.2 oz or 0.002 gal, 1/500 of the total) of glucose in the blood and approximately 45 g (1½ ounces) in the total body water (which includes more than merely blood and will be usually about 60 per cent of the total body weight in men).

Regulation

A body's homeostatic mechanism keeps blood glucose levels within a narrow range. It is composed of several interacting systems, of which hormone regulation is the most important.

There are two types of mutually antagonistic metabolic hormones affecting blood glucose levels:

1. Catabolic hormones (such as glucagon, growth hormone, cortisol and catecholamines) which increase blood glucose.
2. One anabolic hormone (insulin), which decreases blood glucose.

Health effects

If blood sugar levels drop too low, a potentially fatal condition called hypoglycemia develops. Symptoms may include lethargy, impaired mental functioning, irritability, shaking, weakness in arm and leg muscles, sweating and loss of consciousness. Brain damage is even possible. If levels remain too high, appetite is suppressed over the short-term. Long-term hyperglycemia causes many of the long-term health problems associated with diabetes, including eye, kidney, heart disease and nerve damage.

Low blood sugar

Some people report drowsiness or impaired cognitive function several hours after meals, which they believe is related to a drop in blood sugar, or 'low blood sugar'. Mechanisms which restore satisfactory blood glucose levels after hypoglycemia must be quick and effective, because of the immediately serious consequences of insufficient glucose, in the extreme, coma, but also less immediately dangerous, confusion or unsteadiness, amongst many other symptoms. This is because, at least in the short-term, it is far more dangerous to have too little glucose in the blood than too much. In healthy individuals these mechanisms are generally quite effective, and symptomatic hypoglycemia is generally only found in diabetics using insulin or other pharmacological treatment. Such hypoglycemic episodes vary greatly between persons and from time to time, both in severity and swiftness of onset. For severe cases, prompt medical assistance is essential, as damage (to brain and other tissues) and even death will result from sufficiently low blood glucose levels.

Glucose measurement

Sample type: Glucose can be measured in whole blood or serum (i.e. plasma). Historically, blood glucose values were given in terms of whole blood, but most laboratories now measure and report the serum glucose levels. Because red blood cells (erythrocytes) have a higher concentration of protein (e.g. haemoglobin) than serum, serum has a higher water content and consequently more dissolved glucose than does whole blood. To convert from whole-blood glucose, multiplication by 1.15 has been shown to generally give the serum/plasma level.

Collection of blood in clot tubes for serum chemistry analysis permits the metabolism of glucose in the sample by blood cells until separated by centrifugation. Red blood cells, for instance, do not require insulin to intake glucose from the blood. Higher than normal amounts of white or red blood cell counts can lead to excessive glycolysis in the sample with substantial reduction of glucose level if the sample is not processed quickly. Ambient temperature at which the blood sample is kept prior to centrifuging and separation of plasma/serum also affects glucose levels. At refrigerator temperatures, glucose remains relatively stable for several hours in a blood sample. At room temperature (25°C), a loss of 1 to 2 per cent of total glucose per hour should be expected in whole blood samples. Loss of glucose under these conditions can be prevented by using fluoride tubes (i.e. gray-top) since fluoride inhibits glycolysis. However, these should only be used when blood will be transported from one hospital laboratory to another for glucose measurement. Red-top serum separator tubes also preserve glucose in samples after being centrifuged isolating the serum from cells.

Particular care should be given to drawing blood samples from the arm opposite the one in which an intravenous line is inserted, to prevent contamination of the sample with intravenous fluids. Alternatively, blood can be drawn from the same arm with an IV line after the IV has been turned off for at least 5 minutes, and the arm elevated to drain infused fluids away from the vein. Inattention can lead to large errors, since as little as 10 per cent contamination with 5 per cent dextrose (D5W) will elevate glucose in a sample by 500 mg/dl or more. Remember that the actual concentration of glucose in blood is very low, even in the hyperglycemic. Arterial, capillary and venous blood have comparable glucose levels in a fasting individual. After meals venous levels are somewhat lower than capillary or arterial blood, a common estimate is about 10 per cent.

Measurement techniques: Two major methods have been used to measure glucose. The first, still in use in some places, is a chemical method exploiting the nonspecific reducing property of glucose in a reaction with an indicator substance that changes colour when reduced. Since other blood compounds also have reducing properties (e.g. urea, which can be abnormally high in uremic patients), this technique can produce erroneous readings in some situations (5 to 15 mg/dl has been reported). The more recent technique, using enzymes specific to glucose, are less susceptible to this kind of error. The two most common employed enzymes are glucose oxidase and hexokinase.

In either case, the chemical system is commonly contained on a test strip, to which a blood sample is applied, and which is then inserted into the meter for reading. Test strip shapes and their exact chemical composition vary between meter systems and cannot be interchanged. Formerly, some test strips were read (after timing and wiping away the blood sample) by visual comparison against a colour chart printed on the vial label. Strips of this type are still used for urine glucose readings, but for blood glucose levels they are obsolete. Their error rates were, in any case, much higher.

Urine glucose readings, however, taken, are much less useful. In properly functioning kidneys, glucose does not appear in urine until the renal threshold for glucose has been exceeded. This is substantially above any normal glucose level, and so is evidence of an existing severe hyperglycemic condition. However, urine is stored in the bladder and so any glucose in it might have been produced at any time since the last time the bladder was emptied. Since metabolic conditions change rapidly, as a result of any of several factors, this is delayed news and gives no warning of a developing condition. Blood glucose monitoring is far preferable, both clinically and for home monitoring by patients.

Blood glucose laboratory tests: Blood glucose laboratory tests are:

1. Fasting blood sugar (i.e. glucose) test (FBS).
2. Urine glucose test.
3. Two-hour post-prandial blood sugar test (2-hr PPBS).
4. Oral glucose tolerance test (OGTT).
5. Intravenous glucose tolerance test (IVGTT).
6. Glycosylated haemoglobin (HbA$_{1C}$).
7. Self-monitoring of glucose level via patient testing.

Clinical correlation: The fasting blood glucose (FBG) level, which is measured after a fast of 8 hr, is the most commonly used indication of overall glucose homeostasis, largely because disturbing events such as food intake are avoided. Abnormalities in these test results are due to problems in the multiple control mechanism of glucose regulation.

The metabolic response to a carbohydrate challenge is conveniently assessed by a post-prandial glucose level drawn 2 hr after a meal or a glucose load. In addition, the glucose tolerance test, consisting of several timed measurements after a standardised amount of oral glucose intake, is used to aid in the diagnosis of diabetes. It is regarded as the gold standard of clinical tests of the insulin/glucose control system, but is difficult to administer, requiring much time and repeated blood tests. In comparison, the fasting blood glucose level is a much poorer screening test because of the high variability of the experimental conditions such as the carbohydrate content of the last meal and the energy expenditure between the last meal and the measurement.

Actually, many people with prediabetes or diabetes can have a fasting blood glucose below the prediabetic/diabetic threshold if their last meal happened to be low in carbohydrate and they burnt all the related glucose in their blood stream before taking the test.

Error rates for blood glucose measurements systems vary, depending on laboratories, and on the methods used. Colorimetry techniques can be biased by colour changes in test strips (from airborne or finger borne contamination, perhaps) or interference (e.g. tinting contaminants) with light source or the light sensor. Electrical techniques are less susceptible to these errors, though not to others. In home use, the most important issue is not accuracy, but trend. Thus if your meter/test strip system is consistently wrong by 10 per cent, there will be little consequence, as long as changes (e.g. due to exercise or medication adjustments) are properly tracked. In the US, home use blood test meters must be approved by the Federal Food and Drug Administration before they can be sold.

Finally, there are several influences on blood glucose level aside from food intake. Infection, for instance, tends to change blood glucose levels, as does stress either physical or psychological. Exercise, especially if prolonged or long after the most recent meal, will have an effect as well. In the normal person, maintenance of blood glucose at near constant levels will nevertheless be quite effective.

Etymology and use of term: The term 'blood sugar' has colloquial origins. In a physiological context, the term is a misnomer because it refers to glucose, yet other sugars besides glucose are always present. Food contains several different types (e.g. fructose largely from fruits/table sugar/industrial sweeteners), galactose (milk and dairy products), as well as several food additives such as sorbitol, xylose, maltose). But because these other sugars are largely inert with regard to the metabolic control system (i.e. that controlled by insulin secretion), since glucose is the dominant controlling signal for metabolic regulation, the term has gained currency, and is used by medical staff and lay folk alike.

Blood glucose in birds and reptiles: In birds and reptiles the processing of sugars is done differently, the pancreas is slightly more well developed in birds than in mammals, perhaps as a partial compensation for the lack of saliva and chewing. It produces carbohydrate, fat and protein digesting enzymes which are secreted into the small intestine. The liver has two distinct lobes each with its own duct leading into the small intestine. The liver, as in mammals, houses the bile, which in birds however, is acidic and not alkaline as it is in mammals. Many birds do not have a gall bladder to hold the bile, and it is secreted directly into the pancreatic ducts.

cAMP-dependent pathway

In the field of molecular biology, the cAMP-dependent pathway, also known as the adenylyl cyclase pathway, is a G-protein-coupled receptor-triggered signalling cascade used in cell communication.

Mechanism: G-protein-coupled receptors (GPCRs) are a large family of integral membrane proteins that respond to a variety of extracellular stimuli. Each GPCR binds to and is activated by a specific ligand stimulus that ranges in size from small molecule catecholamines, lipids or neurotransmitters to large protein hormones. When a GPCR is activated by its extracellular ligand, a conformational change is induced in the receptor that is transmitted to an attached intracellular heterotrimeric G-protein complex.

The G_s alpha subunit of the stimulated G-protein complex exchanges GDP for GTP and is released from the complex. In a cAMP-dependent pathway, the activated G_s alpha subunit binds to and activates an enzyme called adenylyl cyclase, which, in turn, catalyse the conversion of ATP into cyclic adenosine mono-phosphate (cAMP). Increases in concentration of the second messenger cAMP may lead to the activation of:

1. Cyclic nucleotide-gated ion channels.
2. Exchange proteins activated by cAMP (EPAC) such as RAPGEF3.
3. An enzyme called protein kinase A (PKA).

The PKA enzyme is also known as cAMP-dependent enzyme because it gets activated only if cAMP is present. Once PKA is activated, it phosphorylates a number of other proteins including:

1. Enzymes that convert glycogen into glucose.
2. Enzymes that promote muscle contraction in the heart leading to an increase in heart rate.
3. Transcription factors, which regulate gene expression.

Specificity of signalling between a GPCR and its ultimate molecular target through a cAMP-dependent pathway may be achieved through formation of a multiprotein complex that includes the GPCR, adenylyl cyclase, and the effector protein. In humans, cAMP works by activating protein kinase A (PKA, cAMP-dependent protein kinase), and, thus, further effects mainly depend on cAMP-dependent protein kinase, which vary based on the type of cell.

cAMP-dependent pathway is necessary for many living organisms and life processes. Many different cell responses are mediated by cAMP. These include increase in heart rate, cortisol secretion, and breakdown of glycogen and fat. This pathway can activate enzymes and regulate gene expression. The activation of preexisting enzymes is a much faster process, whereas regulation of gene expression is much longer and can take up to hours. The cAMP pathway is studied through loss of function (inhibition) and gain of function (increase) of cAMP. If cAMP-dependent pathway is not controlled, it can ultimately lead to hyper-proliferation, which may contribute to the development and/or progression of cancer.

Activation: Activated GPCRs cause a conformational change in the attached G-protein complex, which results in the G_s alpha subunit's exchanging GDP for GTP and separation from the beta and gamma subunits. The G_s alpha subunit, in turn, activates adenylyl cyclase, which quickly converts ATP into cAMP. This leads to the activation of the cAMP-dependent pathway. This pathway can also be activated downstream by directly activating adenylyl cyclase or PKA.

Molecules that activate cAMP pathway include:

1. Cholera toxin — increase cAMP level.
2. Forskolin — a diterpine natural product that activates adenylyl cyclase.
3. Caffeine and theophylline inhibit cAMP phosphodiesterase, which leads to an activation of G-proteins that result in the activation of the cAMP pathway.
4. Bucladesine (dibutyryl cAMP, db cAMP) — also a phosphodiesterase inhibitor.
5. Pertussis toxin, which increase cAMP levels by inhibiting Gi to its GDP (inactive) form. This leads to an increase in adenylyl cyclase, therefore increasing cAMP levels, which can lead to an increase in insulin and therefore hypoglycemia.

Deactivation: The G_s alpha subunit slowly catalyses the hydrolysis of GTP to GDP, which in turn deactivates the G_s protein, shutting off the cAMP pathway. The pathway may also be deactivated downstream by directly inhibiting adenylyl cyclase or dephosphorylating the proteins phosphorylated by PKA.

Molecules that inhibit cAMP pathway include:

1. cAMP phosphodiesterase dephosphorylates cAMP into AMP, reducing the cAMP levels.
2. G_i protein, which is a G-protein that inhibits adenylyl cyclase, reducing cAMP levels.

PROTEIN TYROSINE PHOSPHORYLATION AS A MECHANISM FOR SIGNAL TRANSDUCTION

Protein tyrosine phosphatases (PTPs) are a group of enzymes that remove phosphate groups from phosphorylated tyrosine residues on proteins. Together with tyrosine kinases, PTPs regulate the phosphorylation state of many important signalling molecules, such as the MAP kinase family. PTPs are increasingly viewed as integral components of signal transduction cascades, despite less study and understanding compared to tyrosine kinases. PTPs have been implicated in regulation of many cellular processes, including, but not limited to: (i) cell growth, (ii) cellular differentiation, (iii) mitotic cycles, and (iv) oncogenic transformation.

Classification of PTPs

On the basis of the primary structure of their catalytic domains, PTPs are divided into four distinct classes: The class I PTPs, are the largest group of PTPs with 99 members which can be further subdivided into 38 classical PTPs and 61 VH-1 like or dual specific phosphatases (DSPs). The class I classical PTPs can be further subdivided into 21 receptor and 17 non-receptor type PTPs. The DSPs can also be further subdivided, in this case into 7 subfamilies made up of 11 MAPK phosphatases (MPKs), 3 Slingshots, 3 PRLs, 4CDC14s, 19 atypical DSPs, 5 phosphatase and tensin homologs (PTENs) and 16 myotubularins. The class II PTPs contain only one member, low-molecular-weight phosphotyrosine phosphatase (LMPTP). The Class III PTPs contains three members, CDC25 A, B and C and the class IV PTPs contains four members, Eya1-4. Links to all 107 members of the protein tyrosine phosphatase family can be found in the template at the bottom of this section.

Expression pattern

Individual PTPs may be expressed by all cell types or their expression may be strictly tissue specific. Most cells express 30 to 60 per cent of all the PTPs, however, haematopoietic and neuronal cells express a higher humber of PTPs in comparison to other cell types. T cells and B cells of haematopoietic origin express around 60 to 70 different PTPs. The expression of several PTPs is restricted to haematopoietic cells, for example LYP, SHP1, CD45 and HePTP.

Tyrosine Kinase

A tyrosine kinase is an enzyme that can transfer a phosphate group from ATP to a tyrosine residue in a protein. Tyrosine kinases are a subgroup of the larger class of protein kinases. Phosphorylation of proteins by kinases is an important mechanism in signal transduction for regulation of enzyme activity. Most tyrosine kinases have an associated protein tyrosine phosphatase (Fig. 29.10).

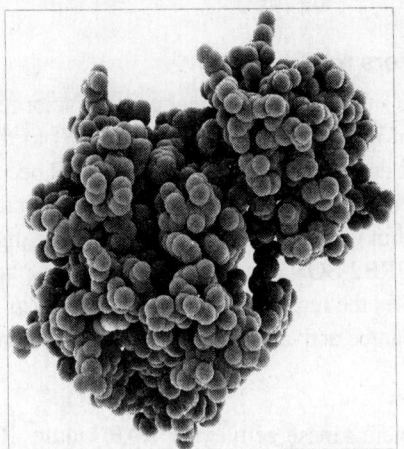

Fig. 29.10: Protein tyrosine phosphatase.

Protein kinases are a group of enzymes that possess a catalytic subunit which transfers the gamma phosphate from nucleotide triphosphates (often ATP) to one or more amino acid residues in a protein substrate side chain, resulting in a conformational change affecting protein function. The enzymes fall into two broad classes, characterised with respect to substrate specificity: serine/threonine specific and tyrosine specific (this domain). The tyrosine kinases are divided into two main families:

1. The transmembrane receptor-linked kinases.
2. Those that are cytoplasmic proteins.

Receptor

Approximately 2000 kinases are known, and more than 90 protein tyrosine kinases (PTKs) have been found in the human genome. They are divided into two classes, receptor and non-receptor PTKs. At present, 58 receptor tyrosine kinases (RTKs) are known, grouped into 20 subfamilies. They play pivotal roles in diverse cellular activities including growth, differentiation, metabolism, adhesion, motility, death. RTKs are composed of an extracellular domain, which is able to bind a specific ligand, a transmembrane domain, and an intracellular catalytic domain, which is able to bind and phosphorylate selected substrates.

Cytoplasmic/non-receptor

In humans, there are 32 cytoplasmic protein tyrosine kinases (EC 2.7.10.2). The first non-receptor tyrosine kinase identified was the *v-Src* oncogenic protein. Most animal cells contain one or more members of the *Src* family of tyrosine kinases. A chicken sarcoma virus was found to carry mutated versions of the normal cellular *Src* gene. The mutated *v-Src* gene has lost the normal built-in inhibition of enzyme activity that is characteristic of cellular SRC (*c-Src*) genes. SRC family members have been found to regulate many cellular processes.

For example, the T-cell antigen receptor leads to intracellular signalling by activation of *Lck* and *Fyn*, two proteins that are structurally similar to *Src*.

MAPK/ERK Pathway

The MAPK/ERK pathway is a signal transduction pathway that couples intracellular responses to the binding of growth factors to cell surface receptors. This pathway is very complex and includes many protein components.

Coupling cell surface receptors to G-proteins

Receptor-linked tyrosine kinases such as the epidermal growth factor receptor (EGFR) are activated by extracellular ligands. Binding of epidermal growth factor (EGF) to the EGFR activates the tyrosine kinase activity of the cytoplasmic domain of the receptor. The EGFR becomes phosphorylated on tyrosine residues. Docking proteins such as GRB2 contain SH2 domains that bind to the phosphotyrosine residues of the activated receptor. GRB2 binds to the guanine nucleotide exchange factor SOS by way of an SH3 domain of GRB2. When the GRB2-SOS complex docks to phosphorylated EGFR, SOS becomes activated. Activated SOS promotes the removal of GDP from *Ras*. *Ras* can then bind GTP and become active. Other small G-proteins can be activated in a similar way, but are not discussed further here.

Kinase cascade

Activated Ras activates the protein kinase activity of RAF kinase. RAF kinase phosphorylates and activates MEK. MEK phosphorylates and activates a mitogen-activated protein kinase (MAPK). RAF, MEK and MAPK are all serine/threonine-selective protein kinases. Technically, RAF, MEK and MAPK are all mitogen-activated kinases, as is MNK. MAPK was originally called 'extracellular signal-regulated kinases' (ERKs) and microtubule-associated protein kinase (MAPK). One of the first proteins known to be phosphorylated by ERK was a microtubule-associated protein. Many additional targets for phosphorylation by MAPK were later found and the protein was renamed 'mitogen-activated protein kinase' (MAPK). The series of kinases from RAF to MEK to MAPK is an example of a protein kinase cascade. Such series of kinases provide opportunities for feedback regulation and signal amplification.

Regulation of translation and transcription

MAPK regulates the activities of several transcription factors. MAPK can phosphorylate C-*myc*. MAPK phosphorylates and activates MNK which in turn phosphorylates CREB. MAPK also regulates the transcription of the *C-Fos* gene. By altering the levels and activities of transcription factors, MAPK leads to altered transcription of genes that are important for the cell cycle. The 22q11, 1q42, and 19p13 genes are associated with schizophrenia, schizo-affective, bipolar and migraines by affecting the ERK pathway.

Clinical significance

The kinase cascade is relevant to many cancers, e.g. Hodgkin disease. The first drug licensed to act on this pathway is sorafenib—a Raf kinase inhibitor. Protein microarray analysis can be used to detect subtle changes in protein activity in signalling pathways.

GTPase-activating protein: GTPase-activating proteins or GAPs or GTPase-accelerating proteins is a family of regulatory proteins whose members can bind to activated G-proteins and stimulate their GTPase activity, with the result of terminating the signalling event. GAPs mediate switching a G-protein on and off. G-proteins are switched from the active, GTP-bound form to the inactive, GDP-bound form by hydrolysis of the GTP through intrinsic GTPase-activity.

It can be reverted (switching the G-protein on again) by guanine nucleotide exchange factors (GEFs). Only the active state of the G-protein can transduce a signal to a reactor chain.

The ability of GAPs to turn off G proteins depends on their local concentration in the cell, and on their own activity state. Both of these are frequently under regulation of one or more signalling pathways, and modified by binding to other regulatory proteins or specific lipids, or by phosphorylation.

An example of a GTPase is the monomer *Ran*, which is found in the cytosol as well as the nucleus. Hydrolysis of GTP by Ran is thought to provide the energy needed to transport nuclear proteins into the cell. Ran is turned on or off by GEFs and GAPs, respectively.

Guanine nucleotide exchange factor: Guanine nucleotide exchange factors (GEFs) are components of intracellular signalling networks. They function as activators of small GTPases. G-proteins function as molecular switches, where the resting (inactive) state they are bound to guanosine dephosphate (GDP) and their activation requires the dissociation of GDP and binding of guanosine triphosphate (GTP), which exists at a approximate 10-fold higher concentration in the cell cytoplasm. GEFs activate G-proteins by promoting this nucleotide exchange. The hundreds of GEFs described thus far exhibit varying degrees of specificity with some being able to activate multiple G-proteins of different families and other only able to activate one specific isoform.

Regulation: The GEF activity of a given protein is provided by one or more protein domains. A tandem placement of a dbl homology (DH) domain followed by a pleckstrin homology (PH) domain forms the minimal functional unit of most GEFs (those of the dbl family). Specifically, DH domain is the catalytic site required for GDP-GTP exchange, while the PH domain contributes to protein-protein, protein-cytoskeleton and protein-lipid intractions to help regulate the GEF's intracellular localisation and catalytic activity. Other accessory/regulatory domains are usually present in the protein displaying complementary, inhibitory or unrelated functions. GEF domains can be found in variety of signalling proteins, many of which are unrelated with respect to structure and physiological function. Examples of GEFs: (i) Son of sevenless (SOS), (ii) dedicator of cytokinesis (DOCK), and (iii) Vav.

Guanosine nucleotide dissociation inhibitors: The guanosine nucleotide dissociation inhibitors (GEIs), bind to the GDP-bound form of Rho and Rab small GTPases and not only prevent exchange (maintaining the small GTPase in an off-state), but also prevent the small GTPase from localising at the membrane, which is their place of action. This inhibition can be removed by the action of a guanine nucleotide exchange factor (GEF).

Insulin Receptor

In molecular biology, the insulin receptor is a transmembrane receptor that is activated by insulin. It belongs to the large class of tyrosine kinase receptors. Two alpha subunits and two beta subunits make up the insulin receptor. The beta subunits pass through the cellular membrane and are linked by disulphide bonds. The alpha and beta subunits are encoded by a single gene (INSR). The insulin receptor has also recently been designated CD220 (cluster of differentiation 220).

Function

Tyrosine kinase receptors, including the insulin receptor, mediate their activity by causing the addition of a phosphate group to particular tyrosines on certain proteins within a cell. The 'substrate' proteins which are phosphorylated by the insulin receptor include a protein called 'IRS-1' for 'insulin receptor substrate 1'. IRS-1 binding and phosphorylation eventually leads to an increase in the high affinity glucose transporter (Glut4) molecules on the outer membrane of insulin-responsive tissues, including muscle cells and adipose tissue, and therefore to an increase in the uptake of glucose from blood into these tissues. Briefly, the glucose transporter Glut4 is transported from cellular vesicles to the cell surface, where it then can mediate the transport of glucose into the cell.

The main activity of activation of the insulin receptor is inducing glucose uptake. For this reason 'insulin insensitivity' or a decrease in insulin receptor signalling, leads to diabetes mellitus type 2 — the cells are unable to take up glucose, and the result is hyperglycemia (an increase in circulating glucose), and all the sequelae which result from diabetes. Patients with insulin resistance may display acanthosis nigricans. A few patients with homozygous mutations in the INSR gene have been described, which causes Donohue syndrome or Leprechaunism.

This autosomal recessive disorder results in a totally non-functional insulin receptor. These patients have low set, often protuberant ears, flared nostrils, thickened lips, and severe growth retardation. In most cases, the outlook for these patients is extremely poor with death occurring within the first year of life. Other mutations of the same gene cause the less severe Rabson-Mendenhall syndrome, in which patients have characteristically abnormal teeth, hypertrophic gingiva (gums) and enlargement of the pineal gland. Both diseases present with fluctuations of the glucose level: after a meal the glucose is initially very high, and then falls rapidly to abnormally low levels.

Regulation of gene expression

The activated IRS-1 acts as a secondary messenger within the cell to stimulate the transcription of insulin-regulated genes. First, the protein Grb2 binds the P-Tyr residue of IRS-1 in its SH2 domain. Grb2 is then able to bind SOS, which in turn catalyses the replacement of bound GDP with GTP on Ras, a G-protein. This protein then begins a phosphorylation cascade, culminating in the activation of mitogen-activated protein kinase (MAPK), which enters the nucleus and phosphorylates various nuclear transcription factors (such as Elk1).

Stimulation of glycogen synthesis

Glycogen synthesis is also stimulated by the insulin receptor via IRS-1. In this case, it is the SH2 domain of PI-3 kinase (PI-3K) that binds the P-Tyr of IRS-1. Now activated, PI-3K can convert the membrane lipid phosphatidylinositol 4,5-bisphosphate (PIP2) to phosphatidylinositol 3,4,5-triphosphate (PIP3). This indirectly activates a protein kinase, PKB (Akt), via phosphorylation. PKB then phosphorylates several target proteins, including glycogen synthase kinase 3 (GSK-3).

Degradation of insulin

Once an insulin molecule has docked onto the receptor and effected its action, it may be released back into the extracellular environment or it may be degraded by the cell. Degradation normally involves endocytosis of the insulin-receptor complex followed by the action of insulin degrading enzyme. Most insulin molecules are degraded by liver cells. It has been estimated that a typical insulin molecule is finally degraded about 71 minutes after its initial release into circulation.

Interactions

Insulin receptor has been shown to interact with ectonucleotide pyrophosphatase/phosphodiesterase 1, PTPN11, GRB10, GRB7, PRKCD, IRS1, SH2B1 and Mothers against decapentaplegic homologue 2.

Insulin receptor substrate

Insulin receptor substrate (IRS) is an important ligand in the insulin response of human cells. IRS-1, for example, is an IRS protein which contains a PTB-domain. In addition, the insulin receptor contains a NPXpY domain. The PTB-domain binds the NPXpY domain. Thus, the insulin receptor binds IRS.

Glucose transporter

Glucose transporters (GLUT or SLC2A family) are a family of membrane proteins found in most mammalian cells. Glucose (Fig. 29.11) is an essential substrate for the metabolism of most cells. Because glucose is a polar molecule, transport through biological membranes requires specific transport proteins.

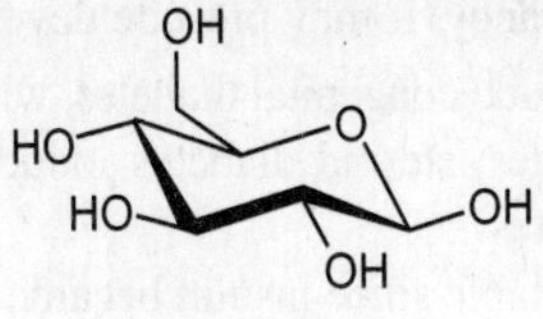

Fig. 29.11: Glucose.

Active transport—cotransporters: Transport of glucose through the apical membrane of intestinal and kidney epithelial cells depends on the presence of secondary active Na^+/glucose symporters, SGLT-1 and SGLT-2, which concentrate glucose inside the cells, using the energy provided by cotransport of Na^+ ions down their electrochemical gradient.

Passive transport—GLUTs: Facilitated diffusion of glucose through the cellular membrane is otherwise catalysed by glucose carriers (protein symbol GLUT, gene symbol SLC2 for solute carrier family 2) that belong to a superfamily of transport facilitators (major facilitator superfamily) including organic anion and cation transporters, yeast hexose transporter, plant hexose/proton symporters, and bacterial sugar/proton symporters. Molecule movement by such transporter proteins occurs by facilitated diffusion. This makes them energy independent, unlike active transporters which often require the presence of ATP to drive their translocation mechanism, and stall if the ATP/ADP ratio drops too low.

GLUTs are integral membrane proteins which contain 12 membrane spanning helices with both the amino and carboxyl termini exposed on the cytoplasmic side of the plasma membrane. GLUT proteins transport glucose and related hexoses according to a model of alternate conformation, which predicts that the transporter exposes a single substrate binding site toward either the outside or the inside of the cell. Binding of glucose to one site provokes a conformational change associated with transport, and releases glucose to the other side of the membrane. The inner and outer glucose-binding sites are probably located in transmembrane segments 9, 10, 11, also, the QLS motif located in the seventh transmembrane segment could be involved in the selection and affinity of transported substrate.

Types: Each glucose transporter isoform plays a specific role in glucose metabolism determined by its pattern of tissue expression, substrate specificity, transport kinetics, and regulated expression in different physiological conditions. To date, 13 members of the GLUT/SLC2 have been identified.

Diabetes mellitus

Diabetes mellitus (DM), often simply referred to as diabetes—is a condition in which a person has a high blood sugar (glucose) level as a result of the body either not producing enough insulin, or because body cells do not properly respond to the insulin that is produced. Insulin is a hormone produced in the pancreas which enables body cells to absorb glucose, to turn into energy. If the body cells do not absorb the glucose, the glucose accumulates in the blood (hyperglycemia), leading to various potential medical complications.

There are many types of diabetes, the most common of which are:

1. Type 1 diabetes results from the body's failure to produce insulin, and presently requires the person to inject insulin.

2. Type 2 diabetes results from insulin resistance, a condition in which cells fail to use insulin properly, sometimes combined with an absolute insulin deficiency.

3. Gestational diabetes is when pregnant women, who have never had diabetes before, have a high blood glucose level during pregnancy. It may precede development of type 2 DM.

Other forms of diabetes mellitus include congenital diabetes, which is due to genetic defects of insulin secretion, cystic fibrosis-related diabetes, steroid diabetes induced by high doses of glucocorticoids, and several forms of monogenic diabetes.

All forms of diabetes have been treatable since insulin became medically available in 1921, and type 2 diabetes can be controlled with tablets, but it is chronic condition that usually cannot be cured. Pancreas transplants have been tried with limited success in type 1 DM, gastric by-pass surgery has been successful in many with morbid obesity and type 2 DM, and gestational diabetes usually resolves after delivery. Diabetes without proper treatments can cause many complications. Acute complications include hypoglycemia, diabetic ketoacidosis or nonketotic hyperosmolar coma. Serious long-term complications include cardiovascular disease, chronic renal failure, retinal damage. Adequate treatment of diabetes is thus important, as well as blood pressure control and lifestyle factors such as smoking cessation and maintaining a healthy body weight.

Most cases of diabetes mellitus fall into the three broad categories of type 1 or type 2 and gestational diabetes. A few other types are described.

The term diabetes, without qualification, usually refers to diabetes mellitus, which roughly translates to excessive sweet urine (known as 'glycosuria'). Several rare conditions are also named diabetes. The most common of these is diabetes insipidus in which large amounts of urine are produced (polyuria), which is not sweet (insipidus meaning 'without taste' in Latin).

Type 1 diabetes: Type 1 diabetes mellitus is characterised by loss of the insulin-producing beta cells of the islets of Langerhans in the pancreas leading to insulin deficiency. This type of diabetes can be further classified as immune-mediated or idiopathic.

Type 2 diabetes: Type 2 diabetes mellitus is characterised by insulin resistance which may be combined with relatively reduced insulin secretion. The defective responsiveness of body tissues to insulin is believed to involve the insulin receptor.

Gestational diabetes: Gestational diabetes mellitus (GDM) resembles type 2 diabetes in several respects, involving a combination of relatively inadequate insulin secretion and responsiveness. It occurs in about 2–5 per cent of all pregnancies and may improve or disappear after delivery. Gestational diabetes is fully treatable but requires careful medical supervision throughout the pregnancy. About 20–50 per cent of affected women develop type 2 diabetes later in life.

Other types: Prediabetes indicates a condition that occurs when a person's blood glucose levels are higher than normal but not high enough for a diagnosis of type 2 diabetes. Many people destined to develop type 2 diabetes spend many years in a state of prediabetes which has been termed 'America's largest healthcare epidemic'.

Signs and symptoms of diabetes mellitus

The classical symptoms of DM are polyuria (frequent urination), polydipsia (increased thirst) and polyphagia (increased hunger). Symptoms may develop quite rapidly (weeks or months) in type 1 diabetes, particularly in children. However, in type 2 diabetes symptoms usually develop much more slowly and may be subtle or completely absent. Type 1 diabetes may also cause a rapid yet significant weight loss (despite normal or even increased eating) and irreducible mental fatigue. All of these symptoms except weight loss can also manifest in type 2 diabetes in patients whose diabetes is poorly controlled, although unexplained weight loss may be experienced at the onset of the disease. Final diagnosis is made by measuring the blood glucose concentration.

When the glucose concentration in the blood is raised beyond its renal threshold (about 10 mmol/l, although this may be altered in certain conditions, such as pregnancy), reabsorption of glucose in the proximal renal tubuli is incomplete, and part of the glucose remains in the urine (glycosuria). This increases the osmotic pressure of the urine and inhibits reabsorption of water by the kidney, resulting in increased urine production (polyuria) and increased fluid loss. Lost blood volume will be replaced osmotically from water held in body cells and other body compartments, causing dehydration and increased thirst.

A rarer but equally severe possibility is hyperosmolar nonketotic state, which is more common in type 2 diabetes and is mainly the result of dehydration due to loss of body water. Often, the patient has been drinking extreme amounts of sugar-containing drinks, leading to a vicious circle in regard to the water loss. A number of skin rashes can occur in diabetes that are collectively known as diabetic dermadromes.

Causes: Type 2 diabetes is determined primarily by lifestyle factors and genes.

Lifestyle: A number of lifestyle factors are known to be important to the development of type 2 diabetes. In one study, those who had high levels of physical activity, a healthy diet, did not smoke, and consumed alcohol in moderation had an 82 per cent lower rate of diabetes. When a normal weight was included the rate was 89 per cent lower.

Medical conditions: Subclinical Cushing's syndrome (cortisol excess) may be associated with DM type 2. The percentage of subclinical Cushing's syndrome in the diabetic population is about 9 per cent. Diabetic patients with a pituitary microadenoma can improve insulin sensitivity by removal of these microadenomas. Hypogonadism is often associated with cortisol excess, and testosterone deficiency is also associated with diabetes mellitus type 2, even if the exact mechanism by which testosterone improve insulin sensitivity is still not known.

Genetics: Both type 1 and type 2 diabetes are partly inherited. Type 1 diabetes may be triggered by certain infections, with some evidence pointing at Coxsackie B4 virus. There is a genetic element in individual susceptibility to some of these triggers which has been traced to particular HLA genotypes (i.e. the genetic 'self' identifiers relied upon by the immune system). However, even in those who have inherited the susceptibility, type 1 diabetes mellitus seems to require an environmental trigger. There is a stronger inheritance pattern for type 2 diabetes. Those with first-degree relatives with type 2 have a much higher risk of developing type 2, increasing with the number of those relatives.

Pathophysiology

Insulin is the principal hormone that regulates uptake of glucose from the blood into most cells (primarily muscle and fat cells, but not central nervous system cells). Therefore deficiency of insulin or the insensitivity of its receptors plays a central role in all forms of diabetes mellitus.

Humans are capable of digesting some carbohydrates, in particular those most common in food, starch, and some disaccharides such as sucrose, are converted within a few hours to simpler forms most notably the monosaccharide glucose, the principal carbohydrate energy source used by the body. The most significant exceptions are fructose, most disaccharides (except sucrose and in some people lactose), and all more complex polysaccharides, with the outstanding exception of starch. The rest are passed on for processing by gut flora largely in the colon. Insulin is released into the blood by beta cells (β-cells), found in the Islets of Langerhans in the pancreas, in response to rising levels of blood glucose, typically after eating. Insulin is used by about two-thirds of the body's cells to absorb glucose from the blood for use as fuel, for conversion to other needed molecules or for storage (Fig. 29.12).

Insulin is also the principal control signal for conversion of glucose to glycogen for internal storage in liver and muscle cells. Lowered glucose levels result both in the reduced release of insulin from the beta cells and in the reverse conversion of glycogen to glucose when glucose levels fall. This is mainly controlled by the hormone glucagon which acts in the opposite manner to insulin. Glucose thus forcibly produced from internal liver cell stores (as glycogen) re-enters the bloodstream, muscle cells lack the necessary export mechanism. Normally liver cells do this when the level of insulin is low (which normally correlates with low levels of blood glucose).

Higher insulin levels increase some anabolic (building up) processes such as cell growth and duplication, protein synthesis, and fat storage. Insulin (or its lack) is the principal signal in converting many of the bidirectional processes of metabolism from a catabolic to an anabolic direction, and vice versa. In particular, a low insulin level is the trigger for entering or leaving ketosis (the fat burning metabolic phase).

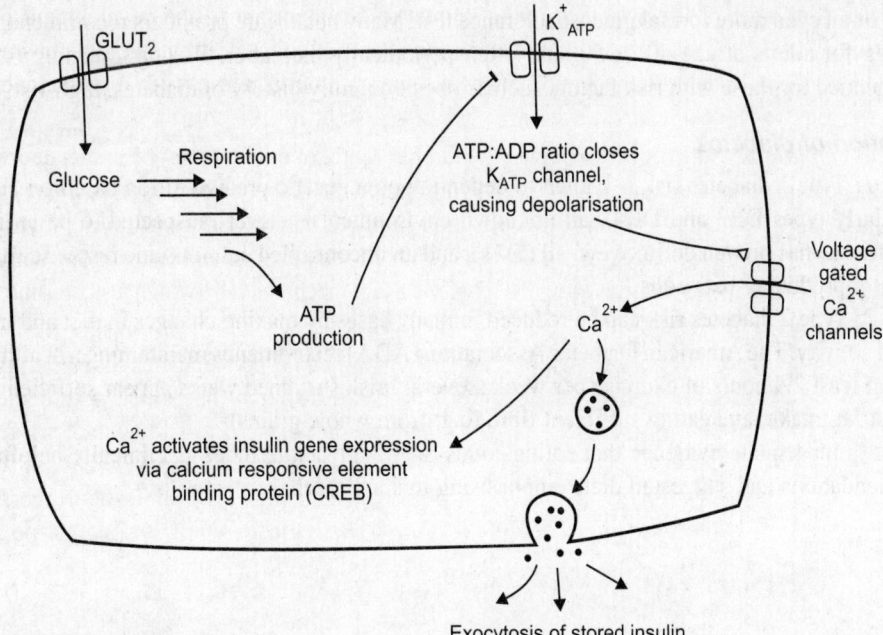

Fig. 29.12: Mechanism of insulin release in normal pancreatic beta cells. Insulin production is more or less constant within the beta cells, irrespective of blood glucose levels. It is stored within vacuoles pending release, via exocytosis, which is primarily triggered by food, chiefly food containing absorbable glucose. The chief trigger is a rise in blood glucose levels after eating.

If the amount of insulin available is insufficient, if cells respond poorly to the effects of insulin (insulin insensitivity or resistance), or if the insulin itself is defective, then glucose will not have its usual effect so that glucose will not be absorbed properly by those body cells that require it nor will it be stored appropriately in the liver and muscles. The net effect is persistent high levels of blood glucose, poor protein synthesis, and other metabolic derangements, such as acidosis.

Diagnosis of diabetes

Diabetes mellitus is characterised by recurrent or persistent hyperglycemia, and is diagnosed by demonstrating any one of the following:

1. Fasting plasma glucose level at or above 7.0 mmol/l (126 mg/dl).
2. Plasma glucose at or above 11.1 mmol/l (200 mg/dl) two hours after a 75 g oral glucose load as in a glucose tolerance test.
3. Symptoms of hyperglycemia and casual plasma glucose at or above 11.1 mmol/l (200 mg/dl).
4. Glycated haemoglobin (haemoglobin A1C) at or above 6.5.

Screening of diabetes

Diabetes screening is recommended for many people at various stages of life, and for those with any of several risk factors. The screening test varies according to circumstances and local policy, and may be a random blood glucose test, a fasting blood glucose test, a blood glucose test two hours after 75 g of glucose or an even more formal glucose tolerance test. Many healthcare providers recommend universal screening for adults at age 40 or 50, and often periodically thereafter. Earlier screening is typically recommended for those with risk factors such as obesity, family history of diabetes, high-risk ethnicity.

Prevention of diabetes

Type 1: Type 1 diabetes risk is known to depend upon a genetic predisposition based on HLA types (particularly types DR3 and DR4), an unknown environmental trigger (suspected to be an infection, although none has proven definitive in all cases), and an uncontrolled autoimmune response that attacks the insulin producing beta cells.

Type 2: Type 2 diabetes risk can be reduced in many cases by making changes in diet and increasing physical activity. The American Diabetes Association (ADA) recommends maintaining a healthy weight, getting at least 2½ hours of exercise per week (several brisk sustained walks appear sufficient), having a modest fat intake, and eating sufficient fibre (e.g. from whole grains).

There is inadequate evidence that eating foods of low glycemic index is clinically helpful despite recommendations and suggested diets emphasising this approach.

Chapter 30

Cancer: Signal Transduction and Oncogenes

INTRODUCTION

The cellular phenotypes are regulated with the signalling pathways consist of molecular interactions. Network of several signalling pathways activates the stem cells and cancer to transit the cellular phonotypes. The molecules in the signalling pathway are epigenetically regulated upon the stimulation, which leads to dynamic changes in cell types such as differentiation of stem cells or malignancy of cancer cells. Considering that the disease status is involved in signalling pathway alteration, the investigation in epigenetic changes to find the targets of therapeutics are clinically of importance.

MEDIATORS OF SIGNALLING PATHWAYS

The stimulation with extracellular substances such as chemicals or molecules in vesicles, and intercellular adhesion molecules start the signalling transduction in the cells. The receptors receive the stimulation and transduce the information to down-stream regulators mainly with conformational changes. The cascade of signalling occurs with phosphorylation of the molecules mediated by several kinases towards nucleus. Vesicles containing microRNA internalise through the membranes and mediate the signalling inside the cells.

Some receptors such as nuclear receptors internalise and directly activate the nucleic signalling. Transcription factors bind to DNA and regulate the expression of genes, which leads to the activation of other signalling pathways. Epigenetic regulation such as methylation and acetylation of DNA modulate the gene transcription, followed by the consequences as cell proliferation or differentiation.

SIGNALLING PATHWAYS IN STEM CELLS

In stem cells, signalling for self-renewal and differentiation balance the cellular phenotypes. Wnt signalling pathway, Hedgehog signalling pathway and Notch signalling pathway are activated in stem cells. For maintaining the stem cells, several molecules such as Nanog, Sox2, and Oct4 (Pou5f1) are important and these molecules are regulated as the consequence of the signalling pathway activation. Cross-talks of several signalling pathways modify the cellular phenotypes in the feedback mechanism, which emphasises the significance of networking of signalling pathways in stem cells.

SIGNALLING PATHWAYS IN CANCER

In general, proliferation signalling is activated and apoptosis signalling is reduced in cancer. The therapeutic targets for cancer include EGF signalling, since the EGF signalling is usually activated in cancer. Another strategy to target cancer is PD1 inhibition with antibodies to regain the anti-cancer immunity with immune cells. The signalling pathways to activate and modulate the immune cells may be of clinical importance for cancer medication. For cancer phenotype identification, gene expression profiling in activated signalling pathways are useful and concise. The diagnosis with microRNA in the blood is practical in clinical setting, and the microRNA signalling pathway will elucidate the cancer metastasis signalling pathways and networking of cancer signalling pathways.

MAPPING OF SIGNALLING PATHWAYS

The expression of the molecules in the signalling pathways is regulated in epigenetic alterations. The mapping of the molecules in terms of the expression and interaction with the other signalling pathways is essential for elucidating the whole picture of signalling pathway networks. Overlapping of timing and location of several signalling pathways in the cells are important for the cross-talk of the signalling pathways. The epigenetic regulation in the signalling pathway network would require the further investigation to target the cancer and stem cell signalling for therapeutics.

CANCER CELLS OFTEN SEND THE WRONG SIGNALS

The human body functions in large part because of billions of chemical signals sent between and inside cells. Healthy cells exchange signals to regulate the immune system, help muscles and organs function, and perform an endless list of biological tasks.[:breakpost:] These signals also dictate how cells grow and divide, and when they shut themselves down to make room for new, healthy cells (called apoptosis)—critical processes that determine everything from how the body heals a skinned knee to how the skin ages to how the brain processes pain.

This constant communication is so fundamental to the body's health and development that when cellular signals go awry, the interference may cause a number of conditions or diseases, such as diabetes—or cancer. In fact, researchers have concluded that many cancers form when these signals are disrupted, diverted or used for other, more harmful uses. These evolving insights have become a key focus of research that has led to a new and emerging line of cancer treatments.

As scientists learn more about how cellular signals work, and what happens when they get mixed up, they have found that intercepting broken cancer cell signals may help the body fight the disease. Some drugs, for instance, are designed to block the signals cancer cells send to evade the immune system. In other cases, cancer cell signalling remains a mystery, and a strong focus of future research. 'We have a great deal to learn about the complexities of cell signalling, evasion of apoptosis, and other mechanisms of cell growth and regulation,' says Dr. Pamela Crilley, Chair of the Department of Medical Oncology at Cancer Treatment Centers of America® (CTCA) and Chief of Medical Oncology at Philadelphia hospital. 'At the same time, there have been important advances in the fields of biology, oncology and immunology that may translate the scientific findings into treatments.'

Getting the Message

A cell receives messages through receptors on its surface. Receptors are like cellular satellite dishes that receive chemical signals via protein molecules, or ligands, from other cells. When a ligand reaches a receptor, it sets off a chain reaction that allows the signal to penetrate the cell surface and reach the thick fluid inside, called cytoplasm. Once inside the cell, the message passes from one enzyme to another along a signalling pathway until it reaches its destination— the nucleus, where every cell's DNA resides. The cell then carries out the instructions encoded in the signal.

In a given day, the body's cells send and receive billions of signals. In some cancer cells, the signals sent to regulate growth or initiate apoptosis get short-circuited, resulting in rapid cell growth that may lead to tumours. For instance, human epidermal growth factor receptor 2 (HER2), found on the surface of normal cells, sends signals that help cells grow. In some breast cancer patients, cells produce too many HER2 receptors, creating an overload of signals that may cause uncontrolled growth.

Overriding Key Signals

While healthy cells communicate to divide and thrive, cancer cells may take over those signalling pathways and use them in harmful ways—to help them grow and metastasise, for example. One of the body's earliest and most important signalling pathways is called hedgehog. Most active before we are born and during childhood, the hedgehog pathway transmits a diverse set of instructions that tell the body how to develop and maintain our organs, skin and bones. As we enter adulthood, the hedgehog pathway all but shuts down—unless it gets turned back on by cancer cells. Once active, the signalling pathway that once helped the body mature as we grew up may now be used to help tumours spread. Scientists in California have linked the reactivation of the hedgehog pathway to gastrointestinal stromal tumours, while researchers in North Carolina have concluded that one of the signals that reactivates the pathway 'has been implicated in many human cancers that account for up to 25 per cent of human cancer deaths.'

If cellular communication is key to helping some tumours develop, it may also be used to reverse the behaviour—and kill the cancer in some instances, scientists believe. Developing drugs designed for a specific receptor, ligand or pathway is at the root of some targeted therapies, used to treat a number of cancers. These drugs are designed to disrupt cell communication by:

Targeting the ligand so it cannot communicate with the receptor. For instance, bevacizumab (Avastin®), used to treat colorectal, breast, kidney and non-small cell lung cancers, as well as some brain tumours, attempts to prevent a specific protein from binding to a receptor that triggers growth signals, aborting the communication that helps the cancer grow and thrive.

Targeting the receptor. Trastuzumab (Herceptin®), for instance, one of the most commonly prescribed drugs for HER2-positive breast cancer, is designed to target defective HER2 proteins receptors and block growth signals.

Targeting the signalling pathway inside the cell. When a receptor is activated, it triggers an enzyme known as a tyrosine kinase, which acts as an on-off switch for many cell signals. Tyrosine kinase inhibitors such as erlotinib (Tarceva®), used to treat some non-small cell lung cancers and pancreatic cancers, are designed to keep that switch in the off position.

The hope is that finding new ways to tap those communications and learning more about the intricacies of signalling pathways will help cancer researchers develop new cancer therapies, Dr. Crilley says. 'Research into the details of signalling pathways,' she says, 'may provide scientists with insights into novel drug therapies that may have an important impact.'

ONCOGENES

As study of the molecular and cellular basis of cancer progresses, it is becoming clear that no two cancers are identical: tumour development is a complex process, and there are many paths to malignancy.

Nevertheless, certain tenets persist: that cancer arises as the result of genetic change, that this leads to loss of control over cellular proliferation, and that usually several genetic errors are required to reach the full neoplastic phenotype. Deregulated cellular proliferation may arise in two main ways: through the loss of genes that normally checkcell growth (the tumour suppressors) or by the gain of function of genes that either promote cellular proliferation or prevent cell death (the oncogenes) (from Greek onkos, tumour). Some cancer-associated genes, for example those involved in DNA repair, do not fall easily into either category, others such as P53 are tumour suppressors in wild-type form, but can act as dominant oncogenes in certain mutant forms. In many instances of adult human cancer, both features – oncogenic activation and loss of tumour suppressor activity – may be identified.

A typical oncogene has dominant activity, and requires only one allele to be activated in order to be oncogenic. An oncogene maybe viral or cellular in origin, a viral oncogene may be unique to the virus, or a homologue of a cellular 'proto-oncogene'. An oncogene can promote transformation *in vitro*, and tumour formation in transgenic animals, further, its deregulation is usually recurrently associated with malignancy. Of over a hundred oncogenes that have been described, many are not entirely typical, but the model remains useful.

Viral-induced Tumours

The concept of cancer-causing genes arose from early observations that viruses can induce tumour formation in animals. Both retroviruses and DNA viruses can carry oncogenes, which often resemble cellular genes. Viruses may also induce tumours through integration into the host genome, bringing a cellular gene under control of a viral promoter, or a virus may promote tumour formation through its suppressive effect on the host immune system. Despite these varied mechanisms, the contribution viruses make to cancer in human and animal populations is relatively small, although the discovery of virally induced tumours has had far-reaching implications for our understanding of oncogenes.

Retroviruses

Rous sarcoma virus (RSV), is a typical acute retrovirus, anRNAvirus that copies itsRNA to DNA by reverse transcription after infection of a cell. The DNA is inserted into the host genome, where it can persist and be inherited by subsequent cell generations. Workon RSV and other acute retroviruses demonstrated not only tumour formation by the viruses, but their ability to transform fibroblasts. Transformation is an *in vitro* phenomenon which has proved a useful assay for oncogenic viruses – and oncogenes themselves. Transformed cells do not respond to growth inhibitory signals such as cell–cell contact, and they have less requirement for growth factors than their untransformed counterparts. They are 'immortal', in that they can proliferate indefinitely, and have an unusually rounded morphology. They thus appear as fast-growing colonies of rounded cells which can be quantified on a culture plate. Studies on a form of mutant RSV that failed to induce transformation led to the identification of the first viral oncogene, *src*.

Oncogenes like *src* are thought to have been captured from the host genome during viral integration, although they have often undergone mutation during their viral passage. While retroviral oncogenes thus have cellular counterparts, the context in which they are carried renders them oncogenic. They are driven by the promoter within the retroviral long terminal repeat (LTR), which produces unregulated, often higher, expression than the normal cellular genes. Furthermore, retroviral oncogenes may encode proteins with properties different to those of the cellular proteins, as a result of mutation. Importantly, retroviral oncogenes are unnecessary for replication of the virus. Indeed, they often carry a survival disadvantage as a result of tumour induction, and in all likelihood are maintained artificially within the experimental environment, with low natural prevalence or significance. Chronic retroviruses generally induce tumour formation by the alternative mechanism of gene insertion, whereby random insertion of the viral genome into the host genome can cause activation of cellular genes, causing them to become oncogenic. Because the process of gene activation is random, and because the resulting gene activation is often lethal for the cell, it can take many years for a tumour to be induced by chronic retroviral infection.

Viral tumours in humans

There are a small number of human malignancies in which a viral aetiology has been demonstrated, or strongly suspected. However, no acute retrovirus has been associated with any human tumour, and only two chronic retroviruses are linked to cancer in humans. Human immunodeficiency virus (HIV) is associated with a number of malignancies through its immunosuppressive effects, which prevent an adequate T-cell response to malignant cells. This is particularly marked when the malignant cells are expressing foreign antigens, for example from other viruses, which would normally provoke a host response. Moreover, HIV can have a more direct effect on tumour formation by inducing capillary growth, contributing to the pathogenesis of Kaposi sarcoma and perhaps facilitating spread of other tumours. Human T cell leukaemia virus type I (HTLV-I), another chronic retrovirus, has been identified as the aetiological agent of adult T-cell leukaemia, endemic in certain areas of the world including central Africa and the Caribbean basin. Only 1–4% of HTLV-I carriers develop T-cell leukaemia, and this only after a latency of 20–30 years.

DNA viruses are also not commonly oncogenic in humans – surprisingly, given their frequency of infection in higher animals, and their tendency to promote cell proliferation. One reason is that malignant transformation confers no survival benefit to the virus. Second, DNA virus replication is accompanied by expression of immunogenic proteins, leading to destruction of the host cell. Where such virus-associated tumours are common, therefore, is in the context of impaired T-cell immunity. For example, tumours associated with immunosuppression due to HIV infection include Epstein–Barr virus (EBV)-associated lymphomas, Human herpes virus 8 (HHV-8)-positive Kaposi sarcoma, and anogenital carcinoma associated with Human papillomavirus (HPV) infection. Third, there are nonimmune mechanisms thought to operate within and between cells that suppress the function of viruses and their oncogene products.

EBV is a lymphotropic herpesvirus, endemic in all human populations but only rarely associated with malignant change. Acute EBV infection can give rise to fatal lymphoproliferation of B cells, and indeed T cells, but only in the context of severe immunosuppression such as exists after bone marrow transplantation, or through rare genetic defects. Similarly, reactivation of latent EBV, leading to lymphoproliferative tumours, may occur with chronic immunosuppression, either iatrogenic (post-transplant) or virus-induced (AIDS-associated). In nonimmunosuppressed patients, Burkitt lymphoma and nasopharyngeal carcinoma have an established association with EBV. Burkitt lymphoma was long suspected to have an infectious cause, due to its geographically limited occurrence, and the link was initially demonstrated by electron microscopic observation of EBV particles in tumour cultures. Some types of Hodgkin disease and some T-cell lymphomas also have an association with the virus.

Other DNA viruses involved in human malignancy include HHV8, another herpesvirus identified from Kaposi sarcoma in acquired immune deficiency syndrome (AIDS) patients, now with an established role in the aetiology of this tumour. HPV, aDNA virus, has over 60 genotypes, 11 of which are associated with human cancers, HPV-16 and 18 being strongly associated with cervical and anal carcinomas.

Similarly, Hepatitis B virus (HBV) was linked with hepatocellular carcinoma through seroepidemiological studies, and a closely related virus was isolated from woodchucks, which causes liver cancer. However, the precise role that Hepatitis B virus plays in human liver cancer remains ill defined, with no oncogenes being clearly identified.

Viral Oncogenes

According to the model, a true viral oncogene demonstrates the ability to transform primary cells *in vitro*, although often cooperation between two oncogenes is required for efficient transformation. It should cause tumour formation in transgenic mice, and be associated with cancers, either in its viral form, or as deregulated expression of a cellular homologue.

Retroviral oncogenes

It seems that all oncogenes carried by retroviruses have a cellular counterpart, although in many cases this has only been identified after discovery of the viral oncogene. Thus the RSV oncogene *src* has a cellular homologue, SRC. Despite the fact that RSV strains are not tumorigenic in mammals, mammalian fibroblasts can be transformed to a malignant phenotype by both *src* and SRC, further, increased SRC expression has been identified in some human cancers, including colon, skin and breast cancers.

Viral oncogenes in humans

Of the virus-associated human tumours mentioned above, only EBV, HHV-8 and HPV possess clearly defined oncogenes. EBV is a complex virus with a large genome, in latent infections, about 11 viral genes are expressed, grouped into the nuclear antigens or EBNAs, and the latent membrane proteins or LMPs. EBNA1 induces tumours in transgenic animals, but not transformation *in vitro*, EBNA2 has transforming properties *in vitro*. It is likely that the oncogenic potential of EBV is the result of the combined contribution of several of these protein products, some of which activate cellular proliferative pathways, and others of which inhibit cell death.

The HHV-8 genome also contains a number of potential oncogenes: here, the protein products are related to cyclin D, interleukins and interferon-responsive factors. Two oncoproteins, E6 and E7, are encoded within the genome of HPV types 16 and 18, these interfere with the function of two important cellular tumour suppressors, p53 and Rb. These oncogenes result in tumour formation in transgenic mice, and cooperate with cellular genes to transform fibroblasts *in vitro*.

Other viral proteins contributing to human cancers are less typical in their role as oncoproteins, or await clearer definition of their function in tumour formation. HBV frequently shows integration during chronic infection, although this is not part of its life cycle. *Cis*-activation of adjacent cellular genes may result from such integration, while transactivating viral proteins such as pX may contribute to aberrant expression of cellular genes. HTLV-I similarly possesses the viral gene, tax, which transactivates the viral LTR through protein–protein interaction. In addition it can transactivate a number of cellular genes, including those encoding cytokines, cytokine receptors and transcription factors, and it is this function that is thought to contribute to malignant transformation. The tax gene cannot, however, induce transformation alone, and there may be other HTLV-I genes, and probably nonviral cellular events, necessary for inducing the malignant T-cell phenotype. Similarly, HIV does not carry a true oncogene, but it does carry the gene Tat that encodes a protein with angiogenic properties, inducing endothelial cell growth, migration and invasion *in vitro*.

Cellular Oncogenes

Viruses have contributed greatly to the present understanding of oncogene function, but have had a less significant role in human oncogenesis. Most oncogenes involved in human tumours are not viral but cellular – genes that are present in the normal genome, which are deregulated or activated by mutation. There are three mechanisms of cellular oncogenic activation: (i) through alteration of the coding sequence by deletion or point mutation, (ii) by increasing the copy number of the gene, and (iii) by chromosomal rearrangement.

Activation by alterations of the coding sequence

Point mutations and intragenic mutations arise as the result of DNA damage caused by chemical agents, or physical agents such as radiation. Because of base changes, the amino acid sequence of an encoded protein is altered, with a corresponding change in function. If the protein is a key player in growth or other signalling pathways, loss of function will have no effect (unless both alleles are affected – as in tumour suppressors), but gain of function may result in accelerated proliferation. A prime example is the Ras family of signalling molecules that become hyperactive as the result of single base substitutions, providing these occur at crucial points in the coding sequence. Activated RAS has been identified in many human tumours, including about 80% of pancreatic and 40% of colorectal carcinomas. Such mutations have been demonstrated to be inducible by chemical toxins or ultraviolet radiation, and there is a viral homologue of activated RAS, carried by the murine sarcoma virus. Activated RAS mediates transformation of fibroblasts in culture, and leads to tumour formation in transgenic animals.

Activation by gene amplification

Amplification as a route to oncogene activation is a poorly understood process in which several megabases of chromosomal material are typically copied in tandem, up to perhaps 50 or 100 times. The resulting DNA is then retained episomally (outside the normal cellular chromosomes), in which case cell division may result in unequal portions of replicated material being passed to the progeny, or it may be reintegrated within a chromosome. Such phenomena have never been described in nonmalignant tissues, and appear to be typical of solid tumours rather than haematological malignancies. Examples of oncogenes activated in this way include EGFR, NEU and CCND1, encoding the epidermal growth factor receptor (EGFR), the related erbB2 receptor and cyclin D1, respectively.

Activation by chromosomal rearrangement

Oncogenes may also be activated through chromosomal rearrangement, i.e. translocations, interstitial deletions or inversions. These tend to result in the gene being brought under new transcriptional control, leading to overexpression, or in the gene being truncated, making it hyperactive, or in the gene being fused to another, leading to a hybrid oncoprotein with functions combining those of both gene partners. Haematological malignancies are particularly associated with chromosomal rearrangements: a well-known example of a fusion gene results from the translocation of ABL on chromosome 9 to the BCR locus on 22. The result, BCR-ABL, produces a new Bcr-Abl fusion protein. This molecular change is very strongly associated with chronic myeloid leukaemia (CML) in which it is frequently the only abnormality. A typical translocation in lymphomas results in a variety of genes, often called B-cell leukaemia/lymphoma genes, (BCL-), being translocated near to one of the immunoglobulin loci, where they are brought under control of the immunoglobulin promoter and/or enhancer. Since the normal lymphocyte expresses high levels of immunoglobulin, any gene translocated to the same locality, such as MYCin Burkitt lymphoma, BCL2 in follicular lymphoma, or CCND1 in mantle cell lymphoma, will also be expressed at high levels.

Virus-associated chromosomal rearrangements

The IgH-MYC translocation, together with similar translocations of MYC to the immunoglobulin light chain loci, are universal findings in Burkitt lymphoma, even in the sporadic cases where EBV is not involved. The close association between a chromosomal translocation and a viral oncogenic effect, however, remains something of a puzzle – are they separate phenomena, both important in the development of lymphoma? If so, non-EBV-related cases are more difficult to explain. Another speculative explanation has been that EBV increases the probability of specific gene translocation, either directly at the gene level, or indirectly by selecting for cells containing that translocation. Interestingly, it has recently been demonstrated that an adenovirus oncogene, E1A, specifically induces a fusion oncogene identical to that found in the human tumour Ewing sarcoma.

Normal Functions of Oncogenes

Both cellular oncogenes and most viral oncogenes derive from normal cellular genes or proto-oncogenes. These genes encode proteins that function in essential cellular pathways: in general, a proto-oncogene is likely to be proproliferative, and/or pro-survival, and/or an inhibitor of differentiation. These functions of a cell are governed by factors in the extracellular environment such as cell–cell contact and growth factors, and signals are relayed from the cell surface to the cell nucleus by signalling cascades. Proto-oncogenes may be divided into broad groups according to their position in such cascades: they may be growth factors, cell surface receptors, membrane transducers, intracellular signalling proteins or transcription factors. The pathways are complex, converging and diverging, and the endpoints – proliferation, survival and state of differentiation are often interdependent. Nevertheless, even an incomplete under-standing of normal proto-oncogene function provides insights into the role of oncogenes in tumorigenesis.

Growth factors and receptors

Cell surface receptors that function in growth regulation fall into several superfamilies. One of these includes the platelet-derived growth factor (PDGF) receptor, the ligand for which has an oncogenic homologue, SIS, which when overexpressed causes excessive signalling through the PDGF pathway. Another of the receptor tyrosine kinase families is the epidermal growth factor (EGF) receptor family. In this case, the gene encoding the EGF receptor itself is amplified in some human tumours, causing it to function as an oncogene. Arelated gene, NEU, is also overexpressed in tumours and has a viral homologue erbB, which encodes a truncated EGF receptor. In this form, the receptor is constitutively active, and does not require ligand binding to function. The EGF receptor, like most growth factor receptors, is a tyrosine kinase, signalling to downstream molecules through membrane-associated binding and phosphorylation.

Membrane transducers

Two important categories of protein that transmit signals from receptors to cytoplasmic molecules are the 'nonreceptor tyrosine kinases' such as the protein encoded by SRC, and GTP-binding proteins or 'G-proteins', such as members of the Ras family. This family is comprised of closely related genes H-RAS, K-RAS and N-RAS, encoding proteins of 21 kDa (hence, p21ras). Each p21ras protein binds one molecule of guanosine triphosphate (GTP) or guanosine diphosphate (GDP), phosphorylation of bound GDP converts p21ras from 'off' mode to 'on' mode, mediating binding and activation of downstream regulators like Raf andMEK. RAS becomes oncogenic usually as the result of point mutations, which prevent the hydrolysis of p21ras-bound GTP, maintaining it permanently in the 'on' position.

Serine/threonine kinases

Further downstream, many molecular mediators function as serine/threonine kinases, each kinase phosphorylating other kinases in cascade fashion. These include the protein product of AKT, the cellular homologue of an avian viral oncogene. The Akt protein is an important cytoplasmic kinase that lies downstream of several growth factor and cytokine receptors, and upstream of cell cycle and apoptotic regulators.

Cell cycle regulators

The proliferation state of the cell is determined by its position in, and passage through, the cell cycle. Passage through the cycle is in turn governed by a number of proteins that take their cues from signalling cascades, allowing the cell to move from one stage to the next. Some of these proteins can function as oncogenes–such as cyclin D1, encoded by CCND1, which normally governs entry of the cell into S phase from G1. When overexpressed as a result of gene amplification or immunoglobulin H (IgH) translocation, the increased cyclin D1 promotes cycling and proliferation.

Inhibitors of apoptosis

In parallel with the mitogenic pathways are the pathways leading to cell death, which must be inhibited in order for malignant proliferation to proceed in exponential fashion. Inhibitors of apoptosis can thus function as oncogenes: the paradigm here is Bcl2, an antiapoptotic molecule bound to the mitochondrial membrane, serving to prevent caspase activation. Bcl2 is overexpressed in many lymphomas.

Transcription factors

The endpoints of mitogenic, cell cycle and apoptotic signalling usually lie within the nucleus, where expression of proteins is altered at the level of transcription. Many pathways converge on transcription factors that promote or inhibit transcription of important genes. Not surprisingly, several of these transcription factors are themselves proto-oncogenes. MYC, for example, encodes an important transcription factor, regulating expression of many genes and being essential for cell cycle progression. Similarly, Fos and Jun proteins are activated by a number of mitogenic pathways. These proteins heterodimerise to each other and to other transcription factors, and thus may act as 'AND' gateways to protein expression, allowing transcription of important genes when several growth signals are present.

Therapeutic Prospects

If activation or deregulation of a proto-oncogene contributes to oncogenesis, then the corollary – that suppressing oncogene function may somehow stop cancer development – is an attractive hypothesis. Indeed, this has been the emphasis of many drug development strategies. There are several levels at which oncogene activity may be tackled: (i) at the level of transcription, where some level of control is re-exerted over oncogene expression, (ii) at translation, where RNA message is inhibited, (iii) through alteration of oncoprotein localisation, stability, or function, (iv) at the level of signal transduction pathways, which may be targeted upstream or downstream of the oncogene, and (v) at the level of immune response, which may be provoked into recognising an abnormal, oncogenic protein.

Intervention in the EGFR signalling pathway

These levels of intervention are well exemplified by the EGFR–p21ras–Raf–MEK–ERK signalling pathway, which contains a number of proteins that may act as, or be replaced by, oncoproteins. Taking the levels of potential therapeutic manipulation described above, the first site for targeting is transcription. Here, preliminary success has been achieved using oligonucleotides that form triple helix structures at the site of promoters for EGF receptor family genes such as NEU (encoding erbB2), inhibiting the start of transcription. Other oligonucleotides are designed to act as decoys, binding to transcription factors in direct competition with the promotors. One level further, oligonucleotides antisense to messenger RNA (mRNA) have proven useful in preventing translation and promoting degradation of mRNA. Clinical trials are already underway using antisense to members of the EGF–p21ras–ERK pathway including RAS in lung cancer patients, and MYC in breast and prostate cancer. Despite problems of variable and unpredictable efficacy, and difficulties in delivering the oligonucleotides to their site of action, some anecdotal success is being reported.

Therapeutic targeting of the oncoproteins themselves may be mediated by antibodies – either extracellular antibodies directed, for example, to the erbB2 receptor (now an approved treatment for breast cancer), or intracellular antibodies ('intrabodies') like the anti-erbB2 single chain antibody (scFv), which has been shown to downregulate erbB2 expression. Activity may also be modified indirectly, using inhibitors of molecular chaperones such as Hsp90, which affects the folding and cellular localisation of both erbB2 and Raf-1, ultimately leading to protein degradation. Similarly, clinical trials are currently underway to look at the effects of inhibitors of farnesyltransferase, which blocks p21ras farnesylation – a posttranscriptional modification essential for its membrane localisation and function. Finally, progress is being made using immunotherapeutic approaches to counter oncogenic members of theEGFR signalling pathways. Thus, T cell responses have been generated to erbB2 and mutant p21ras, both *in vitro* and *in vivo*.

Bcr-Abl as a target for intervention

Another therapeutic oncogene target results from the Bcr-Abl juxtaposition in CML. This molecular translocation gives rise to a novel mRNA and a novel tyrosine kinase: both have been explored as sites for intervention. Antisense oligonucleotides to the hybrid transcript have had apparent effects in early clinical trials, while a tyrosine kinase inhibitor, CGP 57148 (ST1 571), has similarly demonstrated impressive activity, at minimal toxicity, in phase I trials.

Thus, oncogenes are genes that are directly involved in the development of malignancy, and may well be essential for this process. They are often derived from normal cellular genes, or proto-oncogenes, whose functions in cell proliferation, differentiation and survival have become deregulated. Oncogenes may be carried by viruses, or represent cellular genes that have been activated by viruses or by mutation. They usually operate in key cell signalling pathways, and have become important molecular targets for the development of novel anticancer agents, with some preliminary success.

SECTION XI

Cell Death and Cell Renewal

Chapter 31

Cell Death

INTRODUCTION

Soon after the realization that organisms are composed of individual cells, it was noted that cell death is a normal part of development. The first (circa 1840), reported example was cell death in the notochord and adjacent cartilage of metamorphic toads. It has since been recognized that death occurs during the normal development of a wide variety of tissues in metazoans, including humans. Moreover, it has become clear that in addition to proliferation, migration and differentiation, cell death plays an indispensable role in normal embryogenesis. Recent evidence also supports a role for misregulated cell death in a variety of human developmental defects.

Various terms have been used to describe the types of cell death that occur in development and under other conditions. The term 'programmed cell death' is often used in the context of development and makes the point that genetic programs cause predictable death of specific groups of cells under physiologic circumstances. However, all mammalian cells appear to have the potential to die, and thus elaborate molecular mechanisms have evolved to regulate this process and to assure that the proper cells die at the right time and in the right place. In this section we will consider the "canonical" mechanisms that are triggered in cells that lead to their death during development.

Much of the death that occurs during development falls under the general mechanism of 'apoptotic'. The term apoptosis was coined by Kerr, Wylie and Currie in 1972 to distinguish the morphologicfeatures of cells dying under a number of physiologic conditions from the features which occur (termed necrosis) when cells die in response to toxins or physical damage.

Typically, in apoptotic death, the nuclear chromatin condenses, the nucleus and cytoplasmic content of the cell become pyknotic, the DNA is digested by endonucleases and the cell breaks up into membrane limited fragments that are typically engulfed by macrophages. Because the cytoplasmic contents are typically not released in apoptotic death, it generally occurs without inflammation and dead cells disappear from the tissue like 'leaves falling from trees' (the meaning that Kerr, Wylie and Currie wished to convey in the term apoptosis). Another important feature of apoptotic death followed by phagocytosis is that cell components are not released into the circulation and are therefore not available to cause immune responses. This may be particularly important during development to avoid a maternal immune response to embryonic antigens. In contrast, necrotic cell death is distinguished by cell swelling, disintegration of cell membranes and loss of cytoplasmic contents, and random DNA digestion without chromatin condensation. Many cases of developmental cell death have features associated with apoptosis. However, there are also cases in which the morphologic features of dying cells are not necrotic, but also fail to fulfill all the criteria of apoptotic death.

Cell death is the event of a biological cell ceasing to carry out its functions. This may be the result of the natural process of old cells dying and being replaced by new ones, or may result from such factors as disease, localized injury, or the death of the organism of which the cells are part. Kinds of cell death include the following:

Programmed cell death (PCD) is cell death mediated by an intracellular program. PCD is carried out in a regulated process, which usually confers advantage during an organism's life-cycle. For example, the differentiation of fingers and toes in a developing human embryo occurs because cells between the fingers apoptose; the result is that the digits are separate. PCD serves fundamental functions during both plant and metazoa (multicellular animals) tissue development.

Apoptosis or Type I cell-death, and autophagy or Type II cell-death are both forms of programmed cell death, while necrosis is a non-physiological process that occurs as a result of infection or injury. Necrosis is cell death caused by external factors such as trauma or infection, and occurs in several different forms. Recently a form of programmed necrosis, called necroptosis, has been recognized as an alternative form of programmed cell death. It is hypothesized that necroptosis can serve as a cell-death backup to apoptosis when the apoptosis signalling is blocked by endogenous or exogenous factors such as viruses or mutations.

Mitotic catastrophe is a mode of cell death that is due to premature or inappropriate entry of cells into mitosis. It is the most common mode of cell death in cancer cells exposed to ionizing radiation and many other anti-cancer treatments.

FUNCTIONS OF DEVELOPMENTAL CELL DEATH

- Sculpting/shaping structures/morphogenesis: Cell death plays a major role in morphogenesis. This ranges from contributing to creation of cavities and tubes from solid structures, to fusion of tissue masses (such as in formation of the palate, fusion of the neural tube), to sculpting of features such as digits.

- Regulation of cell migration and pattern formation. Death of cells can affect the routes that cells take during migration and thereby affect pattern formation.

- Deletion of unneeded structures. In some cases, vestigial structures are deleted by cell death (example, pronephros and mesonephros). In others, such as the case of the cortical subplate, structures play a transient role and are then eliminated. Cell death also functions in regulation of sexual differentiation by eliminating either the Wolffian or Müllerian ducts.

- Regulation of cell numbers: culling. Particularly for cases in which structures that will eventually interact develop in isolation from one another, cell death functions to provide the appropriate numerical matchup between cell populations. The best defined example is in the nervous system in which development is characterized by large-scale death of neurons.

- Eliminating abnormal, misplaced or harmful cells. DNA damage or problems with DNA replication that affect mitosis triggers cell death. This eliminates cells that may have a compromised genome and that might have the capacity to form tumours. Cell death also eliminates cells that have migrated to the inappropriate place (ectopic cells). Cell death mechanisms are also used to eliminate unneeded cells in the immune system.

- Production of structures without organelles. In some instances, cell-death-like mechanisms function to create somata without nuclei or organelles. Examples include the formation of squamous epithelium from skin keratinocytes and the formation of clear lenses in the eye.

TYPES OF PROGRAMMED CELL DEATH

1. Apoptosis or Type I cell-death.
2. Autophagic or Type II cell-death. (Cytoplasmic: characterised by the formation of large vacuoles that eat away organelles in a specific sequence prior to the destruction of the nucleus.)

Apoptosis

Apoptosis (31.1) is the process of programmed cell death (PCD) that may occur in multi-cellular organisms. Biochemical events lead to characteristic cell changes (morphology) and death. These changes include blebbing, cell shrinkage, nuclear fragmentation, chromatin condensation, and chromosomal DNA fragmentation. It is now thought that- in a developmental context- cells are induced to positively commit suicide whilst in a homeostatic context; the absence of certain survival factors may provide the impetus for suicide. There appears to be some variation in the morphology and indeed the biochemistry of these suicide pathways; some treading the path of 'apoptosis', others following a more generalised pathway to deletion, but both usually being genetically and synthetically motivated. There is some evidence that certain symptoms of 'apoptosis' such as endonuclease activation can be spuriously induced without engaging a genetic cascade, however, presumably true apoptosis and programmed cell death must be genetically mediated. It is also becoming clear that mitosis and apoptosis are toggled or linked in some way and that the balance achieved depends on signals received from appropriate growth or survival factors.

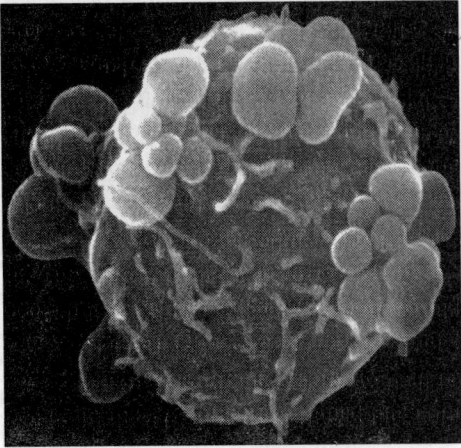

Fig. 31.1: Apoptosis.

Autophagy

Macroautophagy, often referred to as autophagy, is a catabolic process that results in the autophagosomic-lysosomal degradation of bulk cytoplasmic contents, abnormal protein aggregates, and excess or damaged organelles. Autophagy (Fig. 31.2) is generally activated by conditions of nutrient deprivation but has also been associated with physiological as well as pathological processes such as development, differentiation, neurodegenerative diseases, stress, infection and cancer.

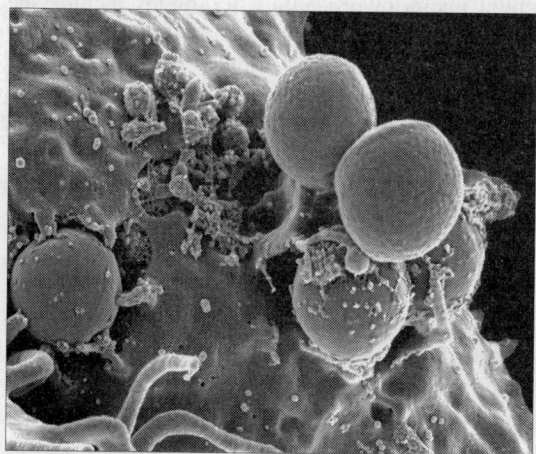

Fig. 31.2: Autophagy.

Mechanism of programmed cell death

A critical regulator of autophagy induction is the kinase mTOR, which when activated, suppresses autophagy and when not activated promotes it. Three related serine/threonine kinases, UNC-51-like kinase -1, -2, and -3 (ULK1, ULK2, UKL3), which play a similar role as the yeast Atg1, act downstream of the mTOR complex. ULK1 and ULK2 form a large complex with the mammalian homolog of an autophagy-related (Atg) gene product (mAtg13) and the scaffold protein FIP200. Class III PI3K complex, containing hVps34, Beclin-1, p150 and Atg14-like protein or ultraviolet irradiation resistance-associated gene (UVRAG), is required for the induction of autophagy.

The ATG genes control the autophagosome formation through ATG12-ATG5 and LC3-II (ATG8-II) complexes. ATG12 is conjugated to ATG5 in a ubiquitin-like reaction that requires ATG7 and ATG10. The Atg12–Atg5 conjugate then interacts non-covalently with ATG16 to form a large complex. LC3/ATG8 is cleaved at its C terminus by ATG4 protease to generate the cytosolic LC3-I. LC3-I is conjugated to phosphatidylethanolamine (PE) also in a ubiquitin-like reaction that requires Atg7 and Atg3. The lipidated form of LC3, known as LC3-II, is attached to the autophagosome membrane.

Autophagy and apoptosis are connected both positively and negatively, and extensive crosstalk exists between the two. During nutrient deficiency, autophagy functions as a pro-survival mechanism, however, excessive autophagy may lead to cell death, a process morphologically distinct from apoptosis. Several pro-apoptotic signals, such as TNF, TRAIL, and FADD, also induce autophagy. Additionally, Bcl-2 inhibits Beclin-1-dependent autophagy, thereby functioning both as a pro-survival and as an anti-autophagic regulator.

Other types of programmed cell death

Besides the above two types of PCD, other pathways have been discovered. Called 'non-apoptotic programmed cell-death' (or 'caspase-independent programmed cell-death' or 'necroptosis'), these alternative routes to death are as efficient as apoptosis and can function as either backup mechanisms or the main type of PCD. Other forms of programmed cell death include anoikis, almost identical to apoptosis except in its induction; cornification, a form of cell death exclusive to the eyes; excitotoxicity; ferroptosis, an iron-dependent form of cell death and Wallerian degeneration.

Necroptosis is a programmed form of necrosis (Fig. 31.3), or inflammatory cell death. Conventionally, necrosis is associated with unprogrammed cell death resulting from cellular damage or infiltration by pathogens, in contrast to orderly, programmed cell death, via., apoptosis.

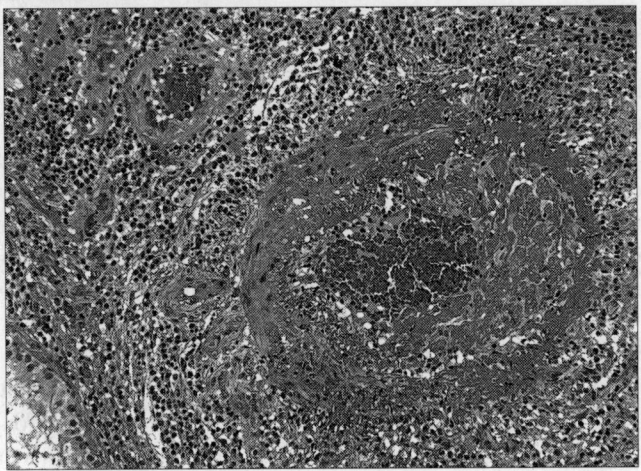

Fig. 31.3: Necrosis.

Eryptosis is a form of suicidal erythrocyte death. Aponecrosis is a hybrid of apoptosis and necrosis and refers to an incomplete apoptotic process that is completed by necrosis. NETosis is the process of cell-death generated by NETs. Plant cells undergo particular processes of PCD similar to autophagic cell death. However, some common features of PCD are highly conserved in both plants and metazoa.

ATROPHIC FACTORS OF PROGRAMMED CELL DEATH

An atrophic factor is a force that causes a cell to die. Only natural forces on the cell are considered to be atrophic factors, whereas, for example, agents of mechanical or chemical abuse or lysis of the cell are considered not to be atrophic factors. Common types of atrophic factors are:

1. Decreased workload.
2. Loss of innervation.
3. Diminished blood supply.
4. Inadequate nutrition.
5. Loss of endocrine stimulation.
6. Senility.
7. Compression.

Role of PCD in the development of the Nervous System

The initial expansion of the developing nervous system is counterbalanced by the removal of neurons and their processes. During the development of the nervous system almost 50% of developing neurons are naturally removed by programmed cell death (PCD). PCD in the nervous system was first recognised in 1896 by John Beard. Since then several theories were proposed to understand its biological significance during neural development.

Role in neural development

PCD in the developing nervous system has been observed in proliferating as well as post-mitotic cells. One theory suggests that PCD is an adaptive mechanism to regulate the number of progenitor cells. In humans, PCD in progenitor cells starts at gestational week 7 and remains until the first trimester. This process of cell death has been identified in the germinal areas of the cerebral cortex, cerebellum, thalamus, brainstem, and spinal cord among other regions. At gestational weeks 19–23, PCD is observed in post-mitotic cells. The prevailing theory explaining this observation is the neurotrophic theory which states that PCD is required to optimise the connection between neurons and their afferent inputs and efferent targets. Another theory proposes that developmental PCD in the nervous system occurs in order to correct for errors in neurons that have migrated ectopically, innervated incorrect targets, or have axons that have gone awry during path finding. It is possible that PCD during the development of the nervous system serves different functions determined by the developmental stage, cell type, and even species.

Neurotrophic theory

The neurotrophic theory is the leading hypothesis used to explain the role of programmed cell death in the developing nervous system. It postulates that in order to ensure optimal innervation of targets, a surplus of neurons is first produced which then compete for limited quantities of protective neurotrophic factors and only a fraction survive while others die by programmed cell death. Furthermore, the theory states that predetermined factors regulate the amount of neurons that survive and the size of the innervating neuronal population directly correlates to the influence of their target field.

The underlying idea that target cells secrete attractive or inducing factors and that their growth cones have a chemotactic sensitivity was first put forth by Santiago Ramon y Cajal in 1892. Cajal presented the idea as an explanation for the 'intelligent force' axons appear to take when finding their target but admitted that he had no empirical data. The theory gained more attraction when experimental manipulation of axon targets yielded death of all innervating neurons. This developed the concept of target derived regulation which became the main tenet in the neurotrophic theory. Experiments that further supported this theory led to the identification of the first neurotrophic factor, nerve growth factor (NGF).

Peripheral versus central nervous system

Different mechanisms regulate PCD in the peripheral nervous system (PNS) versus the central nervous system (CNS). In the PNS, innervation of the target is proportional to the amount of the target-released neurotrophic factors NGF and NT3. Expression of neurotrophin receptors, TrkA and TrkC, is sufficient to induce apoptosis in the absence of their ligands. Therefore, it is speculated that PCD in the PNS is dependent on the release of neurotrophic factors and thus follows the concept of the neurotrophic theory.

Programmed cell death in the CNS is not dependent on external growth factors but instead relies on intrinsically derived cues. In the neocortex, a 4:1 ratio of excitatory to inhibitory interneurons is maintained by apoptotic machinery that appears to be independent of the environment. Supporting evidence came from an experiment where interneuron progenitors were either transplanted into the mouse neocortex or cultured *in vitro*. Transplanted cells died at the age of two weeks, the same age at which endogenous interneurons undergo apoptosis. Regardless of the size of the transplant, the fraction of cells undergoing apoptosis remained constant. Furthermore, disruption of TrkB, a receptor for brain derived neurotrophic factor (Bdnf), did not affect cell death. It has also been shown that in mice null for the proapoptotic factor Bax (Bcl-2-associated X protein) a larger percentage of interneurons survived compared to wild type mice. Together these findings indicate that programmed cell death in the CNS partly exploits Bax-mediated signaling and is independent of BDNF and the environment. Apoptotic mechanisms in the CNS are still not well understood, yet it is thought that apoptosis of interneurons is a self-autonomous process.

Nervous system development in its absence

Programmed cell death can be reduced or eliminated in the developing nervous system by the targeted deletion of pro-apoptotic genes or by the overexpression of anti-apoptotic genes. The absence or reduction of PCD can cause serious anatomical malformations but can also result in minimal consequences depending on the gene targeted, neuronal population, and stage of development. Excess progenitor cell proliferation that leads to gross brain abnormalities is often lethal, as seen in caspase-3 or caspase-9 knockout mice which develop exencephaly in the forebrain. The brainstem, spinal cord, and peripheral ganglia of these mice develop normally, however, suggesting that the involvement of caspases in PCD during development depends on the brain region and cell type. Knockout or inhibition of apoptotic protease activating factor 1 (APAF1), also results in malformations and increased embryonic lethality. Manipulation of apoptosis regulator proteins Bcl-2 and Bax (overexpression of Bcl-2 or deletion of Bax) produces an increase in the number of neurons in certain regions of the nervous system such as the retina, trigeminal nucleus, cerebellum, and spinal cord.

However, PCD of neurons due to Bax deletion or Bcl-2 overexpression does not result in prominent morphological or behavioural abnormalities in mice. For example, mice over expressing Bcl-2 have generally normal motor skills and vision and only show impairment in complex behaviours such as learning and anxiety. The normal behavioural phenotypes of these mice suggest that an adaptive mechanism may be involved to compensate for the excess neurons.

Invertebrates and vertebrates

Learning about PCD in various species is essential in understanding the evolutionary basis and reason for apoptosis in development of the nervous system. During the development of the invertebrate nervous system, PCD plays different roles in different species. The similarity of the asymmetric cell death mechanism in the nematode and the leech indicates that PCD may have an evolutionary significance in the development of the nervous system. In the nematode, PCD occurs in the first hour of development leading to the elimination of 12% of non-gonadal cells including neuronal lineages. Cell death in arthropods occurs first in the nervous system when ectoderm cells differentiate and one daughter cell becomes a neuroblast and the other undergoes apoptosis. Furthermore, sex targeted cell death leads to different neuronal innervation of specific organs in males and females. In Drosophila, PCD is essential in segmentation and specification during development. In contrast to invertebrates, the mechanism of programmed cell death is found to be more conserved in vertebrates. Extensive studies performed on various vertebrates show that PCD of neurons and glia occurs in most parts of the nervous system during development. It has been observed before and during synaptogenesis in the central nervous system as well as the peripheral nervous system. However, there are a few differences between vertebrate species. For example, mammals exhibit extensive arborisation followed by PCD in the retina while birds do not. Although synaptic refinement in vertebrate systems is largely dependent on PCD, other evolutionary mechanisms also play a role.

PCD IN PLANT TISSUE

Programmed cell death in plants has a number of molecular similarities to animal apoptosis, but it also has differences, the most obvious being the presence of a cell wall and the lack of an immune system that removes the pieces of the dead cell. Instead of an immune response, the dying cell synthesises substances to break itself down and places them in a vacuole that ruptures as the cell dies.

In 'APL regulates vascular tissue identity in Arabidopsis', Martin Bonke and his colleagues had stated that one of the two long-distance transport systems in vascular plants (Fig. 31.4), xylem, consists of several cell-types 'the differentiation of which involves deposition of elaborate cell-wall thickenings and programmed cell-death.' The authors emphasise that the products of plant PCD play an important structural role.

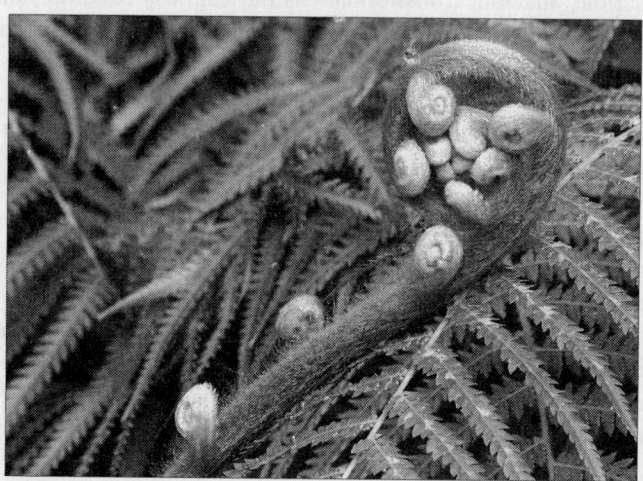

Fig. 31.4: vascular plants.

Basic morphological and biochemical features of PCD have been conserved in both plant and animal kingdoms. It should be noted, however, that specific types of plant cells carry out unique cell-death programs.

These have common features with animal apoptosis—for instance, nuclear DNA degradation—but they also have their own peculiarities, such as nuclear degradation triggered by the collapse of the vacuole in tracheary elements of the xylem. Janneke Balk and Christopher J. Leaver, of the Department of Plant Sciences, University of Oxford, carried out research on mutations in the mitochondrial genome of sun-flower cells. Results of this research suggest that mitochondria play the same key role in vascular plant PCD as in other eukaryotic cells.

PCD in Pollen Prevents Inbreeding

During pollination, plants enforce self-incompatibility (SI) as an important means to prevent self-fertilisation. Research on the corn poppy (Papaver rhoeas) has revealed that proteins in the pistil on which the pollen lands, interact with pollen and trigger PCD in incompatible (i.e., self) pollen. The researchers, Steven G. Thomas and Veronica E. Franklin-Tong, also found that the response involves rapid inhibition of pollen-tube growth, followed by PCD.

PCD in Slime Molds

The social slime mold Dictyostelium discoideum has the peculiarity of either adopting a predatory amoeba-like behaviour in its unicellular form or coalescing into a mobile slug-like form when dispersing the spores that will give birth to the next generation.

The stalk is composed of dead cells that have undergone a type of PCD that shares many features of an autophagic cell-death: Massive vacuoles forming inside cells, a degree of chromatin condensation, but no DNA fragmentation. The structural role of the residues left by the dead cells is reminiscent of the products of PCD in plant tissue.

D. discoideum is a slime mold, part of a branch that might have emerged from eukaryotic ancestors about a billion years before the present. It seems that they emerged after the ancestors of green plants and the ancestors of fungi and animals had differentiated. But, in addition to their place in the evolutionary tree, the fact that PCD has been observed in the humble, simple, six-chromosome *D. discoideum* has additional significance: It permits the study of a developmental PCD path that does not depend on caspases characteristic of apoptosis.

Chapter 32

Stem Cells

INTRODUCTION

Stem cells have the remarkable potential to develop into many different cell types in the body during early life and growth. In addition, in many tissues they serve as a sort of internal repair system, dividing essentially without limit to replenish other cells as long as the person or animal is still alive. When a stem cell divides, each new cell has the potential either to remain a stem cell or become another type of cell with a more specialised function, such as a muscle cell, a red blood cell, or a brain cell.

Stem cells are distinguished from other cell types by two important characteristics. First, they are unspecialised cells capable of renewing themselves through cell division, sometimes after long periods of inactivity. Second, under certain physiologic or experimental conditions, they can be induced to become tissue- or organ-specific cells with special functions. In some organs, such as the gut and bone marrow, stem cells regularly divide to repair and replace worn out or damaged tissues. In other organs, however, such as the pancreas and the heart, stem cells only divide under special conditions.

Until recently, scientists primarily worked with two kinds of stem cells from animals and humans: embryonic stem cells and non-embryonic 'somatic' or 'adult' stem cells. The functions and characteristics of these cells are discussed in this chapter. Scientists discovered ways to derive embryonic stem cells from early mouse embryos in 1981. The detailed study of the biology of mouse stem cells led to the discovery, in 1998, of a method to derive stem cells from human embryos and grow the cells in the laboratory. These cells are called human embryonic stem cells. The embryos used in these studies were created for reproductive purposes through *in vitro* fertilisation procedures. When they were no longer needed for that purpose, they were donated for research with the informed consent of the donor. In 2006, researchers made another breakthrough by identifying conditions that would allow some specialised adult cells to be 'reprogrammed' genetically to assume a stem cell-like state. This new type of stem cell, called induced pluripotent stem cells (IPSCs) is also discussed later in this section.

Stem cells are important for living organisms for many reasons. In the 3- to 5-day-old embryo, called a blastocyst, the inner cells give rise to the entire body of the organism, including all of the many specialised cell types and organs such as the heart, lung, skin, sperm, eggs and other tissues. In some adult tissues, such as bone marrow, muscle, and brain, discrete populations of adult stem cells generate replacements for cells that are lost through normal wear and tear, injury, or disease. Given their unique regenerative abilities, stem cells offer new potentials for treating diseases such as diabetes and heart disease. However, much work remains to be done in the laboratory and the clinic to understand how to use these cells for cell-based therapies to treat disease, which is also referred to as regenerative or reparative medicine.

Laboratory studies of stem cells (Fig. 32.1) enable scientists to learn about the cells' essential properties and what makes them different from specialised cell types. Scientists are already using stem cells in the laboratory to screen new drugs and to develop model systems to study normal growth and identify the causes of birth defects. Research on stem cells continues to advance knowledge about how an organism develops from a single cell and how healthy cells replace damaged cells in adult organisms. Stem cell research is one of the most fascinating areas of contemporary biology, but, as with many expanding fields of scientific inquiry, research on stem cells raises scientific questions as rapidly as it generates new discoveries.

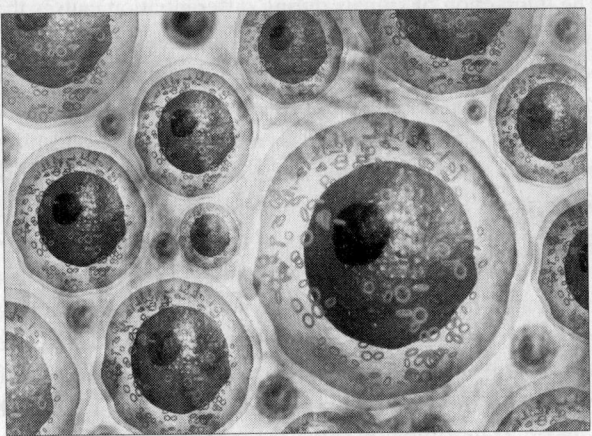

Fig. 32.1: Stem cells.

UNIQUE PROPERTIES OF ALL STEM CELLS

Stem cells differ from other types of cells in the body. All stem cells—regardless of their source—have three general properties: (i) they are capable of dividing and renewing themselves for long periods, (ii) they are unspecialised, and (iii) they can give rise to specialised cell types.

Stem cells are capable of dividing and renewing themselves for long periods: Unlike muscle cells, blood cells, or nerve cells—which do not normally replicate themselves—stem cells may replicate many times, or proliferate. A starting population of stem cells that proliferates for many months in the laboratory can yield millions of cells. If the resulting cells continue to be unspecialised, like the parent stem cells, the cells are said to be capable of long-term self-renewal.

The specific factors and conditions that allow stem cells to remain unspecialised are of great interest to scientists. It has taken many years of trial and error to learn to derive and maintain stem cells in the laboratory without them spontaneously differentiating into specific cell types. For example, it took two decades to learn how to grow human embryonic stem cells in the laboratory following the development of conditions for growing mouse stem cells. Likewise, scientists must first understand the signals that enable a non-embryonic (adult) stem cell population to proliferate and remain unspecialised before they will be able to grow large numbers of unspecialised adult stem cells in the laboratory.

Stem cells are unspecialised: One of the fundamental properties of a stem cell is that it does not have any tissue-specific structures that allow it to perform specialised functions. For example, a stem cell cannot work with its neighbours to pump blood through the body (like a heart muscle cell), and it cannot carry oxygen molecules through the bloodstream (like a red blood cell). However, unspecialised stem cells can give rise to specialised cells, including heart muscle cells, blood cells, or nerve cells.

Stem cells can give rise to specialised cells: When unspecialised stem cells give rise to specialised cells, the process is called differentiation. While differentiating, the cell usually goes through several stages, becoming more specialised at each step. Scientists are just beginning to understand the signals inside and outside cells that trigger each step of the differentiation process. The internal signals are controlled by a cell's genes, which are interspersed across long strands of DNA, and carry coded instructions for all cellular structures and functions. The external signals for cell differentiation include chemicals secreted by other cells, physical contact with neighbouring cells, and certain molecules in the micro environment . The interaction of signals during differentiation causes the cell's DNA to acquire epigenetic marks that restrict DNA expression in the cell and can be passed on through cell division.

Many questions about stem cell differentiation remain. For example, are the internal and external signals for cell differentiation similar for all kinds of stem cells? Can specific sets of signals be identified that promote differentiation into specific cell types? Addressing these questions may lead scientists to find new ways to control stem cell differentiation in the laboratory, thereby growing cells or tissues that can be used for specific purposes such as cell-based therapies or drug screening.

Adult stem cells typically generate the cell types of the tissue in which they reside. For example, a blood-forming adult stem cell in the bone marrow normally gives rise to the many types of blood cells. It is generally accepted that a blood-forming cell in the bone marrow—which is called a hematopoietic stem cell—cannot give rise to the cells of a very different tissue, such as nerve cells in the brain. Experiments over the last several years have purported to show that stem cells from one tissue may give rise to cell types of a completely different tissue. This remains an area of great debate within the research community. This controversy demonstrates the challenges of studying adult stem cells and suggests that additional research using adult stem cells is necessary to understand their full potential as future therapies.

EMBRYONIC STEM CELLS

Embryonic stem cells, as their name suggests, are derived from embryos. Most embryonic stem cells are derived from embryos that develop from eggs that have been fertilised *in vitro*—in an *in vitro* fertilisation clinic—and then donated for research purposes with informed consent of the donors. They are *not* derived from eggs fertilised in a woman's body.

Embryonic Stem Cells Grown in the Laboratory

Growing cells in the laboratory is known as cell culture. Human embryonic stem cells (hESCs) are generated by transferring cells from a preimplantation-stage embryo into a plastic laboratory culture dish that contains a nutrient broth known as culture medium . The cells divide and spread over the surface of the dish. The inner surface of the culture dish is typically coated with mouse embryonic skin cells that have been treated so they will not divide. This coating layer of cells is called a feeder layer . The mouse cells in the bottom of the culture dish provide the cells a sticky surface to which they can attach. Also, the feeder cells release nutrients into the culture medium. Researchers have devised ways to grow embryonic stem cells without mouse feeder cells. This is a significant scientific advance because of the risk that viruses or other macromolecules in the mouse cells may be transmitted to the human cells.

The process of generating an embryonic stem cell line is somewhat inefficient, so lines are not produced each time cells from the preimplantation-stage embryo are placed into a culture dish. However, if the plated cells survive, divide, and multiply enough to crowd the dish, they are removed gently and plated into several fresh culture dishes. The process of re-plating or subculturing the cells is repeated many times and for many months. Each cycle of subculturing the cells is referred to as a passage. Once the cell line is established, the original cells yield millions of embryonic stem cells. Embryonic stem cells that have proliferated in cell culture for six or more months without differentiating, are pluripotent, and appear genetically normal are referred to as an embryonic stem cell line. At any stage in the process, batches of cells can be frozen and shipped to other laboratories for further culture and experimentation.

ADULT STEM CELLS

An adult stem cell is thought to be an undifferentiated cell, found among differentiated cells in a tissue or organ that can renew itself and can differentiate to yield some or all of the major specialised cell types of the tissue or organ. The primary roles of adult stem cells in a living organism are to maintain and repair the tissue in which they are found. Scientists also use the term somatic stem cell instead of adult stem cell, where somatic refers to cells of the body (not the germ cells, sperm or eggs). Unlike embryonic stem cells, which are defined by their origin (cells from the preimplantation-stage embryo), the origin of adult stem cells in some mature tissues is still under investigation.

Research on adult stem cells has generated a great deal of excitement. Scientists have found adult stem cells in many more tissues than they once thought possible. This finding has led researchers and clinicians to ask whether adult stem cells could be used for transplants. In fact, adult hematopoietic, or blood-forming, stem cells from bone marrow have been used in transplants for 40 years. Scientists now have evidence that stem cells exist in the brain and the heart. If the differentiation of adult stem cells can be controlled in the laboratory, these cells may become the basis of transplantation-based therapies.

The history of research on adult stem cells began about 50 years ago. In the 1950s, researchers discovered that the bone marrow contains at least two kinds of stem cells. One population, called hematopoietic stem cells, forms all the types of blood cells in the body. A second population, called bone marrow stromal stem cells (also called mesenchymal stem cells, or skeletal stem cells by some) were discovered a few years later. These non-hematopoietic stem cells make up a small proportion of the stromal cell population in the bone marrow, and can generate bone, cartilage, fat, cells that support the formation of blood, and fibrous connective tissue.

In the 1960s, scientists who were studying rats discovered two regions of the brain that contained dividing cells that ultimately become nerve cells. Despite these reports, most scientists believed that the adult brain could not generate new nerve cells. It was not until the 1990s that scientists agreed that the adult brain does contain stem cells that are able to generate the brain's three major cell types—astrocytes and oligodendrocytes, which are non-neuronal cells, and neurons, or nerve cells.

Identification of Adult Stem Cells

Adult stem cells have been identified in many organs and tissues, including brain, bone marrow, peripheral blood, blood vessels, skeletal muscle, skin, teeth, heart, gut, liver, ovarian epithelium, and testis. They are thought to reside in a specific area of each tissue (called a 'stem cell niche'). In many tissues, current evidence suggests that some types of stem cells are pericytes, cells that compose the outermost layer of small blood vessels. Stem cells may remain quiescent (non-dividing) for long periods of time until they are activated by a normal need for more cells to maintain tissues, or by disease or tissue injury.

Typically, there is a very small number of stem cells in each tissue, and once removed from the body, their capacity to divide is limited, making generation of large quantities of stem cells difficult. Scientists in many laboratories are trying to find better ways to grow large quantities of adult stem cells in cell culture and to manipulate them to generate specific cell types so they can be used to treat injury or disease. Some examples of potential treatments include regenerating bone using cells derived from bone marrow stroma, developing insulin-producing cells for type 1 diabetes, and repairing damaged heart muscle following a heart attack with cardiac muscle cells.

Most adult stem cells are lineage-restricted (multipotent) and are generally referred to by their tissue origin (mesenchymal stem cell, adipose-derived stem cell, endothelial stem cell, dental pulp stem cell, etc.). Stem cell division and differentiation is shown in Fig. 32.1. Adult stem cell treatments have been successfully used for many years to treat leukemia and related bone/blood cancers through bone marrow transplants.

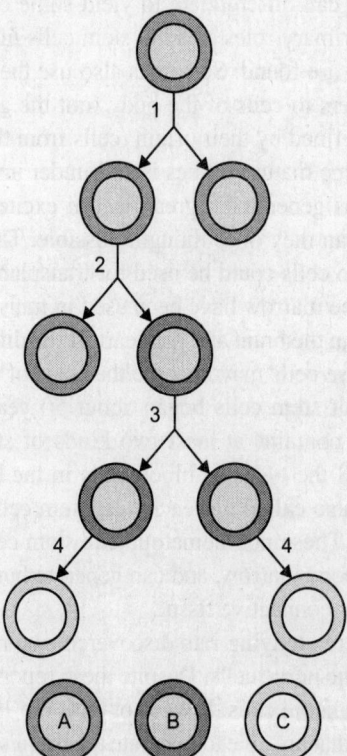

Fig. 32.2: Stem cell division and differentiation. A: stem cell, B: progenitor cell, C: differentiated cell, 1: symmetric stem cell division, 2: asymmetric stem cell division, 3: progenitor division, 4: terminal differentiation.

Tests used to Identify Adult Stem Cells

Scientists often use one or more of the following methods to identify adult stem cells: (i) label the cells in a living tissue with molecular markers and then determine the specialised cell types they generate, (ii) remove the cells from a living animal, label them in cell culture, and transplant them back into another animal to determine whether the cells replace (or repopulate) their tissue of origin.

Adult Stem Cell Differentiation

As indicated above, scientists have reported that adult stem cells occur in many tissues and that they enter normal differentiation pathways to form the specialised cell types of the tissue in which they reside.

Normal differentiation pathways of adult stem cells: In a living animal, adult stem cells are available to divide for a long period, when needed, and can give rise to mature cell types that have characteristic shapes and specialised structures and functions of a particular tissue. The following are examples of differentiation pathways of adult stem cells that have been demonstrated *in vitro* or *in vivo*.

- Hematopoietic stem cells give rise to all the types of blood cells: red blood cells, B lymphocytes, T lymphocytes, natural killer cells, neutrophils, basophils, eosinophils, monocytes, and macrophages.

- Mesenchymal stem cells have been reported to be present in many tissues. Those from bone marrow (bone marrow stromal stem cells, skeletal stem cells) give rise to a variety of cell types: bone cells (osteoblasts and osteocytes), cartilage cells (chondrocytes), fat cells (adipocytes), and stromal cells that support blood formation. However, it is not yet clear how similar or dissimilar mesenchymal cells derived from non-bone marrow sources are to those from bone marrow stroma.

- Neural stem cells in the brain give rise to its three major cell types: nerve cells (neurons) and two categories of non-neuronal cells—astrocytes and oligodendrocytes.

- Epithelial stem cells in the lining of the digestive tract occur in deep crypts and give rise to several cell types: absorptive cells, goblet cells, Paneth cells, and enteroendocrine cells.

- Skin stem cells occur in the basal layer of the epidermis and at the base of hair follicles. The epidermal stem cells give rise to keratinocytes, which migrate to the surface of the skin and form a protective layer. The follicular stem cells can give rise to both the hair follicle and to the epidermis.

Transdifferentiation: A number of experiments have reported that certain adult stem cell types can differentiate into cell types seen in organs or tissues other than those expected from the cells' predicted lineage (i.e. brain stem cells that differentiate into blood cells or blood-forming cells that differentiate into cardiac muscle cells, and so forth). This reported phenomenon is called transdifferentiation.

Although isolated instances of transdifferentiation have been observed in some vertebrate species, whether this phenomenon actually occurs in humans is under debate by the scientific community. Instead of transdifferentiation, the observed instances may involve fusion of a donor cell with a recipient cell. Another possibility is that transplanted stem cells are secreting factors that encourage the recipient's own stem cells to begin the repair process. Even when transdifferentiation has been detected, only a very small percentage of cells undergo the process.

In addition to reprogramming cells to become a specific cell type, it is now possible to reprogramme adult somatic cells to become like embryonic stem cells (induced pluripotent stem cells, iPSCs) through the introduction of embryonic genes. Thus, a source of cells can be generated that are specific to the donor, thereby avoiding issues of histocompatibility, if such cells were to be used for tissue regeneration. However, like embryonic stem cells, determination of the methods by which iPSCs can be completely and reproducibly committed to appropriate cell lineages is still under investigation.

SIMILARITIES AND DIFFERENCES BETWEEN EMBRYONIC AND ADULT STEM CELLS

Human embryonic and adult stem cells each have advantages and disadvantages regarding potential use for cell-based regenerative therapies. One major difference between adult and embryonic stem cells is their different abilities in the number and type of differentiated cell types they can become. Embryonic stem cells can become all cell types of the body because they are pluripotent. Adult stem cells are thought to be limited to differentiating into different cell types of their tissue of origin.

Embryonic stem cells can be grown relatively easily in culture. Adult stem cells are rare in mature tissues, so isolating these cells from an adult tissue is challenging, and methods to expand their numbers in cell culture have not yet been worked out. This is an important distinction, as large numbers of cells are needed for stem cell replacement therapies. Scientists believe that tissues derived from embryonic and adult stem cells may differ in the likelihood of being rejected after transplantation. It is not yet know whether tissues derived from embryonic stem cells would cause transplant rejection, since relatively few clinical trials have tested the safety of transplanted cells derived from hESCS.

Adult stem cells, and tissues derived from them, are currently believed less likely to initiate rejection after transplantation. This is because a patient's own cells could be expanded in culture, coaxed into assuming a specific cell type (differentiation), and then reintroduced into the patient. The use of adult stem cells and tissues derived from the patient's own adult stem cells would mean that the cells are less likely to be rejected by the immune system. This represents a significant advantage, as immune rejection can be circumvented only by continuous administration of immuno suppressive drugs, and the drugs themselves may cause deleterious side effects.

INDUCED PLURIPOTENT STEM CELLS

Induced pluripotent stem cells (iPSCs) are adult cells that have been genetically reprogrammed to an embryonic stem cell–like state by being forced to express genes and factors important for maintaining the defining properties of embryonic stem cells. Although these cells meet the defining criteria for pluripotent stem cells, it is not known if iPSCs and embryonic stem cells differ in clinically significant ways. Mouse iPSCs were first reported in 2006, and human iPSCs were first reported in late 2007. Mouse iPSCs demonstrate important characteristics of pluripotent stem cells, including expressing stem cell markers, forming tumours containing cells from all three germ layers, and being able to contribute to many different tissues when injected into mouse embryos at a very early stage in development. Human iPSCs also express stem cell markers and are capable of generating cells characteristic of all three germ layers.

Although additional research is needed, iPSCs are already useful tools for drug development and modelling of diseases, and scientists hope to use them in transplantation medicine. Viruses are currently used to introduce the reprogramming factors into adult cells, and this process must be carefully controlled and tested before the technique can lead to useful treatments for humans. In animal studies, the virus used to introduce the stem cell factors sometimes causes cancers. Researchers are currently investigating non-viral delivery strategies. In any case, this breakthrough discovery has created a powerful new way to 'dedifferentiate' cells whose developmental fates had been previously assumed to be determined. In addition, tissues derived from iPSCs will be a nearly identical match to the cell donor and thus probably avoid rejection by the immune system. The iPSC strategy creates pluripotent stem cells that, together with studies of other types of pluripotent stem cells, will help researchers learn how to reprogramme cells to repair damaged tissues in the human body.

POTENTIAL USES OF HUMAN STEM CELLS AND THE OBSTACLES THAT MUST BE OVERCOME BEFORE THESE POTENTIAL USES WILL BE REALISED

There are many ways in which human stem cells can be used in research and the clinic. Studies of human embryonic stem cells will yield information about the complex events that occur during human development. A primary goal of this work is to identify how undifferentiated stem cells become the differentiated cells that form the tissues and organs. Scientists know that turning genes on and off is central to this process. Some of the most serious medical conditions, such as cancer and birth defects, are due to abnormal cell division and differentiation. A more complete understanding of the genetic and molecular controls of these processes may yield information about how such diseases arise and suggest new strategies for therapy. Predictably controlling cell proliferation and differentiation requires additional basic research on the molecular and genetic signals that regulate cell division and specialisation. While recent developments with iPS cells suggest some of the specific factors that may be involved, techniques must be devised to introduce these factors safely into the cells and control the processes that are induced by these factors.

Human stem cells are currently being used to test new drugs. New medications are tested for safety on differentiated cells generated from human pluripotent cell lines. Other kinds of cell lines have a long history of being used in this way. Cancer cell lines, for example, are used to screen potential anti-tumour drugs. The availability of pluripotent stem cells would allow drug testing in a wider range of cell types. However, to screen drugs effectively, the conditions must be identical when comparing different drugs. Therefore, scientists will have to be able to precisely control the differentiation of stem cells into the specific cell type on which drugs will be tested. Current knowledge of the signals controlling differentiation falls short of being able to mimic these conditions precisely to generate pure populations of differentiated cells for each drug being tested.

Perhaps the most important potential application of human stem cells is the generation of cells and tissues that could be used for cell-based therapies. Today, donated organs and tissues are often used to replace ailing or destroyed tissue, but the need for transplantable tissues and organs far outweighs the available supply. Stem cells, directed to differentiate into specific cell types, offer the possibility of a renewable source of replacement cells and tissues to treat diseases including Alzheimer's disease, spinal cord injury, stroke, burns, heart disease, diabetes, osteoarthritis, and rheumatoid arthritis.

For example, it may become possible to generate healthy heart muscle cells in the laboratory and then transplant those cells into patients with chronic heart disease. Preliminary research in mice and other animals indicates that bone marrow stromal cells, transplanted into a damaged heart, can have beneficial effects. Whether these cells can generate heart muscle cells or stimulate the growth of new blood vessels that repopulate the heart tissue, or help via some other mechanism is actively under investigation. For example, injected cells may repair by secreting growth factors, rather than actually incorporating into the heart. Promising results from animal studies have served as the basis for a small number of exploratory studies in humans. Other recent studies in cell culture systems indicate that it may be possible to direct the differentiation of embryonic stem cells or adult bone marrow cells into heart muscle cells.

In people who suffer from type 1 diabetes, the cells of the pancreas that normally produce insulin are destroyed by the patient's own immune system. New studies indicate that it may be possible to direct the differentiation of human embryonic stem cells in cell culture to form insulin-producing cells that eventually could be used in transplantation therapy for persons with diabetes.

To realise the promise of novel cell-based therapies for such pervasive and debilitating diseases, scientists must be able to manipulate stem cells so that they possess the necessary characteristics for successful differentiation, transplantation, and engraftment. The following is a list of steps in successful cell-based treatments that scientists will have to learn to control to bring such treatments to the clinic. To be useful for transplant purposes, stem cells must be reproducibly made to:

- Proliferate extensively and generate sufficient quantities of cells for making tissue.

- Differentiate into the desired cell type(s).
- Survive in the recipient after transplant.
- Integrate into the surrounding tissue after transplant.
- Function appropriately for the duration of the recipient's life.
- Avoid harming the recipient in any way.

Also, to avoid the problem of immune rejection, scientists are experimenting with different research strategies to generate tissues that will not be rejected. To summarise, stem cells offer exciting promise for future therapies, but significant technical hurdles remain that will only be overcome through years of intensive research.

STEM CELLS USED IN REGENERATIVE MEDICINE

Advances in stem cell biology have made it possible for organ regeneration to become a reality, and this new technique is poised to enter the field of clinical medicine. The stem cells used in regenerative medicine are classified as embryonic or adult. Neurons, vascular endothelial cells, skeletal muscle cells, cardiomyocytes, osteoblasts, and chondroblasts have already been obtained from stem cells in the laboratory setting. Embryonic stem cells are amenable to mass culture and have versatile pluripotency but tend to be associated with problems in clinical application, including tumorigenesis, immunological rejection, and ethical issues. Since adult stem cells are obtained from the bone marrow of the patient, problems related to donors, ethics, rejection, and tumorigenesis do not apply. However, techniques for the isolation and *in vitro* amplification of adult stem cells have yet to be established, raising issues that await future solutions. For stem cells to be used in the clinical setting, regeneration at the tissue level is necessary, requiring the combined resources of tissue engineering and material science. Regenerative medicine is expected to play a leading role in 21st century medicine. However, the integration of studies from various scientific fields seems necessary for success in this area.

Stem cells that can be used for regenerative medical therapies are broadly divided into two groups: embryonic stem cells (ES cells) obtained from early-stage embryos and adult stem cells that still are present in the adult body. These two types of stem cells have their own particular advantages and disadvantages. Whether one type is superior to the other remains controversial, depending on the type of tissue to which they are to be transplanted. A method of culture has already been established for ES cells, and their particular advantage is that they are capable of differentiating into any type of cell within the body.

Current Status and Problems of Regenerative Medicine using ES Cells

At present, the regeneration of neurons, blood cells, vascular endothelial cells, cardiomyocytes, pigment cells, osteoblasts, and islet cells is feasible or trying to be developed. In theory, ES cells can differentiate into any type of cell in the body. However, in the actual setting, cells that occur in the early stage of development are fairly easy to obtain, whereas those that have undergone advanced differentiation in the late prenatal or postnatal period are more difficult to obtain. In addition, among neurons, large cells such as spinal cord ventral horn cells are considered easier to obtain from ES cells than from adult stem cells. Although ES cells represent a very attractive tool from the viewpoint of tissue regeneration, they are associated with a number of drawbacks. First, because the ES cells used in allogeneic transplantation are obtained from others, rejection reactions cannot be avoided. Immunosuppressive therapy is required to manage the rejection, but such therapy may cause the quality of the patient's life to deteriorate and lead to high, ongoing medical expenditures. Second, if undifferentiated cells are present among the transplanted cells, it is possible that a malignant tumour, teratoma, may form in the tissue undergoing transplantation. In general, rejection reactions are more likely to occur in organs where blood flow is abundant, leading to a higher possibility of cellular infiltration. On the other hand, from clinical experience with the transplantation of fetal midbrain obtained through artificial termination of pregnancy into the nigrostriatum in patients with Parkinson's disease, it has been found that about one month of immuno suppressive therapy is sufficient for cases of transplantation of allogeneic nerve cells into the brain, because lymphocytes cannot cross the blood-brain barrier. Thus, ES cells are presumed to be superior for the regeneration of nerve cells in the central nervous system.

Application of Adult Stem Cells to Regenerative Medicine

Let us now turn to the other type of stem cells, adult stem cells. To begin with, stem cells are known to be characterised by their capacity for self-replication, proliferative potency, and pluripotency. Stem cells are ranked from high to low in terms of the diversity of their ability to differentiate. For example, ES cells, which can differentiate into any type of cell, are given the highest rank, whereas hematopoietic stem cells are ranked in the middle, and cutaneous stem cells are considered low-ranking stem cells or precursor cells. Somatic tissues are formed from endoblasts, mesoblasts, or ectoblasts in the fetal stage. Skin and nerve tissues are derived from ectoblasts, and the stem cells of these tissues are therefore present in local areas. More specifically, cutaneous stem cells are present in the granular layer of the dermis, and neural stem cells are present around the cerebral ventricle of the cerebral hippocampus, where they are responsible for the regeneration of the respective tissues. Visceral organs such as the liver and pancreas are derived from endoblasts, and the stem cells of these tissues are present in the respective organs. If the liver is excised, oval cells or small hepatocytes in the remaining liver proliferate to regenerate the liver.

Various other cells of the body, such as bone, cartilage, fat, ligament, tendon, skeletal muscle, myocardium, and smooth muscle, are derived from mesoblasts. Among the stem cells of these tissues, some exist in muscle, for example, satellite cells, which are low-ranking stem cells found in the skeletal muscle. However, recent studies have revealed that the stem cells of these tissues are present in the bone marrow. As is well known, bone marrow consists mainly of hematopoietic stem cells and other cells of the blood cell series, but cells which are not blood cells are also present in bone marrow. Called bone marrow stromal cells, these cells are known to secrete various cell growth factors and cytokines that control the proliferation and differentiation of the blood cell series. In recent years, it has become apparent that mesenchymal stem cells in the bone marrow with pluripotent capacity are present among marrow stromal cells. It had been reported by the early 1990s that mesenchymal stem cells differentiate into osteoblasts, chondroblasts, and adipocytes, and these cells began to be referred to as mesenchymal in the sense of mesoblast-derived stem cells. Since mesenchymal stem cells are stem cells for mesoblastderived cells, we wondered whether they could differentiate to become cardiomyocytes, and we carried out studies along this line. We demonstrated that cardiomyocytes that beat regularly by themselves could be obtained from mesenchymal stem cells. It has also been reported that mesenchymal stem cells can differentiate into mesoblast-derived tissues such as tendon and ligament.

At this point, it is important to determine to what extent these stem cells in bone marrow are pluripotent and how far they can differentiate. Results were reported in the US last year of an autopsy case of leukemia in a female patient who died after the transplantation of bone marrow from a male donor. In this patient, cells possessing the Y chromosome derived from the male donor were found in liver, skeletal muscle, and the intestinal tract. Thus, it became apparent that adult stem cells can differentiate not only into mesoblast- but also into endoblast-derived organs. A more recent study demonstrated that mesenchymal stem cells can differentiate into ectoblastderived nerve cells. Therefore, the expression 'mesenchymal' is no longer accurate, and these cells have been called adult stem cells because they can differentiate to become tissues derived from any germ layer.

To sum up, regenerative medicine has become an important focus of the medical profession in the 21st century. However, the success of this type of medical care will require the cooperation of various fields of science, including molecular biology, developmental biology, embryology, anatomy, tissue engineering, and material science. People have high expectations of regenerative medicine. It is therefore important that basic research and translational research that applies the results of basic research continue to make progress.

SECTION XII

Cancer Its Causes and Cure

Chapter 33

Cancer

INTRODUCTION

Cancer can be defined as a disease in which a group of abnormal cells grow uncontrollably by disregarding the normal rules of cell division. Normal cells are constantly subject to signals that dictate whether the cell should divide, differentiate into another cell or die. Cancer cells develop a degree of autonomy from these signals, resulting in uncontrolled growth and proliferation. If this proliferation is allowed to continue and spread, it can be fatal. In fact, almost 90% of cancer-related deaths are due to tumour spreading a process called metastasis. The foundation of modern cancer biology rests on a simple principle virtually all mammalian cells share similar molecular networks that control cell proliferation, differentiation and cell death. The prevailing theory, which underpins research into the genesis and treatment of cancer, is that normal cells are transformed into cancers as a result of changes in these networks at the molecular, biochemical and cellular level, and for each cell there is a finite number of ways this disruption can occur.

TUMOUR VIRUSES

Viruses are capable of causing a wide variety of human diseases, ranging from rabies to smallpox to the common cold. The great majority of these infectious agents do harm through their ability to multiply inside infected host cells, to kill these cells, and to release progeny virus particles that proceed to infect other hosts nearby. The cytopathic (cell-killing) effects of viruses, together with their ability to spread rapidly throughout a tissue, enable these agents to leave a wide swath of destruction in their wake. But the peculiarities of certain viral replication cycles may on occasion yield quite another outcome. Rather than killing infected cells, some viruses may, quite paradoxically, force their hosts to thrive, indeed, to proliferate uncontrollably. In so doing, such viruses—often called tumour viruses—can create cancer.

The cancer-causing powers of tumour viruses drove many researchers to ask precisely how they succeed in creating disease. Most of these viruses possess relatively simple genomes containing small numbers of viral genes, yet some were found able to overwhelm an infected cell and its vastly more complex genome and to redirect cell growth in new directions. Such behaviour indicated that tumour viruses have developed extremely potent genes to perturb the complex regulatory circuitry of the host cells that they infect.

481

By studying tumour viruses and their mechanisms of action, researchers changed the entire mindset of cancer research. Cancer became a disease of genes and thus a condition that was susceptible to analysis by the tools of molecular biology and genetics. When this story began, no one anticipated how obscure tumour viruses would one day revolutionise the study of human cancer pathogenesis.

Generally, tumour viruses cause little or no disease after infection in their hosts, or cause non-neoplastic diseases such as acute hepatitis for hepatitis B virus or mononucleosis for Epstein–Barr virus. A minority of persons (or animals) will go on to develop cancers after infection. This has complicated efforts to determine whether or not a given virus causes cancer. The well-known Koch's postulates, 19th-century constructs developed by Robert Koch to establish the likelihood that Bacillus anthracis will cause anthrax disease, are not applicable to viral diseases. (Firstly, this is because viruses cannot truly be isolated in pure culture—even stringent isolation techniques cannot exclude undetected contaminating viruses with similar density characteristics, and viruses must be grown on cells. Secondly, asymptomatic virus infection and carriage is the norm for most tumour viruses, which violates Koch's third principle. Relman and Fredericks have described the difficulties in applying Koch's postulates to virus-induced cancers. Finally, the host restriction for human viruses makes it unethical to experimentally transmit a suspected cancer virus.) Other measures, such as A. B. Hill's criteria, are more relevant to cancer virology but also have some limitations in determining causality. Tumour viruses come in a variety of forms: Viruses with a DNA genome, such as adenovirus (Fig. 33.1), and viruses with an RNA genome, like the Hepatitis C virus (HCV), can cause cancers, as can retroviruses having both DNA and RNA genomes (Human T-lymphotropic virus and hepatitis B virus, which normally replicates as a mixed double and single-stranded DNA virus but also has a retroviral replication component).

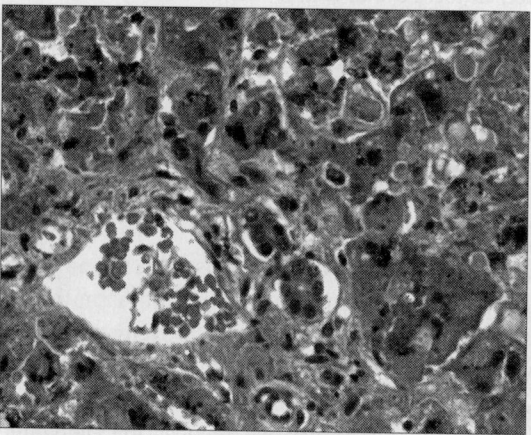

Fig. 33.1: Adenovirus.

In many cases, tumour viruses do not cause cancer in their native hosts but only in dead-end species. For example, adenoviruses do not cause cancer in humans but are instead responsible for colds, conjunctivitis and other acute illnesses. They only become tumorigenic when infected into certain rodent species, such as Syrian hamsters. Some viruses are tumorigenic when they infect a cell and persist as circular episomes or plasmids, replicating separately from host cell DNA (Epstein–Barr virus and Kaposi's sarcoma-associated herpesvirus). Other viruses are only carcinogenic when they integrate into the host cell genome as part of a biological accident, such as polyomaviruses and papillomaviruses. A direct oncogenic viral mechanism involves either insertion of additional viral oncogenic genes into the host cell or to enhance already existing oncogenic genes (proto-oncogenes) in the genome. Indirect viral oncogenicity involves chronic nonspecific inflammation occurring over decades of infection, as is the case for HCV-induced liver cancer. These two mechanisms differ in their biology and epidemiology: direct tumour viruses must have at least one virus copy in every tumour cell expressing at least one protein or RNA that is causing the cell to become cancerous. Because foreign virus antigens are expressed in these tumours, persons who are immuno suppressed such as AIDS or transplant patients are at higher risk for these types of cancers. Chronic indirect tumour viruses, on the other hand, can be lost (at least theoretically) from a mature tumour that has accumulated sufficient mutations and growth conditions (hyperplasia) from the chronic inflammation of viral infection. In this latter case, it is controversial but at least theoretically possible that an indirect tumour virus could undergo 'hit-and-run' and so the virus would be lost from the clinically diagnosed tumour. In practical terms, this is an uncommon occurrence if it does occur.

CANCER IS CLONAL IN ORIGIN

Current dogma states that cancer is a multi-gene, multi-step disease originating from a single abnormal cell (clonal origin) with an altered DNA sequence (mutation). Uncontrolled proliferation of these abnormal cells is followed by a second mutation leading to the mildly aberrant stage. Successive rounds of mutation and selective expansion of these cells results in the formation of a tumour mass. Subsequent rounds of mutation and expansion leads to tumour growth and progression, which eventually breaks through the basal membrane barrier surrounding tissues and spreads to other parts of the body (metastasis). Death as a result of cancer is due to the invading, eroding and spread of tumours into normal tissues due to uncontrolled clonal expansion of these somatic cells.

INSIGHTS INTO CANCER

Initiation and progression of cancer depends on both external factors in the environment (tobacco, chemicals, radiation and infectious organisms) and factors within the cell (inherited mutations, hormones, immune conditions, and mutations that occur from metabolism). These factors can act together or in sequence, resulting in abnormal cell behaviour and excessive proliferation. As a result, cell masses grow and expand, affecting surrounding normal tissues (such as in the brain), and can also spread to other locations in the body (metastasis). However, it is important to remember that most common cancers take months and years for these DNA mutations to accumulate and result in a detectable cancer. Cancers arise approximately in one among every 3 individuals. DNA mutations arise normally at a frequency of 1 in every 20 million per gene per cell division. The average number of cells formed in any individual during an average lifetime is 10^{16} (10 million cells being replaced every second!). It would therefore be logical to assume that human populations anywhere in the world would show similar frequencies of cancer. However, cancer incidence rates (number of individuals diagnosed) vary dramatically across countries. Evidently, some factors seem to intervene to dramatically increase cancer incidences in some populations. The obvious inference is that contributory factors that cause cancer are either hereditary or environmental. It means that either certain populations carry a large number of cancer-susceptibility genes or that the environment in which populations live largely contribute to the cancer incidence rates.

CAUSES OF CANCER

Cancer is caused by accumulated damage to genes. Such changes may be due to chance or to exposure to a cancer causing substance. The substances that cause cancer are called carcinogens. A carcinogen may be a chemical substance, such as certain molecules in tobacco smoke.

The cause of cancer may be environmental agents, viral or genetic factors. We can roughly divide cancer risk factors into the following groups:

- Biological or internal factors, such as age, gender, inherited genetic defects and skin type.
- Environmental exposure, for instance to radon and UV radiation, and fine particulate matter.
- Occupational risk factors, including carcinogens such as many chemicals, radioactive materials and asbestos.
- Lifestyle-related factors.

Lifestyle-related factors that cause cancer include:

- Tobacco
- Alcohol
- UV radiation in sunlight
- Some food-related factors, such as nitrites and poly aromatic hydrocarbons generated by barbecuing food.

FACTORS INFLUENCING CANCER DEVELOPMENT

A number of intrinsic (biological) and external factors are associated with the development of cancers. The intrinsic factors include the age and hormonal status of the individual, family history and genetic predisposition. The extraneous factors include diet and life style, individuals habits like smoking and alcohol use, exposure to toxic chemicals and radiation, some infections, etc. Several external factors, including asbestos, many chemicals, dyes, food additives, vehicular emissions, act as promoters in carcinogenesis.

Biological Factors

Age and hormonal status

Cancer is considered to be an old age disease. Some types of cancers are almost entirely found in people above 50–55 years, e.g. prostate cancer. Similarly cervix cancer in women are more commonly detected at the peri- or post-menopausal ages. However, no age group is immune to this disease. Hormonal factors play an important role in the development of gender-specific cancers, e.g. estrogen in cancers of ovary and uterus in female.

Family history

Some cancers are indicated to have a link with family occurrence. For example, women whose close relatives like grandmother, mother, maternal aunt or sister has suffered from breast cancer, are found to run about 3 times higher risk of developing breast cancer than those who do not have such a family history. Similarly, cancers of the uterine cervix (females) and of prostate (males) are also thought to have a familial connection.

Genetic predisposition

Certain genetic conditions are known to predispose the individual to cancer. For example, individuals with genetic conditions like xeroderma pigmentosum, ataxia telangiectasia, Bloom's syndrome, and Fanconi's anaemia are found to be highly susceptible to different types of cancer.

External factors

Diet, alcohol, and tobacco use: More than 50% of all cancers are related to the diet and individual habits like alcoholism, tobacco chewing and smoking. High fat diet and obesity are associated with breast cancer. A positive correlation has been reported between age-adjusted breast cancer mortality rates and the average per capita fat consumption in a given nation on a daily basis. Similarly, deep-fried and burnt food and preserved (high salt) food are associated with increase in gastric cancer incidence. Regular consumption of food low in fibre content and rich in animal fat increased the risk of cancers of stomach and oesophagus. High intake of red meat and low fibre diet has been considered to be the cause of the high incidence of gastric cancer in the USA. The role of cigarette smoking in lung cancer is established. Tobacco smoke contains a chemical, nitrosamine, which can induce neoplastic changes in the lung cells. Non-smoking tobacco habits, like chewing, are found to greatly increase the cancers of the upper alimentary tract and buccal mucosa. India has the highest incidence of oral cancers in the world, which is correlated with the tobacco chewing habit. Alcoholism is found to increase the risk of liver and bladder cancers. Smoking combined with alcohol consumption poses a higher risk of cancers of the breast, oesophagus, liver, stomach and urinary bladder. Alcoholism along with hepatitis B virus infection is a more serious risk factor in liver cancer (Fig. 33.2).

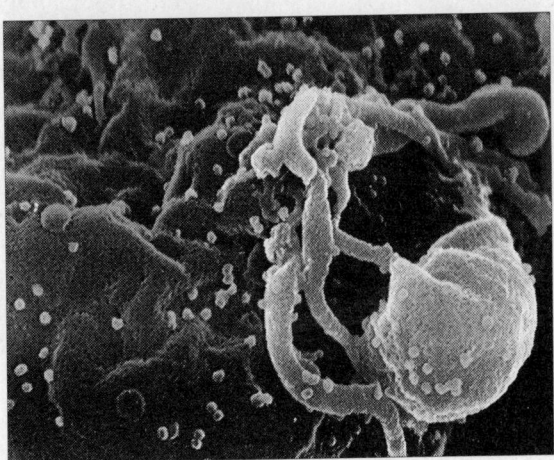

Fig. 33.2: Liver cancer.

Radiation and cancer

Ionising radiation is an established carcinogen, having both initiating and promoting effects. The positive correlation between ionising radiation and carcinogenesis has been established from the studies on the early radiologists, radium dial painters and atom bomb victims of Japan. A positive association has been seen in the increase in childhood cancers and obstetric X-ray exposures of the mother. Tumours induced by radiation have relatively long latencies, which vary in different species as a more or less constant function. Within a given species the latency varies also with age at the time of irradiation and with the type of neoplasm induced. The age differences in latencies appear to be related to similar age differences in the rates of corresponding spontaneous leukemias. The risk of adult type of malignancies tend to increase progressively with time after irradiation, in parallel with the age-dependent increase in the underlying base-line incidence.

Viruses and cancer

Oncoviruses play an important role in specific human cancers, e.g. human papilloma virus in cervix cancer, and certain skin cancers, Epstein-Barr virus in Burkitt lymphoma and nasopharyngeal carcinoma, hepatitis B virus in hepatocellular carcinoma, human T-cell leukemia virus in leukemia. The viruses are of two types: DNA viruses which incorporate into the cellular genome and the retroviruses (RNA viruses) which cause transformation of cellular genome, leading to malignant changes in the infected cell.

Role of free radicals

Reactive oxygen species (ROS) and other free radicals are produced in the body, both during the normal metabolic process as well as by interaction with external toxic agents, for example, radiation and toxic chemicals. They include superoxide anions, hydroxyl radicals, peroxy radicals and hydroperoxides. These interact with DNA and produce gene mutations and chromosomal aberrations, leading to cell transformation. Free radicals are considered to have a major role in the induction of cancers by chemicals and radiation. Several factors of our modern life style, e.g. excess alcohol consumption, tobacco chewing and smoking habits, exposure to toxic chemicals and radiations, all add to the free radical production in the body and increase the risk of cancer.

Lifestyles can Reduce the Risk of Cancer

Lifestyles are important factors in the formation of many types of cancer. Behaviour and choice can affect our own cancer risks. But when it comes to individual cancers it is not possible to say for sure what causes the cancer. Healthy lifestyles can prevent cancer. Everyone should exercise regularly and have a varied diet. People need to eat plenty of plant products and fibre, and only very little red meat and saturated fat. Things to avoid are smoking, drinking and too much exposure to the Sun.

Cancer causing factors related to work and living environments include:

- Asbestos fibres.
- Tar and pitch.
- Polynuclear hydrocarbons (e.g. benzopyrene).
- Some metal compounds.
- Some plastic chemicals (e.g. Vinyl chloride).

Bacteria and viruses can cause cancer:

- Helicobacter pylori (H. pylori, which causes gastritis).
- HBV, HCV (hepatitis viruses that cause hepatitis).
- HPV (human papilloma virus, papilloma virus, which causes changes, e.g. Cervical cells).
- EBV (Epstein-Barr virus, the herpes virus that causes inflammation of the throat lymphoid).

Radiation can cause cancer:

- Ionising radiation (e.g. X-ray radiation, soil radon).
- Non-ionised radiation (the Sun ultraviolet radiation).

Some drugs may increase the risk of cancer:

- Certain antineoplastic agents.
- Certain hormones.
- Medicines that cause immune deficiency.

In 5–10% of breast cancer genetic predisposition plays an important role in the emergence of the disease.

Cancer Genetics

According to current estimates, only about one in 10 cases of cancer is associated with hereditary predisposition. Cancer is a common disease, and almost every family has a number of members who suffer from cancer. However, this does not generally mean that families have a hereditary predisposition to cancer. The vast majority of cancer cases originate from the combined effect of hereditary as well as external influences, such as environmental and lifestyle factors.

Cancer is not inherited. It is only the genetic defect that can lead to cancer that is inherited, which means that the predisposition to getting cancer, or increased risk, can be inherited. However, this is not common. According to current estimates, only about one in 10 cases of cancer is associated with hereditary predisposition. An inherited genetic defect is not necessarily passed on to all members of the same family, and not everyone who receives the same defective gene will develop cancer. It is also worth remembering that the genetic changes that occur in cancerous tumours are not passed on genetically to one's offspring.

Identification of Cancer Hereditary

A genetic disposition to cancer can be identified by the onset of cancer occurring at a very young age or that many closely related members of the same family suffer from the same type of cancer. The genetic defects that incur a predisposition to cancer are varied. They can be rare, they may involve genetic changes that pose a high cancer risk, or ones that carry only a low risk, or then somewhere in between. Now-a-days, we know about some of the genetic defects that carry a bigger cancer risk, but not all. Many genes are still being investigated.

Hereditary breast cancer

Breast cancer is the most common form of cancer among women. Nearly 5000 women and some 20 men fall ill with the disease. From what we know at present, about 10 per cent of breast cancer is hereditary. The best-known genes that carry a high risk of causing breast and ovarian cancer are the BRCA1 and BRCA2 genes. There is also a susceptibility gene, which is linked to a moderate risk of breast cancer.

It is good to find out about one's inherited breast cancer predisposition if

- At least three of four relatives from the same side of the family have had breast or ovarian cancer.
- A close relative had cancer at a young age.
- There has been both breast and ovarian cancer in the same family.
- A man in one's family has had breast cancer.

Hereditary colorectal cancer

About two-three per cent of the new cases of colorectal cancer detected each year are hereditary.

We refer to hereditary colorectal cancer if:

- At least three close family relatives have had colorectal cancer and at least one of them is under 50 years old.
- There has been, in addition to colorectal cancer, endometrial, small bowel, urethral or renal pelvis cancer among close family relatives.

There are about 250 extended families in Finland in which gene defect causing a predisposition to hereditary non-polyposis colorectal cancer (Lynch Syndrome) has been detected.

Detecting Cancer with Gene Test

Cancer cannot be found using gene testing, but with the help of current genetics research we can detect some cancer-predisposing gene defects. At present, there is no simple genetic test for those interested in being tested. Genetic tests are only used when there is clear evidence of a possible hereditary predisposition to cancer.

IDENTIFICATION AND HISTOPATHOLOGY OF CANCERS

Why do we need to identify and classify cancers? There are several benefits to identifying and classifying cancers using histological sections and staining methodology

1. Diagnosis: Microscopic observation helps determine whether the tumour tissue is benign (harmless) or malignant (potentially fatal). Gross cellular morphology and tissue specific markers are used to classify cancerous cells.

2. Therapy: Pathology can be used as a confirmation or in prognosis, e.g. has the surgeon removed the entire tumour? Or was the treatment effective in eliminating tumours? Or what is the rate of progression of the cancer? Progression can be predicted by histotyping, e.g. patients with simple hyperplasia in the uterine epithelium have <1% chance of developing cancer compared 82% risk in patients with atypical hyperplasia.

3. Cellular origin (histogenesis): Determining the origins of the tumour by histopathological classification of tissue is useful in (a) identifying whether the tumour is a primary or secondary tumour, e.g. a liver tumour may have metastasised from elsewhere or (b) source of origin of the tumour, e.g. lung cancer due to smoking is epithelial (lung carcinoma) but due to asbestos exposure is mesothelial.

HALLMARKS OF CANCER

DNA mutations result in defects in the regulatory circuits of a cell, which disrupt normal cell proliferation behaviour. However the complexity of this disease is not as simple at the cellular and molecular level. Individual cell behaviour is not autonomous, and it usually relies on external signals from surrounding cells in the tissue or micro environment. There are more than 100 distinct types of cancers and any specific organ can contain tumours of more than one subtype. This provokes several questions. How many of these regulatory circuits need to be broken to transform a normal cell into a cancerous one? Is there a common regulatory circuit that is broken among different types of cancers? Which of these circuits are broken inside a cell and which of these are linked to external signals from neighbouring cells in the tissue? The answer to these questions can be summarised in a heterotypic model, manifested as the six common changes in cell physiology that results in cancer. This model looks at tumours as complex tissues, in which cancer cells recruit and use normal cells in order to enhance their own survival and proliferation. The 6 hallmarks of this currently accepted model can be described using a traffic light analogy.

1. Immortality: Continuous cell division and limitless replication.
2. Produce 'Go' signals (growth factors from oncogenes).
3. Override 'Stop' signals (anti-growth signals from tumour suppressor genes).
4. Resistance to cell death (apoptosis).
5. Angiogenesis: Induction of new blood vessel growth.
6. Metastasis: Spread to other sites.

CHEMOTHERAPY

Chemotherapy is the treatment of cancer by means of chemicals that kill cancer cells. These 'anti-cancer' drugs destroy cancer cells by stopping their growth and reproduction. Unfortunately, normal healthy cells are also affected and this causes the well-known side effects of chemotherapy. The normal healthy cells have an organised cell structure and repair mechanisms in place. This results in them being able to reproduce new normal tissue after chemotherapy. Often, two or more drugs are given. This is called combination chemotherapy and forms the basis of most of chemotherapy today. The rationale is that the different drugs enhance each other's effect and create a better effect combined than if they were used as single agents. Different chemotherapy drugs are chosen so that they do not have the same side effects on tissue, in order for the side effects to be minimised.

Chemotherapy can have different goals:

• To cure cancer.
• To control the growth of cancer.
• To alleviate symptoms such as pain caused by cancer.

Chemotherapy can be used as a single treatment modality, but is also commonly used in combination with surgery, radiotherapy and biological treatment in order to:

• Shrink a tumour before radiotherapy or surgery. This is called neo-adjuvant therapy.
• Destroy any remaining cancer cells after surgery or radiotherapy. This is called adjuvant therapy.
• Enhance the effect of radiotherapy and biological therapy.
• Destroy recurring cancer or destroy cancer that has spread to other parts of the body.

PLANNING OF CHEMOTHERAPY TREATMENT

Each treatment plan is tailor-made to suit every individual and will depend on:

• The type of cancer.
• The area of the body where the cancer is.
• The stage of the development of the cancer, e.g. the size of the tumour in the affected organ.
• Has there been any spread to the rest of the body?
• How the cancer influences the functioning of your body.
• Your general health.
• The purpose of the treatment, either curative or to relieve symptoms.

Clinical trials, also called treatment studies or research studies, test new treatment regimes. These could include new drugs, new approaches to surgery or radiotherapy or new treatments such as gene therapy. The purpose of this research is to find better methods of treatment for cancer patients.

Administration of Chemotherapy

Chemotherapy can be given in different ways, namely: intravenous (into a vein), orally (in pill form) or an injection under the skin or into muscle. In some cases it can be applied to the skin.

Intravenous administration

This is the most common method of administration. A thin needle is inserted into a vein on the hand or lower arm. This needle is removed once the chemotherapy has been completed. Chemotherapy can also be given intravenously by means of catheters, ports and pumps. A port is a round plastic or metal chamber that is placed under the skin. It is connected via a thin tube to one of the major vessels in the chest cavity. This method is more permanent and can be used for as long as necessary.

Oral administration

The chemotherapy is given in the form of a pill or capsule

Injection: A needle and syringe deliver the chemotherapy drug either intramuscularly (into a muscle) or subcutaneously. Most patients receive chemotherapy as out-patients in the oncology unit and do not need to be admitted to hospital. Sometimes, it may be necessary for hospital admission for certain chemotherapy regimes.

Chemotherapy given and how long does it take

This is decided by:
- The type of cancer.
- The goal of the treatment, either curative or to relieve symptoms.
- The different chemotherapy drugs.
- How your body copes with the chemotherapy.

Chemotherapy can be given daily, weekly or monthly. It is given in cycles where treatment is alternated with rest periods. It is important to keep to the chemotherapy schedule in order to get the optimum results.

CHEMORADIATION

Chemoradiation involves a combination of treatments given together: Chemotherapy and radiotherapy. Chemotherapy is a form of drug treatment given to treat or control cancer cells, while radiotherapy is the use of precise, accurately measured doses of radiation (X-ray beams) directed to a specific area to treat cancer cells.

Chemoradiation can be used to treat all types of oesophageal cancers, but has a specific, defined role in squamous cell cancer. It can be used either as an alternative to surgery, or when a tumour cannot be surgically removed. The chemotherapy increases the sensitivity of the cancer cells to radiation and it is known as a radiosensitiser.

Chemotherapy is usually given by an injection directly into a vein, usually by an infusion or drip. Chemotherapy drugs can sometimes be given orally in a tablet form. The intravenous chemotherapy is usually given in the first and last week of treatment. Radiation therapy is given as an out-patient. Some chemotherapy infusions will require an overnight stay in hospital to hydrate the patient and monitor their urine output. The commonly drugs used for chemoradiation to treat cancer of the oesophagus are *cis* platin and 5 Fluoro-uracil or Capecitabine. Treatment usually ranges from 5 to 6 weeks depending on the duration of the radiotherapy. When radiation and chemotherapy are given in combination it is likely that the side effects will increase.

TUMOUR SUPPRESSOR

A tumour suppressor gene, or antioncogene, is a gene that protects a cell from one step on the path to cancer. When this gene mutates to cause a loss or reduction in its function, the cell can progress to cancer, usually in combination with other genetic changes. The loss of these genes may be even more important than proto-oncogene/oncogene activation for the formation of many kinds of human cancer cells. Tumour suppressor genes can be grouped into categories including caretaker genes, gatekeeper genes, and landscaper genes, the classification schemes are evolving as medicine advances, learning from fields including molecular biology, genetics, and epigenetics.

Functions of Tumour Suppressor

Tumour suppressor genes, or more precisely, the proteins for which they code, either have a damping or repressive effect on the regulation of the cell cycle or promote apoptosis, and sometimes do both.

The functions of tumour suppressor proteins fall into several categories including the following:

- Repression of genes that are essential for the continuing of the cell cycle. If these genes are not expressed, the cell cycle does not continue, effectively inhibiting cell division.
- Coupling the cell cycle to DNA damage. As long as there is damaged DNA in the cell, it should not divide. If the damage can be repaired, the cell cycle can continue.
- If the damage cannot be repaired, the cell should initiate apoptosis (programmed cell death) to remove the threat it poses for the greater good of the organisms produced.
- Some proteins involved in cell adhesion prevent tumour cells from dispersing, block loss of contact inhibition, and inhibit metastasis. These proteins are known as metastasis suppressors.
- DNA repair proteins are usually classified as tumour suppressors as well, as mutations in their genes increase the risk of cancer, for example mutations in HNPCC, MEN1 and BRCA. Furthermore, increased mutation rate from decreased DNA repair leads to increased inactivation of other tumour suppressors and activation of oncogenes.

Examples of Tumour Suppressor

The first tumour suppressor protein discovered was the retinoblastoma protein (pRb) in human retinoblastoma. however, recent evidence has also implicated pRb as a tumour-survival factor. Another important tumour suppressor is the p53 tumour-suppressor protein encoded by the TP53 gene. Homozygous loss of p53 is found in 65% of colon cancers, 30–50% of breast cancers, and 50% of lung cancers. Mutated p53 is also involved in the pathophysiology of leukemias, lymphomas, sarcomas, and neurogenic tumours. Abnormalities of the p53 gene can be inherited in Li-Fraumeni syndrome (LFS), which increases the risk of developing various types of cancers.

PTEN acts by opposing the action of PI3K, which is essential for anti-apoptotic, pro-tumorogenic Akt activation. As costs of DNA sequencing have diminished, many cancers have now been sequenced for the first time, revealing novel tumour suppressors. Among the most frequently mutated genes are components of the SWI/SNF chromatin remodelling complex, which are lost in about 20% of tumours. Other examples of tumour suppressors include pVHL, APC, CD95, ST5, YPEL3, ST7, and ST14.

CELLULAR DEFENSE MECHANISMS IN RELATION TO CANCER PREVENTION AND CARCINOGENESIS

Normal cells are naturally equipped with efficient defense mechanisms that work at different levels.

Antioxidants

The cells synthesise their own defense molecules, which include the non-protein thiol gluthathione, and antioxidant enzymes like superoxide dismutase, catalase, glutathione peroxidase, reductase and S-transferases. These scavenge the ROS before they can reach the target molecules in the cell and thus protect against their attack on the vital molecules like DNA. Thus they serve as the biological watchdogs in safeguarding against free radical induced initiating changes, mutations and chromosomal aberrations.

Many dietary ingredients like green vegetables, fruits, tea, spices and some diet supplements contain antioxidants. These include the vitamins A, C, and E, beta-carotene, alpha-tocopherol, ascorbic acid, flavonoids, lycopenes, curcumins and enzymes like caspasine. They act as chemo-preventers by scavenging free radicals and enhancing cellular defense through their adaptogenic properties.

DNA Repair

Damage to cellular DNA is the crucial early event in the neoplastic transformation of a cell. The DNA lesions may include altered bases, covalent binding of bulky adducts, inter- and intra-strand cross-links and generation of strand breaks. A range of alkylated products is formed in DNA by exposure to nitroso-compounds and other alkylating agents. Ionising radiation and many genotoxic chemicals generate free radicals, which interact with DNA and produce different lesions ranging from base damage, deletions and complex and multiple lesions. Most normal cells possess a high capacity for repair of DNA damage. However, efficient repair depends on the type of damage, its severity and the time available for repair. The base damage and single strand breaks are repaired fast and without error, restoring the molecular structure. But double strand breaks and multiple breaks and local cluster lesions are not properly repaired and often contain errors (error-prone repair or misrepair), leading to cell death or cell survival with abnormal gene functions and chromosomal abnormalities which are associated with malignant cell transformation. DNA repair involves a number of genes, the products of which operate in a co-ordinated manner to form repair pathways that control restitution of DNA structure.

Apoptosis or programmed cell death is an important mechanism of cellular defense in reducing the risks of error-prone repair. Cells with DNA damage undergo apoptosis, thus preventing these cells from surviving and entering the proliferating cell pool and, thereby, preventing the possibility of tumour development. Apoptosis is a genetically controlled process involving p53, bcl2 and other genes. Mutations in p53 can block the tumour-suppressive effect by eliminating apoptosis, and thus, allowing the damaged cells to survive and undergo proliferation. Some of the gene products that control cell cycle also influence apoptotic tendencies, e.g. c-myc, pRb, Tp53.

ROLE OF DIET IN CANCER CONTROL

Doll and Peto were the first to point out an association between dietary constituents and cancer. A vegetarian diet is considered to be beneficial in reducing cancer incidence. Epidemiological studies have suggested that diets rich in vegetables, and fruits reduces the risk of certain cancers. For example, diets rich in fibre, vitamins A,C, and E, beta-carotene, retinols, alpha-tocopherol, polyphenols, and flavonoids, and minerals like selenium and zinc, have cancer chemopreventive effect. Fruits and vegetables are rich sources of chemopreventive chemicals. These include inhibitors of carcinogen formation, blocking agents (block conversion of procarcinogens to carcinogens), stimulators of detoxifying system, trapping agents (trap and eliminate potential carcinogens) and suppressing agents (suppress the different steps of the metabolic pathway leading to cancer). A study in China showed a high incidence of oesophageal and gastric cancers in a population whose diet is deficient in beta-carotene and vitamins C and E. An interventional programme, where the diet was supplemented with beta-carotenes, vitamin E and selenium, produced a 20% reduction in the stomach cancer mortality over a period 5 years.

Chapter 34

Molecular Approaches to Cancer Treatment

INTRODUCTION

Colorectal cancer is an important disease of the modern world, generating significant mortality and morbidity rates. Its therapy, although considerably improved, continues to be unhelpful for a large percentage of patients, especially for those in advanced stages. This justifies the efforts toward producing new therapies, as well as for stratifying patients according to risk factors and prediction of therapeutic response. In this respect, the contributions of modern science are essential for defining the most intimate mechanisms and players of tumorigenesis and for proposing new biomarkers. The study of antitumor immune responses has revealed new insights into the tumor microenvironment, leading to the development of vaccines and adoptive transfer of immunocompetent cells. Circulating tumor cells are a real opportunity to detect early relapses and to define risk categories, while miRNAs, a family of small non-coding RNA implicated in regulation of gene expression, evolved as a new class of biomarkers with high potential for diagnosis, prognosis and prediction of colorectal cancers.

Colorectal cancer (CRC) represents the fourth death cause in the world, with over 600,000 deaths per year, of which almost 70% in poorer countries. Although the treatment of CRC definitely improved during the past decades, there are patients who do not benefit from the current therapeutic schemes, especially in advanced stages. This justifies the intensive research conducted to establish the prognostic and predictive role of biological markers. This chapter summarises the latest contributions of antitumor immunology, morphopathology of circulating tumor cells, and microRNA assessment in identifying novel biomarkers for CRC. The chapter also discusses new therapies which have emerged as alternatives to conventional approaches.

IMMUNOLOGICAL MARKERS AND THERAPIES FOR COLORECTAL CANCER

An important number of cells and molecules of the immune system are now correlated with survival and response to different therapies, due to a large body of data provided by numerous studies performed during the past decades. First of all, the presence of tumor-infiltrating lymphocytes (TILs) was recognised as an independent prognostic factor in CRC since 1987. Jass and others observed a direct relation between the number of TILs and survival, and an inverse relation between the presence of TILs and tumor stage. In another study done by Phil and others, the density and type of local lymph nodes-infiltrating lymphocytes (Fig. 34.1) were proved to exert an influence on survival, establishing a direct link between the antineoplastic immune response mounted by the organism and the tumor evolution. More recently, the researchers are not focused on TILs as a whole, but on their subtypes, knowing that CD4+ T helper cells, CD8+ T cytotoxic cells, and regulatory T cells (Tregs) play different roles in oncologic surveillance.

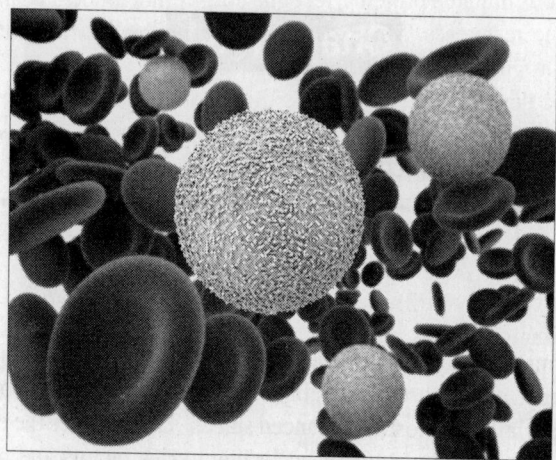

Fig. 34.1: Lymphocytes.

CD8+ cytotoxic T lymphocytes can kill tumoral cells by recognising the tumor specific antigens presented in the context of MHC class I molecules. In a study conducted on 602 early-stage (TNM I and II) CRC, the density of intratumoral CD8+T cells with memory phenotype (CD45RO+) proved to be a very good prognostic marker, since recurrence rates were 4.8% versus 75% (p<0.0001) in high and, respectively, low density CD8+CD45RO+ T cells CRC. Similar studies have shown that CRC free of early metastatic invasion had important infiltrates of CD8+ T cells.

Regulatory T cells are characterised by their ability to inhibit the auto-reactive and unwanted immune responses. Their role was better understood in the last decade, when it became clear that an immune response is the result of a complex balance between action and suppression. As would be expected, Tregs are detrimental in oncologic surveillance, inducing poor clinical outcomes if accumulated in large quantities in solid tumors. Regarding the impact of Tregs in CRC, there has been a large debate over the latter years, whether these types of cells, if considerably accumulated in tumors, are connected, or not, with a poor clinical outcome. The initial assumption, that Tregs are detrimental in CRC, was questioned by several reports published beginning with 2005. In 2009, a study conducted on 967 patients diagnosed with stage II and III CRC, evaluated by immunohistochemistry the presence of intratumoral FoxP3+ Tregs, concluding – by multivariate analysis – that a high density of these cells is positively correlated with survival. Treg cells would thus be granted the value of a positive prognostic marker in CRC patients. A possible explanation for this apparent paradox would be the fact that CRC develops in a septic environment, and bacterial products from the intestinal lumen would act as stimulators of inflammation, chronic inflammation being incriminated as a risk factor developing CRC. In 2010, Frey and others demonstrated, on a cohort of 1420 patients with nonmetastatic CRC, that the presence of Tregs, characterised by the CD4+FoxP3+ combination, is an independent prognostic marker in MMR

(*Mismatch Repair*) genes-proficient CRC, both in univariate and multivariate analysis, according to this study, CD4+FoxP3+ Tregs correlate with better survival rates. In MMR-deficient CRC, this correlation was kept only in univariate statistical analysis, which has triggered live debates, especially after several researchers failed to identify the above mentioned correlations in their studies. Stratification of CRC patients according to the status of MMR genes in this type of studies is performed due to the fact that a deficiency of DNA mismatch repair genes generates an advanced genomic instability, leading to the appearance of numerous mutated proteins, recognised as tumor associated antigens (TAA), capable of inducing livelier immune responses. MMR-deficient patients have better survival, and this is why the confirmation of novel prognostic markers in CRC takes into account the MMR state. In conclusion, involvement of Tregs in the development of CRC is still under debate, and their function as prognostic markers is yet to be ascertained.

Myeloid-derived suppressor cells (MDSC) are classically identified based on the CD11b+CD14-CD33+ phenotype. MDSC inhibit anti-tumor immune responses, they can reach 10 times higher numbers than normal in the peripheral blood of oncologic patients. Recently, a new molecular marker was proposed for identification of these cells: S100A9. They can have double origin – myeloid or monocyte – and are capable of inhibiting cytotoxic T lymphocytes. Their number increases progressively, from stage I to stage IV of a tumor, metastatic patients presenting with the highest numbers of MDSC in peripheral blood. The role of MDSC as prognostic markers in CRC has not yet been fully established.

β2-microglobulin stabilises the MHC-I complex, when the tumor associated antigens are presented to CD8+ T lymphocytes by tumor cells. Downregulation of *β2*- microglobulin expression in neoplasias is one of the many evasion strategies observed in CRC, as well as in other malignancies or chronic viral infections. Yet tumors which completely suppress *β2*-microglobulin synthesis and, implicitly, MHC class I assembly, become the target of NK cells. Therefore, it is not surprising to observe that, in CRC patients, an intermediate expression of MHC-I is associated with reduced survival, indicating that tumors which downregulate the expression of HLA class I molecules without fully suppressing it, can avoid cytotoxicity caused by T cells and NK cells.

Immunotherapy in CRC has a history of over one hundred years, at its beginnings, non-specific immune stimulators such as the Coley extract (heat-inactivated extract of Streptococcus and Serratia) were used to boost the anti-oncogenic immune response. During the past decades, clinical trials have tested numerous immunotherapies, ranging from nonspecific to specific – vaccines and monoclonal antibodies. Among the first agents used in a clinical setting, we must mention interleukin 2 (IL-2), a stimulator of T cells. A meta-analysis targeting publications between 1990 and 2004 has shown that IL-2 is efficient only if associated with standard therapy, in early stages of metastatic colorectal cancer (mCRC).

Antitumor Vaccination

CRC was not initially described as an immunogenic tumor, but recent studies have demonstrated the existence of an antitumor immune response in this case, too: the presence and number of intratumoral T cells is inversely correlated with the tumor stage, and directly correlated with overall survival (OS). Clinical and immunological responses to specific active immunotherapy in CRC were assessed by a meta-analysis including 32 clinical trials and 527 patients. The clinical benefit rate was 11.2%. Antitumor responses were detected in 59% of treated patients. Cell-mediated antitumor responses were present in 44% of patients. In a more recent study, a βHCG-based (beta-Human Chorionic Gonadotropin plays the surprising role of Tumor specific antigen – TSA in CRC) vaccine which was administered to 77 patients with mCRC, in a phase II clinical trial: 73% of patients developed anti-βHCG antibodies post-immunisation, and higher antibody titers were correlated with increased OS.

Indoleamine 2,3-dioxygenase (IDO) is an enzyme involved in the metabolism of tryptophan, with immunosuppressive effects – inhibits lymphocyte proliferation – and is produced by Tregs. Tryptophan is required for active immune responses and it is intensely degraded by IDO. In CRC patients, an upregulation of IDO was noted in a subset of dendritic cells (plasmacytoid DC) and in some tumor cells. Vaccination with peptides resulted from IDO fragmentation, induces a cell-mediated immune response based on specific anti-tumor cytotoxic T cells or tolerogenic DC. In a similar fashion, it can be speculated the induction of active immunity toward other immunosuppressive molecules such as TGF-β (Transforming Growth Factor Beta). In a mini-study enrolling 19 CRC patients, vaccination with a synthetic peptide TGFβRII-like, in association with GM-CSF (Granulocyte-Macrophage Colony Stimulating Factor) as a booster of antigen presenting cells, managed to induce an antitumor immune response in all 19 patients.

Another antigenic molecule for CRC, the glycoprotein MUC1, was speculated as tumor antigen in CRC patients. L-BLP25, a molecule inducing anti-MUC1 responses, is currently being tested in association with chemotherapy in metastatic CRC. After complete resection of primary tumor and all liver metastasis, the patients are randomised 2:1 to receive either L-BLP25 or placebo.

Adoptive cell therapy

In adoptive immunotherapy, T lymphocytes are harvested from the host, conditioned *ex vivo* by stimulation with tumor extracts, expanded and reinjected. T cells obtained in this manner are generally CD8+ memory T cells. There are many attempts of adoptive immunotherapy in CRC, of which we are presenting two studies which appear to be more promising. Karlsson and collaborators have harvested T cells from sentinel lymph nodes in 16 patients with stage II-IV CRC, after conditioning and reinjection, 8 patients from the study group were also subjected to chemotherapy. Among patients with disease in stage IV, the outcome was: 4 stable disease, 1 partial response, and 4 complete remissions. There was also a significant increase of OS (2.6 versus 0.8 years). Patients in stages II-III were recurrence-free at 3 years, with the exception of one patient who presented with liver metastases at 6 months.

A second clinical trial has combined immunotherapy with chemotherapy to increase the chance of a successful intervention. Correale and others conducted a phase II clinical trial on 47 patients with pretreated mCRC. The patients were administered the GOLFIG combination (FOLFOX + gemcytabine + IL-2 + GM-CSF), with promising results: 10 complete remissions, 16 partial remissions and 16 patients with stable disease. The survival indices were as follows: overall response rate – 43%, time to progression – 12.26 months, OS – 18.76 months.

These encouraging results have prompted the Italian group to start a phase III trial entitled GOLFIG-2, which is ongoing, comparing GOLFIG with FOLFOX-4 (oxaliplatin, 5-fluorouracil, leucovorin) in the first line of treatment of mCRC patients. High CD8+ T cells CCR7+ tumor infiltration score has already emerged as a favourable prognostic factor for mCRC in this new trial.

Circulating Tumor Cells

An essential element in CRC progress is the process of metastasis. This implies malignant cells leaving the primary tumor and migrating to distant organs, using the vascular or lymphatic system. The presence, in the blood, of cells with morphologic similarities to primary tumor cells, was first spotted by the Australian pathologist T. Ashworth more than 100 years ago.

Only recently have the cellular detection methods enabled the isolation of circulating tumor cells (CTC) by reproducible manner, thus allowing the assessment of their role in the clinical evolution of patients. The studies performed at present for CTC identification have proven that these cells have an important role in establishing the diagnosis, prognosis, or in monitoring of recurrences and therapeutic response for patients with CRC, breast and prostate cancer. Existing methods are limited in terms of predicting the clinical evolution of CRC patients or response to therapy, which makes CTC determination a potentially valuable tool for providing new information in this respect.

CTC isolation methods

Few CTC isolation methods are used today for CRC patients, each of them presenting advantages and disadvantages, they are mainly based on the different morphological and molecular characteristics of epithelialderived CTC, as opposed to blood cells. At present, most studies are performed using the immunomagnetic separation (IMS) method. This can be achieved by using a classic separation system (MACS, Miltenyi Biotec), or an automatic one (CellSearch, Veridex™), the latter being approved by the FDA. The automatic method uses microbeads covered by anti-EpCAM (Epithelial Cell Adhesion Molecule) antibodies for the isolation of epithelial cells from peripheral blood. Afterwards, the isolated cells are identified by positivity for CKs (cytokeratins) 8, 18, 19 and DAPI (4',6-diamidino-2-phenylindole), and negativity for CD45. This technique presents the advantages of a high sensitivity and specificity, as well as reproducibility. Being commercially available and approved by the FDA, it is currently used in most of the clinical studies with large numbers of patients.

Nevertheless, it also presents a few disadvantages such as selection of a small number of EpCAM-expressing cells, and the impossibility of their subsequent molecular analysis. Another method, based on the size difference between epithelial cells and blood cells, is ISET (Isolation by Size of Epithelial Tumor cells). In this case, filters with pores of about 8 micrometers are used to obtain a mechanical separation of CTC. It is a quick and easy method, it does not destroy the cells, enabling their further molecular analysis. In terms of disadvantages it has a low specificity, but it also retains cells in epithelial–mesenchymal transition, which do not express EpCAM.

Apart from the gene amplification technique, other methods used to confirm isolated cells as CTC rely on identifying certain morphological characteristics of the cell, which requires the experience of a trained pathologist. From this point of view, it was agreed upon several criteria for CTC identification: presence of cytoplasm, irregular nuclear membrane, size of nucleus (>24 micrometers), anisonucleosis (ratio>0.5), an increased nucleo-cytoplasmic ratio and the presence of grouped cells. Depending on such criteria, the cells are categorised in: malignant – 4 criteria, non-determined malignant potential – 2 criteria, and benignant – absence of all criteria. For an accurate identification, several molecular criteria were added (e.g. positivity for CK 8, 18, 19).

Following isolation, PCR (Polymerase Chain Reaction) assays are efficient *in vitro* assays for amplification of RNA sequences specific for the epithelial phenotype or for stem cells, in order to obtain a molecular characterisation of CTC but do not distinguish between viable and nonviable cells and do not allow further molecular analysis of the isolated cells.

Clinical studies

The first study showing a correlation between CTC disseminated in the bone marrow and the prognosis of CRC patients was published more than two decades ago. The following studies confirmed the initial results, but they were heterogeneous in respect of detection methods, therefore a standardisation of

CTC detection methodologies is mandatory for achieving comparability and validation of large scale studies. Regarding the clinical studies which have been so far conducted, there is a difference between those enrolling patients with CRC stage I-III, on one hand, and metastatic stage IV, on the other hand. For stages I-III CRC, the number of isolated CTC is lower, which makes the methods used more sensitive, most of them being based on the PCR technique. Even so, the CTC presence was correlated with poor disease-free survival and overall survival.

Metastatic colon cancer has been the subject of even more studies, those including the highest number of patients and is focused on two of the most important, conducted by Cohen and others (430 patients) and Tol and others (467 patients). Presence of CTC in the patients' blood (3 CTC/7.5 ml) was linked in both studies with lower PFS (progression-free survival) and OS, confirming the prognostic value of CTC in CRC. Concerning the response to treatment, the patients who became negative for CTC after 3-5 weeks (Cohen study) or 1-2 weeks (Tol study, Cairo-2) had a better PFS than those who remained CTC-positive during these intervals, stating the CTC as a predictive marker, as well. Unlike other tumors, such as, for example, lung, breast or prostate, for which the threshold of CTC positivity is considered to be at least 5 CTC/7.5 ml blood, in CRC this was established at only 3 CTC/7.5 ml. This is due to two facts: (i) the liver acts as a 'filter' for CTC from colorectal tumors, leaving fewer to escape in the systemic circulation, (ii) CRC-derived CTC are present more as groups, rather than isolated cells. Other studies, with smaller number of patients, have produced similar results, indicating the value of CTC assessment in the management of patients suffering from metastatic CRC.

An interesting study has attempted to evaluate the relationship between the type of hepatic metastases ablation and the number of CTC, in patients with stage IV CRC. The data collected by this group showed that the CTC number drops when the ablation is made surgically, unlike radiofrequency ablation, when the CTC number increases. If the presence and especially the CTC number were proven to have an impact upon OS and PFS, it remains yet to establish the CTC role in indicating and monitoring systemic chemotherapy. This would be clinically significant, because from stage II CRC patients 25% will progress, and chemotherapy would be useful in their case.

Whereas at present there are no means of identifying these patients, highlighting CTC could serve as a guide for the therapeutic decision. Additionally, in those patients who already have an indication for systemic treatment, choosing the type and dosage of chemotherapy could be assisted by CTC determination at different time points.

MicroRNAs AS NEW MOLECULAR TOOLS FOR CLINICAL APPLICATIONS

MicroRNAs (miRNAs) represent small non-coding RNAs of about 22-nucleotides (nt), transcribed from individual genes, mostly located in intergenic regions, in introns of protein coding genes or in introns and exons of non-coding genes. miRNAs are processed from stem-loop precursors into miRNA. One strand of these duplexes is usually incorporated into the RNA-induced silencing complex (RISC) which interacts with the 3'untranslated region (3'-UTR) of the mRNA targets, inducing translational repression or mRNA (messenger RNA) cleavage. Generally, miRNAs are involved in negative regulation of gene expression at the post-transcriptional level, but there have been reports about positive regulation of gene expression mediated by miRNAs. Their activities are involved in many crucial biological processes, including metabolism, survival, differentiation, apoptosis and proliferation.

A considerable advantage of implementing miRNAs as novel molecular tools derives from the fact that a single miRNA can target and regulate the expression of hundreds of mRNAs. Therefore, it is easier to work with a small number of miRNAs than with mRNAs to discover biomarkers of interest with higher sensitivity and specificity. The data obtained by genomic high-throughput technologies provide specific profiles of up-regulated and down-regulated miRNAs for many cancer types. Another advantage of miRNAs is their high stability and resistance to storage and handling, including archived formalin fixed paraffin embedded (FFPE) tissues and body fluids.

Several methods including quantitative real-time PCR (qRT-PCR), miRNA-microarray and deep sequencing (next-generation sequencing) are currently available for miRNA detection. Generally, qRT-PCR is used to evaluate a small number of miRNAs, while miRNA-microarray and next-generation sequencing are used for assessing comprehensively screening panels of miRNA. Even if qRT-PCR is considered the most sensitive and reproducible method for miRNA quantification, there are some limitations regarding the consensus about housekeeper miRNAs or endogenous controls used for normalisation. The common controls used for miRNAs quantification are: U6 small nuclear RNA (RNU6B), 5SrRNA, let-7a, mir-16, mir-345, mir-16, mir-223.

miRNAs in Colorectal Pathology

MiRNAs in CRC diagnosis

Now-a-days, early diagnosis of CRC is based on colonoscopy and fecal occult blood test (FOBT). Colonoscopy represents the most reliable method for CRC detection, but has a major drawback due to its invasive nature. Instead, FOBT represents a widespread CRC noninvasive test, but has low sensitivity especially for pre-neoplastic lesions. Thus, it is necessary to identify a new class of noninvasive biomarkers for early detection of CRC, miRNAs being regarded as valuable candidates to this challenge. miRNAs could influence colorectal carcinogenesis by direct regulation of their mRNA targets, represented by oncogenes or tumor suppressor genes. Wnt/β-catenin, PI3K, KRAS, p53 or regulators of extracellular signals are the most important pathways mediated by miRNAs.

Identification of miRNAs in the body fluids has followed the discovery of tissue miRNAs. The studies on serum or plasma from patients suffering from CRC are relatively recent and suggest the possible use of miRNAs as novel noninvasive biomarkers for cancer detection. In one of these studies, Pu and others have analysed plasma miR-21, miR-221 and miR-222 as possible noninvasive biomarkers for CRC diagnosis: 103 CRC patients and 37 healthy subjects, as controls, were included in the study. Smith and others identified miR-221 as potential biomarker for differentiating CRC patients from controls. miR-221 was proposed as a significant prognostic factor for poor OS in CRC patients, its level being well correlated with p53 expression. In another study, Huang and others identified miR-29a and miR-92a as noninvasive biomarkers for early detection of CRC versus advanced adenoma. Collin and others reported increased levels of miR-135b, miR-95, miR-222, miR-17-3p, and miR-92 in the plasma of CRC patients when compared with plasma of healthy subjects. They showed that miR-92 plasma levels can distinguish patients with CRC from gastric cancer, inflammatory bowel disease (IBD) and healthy subjects, with 89% sensitivity and 70% specificity. Cheng and others tried to correlate CRC stage of evolution with plasma levels of three miRNA types: miR-21, miR-92, and miR-141. They found that only miR-141 was significantly associated with stage IV CRC versus other stages, with 77.1% sensitivity and 89.7% specificity. Smith and others proposed a more accurate screening program for CRC patients, combining the miR-141 level with the CEA test.

Link and others identified an alternative miRNA test using fecal samples. They found that miR-21 and miR-106a are up-regulated in CRC fecal samples compared with healthy subjects and the expression of these two miRNAs decreases with advanced stages.

Role of miRNAs in CRC prognosis

Xi and others reported for the first time the utility of miRNAs in CRC prognosis. They found that a high level of miR-200c in CRC is significantly correlated with patient survival. In a miRNA-microarray study, the group of Motoyoma identified miR-18 as being involved in CRC prognosis. They reported that CRC patients with high levels of miR-18 have a poorer clinical prognosis compared to the low expression group. Moreover, high levels of miR-21, which acts as a putative oncogene, were correlated with poor survival in CRC patients. Schepeler and others reported a molecular signature based on four miRNAs (miR-142-3p, miR-212, miR-151, miR-144), used for predicting tumor recurrence in stage II colon cancer. Even if these data reveal a significant potential for miRNAs as prognostic markers in CRC, larger studies are needed to strengthen these facts.

Predicting treatment response in CRC based on miRNAs

An important step in CRC treatment involves modulating the response of CRC cells to chemotherapeutic drugs. Song and others reported miR-192, miR-215 and miR-140 as being involved in modulation of chemoresistance of CRC cells. Overexpression of miR-192 led to inhibition of dihydrofolate reductase (DHFR) and an increased chemosensitivity of CRC to methotrexate (MTX). The authors also found that overexpression of miR-215 could lead to an increased chemoresistance to MTX and tomudex (TDX), and overexpression of miR-140 is linked with increased chemoresistance to MTX and 5-fluorouracil (5-FU). In another study, Wang and others reported that the inhibition of miR-31 in CRC could increase the sensitivity to 5-FU at an early stage.

Other strategies for boosting chemo-responsiveness in CRC cells are based on increasing the tumor suppressor-like activity and/or on repressing the oncogenic-like activity of miRNAs. In this respect, the overexpression of miR-143 and miR-34a in CRC cell lines have led to increased chemosensitivity to 5-FU. Li and others have shown that overexpression of miR-22 in p53-mutated CRC cell lines has increased the chemosensitivity to paclitaxel. The inhibition of miR-21, which acts as a potential oncogene, may improve the response to CRC therapy.

To sum up, the immunologic approach shifts the focus from the tumour towards the other major protagonist involved in oncogenesis, namely the immune system of the host. Antitumor immunity can offer clinically significant biomarkers, and opportunities for improving existing therapies. CTC isolation and molecular analysis could open new perspectives in understanding the metastatic process, leading to the development of new treatments or to the customisation of those already existent. The high stability of miRNAs renders them important candidates for a new class of biomarkers, potentially useful for improving diagnosis, prognosis and prediction in CRC. Larger studies are required to validate the clinical usefulness of these biomarkers in colorectal carcinoma, their role as prognostic or predictive factors, either alone or in combination with other known markers.

References

Adams, J.L., and Roberts, K.J., *Molecular Biology of the Cell*, Garland Science, Taylor & Francis Group, London.

Brown, M.E., *Molecular Biology of Cell*, Marcel Dekker, New York.

Collin, R.K., *Cell Biology*, Cambridge University Press, Cambridge.

Didier, M.B., *Lichen Physiology and Cell Biology*, Kluwer Academic/Plenum Publishers, New York.

David, K.N., *Fundamental of Cell Biology*, Peragam, Oxford.

Eklun, R.W, *Plant Cell and Its Growth*, Academic Press, London.

Frische, B., *DNA Molecular Gymnastics*, Marcel Dekker Inc., New York.

George Plopper, *Principles of Cell Biology*, Jones and Bartlett Publishers, Inc, United States.

Hall, D.R., *Molecular Neurobiology*, Humana Press Inc., New Jersey.

Harvey Lodish, *Molecular Cell Biology*, W. H. Freeman and Company, New York.

Jetten, N.S., *Gene regulation by MicroRNAs*, McGraw Hill, Columbus, Ohio, USA.

Karp, G.C., *Cell and Molecular Biology*, John Wiley & Sons Inc., New York.

Keith, V.G, *Nucleus and Gene Expression*, Pergamon Press, Oxford, New York.

Lewis, D.A, *Ten Commandments of Enzymology*, Science Publishers, New York.

Liebier, F.T, *Biology of Cancer*, Tata McGraw Hill, New York.

Machacon, L.M, *Cell and Molecular Immunology*, Oxford University Press, Oxford.

Martin Raff,, *Molecular Cell Biology*, McGraw-Hills, New York.

Nelson, D.L., *Lehninger, Principles of Biochemistry*, W. H. Freeman and Company, New York.

Pinto, B.C., *The Cell*, Science Publishers, New York.

Peter Walter, *Molecular Biology*, Applied Science Publishers, London.

Phat Dinh, *DNA and Cell Biology*, Mary Ann Liebert, Inc., Publishers, New York.

Reeve, O.M., *Membranes and Their Applications*, Prentice-Hall of India Pvt. Ltd., New Delhi.

Sadava, D.E., *Cell Biology: Organelle Structure and Function*, Jones and Bartlett Publishers, Boston.

Shoshkes, C.R., *DNA and Cell Biology*, Mary Ann Liebert, Inc., Publishers, New York.

Smith, W.D., *Microbial Biotechnology*, John Wiley & Sons, New York.

Tellez, P.E., *Gene Expression*, Affiliated East-West Press, Pvt. Ltd. Moscow

Umetsu, P.N, *Biology and Biotechnology*, Plenum Publishing Corporation, London.

Voet, D., *Biochemistry*, Tata McGraw Hill, New York.

Watson, K.C., *Replication and Repair of DNA*, Routledge, New York.

Wrobel, A.P, *Energy and Metabolism*, Ellis Harwood, New York.

Zeikus, J.G., *Mitochondrion and Bioenergetics*, Marcel Dekker Inc., New York.

Index